MEDICAL RADIOLOGY

Diagnostic Imaging and Radiation Oncology

Springer
Berlin
Heidelberg
New York
Barcelona
Budapest
Hong Kong
London
Milan
Paris
Santa Clara
Singapore
Tokyo

Helmut W. Vahrson (Ed.)

Radiation Oncology of Gynecological Cancers

With Contributions by

I.A. Adamietz · J. Bahnsen · M.W. Beckmann · H.G. Bender · H.D. Böttcher
L.W. Brady · D. Carstens · G. Crombach · R.G. Dale · M.F. Dzeda · G. Emons
H.J. Frischbier · A. Gerbaulet · C. Haie-Meder · M. Herbolsheimer · R.D. Hunter
H. Jacobs · H. Junkermann · U. Karck · D. Kieback · P.G. Knapstein
R. Kreienberg · H. Kucera · H.-A. Ladner · S. Ladner · E. Lartigau · W.A. Longton
M. Maher · H. Marsiglia · B. Micaily · K. Morita · R.F. Mould · D. Niederacher
U. Nitz · D.M. Ostapovicz · C.A. Perez · R. Pfab · A. Pfleiderer · G. Rauthe
K. Rotte · B. Schopohl · I. Schreer · K.-D. Schulz · V. Stelte · D. Timmerman
H.W. Vahrson · I.B. Vergote · D. von Fournier · W. Weikel

Foreword by

Luther W. Brady and Hans-Peter Heilmann

Springer

Professor Dr. HELMUT W. VAHRSON
Leiter der Abteilung für Gynäkologische Radiologie
und Strahlentherapie, Frauenklinik
Klinikum der Justus-Liebig-Universität
Klinikstraße 32, 35385 Gießen, Germany

MEDICAL RADIOLOGY · Diagnostic Imaging and Radiation Oncology

Continuation of
Handbuch der medizinischen Radiologie
Encyclopedia of Medical Radiology

With 185 Figures in 245 Separate Illustrations and 199 Tables

ISSN 0942-5373
ISBN 3-540-56768-2 Springer-Verlag Berlin Heidelberg New York

Library of Congress Cataloging-in-Publication Data.
Radiation oncology of gynecological cancers/H.W. Vahrson, ed.; with contributions by I.A. Adamietz . . . [et al.]; foreword by Luther W. Brady and Hans-Peter Heilmann. p. cm. – (Medical radiology) Includes bibliographical references and index.
ISBN 3-540-56768-2 (alk. paper)
1. Generative organs, Female–Cancer–Radiotherapy. 2. Generative organs, Female–Cancer-Imaging. 3. Radioisotope brachytherapy. I. Vahrson, H.W. (Helmut). II. Adamietz, I.A. III. Series. [DNLM: 1. Genital Neoplasms, Female–radiotherapy. 2. Genital Neoplasms, Female–surgery. 3. Genital Neoplasms, Female–drug therapy. WP 145 R1285 1997] RC280.G5R326 1997 616.99′4650642–dc21 96-29741

Printed in Germany

Cover design: de'blik, Berlin
Typesetting: Best-set Typesetter Ltd., Hong Kong

SPIN: 10061472 21/3135 – 5 4 3 2 1 0 – Printed on acid-free paper

Foreword

The incidence, diagnosis, and treatment of gynecologic cancer have undergone major changes during the past 20 years. In addition to significant changes in the incidence of the diseases, there has been extensive application of new technologies in the field.

- While the incidence of invasive cancers of the cervix has diminished sharply, there has been a marked increase in the number of patients presenting with in situ carcinomas of the cervix. This has resulted primarily from better education but also from the regular use of Papanicolaou screening for early diagnosis. This trend has been associated with a major shift from late stage disease to early stage disease, which has led to more effective utilization of surgical techniques in primary management, with less emphasis on radiation therapy techniques. Almost invariably, in situ cancers of the cervix can be cured by surgical management, and high cure rates can be achieved by surgical techniques in early invasive cancers of the cervix. Therefore, more patients are receiving definitive surgical management rather than definitive radiation therapy management.
- Because of its tendency to present at an early stage, cancer of the endometrium is now more commonly managed by surgical techniques. Postoperative radiation therapy is used when there is persistent residual disease following surgery, a more advanced disease stage than indicated by preliminary study, transection or spillage of tumor during the operative procedure, or positive cytology at the time of the original surgery.
- More precise programs for management of carcinoma of the vulva have been outlined, with emphasis on surgical management for early stage invasive cancers and radiation therapy with or without surgery for more advanced stage disease.
- Increasing emphasis is being placed on the use of chemotherapy techniques following surgery in the management of patients with cancer of the ovary; by contrast, radiation therapy is being relegated to the treatment of recurrent disease, more advanced disease or special forms of metastatic disease.
- There have been advances in the workup to identify those patients with primary malignant disease of the vagina, and treatment techniques primarily involving radiation therapy have been developed.
- It has been recognized that patients with carcinomas of the fallopian tube present unique and complicated problems with regard to management.
- More appropriate techniques have been defined for the management of female patients with carcinomas of the urethra, with emphasis on interstitial radiation therapy techniques.

In spite of the more widespread utilization of surgical management with or without pre-/postoperative radiation therapy, primary radiation therapy, and chemotherapy, local-regional recurrence remains a significant problem in gynecologic cancer, accounting for 50%–60% of failures of primary treatment regimens.

This volume, edited by Professor Helmut W. Vahrson, deals effectively with these important issues in gynecologic cancer, and contributes significantly to the definition of appropriate treatment programs for each of the major tumor sites.

Philadelphia/Hamburg
July 1997

Luther W. Brady
Hans-Peter Heilmann

Preface

The management of patients with gynecological cancer has undergone far-reaching changes. Today, radical surgery is being used more commonly in patients with cancer of the cervix and endometrium, including older patients who were formerly treated with radiation therapy; this has occurred because of better perioperative care, better anesthesia, and better general medical management. More effective chemotherapeutic agents have been introduced, and some, particularly platinum compounds and taxol, have been associated with long-term survival. Trials with combined radiation therapy and chemotherapy are being conducted more actively in advanced stages of cervical cancer or are replacing sole radiation therapy or chemotherapy in ovarian cancer.

At the same time, radiation therapy techniques have become more sophisticated, with three-dimensional reconstructed treatment planning and delivery being more commonly utilized today than 5 years ago. This allows for more precise definition of the tumor extent by computed technological techniques with contrast material, and the use of three-dimensional reconstruction of the treatment program with non-coplanar fields in order to avoid complications from the inclusion of small bowel, bladder, or rectum. Manual radium brachytherapy, used worldwide until recently, has been replaced by modern remotely controlled afterloading techniques. On the other hand, source-dependent low-, medium-, and high-dose-rate regimens are still under study, and it remains a matter of controversy as to which is better. Biological considerations with regard to the reduction of the acute and late complications of treatment have had a considerable influence on the move toward multiple fractions with teletherapy and brachytherapy remote-controlled afterloading techniques. Quality of life has emerged as a major concern in any treatment program, the emphasis being on achieving satisfactory quality of life without any reduction in the long-term survival or cure rates.

In Germany, formerly independent Departments of Gynecological Radiation Therapy are now being merged into Departments of Radiation Oncology, and the diagnostic components of these departments merged into Departments of Diagnostic Radiology. In the near future this development will have been completed. Therefore, the present volume clearly represents a significant opportunity to preserve the experience and knowledge of experts on gynecological radiation oncology. The approach adopted in this volume differs from that in other books on the same subject, in that knowledge and recent developments in surgery and chemotherapy, as well as radiation oncology, are presented. Leading gynecological surgeons discuss the role for surgery in the management of patients with cancer of the cervix and the vulva as an alternative to radiation therapy techniques. Therefore, the reader is provided with information on the entire field of treatment for female genital cancers. The individual chapters are all written by experts who have achieved international recognition for their work.

The editor expresses his deep debt of gratitude to the late Professor Richard K. Kepp (1912–1984), Director of the Universitäts-Frauenklinik Giessen, and Professor W. Dietrich Hofmann (born in 1925), of the same institution. Professor Kepp wrote *Grundlagen der Strahlentherapie* and *Gynäkologische Strahlentherapie* (published in 1952 by G. Thieme, Stuttgart), while Professor Hofmann is the author of *Klinik der Gynäkologischen Strahlentherapie* (published in 1963 by Urban & Schwarzenberg, München/Berlin).

The editor expresses his sincere appreciation to the various authors for their cooperation and to Mrs. Berger and Mrs. Schneider, who transcribed the chapters and managed the correspondence. The volume is dedicated to my wife, Frauke, who agreed to my frequent absence, without which this volume could not have been accomplished.

I wish to express my thanks to Mr. Rick Mills (Nottingham, UK), who reviewed and thoroughly corrected all of the contributions to this volume, ensuring that they are all of a high linguistic standard.

Gießen, July 1997 Helmut W. Vahrson

Contents

1 The Historical Roots of Modern Brachytherapy for Cervical and Endometrial Cancer

R.F. MOULD

CONTENTS

1.1 Introduction

The very first roots of gynaecological brachytherapy can be traced to the discovery of radioactivity by Henri Becquerel in 1896, which led to the discovery of radium in 1898 by Marie and Pierre Curie. However, radium therapy, which for many years was the only form of brachytherapy apart from applications using its short half-life gaseous daughter product radon, began with surface applications using radium plaques/moulds for squamous cell and basal cell carcinomas of the face. The first successful treatment for cancer using this technique was documented in Stockholm in the year 1899 (MOULD 1993).

The use of radium then progressed to applications within natural body cavities (intracavitary brachytherapy), such as the vagina, uterus and rectum. Two of the earliest commentaries on the gynaecological use of radium in the United States and in Europe appeared in 1904 and 1910, respectively: "A glass capsule of radium inserted directly into the tissue.... Radium is a very convenient substance at a point where the application of X-rays is impossible or exceedingly difficult" (PUSEY and CALDWELL 1904). "Radium is of great service in various affections of the uterus.... Cylindrical and flat applicators are equally useful in gynaecology.... The first paper of any importance on the subject of gynaecological radium therapy was by Robert Abbe in 1905" (WICKHAM and DEGRAIS 1910). Abbe was the first to cure a cervix cancer by radium in 1905; in 1914 he reported on this case.

Interstitial brachytherapy was suggested in 1903 by the inventor of the telephone, Alexander Graham Bell, using the following wording: "The Crookes' tube, from which the Röntgen rays are emitted is of course too bulky to be admitted into the middle of a mass of cancer, but there is no reason why a tiny fragment of radium sealed in a fine glass tube should not be directly inserted into the very heart of the cancer, thus acting directly upon the diseased material." However, it is also of interest to note that VOLTZ (1930), in his textbook "*Die Strahlenbehandlung der weiblichen Genitalcarcinome, Methoden und Ergebnisse*", states that Deutsch of Munich in the year 1902 was the first to treat uterine carcinoma with x-rays and that in 1903 Döderlein of Tübingen (and later of Munich) was the first to use radium for the treatment of inoperable cancer of the cervix.

Nevertheless, it was not until 1914 that an illustrated case of interstitial brachytherapy appeared in the medical literature. In that year, two such cases were reported by Stevenson and Joly from Dublin, Ireland, these concerning the treatment of a parotid tumour and a fibrous scar (MOULD 1993). Interstitial applications in gynaecology have been relatively limited, although CADE (1929) described two approaches: needling via the vagina and intraabdominal irradiation, an early form of intraoperative brachytherapy. One of the problems with radium needles was that their lengths were limited, although this was overcome in the 1960s when tantalum-182 (the predecessor of iridium-192) wires became available and a two-plane manual afterloading technique became practical. In the 1990s the use of interstitial brachytherapy is limited to bulky cervical tumours and a technique involving a template such as the MUPIT design of Martinez.

More than half a century after the first gynaecological use of radium, Ulrich Henschke pioneered

R.F. MOULD, MSc, PhD, CPhys, FInstP, FIPSM, FIMA, FIS, Scientific Consultant, 41 Ewhurst Avenue, Sanderstead, South Croydon, Surrey, CR2 ODH, UK the use of manual gynaecological afterloading with his 1964 paper with Hilaris and Mahan, entitled *Remote Afterloading with Intracavitary Applicators*; this was followed in 1966 by a report on a truly remote controlled afterloading device (Henschke et al. 1966). However, the principle of (manual) afterloading had been described much earlier in Europe and the United States, as can be seen from the following quotations:

1. "To increase the effectiveness of radium for deeper seated conditions quite significantly without causing undesirable effects on the skin. ... Intratumoural application by inserting the radium which is in the drilled tip of a small aluminium rod, with the help of a previously inserted trepan" (H. Strebel, Munich, in the *Deutsche Medizinal Zeitung*, 1903). Strebel appears to have been a dermatologist and was the author of the chapter on radiotherapy in the 1903 Dessauer and Wiesner textbook *Leitfaden des Röntgen-Verfahrens*.
2. "A very ingenious method of introducing radium into the tumour.... Applicator tubes of celluloid or rubber were used because of the fragile nature of the radium sources" (Robert Abbe in *JAMA* in 1906 and in *The Archives of The Roentgen Ray* in 1910). Abbe was a New York surgeon who was also one of the early experimentalists in the field of radiation biology; in 1904, he quantified time-dose factors for radium gamma-rays using germinative seedlings (Mould 1993).

The basis of modern brachytherapy, albeit incomplete, was therefore present in the literature before the end of the first decade of the twentieth century. To a certain extent it remained only to synthesise experience into standard systems (such as those of Paris, Manchester and Stockholm for cancer of the cervix and that of Heyman, also in Stockholm, for endometrial cancer), to develop technology (such as applicator design), to improve (originally non-existent) radiation protection and to manufacture radionuclides to replace radium which could eventually be produced as the miniature radioactive sources.

The following sections cover most of the major advances in gynaecological brachytherapy from the 1920s following the initial work described above, which in the decade 1910–1920 fell into disuse to a certain extent due to the then enormously high cost of radium, the realisation following the early "cures" that the results of radium therapy were largely temporary, World War I, and the resistance (which lasted well into the 1930s) of the gynaecological surgeons, who believed that radium was not a viable alternative to surgery.

1.2 Systems for Cancer of the Cervix

Five major centres developed techniques which were adopted by many centres throughout the world: Paris (1920s), Stockholm (1920s), Manchester (1930s), Munich (1940s) and the M.D. Anderson, Houston (1960s: the Fletcher system). Of these, both the Manchester and the Fletcher system were in effect direct descendents of the Paris system. In addition, in German-speaking countries, the Munich "pin and plate" system (pin referring to the uterine tube and plate to the vaginal applicator), which had its origins in Heidelberg around 1910 (von Seuffert 1929), was also widely used (Ries and Breitner 1959). Table 1.1 summarises the original treatment schedules for the Paris, Stockholm, Munich and Manchester systems (see also Figs. 1.1 and 1.2).

Since the original systems were described, there have been many variations in terms of dose fraction-

Table 1.1. Summary of the Paris, Stockholm, Munich and Manchester systems

Paris system
Continuous treatment for 120 h
Uterine tube of 33.3 mg radium
Two cylindrical vaginal cork applicators: 13.3 mg radium each
Stockholm system
Three insertions each of 22 h, separated by 1–2 weeks
Uterine tube of 50 mg radium
Two vaginal silver boxes containing a total of 60–80 mg radium
Munich system
Individualized treatment with three insertions each of 24 h, separated by 2 weeks
Intrauterine tube (of 20–50 mg radium dependent on intrauterine length) fixed to small, medium or large round plate (of 30–40 mg radium)
Direct dose measurement in bladder and rectum not to exceed tolerance dose of 6000 (–8000) r ruled and confined the treatment
Manchester system
Two insertions each of 72 h delivered over 10 days
Three uterine sources were available and the choice depended on the length of the uterine cavity. Source activities were 35, 25 and 20 mg radium for uterine lengths of 6, 4 and 2 cm
Large, medium and small vaginal ovoids were available with activities of 22.5, 20 and 17.5 mg radium, respectively

ation and design modifications to the applicators. Including the designs for manual and remote afterloading and for low-dose-rate (LDR) and high-dose-rate (HDR) applications, there must have been at least 300 different types of applicator available during the last 100 years. One applicator which has had popular appeal is the ring applicator; some consider that this applicator was designed in the remote afterloading era to duplicate a pair of Stockholm vaginal boxes, but in fact this design had been available many years earlier (Fig. 1.3).

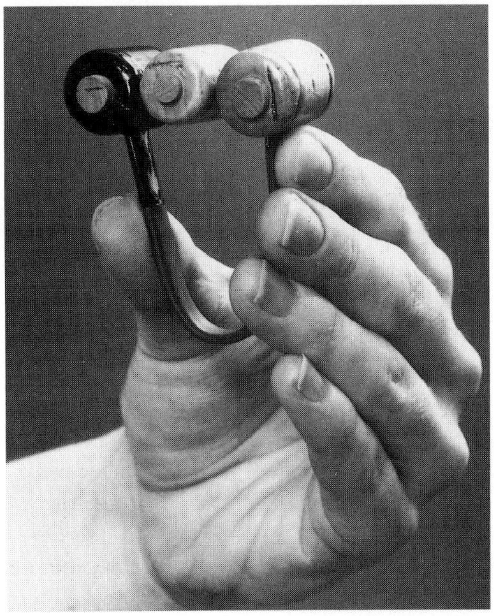

Fig. 1.1. Paris system cork vaginal applicators: two or three could be used, with the lateral pair being joined together with a flexible spring

One of the advantages of the early designs of the Munich and Fletcher-Suit-Delclos applicators was their geometrical rigidity. The accuracy of applicator positioning with such as the Manchester and Stockholm techniques, where the ovoids were not fixed together, depended to a large extent on the skill of the physician making the radium insertion with the use of gauze packing. Figure 1.4 shows an AP radiograph of a Manchester insertion and it is well recorded that the vaginal ovoids were sometimes positioned 180° differently compared with Fig. 1.4. The AP radiograph in Fig. 1.5 is for a pre-loaded radium Fletcher applicator (1960s) in which the ovoids could be positioned by using a hinged fixing mechanism (not seen in the radiograph). This was a great improvement, as was the incorporation of tungsten rectal shielding into the Fletcher ovoids. When the first manual afterloading Fletcher applicators were designed (Fig. 1.6), the intrauterine tube was also clamped to the ovoid arrangement, thus guaranteeing much greater positional accuracy of the sources. A further improvement in the accuracy of positioning came with HDR remote afterloading, because of the very short treatment times during

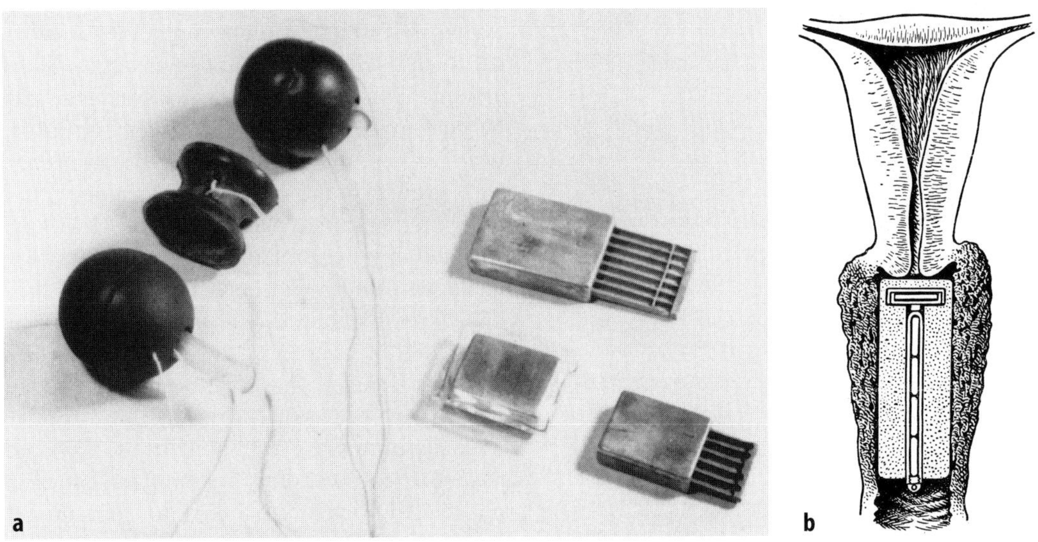

Fig. 1.2. **a** Manchester vaginal ovoids and Stockholm vaginal boxes. **b** Munich system pin and plate applicator. Unlike those of the Paris, Manchester and Stockholm systems, the Munich applicator arrangement had the uterine source attached by a screw thread to the vaginal plate. The illustration shown here (Voltz 1930) illustrates how the system could equally well be used to treat vaginal disease. The "uterine pin" in this situation was positioned in the vagina, rather than in the uterus, and the entire applicator was placed within a cork cylinder to ensure central positioning

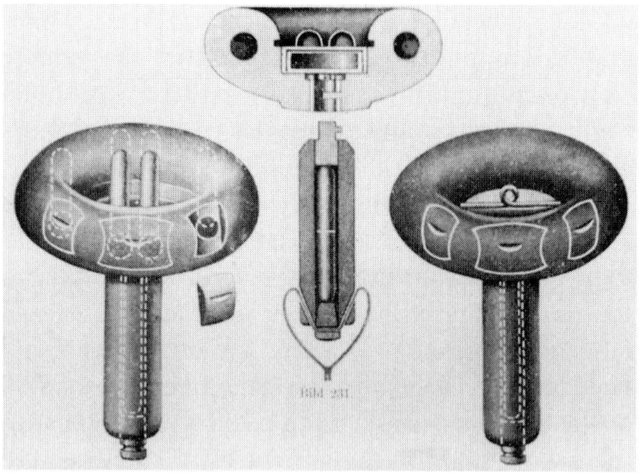

Fig. 1.3. An early design of a ring applicator (VON SEUFFERT 1929). In the 1990s the ring applicator is widely used with both LDR and HDR remote afterloading systems

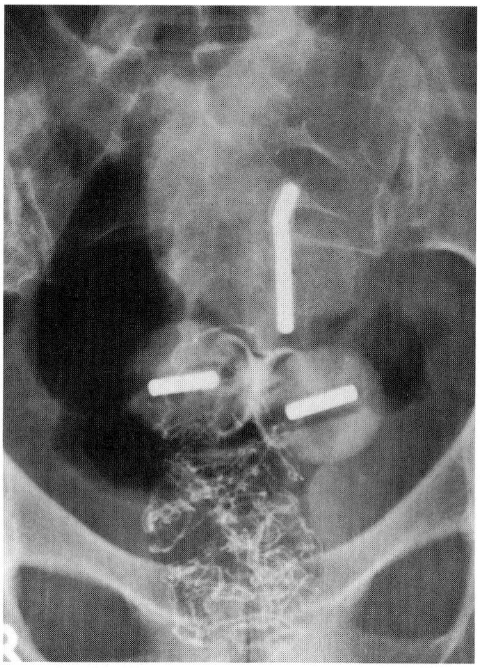

Fig. 1.4. AP radiograph of a Manchester pre-loaded radium insertion (1960s)

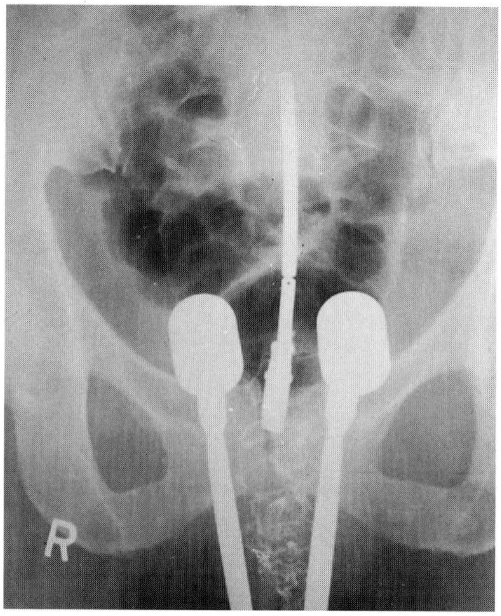

Fig. 1.5. AP radiograph of a Fletcher pre-loaded radium insertion (1960s)

which there was no opportunity for movement of the applicators.

1.3 Dosimetry

For many years the standard unit of dosage was the milligram-hour, but this was eventually replaced by the roentgen when the ICRU 1937 recommendation that this unit be used for both x-rays and gamma rays was finally accepted. However, the dosimetry for the Manchester system was often only the well-known point A, with an additional point B sometimes used. Nevertheless, some dosimetry was occasionally undertaken, and Fig. 1.7 is from Brussels (MURDOCH 1931) for the Paris cork applicator system, with the dosimetry units measured in ergs/cc. In this particular instance an argon-filled ionisation chamber was used which was later shown to be inaccurate (MOULD 1993); even so, the familiar pear shape of the distribution is clearly seen.

A growth point in dosimetry came with digital computer treatment planning, although in some centres, notably the Royal Marsden Hospital, London, analogue devices had been developed in the 1940s and 1950s to obtain three-dimensional distributions for a radium insertion. However, the author knows from experience that these methods required a physicist working an entire day to obtain the final dose distribution! Fortunately, these days are long past. Current planning systems are extremely sophisticated; some are linked to computed tomographic and magnetic resonance imaging devices, and far more accurate dosimetry can be achieved than could ever have been envisaged even as recently as the 1960s.

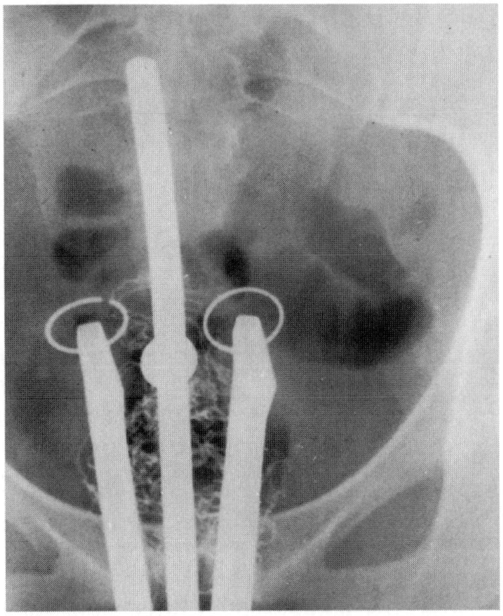

Fig. 1.6. AP radiograph of a Fletcher manually afterloaded radium insertion (1960s)

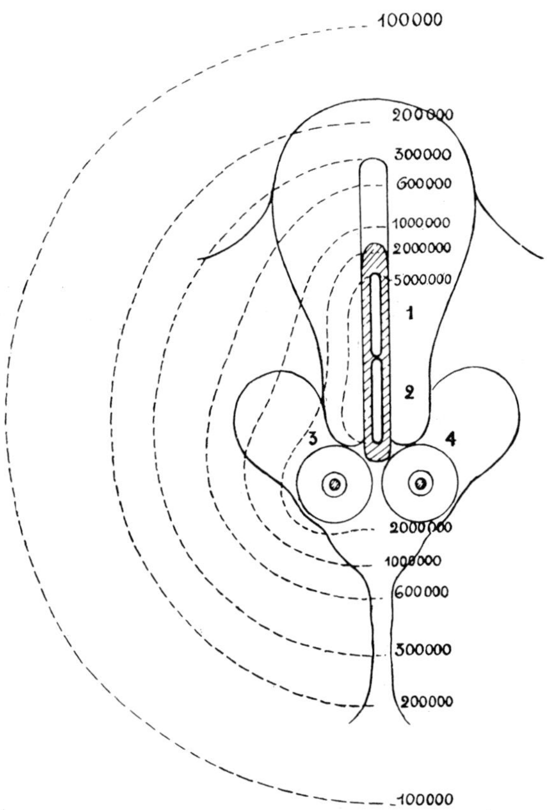

Fig. 1.7. Isodose distribution for the Paris system. It was stated by MURDOCH (1931) that the uterine mucosa absorbs up to 5 000 000 ergs/cc

We are now also entering the era of biological dosimetry and can expect an increasing number of centres to specify "dose" in terms of iso(biological) effect curves and surfaces rather than in terms of isodose distributions. This has been helped by the development of radiobiological modelling, commencing with the Ellis NSD concept via TDF and CRE models to the currently most useful model: the linear quadratic. It has long been recognised that the simple arithmetic addition of "brachytherapy Gy" to "teletherapy Gy" for a protocol involving both brachytherapy and teletherapy (as do the majority of cervical carcinoma protocols except for some stage I cases) is not really meaningful. However, before the availability of radiobiological modelling on a relatively wide scale, this was all that could be achieved. One recent example of the use of radiobiological modelling relevant to gynaecological cancer is the paper by JONES and BLEASDALE (1994).

Dose-volume histograms are relevant to interstitial brachytherapy and are extremely useful in assessing "implant quality". MEERTENS et al. (1994) have reviewed the spectrum of indices related to the uniformity of the dose distribution and also dosimetric parameters for the description of the quality of a brachytherapy application: coverage index, external volume index, relative dose homogeneity index, overdose volume index and sum index. Just as quality of life scales and performance status scales such as Karnofsky and ECOG are now a routine part of treatment assessment, the future will probably also bring with it routine assessments of the quality of a brachytherapy application.

1.4 Heyman Packing for Cancer of the Endometrium

The standard technique for many years was the Heyman packing method developed at the Radiumhemmet, Stockholm in the 1930s. The Heyman apparatus (Fig. 1.8) consisted of a series of curved steel rods containing a radium capsule at one end which was fixed to the rod by a taut steel wire. At the other end of the rod was a release mechanism so that after the radium capsule had been inserted into position the rod could be withdrawn. The steel wire, no longer taut, was used at the end of treatment to withdraw the radium capsule.

The aim of the physician was to pack as many of these small capsules into the uterus as possible. The

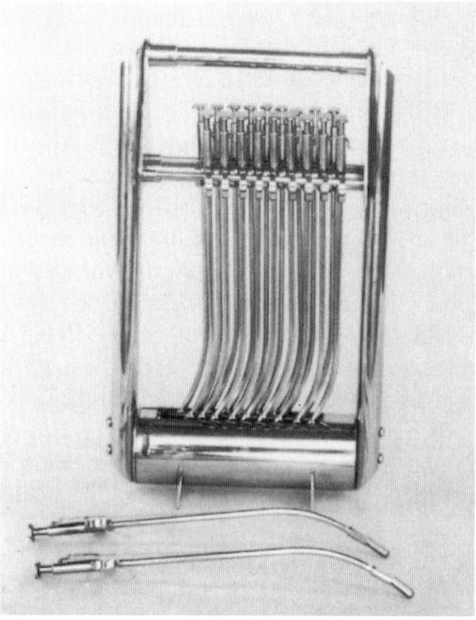

Fig. 1.8. Heyman apparatus for the treatment of endometrial cancer using a series of small capsules of radium

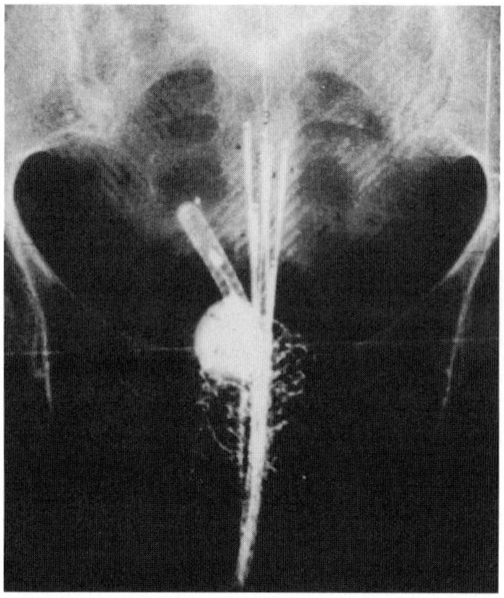

Fig. 1.9. AP radiograph of the Rotte microSelectron-HDR technique using a catheter bundle (ROTTE 1990)

modern equivalent of this technique is that designed by ROTTE (1990) in Würzburg (Fig. 1.9); the latter uses a microSelectron-HDR remote afterloader with a bundle of catheters into which the miniature iridium-192 stepping source can be programmed. Previous afterloading techniques using rigid applicators, such as the Y-shaped applicator, failed to reproduce the Heyman packing technique.

1.5 Radiation Protection

The principle of afterloading as proposed by Strebel in 1904 and Abbe in 1910 was not for the purposes of radiation protection. However, it was for this reason that Henschke commenced the use of afterloading in modern times, eventually in the 1960s developing his remote-controlled afterloading device using a cycling cobalt-60 source (Fig. 1.10). However, manual afterloading became widespread before remote afterloaders, in part due to the later technological developments and in part due to cost, and Fig. 1.6 illustrates the use of an early Fletcher manual afterloading technique. Some protection, though, still had to be used, and Fig. 1.11 shows a typical moveable lead shield for use by nurses: the curved design at the top and the two cutaway areas were devised so as to allow the nurse to lean over the patient and to give free access to her arms.

1.6 Radioactive Isotopes

Radium was replaced by a series of artificially produced radioactive isotopes including cobalt-60, tantalum-182, caesium-137 and finally iridium-192. The use of a radionuclide in brachytherapy depends in part on its specific activity: whether it can be produced in wire form and whether it can be produced as a miniature source with a high activity. Figure 1.12 shows typical radium tubes and needles from Amersham; these were termed G-tubes and were 2 cm in geometrical length but could be purchased containing different activities such as 10 mg, 15 mg, 20 mg and 25 mg radium. They were eventually replaced by caesium-137 tubes containing a radium-equivalent activity for this 33-year half-life radionuclide.

However, it was the development of miniaturised iridium-192 sources that revolutionised remote afterloading and the concept of a high (10 Ci iridium-192) activity stepping source became a reality with all the associated advantages of HDR techniques (including outpatient treatment) and optimisation. Figure 1.13 gives the dimensions of the microSelectron-HDR iridium-192 source of the 1990s for comparison with Fig. 1.12.

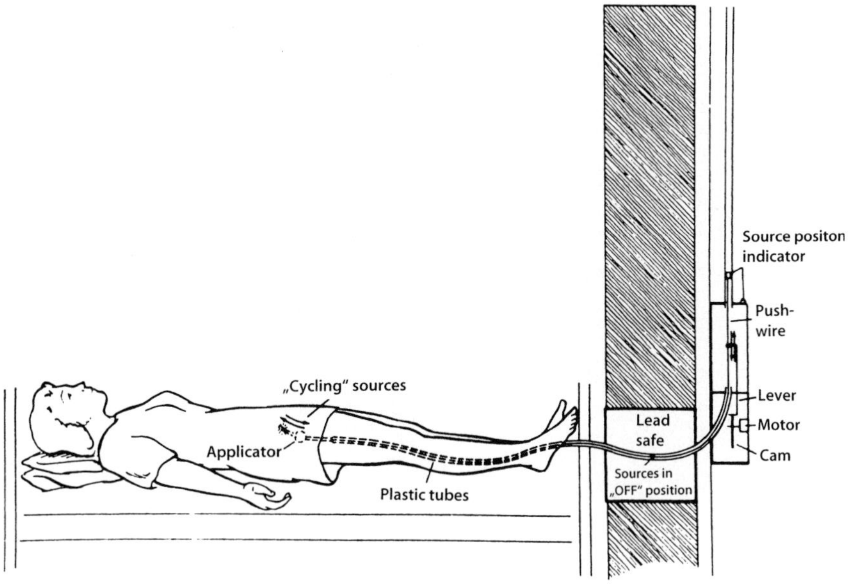

Fig. 1.10. The Henschke remote afterloader. This was in fact not the very first remote afterloader: that was designed by Walstam of Stockholm, who first reported on his proposal in 1962. His design consisted of a three-linked source system of three 50-mg and one 9-mg radium tubes. (Mould 1993)

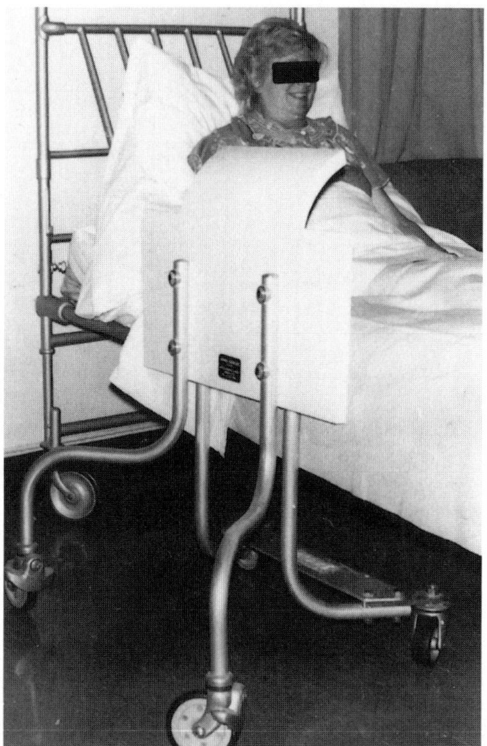

Fig. 1.11. Lead bed shield for nursing protection during manual afterloading treatment for cancer of the cervix (1960s)

1.7 Remote Afterloading and Dose Rate

Several designs of remote afterloader followed the early work of Henschke and Walstam and devices were produced in several countries: TEM/Cathetron (UK), GammaMed/Sauerwein, Buchler and Decatron (Germany), Nucletron/Selectron (The Netherlands), Brachytron (Canada) and Ralstron (Japan). However, the remote afterloading devices now used in gynaecological brachytherapy are (with computer treatment planning) the current endpoint of the 1990s in the development of gynaecological brachytherapy. Both HDR and LDR systems (Table 1.2) are in current use and several clinical trials/surveys are taking place to determine whether survival and local recurrence rates and morbidity rates are the same or different for LDR and HDR. For example, the recent *International Review on Patterns of Care in Cancer of the Cervix* reviewed data from 56 centres treating a total of more than 17000 patients with HDR brachytherapy (Orton et al. 1991) and compared these data with those for LDR from the centres, from the FIGO Report Volume 21 (1991) and from the French Cooperative Group of nine centres (Horiot et al. 1988). Their conclusions were summarised (Orton and Somnay 1994) as follows: "HDR cervical cancer brachytherapy can be as successful as the best achieved with LDR as far as five-year survival is concerned. With respect to

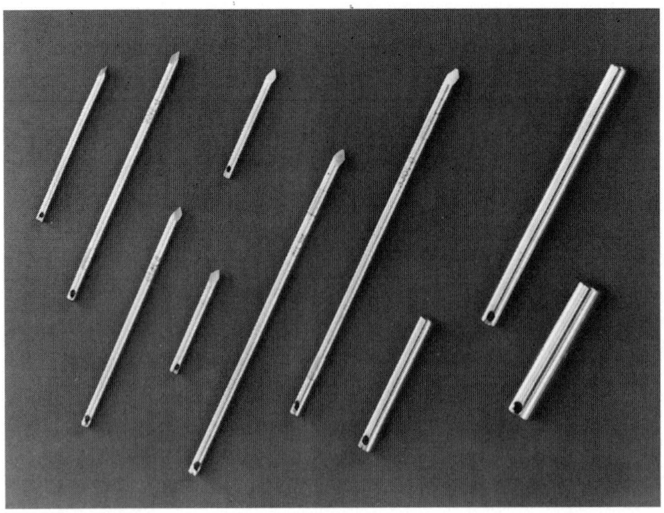

Fig. 1.12. Radium tubes and needles manufactured by the Radiochemical Centre, Amersham, England

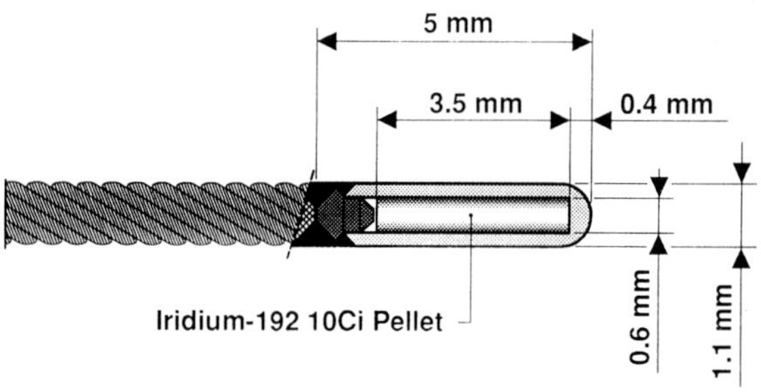

Fig. 1.13. The iridium-192 stepping source of the microSelectron-HDR remote afterloader

Table 1.2. Dose rate definitions from the ICRU Report No. 38 (1985)

Low dose rate (LDR):	0.4–2.0 Gy/h
Medium dose rate (MDR):	2–12 Gy/h
High dose rate (HDR):	Exceeding 2 Gy/min

morbidity, HDR can be significantly better than LDR, especially if the dose per fraction to point A is kept low."

There is still progress to be made in the comparison of LDR and HDR and also in the development of treatment planning software, but such advances have already been made that it is doubtful whether the early pioneers of gynaecological radium brachytherapy would have recognised the techniques of today. It is therefore appropriate to end this chapter with the first ever published photograph of an applicator system for cancer of the cervix, dating from 1905, i.e. that of Wickham and Degrais of St. Louis Hospital, Paris (Fig. 1.14), remembering the Wick-

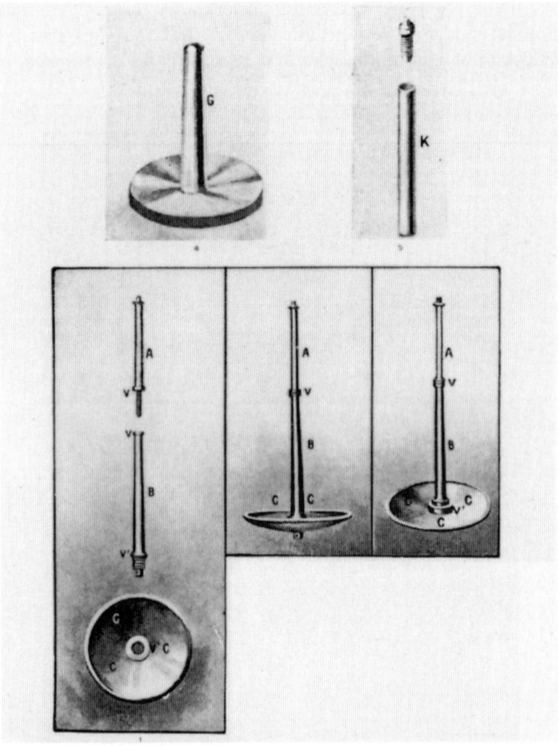

Fig. 1.14. Cancer of the cervix applicator of 1905. "Three parts form the apparatus. The base is screwed on. The depression on the rods A and B are intended to be filled with radiferous varnish. The varnish deposited in depression C is independent of the centre of the cup. The end which passes through cup C is perforated for the insertion of a band. The stem is inserted in the uterus: as a whole if it is desired to treat the body, or without part A for the cervix alone. The cup is applied to the cervix." At the *top right* is a lead or silver screen which fits onto the stem and cup. (From Wickham and Degrais 1910)

ham and Degrais quotation in the Introduction to this brief historical review.

References

Abbè R (1914) Die Anwendung von Radium bei Karzinom und Sarkom. Strahlentherapie 4:27

Cade S (1929) Radium treatment of cancer. Churchill, London

FIGO (1991) Annual report of the results of treatment in gynaecological cancer, 21. Radiumhemmet, Stockholm

Henschke UK, Hilaris BS, Mahan DG (1966) Intracavitary radiation therapy of uterine cancer by remote afterloading with cycling sources. Am J Roentgenol 96:45

Horiot JC, Pigneaux J, Pourquier H, et al. (1988) Radiotherapy alone in carcinoma of the intact cervix according to GH guidelines: a French cooperative study of 1383 cases. Int J Radiat Oncol Biol Phys 14:605–611

Jones B, Bleasdale C (1994) Effect of overall time when radiotherapy includes teletherapy and brachytherapy: a mathematical model. Br J Radiol 67:63–70

Meertens H, Borger J, Steggerda M, Blom A (1994) Evaluation and optimisation of interstitial brachytherapy dose distributions. In: Mould RF, Battermann JJ, Martinez AA, Speiser BL (eds) Brachytherapy from radium to optimization. Nucletron, Veenendaal, pp 300–306

Mould RF (1993) A century of X-rays and radioactivity in medicine with emphasis on the photographic records of the early years. Institute of Physics Publishing, Bristol

Murdoch J (1931) Dosage in radium therapy. Br J Radiol 4:256

Orton CG, Somnay A (1994) Results of an international review on patterns of care in cancer of the cervix. In: Mould RF, Battermann JJ, Martinez AA, Speiser BL (eds) Brachytherapy from radium to optimization. Nucletron, Veenendaal, pp 49–54

Orton CG, Seyedsadr M, Somnay A (1991) Comparison of high and low dose rate remote afterloading for cervix cancer and the importance of fractionation. Int J Radiat Oncol Biol Phys 21:1425–1434

Pusey WA, Caldwell EW (1904) The practical applications of the Röntgen rays in therapeutics and diagnosis, 2nd edn. Saunders, Philadelphia

Ries J, Breitner J (1959) Strahlenbehandlung in der Gynäkologie. Sonderband Strahlentherapie 40, Urban and Schwarzenberg, München

Rotte K (1990) Technique and results of HDR afterloading in cancer of the endometrium. In: Martinez AA, Orton CG, Mould RF (eds) Brachytherapy HDR and LDR. Nucletron, Columbia, p 68

Voltz F (1930) Die Strahlenbehandlung der weiblichen Genitalcarcinome, Methoden und Ergebnisse. Sonderband Strahlentherapie 13, Urban und Schwarzenberg, Berlin

von Seuffert E (1929) Die Radiumbehandlung maligner Neubildungen in der Gynäkologie. In: Meyer H, Gauss CJ (eds) Lehrbuch der Strahlentherapie, volume IV, Gynäkologie. Urban and Schwarzenberg, München

Walstam R (1962) Remotely controlled afterloading radiotherapy apparatus. Phys Med Biol 7:225

Wickham L, Degrais M (1910) Radiumtherapy. Cassell, London

Basics

2 Radiobiological Considerations in Gynaecological Radiotherapy

R.G. DALE

CONTENTS

2.1 Introduction

Gynaecological radiotherapy normally involves the use of various combinations of external beam irradiation and brachytherapy, the latter component of which may be fractionated, and delivered at low, medium or high dose rate. A wide variety of treatment techniques have evolved and in recent years there has been a move towards the use of remote-controlled afterloading systems with which to deliver the brachytherapy component. Gynaecological radiotherapy is therefore a subject of major radiobiological significance, but analytically is complicated by the fact that irradiated volumes can vary considerably, and by the presence of the unavoidable dose gradients associated with all types of brachytherapy. Nevertheless, there have emerged some fairly clear radiobiological principles which, although not yet capable of being used for the routine optimisation of gynaecological radiotherapy, can at least throw light on the identification of relatively "safe" techniques.

Early attempts at quantification of biological effects used empirical power-law models (e.g. KIRK et al. 1972; ORTON and ELLIS 1973) which sought to express biological effect in terms of the total physical dose, dose rate, number of fractions, overall time etc. A number of drawbacks have been identified with such models, and these have been widely documented (e.g. LIVERSAGE 1971; JOINER 1993). The most significant problem with the power law approach, apart from its empirical foundations, rests with the fact that there are no clearly identifiable tissue-specific parameters to use with such models. It is well established that, for a given total dose, changes in fractionation, dose rate etc. lead to changes in biological effect, the magnitude of which will depend on the nature of the tissue irradiated. Since clinical radiation doses are ultimately limited by the biological tolerance of the critical normal tissues, a clear understanding of the differences in response between normal and malignant tissues is an essential component of radiobiological understanding. Although power-law models were originally introduced with the intention of later identifying and incorporating tissue-specific parameters, this essential development did not occur.

This chapter will review the radiobiology of gynaecological radiotherapy entirely in terms of the the more recent linear-quadratic (LQ) model. The possible advantages of an LQ-type model were originally outlined by FOWLER and STERN (1960), but it was the comprehensive relaunch of the idea by BARENDSEN (1982) which led to the model becoming the focus of extensive interest and attention. The LQ formulation may be developed from rigorous biophysical considerations, rather than empirical clinical observations, and is therefore more closely identified with the parameters which are likely to influence biological response (KELLERER and ROSSI 1972; CHADWICK and LEENHOUTS 1973).

Although the biophysical origins of LQ-type formulations need not be discussed here, it is useful to appreciate that, through its application, macroscopic clinical observations can, in principle, be related to microscopic radiation events taking place at the

R.G. DALE, PhD, FInstP, FIPEM, Department of Radiation Physics and Radiobiology, Charing Cross Hospital, Fulham Palace Road, London, W6 8RF, UK intracellular level, especially in relation to radiation-induced DNA damage and repair.

2.2 Quantification of Biological Effect: The Concept of Biologically Effective Dose

In its simplest form, the LQ model considers that radiation damage at the cellular level can result from one of two separate, yet concurrent, processes.

In the first of these processes the damage is assumed to result from one interaction between the radiation and the critical target in the cell nucleus. The amount of biological damage therefore varies linearly with dose, i.e. doubling the dose produces twice the damage, etc., and, most importantly, is independent of the dose rate. This mechanism of irreparable damage production is referred to as the "single-hit" process, and damage produced in this way is called the α-component, or type A damage (Dale 1985; Thames 1985). If the probability that a cell will undergo a type A event is α, then, for a single dose (d):

$$\text{Type A damage} = \alpha d.$$

In the second process the damage is assumed to result from an interaction between two quite separate radiation interactions within the critical target. The individual interactions are said to be sublethal (as, by themselves, they are insufficiently toxic to kill the cell), but an interaction between two sublethal lesions is considered lethal. In this case the amount of damage varies with the square of the dose, i.e. doubling the dose produces four times as much damage, etc. This mechanism of damage production is referred to as the "two-hit" process, and the damage so produced is called the β-component, or type B damage (Dale 1985). If the probability that a cell will undergo a type B event is β, then for a single dose (d):

$$\text{Type B damage} = \beta d^2.$$

The total amount of radiation damage to the cell is the summation of these two components, and is clearly dependent on the dose delivered and on the relative propensity of the critical target to undergo the single-hit or two-hit process, as determined by the individual values of α and β.

The total damage created by a dose d, is therefore given as:

$$\text{Total damage} = \text{Type A} + \text{Type B} = \alpha d + \beta d^2. \tag{2.1}$$

At this stage it is assumed that the time taken to deliver the dose (d) is short, and that the type A and B damage is consequently produced "instantaneously". As will be discussed later, in cases where the radiation delivery cannot be classed as "instantaneous" the expression for the amount of type B damage is more complex. In terms of clinically observable effects on particular tissues, it is conventionally assumed that the magnitude of the observed effect (e.g. tumour cell kill or loss of organ function) is related to the surviving fraction (S) of cells. Surviving fraction decreases as an exponential function of the total damage, i.e.:

$$S = \exp(-\text{Type A damage}) \times \exp(-\text{Type B damage}),$$

i.e. $$S = \exp\left(-\alpha d - \beta d^2\right)$$

or: $$\ln(S) = -\alpha d - \beta d^2.$$

(The negative signs indicate that S decreases as d increases.)

It will now be seen that the total cellular damage referred to in Eq. 2.1 is identical to $-\ln(S)$, because:

$$-\ln(S) = \alpha d + \beta d^2. \tag{2.2}$$

Equation 2.2 is the usual starting point with which to discuss the LQ formulation, so-called because, irrespective of the type of radiotherapy involved, it always consists of a linear and a quadratic radiation damage component, the influence of each being governed by the respective magnitudes of α and β.

Because the surviving fraction (S_N) resulting from N well-spaced irradiations of dose (d) may be found simply by summing the log survivals associated with each individual irradiation we have, for N fractions:

$$-\ln(S_N) = N\cdot\left(\alpha d + \beta d^2\right) = N\alpha d + N\beta d^2. \tag{2.3}$$

By dividing both sides of Eq. 2.3 by α we can derive an expression called the biologically effective dose (BED), i.e.:

$$\text{BED} = -\ln(S_N)/\alpha = N\cdot d + d^2/(\alpha/\beta),$$

i.e. $$\text{BED} = Nd\cdot\left[1 + d/(\alpha/\beta)\right]. \tag{2.4}$$

The BED concept is useful in many practical applications of the LQ model. It was originally introduced by Barendsen (1982), at which time it was referred to as the extrapolated response dose (ERD). Because the ERD was essentially representative of a biological dose, it was renamed and given its present symbol (BED) by FOWLER (1989).

Equation 2.4 is the simplest definition of BED and applies in the case of N well-spaced fractions delivered to tissues which have a negligible rate of growth during the time taken to deliver all N fractions. This is probably the case with most late-responding normal tissues.

For acute-responding normal tissues, or tumours, for both of which there is likely to be relatively rapid clonogenic proliferation during the course of a radiotherapy treatment, Eq. 2.4 may be modified to allow for the effects of such proliferation (TRAVIS and TUCKER 1987; WHELDON and AMIN 1988),

$$\text{i.e.}\quad \text{BED} = Nd\cdot\left[1+d/(\alpha/\beta)\right]-0.693T/\alpha T_{pot}, \qquad (2.5)$$

where T is the overall time taken to deliver the treatment and T_{pot} is the potential doubling time of the clonogens. It will be appreciated from the form of Eq. 2.5 that, because the repopulation factor appears as a subtractive factor, tumour BEDs are most likely to be compromised by using prolonged treatment times when treating those tumours which combine a low radiosensitivity (α) and a rapid growth rate (small value of T_{pot}).

In words, the BED definition may be committed to memory as:

$$\text{BED} = (\text{Total Dose} \times \text{Relative Effectiveness}) - \text{Repopulation Factor}$$

and symbolically as:

$$\text{BED} = (\text{TD} \times \text{RE}) - \text{RF} \qquad (2.6)$$

The relative effectiveness (RE) is the factor which determines the biological effectiveness of the delivered total dose (TD) in the absence of repopulation. The mathematical definition of RE will depend on the type of radiotherapy involved, and in some cases can be very complex, but it will always incorporate the ratio α/β, which is expressed in units of Gy. In the case of fractionated radiotherapy we have (from both Eqs. 2.4 and 2.5):

$$\text{RE} = 1 + d/(\alpha/\beta).$$

As with the BED, the underlying conceptual significance of RE is important. It is the factor which takes into account those aspects of the pattern of radiation delivery which most influence the biological outcome and which (unlike the α/β ratio, which is essentially a fixed biological parameter) are under the control of the prescribing physician. For fractionated high-dose-rate (HDR) radiotherapy the important treatment parameter is d, the dose/fraction; for protracted irradiation the important treatment parameter is the dose rate (R), these being the two simplest examples. In all cases it is important to note that the RE can never assume a value less than unity.

As BEDs can only be calculated by using a particular value of α/β in the corresponding RE equation, it has become commonplace to place a suffix after the BED symbol in order to indicate the value of α/β which is being assumed, e.g. BED_3, BED_{10}, etc. That same convention will be adopted in this chapter.

The repopulation factor (RF) in Eq. 2.6 is normally taken to be zero for late-reacting normal tissues. For tumours the definition of RF is given by:

$$\text{RF} = 0.693T/\alpha T_{pot}$$

as has been used in Eq. 2.5.

For any pattern of radiation treatment, BED is assumed to be a measure of the gross biological effect on a specified tissue. Because BED is an additive quantity, the total biological effect resulting from combining together different types of radiotherapy can be found by summing the BED values associated with each individual component. Because gynaecological radiotherapy often involves both external beam and brachytherapy techniques, the BED concept, when used with a modicum of caution, is of value in assessing and intercomparing the summed radiobiological effects associated with various treatment regimens.

2.3 Fractionation Factors (α/β Ratios)

It was shown in Sect. 2.2 how the BED received by a specified tissue is influenced by the RE, which in turn is a function of the α/β ratio for that tissue. The incorporation of tissue-specific α/β ratios is therefore one of the most significant features of the LQ method, and the one which most obviously sets it apart from the earlier power-law models. Thus, even in a uniformly irradiated volume encompassing a number of different organs the biological doses (BEDs) will vary from one organ to another, even though they are each subjected to the same physical dose, number of fractions and dose/fraction.

α/β ratios are important because they reflect the shape of the underlying dose-response curve. Because the "sparing" effect of fractionation is itself dependent on the dose-response relationship, it is clear that α/β ratios must exert an important influence on the effects of changing fractionation. For this reason they are sometimes referred to as fractionation factors.

All types of radical radiotherapy ultimately aim to produce as much damage to the tumour as possible, whilst minimising damage to critical (late-reacting) normal tissues, i.e. they seek to achieve the highest possible therapeutic ratio. Knowledge of the late-normal tissue and tumour α/β ratio is therefore of major importance, as these parameters may be used to define patterns of radiation delivery which might lead to an improved therapeutic ratio.

The magnitude of the late-normal and tumour α/β ratios are under continual review (for a recent summary see JOINER 1993). As a generalisation, late-reacting normal tissues are associated with fractionation factors in the approximate range 0.5–6 Gy, with a mean value of between 3 and 4 Gy. For early-reacting tissues and human tumours the spread of α/β values is larger, and they are generally higher than those for the late-reacting tissues, typically being in the range 5–20 Gy. Important exceptions to this general rule are melanoma and liposarcoma, which possess α/β values of ~0.5 Gy. The magnitude of any sparing induced by fractionation is directly related to the shape of the underlying dose-response curve, and hence the α/β ratio. Figures 2.1 and 2.2 respectively illustrate the principle involved for late- and early-responding tissues. As the dose/fraction is decreased, and the number of fractions increased, the sparing produced by any particular total dose is seen to increase with the degree of fractionation. However, for a given total dose, the amount of sparing depends on the "curviness" of the basic dose-response curve – those associated with late-responding normal tissues (generally small α/β ratios) possess relatively more downward curvature, as shown in Fig. 2.1, and therefore demonstrate a relatively large amount of sparing with increasing fractionation. For tumours (larger α/β ratios) the sparing effect is still present but, relative to a late-responding tissue, it is reduced on account of the smaller curvature associated with the underlying dose-response curve, as demonstrated in Fig. 2.2. In the chosen example these effects are most clearly seen by observing how, after a total dose of 10 Gy, the differences between the resultant cell survival, as fraction number is increased, are much greater for the late-reacting tissue (Fig. 2.1) than for the tumour (Fig. 2.2).

It is precisely this effect which has given rise to the notion that hyperfractionation, using smaller than usual doses/fraction in the same overall treatment time, is likely to favourably increase the damage differential between tumour and normal tissue. Conversely, the use of a relatively small number of fractions, each with a large dose/fraction. is likely to lead to a therapeutic detriment. Since the majority of HDR applications in gynaecological brachytherapy involve small numbers of fractions, this is clearly a pertinent point, and one which will be discussed in more detail in Sect. 2.6.

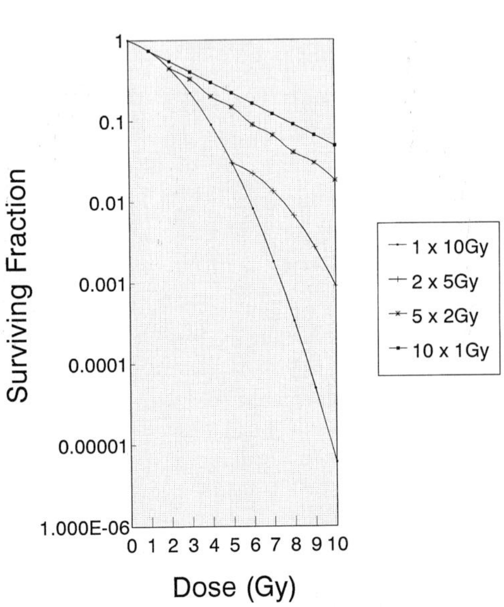

Fig. 2.1. Sparing effect of HDR fractionation on late-reacting normal tissue. The assumed α/β ratio is 2 Gy

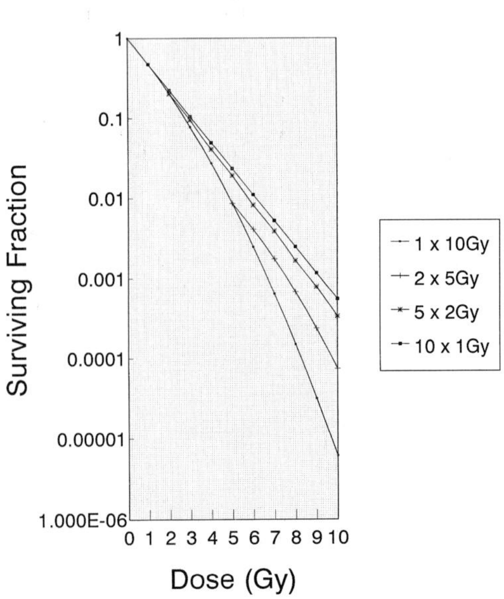

Fig. 2.2. Sparing effect of HDR fractionation on tumour/early-reacting normal tissue. The assumed α/β ratio is 14 Gy

2.4 Sublethal Damage Recovery

The type B (β-component) of lethal radiation damage is believed to result from an interaction between two independent (sublethal) radiation events within a critical target. The sublethal damage is reparable, generally with a recovery half-life of 0.5–3h. Type B damage only occurs if the damage resulting from the first event remains unrepaired at the time of the second event – the longer the time interval between the two events the less likely it will be that a lethal type B interaction can take place.

In fractionated radiotherapy involving fractions of short duration and reasonably long gaps between the fractions (e.g. conventional external beam therapy or HDR brachytherapy), any sublethal damage remaining after each fraction is fully repaired by the time the next fraction is delivered. However, if the interval between fractions if reduced to (say) 3h, there will always remain some unrepaired sublethal damage at the time of each subsequent fraction delivery, as a result of which the total amount of type B damage will be increased. When the inter-fraction intervals between all the fractions are made to be short, the increased type B damage tends to "snowball" throughout the entire treatment, with the result that a given physical dose becomes much more damaging. For this reason the use of hyperfractionated treatments (i.e. those involving two or more fractions per day) should only be adopted if the gap between fractions can be made to be at least 6h (Thames 1984; Fowler 1988).

It is not difficult to see how treatments involving continuous irradiation can be considered as consisting of a hypothetically large number of small dose fractions given at close time intervals, in which case the sublethal damage repair both during and between each fraction delivery will have an influence on overall biological effect. As the number of hypothetical fractions gets larger, the associated dose/fraction becomes correspondingly smaller, and it might be predicted that continuous low-dose-rate (CLDR) treatments might demonstrate some of the sparing characteristics associated with hyperfractionation. In fact this is exactly the case, and the LQ model helps to understand the close conceptual link which exists between the tissue sparing associated with CLDR and fractionated HDR treatments.

Figures 2.3 and 2.4 diagrammatically illustrate the variations in the sparing effect as dose rate is systematically reduced. Once again, the amount of sparing achievable will be governed not only by the dose rate but also by the α/β ratio. In this context the similarities between Figs. 2.3 and 2.4, and their respective fractionated counterparts, Figs. 2.1 and 2.2, are very clear.

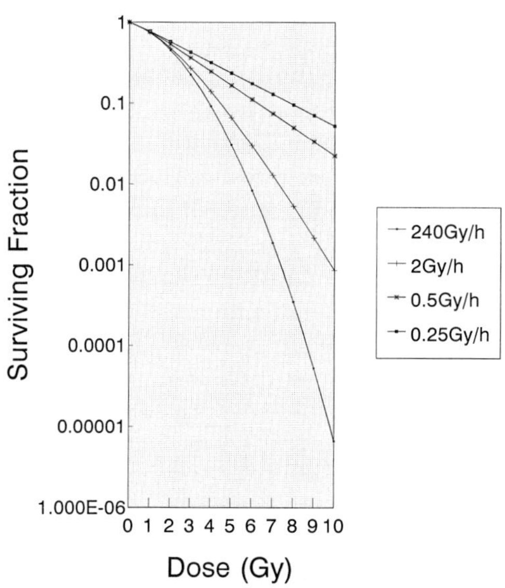

Fig. 2.3. Sparing effect of reducing dose rate on late-reacting tissue. The assumed α/β ratio is 2 Gy

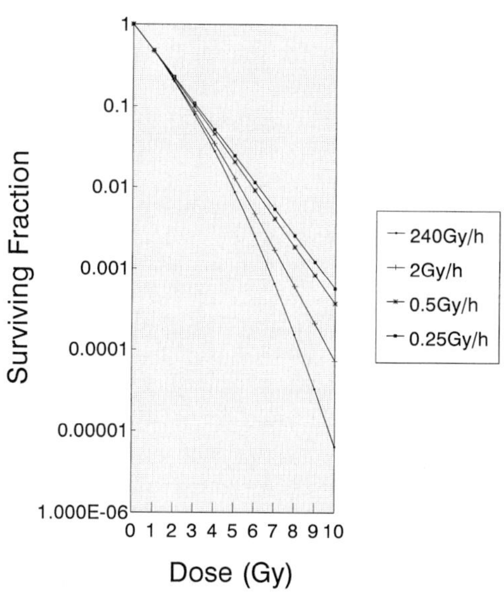

Fig. 2.4. Sparing effect of reducing dose rate on tumour/early-reacting tissue. The assumed α/β ratio is 14 Gy

2.5 The Effects of Changes in Dose-Rate

As discussed in the previous section, the phenomenon of sublethal damage repair is of little direct relevance to fractionated HDR irradiation, for which the duration of each fraction is a few minutes or less. However, it becomes of major importance when treatment times are protracted, i.e. when the irradiation time is comparable with, or longer than, the recovery half-life. For a given dose, treatment times are determined by the dose rate of the applied radiation, and an appreciation of the sublethal damage repair process is therefore essential to understanding why dose rate effects exist.

As dose rate is reduced, the number of radiation interactions within the critical targets in any time period also reduces. Lethal events resulting from type A damage will continue to occur and will be proportional to the total dose delivered, irrespective of the dose rate.

Sublethally damaged cells will also continue to be produced but, at low dose rates, they are more likely to repair themselves during the irradiation. Because they are repairing, and because of the reduced rate at which subsequent sublethal lesions are being produced, the number of type B interactions is also reduced. The amount of type B damage is therefore dependent, in a fairly complex way, on the dose rate. At very low dose rates virtually all of the damage produced is type A, the type B process becoming insignificant. This explains why the LDR curves in Figs. 2.3 and 2.4 become straighter as dose rate is reduced: the cell kill due to type B damage becomes relatively less important.

The associated LQ equation for calculating BEDs at low dose rate, when treatment times are relatively long, is:

$$BED = RT \cdot \left[1 + 2R/\mu(\alpha/\beta)\right], \tag{2.7}$$

where R is the dose rate, T the treatment time, and μ the recovery constant. (μ is related to the recovery half-life, $T_{1/2}$, by $\mu = 0.693/T_{1/2}$.) When the treatment time is only of the order of a few hours, other, more complex equations, should be used in place of Eq. 2.7 (Dale 1985).

The above discussion may help to clarify the point that dose rate effects are essentially time effects looked at from a different perspective. In conventional HDR fractionated radiotherapy the time gap between each fraction allows the sublethal damage which exists after each irradiation to fully recover before delivery of the next fraction. In CLDR it is the duration of the treatment itself which governs how much recovery can occur and, for a specified total dose, the treatment duration is obviously dependent on the dose rate. If the dose rate is high then treatment time is likely to be short, thus allowing little opportunity for sublethal recovery during irradiation. If the dose rate is low then treatment time will be long, allowing more opportunity for recovery during irradiation and an associated reduction in cell kill. It therefore seems logical that the definitions of LDR and HDR should centre more on the time taken to deliver a particular dose of radiation, rather than the dose rate per se.

The evolving view is that HDR treatments may be defined as those which allow the dose to be delivered in a time which is short compared with the recovery half-life. Conversely, CLDR treatments are those which cause the dose to be delivered in a time span which is long in comparison with the recovery half-life. Since half-lives are typically in the range 0.5–3 h, it would seem logical to class HDR treatments as those which take only a few minutes, and LDR treatments as those which take many hours. The supplementary question then is: How should we quantitatively define a few minutes, or many hours?

This point has been addressed elsewhere (Orton et al. 1994), using a range of likely radiobiological parameters, with the result that a more rigid definition of HDR is a treatment that takes about 30 min or less for the delivery, while LDR is one which takes about 14 h or more for its delivery. It should be noted that medium-dose-rate (MDR) treatments, i.e. those delivered over a period of a few hours, are likely to be the most unpredictable in their effects, because the variation of BED with treatment time is most rapid for those treatment times which are comparable with the tissue recovery half-lives. This could mean, for example, that treatment time corrections based only on a straightforward compensation for source decay might be especially unreliable (in radiobiological terms) in the case of MDR treatments.

Whatever the merits and demerits of such theoretical definitions of HDR, MDR and LDR, it is important to realise that there is almost certainly no sharp distinction between one category and the next, even though some publications continue to suggest that this is the case. This point is perhaps more clearly demonstrated by reference to Fig. 2.5, which, for a single dose of 5 Gy, shows how the relative effectiveness (RE) on a tumour/early-reacting tissue changes as the dose rate is decreased, and the treatment time increases. The changes in RE (and hence, the magnitude of the dose rate effect) are seen to be

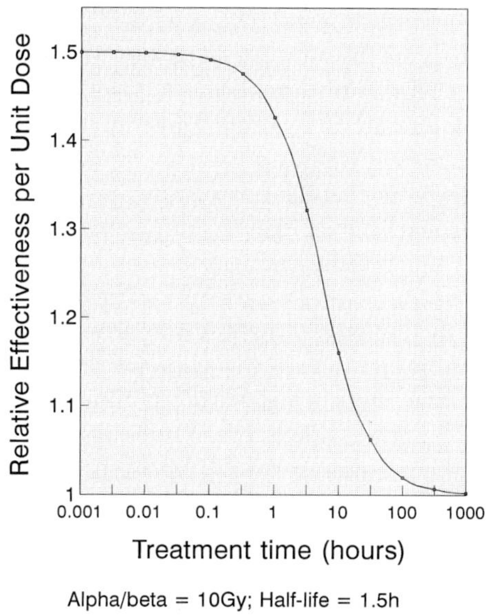

Fig. 2.5. Decrease in the relative effectiveness (RE) of a single dose of 5 Gy with increasing treatment time. The change in RE with time (and hence, the magnitude of the dose rate effect), is smallest when the treatment time is either relatively short (seconds/minutes) or very long (many tens of hours). The biggest changes in RE occur for middle-range variations in treatment times. The assumed parameters are α/β = 10 Gy, recovery half-life-1.5 h. For smaller α/β ratios the curve is expanded in the vertical direction; for smaller half-lives the curve is contracted in the horizontal direction

smallest when the irradiation time is either very small or very large in comparison with the recovery half-life.

2.6 The Design of HDR Treatments to Replace an Existing LDR Treatment

One of the key features of the LQ model is that it allows a more systematic radiobiological inter-comparison between different types of treatment. Because the main parameters (α/β and μ) are tissue-specific, such intercomparisons also allow there to be an assessment of the likely change in therapeutic ratio when switching between treatments. One of the main applications of LQ methodology, spurred on by the increasing availability of remote after-loading units, has been the design of fractionated HDR treatments which can replace existing CLDR techniques. The principles involved will now be briefly discussed.

Suppose an existing CLDR treatment involves the delivery, to the tumour dose reference point, of 40 Gy in 48 h, i.e. at a dose rate of 0.83 Gy h^{-1}. What are the equivalent fractionated HDR regimens? Bearing in mind that LQ equations must be tissue-specific, the question we are initially asking is: What fractionated HDR treatments deliver the same tumour BED as the existing LDR regimen? Assuming values of α/β = 10 Gy and μ = 0.5 h^{-1}, and neglecting any repopulation occurring in the short treatment period of 48 h, we have for the LDR treatment (from Eq. 2.7):

$$BED_{10} = 40 \times \left[1+2 \times 0.83/(10 \times 0.5)\right] = 53.3\,Gy.$$

This biological dose of 53.3 Gy to the tumour now becomes the "target" figure for the fractionated HDR treatments if we wish to maintain the effect on the tumour. Equation 2.4 may now be used to find how specific numbers of fractions and dose/fraction can be combined together to produce a specified BED. In this case, assuming that the fractionated brachytherapy can be given in a short enough time period to allow tumour repopulation effects to be neglected:

$$Nd \cdot \left[1+d/10\right] = 53.3.$$

This relationship can be solved by assuming various values of N (2, 4, 6, etc.) and finding the corresponding values of d. The first three columns in Table 2.1 show the result of this exercise.

It will be seen in column 3 that, for 12 or less fractions, the HDR regimens require the delivery of a

Table 2.1. The number of fractions (N) and HDR dose/fraction (d) required to maintain the same tumour effect as an LDR regimen delivering 40 Gy/48 h. The assumed tumour parameters are α/β = 10 Gy and μ = 0.5 h^{-1}. The BED_3 is the biological dose to late-reacting normal tissues (assumed α/β = 3 Gy, μ = 0.5 h^{-1}) for each combination of N and d. (For comparison, the BED_3 associated with the original LDR treatment is 84.4 Gy.) The final column shows how more favourable values of BED_3 are achieved when, relative to the tumour, the dose/fraction (and hence total dose) to the late-responding tissues is reduced by 10% as a result of source repositioning and/or shielding

Number of fractions N	Dose/ fraction d (Gy)	Total dose Nd (Gy)	BED_3 (Gy)	BED_3 (Gy) (with 10% extra sparing)
2	12.07	24.15	121.3	100.4
4	7.58	30.32	106.9	89.3
6	5.67	34.02	98.3	82.7
8	4.57	36.58	92.3	78.1
10	3.85	38.49	87.9	74.6
12	3.33	39.98	84.4	71.9
14	2.94	41.18	81.6	69.8
16	2.64	42.18	79.2	68.0
18	2.39	43.02	77.3	66.5
20	2.19	43.74	75.6	65.2

total dose which is lower than in the CLDR case. This is one of the characteristics of HDR brachytherapy; the total doses required for given biological endpoints are generally lower than with LDR, the reduction being much more pronounced for very small fraction numbers. Conversely, for more than 12 fractions the total dose at HDR needs to be higher than with CLDR.

What about the effects of these HDR regimens on late-reacting normal tissues? If we assume for the moment that the point A dose is representative of the dose to these tissues also, then, by reworking Eq. 2.4 with an assumed late-reacting α/β ratio of 3 Gy and a μ value of 0.5 Gy h^{-1}, we have:

$$BED_3 = 40 \times \left[1+2 \times 0.83/(3 \times 0.5)\right] = 84.3\,\text{Gy}.$$

Ideally, all of the fractionated HDR alternatives listed in Table 2.1 should also deliver a BED_3 of 84.3 Gy. Inspection of column 4 of Table 2.1 shows that this is not so; for 12 fractions or less the late-reacting biological dose is increased by the use of HDR, i.e. the therapeutic ratio, relative to the original LDR regimen, has been compromised. For more than 12 fractions the therapeutic ratio is improved. Also, for the particular radiobiological parameters assumed here, it is only at 12 fractions that equivalence is obtained for both types of tissue, and it will be noted that only with 12 fractions is the HDR dose exactly the same as that in the original LDR regimen.

In this chosen example, what is so special about 12 fractions? The answer to this question can be found by reference to LIVERSAGE (1969), who looked at the conditions for equivalence between HDR and CLDR. Liversage found that, provided the tumour and late-reacting recovery constants were the same, the condition for equal radiobiological effect on all tissues would be achieved if an LDR treatment of duration T hours were to be replaced by a fractionated scheme delivering the same dose in N fractions, where N is calculated from $N = \mu T/2$. In the above example we have chosen $\mu = 0.5\,\text{h}^{-1}$ and $T = 48\,\text{h}$, i.e. the theoretical point for complete equivalence is when the original LDR dose (40 Gy) is given in $0.5 \times 48/2 = 12$ fractions, which is exactly what Table 2.1 shows.

The remarkable aspect of this result is that the Liversage method was based on a quite different starting point, and predated the LQ approach by several years. The LQ model arrives at the same mathematical condition for equivalence (DALE 1985), and clarifies the point that, when the Liversage equation for equivalence between CLDR and HDR is satisfied, the α/β ratios are no longer significant, i.e. radiobiological effects on all tissues can remain unchanged in giving the same dose at HDR as with LDR, provided the μ values are the same for all tissues. The principle is the same for all total doses, i.e. 60 Gy/72 h at CLDR would require the 60 Gy to be delivered in $0.5 \times 72/2 = 16$ fractions at HDR.

On this basis, therefore, it would appear that HDR in gynaecology is only likely to be a viable alternative to CLDR if it is delivered with a prohibitively large number of fractions. Two points can be made about this. Firstly, the above analysis assumes that the recovery constants (μ) are the same for both tumour and late-reacting normal tissue. If tumours repair faster than normal tissues (i.e. if tumour μ values are higher) then the situation is improved, with fewer than 12 fractions being required in the above example. As a general rule experimental evidence suggests that tumours do repair faster than late-reacting tissues (BRENNER and HALL 1991a).

Secondly (and perhaps more importantly), the assumption has been made that the tumour and critical normal tissues are each subjected to the same total dose and dose/fraction. For gynaecological brachytherapy in particular this is not usually the case; careful geometrical placement of the HDR applicators, together with packing and/or retraction, can cause both the bladder and the rectum to receive considerably less radiation than the tumour. This has the immediate advantage of lowering both the dose and the dose/fraction received by the normal tissues, causing the normal tissue BED to fall by a proportionately greater amount.

This effect has been discussed by a number of authors (e.g. BRENNER and HALL 1991a; STITT et al. 1992). In particular, DALE (1990) has shown how even very modest additional reductions in the normal tissue dose at HDR can allow such techniques to be satisfactorily performed with more realistic fraction numbers. To illustrate this point, the BED_3 values in Table 2.1 have been recalculated on the basis that, at HDR, the normal tissues can be made to receive 10% less dose than the tumour. The results are compiled in the last column, and it is seen that the number of fractions required for equivalence falls from 12 to a more practical figure of about 5.

The important point to bear in mind is that, in the majority of cases, the radiobiological parameters will not be known with any degree of certainty. It is therefore not yet possible to devise optimised brachytherapy treatments to suit individual patients, in which case the use of very small fraction numbers and/or doses/fraction in excess of about 7.5 Gy are best avoided (ORTON et al. 1991). It is also perhaps wrong always to attempt to design new HDR treatments to radiobiologically match their LDR counterparts. Although the principle of LDR is radiobiologically sound, a wide variety of LDR regimens have been developed over the years for treating gynaecological malignancies, not all of which would necessarily be classed as "gold standard". Remote HDR afterloading provides more scope for accurate and reproducible source positioning than is normally possible with LDR techniques, and the importance of this physical advantage should not be underrated.

2.7 Special Considerations for Gynaecological Applications: Dose Gradients

Although the application of the LQ model to brachytherapy is, in analytical terms, relatively straightforward, there are some subtle aspects which must always be borne in mind. It is inherently assumed in the basic LQ calculations discussed in this chapter that there is dose uniformity throughout the various irradiated organs, i.e. that the calculated BED is representative of the BED to the entire organ. In brachytherapy this is never true: the BED gradients will in fact be even steeper than the associated physical dose gradients. The immediate implication of this is that radiobiological intercomparisons of treatments from different centres can only be useful if the BEDs are specified at common anatomical sites and if the irradiation geometries are reasonably similar. Whatever the reference point in gynaecological brachytherapy, it is useful to remember that the chosen point is part of a three-dimensional iso-biological effect surface which surrounds the treatment sources (Deehan and O'Donoghue 1994). Therefore, all sites within that surface will receive higher biological doses, and the observed clinical effects will be the result of an integrated biological response within the contained volume, because the true biological dose received by the enclosed tissues will be greater than that calculated at the reference point. The irradiated volume is especially important in relation to normal tissue effects, and it is for these in particular that care is required in ensuring that similar anatomical reference points are selected. In terms of tumour cure the volume effect is probably of less significance. Provided a curative dose is always prescribed to the outermost extent of the tumour then the tumour cure probability ought not to vary between patients, even though the tumour volumes themselves may vary. Treatment intercomparisons might therefore be based on tumour doses existing at the (variable) position of the tumour surface, whilst normal tissue doses should be selected from (non-variable) geometrical sites.

Integrated biological response models are already being developed, and it is likely that these, when used in conjunction with dose-volume histograms, will in future play an increasingly important role in refining the intercomparison of brachytherapy treatments.

2.8 Pulsed-Dose Rate Brachytherapy

Pulsed-dose rate (PDR) brachytherapy is another suggested replacement for conventional CLDR techniques, in which the continuous low dose rate is replaced by one pulsed exposure of about 10 min duration in each hour. The overall duration of a PDR technique would normally be similar to that of the CLDR technique which it replaces. The radiation delivery is by means of a single stepping source (iridium-192) of intermediate activity, and it is clear that the advent of PDR would not have been possible without the associated technology required to automatically and repeatedly carry out a complex series of source movements.

The radiobiology of PDR has been investigated by Brenner and Hall (1991b) and Fowler and Mount (1992), using previously derived radiobiological equations for closely spaced non-instantaneous fractions (Dale et al. 1988; Nilsson et al. 1990). The dose rate associated with each pulse is relatively high (typically 3 Gy/h), but the averaged dose rate in any one hour is similar to that in the CLDR treatment which is being replaced. Because the duration of each pulse is short, and is followed by an interval which is sufficiently long to allow some repair, it is theoretically possible that the treatment can be designed in such a way that the amount of repair between all of the fractions can be made to closely match that occurring in the CLDR regimen.

The advantage of PDR is that it eradicates the radiation protection risks for nursing staff, visitors, etc. which are associated with CLDR. However, the technique requires a well-protected room, and the logistic problems for patients being treated for a few minutes in each hour over a period of several days have yet to be properly assessed. Early clinical results indicate that the acute toxicity with PDR is similar to that expected with CLDR, but only if the prescribed pulsing techniques are closely adhered to (e.g. SWIFT et al. 1994).

There is also the question of cost effectiveness. PDR patients can only be treated as in-patients and, in general, a single PDR afterloading unit would not be able to treat as many patients as a single HDR unit delivering fractionated brachytherapy. As a consequence there might be a temptation to modify PDR schedules in order to allow longer "radiation-free" intervals. Such a step might have deleterious consequences for the treatment outcome, because the theoretical analysis which suggests that PDR is feasible is more critically dependent on the radiobiological assumptions than perhaps any other type of radiation treatment.

2.9 Possible Future Developments

Within the past few years more concerted efforts have been made to use radiobiological models prospectively, as well as retrospectively. This opens up the possibility of using models more adventurously, e.g. in the design of tailored treatments to suit individual patients. The fuller application of such a process will necessarily depend on the more widespread availability of serial imaging and predictive assay techniques in radiotherapy departments. Specific areas of interest for gynaecological treatments are likely to be:

1. Using a knowledge of tumour growth kinetics to decide whether or not the external beam component needs to be accelerated and/or hyperfractionated, or whether once-daily fractionation is adequate (DALE 1989; FOWLER 1990).
2. Using a knowledge of tumour shrinkage rates and potential doubling times to ascertain the optimum time intervals between brachytherapy fractions, and to decide whether to place the brachytherapy component within the external beam schedule or to delay it until later. A preliminary assessment of the radiobiological issues involved in such decisions has already been undertaken (JONES and BLEASDALE 1994; JONES et al. 1994).
3. A linking between the physical information obtained from dose-volume histograms with overall biological response.

References

Barendsen GW (1982) Dose fractionation, dose rate and isoeffect relationships for normal tissue response. Int J Radiat Oncol Biol Phys 8:1981–1997

Brenner DJ, Hall EJ (1991a) Fractionated high dose-rate versus low dose-rate regimens for intracavitary brachytherapy of the cervix. Br J Radiol 64:133–141

Brenner DJ, Hall EJ (1991b) Conditions for the equivalence of continuous to pulsed low dose-rate brachytherapy. Int J Radiat Oncol Biol Phys 20:181–190

Chadwick KH, Leenhouts HP (1973) A molecular theory of cell survival. Phys Med Biol 18:78–87

Dale RG (1985) The application of the linear-quadratic dose-effect equation to fractionated and protracted radiotherapy. Br J Radiol 58:515–528

Dale RG (1989) Time-dependent tumour repopulation factors in linear-quadratic equations – implications for treatment. Radiother Oncol 15:371–382

Dale RG (1990) The use of small fraction numbers in high dose-rate gynaecological afterloading: some radiobiological considerations. Br J Radiol 63:290–294

Dale RG, Huczkowski J, Trott KR (1988) Possible dose-rate dependence of recovery kinetics as deduced from a preliminary analysis of the effects of fractionated irradiations at varying dose-rates. Br J Radiol 61:153–157

Deehan C, O'Donoghue JA (1994) Biological equivalence of LDR and HDR brachytherapy. In: Mould RF, Batterman JJ, Martinez AA, Speiser BL (eds) Brachytherapy-from radium to optimization. Nucletron International BV, pp 19–33

Ellis F (1969) Dose, time and fractionation: a clinical hypothesis. Clin Radiol 20:1–7

Fowler JF (1988) Intervals between multiple fractions per day. Acta Oncol 27:181–183

Fowler JF (1989) The linear-quadratic formula and progress in fractionated radiotherapy. Br J Radiol 62:679–694

Fowler JF (1990) How worthwhile are short schedules in radiotherapy? A series of exploratory calculations. Radiother Oncol 18:165–181

Fowler JF, Mount M (1992) Pulsed brachytherapy: the conditions for no significant loss of therapeutic ratio compared with traditional low dose-rate brachytherapy. Int J Radiat Oncol Biol Phys 23:661–669

Fowler JF, Stern BE (1960) Dose-rate effects: some theoretical and practical considerations. Br J Radiol 33:389–395

Joiner MC (1993) Linear-quadratic approach to fractionation. In: Steel GG (ed) Basic clinical radiobiology. Edward Arnold, London, pp 55–64

Jones B, Bleasdale C (1994) Effect of overall time when radiotherapy includes teletherapy and brachytherapy: a mathematical model. Br J Radiol 67:63–70

Jones B, Dale RG, Bleasdale C, Tan LT, Davies M (1994) A mathematical model of intraluminal and intracavitary brachytherapy. Br J Radiol 67:805–812

Kellerer AM, Rossi HH (1972) The theory of dual radiation action. Curr Top Radiat Res Q 8:85–158

Kirk J, Gray WM, Watson R (1972) Cumulative radiation effect. 1. Fractionated treatment regimes. Clin Radiol 22:145–155

Liversage WE (1969) A general formula for equating protracted and acute regimes of radiation. Br J Radiol 42:432–440

Liversage WE (1971) A critical look at the ret. Br J Radiol 44:91–100

Nilsson P, Thames HD, Joiner MC (1990) A generalized formulation of the "incomplete-repair" model for cell survival and tissue response to fractionated low dose-rate irradiation. Int J Radiat Biol 57:127–142

Orton CG, Ellis F (1973) A simplification in the use of the NSD concept in practical radiotherapy. Br J Radiol 46:529–537

Orton CG, Seyedsadr M, Somnay A (1991) Comparison of high and low dose-rate remote afterloading for cervix cancer and the importance of fractination. Int J Radiat Oncol Biol Phys 21:1425–1434

Orton CG, Brenner DJ, Dale RG, Fowler JF (1994) Radiobiology. In: Nag S (ed) High dose-rate brachytherapy: a textbook. Futura, Mt. Kisco, NY, pp 11–25

Steel GG (1993) The dose-rate effect: brachytherapy. In: Steel GG (ed) Basic clinical radiobiology. Edward Arnold, London, pp 120–129

Steel GG, Kelland LR, Peacock JH (1989) The radiobiological basis for low dose-rate radiotherapy. In: Mould RF (ed) Brachytherapy 2. Nucletron International BV, Veenendal, pp 15–25

Stitt JA, Fowler JF, Thomadsen BR, et al. (1992) High dose-rate intracavitary brachytherapy for carcinoma of the cervix: the Madison System. 1. Clinical and radiobiological considerations. Int J Radiat Oncol Biol Phys 24:335–348

Swift PS, Fu KK, Phillips TL, Roberts LW, Weaver KA (1994) Pulsed LDR interstitial and intracavitary therapy; clinical experience at UCSF, San Francisco, USA. In: Mount M (ed) Pulsed dose-rate brachytherapy. Radiobiology and initial clinical results. Nucletron Special Report Number 5, pp 29–31

Thames HD (1984) Effect-independent measures of tissue responses to fractionated irradiation. Int J Radiat Oncol Biol Physics 45:1–10

Thames HD (1985) An "incomplete-repair" model for survival after fractionated and continuous irradiations. Int J Radiat Biol 47:319–339

Travis EL, Tucker SL (1987) Isoeffect models and fractionated radiation therapy. Int J Radiat Oncol Biol Phys 13:283–287

Wheldon TE, Amin AE (1988) The linear-quadratic model (letter). Br J Radiol 61:700–703

3 Diagnostic Workup and Staging

H. JUNKERMANN and D. VON FOURNIER with contributions from H.W. VAHRSON

CONTENTS

3.1 Introduction

Before commencing therapy of a gynecological carcinoma it is necessary to obtain, as precisely as possible, an overview of the type of tumor and its extension in order to adjust the therapy optimally to the aggressiveness of the tumor and its pattern of spread.

H. JUNKERMANN, MD, Abteilung für Gynäkologische Radiologie, Radiologische Universitätsklinik, Bereich Frauenklinik, Voßstraße 9, D-69115 Heidelberg, Germany
D. VON FOURNIER, MD, Professor, Abteilung für Gynäkologische Radiologie, Radiologische Universitätsklinik, Bereich Frauenklinik, Voßstraße 9, D-69115 Heidelberg, Germany

3.2 Clinical Examination

In the majority of patients with gynecological carcinomas, clinical examination is of paramount importance because the affected organ systems can be approached by direct inspection and/or palpation. For that part of the genital region which can be approached by inspection or palpation, the clinical examination provides basic information that cannot be gathered by instrumental imaging methods. Clinical examination should not encompass the local situation in the genital region alone; rather at the same time a gross general examination should be done in order to assess the general state of health and to exclude concomitant diseases, which may be important for the therapeutic decision.

The gynecological examination begins with a careful inspection of the external genitalia on the gynecological chair. The vulva, the perineum, and the perianal region are inspected. The introitus of the vagina is inspected after gently pulling the labia apart. Palpation of the inguinal lymph nodes should be done. By distending the vagina with specula, its walls may be carefully inspected and the cervix is displayed. A Papanicolaou smear of the cervix should be taken before initiating therapy of a genital carcinoma, because multilocular development of cancer is possible. After inspection, bimanual palpation is performed to estimate the size, form, consistency, and moveability of the uterus and the adnexal regions on both sides. The reliability of this examination depends very much on the constitution (adiposity) of the patient and her ability to cooperate (relaxation of the abdominal wall). The examination is concluded by rectal palpation, which does not only serve to evaluate the rectal wall itself: in particular, the circumference of the cervix uteri and the parametria are best examined by this method. Documentation of the results of the clinical examination is preferably done as a small sketch.

3.3 Methods of Morphological Diagnosis

3.3.1 Cytology

Exfoliative cytology of the cervix has had a major impact on the prevention of invasive cervical carcinoma. In the clinical situation its value mainly resides in the fact that a negative smear of the cervix largely excludes involvement of the macroscopically normal cervix uteri. Therefore a cervical smear should be taken in the pretherapeutic staging examination of any genital carcinoma. If a clinically suspicious lesion is found, a histological examination is necessary irrespective of the result of exfoliative cytology.

While fine-needle biopsy has not found a place in the evaluation of primary tumors of the female genital organs, it is a valuable method in experienced hands to investigate metastatic spread to lymph nodes in the inguinal and para-aortic regions, as well as to confirm metastasis in the liver and lung or meningiosis carcinomatosa. In the para-aortic region fine-needle aspiration is done under CT guidance, while in the liver ultrasound guidance is preferred, if the lesion can be localized using ultrasound.

For adequate interpretation of the cytological smears the cytologist should have full knowledge of the clinical and – if available – histological information.

3.3.2 Histology

Histological confirmation is the standard in the diagnosis of any gynecological malignant disease.

Vulvar, vaginal, or cervical lesions can be easily biopsied using punch biopsy without anesthesia or with local anesthesia only. To obtain representative material, especially in larger lesions, it is necessary to perform the biopsy from the invasive front of the tumor, otherwise necrotic and inconclusive material may be collected.

If a tumor is suspected in the cervical canal or in the uterus, dilatation and curettage is performed, usually with the patient under general anesthesia, because this allows for a better clinical staging examination of the internal genitalia. If a malignant tumor is suspected, curettage should always be performed separately from the cervical canal and the uterine cavity (fractionated curettage) in order to assess cervical and/or intracavitary extension of the tumor.

Conization of the cervix is done for diagnostic reasons, if cervical cytology gives a suspicious result and clinically or colposcopically the lesion cannot be located for a guided biopsy. Conization can also be used therapeutically if the smear is suggestive of carcinoma in situ and a young woman wants to retain her reproductive capacity. It is not a method to confirm clinically overt lesions, because the morbidity of the procedure (bleeding, infection) is higher than the complications of guided punch biopsy and time elapses until definite therapy can be carried out.

Diagnostic laparoscopy or laparotomy has to be done to confirm the diagnosis of a suspected tumor of the upper genitalia (tubes and ovaries). Staging laparotomy is also sometimes done to assess the operability of cervical carcinoma, because of the known inaccuracy of clinical staging. However, no consensus has been reached on the indications for staging laparotomies or on the question of when a pelvic tumor is to be regarded as inoperable. If a staging laparotomy is performed, it should be kept in mind that a transperitoneal staging operation increases the complication rate of later para-aortic irradiation (Rotman et al. 1990).

3.4 Blood Chemistry

Red and white blood cell count, platelet count, liver tests, and especially renal function tests should always be done in patients with gynecological carcinoma. Because of the possibility of obstructive nephropathy due to pelvic tumors, a careful evaluation of renal function is especially important.

3.5 Tumor Markers

The value of tumor markers in the primary diagnosis of gynecological tumors is limited. The determination of CA-125 can be helpful in the sometimes difficult preoperative differential diagnosis of ovarian tumors in postmenopausal women. HCG is a sensitive and specific marker for trophoblastic tumors. High HCG values are considered a risk factor. The importance of tumor markers for therapeutic monitoring and follow-up will be discussed under the different tumor entities.

3.6 Imaging Procedures

3.6.1 Conventional Roentgenography

Conventional X-ray films of the thorax should be obtained routinely in all patients with malignant tumors in order to exclude pulmonary metastasis. In gynecological tumors urography is of special importance because of the possibility of involvement of the urinary system. Intravenous urography allows not only the detection of obstructive uropathy with high sensitivity but also pre-operative diagnosis of anomalies of the urinary system (renal dystopia, anomalies of the ureters). This is of special importance if operative therapy is planned.

Contrast enemas can be helpful in the differential diagnosis between gynecological and colorectal tumors. They also can be used to exclude secondary involvement of the rectum. Today, however, their use has largely been overtaken by endoscopic investigations.

In the case of symptomatic bone metastasis, conventional roentgenography reveals whether a fracture of the affected bone is impending or even has taken place.

3.6.2 Lymphography

Since the advent of computer tomography (CT) lymphography has been used less frequently because it is rather tedious to perform. In experienced hands, however, lymphography is the most sensitive imaging method for the detection of lymphatic spread. While CT relies on the size of the lymph node, lymphography detects architectural changes before the node is enlarged and thus has a potentially much higher sensitivity (Fig. 3.1).

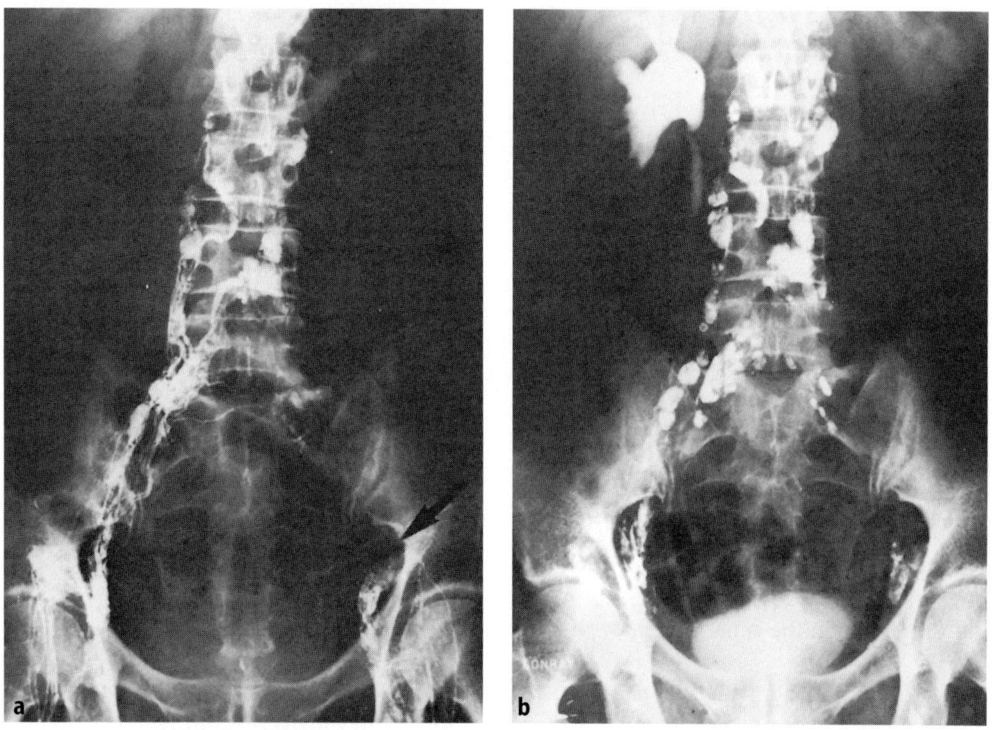

Fig. 3.1 a,b. Lymphography in a patient presenting with edema of the left lower limb 3 years after irradiation of a cervical cancer stage IIIb. **a** Lymphangiogram with complete lymphatic obstruction (*arrow*) at the level of the lower external iliac lymph nodes. **b** Lymphadenogram and urogram of the same patient. Incomplete metastatic imaging of the lower external iliac lymph nodes; there is loss of three external iliac and some of the communal lymph nodes. The urogram reveals complete obstruction of the left ureter with a nonfunctioning kidney and beginning urinary retention on the right side. (From Vahrson 1976)

Besides the tedious manipulation required to puncture lymph vessels, there are two drawbacks to lymphography:

1. Important lymph nodes situated along the iliac internal vessels cannot be demonstrated by pedal lymphography.
2. The interpretation of the lymphograms needs considerable experience, because both metastases and degenerative lesions following inflammatory reactions may show up as defects in the contrast filling of the lymph node. The comparison of lymphangiograms and lymphadenograms helps in the differentiation. Metastases typically show obstruction of the flow of the contrast medium, while degenerative lesions do not show such obstruction.

Experienced lymphographers can reach an accuracy of 90% (Kindermann et al. 1970). Thus the accuracy of lymphography in experienced hands is only exceeded by that of diagnostic biopsy.

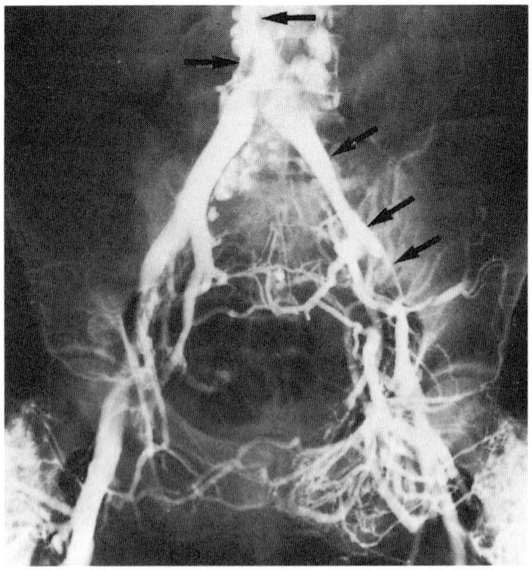

Fig. 3.2. Ossovenogram of the same patient as in Fig. 3.1 There is complete obstruction of the left v. iliaca externa and v. iliaca interna. Blood flow is sustained by collateral veins to the right side and to the left v. iliaca communis. There is hourglass constriction of the left v. iliaca communis and lateral impressions of the inferior vena cava (*arrows*). (From Vahrson 1976)

3.6.3 Pertrochanteric Ossovenography and Phlebography

H.W. Vahrson

In advanced recurrences of cervical cancer, so-called lymphedema of one or both lower limbs may occur. In such cases, lymphography shows complete obstruction of all lymphatic vessels at the lower a. iliaca externa level (Fig. 3.1a) and missing lymph nodes from a. iliaca externa to the a. iliaca communis (Fig. 3.1b). Lymphography should then be complemented by pertrochanteric ossovenography (a technique in which contrast medium is instilled using a special cannula, which has been hammered into the trochanter major, to visualize the venous system of the pelvis and inferior vena cava) (Fig. 3.2) or pedal phlebography and urography to determine with certainty the nature of the disease, which presents with obstruction of lymphatic vessels, pelvic veins, and the ureter in the same region of the true pelvis.

In a series of 30 patients with "lymphedema" of the lower limb, Vahrson (1972, 1976) could demonstrate that lymphatic vessel obstruction does not lead to lymphedema as long as the lymphovenous anastomoses are intact. Only if the pelvic veins (v. iliaca externa, interna, and/or communis) are obstructed does edema occur. Additional urography may also demonstrate obstruction of the ureter on the same side. Therefore we called this disease entity combined obstructive edema, which is pathognomonic for pelvic metastasis. Pertrochanteric ossovenography is a very time-consuming and expensive examination (general anesthesia required) but it gives much better contrast in the x-ray series than the usual pedal phlebography.

3.6.4 Ultrasonography

Ultrasonography is an inexpensive method to evaluate the extent of pelvic disease. It has the advantage of allowing arbitrary imaging planes. On the other hand, interpretation is very much dependent on the expertise of the examiner and reproducible documentation is difficult.

3.6.4.1 Abdominal Ultrasonography

The value of abdominal ultrasonography in gynecological cancers lies mainly in the evaluation of ascites and large ovarian tumors. The pelvis itself can be better visualized using endovaginal or endorectal probes.

Evaluation of the liver can be efficiently done by ultrasonography when a genital tumor is suspected to have metastasized into the liver.

Obstructive uropathy can be evaluated using ultrasonography, especially if the kidney function is impaired, precluding intravenous urography (FRÖHLICH et al. 1991). Intravenous urography, however, is preferred for its ability to delineate the course of the ureters.

3.6.4.2 Intracavitary Ultrasonography

With the development of small intracavitary probes, intravaginal ultrasonography has largely superseded abdominal ultrasonography for the evaluation of intrapelvic disease. Its advantages are high resolution and the avoidance of the inconvenience of the full bladder that is needed as an acoustic window for the transabdominal visualization of intrapelvic organs. However, in patients with exophytic tumors and in old women with a shrunken vagina intravaginal ultrasonography may not be possible.

Transrectal ultrasonography (TRUS) has been advocated for imaging of cervical tumors and parametrial extension (INNOCENTI et al. 1992; GITSCH et al. 1993). Its accuracy in the detection of parametrial invasion seems to be better than that of palpation by an experienced gynecological surgeon and also superior to that of CT. It can be used as an adjunct to clinical examination in radiological treatment planning because it allows objective measurement of the diameter of cervical tumors (MAGEE et al. 1991), which may be important in planning the relative roles of percutaneous and intracavitary irradiation. By objectively showing the length of the uterine cavity and the position of the uterus, TRUS helps to avoid perforation and irradiation with misplaced applicators in intrauterine insertions for brachytherapy, especially in adipose patients, in whom the effectiveness of bimanual palpation is often limited. Hysterosonography also has been advocated as a method which allows estimation of the depth of tumorous infiltration of the myometrium in endometrial carcinoma (HÖTZINGER and BECKER 1984).

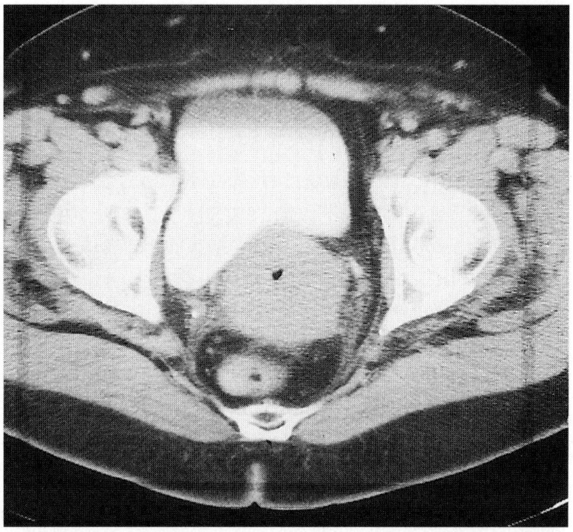

Fig. 3.3. CT of a stage III cervical cancer. Axial plane through the enlarged cervix. Tumor and surrounding healthy tissue cannot be distinguished

3.6.5 Computed Tomography

Computed tomography has found wide acceptance in the preoperative staging of gynecological tumors. A major advantage in comparison with ultrasonography is the systematic imaging in parallel axial planes. Observer variability is therefore of little importance compared with ultrasonography. The disadvantage of CT is that there is little contrast between normal and tumorous uterine tissues (Fig. 3.3). Because of partial volume effects its ability to evaluate bladder or rectal involvement is limited. The value of CT in pretherapeutic staging of gynecological tumors resides mainly in its ability to demonstrate extrauterine disease, especially nodal involvement in the upper part of the pelvis and the retroperitoneum (Fig. 3.4), which cannot be reached by the palpating finger. Micrometastatic disease, however, cannot be detected and lymph node enlargement is an unspecific sign of tumorous spread. Thus the value of this method is limited in those cases where staging or therapeutic laparotomy is planned anyway.

3.6.6 Magnetic Resonance Imaging

Magnetic resonance imaging (MRI) has proven in recent years to be the most exact imaging modality in pelvic tumors (HRICAK et al. 1985). Its advantage in comparison with CT is the superior tissue contrast and the possibility of choosing different planes, such as sagittal or frontal planes, thus giving a better overview of the pelvic organs and reducing the impact of partial volume effects. MRI allows the delineation of the volume of cervical tumors in relation to the normal uterine tissues (LIEN et al. 1991a,b) (Fig. 3.5a). This method allows differentiation between tumorous and benign parauterine tissue using T2-weighted images (YAMASHITA et al. 1993; SIRONI et al. 1991), thus yielding an improvement of parametrial staging. In difficult cases contrast enhancement with gadolinium seems to be superior to T2-weighted imaging (HRICAK et al. 1991; YAMASHITA et al. 1993) (Figs. 3.5, 3.6). The accuracy of the imaging of the tumor within the surrounding tissues allows improved treatment planning, especially for brachytherapy in cervical and endometrial carcinoma. For cervical carcinoma, HRICAK et al. (1996) have shown that in spite of the high cost of the method, staging with MRI is cheaper than conventional staging, because a number of cheaper studies are rendered unnecessary.

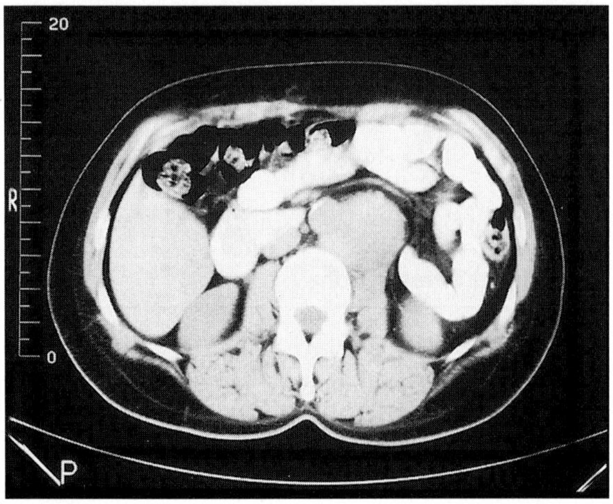

Fig. 3.4. Retroperitoneal CT of patient 2 years after primary therapy of cervical carcinoma. A large para-aortic lymph node is present

In endometrial carcinoma MRI allows pretherapeutic evaluation of the depth of myometrial invasion (SIRONI et al. 1992; MINDERHOUD-BASSIE et al. 1995), though with large polypoid tumors the accuracy is reduced (LIEN et al. 1991b; SCOUTT et al. 1995). The clinical importance of the information provided by MRI, however, is limited, because endometrial carcinoma of stage I is generally treated surgically; the same information thus can be obtained intraoperatively. MRI allows reliable detection of spread to the cervix, which has important therapeutic implications. In ovarian carcinomas MRI has only marginal advantages over CT.

In contrast to CT, MRI can differentiate between tumorous or fibrotic enlargement of lymph nodes, a question which is of less importance in the primary staging than in the evaluation of recurrences (HAWIGHORST et al. 1996).

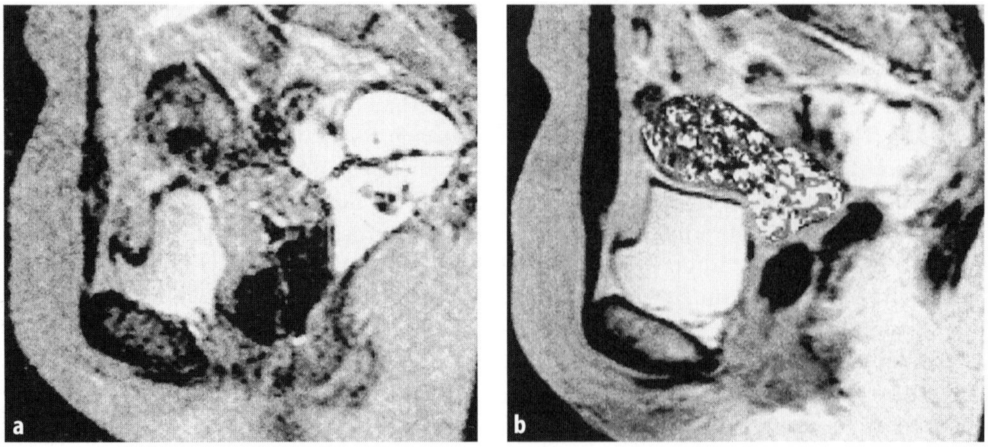

Fig. 3.5 a,b. Sagittal plane through the pelvis of a woman with stage IB cervical cancer. **a** T2-weighted image allows distinction of cervical tumor and healthy uterine tissue. Delineation of the bladder wall is difficult. **b** Dynamic contrast imaging with pharmacodynamic color mapping rules out infiltration of the bladder wall (surgically confirmed). (Courtesy of Dr. HAWIGHORST, DKFZ Heidelberg)

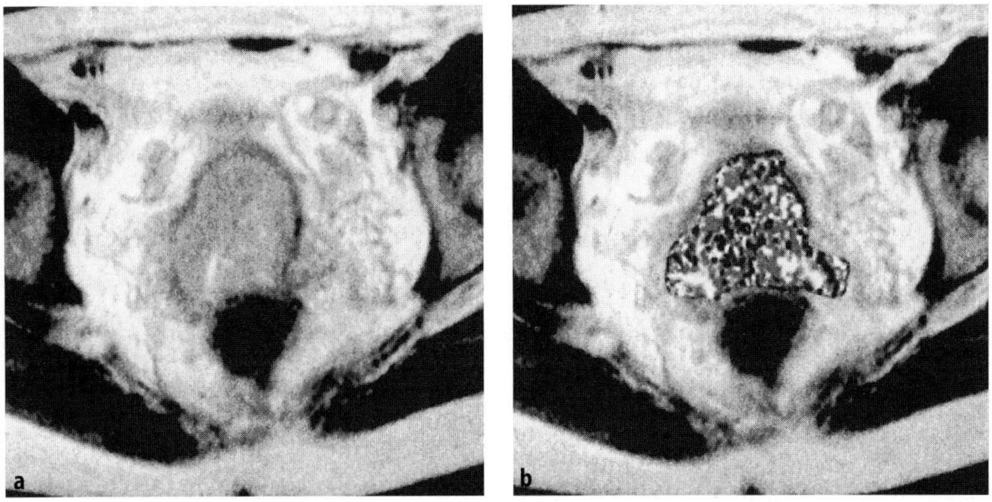

Fig. 3.6 a,b. Axial plane through the uterus of a woman with stage IIB cervical cancer. **a** T2-weighted images show infiltration of both parametria. **b** Dynamic contrast imaging with pharmacodynamic color mapping shows superior delineation of parametrial extension (surgically confirmed). (Courtesy of Dr. HAWIGHORST, DKFZ Heidelberg)

3.6.7 Scintigraphy

Scintigraphic methods are of little importance for the investigation of primary pelvic tumors. Immune scintigraphy with OC 125 is able to localize recurrences of ovarian carcinomas if the tumor marker CA-125 rises and other methods are not able to localize the recurrence. In certain cases this may have implications for therapy (surgery vs radiotherapy vs systemic therapy). The method, however, is still at an experimental stage and not widely available (BAUM et al. 1989).

Renal scintigraphy is used to assess the function of the kidney if the ureter is obstructed, in order to determine whether an effort at recanalization is worthwhile.

Bone scintigraphy is not routinely used in patients with gynecological tumors because the prevalence of bone metastasis is low. It is reserved for cases with symptomatic bone disease.

3.6.8 Hysterography with an Indwelling Applicator

H.W. VAHRSON

The transformation of Heyman's radium packing method into an adequate high-dose-rate (HDR) or low-dose-rate (LDR) afterloading technique, as used in Würzburg (see Chap. 10), requires very sophisticated technique, time and qualified staff, which may not be available in every center.

Hysterography employing the usual technique (occlusion of the cervical canal by a cone and injection of contrast medium with moderate pressure) prior to brachytherapy with radium was initially the subject of controversy but was emphasized as a routine measure by FRISCHKORN as long ago as 1976.

For the users of HDR devices with one or two moving sources in steel applicators we developed a simple method of hysterography with an indwelling applicator to distinguish cavities suitable for brachytherapy from those not suited for this treatment. The method was first described by ROTH and VAHRSON (1984), ROTH et al. (1985), and VAHRSON (1992) from Giessen and by HAASE (1987, 1989) from Karlsruhe.

3.6.8.1 Materials and Methods

The appropriate time for hysterography with an indwelling applicator is after the first intracavitary treatment using a dose of 6–10 Gy (with a distance of 2 cm) or after adequate central percutaneous irradiation. This pretreatment provides for occlusion of the fallopian tubes and prevents intraperitoneal spread of tumor cells, if the tumor itself does not already obstruct the tubes.

The materials required are: a 20-ml syringe, a flexible venous catheter which can be attached to the syringe [we use a Cavafix v. jugularis type 45 cm × 0.8 × 1.4 mm/18 G (B. BRAUN Melsungen AG, D-34212 Melsungen, Germany)], and 10–20 ml of usual water-soluble contrast medium 60% (as used for angiography or urography).

After clamping of the portio vaginalis and cervical dilatation (up to Hegar stick 5.5 for an applicator of 5 mm diameter), the venous catheter is placed into the uterine cavity as measured with the probe. The catheter should be filled with contrast medium before insertion. The afterloading applicator is then inserted and brought into position without a stopper or plate before the surface of the portio to avoid breakage of the catheter. Fixation of the catheter to the applicator by means of a thin adhesive tape may be easier in some cases. A clamp must be kept at the portio. Cautious packing with gauze can then be done around the applicator, clamp and catheter in the center. This arrangement allows the applicator to be pushed into or turned within the uterine cavity (while holding tight the clamp) without reinsertion.

After testing the passage of contrast medium and possible brief withdrawal of the catheter, 7–10 ml contrast medium is slowly injected under an x-ray unit which allows exposures in anteroposterior and lateral views. Passage of the contrast medium into the peritoneal cavity is nearly excluded, as no intrauterine pressure can be established because of the open cervical canal which allows the liquid to flow out immediately.

3.6.8.2 Results

During more than 10 years' experience this method has proved its usefulness and safety, with freedom from complications. It is therefore a routine procedure in every case in which primary HDR afterloading brachytherapy is employed for endometrial cancer. We can subdivide the results into four categories:

1. Ideal central position of the applicator within a narrow and/or symmetrical uterine cavity. No correction of the applicator position is necessary for adequate irradiation (Fig. 3.7).
2. Intracervical or eccentric position of the applicator in a more extended and/or deformed uterine cavity. Either one applicator with a special curve and 180° turnaround after half-time or a symmetrically curved twin applicator or differently curved applicators for both tubal angles are required. An adequate irradiation of the uterine wall and the tubular angles can be achieved (Fig. 3.8).
3. Hysterography reveals an unexpected perforation of the uterus. The anatomical situation must be clarified by hysterography or by laparoscopy. Nevertheless, brachytherapy can be performed if the applicator can be correctly inserted (see Fig. 3.10).
4. No access is possible from the cervical canal to the uterine cavity or there is extreme and uncorrectable displacement of the applicator at the wall of an enlarged uterine cavity. No adequate intracavitary treatment is then possible (see Figs. 3.11–3.13).

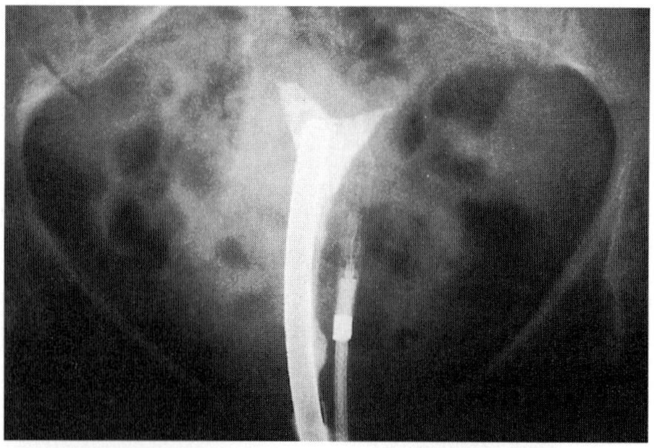

Fig. 3.7. Anteroposterior hysterogram showing narrow cavity tubal corners within 1 cm from the applicator

Roughly 50% of cavities are ideal or nearly ideal for intracavitary brachytherapy and can be irradiated with a single steel applicator delivering a sufficient dose to the myometrium and tubal angles. Of the remaining cases, 40% need a special applicator arrangement, for instance differently curved applicators for each side of the cavity, either simultaneously or in consecutive sessions, or a twin applicator. To this category belong cases in which the applicator is only placed into an abnormally long cervical canal (Fig. 3.9) or in which hysterography reveals a perforation (Fig. 3.10). It must be stressed that a considerable percentage of such patients suffer local recurrence when only one usual applicator is inserted centrally into the cavity. The final 10% of cases, which represent an absolute contraindication to intracavitary brachytherapy, include: (a) balloon-shaped cavity (Fig. 3.11), (b) obstruction of the cervix/isthmus uteri, (c) sharp-cornered deviation between the cervical canal and the cavum uteri (Fig.

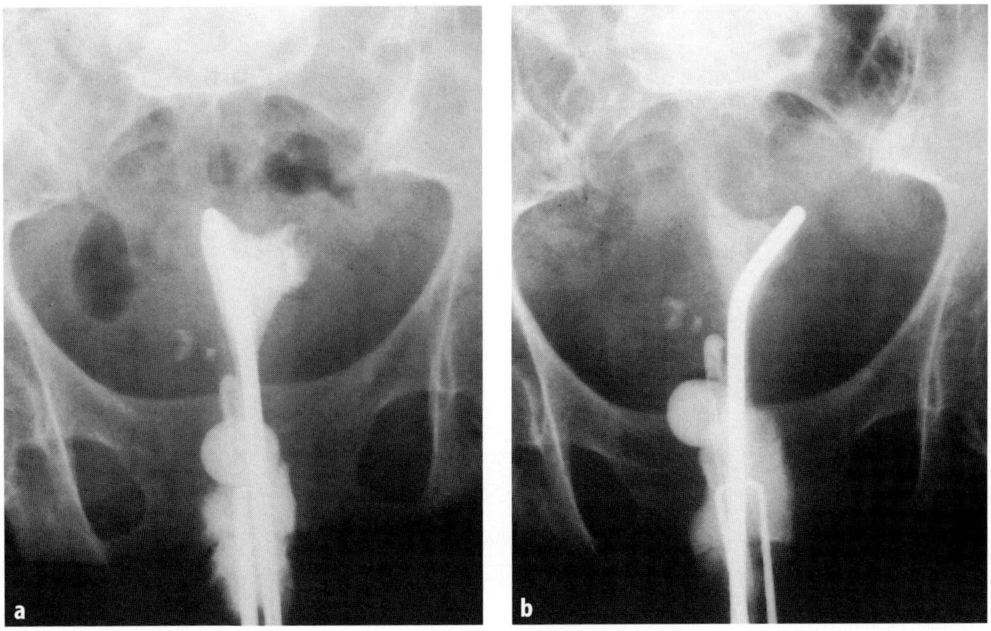

Fig. 3.8. a Anteroposterior hysterogram showing a nearly symmetrical cavity with a wide distance from the central applicator to the left corner. b Anteroposterior hysterogram after replacement of the former applicator by a 45° curved applicator in the left corner position

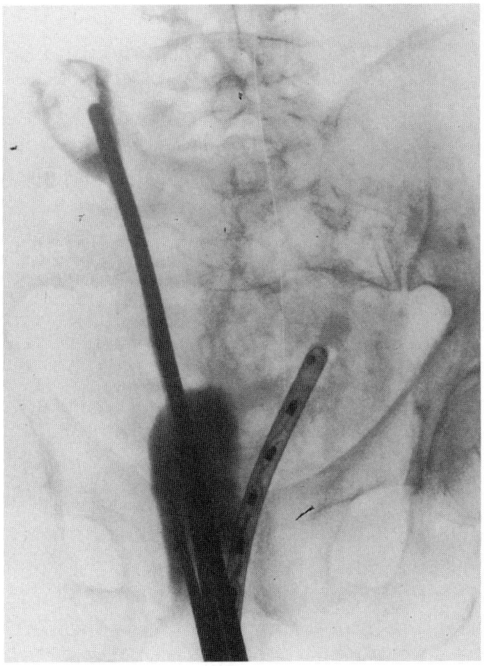

Fig. 3.9. Anteroposterior hysterogram showing an extremely long cervical canal with the uterine cavity located at the right os ilium; the tip of the catheter is sticking in the lower cavity. Lubrification by the contrast medium allowed the tip to be pushed into the upper cavity (probe length 13 cm!)

3.12), (d) hyperanteflexio or hyperretroflexio uteri with enlarged cavity, (e) "interpositio uteri" (obsolete former surgery, Fig. 3.13) and (f) extreme deformation of the cavity (subserous myomas). To exclude these patients from intracavitary irradiation, hysterography with an indwelling applicator is essential.

Most of these patients must be transferred to surgery even when surgery has a high risk. Although one afterloading treatment has been done prior to surgery, the surgical procedure is not adversely influenced by this brachytherapy. Only if the patient refuses to undergo surgery may an attempt be made to irradiate the uterus with doses of 60–70 Gy by means of a pendulum, box or opposing field technique; the results will, however, be inferior to those achieved by surgical intervention.

3.7 Rules of Final Staging (FIGO, TNM)

Two systems of staging of gynecological tumors have found worldwide acceptance, the FIGO system and the TNM system. The FIGO system originates from an initiative of the League of Nations in the late 1920s. This initiative resulted in 1937 in the publication of the "First Annual report of the results of

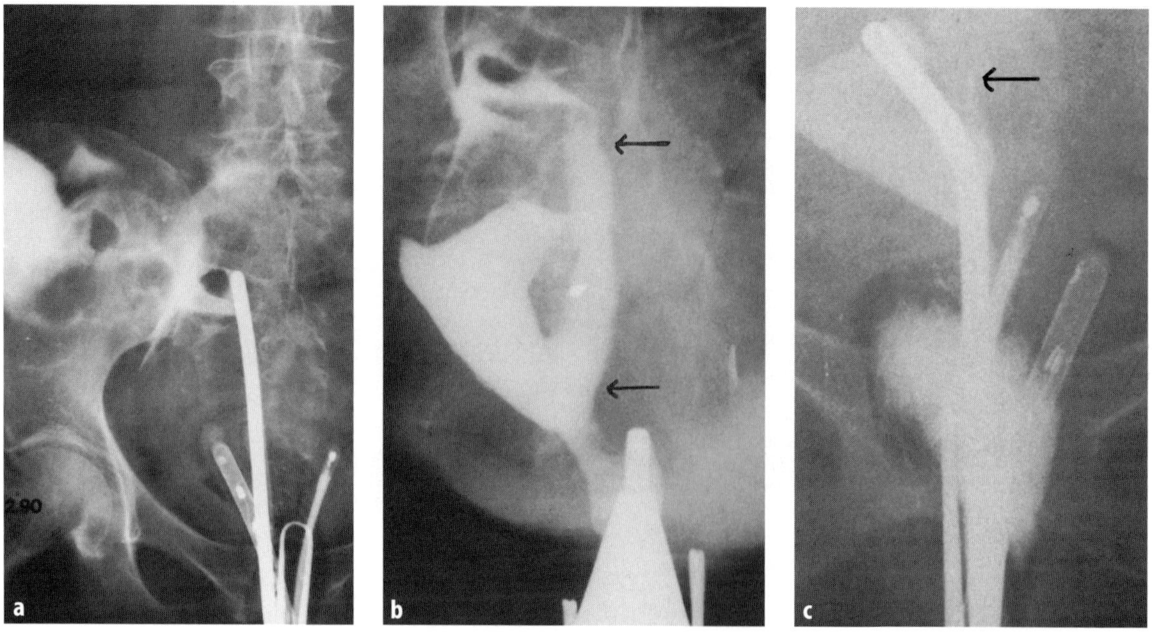

Fig. 3.10. **a** Anteroposterior hysterogram revealing perforation of the uterus. There is massive inflow of contrast medium into the peritoneal cavity; the uterine cavity is not visible. **b** Anteroposterior hysterogram, repeated with the usual technique (occluding cone and injection of contrast medium with pressure), revealing dextroflexio uteri and a straight perforating channel at the os internum (*arrows*). **c** Anteroposterior hysterogram 7 days later. The perforating canal is closed (*arrow*) and the applicator is in the correct uterine position

radiological treatment in cancer of the cervix." The principal aim of the FIGO system has been to enable comparison of the results of radiotherapy between different institutions. The basis for the staging is simple clinical investigations which are available at every contributing institution throughout the world: palpation, inspection, colposcopy, endocervical curettage, hysteroscopy, cystoscopy, proctoscopy, and intravenous urography. Examinations like CT, MRI, scintigraphy, and lymphography, which are not available at every institution, may be performed, but the results of these additional studies should not influence the staging in order to ensure comparability between international centers. Results of 117 contributors based on this staging system have been published in the 22nd volume of the "Annual report on the results of treatment in gynecological cancer" (Petterson 1994). In 1958 the International Federation of Gynecology and Obstetrics (FIGO) assumed patronage for these reports, which have been issued at 3-yearly intervals since.

In 1954 the International Union Against Cancer (UICC) appointed a committee with the task of establishing rules for the classification and clinical staging of malignant tumors and for the presentation of therapeutic results. A TNM classification for carcinoma of the cervix was proposed by this committee in 1966, which took into consideration the experience gained from the FIGO stage grouping.

The close collaboration between the TNM committee of the UICC and the cancer committee of the FIGO has ensured that current staging definitions of gynecological carcinoma are concordant. However, while the FIGO system has been developed from primarily clinical staging systems used for the pretreatment staging of radiotherapeutically treated cancers, the TNM system, according to its system of prefixes and suffixes, differentiates between different levels of evidence. For instance, it allows for detailed description of the pathological results in surgically treated cervical carcinomas.

In accordance with the changing use of treatment options (shift from radiotherapy to surgery), FIGO decided in 1988 to make corpus cancer a surgically staged entity. Only for cases not treated by primary operation is clinical staging still recommended. The TNM system allows for clinical investigation including advanced imaging methods like MRI and ultrasonography using the same categories as are used for pathological staging. Therefore the clinical staging of FIGO and TNM is not congruent in stage I in contrast to surgical/pathological staging. Note that while para-aortic lymph nodes are not considered regional lymph nodes in cervical carcinomas, they are regional lymph nodes in corpus carcinoma. Thus para-aortic lymph node metastasis is not considered distant metastasis in corpus carcinoma, while it is considered distant metastasis in cervical carcinoma.

In ovarian tumors staging is based on clinical examination and surgical exploration because clinical evaluation alone is usually not adequate to describe the spread of the tumor. A close correlation in all stages is present between the FIGO and TNM stages.

In vulvar and vaginal carcinoma the classifications of FIGO and TNM are congruent.

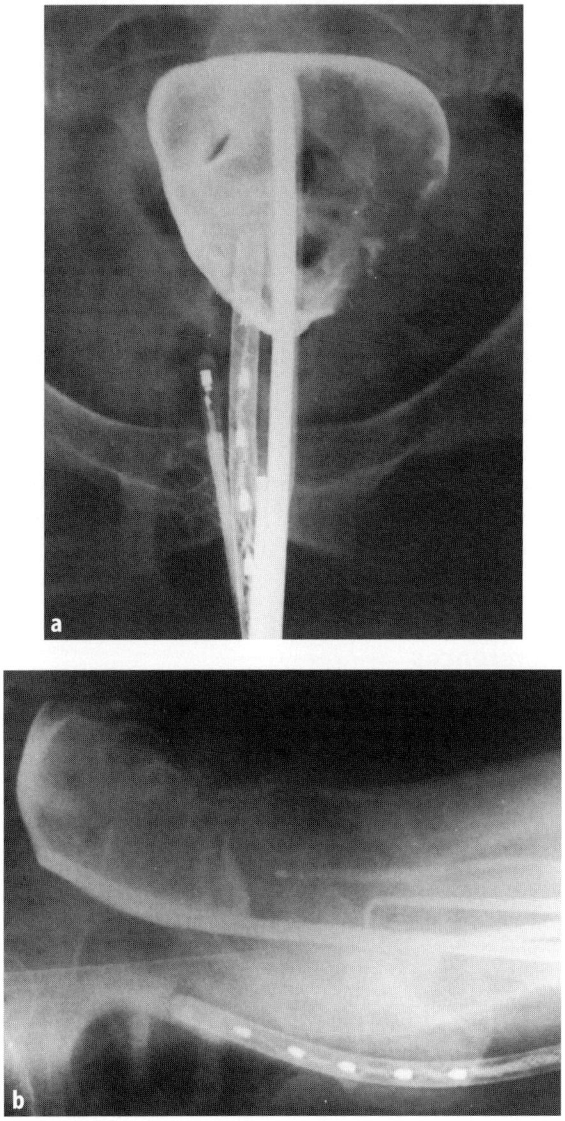

Fig. 3.11. a Anteroposterior hysterogram revealing a balloon-shaped cavity with a central applicator. **b** Lateral hysterogram: a curved applicator is in contact with the posterior wall of the cavity. There is no chance of delivering a sufficient dose to the anterior uterine wall

In 1991 FIGO established a staging system for cancer of the fallopian tube, similar to that for ovarian cancer. Also a new staging system for gestational trophoblastic tumors was recommended, which includes the risk factors high HCG levels (>100 000 IU/l) and duration of disease since last pregnancy (>6 months).

3.8 Follow-up

Systematic follow-up of patients after tumor therapy has the following objectives: (a) evaluation of the effectiveness of the therapy used; (b) detection of therapeutic side-effects and instigation of adequate treatment; (c) counselling of the patient regarding

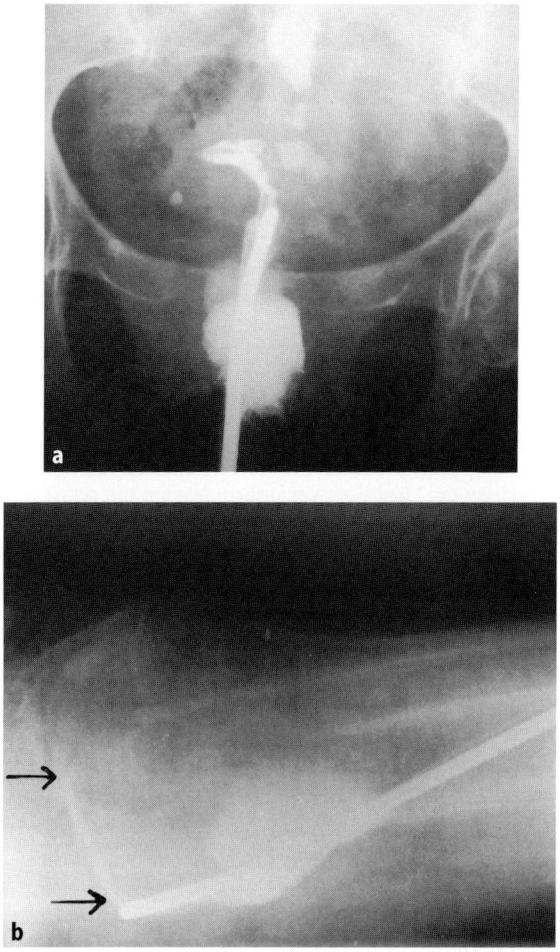

Fig. 3.12. a Anteroposterior hysterogram demonstrating a small cavity with the applicator tip stuck at the os internum. **b** Lateral hysterogram revealing rectangular deviation at the os internum (*arrows*) which could not be straightened by pulling at the clamp

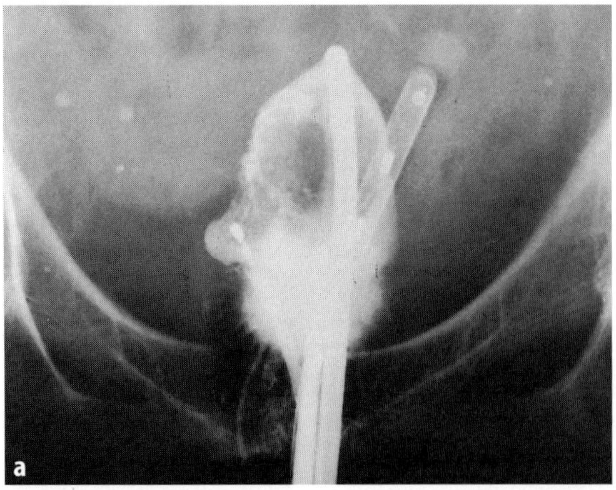

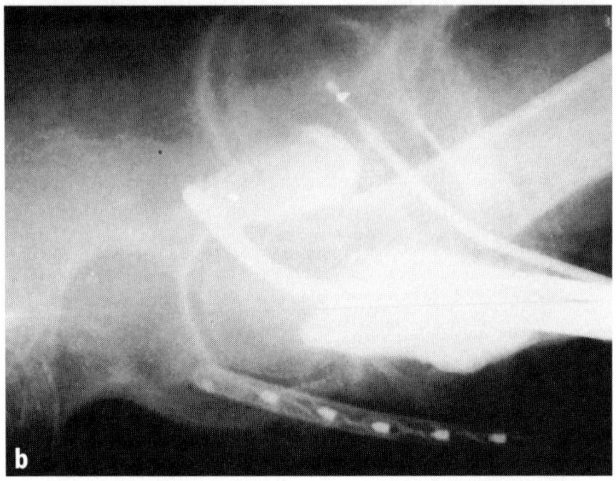

Fig. 3.13. **a** Anteroposterior hysterogram showing superposition of the cervical canal and applicator with an inverse position of the cavity. **b** Lateral hysterogram showing acute-angled deviation between the cervix and corpus uteri due to an "interpositio uteri" as treatment of a descensus uteri et vaginae many years previously. However, in fact an "interpositio corporis uteri" had been performed, leaving the cervix in a normal position

the necessary adaptation of life-style and psychological counselling; (d) early detection of metastasis and/ or recurrence, while treatment may be still effective.

In the past systematic follow-up with sumptuous laboratory and imaging methods has been propagated as a means of improving the results of cancer treatment. Today newer results have cast some doubt on the effectiveness of this approach. It is now generally held that the use of systematic investigations for the "early" detection of distant metastasis in most tumor entities has no measurable effect. In breast cancer patients randomized studies with systematic follow-up have not shown improvement in the course of the disease. Therefore the intent of the follow-up investigations should be focused on the detection of local recurrence, which may often be treated effectively, improving quality of life even if mortality can no longer be influenced. Also from a palliative point of view early symptoms of recurrence should be taken seriously in order to avoid disabling destruction by tumor, for instance by bone metastasis.

In genital tumors screening for recurrence relies heavily on clinical examination. The experienced examiner reserves elaborate imaging methods for cases with suspicious findings or symptoms. It is also not useful to apply expensive laboratory methods like tumor markers as screening tests, because the early detection of distant metastasis does not confer any benefit to patients. One has to consider that these tests also may do harm, because of the consequences of false-positive results as well as the psychological sequelae of knowing the diagnosis earlier without being able to influence the prognosis.

Systematic follow-up examinations should be scheduled according to the risk of development of local recurrence and therapeutic sequelae. Both develop preferentially in the first 2 years after treatment, then with rapidly diminishing frequency. A first visit should be scheduled 4–6 weeks after the treatment has been completed. Three-monthly visits are recommended for the first 2 years if no problems arise. Later the intervals are gradually lengthened until after 5 years patients who are apparently tumor free should resume the regular prophylactic visits as recommended for healthy women in the same age group.

References

Baum R, Chatal JF, Fumoleau P, et al. (1989) Results of a European multicenter study on immunoscintigraphy with In-111-DTPA OC 125 F(ab') in gynecological tumors. In: Schmidt HAE, Buraggi GL (eds) Trends and possibilities in nuclear medicine. Schattauer, Stuttgart, pp 679–682

Frischkorn R (1976) Gynäkologische Strahlentherapie. In: Schwalm H, Döderlein G, Wulf KH (eds) Klinik der Frauenheilkunde und Geburtshilfe, vol II, Suppl. Urban & Schwarzenberg, München, p 664

Fröhlich EP, Bex P, Nissenbaum MM, Epstein BM, Sonnendecker EW (1991) Comparison between renal ultrasonography and excretory urography in cervical cancer. Int J Gynaecol Obstet 34:49–54

Gitsch G, Deutinger J, Reinthaller A, Breitenecker G, Bernaschek G (1993) Cervical cancer: the diagnostic value of rectosonography for the judgement of parametrial invasion in regard of inflammatory stromal reaction. Br J Obstet Gynaecol 100:696–697

Haase W (1987) Hysterographie bei der Afterloading-Technik des Korpuskarzinoms. In: Hammer J, Kärcher KH (eds) Fortschritte in der interstitiellen und intrakavitären Strahlentherapie. (Jahrestagung der Österreichische

Gesellschaft für Radioonkologie, Radiobiologie und Medizinische Radiophysik). Zuckschwerdt, München, pp 241–245

Haase W (1989) Hysterography as part of the afterloading therapy of endometrial carcinoma. In: Kutzner J (ed) Afterloading brachytherapy. (International meeting on remote controlled afterloading in cancer treatment, Wuhan, People's Republic of China, 1988). Zuckschwerdt, München

Hawighorst H, Knapstein PG, Schaeffer U, Knopp MV, Brix G, Hoffmann U, Zuna I, Essig M, van Kaick G (1996) Pelvic lesions in patients with treated cervical carcinoma: efficacy of pharmacokinetic analysis of dynamic MR images in distinguishing recurrent tumors from benign conditions. AJR Am J Roentgenol 166:401–408

Hötzinger H, Becker H (1984) Intrauterine Ultraschalltomographie (IUT): Vergleich mit makroskopischen Präparatschnitten. Geburtshilfe Frauenheilkd 44:219–224

Hricak H, Lacey C, Schriock E, Fisher MR, Amparo E, Dooms G, Jaffe R (1985) Gynecologic masses: value of magnetic resonance imaging. Am J Obstet Gynecol 153:31–37

Hricak H, Hamm B, Semelka RC, Cann CE, Nauert T, Secaf E, Stern JL, Wolf KJ (1991) Carcinoma of the uterus: use of gadopentetate dimeglumine in MR imaging. Radiology 181:95–106

Hricak H, Quivey JM, Campos Z, Gildengorin V, Hindmarsh T, Bis KG, Stern JL, Phillips TL (1993) Carcinoma of the cervix: predictive value of clinical and magnetic resonance (MR) imaging assessment of prognostic factors. Int J Radiat Oncol Biol Phys 27:791–801

Hricak H, Powell CB, Yu KK, Washington E, Subak LL, Stern JL, Cisternas MG, Arenson RL (1996) Invasive cervical carcinoma: role of MR imaging in pretreatment work-up – cost minimization and diagnostic efficacy analysis. Radiology 198:403–409

Innocenti P, Pulli F, Savino L, Nicolucci A, Pandimiglio A, Menchi I, Massi G (1992) Staging of cervical cancer: reliability of transrectal US. Radiology 185:201–205

Kindermann G, Gerteis W, Weishaar J (1970) [Achievement of lymphography in the recognition of cervix carcinoma metastases.] Was leistet die Lymphographie in der Erkennung von Metastasen beim Zervixkarzinom? Geburtshilfe Frauenheilkd 30:444–452.

Lien HH, Blomlie V, Kjorstad K, Abeler V, Kaalhus O (1991a) Clinical stage I carcinoma of the cervix: value of MR imaging in determining degree of invasiveness. AJR Am J Roentgenol 156:1191–1194

Lien HH, Blomlie V, Trope C, Kaern J, Abeler VM (1991b) Cancer of the endometrium: value of MR imaging in determining depth of invasion into the myometrium. AJR Am J Roentgenol 157:1221–1223

Magee BJ, Logue JP, Swindell R, McHugh D (1991) Tumour size as a prognostic factor in carcinoma of the cervix: assessment by transrectal ultrasound. Br J Radiol 64:812–815

Minderhoud-Bassie W, Treurniet FE, Koops W, Chadha Ajwani S, Hage JC, Huikeshoven FJ (1995) Magnetic resonance imaging (MRI) in endometrial carcinoma; preoperative estimation of depth of myometrial invasion. Acta Obstet Gynecol Scand 74:827–831

Petterson F (1994) Annual report on the results of treatment in gynecological cancer. 22

Roth G, Vahrson H (1984) Erste 5-Jahres-Ergebnisse der primären und postoperativen High-dose-rate Iridium-Bestrahlung des Korpuskarzinoms. In: Kucera H (ed) Symposium "High Dose Rate Afterloading Technique" – 4th Afterloading Buchler Anwendertreffen, Wien 1984. Buchler, Braunschweig

Roth G, Vahrson H, Rauthe G (1985) Hysterographie bei liegendem Afterloading-Applikator. Strahlentherapie 161: 336–342

Rotman M, Choi K, Guse C, Marcial V, Hornback N, John M, Guze C [corrected to Guse C] (1990) Prophylactic irradiation of the para-aortic lymph node chain in stage IIB and bulky stage IB carcinoma of the cervix, initial treatment results of RTOG 7920 [published erratum appears in Int J Radiat Oncol Biol Phys (1991) 20:193. Int J Radiat Oncol Biol Phys 19:513–521

Scoutt LM, McCarthy SM, Slynn SD, Lange RC, Long F, Smith RC, Chambers SK, Kohorn E, Schwartz P, Chambers JT (1995) Clinical stage I endometrial carcinoma: pitfalls in preoperative assessment with MR imaging. Work in progress. Radiology 194:567–572

Sironi S, Belloni C, Taccagni GL, DelMaschio A (1991) Carcinoma of the cervix: value of MR imaging in detecting parametrial involvement. AJR Am J Roentgenol 156:753–756

Sironi S, Colombo E, Villa G, Taccagni G, Belloni C, Garancini P, DelMaschio A (1992) Myometrial invasion by endometrial carcinoma: assessment with plain and gadolinium-enhanced MR imaging. Radiology 185:207–212

Vahrson H (1972) Das sogenannte Lymphödem der unteren Extremität nach gynäkologischer Strahlentherapie. Strahlentherapie 143:172–178

Vahrson H (1976) Der Wert der Ossovenographie beim fortgeschrittenen Genitalkarzinom der Frau. Ein Beitrag zur Diagnose des kombinierten Stauungsödems. Röntgen-Bl 29:341–349

Vahrson H (1992) Die primäre HDR-AL-Bestrahlung des Endometriumkarzinoms, Probleme, Technik, Ergebnisse. In: Grimm D, Eichhorn M, Hänsgen G (eds) Fortschritte in der intrakavitären und interstitiellen Afterloadingtherapie. Isotopentechnik Sauerwein, Haan, pp 63–74

Yamashita Y, Mizutani H, Torashima M, Takahashi M, Miyazaki K, Okamura H, Ushijima H, Ohtake H, Tokunaga T (1993) Assessment of myometrial invasion by endometrial carcinoma: transvaginal sonography vs contrast-enhanced MR imaging. AJR Am J Roentgenol 161:595–599

4 Radiation Planning in Female Genital Cancers

H.D. Böttcher, I.A. Adamietz, and B. Schopohl

CONTENTS

4.1 Therapy Planning Systems

Treatment planning comprises the establishment of a general procedural strategy which may entail radiation therapy alone or in conjunction with other methods. Treatment planning is based on the clinical evaluation of tumoral disease, which takes into consideration the malignancy of the disease as well as the toxicity of the treatment measures. The tumor location, its size, histological aspects, infiltration into neighboring tissues, the presence of metastases, and the clinical and psychological state of the patient must all be considered during treatment planning. The aim of the treatment, whether curative or palliative, must always be explicitly defined. The potential impact of treatment on the patient's quality of life should influence therapeutic decisions; this requires experience in gynecological oncology and in the assessment of its therapeutic range.

Treatment planning takes place in cooperation with the radiation oncologist and the physicist. The aim of the treatment is to destroy or inactivate the tumor while causing no damage to healthy tissues and while influencing the well-being of the patient as little as possible. Although in reality this ideal is fulfilled in very few cases and only under very favorable conditions and with careful treatment planning, it is generally possible to come close to achieving this goal.

The duties of the physician include assessment of the extent of tumor spread, localization of the tumor, establishment of the treatment volume, identification of the regions at risk, and prescription of daily dose, total dose, and fractionation mode. After the treatment plan has been calculated and established by the physicist, it must be prescribed and implemented by the physician.

In order to maximize the effect of treatment on the tumor and to minimize the risk of complications, the radiation therapist must consider several factors. Unfortunately, the radiosensitivity cannot be equated with the radiocurability: the radiosensitivity depends on the reaction of each tumor cell to irradiation, while radiocurability refers to the therapeutic range of the treatment, which depends on the different sensitivities of the normal tissue and tumor tissue. Most gynecological tumors are curable because the therapeutic schemes and techniques used in daily routine provide maximum shielding of normal tissues.

High-energy radiation units (cobalt-60, linear accelerator) make it possible to carry out curative radiation therapy with sufficient depth dose. Durrance et al. (1969) reported that the risk of

H.D. Böttcher, MD, Professor, Leiter der Abteilung für Strahlentherapie und Onkologie, Klinik und Poliklinik, Johann Wolfgang Goethe-Universität, Theodor-Stern-Kai 7, D-60590 Frankfurt am Main, Germany
A. Adamietz, MD, Professor, Leitender Oberarzt der Abteilung für Strahlentherapie und Onkologie, Klinik und Poliklinik, Johann Wolfgang Goethe-Universität, Theodor-Stern-Kai 7, D-60590 Frankfurt am Main, Germany
B. Schopohl, MD, Professor, Oberarzt der Abteilung für Strahlentherapie und Onkologie, Klinik und Poliklinik, Johann Wolfgang Goethe-Universität, Theodor-Stern-Kai 7, D-60590 Frankfurt am Main, Germany

pelvic recurrences in women with cervical cancer in stage II or III was reduced by 50% after the introduction of megavoltage units. KUROHARA et al. (1979) compared two patient categories irradiated at an orthovoltage or at a high-voltage unit and found the survival rate to be distinctly better after irradiation with the high-voltage unit. JOHNS (1976) reported increased survival in women with stage III cervical cancer who were treated with a betatron unit (23-MV photons) in comparison with a population treated with a cobalt unit. The initially widespread assumption that improved local control in the region of the small pelvis might be linked to an increased risk of developing distant metastases could not be verified (KATZ and DAVIES 1980).

Decisions concerning the size of the volume to be irradiated may be based on computed tomography, lymphangiography, fine-needle puncture or surgical staging. (The diagnostic workup has been described elsewhere.)

4.1.1 Treatment Time

Although several combinations of the daily single doses, the total doses, and the breaks between therapy blocks have been reported, single daily irradiation five times a week remains the classical fractionation scheme. It has been well verified that local tumor control increases with enlargement of the total radiation dose. According to BROWN (1985), a dose increase of 10% is required for an improvement in the local control rate by about 20% in cervical cancer. The minimization of delay and shortening of the duration of the total treatment period are important factors in radiation therapy. Generally, delays in treatment or a long treatment period are not reasonable, although better than interruption of therapy. It is known that during therapy a number of tumors alter their proliferative character (accelerated repopulation). After 1–3 weeks of treatment, the tumor doubling time can be reduced from 100 to 3 days (FOWLER and HARARI 1993). At the same time the spontaneous rate of tumor cell loss falls to 0 (there are values of up to 95% before the beginning of therapy). The interruption of treatment can therefore be associated with rapid tumor restitution and therapeutic failure. FYLES et al. (1992) examined the influence of the length of treatment on local pelvic control in 830 patients with cervical cancer. There was a 1% worsening in local control for each day of extended treatment over 30 days. This study emphasized the significance of an accelerated repopulation of tumors. In a new patterns of care study, LANCIANO et al. (1993) pointed out that a distinct worsening of the results by about 14% (pertaining to survival and local control) occurred when the total treatment time was increased from 6 to 10 weeks. This effect was seen especially in females with stage III cervical cancer. Lengthening of treatment time had no influence on the risk of later complications.

4.1.2 Single Dose and Fractionation

The value of the single dose is significant. It is known that doses above 2 Gy increase the potential risk of complications without greater tumor cell inactivation. It has previously been reported that tissues reacting very slowly to radiation (tissues with a tendency to develop fistulas or necrosis, e.g., the vagina) possess the ability to repair sublethal radiation-induced damage. This ability is lost when the single dose is increased to a certain point. By contrast, tissues with a high proliferation rate (e.g., the mucous membrane of the intestine) have practically no ability to repair sublethal radiation-induced damage, regardless of the size of the single dose (FOWLER and HARARI 1993).

Studies with *hypofractionated doses* (high single doses applied less often than 5 times a week) in patients with cervical cancers have yielded distinctly different results. MARCIAL and BOSCH (1968) investigated the 2-year survival rate and acute and late reactions in two groups of patients – one receiving 2.5 Gy three times a week and the other 1.5 Gy 5 times a week – and found no differences between the groups. One has to take into consideration, however, that 1.5 Gy applied 5 times a week is not a standard fractionation. Many of these females also received brachytherapy, and in this case the local control at the small pelvis was distinctly lower. BROWDE et al. (1984) reported that conventional fractionation is clearly more effective than a single radiation dose per week. Even though the differences did not prove statistically significant, the rate of late complications in females treated once a week was four times as high. DEORE et al. (1992) performed a retrospective analysis of the results of hypofractionation with respect to rectal or rectosigmoid complications in 203 females with stage IIIB cervical cancer, and found that the incidence of severe complications (grade II or III) increased from 8.2% following daily treatment with 2 Gy to 33.3% following single weekly treatment with 5.4 Gy. The application of hypofractionation has also been shown in other studies to be associated with increased risk of several late effects (Cox 1985).

In special cases (especially in cases of uterine bleeding in advanced disease), *single pelvic irradiation*, a variation of high hypofractionation, has been suggested as a palliative measure. In a non-randomized study, Chase et al. (1984) reported palliative success with single irradiation with 10 Gy. Hodson and Krepart (1983) reported that single irradiation with 10 Gy, when repeated three times, each time after a 1-month interval, is very well tolerated and has a very good palliative effect.

The results of Marcial et al. (1983) indicate that a *split-course treatment* with a higher single dose (2.5 Gy) can produce the same therapeutic results without increasing the late complication rate. When using this scheme, teletherapy can be completed within a shorter time. This plays a significant role in selected elderly patients or females in a generally poor condition. It should, however, be emphasized that the data from Marcial et al. (1983) could not be verified.

Current radiobiological knowledge allows the application of a high total dose without a danger of late complications. Hyperfractionation (the use of smaller single doses: 1.1–1.6 Gy) can produce about a 10% increase in the biologically effective total dose and a better inactivation of tumor cells (Fowler and Harari et al. 1993). The application of several radiation doses per day with a minimum interval of 4–6 h allows a redistribution of tumor cells with minimum repair of sublethal radiation-induced damage (Stehmann and Bundy 1993). For this reason a correctly planned hyperfractionation (for example 1.6 Gy twice a day) should reduce the risk of late effects through the possibility of repairing sublethal radiation-induced damage in normal cells. As expected, hyperfractionation increases the frequency of early radiation effects, which allows a high dose escalation in females with cervical cancer (Varghese et al. 1992). Komaki et al. (1994) reported the results of the phase I–II RTOG study, which examined a hyperfractionation scheme in cervical cancer. Total parametrial doses 10% higher than normal, combined with brachytherapy, were much better tolerated by patients who received hyperfractionated therapy than by patients receiving the classical fractionation. This effect was independent of tumor stage.

Accelerated fractionation (reduction in the overall time without a significant change in dose per fraction or total dose) shortens the total treatment duration, thereby preventing the proliferation of tumor cells during an extended treatment (Fowler and Harari 1993). However, it has to be borne in mind that the strong acute effects of accelerated fractionation may restrict the continuation of treatment (Fowler and Harari 1993). In most clinical studies, accelerated hyperfractionation is applied with a slightly increased total dose (1.2 Gy twice a day). Although the efficacy of accelerated fractionation schemes for certain tumor types has been well documented, its role in the treatment of gynecological tumors remains to be clarified (Withers 1985; Fowler and Harari 1993). In other tumors, hyperfractionation and accelerated fractionation produce a high incidence of acute as well as late effects (Ang and Peters 1994).

It has been demonstrated that the efficacy of radiation therapy can best be evaluated by means of clinical examination. Coloscopy or determination of copper and ferritin levels in serum provides no further information (Choo et al. 1984). On the other hand the SCC antigen can indicate tumor growth in the absence of pathological clinical findings. West et al. (1991) reported on the prediction of radiation effect on the basis of the radiation sensitivity of cell cultures following irradiation with 2 Gy. However, upon increasing the single dose in daily routine survival times other than those predicted were observed (in more than 55% of the cases).

4.1.3 Planning Systems

The duties of radiation physicists include the selection of radiation type and radiation quality, the calculation and optimization of dose distribution, controlling the production of shields and compensators, and dose measurements in patients.

With modern planning systems it is possible to calculate the dose distribution in the body two- and three-dimensionally. The body cross-sectional values and organ slices are fed into the planning system by means of an on-line or off-line procedure. The single volumes (treatment volume, risk volume, etc.) are defined at a suitable peripheral terminal and the information is transferred to the central computing unit of the planning system. In order to calculate the dose distribution, the body thickness, tissue-air ratio, and backscattering must be taken into consideration. Body cross-sections with inhomogeneities, isodoses, and geometrical characteristics of the radiation field are displayed on the screen or as a hard copy.

The combination of a treatment planning system with computed tomography (CT) offers a series of advantages. It allows individualization of treatment planning through exact localization of the tumor and critical organs. Application of body cross-sections from computed tomographs in the radiation treatment system takes place automatically, and target volume contours and important inhomogeneities are also transported into the radiation system.

Modern planning systems differ from each other in several respects. In gynecological radio-oncology the ability to combine teletherapy and brachytherapy plays a very important role. The treatment planning computer plays a pivotal role in modern radiation therapy because it allows the radiation oncologist to plan complex treatments similar to those presented in the previous section. DOPPKE and GOITEIN (1988) reported that in an intradepartmental survey of the usefulness of isodose computations, they were considered essential in 27% of the treatments and "very useful" in 31%. Current commercial systems can use CT images for dose-heterogeneity-corrected calculations, in some instances including the effects of the target volumes and critical organs in planes adjacent to the central axis. Major innovations are being made in treatment planning computations as more powerful computers become affordable and improved dose algorithms are developed.

There are, however, limitations in current state-of-the-art treatment planning computers (GOITEIN 1982). Isodose computations generally fail to reflect the true two-dimensional field shaping achieved with secondary blocking, and the isodose curves used only approximate correct square or rectangular fields. Dose computation in the build-up and build-down regions is not well modeled, and the effects of oblique incidence in the build-up region are usually neglected. Therefore, in most two-dimensional cross-sectional isodose computations, the isodose lines between the entry surface and d_{max} are only approximate. Actual surface doses generally are not included as part of the dose-calculation algorithm (GLASGOW and PURDY 1992).

Although the dosimetry of full-shield and partial-transmission blocks is represented with reasonable accuracy, missing tissue compensators are usually represented as the patient's surface rather than in their true location away from the patient's surface. Therefore, isodose computations that include these compensators are somewhat approximate, particularly near the surface. Methods of comparing different isodose computations to select the best treatment plan are usually limited to comparing maximum, minimum, and average doses for most systems. Nevertheless, the radiation therapy treatment planning computer is a valuable tool that must be available in all facilities with high-energy linacs with multiple radiation beam capabilities.

Calculation of the dose after an enclosed intracavitary implant was in the past performed with the aid of two radiographs in the anteroposterior and lateral projections. In the early 1980s, reports were published which referred to the advantages of other methods such as ultrasonography or CT for treatment planning (LEE 1989; GOITEIN 1985). Newer data revealed the superiority of computed tomographically aided planning of intracavitary therapy. In certain situations, the dose in specific organs can be reduced by means of CT simulation (vertebral column, small and large intestine, kidneys) (MUNZENRIDER et al. 1991). Moreover, CT shows superiority in determining the maximum dose in normal tissue, and improves the estimation of the optimum dose to the tumor (LICHTER and TEN HAKEN 1994). Magnetic resonance (MR) imaging possibly also allows the prediction of tumor radiation sensitivity and facilitates the follow-up of late responders (FLUECKINGER et al. 1992).

While it is important for most other malignant tumors, computerized treatment planning does not yet play a significant role in gynecological tumors. Two reasons may be held responsible for this: Firstly, radiation therapy of most gynecological tumors is hardly possible without intracavitary therapy. Although the latter contributes significantly to the good results of radiotherapy, it is very difficult to integrate it into the CT planning, especially in combination with teletherapy. Secondly, staging of many gynecological tumors depends foremost on the clinical examination, and above all on the findings of palpation, whereas the staging of other tumors depends on intraoperative findings. The role of CT in staging is considered by most gynecologists to be of little significance. Since there are no significant interindividual variations in the dimensions of the female pelvis, standard radiation treatment plans can be used without any negative impact on treatment quality.

HOBDAY et al. were, however, able to prove in 1979 that in comparison with conventional planning, computerized therapy planning produced alterations in treatment plans in 40% of patients with uterine tumors. BADCOCK (1983) found that in the case of pelvic tumors, a 40% increase in the exactness of the assessment of the target volume is achieved by means of CT. Brizel et al. (1974), Munzenrider et al. (1977), and Goitein et al. (1979) reported similar figures. Besides the exact estimation of the target volume, CT-associated treatment planning facilitates the protection of healthy tissue during radiation therapy of gynecological pelvic tumors and produces a more exact dose estimation.

4.2 Therapy Simulators

The radiation oncologist has access to a variety of imaging modalities for target volume localization. The classic techniques of radiography and fluoroscopy, combined in a radiation therapy simulator that mimics the geometries of actual therapy units, may be augmented with CT, nuclear medicine scanning, ultrasonography, MR imaging, and CT simulators.

The modern simulator mimics the functions and allows the motions of a therapy unit. Gantry arms are rigid to support heavy shielding blocks and simulated electron cones; couch widths are similar to therapy unit couch widths; and operating consoles feature digital displays of parameters and programmable settings for source-axis distance, gantry angles, and field sizes. Some units feature automatic exposure control for improved radiographic techniques (Day and Harrison 1983; Doppke 1987). A radiation therapy simulator is necessary in any facility using state-of-the-art methods of radiation therapy. Simulators are cost effective and allow more efficient use of the therapy units for actual treatment of patients (Mizer et al. 1986). A special report by the British Institute of Radiology concluded that two simulators can support about five therapy units and allow the therapy units to be used fully for patient treatment (Bomford et al. 1976).

Through traditional radiographic (or fluoroscopic) methods using radiopaque rulers placed or projected on the patient's surface, dimensions of treatment areas on films are ascertained, and target volumes are selected. Bentel et al. (1989) demonstrated excellent site-specific examples of simulation procedures. Multiple off-axis CT images can be obtained, and the target area, critical organs, and heterogeneities can be defined in each plane (Lichter et al. 1983). Conventional transverse CT images are now supplemented with sagittal or other desired planes reconstructed from the transverse scans. The CT numbers are correlated with the electron densities of the tissues imaged and used to calculate the dose, accounting for heterogeneities. For CT scans used in treatment planning, the patient's position should be identical to the position to be used during radiation therapy. Numerous studies have documented the improvements in target volume localization and dose distributions achieved with the anatomic data obtained from CT scans (Prasad et al. 1981).

A CT unit with many of the characteristics of a radiation therapy simulator features beam's eye view display, which allows the anatomy to be viewed from the perspective of the radiation beam, permits field shaping electronically at the graphics display station, and allows computer-controlled marking of treatment fields on the patient's skin surface (Galvin et al. 1982). Dedicated CT simulators integrate a CT scanner designed for radiation therapy with a radiation therapy planning computer and many other advanced image manipulation and viewing advantages (Galvin et al. 1987; Smith et al. 1987). However, current CT simulators do not allow verification of the actual shielding blocks, an important process in conventional simulation.

During tumor localization, the desired position of the patient must be considered relative to the incident beams and the patient's ability to reproduce this position throughout the radiation therapy course. Factors affecting daily positioning of a patient include the patient's age, general health, weight, and anatomical site under treatment; obese patients are the most difficult to position. Haus and Marks (1973) observed that about a third of the localization errors in treating pelvic portals were caused by patient movement. Although modern imaging technologies allow the radiation oncologist millimeter precision in tumor localization and target volume definition, the daily positioning of the patient usually depends on less accurate visual alignment techniques, precise to only several millimeters. More accurate and precise positioning is achievable with casting and immobilization techniques, but these methods are relatively expensive, prolong simulation, and usually are employed only for the most difficult cases.

The devices commonly used to position a patient are the treatment machine field localization light and distance indicator and the lateral and overhead laser alignment lights, which provide transverse, coronal, and sagittal light lines on the patient. Visible skin marks, skin marks visible only under an ultraviolet light, India ink tattoos, and plastic shells are used for field delineation by most radiation oncologists (Watkins 1986). A host of positioning pillows and supports are available. These are designed for irradiation of specific anatomical sites and can be used, often with restraining straps, to achieve immobilization during radiation therapy.

Molding techniques may be divided into those that require a cast of the anatomical site to be immobilized and those that use materials that can be formed directly over and around the site without the preparation of a cast. The former include traditional plaster casting techniques, impression compounds, and transparent plastic shells formed over a cast with a vacuum device (DeVereux et al. 1976). Watkins (1986, 1981) gives excellent descriptions of both methods. Plastic shells filled with tissue-equivalent materials can be used to confirm the patient's dosimetry. Shell techniques use thermal plastics that, after being placed in warm water and draped over the site, harden by cooling (Gerber et al. 1982; Mondalek and Orton 1982). Polyurethane foams that harden after chemical mixing in a frame surrounding the site are widely used (Mondalek and Orton 1982). Vacuum-formed molds for adults are available, although cost and ease of preparation are probably the major considerations influencing their use.

The selection of radiation beams, their entry and exit points on the patient, and their shapes in the planes perpendicular and parallel to their incident direction is the crucial step in treatment simulation. Beam direction on conventional simulators and therapy units is determined by an optical system that projects a light field and cross hair onto the skin surface to indicate the entry point of the beam. The distance to the skin surface is measured with an optical distance indicator; mechanical distance indicators are usually reserved for confirming the accuracy of the optical distance indicator. Beam edges are outlined with radiopaque markers. Lead beads or wires that project 1 cm apart at 100 cm, with every fifth centimeter marked, are useful on simulation localization radiographs for direct field size measurements and on therapy units (Van De Geijn et al. 1982). Laser light and back pointers are commonly available to identify the beam exit point.

Secondary beam shaping blocks made from lead sheets or bricks, lead shot in a mold, or low-melting-point bismuth alloys are placed beneath the primary collimators (Kuisk 1973; Maruyama et al. 1969; Powers et al. 1973; Purdy 1983). Using a radiograph from the simulator, the radiation oncologist outlines the transverse field dimensions of the treatment volume on a film. The film is placed on a view box, and a heated wire cuts the desired shape out of a foam block above the view box to form a mold into which the shielding material is placed. The latest technology allows the desired field shape to be digitized from a film or other computer hard copy into a computer, which operates a numerically controlled milling machine or wire cutter that produces the desired mold. Low-melting-point bismuth alloys currently are the most popular materials for secondary collimation for both x-ray and electron beams (Huen et al. 1979; Purdy 1983). After solidification, the completed-block edges are smoothed; the block is mounted on a tray that can be attached beneath the primary collimators of the simulator and therapy unit. After the patient's therapy course is completed, the block is melted for reuse. The bismuth alloys offer greater safety to personnel than similar systems using molten lead (Demeyer et al. 1986; Glasgow and Reeves 1980).

Pseudoblocks constructed from thin lead or foam with the field edges coated with a radiopaque substance and identical in shape to transverse field shaping blocks may be attached directly to the simulator for verification of the desired field shape, if the simulator does not tolerate the weight of the actual treatment blocks (Paliwal and Asp 1976).

During measurements of topography and anatomic diameter, the patient should be in the desired treatment position, because the patient's position alters the diameter of some anatomical regions. Plaster cast strips, lead (solder) wire, flexible curves, or other devices, combined with anatomical thickness measurements using calipers, are common methods of measuring topography (Day and Harrison 1983; Sternick 1983; Weller and Glasgow 1982). Normally, the shape registration device is placed over the anatomical region and transferred to graph paper, onto which the shape is traced (Gerbi 1985; Sternick 1983). Newer manual methods include sonic digitizers and a magnetic stylus that traces over the patient to obtain the contour (Amols et al. 1988; Boyer and Goitein 1980). Anatomical diameters measured are also recorded on the diagram, and the entry and exit points of the beams and their field edges are marked for isodose computations. The outlines of the tumor, target volume, and internal organs of interest are added to the diagram from information obtained from orthogonal films, CT scans, and other imaging modalities or from anatomical atlases if other means are not available.

Employing the power of computer work stations and images available from the CT or MR scans, the radiation oncologist can delineate internal and external contours. Automatic contouring uses edge detection differences in CT numbers to distinguish tissue or bone from air volumes. Anatomical diameter is obtained from the images. From these procedures, the radiation oncologist determines (a) the external topography, (b) tumor, target, treatment, and irradiated volumes, (c) critical organs, and (d) heterogeneities in all three dimensions of the patient.

Frequently, the target volume is immediately above, behind, or adjacent to critical organ, and the radiation therapist faces the difficult task of treating the target volume while maintaining the dose to the critical organ below some tolerance level. Each increase in the field size results in an increased risk of complications. Although individualized therapy should be the aim, the irradiation of gynecological tumors with opposing posterior and anterior fields with a size of 15 × 15 or 16 × 16 cm is a classical solution. Treatment is carried out daily with single doses of 1.8–2 Gy; energies between 6 and 18 MV are prefered. Dose distribution can be improved by the use of additional lateral pelvic fields (box technique), especially in patients with anteroposterior pelvic diameters of more than 24 cm. All fields should be fitted into individually made satellites. The upper limit of the pelvic field is usually the upper edge of the fifth lumbal vertebra. The common iliac lymph nodes must be included in this volume. During treatment of larger volumes or during the use of extended fields (e.g., including para-aortic lymph nodes), a reduction in the total dose is required. In this way the risk of severe gastrointestinal complications can be reduced. The use of high-energy units and a four-field treatment can also reduce the risk. Smit (1991) suggested proton therapy as a therapeutic option and discussed the possibility of a potential reduction of treatment volume by about 60% and a simultaneous increase in total dose by approximately 20%. Three-dimensional CT simulation and three-dimensional treatment planning seem equally to reduce the treatment volume (Shingleton and Orr 1995).

Herbert et al. (1991) reported on a population of 115 women who received radiation therapy after laparotomy and whose small intestine was visualized by means of barium sulfate during simulation. It was found that the small intestine could be localized and that this procedure allowed a minimization of the total dose to the region of the intestine. Treatment simulation resulted in alteration of therapy in about 40% of the study population. Visualization during simulation and treatment planning showed a close correlation with a reduction in both the incidence of diarrhoea and long-term radiation-induced complications. In addition, smaller field sizes were associated with a lower complication rate. Treatment in the prone position with a special positioning system can also reduce intestinal side-effects (Shanahan et al. 1989). The sequence of the radiation fields can be ascertained traditionally through palpation of the percutaneous anatomical orientation points that can be found in conjunction with the radiological imaging of bone structures. However, Greer et al. (1990) reported that intraoperative measurements show a wide deviation from the palpable percutaneous anatomical orientation points. The mean level of the aortic bifurcation was shown intraoperatively to be approximately 6.7 cm above the lumbosacral prominence. The division of the common iliac artery was shown to be 1.7 cm above this point on the left side and 1.4 cm above it on the right. In 87% of the patients the aortic bifurcation could be localized cranially from the lumbosacral prominence. One may conclude from this study that the upper limit of the pelvic fields is at the level of the intervertebral space L4–5. It could then be guaranteed that the confluent region is encompassed. The lateral fields should in any case include the entire anterior sacral region in order to encompass the sacral and cardinal ligaments. The field size especially should be determined by the actual spread of disease. The continuous improvement in CT and other imaging procedures is theoretically increasing the possibility of encompassing all these structures within the treatment volume. A very good aid might be the intraoperative placement of titanium clips in regions which play a special role in the subsequent radiation therapy.

4.3 Reference Points

The reference points are decisive for the prescription of irradiation treatment. Today, physical radiation treatment planning is based on the recommendations of the International Commission on Radiation Units and Measurements (ICRU). In 1978, the ICRU published Report 29, *Dose Specification for Reporting External Beam Therapy with Photons and Electrons* (ICRU 1978), in 1985 Report 38, *Dose and Volume Specification for Reporting Intracavitary Therapy in Gynecology* (ICRU 1985), and in 1993 Report 50, *Prescribing, Recording, and Reporting Photon Beam Therapy* (ICRU 1993). The principal subject of Report 38 (1985) was dose and volume specification for the intracavitary treatment of cervical carcinoma.

Intracavitary therapy is often used in combination with external beam therapy. For this reason, the same terminology has been recommended for both fields. In particular, it would be desirable, whenever possible, to use the concepts of target volume, treatment volume, and irradiated volume as defined for external beam therapy.

The volume definitions given in ICRU Report for external beam therapy (Report 29) are modified where necessary for intracavitary therapy situations. The *target volume* contains those tissues that are to be irradiated to a specified absorbed dose according to a specified time-dose pattern. In tumor therapy, the target volume encompasses the space occupied by the tumor and possibly infiltrated tissue. For any given situation, there may be more than one target volume. This is particularly the case for the treatment of gynecological carcinomas where, depending on the extent of disease, some target volumes may be treated partly or totally by an intracavitary application, while others are treated mainly by external beam therapy.

The target volume must always be described, independently of the dose distribution, in terms of the patient's anatomy, topography, and tumor volume. For the purpose of reporting intracavitary treatment, that part of the target volume which has to be irradiated by means of intracavitary application should be described separately. It should also be stated whether this volume will receive treatment only by intracavitary application or by both modalities.

The *treatment volume* is defined as the volume enclosed by a relevant isodose surface selected by the radiotherapist, and encompasses at least the target volume. It is necessary to include the target volume within the treatment volume. The *irradiated volume* is that volume, larger than the treatment volume, which receives an absorbed dose considered to be significant in relation to tissue tolerance (e.g., 50% of the reference dose). In parallel, we refer to reference systems as areas in which the given dose is valid. The *reference volume* is defined as the volume enclosed by the reference isodose surface. The treatment dose defining the treatment volume may be equal to or different from the reference dose level. The reference point is a point within the target volume in which a fixed energy dose can be approached. The reference range is consequently an isodose area within or enclosing the target volume, in which the fixed energy dose (reference dose) must be attained. For reporting intracavitary therapy, it is necessary to determine the dimensions of the reference volume.

Dose peaks ("hot spots") refer to areas outside the treatment volume in which the reference dose is exceeded. Organs at risk are those radiosensitive organs in or near the target volume which influence treatment planning and/or the prescribed dose. The risk areas are nontumoral tissues or regions within the irradiated volume which are so radiosensitive that irradiation of these tissues (regions of high risk of radiation-induced side effects) could result in unwanted side-effects. A risk organ is therefore an organ that is *part of the risk area*.

The requirements faced by the radiation oncologist during intracavitary brachytherapy can be explained by reference to cervical carcinoma. Based on clinical experience, different systems have been proposed for the treatment of this entity. Three basic systems have been developed: the Stockholm system (Kottmeier 1964), the Paris system (Lamarque and Coliez 1951), and the Manchester system (Paterson 1948) (Fig. 4.1). As used here, the term "system" denotes a set of rules taking into account the source strengths, geometry, and method of application in order to obtain suitable dose distributions over the volumes to be treated. The specification of the source used in the system must always include a description of the kind of radionuclide, reference air kerma rates and its shape, filtration, etc.

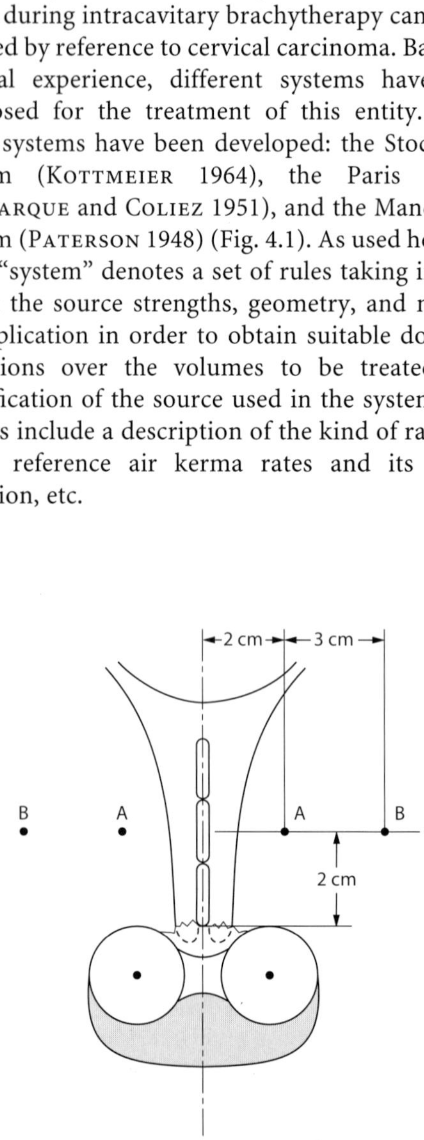

Fig. 4.1. The Manchester system. Definition of points *A* and *B*. In the classical Manchester system, point *A* is defined as a point 2 cm lateral to the central canal of the uterus and 2 cm up from the mucous membrane of the lateral fornix, in the axis of the uterus. Point *B* is defined as being in the transverse axis through A, 5 cm from the midline

In the case of simulation of a linear source by a set of point sources, the activity of these point sources and their separation must be indicated. When moving sources are used to simulate a set of different sources in fixed position, in order to produce an appropriate dose distribution the type of movement (step by step, unidirectional, or oscillation) and speed in different sections of the applicator or the dwell times of the source at different positions should be indicated.

The description of the applicator should include information on the rigidness and shape (e.g., rigid uterine source with fixed curvature), the connection between vaginal and uterine applicators, the type of vaginal sources, the number and orientation of line sources, special sources, and high atomic number shielding materials in the vaginal applicator. Several reference points are in current use. Some are relatively close to the sources and related either to the sources or to the organs at risk; others are relatively far from the sources and are related to bony structures. Reference points close to the sources and related to the sources are located in a region where the dose gradient is high; any inaccuracy in the determination of distance results in large uncertainties in the absorbed doses evaluated at these points. Such points are presently not recommended. Reference points for the expression of the absorbed dose to the bladder and to the rectum have been proposed by Chassagne and Horiot (1977). The bladder reference point is obtained as follows with help of a Foley catheter.[1] The balloon must be filled with 7 cm^3 of radio-opaque fluid. The catheter is pulled downwards to bring the balloon against the urethra. The reference point is taken on this line at the posterior surface of the balloon (Fig. 4.2). On the frontal radiograph, the reference point is taken at the center of the balloon. The reference point for the rectal dose is obtained as follows. On the lateral radiograph, an anteroposterior line is drawn from the lower end of the intrauterine source (or from the middle of the intravaginal sources). The point is located on this line 5 mm behind the posterior vaginal wall. On the AP radiograph, this reference point is at the lower end of uterine source or at the middle of the intravaginal source.

With the help of CT-aided multidimensional dose estimation, Schoeppel et al. (1990) were able to show on orthogonal films that the rectal dose had exceeded the estimation 1.6 times. In several situations, this dose was higher than that at point A. The maximum rectal dose (about 2.5 times higher) was estimated *below* the vaginal fornix. Regardless of the differences in the treatment or dose estimation, correct placement of catheter and radiation source is of great significance. Jampolis et al. (1975) found that local (central) recurrences, especially in lower tumor stages, could retrospectively always be attributed to misplacement. Correct packing of the vagina with gauze allows reduction of the dose to the anterior rectal wall by about 12% (Shingleton and Orr 1995). A slight change in catheter placement can produce a significant change in the tumor dose. Corn et al. (1993) examined the influence of misplacement during low-dose-rate brachytherapy. Deviations from the planned dose were generally very small and had little influence on healing or complications. By contrast, the short duration of high-dose-rate treatment is very critical in this respect since it limits the possibility of adjusting the dose.

It is known that considerable differences exist with respect to physical planning among different radiation therapy centers. The reference point recommended by the ICRU report number 38 in the region of the bladder neck seems to be inadequate for the estimation of the bladder dose. A *dose excess* of up to 63% in the region of the bladder, as compared to the bladder neck, could be observed using several dosimeters. In 17.5% of all examined intracavitary treatment, the radiation dose to the base of bladder was shown to be two times *higher* than had been estimated with the reference point (Shingleton and Orr 1995).

Reference points related to bony structures are used for dose estimation to the iliac lymph nodes

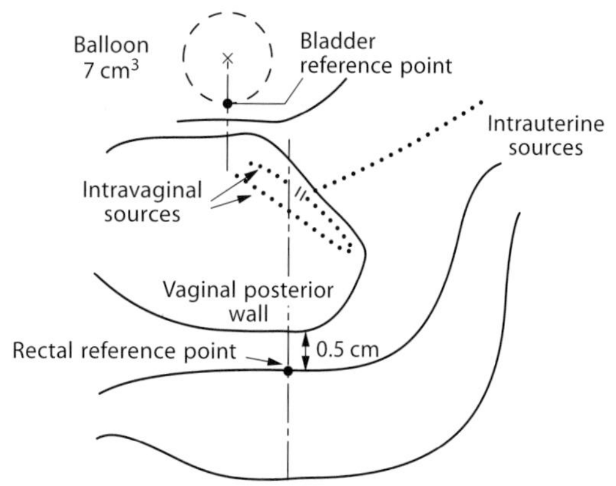

Fig. 4.2. Determination of the reference points for the bladder and rectum according to ICRU 38

[1] Since 1994 a special teflon polyvinyl catheter for gynecological brachytherapy has been produced by Rüsch. It contains three channels, one of which is adapted to the bladder chamber for measurements according to ICRU vol 38.

and to the pelvic wall. The pelvic wall reference point can be visualized on an AP and a lateral radiograph and related to fixed bony structures. This point is intended to be representative of the absorbed dose at the distal part of the parametrium, at the obturator lymph nodes (Fig. 4.3).

The cumulative radiation therapy dose during treatment of uterine tumors results in most cases from the combination of external beam radiation and brachytherapy. It is generally known that the required inactivation doses differ for a tumor of 2 cm diameter and a tumor of 6 cm diameter. Therefore the use of specific reference points and reference volumes is a valuable aid in determining the total doses in the pelvis and to the tumor and for the optimization of the therapeutic range. HANKS et al. (1983) suggested alternative planning systems in order to facilitate asymmetric irradiation of the pelvic region. Paramedian reference points and right and left lateral reference points were defined independently of each other. This system, however, did not receive wide acceptance. The reference volume and reference points from the ICRU report number 38 are better for the planning and documentation of intracavitary irradiation in order to compare the different special techniques.

4.4 Critical Organs and Doses

The therapeutic range of irradiation during treatment of gynecological tumors is relatively narrow. The tolerance doses of the risk organs, and especially of the intestine (Table 4.1), significantly influence this range.

The radiation sensitivity of a tumor depends more on its size than on the histology. It is therefore comprehensible that the potentially curative radiation dose increases with enlargement of the tumor mass (FLETCHER 1973). The size of the therapeutic dose is of special importance when viewed in the context of

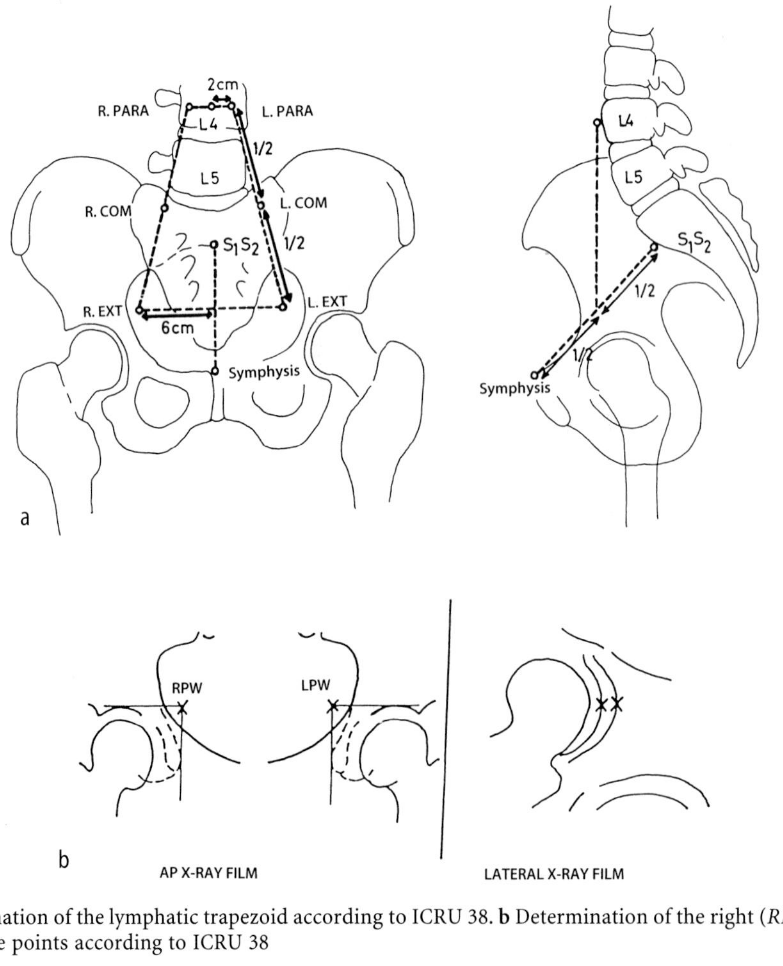

Fig. 4.3. **a** Determination of the lymphatic trapezoid according to ICRU 38. **b** Determination of the right (*RPW*) and left (*LPW*) pelvic wall reference points according to ICRU 38

Table 4.1. Radiation tolerance levels of abdominopelvic organs. (Modified from RUBIN et al. 1975)

Biological significance	Organ	Type of injury or disease	TD 5/5 (Gy)	TD 50/5 (Gy)	Whole or partial organ (field size or length)
Class I	Bone marrow	Aplasia, pancytopenia	2.5	4.5	Whole
			25	40	Segmental
	Liver	Acute and toxic	25	40	Whole
		hepatitis	15	20	Whole (strip)
	Intestine	Ulcer, perforation,	45	55	400 cm^2
		hemorrhage	50	65	100 cm^2
	Spinal cord	Infarction, necrosis	45	55	10 cm
	Kidney	Acute and chronic	20	25	Whole
		nephrosclerosis	15	20	Whole (strip)
Class II	Skin	Dermatitis	55	70	100 cm^2
	Rectum	Ulcer, stricture	60	80	100 cm^2
	Bladder	Contracture	60	80	Whole
	Ureter	Stricture	75	100	5–10 cm
	Ovary	Sterilization	2–3	6–12	Whole
	Bone (adult)	Fracture, sclerosis	60	100	10 cm^2
Class III	Muscle (adult)	Fibrosis	60	80	Whole
	Large arteries	Sclerosis	>80	>100	10 cm^2
	Uterus	Necrosis, perforation	>100	>200	Whole
	Vagina	Ulcer, fistula	90	>100	Whole

the tolerance of the surrounding pelvic and abdominal structures. The tolerance of the vagina, the cervix, uterus, and both ureters is relatively high when blood supply is intact (ALFERT and GILLENWATER 1972). During treatment planning, however, it must be taken into account that the potential curative dose for squamous cell carcinoma of the cervix of more than 4 cm in diameter entails a 50% probability of radiation-induced damage, especially to the intact bladder and rectum. It is therefore not surprising that the cure of gynecological malignancies is often associated with progressive arteritis and fibrosis of the surrounding tissue.

The first radiation-induced changes in the region of the intestinal epithelium are a reduced mitotic rate, degeneration of epithelial cells in the region of Lieberkuhn's crypts (RUBIN and CASARETT 1968; WHITE 1975), microulcerations, edema of the submucosa, inflammatory infiltrates, and dilatation of the capillaries. These processes develop on the basis of reduced absorptive function, accompanied by excessive mucosal secretions and occasional bleedings. At the end of the radiation series or shortly afterwards one can observe increased fibrosis of tissue and progressive obliterative arteritis.

The early radiation-induced changes of the bladder are characterized by the degeneration of radiosensitive epithelial cells, reduction of mitotic activity, congestion of vessels, and edema (SURESH et al. 1993). Changes in the region of the bladder are most severe directly after the end of radiation therapy. The development of fibrosis in the wall of the bladder occurs later. The tolerance dose of both kidneys is significant during irradiation of para-aortic fields as well as total abdomen irradiation. Irradiation with 20 Gy is associated with therapy-resistant nephritis which may result in functional arrest. The liver also shows a comparable radiosensitivity: irradiation of this region with 20–30 Gy may similarly result in hepatitis refractory to therapy. This can be detected relatively easily through the increase in the liver enzyme level in serum.

During irradiation of gynecological tumors, skeletal portions are almost always found within the irradiated volume. Although the tolerance dose of the bone is relatively high, during treatment planning one should take into account the possibility that any bone defects or fractures existing before therapy will worsen after irradiation.

Irradiation of the vagina causes a loss of mitotic activity of the epithelium. However, this very rarely causes an interruption of its continuity and produces few symptoms. On the other hand, late effects such as fibrosis, cicatricial changes, or a change in the vaginal form are often linked with symptoms (ABITBOL and DAVENPORT 1974). Change in the vaginal structure is often associated with pain or dyspareunia (HINTZ et al. 1981). However, early application of intravaginal ointments and early commencement of sexual intercourse combined with manual disconnection of intravaginal adhesions can reduce the severity and the incidence of radiation-induced vaginal side-effects. Intravenous infusions of substances supporting tissue regeneration accelerate ulcer healing and prevent the occurrence of fistulas.

The function of the ovaries is almost always reduced after pelvic irradiation (Janson et al. 1981). It is therefore assumed that women over 40 years of age could have an functional arrest of the ovaries after the application of 6 Gy. However, doses over 20 Gy are necessary to produce the same effect in most women of childbearing age (Orr et al. 1993).

In order to maintain the function of the ovaries, a pretherapeutic transposition could be considered (Nahhas et al. 1971; Pitkin and VanVoorhis 1971). However, transposition of one or both of the ovaries should be restricted to special rare situations in young women, when a reduction of the irradiated pelvic volume (lower cranial border of the field!) is possible and metastases in the ovaries are excluded or unlikely. The risk increases with the stage of disease (Sutton 1992; Koki et al. 1991). Many women who have undergone ovarian transposition must be treated for ovarian cysts or other, mostly endocrinological problems after radiation therapy. Chambers et al. (1991) reported the conservation of ovarian function in 71% of females after ovarian transposition and pelvic irradiation. The incidence of menopause increased especially in women who received a scattering dose of more than 3 Gy and in cases where, during transposition, the ovaries were fixed below the pelvic crest. An increased number of surgical interventions on the ovaries were also required in this group.

External beam irradiation and intracervical brachytherapy cause atrophy of the endometrium. However, if the total radiation dose remains below 60 Gy, the irradiated endometrium usually responds to hormonal stimulation (Larson et al. 1990). It has been assumed that in approximately 25% of patients, endometrial sensitivity to exogenous hormones is maintained (McKay et al. 1990). However, continuous administration of estrogens could potentially favour the development of precancerosis or endometrial cancer. Therefore, today combinations of estrogen and gestagen are the therapy of choice for hormonal substitution. Under certain circumstances, radiation-induced stenosis of the cervix may prevent extrauterine bleeding and a known biological sign of progressive tumors may consequently go unnoticed.

4.5 Radiation Volume and Dose Dependence

4.5.1 Shielding

Lack of care in the local application of higher radiation doses by means of brachytherapy in combination with external beam radiation therapy can result in a vesicovaginal or a rectovaginal fistula (Montana et al. 1986). In the small pelvis, it is especially important to minimize the dose in the region of the small intestine, the rectal mucosa, and the bladder.

Protection of areas already exposed to radiation therapy must be ensured with sufficient exactness. Shielding by means of individualized satellite blocks as well as costly computerized planning, during which the spatial distribution of the applied external beam dose must be adjusted to the isodoses of brachytherapy, cannot solve this problem satisfactorily. Doses to critical organs may be limited by using a full shield (e.g., 3.125% transmission) or a partial transmission shield (permitting a 50% transmission).

The true percentage dose level is usually greater than the percentage stated because of scatter radiation beneath the blocks from adjacent unshielded portions of the field, and the dose level generally increases with depth as more radiation scatters into the volume beneath the shield. The exact transmission is a function of block material layer, thickness, field size, and energy. These blocks change the energy characteristics of the beam in a complex manner (El-Khatib et al. 1987). Thus, it may be better to use a full shield for the second half of the course instead of using a partial shield during the full course. Although lead can be used, low-melting-point bismuth alloys that can be easily shaped to cover a critical organ are widely used for construction of organ shields (Campbell and Loyd 1984; Huen et al. 1979). Mass attenuation, linear attenuation, and mass energy absorption coefficients are now available for these alloys (El-Khatib et al. 1987). Most organ shields are static, simply being placed on the shielding tray attached to the therapy unit; however, gravity-oriented shields have been developed (Engler et al. 1984; Promos and Goldson 1981). An organ shield must be properly positioned to cover the organ, and the radiation oncologist must ensure that it is properly constructed. Organ shields do perturb the beam and beam output.

The most common form of beam modification is shaping the beam transversely in the plane at 90° with respect to the direction of the beam. The fixed circular, square, and rectangular cones commonly found on orthovoltage units were replaced on cobalt units and linear accelerators (linacs) by paired variable collimators that move symmetrically toward or away from the central axis of the beam. Some modern linacs now allow one pair or both pairs of opposing collimators to operate independently, which permits rectangular fields to be formed off the central axis and allows primary collimator shielding at midfield and beyond (KHAN et al. 1986; KLEMP et al. 1988; LOSHEK 1984).

Multileaf collimators that allow true transverse field shaping without adding a secondary blocking system are an expensive option. They are currently being offered on some medical accelerators (BRAHME et al. 1983; KÄLLMAN et al. 1988). They also allow dynamic conformational therapy (TAKAHASHI et al. 1983) (e.g., changes of field shape during therapy, often while the gantry rotates). Such conformational radiation therapy is ideal for implementing three-dimensional treatment planning (TAKAHASHI 1965).

4.5.2 Combination of Intracavitary/Interstitial Brachytherapy and External Beam Therapy

Sequential external beam radiation and brachytherapy must be planned individually. The anatomical changes in the region of gynecological organs are decisive for planning combined therapy. A narrow vagina or an asymmetrical cicatricial vaginal stump limit the use of brachytherapy. An increase in the external beam radiation components might also cause further strictures. Therefore the scheme of combined gynecological treatment must be flexible in order to combine the external beam irradiation and brachytherapy optimally, in accordance with the clinical situation.

In cervical cancer stage Ia (≥5 mm depth of infiltration, ≥8 mm surface or other diameter) sole hysterectomy is the therapy of choice. In cases of local inoperability or inoperability due to the poor general condition of the patient or other coexisting nonmalignant diseases, the equivalent is sole intracavitary therapy. Sole brachytherapy is supported by HAMBERGER (1980), who reported a 100% cure rate in 41 patients (≥3 mm depth of infiltration), GRIGSBY and PEREZ (1991), with 100% local control in 55 patients in stage 0 or Ia, and KOLSTADT (1989), who found no recurrence in 140 females with stage Ia disease.

In cervical cancer stage Ib the risk of lymph node metastases increases with the diameter or volume of the cancer. Therefore, it should preferably be treated with combined brachy- and teletherapy. The strategy must take account of the results of sole brachytherapy in stage Ib published by HAMBERGER (1980), who found a 5-year survival rate of 96% and only 1% complications in 93 patients (≥4 cm diameter) after 60 Gy, and KIM et al. (1988), who reported a 15% recurrence rate (9% pelvic, 6% distant).

While brachytherapy is predominantly used in stages Ia and Ib, its ability to achieve a curative effect decreases rapidly in stages IIb and IIIb, and percutaneous irradiation is the preferred technique. In stages IIIb and IVa, brachytherapy can be completely omitted in favor of a high-dose teletherapy regimen (ULMER and FRISCHBIER 1982), or added as a boost only. Nevertheless, percutaneous irradiation, however highly sophisticated, can never imitate the huge central intracavitary dose in its steep decrease towards the surrounding tissues.

Several variations of intracavitary treatment have been recommended. They differ from each other with respect to the irradiated areas, the total dose, the type of intracavitary irradiation, and the treatment method. Efforts to standardize the biological equivalence of intracavitary and external beam irradiation have thus far been unsuccessful. An optimum method for recalculation of the biological effect of both methods remains to be defined. It is consequently evident that simple addition of the doses of brachytherapy and external beam irradiation is not correct. For this reason several treatment schemes are based on long years of clinical experience; these maintain the target doses to the reference regions within a narrow therapeutic range and guarantee a good cure rate and reduced complication rate.

CORN et al. (1994) analyzed the effects of the technical exactness during intracavitary brachytherapy in 66 females with cervical cancer. They found only 8 out of 66 implants to be ideal. The implants were completely unacceptable in 17 patients, and were described as sufficient in 41. A multivariate statistical analysis clearly showed that the technical exactness was the most important prognostic factor for local control. Survival among patients with qualitatively insufficient implants tended to be poorer (5-year survival 40% vs 60%).

The radiobiological effect of continuous irradiation at a low dose rate during intracavitary irradiation cannot be compared with the effect of external beam irradiation at a higher dose rate (Allen and Reddi 1980). It is known that low-dose-rate (LDR) brachytherapy is characterized by a low oxygen enhancement factor which is responsible for the reduction of the repair of sublethal radiation damage. During recent years, high-dose-rate (HDR) brachytherapy has gained wide acceptance. The short irradiation time with this method is especially advantageous. Comparison of the radiobiological effect of HDR and LDR treatment is very complicated (Joslin 1990) (for discussion of the influence of dose rate and replacement of LDR by HDR treatment, see Chap. 2, Sects. 2.5 and 2.6). As a result of the several advantages of the HDR units, one may assume that further dissemination of this technique will occur (Bastin et al. 1993; Eifel 1992).

Several decades of experience with thousands of patients have resulted in a variety of dose combinations of teletherapy and brachytherapy. A survey by Brenner et al. (1991) revealed the existence of at least 23 different schemes for LDR brachytherapy and external beam radiation therapy. Diverse opinions have arisen as to the number of brachytherapy applications that are necessary. In a patterns of care study, Coia et al. (1990) analyzed 565 women with cervical cancer after treatment with LDR brachytherapy. After 4 years it was observed that women who had received two or more intracavitary applications had significantly better local control (29% vs 17%) and survival (73% vs 50%). Further studies in this area (e.g., Lanciano and Corn 1992) have demonstrated the significance of intracavitary therapy. However, it has not been observed that several applications are beneficial. The division of LDR intracavitary brachytherapy into two fractions increases the paracervical dose, improves the local control in the pelvis, reduces the distal recurrence rate, and improves the survival rate (Marcial et al. 1991). Controversy exists as to the benefit of higher fractionation schemes during intracavitary irradiation for all stages of cervical cancer (Marcial et al. 1991; Kraiphibul et al. 1992).

Several factors support the application of HDR brachytherapy. The possibility of treating outpatients, the reduction in or avoidance of anesthesia, the constant radiation geometry during the treatment, and the minimization of radiation exposure of personnel are often-cited advantages. According to Jones et al. (1990), radiation exposure of nurses could be reduced from 19 mSv to 2.4 mSv by means of HDR afterloading.

There is still an ongoing discussion about LDR versus HDR afterloading brachytherapy. These methods have proven to be equivalent in terms of cure rates and complications, but the technical advantages, the short dwell times (improving patient comfort), the exact radiation geometry and economic reasons favor HDR brachytherapy. It is a fact that the HDR system spread extremely rapidly in the late 1970s and early 1980s in Japan, where in 1985 150 HDR afterloading devices were working and more than 80% of patients who underwent brachytherapy for uterine cancer were treated with HDR afterloading (Hashimoto and Ito 1988). A similar development was reported from West Germany, where in 1986 about 100 afterloading devices were in use or installed, most of them with HDR sources (Vahrson and Glaser 1988).

It has to be emphasized once more that the interval between therapy modalities must remain short. However, such intervals are better than a treatment interruption, which allows an increase in tumor volume due to accelerated proliferation of tumor cells (Fowler and Harari 1993). It has already been observed for LDR brachytherapy that intervals of more than 14 days between single sessions increase the risk of recurrence (Bosch and Marcial 1967).

Homogeneous irradiation of the pelvis, encompassing the pelvic lymph drainage in more advanced tumor stages, is the first step in combined primary irradiation of cervical and endometrial carcinomas. Total doses of 45–50 Gy are aimed at. Single doses of 1.8–2.0 Gy applied five times a week must not be exceeded. The so-called box-field technique can be applied, and provides the advantage of using individual satellite apertures to demarcate the radiation fields. This technique, however, requires radiation units with high-energy photons (more than 4–6 MeV). After approaching the planned dose, a boost dose is given to the tumor region. In cases where intracavitary brachytherapy is not possible, external beam irradiation with a reduced target volume is carried out.

Higher radiation doses and intracavitary therapy generally achieve improved local control in women with stage II and III cervical cancer. However, according to the experience of Perez et al. (1986), irradiation doses exceeding 70 Gy at point A do not result in any improvement in patients with stage IB cervical cancer. It could also be demonstrated in a patterns of care study that local control in the irradiated volume shows dose dependency only in stage III disease (Coia et al. 1990). The lowest recurrence rate was seen in women who received doses of more than 85 Gy at point A. However, in this study it was impossible to establish a dose dependency in the lateral PCS or P points. Reports from different institutions indicate that an adequate combination of megavoltage therapy and brachytherapy, taking special problem regions into consideration, yields excellent results. This combination differs distinctly from one institution to another. Most centers apply 70–85 Gy to the paracervical region (point A) and 60 Gy to the pelvic wall (point B). In this way, the bladder and rectal dose can be reduced to 60 Gy. The treatment strategy of Brady and Perez (1992) comprised primary irradiation and LDR intracavitary therapy. With this approach, curative rates of cervical cancer of 80%–90% in stage I, 60%–70% in stage II, and 30%–50% in stage III may be expected (Berek et al. 1988). However, only 5%–10% of patients with stage IV disease can be cured; in this context one certainly has to bear in mind that 30% of all patients with stage IV disease have a long period of survival. In order to approach the aforementioned figures, the radiotherapist must pay great attention to the exactness of the procedure and the quality control during irradiation (Kapp 1983; Kapp et al. 1983).

Vahrson and Römer (1988) combined brachytherapy and external beam irradiation in cervical carcinoma of stages Ib–IV. In stages Ib and IIb, biaxial bisegmental pendulum irradiation was preferred when there was no evidence or a low risk of metastases outside the small pelvis. The same institution today applies 48 Gy to the parametrium (B-line 5 cm from central axis) given in three weekly fractions of 3 Gy over 5 weeks, and 40 Gy to the A-line (2 cm from central axis) applied by HDR afterloading 5 × 8 Gy at weekly intervals. The sum doses are 78 Gy to the A-line and 60 Gy to the B-line (H. Vahrson, personal communication).

4.6 Standard Techniques and Individualization of Radiotherapy

4.6.1 Cervical Carcinoma

Satisfactory radiation planning is dependent upon precise knowledge of tumor spread. Cervical carcinoma can spread per continuitatem into the parametrium, vagina, bladder, and rectum. The diagnosis can be almost completely established by means of clinical examination; however, ureteral stenosis and hydronephrosis need to be established by urography or ultrasonography and bladder and rectal infiltrations are identified by means of cystoscopy and rectoscopy.

Computed tomography can contribute to the recognition of parametrial involvement, especially in very adipose patients in whom tumoral disease and inflammatory infiltration cannot be distinguished by means of clinical palpation. Spread to the bladder and rectum can be diagnosed with greater certainty with CT. The main indication for the technique, however, is the evaluation of the common iliac lymph nodes and para-aortic lymph nodes, which cannot be palpated. Computed tomography supplements the information provided by the less commonly performed lymphangiography, with which the internal iliac lymph nodes and presacral lymph nodes cannot be evaluated.

External beam radiation therapy must include the regions of direct local tumor spread and the regional lymph nodes (Table 4.2). The frequency of involvement of the pelvic lymph nodes is stage dependent (see Chap. 9). For treatment planning all pelvic lymph nodes must be evaluated, even in the early stages of disease. The controversial irradiation of the para-aortic lymph nodes is recommended in cases of histologically confirmed involvement (Sevin 1986) or involvement of highly localized common iliac lymph nodes or when staging laparotomy has not been performed and distinct enlargement of lymph nodes is seen in CT. While no studies have been reported on other cases, the potential therapeutic benefit should take precedence over the increased rate of side-effects (Lindner 1992).

The target volume during primary and postoperative external beam radiotherapy is identical. The

Table 4.2. Probability of lymph node infiltration in patients with cervical carcinoma, according to stage of disease. (Modified from Bohndorf and Richter 1992)

	Pelvic lymph nodes	Para-aortic lymph nodes
Ib	11%–30%	5%–8%
IIa	23%	12%–14%
IIb	38%	22%–24%
II	20%–40%	8%–25%
III	40%–67%	30%–35%
IV	52%	36%–45%

external beam irradiation is usually performed in the supine position. In order to protect the small intestine, some authors advocate external beam irradiation in the prone position with a fully filled bladder (LINDNER 1992). Planning CT must be performed under the same conditions. A flat CT couch and a lateral laser are employed for positioning. After drawing a topogram, slices are obtained from the ischiadic tuber up to the upper plate of L4 (L4–5 in lower tumor stage), optimally at intervals of 1 cm. Treatment planning is assisted by (a) visualization of the small intestine, (b) the use of oral iodinated contrast medium, (c) visualization of the rectosigmoid, and (d) placement of lead marks or contrast medium in the portio vaginalis/cervical canal or the vagina.

In the treatment of invasive carcinoma of the uterine cervix, it is important to deliver adequate doses of radiation to the pelvic lymph nodes. For stage IB disease, 16 cm × 16 cm fields at the isocenter are sufficient. For patients with stages IIA, IIB, or IVA carcinoma, 16 cm × 20 cm fields are required to cover all of the common iliac nodes in addition to the cephalad half of the vagina. A 2-cm margin lateral to the bony pelvis is adequate (Fig. 4.4). If no vaginal extension is present, the lower margin of the portal is situated at the inferior border of the obturator foramina. When the vagina is involved, the entire length of this organ should be treated down to the introitus. It is very important to identify the distal extension of the tumor at the time of simulation by placing a radiopaque clip or bead on the vaginal wall or inserting a Hegar stick or a small rod with a radiopaque marker in the vagina. In these patients the portals may be modified to cover the inguinal lymph nodes because of the increased probability of metastases (PEREZ 1992a).

The slice level of the central ray is selected to optimize treatment planning, and the corresponding target volume is drawn onto each slice. This procedure offers a more exact and more individualized estimation of the target volume than the simulation of fields with standardized skeletal boundaries. The physical radiation planning is carried out after determination of risk organs (bladder, rectum, caudal dystopic kidneys, and the heads and necks of the femora). A four-field box technique (Fig. 4.5a) is best for postoperative radiation therapy or for the commencement of combined primary radiation therapy in advanced stages of disease or when there is no acute bleeding, since the subcutaneous tissue is better shielded by this method and the 100% isodose volumes are clearly kept to a minimum (Table 4.3). An alternative is the already mentioned technique of biaxial telecobalt pendulum irradiation as performed by ULMER and FRISCHBIER (1982) (Fig. 4.5b). Opposed field irradiation alone is indicated only when intracavitary therapy is carried out in parallel, due to the potentially better shielding of the median structures. This technique is also used for intracavitary radiation therapy in the supine position. Due to the different sizes of the target volumes at the different CT levels, individual absorbers must be estimated using planning CT and the measurements must be given to the mechanical workshop. In order to optimize protection of healthy tissue, an

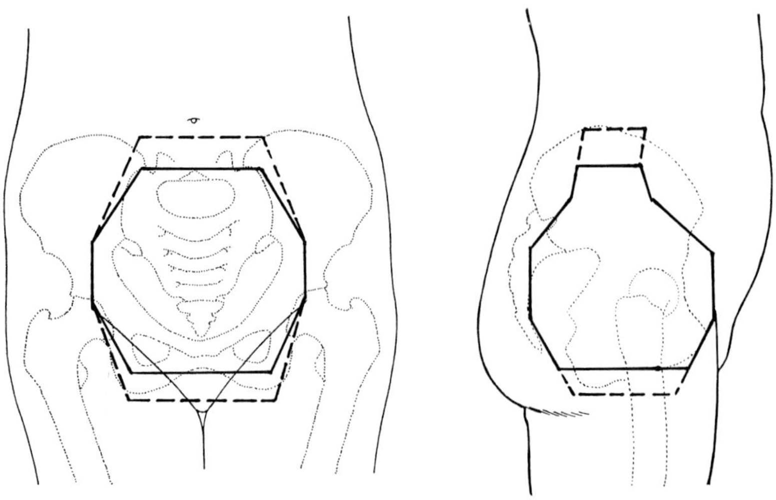

Fig. 4.4. Diagram of the pelvic portals used in external beam irradiation of carcinoma of the uterine cervix. The standard portal for stage IB tumors is outlined by the *solid line*. When the common iliac nodes are to be covered, the upper margin is extended to the L4–5 space. If there is extension of a vaginal tumor, the lower margin of the field is drawn at the introitus

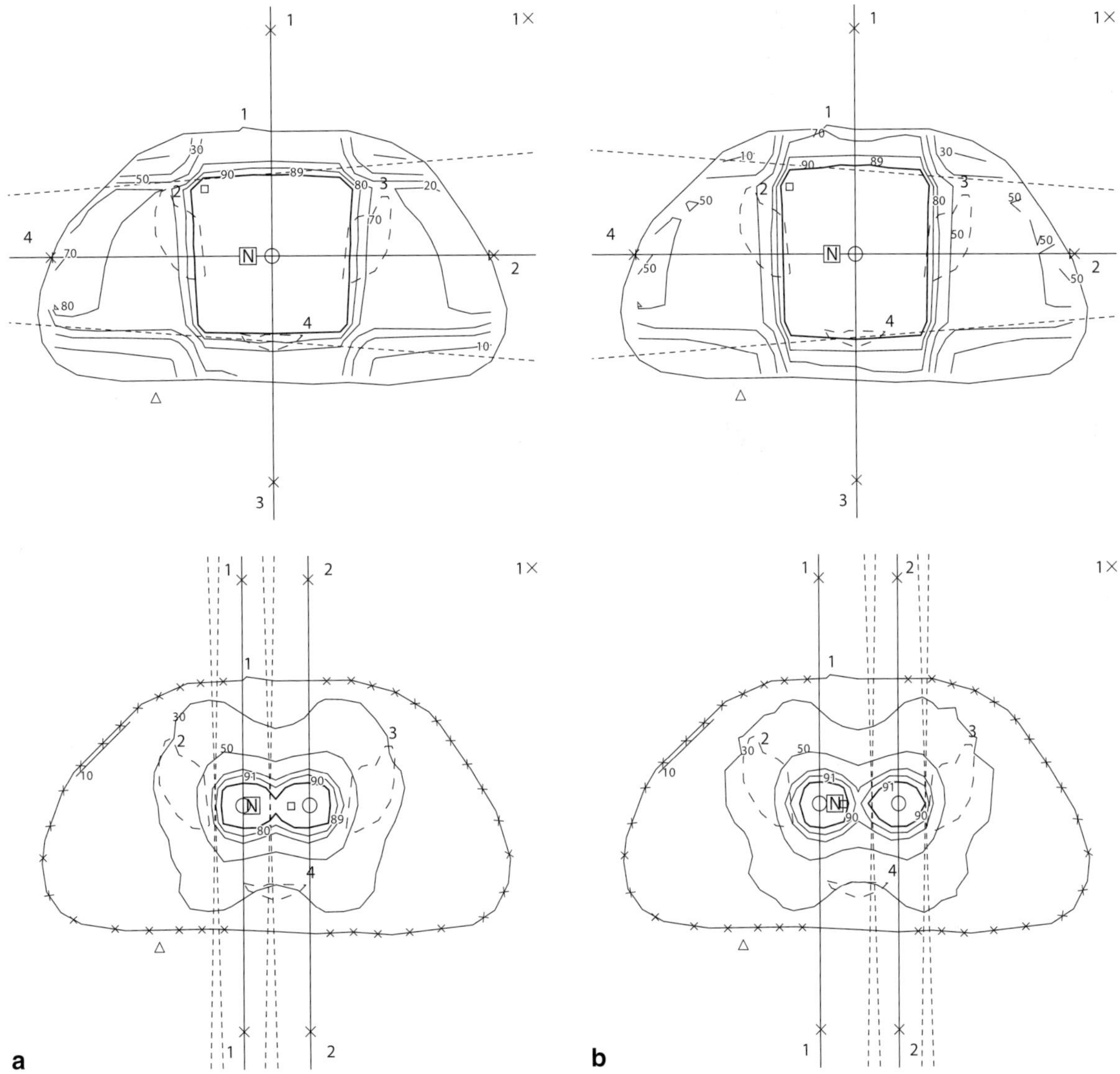

Fig. 4.5. **a** Isodose distribution in the pelvis through parallel opposed anterior and posterior fields and through lateral fields using 6-MV photon beams with equal weighting (*above*) and 2 to 1 weighting favoring the anterior and posterior fields (*below*). **b** Isodose distribution in the pelvis through biaxial bisegmental pendulum external irradiation using ^{60}Co photon beams. Optimization of the dose distribution is achieved by changing the distance between the pendulum axes. *Above* distance = 5 cm; *below* distance = 7 cm

Table 4.3. Comparison of volume dose in relation to the technique of external beam irradiation of the pelvis. (Modified from Bohndorf and Richter 1992)

Type of external beam irradiation	Tumor dose	Intestinal dose	Integral dose
12-MV photon beam, parallel opposed fields	102.2%	90.1%	53.2%
12-MV photon beam, four-field technique, individual absorber	106.3%	80.0%	49.6%
Biaxial ^{60}Co-rotational moving field	105.5%	93.4%	75.9%

alternative to the four-field technique is the above-mentioned biaxial rotational irradiation (Vahrson and Römer 1988). Biaxial bisegmental pendulum irradiation requires no central shielding when external beam treatment is combined with brachytherapy. The planning of the optimum dose distribution is performed by changing the position of the rotation axes. Although tissue inhomogeneities which can be easily assessed by CT for the purpose of exact dose estimation do not play a significant role in the pelvis, the measurements of radiation exposure of the small intestine within the target volume estimated with modern planning CT demonstrated slightly increased values for this technique.

During irradiation of the para-aortic lymph nodes a large opposing field including the pelvic and para-aortic region ("chimney field") has been recommended (usually up to Th12) in order to reduce problems of field contact (Fig. 4.6). After about 30 Gy, AP-PA one-field irradiation of the pelvis and the para-aortic lymph nodes is replaced by rotational irradiation or a three-field technique in order to protect the spinal cord. Dorsal shielding of the spinal cord is not recommended because of significant dose inhomogeneity within the prevertebral target volume. After plotting the isodoses at the different CT levels, the complete image information must always be available and known. Before simulation, the physical plan must be proved and accepted by the radiation therapist with regard to SSD and SAD factors, different gantry angles, the estimation of the isocenter in the body of the patient, and the ability to position and draw irradiation fields on the patient's skin using laser lines. Identical positioning at the simulator, at CT, and at the radiation unit is essential.

The choice of intracavitary target volume in cases of cervical carcinoma without surgical intervention is based primarily on the findings of palpation and on the possibility of catheterizing the cervical canal.

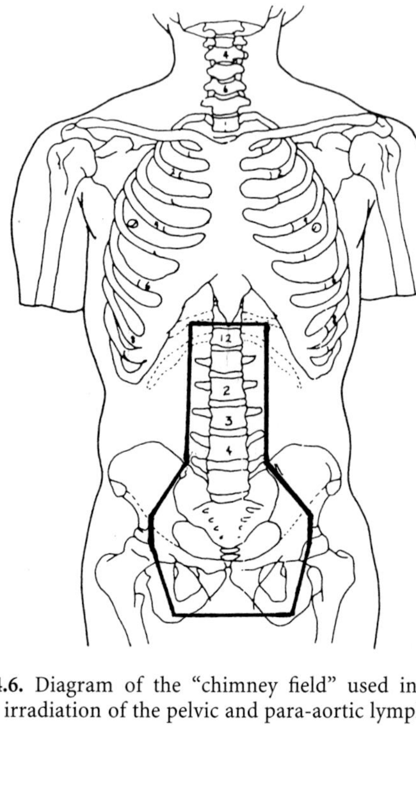

Fig. 4.6. Diagram of the "chimney field" used in external beam irradiation of the pelvic and para-aortic lymph nodes

Since the tumor may occur multicentrically or in the uterine cavity, the cervix, the fornix vaginae, and the entire uterine cavity should be assessed. Rotational symmetrical isodoses in pear-shaped form around the curved intrauterine applicator are chosen in certain cases, including during the use of ovoids in the fornix vaginae or of plate-like ring-shaped applicators with specifically formed isodoses. These are, however, defined by the form and position of the applicator as well as the tumor spread. CT can be employed for localization of the contours of the uterus (Schmidt et al. 1986) through the intrauterine placement of a dummy applicator, the acquisition of CT slices, and transferral of the afterloading isodoses to the CT slices (using the planning system of by hand). One can then recognize, for example, whether the selected isodose in very voluminous portions encloses the tumor completely. MR slices in several projections are, however, more suitable for this purpose. Since afterloading irradiation can only be carried out in the supine position, the position of the legs must be changed from the lithotomy to the horizontal position after application in order to offer a better match with external beam irradiation. The corresponding CT or MR slices must be acquired in the same position.

Primary irradiation of cervical carcinoma practically always involves combined external beam and intracavitary irradiation. In the early disease stages emphasis is placed on intracavitary therapy, whereas at advanced stages greater priority is given to external beam irradiation (external beam irradiation alone is used in stage IV disease). As already mentioned, the optimum geometric balance between intracavitary and external beam therapy varies interinstitutionally. At least during a part of the teletherapy, the middle portion of high radiation exposure from intracavitary therapy (especially the risk organs rectum and bladder) is shielded from the external beam target volume. This is achieved by means of a bell-shaped individual absorber which is fitted into the afterloading target volume isodose and which guarantees a smooth transition of dose in the central region and other areas of the small pelvis (Perez 1992a).

Computed tomography is not necessarily required for adaptation of the target volume, since external beam irradiation is also carried out at the start of intracavitary irradiation using the opposing field technique. CT may, however, be useful. Nowadays, planning CT is capable of estimating summation doses of all irradiation sections, taking into account the middle block attenuation. Underdoses in parametrial regions of the opposite side are observed, for example, by virtue of the steep dose reduction (L/R^2 law) in cases where, due to tumor-induced fixation of the uterus, the afterloading applicator cannot be placed centrally in the pelvis. Such underdoses can and must be compensated in the plan by means of special techniques. The physical summation doses are naturally affected by disregarding the radiobiological differences between external beam and intracavitary radiotherapy.

Pelvic recurrences of cervical carcinomas may occur after surgical, radiotherapeutic, or combined therapy. In some cases such recurrences occur simultaneously with distant metastases. In addition, isolated recurrences in the para-aortic lymph nodes are possible. The percentage of pelvic recurrences increases from approximately 6% in stage IB to about 35% in stage III. CT plays a considerable role in the diagnosis of recurrences with a high localization. Exenteration is the therapy of choice for an isolated pelvic recurrence following primary irradiation of a complete dose, assuming that the general condition of the patient permits such a course of action (5-year survival rate following exenteration: 20%–45%). In the absence of the clinical prerequisites and/or the agreement of the patient, limited irradiation must be considered. CT planning is essential in the case of pelvic wall recurrences after primary sole surgery. A three- or four-field technique is often used to apply the dose to the recurrence target volume. Boost irradiation can be performed by means of interstitial afterloading.

4.6.2 Endometrial Carcinoma

Carcinoma of the corpus uteri spreads through direct infiltration into the cervix, the parametrium, the adnexa, the vagina, and eventually the bladder and rectum. Lymph node involvement may occur from the median and cranial thirds of the corpus into the parametrial lymph node, the internal and external iliac lymph nodes, and rarely the common iliac lymph nodes, and from there into the para-aortic and the presacral lymph nodes. From the cranial third of the corpus, lymph drainage can occur along the ovarian artery directly into the para-aortic lymph nodes, or along the round ligament into the superficial inguinal lymph nodes. After the tumor has spread into the cervix, the parametrial lymph nodes are most often involved.

The therapy of choice is bilateral adnexectomy and hysterectomy, often combined with pelvic and para-aortic lymphadenectomy. Postoperative intracavitary therapy of the vagina is used in order to reduce the vaginal recurrence rate independently of the tumor grading. Additional external beam irradiation of the small pelvis is usually carried out (a) when there is infiltration of the myometrium to a depth of more than a third in patients with G2 and G3 tumors, (b) in the presence of special histological types, and (c) when lymph node metastases are detected. The results of the Annual Report, volume 20 (Petterson 1988), support this approach, as do the randomized studies of Piver et al. (1979), Aalders et al. (1980), and Kucera et al. (1989).

The regional lymph nodes are involved with different frequencies according to grading, stage and depth of infiltration of the myometrium (Table 4.4). When external beam irradiation is subsequently indicated, all pelvic lymph nodes must be encompassed in the target volume. When findings are nonpathological, the inguinal lymph nodes are not irradiated since they are rarely involved. The external beam target volume is identical with that for cervical carcinoma, and steps in CT planning follow the same pattern.

A reduction of the rate of side-effects can be achieved through individualized box irradiation. The question as to whether the para-aortic lymph nodes should be encompassed has not yet been resolved. In the presence of tumor involvement of the upper third of the uterus and histologically proven involvement of the pelvis and the para-aortic lymph nodes, the prevailing tendency is to perform adjuvant irradiation of the para-aortic lymph nodes, which are firstly encompassed in a "chimney field" and subsequently receive an isolated irradiation so as to avoid under- or overdosage. Optimal shielding of the endangered small intestine as

Table 4.4. Probability of lymph node infiltration in patients with endometrial carcinoma. (Modified from Lindner 1992)

	Pelvis	Para-aortic region
In relation to stage (FIGO)		
I	16%–18%	4%–12%
II	15%–35%	10%
In relation to depth of infiltration of myometrium		
<1/3	2%–7%	1.1%–2.5%
<1/3	18%–36%	12%–17%
In relation to grading		
G1–G2	3%–11%	1%–5%
G3	25%–36%	18%–29%

well as of the spinal cord and kidneys is achieved by means of CT planning of rotational and multiple field irradiation.

The combination of intracavitary irradiation of the vaginal fornix with teletherapy of the pelvis causes less problems because of the small intracavitary volume. Shielding of this rotational symmetrical volume can be carried out when necessary, simply with a simulator corresponding to the afterloading localization imaging. When patients are referred for primary irradiation because of inoperability, priority is given to the intracavitary treatment. After accurate clinical staging (fractionated currettage), a stage I endometrial cancer can be treated with sole intrauterine brachytherapy. Percutaneous irradiation should be added in stage II and more advanced stages (Vahrson 1991). The classical packing method of Heymann has been replaced by various applicators designed for afterloading techniques (see Chap. 10). Imaging of the uterine cavity by open hysterography with an indwelling applicator is of great help in adapting the applicator to the cavity. However, assessment of the uterine wall thickness is not possible with this method; for this purpose, tomograms are very helpful (more so than sonograms). The position of a dummy applicator in relation to the uterine surface after intrauterine placement is optimally shown by acquiring several transverse sections. The target volume isodose, which is standardized, for example, at a point 1 cm lateral to the median uterine axis, can be selected individually. The brachytherapy volume can be optimally adapted only in very old patients with nonirradiated external beam target volumes.

In case of recurrence in the pelvis or in the para-aortic lymph nodes, definitive radiation treatment should be planned on the basis of CT imaging when reoperation is not possible. Five-year survival rates of 30%–35% can be achieved when gestagens are given in addition.

4.6.3 Ovarian Carcinoma

After complete tumor extirpation (or at least extensive debulking to <2 cm residual tumor), postoperative irradiation of so-called intermediate-risk tumors (Dembo and Bush 1982) and low-risk tumors (with the exception of the Ia–b, G1 tumors) is an alternative to chemotherapy. The target volume must correspond to the mode of spread and the Toronto results of the entire peritoneal cavity, including the liver and the entire diaphragm (Dembo 1985). The target volume is defined by means of simulation, and the irradiation is delivered by means of opposing fields (when possible isocentric). CT, which initially plays no role in planning, may serve as a means for the total assessment of all peritoneal levels, after marking the blocks (elimination of basal pulmonary sections, lateral soft tissues, and skeletal tissues in the pelvis) (La Rouere et al. 1989).

The patterns of spread of ovarian carcinoma necessitate irradiation of the entire peritoneal cavity. Total abdominal irradiation is followed by a boost to the small pelvis, which again can be optimally planned by means of CT. Boost irradiation of the para-aortic lymph nodes and the diaphragm, the effectiveness of which is controversial, is planned with the simulator using opposing fields. When larger tumor residues are present following surgery, a second-look operation can be performed after postoperative chemotherapy, and limited irradiation is given after marking the residues with clips. CT planning is then essential in order to shield risk organs (especially the small intestine, kidneys, etc.). Good palliative effects can be achieved by this approach.

External beam irradiation is given only with megavoltage equipment. When abdominopelvic irradiation is used, the distance from the target to skin should be sufficient (100–180 cm) to cover the volume from below the pelvic floor to above the diaphragm. During simulation, with the aid of fluoroscopy it should be ascertained that the portals include both diaphragms with 1- to 2-cm margins on both inspiration and expiration. Laterally, the border is beyond the peritoneal line. Marking of the lateral field border should be performed very carefully because the peritoneal cavity tends to be displaced to the side and bony structures become inadequate landmarks. Two techniques have most often been described: the cobalt-60 moving strip (Delclos and Dembo 1978; Dembo et al. 1979; Perez et al. 1978) and treatment by open fields (AP-PA) (Delclos and Quinlan 1969; Delclos and Smith 1975; Townsend et al. 1979; Young et al. 1982). With both techniques the pelvis is boosted by an additional pelvic field, by a field within a field, or by the addition of lateral fields to the pelvis (four-field technique) (Fig. 4.7). Fuks (1975) calculated a nominal single dose or time-dose fractionation (TDF), indicating that both techniques are essentially the same. Townsend et al. (1979) compared radiation sites, dosages, and survival rates. The total dose given to the total abdomen ranges from 15 to

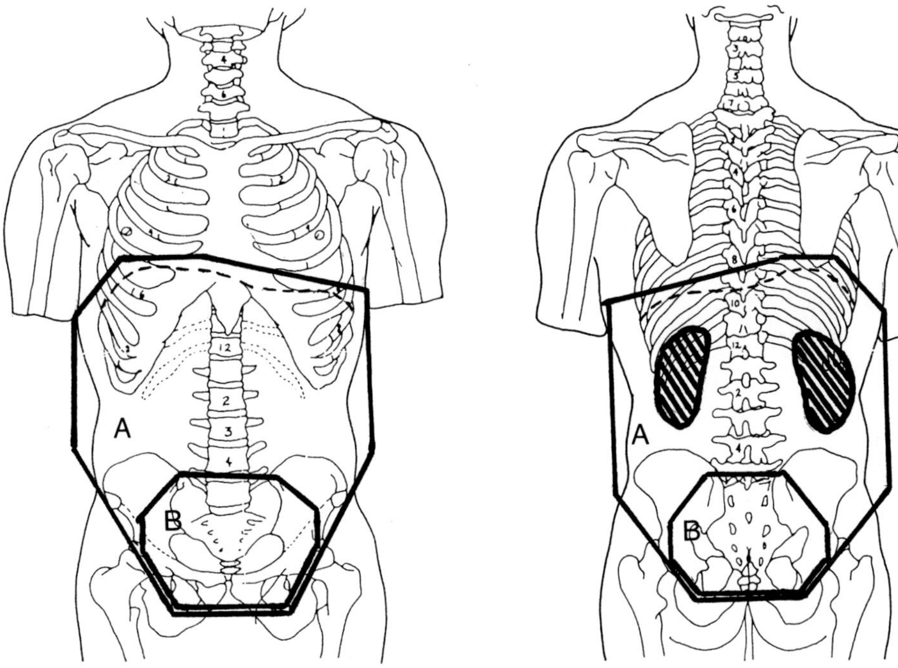

Fig. 4.7. Diagram of abdominal and pelvic portals used sequentially in external beam irradiation of ovarian carcinoma. *A*, abdominal portal; *B* pelvic portal

40 Gy (usually 30 Gy), while the total dose to the pelvis varies from 20 to 60 Gy.

In the moving strip technique, lines 2.5 cm apart are marked on the front and back of the patient. On the first day, a single strip is treated on the front and an identical opposite field is irradiated from the back. Thereafter, one 2.5-cm-wide strip is added daily until four strips have been irradiated from both the front and the back. This 10-cm strip is then moved up by 2.5 cm each day until the last strip is reached. The field is then reduced by one strip of 2.5 cm until on the last day a single 2.5-cm strip is irradiated (DELCLOS and DEMBO 1978). With this technique a tumor dose of 28 Gy in the midplane of the abdomen is delivered in eight treatments in 10–12 days. The liver is routinely shielded on the AP-PA strips and the kidneys only on the PA strips using blocks with different half-value layers (DELCLOS and QUINLAN 1969; PEREZ et al. 1978). Either before or after the abdominopelvic irradiation described above, the pelvis is boosted with a photon beam. AP-PA 15 × 15 cm portals to a dose of approximately 30 Gy are used.

With the open-field technique, the whole abdomen and pelvis including the diaphragm are treated daily AP-PA. The inferior margin extends below the obturator foramen, and lateral borders extend beyond the peritoneum (Fig. 4.8). A dose of 30 Gy is given in 5–6 weeks (1.5 Gy per fraction); the kidneys are shielded posteriorly at 18 Gy, and the liver is shielded in the anterior portal (TOWNSEND et al. 1979).

The abdominopelvic irradiation regimen at the Princess Margaret Hospital, Toronto, as reported by DEMBO (1985) consisted in pelvic irradiation of 22.5 Gy in 10 fractions (15 × 15 cm) followed immediately by a midplane dose of 22.5 Gy in 22 fractions, i.e., 1 Gy per fraction, delivered using the open-field technique.

The MARTINEZ technique (MARTINEZ et al. 1985) consists of three phases. In the first phase the entire peritoneal cavity is treated. The field extends from 1 cm above the diaphragm to the ischial tuberosity and laterally to cover the peritoneal reflexions with at least a 2-cm margin. At 10 Gy, 100% kidney blocks are introduced posteriorly only, and at 15 Gy, 50% transmission liver blocks are placed anteriorly and posteriorly. Anterior and posterior fields are treated daily (5 days/week) to a midplane dose of 15 Gy. The upper abdomen and pelvis receive 30 Gy each; the liver receives 22.5 Gy and the kidneys, 20 Gy. During the second phase, the medial half of the diaphragm, the para-aortic nodes, and the true pelvis are treated by anterior and posterior fields. Eight fractions of

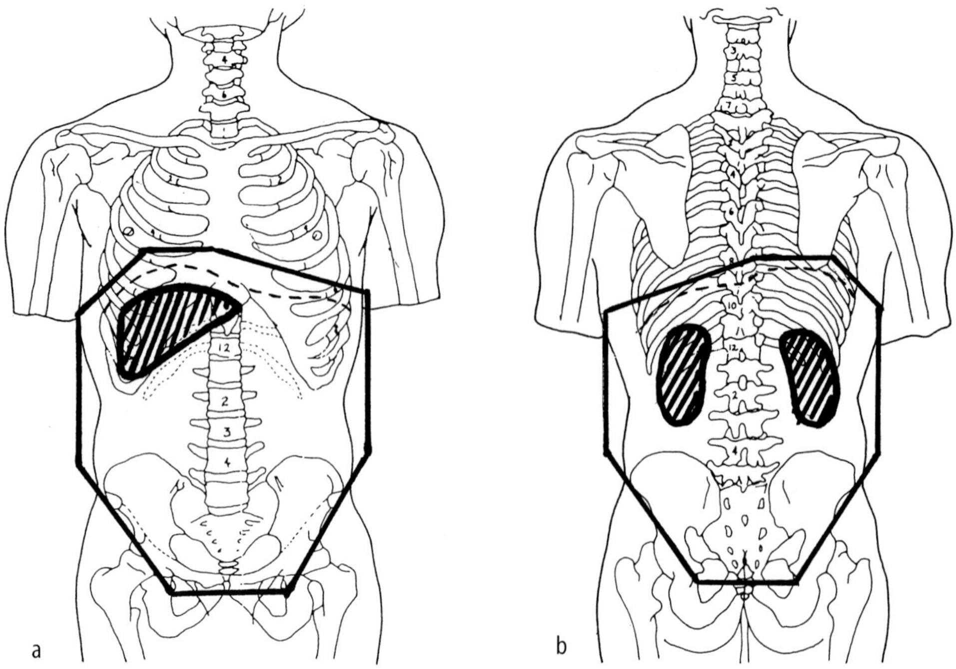

Fig. 4.8 a,b. Diagram of abdominal portals used in external beam irradiation of ovarian carcinoma. Due to the risk area located subphrenically, only a part of the liver can be shielded. The kidney shields are planned for posterior portals. **a** anteroposterior beam direction; **b** posteroanterior beam direction

1.5 Gy are given to this area, to a total dose of 42 Gy. In the third and final phase, the true pelvis is treated with opposing fields. A midplane dose of 18 Gy is given five times to a total dose of 51 Gy. A modification of this technique is now used for patients thought to be at increased risk for late bowel injury. With the modified technique the pelvis receives a total radiation dose of 49.5 Gy, the para-aortic and diaphragm 40.5 Gy, and the abdomen 25.5 Gy (Schray et al. 1989).

Kuten et al. (1988) described a split-field technique in which the lower abdomen received 30 Gy in 3 weeks followed by the same dose to the upper abdomen. The fields were separated by a calculated gap that met at the midplane and provided approximately a homogeneous dose (maximum dose peak in the gap was 157% of the reference dose). The kidneys were shielded from the posterior side and the liver both anteriorly and posteriorly.

Kong et al. (1988) describe a split-course hyperfractionated technique. The entire peritoneal cavity was treated as previously described. Two fractions of 1 Gy each were given daily with at least a 4-h interval between them. A total of 15 Gy was given over 1.5 weeks. After a rest of 3 weeks the same course was repeated. The kidneys were protected with two half-value layer shields from the beginning to limit the renal dose to 20 Gy. The total dose to the right lobe of the liver was limited to less than 28 Gy by using anterior and posterior lead shields during the last three fractions.

4.6.4 Vaginal Carcinoma

Since surgery in patients with vaginal carcinoma often requires resection of neighboring organs (bladder, urethra, and/or rectum) and since such resection is not without risk in older patients, radiation therapy is the therapy of choice. Intracavitary and external beam radiation treatments are combined, whereby emphasis is laid on afterloadings especially in early stages of disease, and sole use of external beam irradiation is preferred in patients with advanced tumors or a risk of development of fistulas.

Several authors have discussed the complex management of patients with carcinoma of the vagina and the need for individualized radiation therapy techniques. Perez (1992b) reported a correlation between the doses of radiation given to patients with vaginal carcinomas of various stages and the probability of local tumor control. Paravaginal or parametrial interstitial implants or both should be considered when residual tumor is present after the planned external and intracavitary therapy has been completed. Additional doses of 20–30 Gy to a limited volume are usually well tolerated.

In planning external beam therapy, especially when the tumor is located in the upper third of the vagina, the entire region cranially up to the common iliac lymph nodes must be assessed. When a tumor infiltrates the lower third of the vagina, the entire inguinal region must be evaluated. Planning of primary external beam irradiation in the prone position is carried out by means of CT (slice thickness 5 mm, table feed 1 cm). After establishing the target volume in each scan, the most favorable field sequence and the optimum individual absorber are estimated. When solely external beam irradiation is performed, the boost must be planned with CT after marking the tumor location with clips or similar structures. Usually the boost is applied by intracavitary therapy in the case of advanced tumors, and possibly also by interstitial therapy. Using external beam, the boost regions are irradiated in the supine position with opposing fields of further irradiated external beam target volume (in order to obtain a sufficient dose in the paravaginal region). Estimation of the physical summation isodoses from intracavitary and external beam irradiation in different CT cross-sections enables one to evaluate the adequacy of the dose in this region with a high risk of recurrence.

The technical approach to vaginal carcinoma is similar to that for carcinoma of the uterine cervix. External beam irradiation should be administered using AP-PA pelvic portals that encompass the entire vagina down to the introitus and the pelvic lymph nodes to the upper portion of the common iliac chain. Portals of 15 cm × 15 cm or 15 cm × 18 cm at the skin are usually adequate. When tumors involve the middle or lower third of the vagina, the inguinal and adjacent femoral lymph nodes should be electively treated, which requires a modification of the standard portals. For patients with clinically palpable nodes, additional doses of 15 Gy (calculated for a depth of 3–5 cm) are necessary with reduced portals. These doses can be achieved using unequal loadings of external beam photon irradiation. In the presence of palpable lymph nodes, a 2-cm bolus should be used. If necessary, reduced AP portals are used to deliver a boost dose to the inguinal nodes with electrons. Special attention is needed to avoid overlapping areas. After a specified tumor dose is delivered to the whole pelvis (20–40 Gy, depending on the extent of the tumor), a midline rectangular or wedge block is interposed, and additional irradiation is given to the parametrial tissues.

Intracavitary therapy is carried out using vaginal cylinders including cesium-137 or iridium-192 (Glaser et al. 1985). The largest possible diameter should be used to smoothen the vaginal folds and improve the ratio of mucosal to tumor dose. Depending on the extent and thickness of the tumor, single plane, double plane, or volume implants should be planned.

4.6.5 Carcinoma of the Vulva

Although carcinoma of the vulva occurs mainly in elderly women, radical vulvectomy with inguinal lymphadenectomy is the most common therapy. Referrals to the radio-oncologist are the result of inoperability or the rejection of further surgery after tumor excision, partial or complete simple vulvectomy, or recurrences (see also Chap. 6).

After standard surgery, when inguinal lymph nodes are certainly affected, external beam irradiation of the pelvic lymph nodes is recommended. In comparison to additional surgery, this produced more favorable results in the GOG study (Homesley et al. 1986). The CT radiation planning is performed similarly to that for endometrial carcinoma following surgery. However, the common iliac lymph nodes must not be included in the target volume, with the exception of enlarged lymph nodes found by CT. When only a simplified vulvectomy or a radical vulvectomy without lymphadenectomy is possible, both inguinal regions must be irradiated with ventral stationary fields (photons or electrons). In the presence of clinically palpable inguinal and pelvic lymph nodes, external beam irradiation is also necessary. If the patient rejects surgery, combined irradiation of the vulva and inguinal and pelvic lymph nodes is performed without combination of single fields. Such a technique reduces the volume dose and also the dose to the bone marrow in comparison to opposing field irradiation planned solely with the simulator. In such cases, the inguinal lymph nodes may also be included in the ventral field and later boosted with electrons.

The patient should be treated in the supine "frog leg" position, with the knees apart and feet together. A cast in the treatment position facilitates daily repositioning. During simulation, wires or comparable devices should be used to identify the vulva and inguinal regions on radiographs. With tumors involving the urethra, a urethral catheter, if tolerated by the patient, may aid in tumor localization. Because of the sloping surface of the perineum, higher doses may be delivered to this area when the tumor dose is calculated at the central axis of the portal. During simulation, consideration should be given to designing and constructing compensating filters to achieve a more homogeneous dose in the entire target volume.

Depending on the available equipment, either an AP-PA beam or an electron beam can be used. If only the vulva and the inguinofemoral lymph nodes are treated, cobalt-60, 4- to 6-MV photons, or even electrons through an anterior portal may be adequate. Care should be taken to deliver appropriate doses to the femoral nodes and the deep pelvic nodes, too. Although dry or moist desquamation is frequently observed, the use of bolus in areas potentially involved by tumor is advocated by some authors (Perez and Grigsby 1992).

When elderly patients receive only palliation, a tangential external photon beam is applied to the vulva instead of electrons. In the authors' experience, this results in fewer side-effects with a consequent reduction in the frequency with which therapy is interrupted.

References

Aalders JG, Abeler V, Kolstad P, Onsrud K (1980) Postoperative external irradiation and prognostic parameters in stage I endometrial carcinoma. Obstet Gynecol 56:419

Abitbol MM, Davenport JH (1974) The irradiated vagina. Obstet Gynecol 44:249

Alfert HJ, Gillenwater JY (1972) The consequences of ureteral irradiation with special references to subsequent ureteral injury. J Urol 107:369

Allen WE Jr, Reddi RP (1980) Simplified irradiation dosimetry in carcinoma of the cervix (external irradiation and one radium insertion). J Natl Med Assoc 72:361

Amols HI, Reinstein LE, Baldwin BC (1988) A computerized tissue compensator (abstract). Phys Med Biol 33:51

Ang KK, Peters LJ (1994) Altered fractionation in radiation oncology. Principles and practice of oncology, vol 8. Lippincott, Philadelphia

Badcock PC (1983) The role of CT-scanning in the radiotherapy planning of pelvic tumors. Int J Radiat Oncol Biol Phys 9:905

Bastin K, Buchler D, Stitt J, et al. (1993) Resource utilization. High dose rate versus low dose rate brachytherapy for gynecologic cancer. Am J Clin Oncol 16:256

Bentel GC, Nelson CE, Noell KT (1989) Treatment planning and dose calculation in radiation oncology, 4th edn. Pergamon Press, New York

Berek JS, Hacker NF, Hatch KD, Young RC (1988) Uterine corpus and cervical cancer. Curr Probl Cancer XII:65

Bohndorf B, Richter J (1992) Computertomographie und Bestrahlungsplanung in der Radioonkologie. Biermann, Zülpig

Bomford CK, Craig LM, Hanna FA, et al. (1976) Treatment simulators. Special report no 10. British Institute of Radiology, London

Bosch A, Marcial VA (1967) Evaluation of the time interval between external irradiation and intracavitary curietherapy in carcinoma of the uterine cervix: influence on curability. Radiology 88:563

Boyer A, Goitein M (1980) Simulator mounted Moiré topography camera for constructing compensator filters. Med Phys 7:19

Brady LW, Perez CA (1992) Principals and practice of radiation oncology, 2nd edn. Lippincott, Philadelphia, p 1162

Brahme A, Eenmma J, Lindback S, et al. (1983) Neutron beam characteristics from 50-MeV protons on beryllium using a continuously variable multileaf collimator. Radiother Oncol 1:65

Brenner DJ, Huang Y, Hall EJ (1991) Fractionated high dose rate versus low dose rate regimens for intracavitary brachytherapy of the cervix: equivalent regimens for combined brachytherapy and external irradiation. Int J Radiat Oncol Biol Phys 21:1415

Brizel HE, Livingston PA, Grayson EV (1974) Radiotherapeutic applications of pelvic computed tomography. J Comput Assist Tomogr 4:453

Browde S, Nissenbaum M, DeMoor NG (1984) High dose weekly fractionation radiotherapy in advanced cancer of the uterine cervix. South Afr Med J 66:11

Brown JM (1985) Sensitizers and protectors in radiotherapy. Cancer 55:2222

Campbell DW, Loyd MD (1984) Correcting for field shaping blocks used with Varian's electron beam applicator system. Am Assoc Med Dosim J 9:6

Chambers SK, Chambers JT, Kier R, Peschel RE (1991) Sequelae of lateral ovarian transposition in irradiated cervical cancer patients. Int J Radiat Oncol Biol Phys 20:1305

Chase W, Fowler WC, Currie JL, et al. (1984) Single-fraction palliative pelvic radiation therapy in gynecologic oncology: 1000 rads. Am J Obstet Gynecol 148:701

Chassagne D, Horiot JC (1977) Propositions pour une définition commune des points de référence en curiethérapie gynécologique. J Radiol 58:781

Choo YC, Hsu C, Ma HK (1984) The assessment of radioresponse of cervical carcinoma by colposcopy. Gynecol Oncol 18:28

Coia L, Won M, Lanciano R, Marcial VA, Martz K, Hanks G (1990) The patterns of care outcome study for cancer of the uterine cervix. Results of the second national practice survey. Cancer 66:2451

Corn BW, Galvin JM, Soffen EM, et al. (1993) Positional stability of sources during low dose rate brachytherapy for cervical carcinoma. Int J Radiat Oncol Biol Phys 26:513

Corn BW, Hanlon AL, Pajak TF, et al. (1994) Technically accurate intracavitary insertions improve pelvic control and survival among patients with locally advanced carcinoma of the uterine cervix. Gynecol Oncol 53:294

Cox JD (1985) Large dose fractionation (hypofractionation). Cancer 55:2105

Day MJ, Harrison RM (1983) Cross sectional information and treatment simulation. In: Bleehen NM, Glatstein E, Haybittle JL (eds) Radiation therapy planning. Dekker, New York

Delclos L, Dembo AJ (1978) Ovaries. In: Fletcher GH (ed) Textbook of radiotherapy. Lea & Febiger, Philadelphia, pp 834–851

Delclos L, Quinlan EJ (1969) Malignant tumors of the ovary managed with postoperative megavoltage irradiation. Radiology 93:659–663

Delclos L, Smith JP (1975) Ovarian cancer with special regard to types of radiotherapy. Cancer Inst Monogr 42:129–135

Dembo AJ (1985) Abdominopelvic radiotherapy in ovarian cancer: a 10 year experience. Cancer 55:2285–2290

Dembo AJ, Bush RS (1982) Choice of postoperative therapy based on prognostic factors. Int J Radiat Oncol Biol Phys 8:893

Dembo AJ, Bush RS, Beale FA, et al. (1979) The Princess Margaret Hospital study of ovarian cancer: stages I, II and asymptomatic III. Cancer Treat Rep 63:249–254

Demeyer CL, Whitehead LW, Jacobson AP, et al. (1986) Potential exposure to metal fumes, particulates, and organic vapors during radiotherapy shielding block fabrication. Med Phys 13:748

Deore SM, Viswanathan PS, Shrivastava SK, et al. (1992) Predictive role of TDF values in late rectal recto-sigmoid complications in irradiation treatment of cervix cancer. Int J Radiat Oncol Biol Phys 24:217

DeVereux C, Grundy G, Littman P (1976) Plastic molds for patient immobilization. Int J Radiat Oncol Biol Phys 1:553

Doppke KP (1987) X-ray simulator developments and evaluation for radiation therapy. In: Kereiakes JG, Elson HR, Born CG (eds) Radiation oncology physics – 1986. American Institute of Physics, New York

Doppke KP, Goitein M (1988) A survey of the information gained from planning treatment computer. Med Phys 15:258

Durrance FY, Fletcher GH, Rutledge F (1969) Analysis of central recurrent disease in stage I and II squamous cell carcinomas of the cervix on intact uterus. Am J Roentgenol 106:831

Eifel PJ (1992) High dose rate brachytherapy for carcinoma of the cervix: high tech or high risk? Int J Radiat Oncol Biol Phys 24:383

El-Khatib E, Podgorsak EB, Pla C (1987) Broad beam and narrow beam attenuation in Lipowitz's metal. Med Phys 14:135

Engler MJ, Herskovic AM, Proimos BS (1984) Dosimetry of rotational photon fields with gravity-oriented eye blocks. Int J Radiat Oncol Biol Phys 10:431

Fletcher GH (1973) Clinical dose response curves of human malignant epithelial tumours. Br J Radiol 46:1

Flueckinger F, Ebner F, Poschauko H, et al. (1992) Cervical cancer: serial MR imaging before and after primary radiation therapy – a 2-year follow-up study. Radiology 184:89

Fowler JF, Harari PM (1993) Hyperfractionation's promise in cancer treatment. Contemp Oncol 3:14

Fuks Z (1975) External radiotherapy of ovarian cancer: standard approaches and new frontiers. Semin Oncol 2:253

Fyles A, Keane TJ, Barton M, Simm J (1992) The effect of treatment duration in the local control of cervix cancer. Radiother Oncol 25:273

Galvin JM, Heidtman B, Cheng E, et al. (1982) The use of a CT scanner specially designed to perform the functions of a radiation therapy treatment unit simulator. Med Phys 9:615

Galvin JM, Turrisi AT, Cheng E (1987) Treatment simulation using a CT unit. In: Kereiakes JG, Elson HR, Born CG (eds) Radiation oncology physics – 1986. American Institute of Physics, New York

Gerber RL, Marks JE, Purdy JA (1982) The use of thermal plastics for immobilization of patients during radiotherapy. Int J Radiat Oncol Biol Phys 8:1461

Gerbi BJ (1985) Compensating filter design using radiographic stereo shift information. Med Phys 12:646

Glaser FH, Grimm D, Haensgen G, Rauh G, Schuchardt K (1985) Klinische Erfahrungen bei der Afterloading-Kurzzeittherapie im Vergleich zur konventionellen Brachytherapy bei der Behandlung gynäkologischer Tumoren. Strahlentherapie 161:459

Glasgow GP, Purdy JA (1992) External beam dosimetry and treatment planning. In: Perez CA, Brady LW (eds) Principles and practice of radiation oncology, 2nd edn. Lippincott, Philadelphia, pp 208–245

Glasgow GP, Reeves GI (1980) Safety considerations during the production of radiation therapy shielding blocks from low melting temperature bismuth alloys. Proceedings of the Health Physics Society Mid-Year Symposium on Medical Physics, Hyanis, MA

Goitein M (1982) Limitations of two dimensional treatment planning programs. Med Phys 9:580

Goitein M (1985) Future prospects in planning radiation therapy. Cancer 55:2234

Goitein M, Wittenberg J, Mendiondo M, et al. (1979) The value of CT-scanning in radiation therapy treatment planning: a prospective study. Int J Radiat Oncol Biol Phys 5:1787

Greer BE, Koh W-J, Figge DC, et al. (1990) Gynecologic radiotherapy fields defined by intraoperative measurements. Gynecol Oncol 38:421

Grigsby PW, Perez CA (1991) Radiotherapy alone for medically inoperable carcinoma of the cervix: stage IA and carcinoma in situ. Int J Radiat Oncol Biol Phys 21:375

Hamberger AD (1980) Long term results of radium therapy in cervical cancer. Int J Radiat Oncol Biol Phys 6:647

Hanks GE, Herring DF, Kramer S (1983) Patterns of care outcome studies: results of the national practice in cancer of the cervix. Cancer 51:959

Hashimoto H, Ito H (1988) History and development of HDR-afterloading in Japan. In: Vahrson H, Rauthe G (eds) High dose rate afterloading in the treatment of cancer of the uterus, breast and rectum. Suppl. Strahlentherapie und Onkologie, vol 82. Urban & Schwarzenberg, München, p 10

Haus AG, Marks JE (1973) Detection and evaluation of localization errors in patient radiation therapy. Invest Radiol 8:384

Herbert SH, Curran WJ Jr, Solin LJ, et al. (1991) Decreasing gastrointestinal morbidity with the use of small bowel contrast during treatment planning for pelvic irradiation. Int J Radiat Oncol Biol Phys 20:835

Hintz BL, Kagan AR, Gilbert HA, et al. (1981) Systemic absorption of conjugated estrogenic cream by the irradiated vagina. Gynecol Oncol 12:75

Hobday P, Hodson NJ, Husband J, MacDonald JS (1979) Computed tomography applied to radiotherapy treatment planning: techniques and results. Radiology 133:477

Hodson DI, Krepart GV (1983) Once monthly radiotherapy for the palliation of pelvic gynecological malignancy. Gynecol Oncol 16:112

Homesley HD, Bundy BN, Sedlis A, Adcock L (1986) Radiation therapy versus pelvic node resection for carcinoma of the vulva with positive groin nodes. Obstet Gynecol 68:733

Huen A, Findley DO, Skov DD (1979) Attenuation in Lipowitz's metal of x-rays produced at 2, 4, 10, and 18 MV and gamma rays from cobalt-60. Med Phys 6:147

Jampolis S, Andras EJ, Fletcher GH (1975) Analysis of sites and causes of failures of irradiation in invasive squamous cell carcinoma of the intact uterine cervix. Radiology 115:681

Janson PO, Jansson I, Skryten A, et al. (1981) Ovarian endocrine function in young women undergoing radiotherapy for carcinoma of the cervix. Gynecol Oncol 11:218

Johns HE (1976) Optimization of energy and equipment. In: Kramer S, Sunthralingam N, Zinninger GF (eds) High-energy photons and electrons. John Wiley, New York, p 33

Jones RD, Symonds RP, Miller RG, et al. (1990) A comparison of remote afterloading and manually inserted cesium in the treatment of carcinoma of the cervix. Clin Oncol (R Coll Radiol) 2:193

Joslin CAF (1990) Brachytherapy: a clinical dilemma. Int J Radiat Oncol Biol Phys 19:801

Källman P, Lind B, Eklöf A, Brahme A (1988) Shaping of arbitrary dose distributions by dynamic multileaf collimation. Phys Med Biol 33:1291

Kapp DS (1983) The role of the radiation oncologist in the management of gynecologic cancer. Cancer 51:2485

Kapp DS, Fischer D, Gutierrez G, Kohorn EI, Schwartz PE (1983) Pretreatment prognostic factors in carcinoma of the uterine cervix: a multivariable analysis of the effect of age, stage, histology and blood counts on survival. Int J Radiat Oncol Biol Phys 9:445

Katz HJ, Davies JNP (1980) Death from cervix uteri carcinoma: the changing pattern. Gynecol Oncol 9:86

Khan FM, Gerbi BJ, Deibel FC (1986) Dosimetry of asymmetric x-ray collimators. Med Phys 13:936

Kim RY, Salter MM, Weppelmann B, Brascho DJ (1988) Analysis of treatment modalities and their failures in stage IB cancer of the cervix. Int J Radiat Oncol Biol Phys 15:831

Klemp PFB, Perry AM, Hedland-Thomas B, et al. (1988) Commissioning of a linear accelerator with independent jaws: computerized data collection and transfer to a planning computer. Phys Med Biol 33:865

Kolstadt P (1989) Followup study of 232 patients with stage IAa and 411 patients with stage IA2 squamous cell carcinoma of the cervix (microinvasive carcinoma). Gynecol Oncol 33:265

Komaki R, Pajak TF, Marcial VA, et al. (1994) Twice-daily fractionation of external irradiation with brachytherapy in bulky carcinoma of the cervix. Cancer 73:2619

Kong JJS, Peters LJ, Wharton JT, et al. (1988) Hyperfractionated split course whole abdominal radiotherapy for ovarian carcinoma: tolerance and toxicity. Int J Radiat Oncol Biol Phys 14:737

Kottmeier HL (1964) Surgical and radiation treatment of carcinoma of the uterine cervix. Acta Obstet Gynecol Scand (Suppl 2) 43:1

Kraiphibul P, Srisupundit S, Pridsowidol O, et al. (1992) Results of treatment in stage IIB squamous cell carcinoma of the uterine cervix: comparison between two and one cavitary insertion. Gynecol Oncol 45:160

Kucera H, Vavra N, Weghaupt K (1989) Zum Wert der postoperativen Bestrahlung beim Endometriumkarzinom im pathohistologischen Stadium I. Geburtsh Frauenklinik 49:618–624

Kuisk H (1973) New methods to facilitate radiotherapy planning and treatment, including a method for fast production of solid lead blocks with diverging wall for cobalt-60 beam. AJR 117:161

Kurohara SS, DiSaia P, Kurohara J, et al. (1979) Uterine cervical cancer: treatment with megavoltage radiation results and afterloading intracavitary techniques. Am J Radiol 133:293

Kuten A, Stein M, Steiner MD, et al. (1988) Whole abdominal irradiation following chemotherapy in advanced ovarian carcinoma. Int J Radiat Oncol Biol Phys 14:273

La Rouere J, Perez-Tamayo C, Fraass B, et al. (1989) Optimal coverage of peritoneal surface in whole abdominal radiation for ovarian neoplasma. Int J Radiat Oncol Biol Phys 17:607

Lamarque P, Coliez R (1951) Les cancers des organes génitaux de la femme. In: Delherm L (ed) Electroradiothérapie. Masson, Paris, p 2549

Lanciano RM, Corn BW (1992) Radiotherapy for gynecologic malignancies. Curr Opin Oncol 4:930

Lanciano RM, Pajak TF, Martz K, Hanks GE (1993) The influence of treatment time on outcome for squamous cell cancer of the cervix treated with radiation: a patterns-of-care study. Int J Radiat Oncol Biol Phys 25:391

Larson JE, Whitney CW, Zaino R, et al. (1990) Case report: endometrial response to endogenous hormones after pelvic irradiation for genital malignancies. Gynecol Oncol 36:106

Lee JKT (1989) Computed body tomography. Raven Press, New York

Lichter AS, Ten Haken RK (1994) Three-dimensional treatment planning and conformal radiation dose delivery. Principles and practice of oncology updates, vol 8(5). Lippincott, Philadelphia

Lichter AS, Frass BA, Van de Geijn J, et al. (1983) An overview of clinical requirements and clinical utility of computer tomography based radiotherapy treatment planning. In: Ling CC, Rodgers CC, Morton RJ (eds) Computed Tomography in Radiation Therapy. Raven Press, New York

Lindner H (1992) CT in der Bestrahlungsplanung von gynäkologischen Tumoren. In: Bohndorf W, Richter J (eds) Computertomographie und Bestrahlungsplanung in der Radioonkologie. Biermann, Zülpich, pp 163–176

Loshek DD (1984) Applications and physics of the independent collimator feature of the Varian Clinac 2500. 10th Varian Users Meeting, Palm Springs, CA, April 15–17

Marcial LV, Marcial VA, Krall JV, et al. (1991) Comparison of 1 vs. 2 or more intracavitary brachytherapy applications in the management of carcinoma of the cervix, with irradiation alone. Int J Radiat Oncol Biol Phys 20:81

Marcial VA, Bosch A (1968) Fractionation in radiation therapy of carcinoma of the uterine cervix. Results of a prospective study of 3 vs. 5 fractions per week. Front Radiat Ther Oncol 3:238

Marcial VA, Amato DA, Marks RD, et al. (1983) Split course versus continuous pelvic irradiation in carcinoma of the uterine cervix: a prospective randomized clinical trial of the radiation therapy oncology group. Int J Radiat Oncol Biol Phys 9:431

Martinez A, Schray MF, Howes AE, et al. (1985) Postoperative radiation therapy for epithelial ovarian cancer: the curative role based on a 24-year experience. J Clin Oncol 3:901

Maruyama Y, Moore VC, Burns D, et al. (1969) Individualized lung shields from lead shot in plastic. Radiology 92:634

McKay MJ, Bull CA, Houghton CR, Langlands AO (1990) Letter to the editor. Gynecol Oncol 39:236

Mizer S, Scheller RR, Deye JA (1986) Radiation therapy simulation workbook. Pergamon Press, New York

Mondalek PM, Orton CG (1982) Transmission and build-up characteristics of polyurethane-foam immobilization devices. Treat Plan 7:5
Montana GS, Fowler WC, Varia MA, et al. (1986) Carcinoma of the cervix, stage III: results of radiation therapy. Cancer 57:148
Munzenrider JE, Pilepich M, Rene-Ferrero JB, et al. (1977) Use of bodyscanner in radiotherapy treatment planning. Cancer 40:170
Munzenrider JE, Coppke KP, et al. (1991) Three-dimensional treatment planning for paraaortic node irradiation in patients with cervical cancer. Int J Radiat Oncol Biol Phys 21:229
Nahhas WA, Nisce LZ, D'Angio CJ, Lewis JL Jr (1971) Lateral ovarian transposition. Obstet Gynecol 38:785
Orr JW Jr, Barret JM, Holloway RW (1993) Neoplasia in pregnancy. In: Moore TR, Reiter RC, Reban RW, Baker W (eds) Gynecology and obstetrics: a longitudinal approach. Churchill Livingstone, New York
Paliwal BR, Asp L (1976) A technique to evaluate styrofoam cutouts used in irregular field shaping. Int J Radiat Oncol Biol Phys 1:791
Paterson R (1948) The treatment of malignant disease by radium and x-rays. Edward Arnold, London
Perez CA (1992a) Uterine cervix. In: Perez CA, Brady LW (eds) Principles and practice of radiation oncology, 2nd edn. Lippincott, Philadelphia, pp 1143–1202
Perez CA (1992b) Vagina. In: Perez CA, Brady LW (eds) Principles and practice of radiation oncology, 2nd edn. Lippincott, Philadelphia, pp 1258–1272
Perez CA, Grigsby PW (1992) Vulva. In: Perez CA, Brady LW (eds) Principles and practice of radiation oncology, 2nd edn. Lippincott, Philadelphia, pp 1273–1289
Perez CA, Korba A, Zivnuska F, et al. (1978) ^{60}Co moving strip technique management of carcinoma of the ovary: analysis of tumor control and morbidity. Int J Radiat Oncol Biol Phys 4:379–388
Perez CA, Camel RM, Kuske RR, et al. (1986) Radiation therapy alone in the treatment of carcinoma of the uterine cervix: a 20-year experience. Gynecol Oncol 23:127
Petterson F (1988) Annual report on the results of treatment in gynecological cancer, 20. Radiumhemmet, Stockholm
Pitkin RM, VanVoorhis LW (1971) Postirradiation vaginitis: an evaluation of prophylaxis with topical estrogen. Radiology 99:417
Piver MS, Yazigi R, Blumenson L, Tsukada Y (1979) A prospective trial comparing hysterectomy plus vaginal radium and uterine radium plus hysterectomy in stage I endometrial carcinoma. Obstet Gynecol 54:85
Powers WE, Kinzie JK, Demidecki AJ, et al. (1973) A new system of field shaping for external-beam radiation therapy. Radiology 108:407
Prasad S, Pilepich MV, Perez CA (1981) Contribution of CT to quantitative radiation therapy planning. Am J Radiol 136:123
Promos BS, Goldson AL (1981) Dynamic dose shaping by gravity oriented absorbers for total lymph node irradiation. Int J Radiat Oncol Biol Phys 7:973
Purdy JA (1983) Secondary field shaping. In: Wright AE, Boyer AL (eds) Advances in radiation therapy treatment planning. American Institute of Physics, New York
Rubin P, Casarett GW (1968) Clinical radiation pathology, vol II. Sounders, Philadelphia, p 919
Rubin P, Constine LS, Nelson DF (1992) Late effects of cancer treatment: radiation and drug toxicity. In: Perez CA, Brady LW (eds) Principles and practice of radiation oncology, 2nd edn. Lippincott, Philadelphia, pp 124–161
Rubin P, Cooper R, Phillips TL (1975) Radiation biology and radiation pathology syllabus (Set R.T. 1 Radiation oncology). American College of Radiology, Chicago
Schmidt BG, Kölbel K, Hübener K-H (1986) Computertomographische Uteruslokalisation zur Optimierung der primär kombinierten Strahlentherapie inoperabler Gebärmutterhalskrebse. Strahlenther Onkol 162:469
Schoeppel SL, LaVigne ML, McShan D, et al. (1990) 3-D treatment planning of intracavitary gynecologic implants: analysis of ten cases and implications for dose specifications. Int J Radiat Oncol Biol Phys 19(Suppl):129
Schray MF, Martinez A, Howes AE (1989) Toxicity of openfield whole abdominal irradiation as primary postoperative treatment in gynecologic malignancy. Int J Radiat Oncol Biol Phys 16:397
Sevin B-U (1986) Prätherapeutische Staging-Laparotomie beim Cervixcarcinom. Gynäkologe 19:62
Shanahan TG, Mehta MP, Gehring MA, et al. (1989) Minimization of small bowel volume utilizing costumized "belly board" mold. Int J Radiat Oncol Biol Phys 17:187
Shingleton HM, Orr JW Jr (1995) Cancer of the cervix. Lippincott, Philadelphia
Smit BM (1991) Prospects for proton therapy in carcinoma of the cervix. Int J Radiat Oncol Biol Phys 22:349
Smith RM, Sanfilippo LJ, Stiedley KD, et al. (1987) Clinical patterns of use of a CT-based simulator. Med Dosim 12:17
Stehmann FB, Bundy BN (1993) Carcinoma of the cervix treated with chemotherapy and radiation therapy. Cooperative studies in the gynecologic oncology group. Cancer 71:1697
Sternick ES (1983) Spherical contouring techniques. In: Wright A, Boyer A (eds) Advances in radiation therapy treatment planning. American Institute of Physics, New York
Suresh UR, Smith VJ, Lupton EW, Haboubi NY (1993) Radiation disease of the urinary tract: histological features of 18 cases. J Clin Pathol 46:228
Sutton G, Bundy B, Delgado G, et al. (1992) Ovarian metastases in stage IB carcinoma of the cervix: a Gynecologic Oncology Group study. Am J Obstet Gynecol 166:50
Takahashi K, Purdy JA, Liu YY (1983) Treatment planning system for conformation radiotherapy. Radiology 147:567
Takahashi S (1965) Conformational radiotherapy. Acta Radiol Suppl (Stockh) 242:1
Toki N, Tsukamoto N, Kaku T, et al. (1991) Microscopic ovarian metastasis of the uterine cervical cancer. Gynecol Oncol 41:46
Townsend R, Glassburn JR, Brady LW, Rowland J (1979) Whole abdominal irradiation for carcinoma of the ovary. Cancer Clin Trials 2:351–358
Ulmer HU, Frischbier H-J (1982) Die ausschließliche perkutane Strahlenbehandlung fortgeschrittener Kollumkarzinome. Geburtsh Frauenklinik 42:243–344
Vahrson H (1991) Die Strahlentherapie des Korpuskarzinoms. In: Künzel W, Kirschbaum M (eds) Giessener Gynäkologische Fortbildung. Springer, Berlin Heidelberg New York, pp 162–179
Vahrson H, Glaser FH (1988) History of HDR-afterloading in brachytherapy. In: Vahrson H, Rauthe G (eds) High dose rate afterloading in the treatment of cancer of the uterus, breast and rectum. Suppl. Strahlentherapie und Onkologie, vol 82. Urban & Schwarzenberg, München, p 2
Vahrson H, Römer G (1988) 5-year results with HDR-afterloading in cervix cancer: dependence on fractionation

and dose. In: Vahrson H, Rauthe G (eds) High dose rate afterloading in the treatment of cancer of the uterus, breast and rectum. Urban & Schwarzenberg, Munchen, pp 139–146

Van de Geijn J, Harrington FS, Fraass B (1982) A graticule for evaluation of megavoltage x-ray port films. Int J Radiat Oncol Biol Phys 8:1999

Varghese CV, Rangad F, Jose CC, et al. (1992) Hyperfractionation in advanced carcinoma of the uterine cervix: a preliminary report. Int J Radiat Oncol Biol Phys 23:393

Watkins DMB (1981) Radiation therapy mold technology. Pergamon Press, Toronto

Watkins DMB (1986) Beam direction shells in the treatment planning of head and neck cancer. Med Dosim 11:45

Weller MK, Glasgow GP (1982) The flexible curve, a useful contouring device. Treat Plan 7:8

West CM, Davidson SE, Hendry JH, Hunter RD (1991) Prediction of cervical carcinoma response to radiotherapy. Letter. Lancet 338:818

White AC (1975) An atlas of radiation histopathology. Technical Information Center, U.S. Energy Research and Developmental Administration, Washington DC

Withers HR (1985) Biologic basis for altered fractionation schemes. Cancer 55:2086

Young RC, Knapp RC, Perez CA, et al. (1982) Cancer of the ovary. In: DeVita VT, Hellman S, Rosenberg SA (eds) Cancer: principles and practices of oncology. Lippincott, Philadelphia, pp 884–913

Special Report

5 Cancer of the Vulva

J. BAHNSEN and H.J. FRISCHBIER

CONTENTS

J. BAHNSEN, MD, PhD, Professor, Abteilung für Gynäkologische Radiologie, Frauenklinik, Universitätskrankenhaus Eppendorf, Martinistraße 52, D-20251 Hamburg, Germany

H.J. FRISCHBIER, MD, PhD, Professor, Klövensteenweg 64, D-22559 Hamburg-Rissen, Germany

5.1 Epidemiology and Risk Factors

Tumors of the vulva constitute about 3.5% of all genital tract tumors. The age-adjusted incidence for squamous cell cancer is 1.39 per 100000 women (HENSON and TARONE 1977). The incidence of invasive cancer of the vulva rises with age, so that at the age of 75 the incidence is 19.8 in 100000 women (REAGAN and NG 1988). The mean age of patients at presentation is 68–70 years (SCHMIDT et al. 1992; KUCERA and WEGHAUPT 1988). In the 21st Annual Report (PETTERSSON 1991), 75.2% of patients were 60 years of age or older, and 51.4%, 70 years or older. In 367 cases of preinvasive lesions (vulvar intraepithelial neoplasia, VIN) the mean age was significantly lower, i.e., 51.1 years (PETTERSSON 1991).

MACK and CASAGRANDE (1981) noted an incidence in women of the lowest social class three times greater than in the highest social class. Employment in the laundering and cleaning industries may increase the risk of vulvar cancer.

There is an association between vulvar cancer and diabetes mellitus [according to SCHMIDT et al. (1992), 30% of patients have diabetes]; this association is, however, partly due to the advanced age of the patients.

An association with vulvar carcinoma is seen in sexually transmitted diseases like lymphogranuloma venereum, syphilis, herpesvirus type II, and condylomata acuminata. The cervix is the most common site of second primary tumors. This suggests the possibility of a common pathogenetic factor. A prior history of leukoplakia or inflammation of the vulva has been reported to be associated with vulvar carcinoma. Condylomata acuminata are found in 5%–10% of patients with vulvar carcinoma.

Some vulvar diseases can alter the risk of invasive carcinoma (preinvasive lesions like VIN, Bowen's disease, Paget's disease, and precursors of melanoma are discussed in Chap. 6). Benign, white lesions of the vulva are named by a great number of confusing terms such as kraurosis vulvae, atrophic vulvitis, leukoplakia, and lichen sclerosus et atrophicus. The International Society for the Study of Vulvar Diseases (ISSVD) coined the term dystrophy for all these entities, characterized by disorders of epithelial growth and nutrition.

One can distinguish two varieties of dystrophy: (a) hyperplastic dystrophy and (b) lichen sclerosus. In addition a mixed dystrophy is possible.

Hyperplastic dystrophy is characterized by thick gray or white plaques. The histological appearance consists of elongation and blunting of the epithelial folds. Chronic inflammation and hyperkeratosis are usually present. The most frequent symptoms are itching and the discovery of a lump.

In lichen sclerosus the squamous epithelium is thinned and loses the epithelial folds (rete ridges). Affected women have pruritus and often stenosis of the introitus.

The most important subclassification is that into lesions with and without atypia. If there is no atypia, progression to invasive carcinoma will not occur. The incidence of invasive cancer depends on the degree of atypia. To distinguish lesions with and lesions without atypia, a Keyes dermatological punch can be easily performed under local anesthesia. A major problem is selection of the right tissue for biopsy, as atypia may exist in limited regions only. Multifocal lesions occur in 10% of patients. Toluidine blue staining is frequently used for selection of the biopsy site; unfortunately, however, false-positive and false-negative results limit the use of this method. As an alternative, application of 3% acetic acid in combination with careful inspection with magnification is recommended for the detection of early vulvar lesions. Indications for biopsy are ulcerated lesions, marked discoloration, and thickening of the skin.

Although vulvar dystrophies are commonly found in association with vulvar carcinoma, they infrequently progress to invasive cancer if left untreated. Thus the rate of progression of dystrophic lesions to invasive cancer is low compared with that of VIN (see Sect. 6.1 in Chap. 6). Patients with invasive vulvar cancer and prior dystrophy have lower tumor stages than those without prior dystrophy (Figge et al. 1985): with prior dystrophy, 56% of the cases were FIGO stage I, versus 28% without. This may be due to earlier detection of the cancer during the control of the dystrophy.

5.2 Topographic Anatomy and Patterns of Spread

The external female genitalia include the mons pubis, the labia majora and minora, the clitoris with its prepuce and frenulum, and the vestibule into which open the orifices of Skene's and Bartholin's glands. The vestibule may occasionally contain scattered mucin-producing glands, the glandulae vestibulares minores. The mons pubis and the lateral aspects of the labia majora bear hair follicles with sebaceous and apocrine glands. On the external and internal surfaces of both the labia majores and the labia minora, sebaceous glands are particularly numerous. The labia minora and the inner aspect of the labia majora are the only areas of the human body in which sebaceous glands develop without concomitant hair formation.

The arterial supply is from the internal pudendal artery. This vessel derives from the hypogastric artery. The venous drainage accompanies the arterial vessels.

The lymphatic vessels travel along the length of the labium. The direction of flow is from the labium minus to the labium majus. The superficial external pudendal lymphatic vessels drain to the superficial femoral nodes. The boundary line of lymphatic drainage to the superficial iliac nodes is formed by the genitocrural folds, the mons pubis, the anus, the hymen, and the lower third of the urethra. The lymphatics subsequently penetrate the cribriform fascia and reach the deep femoral nodes. The inguinal canal serves as a portal to the intrapelvic lymph nodes. These nodes lie extraperitoneally on the side wall of the pelvis.

The superficial inguinal nodes are arranged into two groups: The upper group, usually six or seven in number, form a chain immediately below and arranged along the line of the inguinal ligament and superficial to the fascia lata. The lower group, sometimes called the superficial subinguinal or superficial femoral, and usually four or five in number, lie vertically along the terminal part of the great saphenous vein before it enters the femoral vein, at the saphenous opening. The deep inguinal nodes, one to three in number, are placed deep to the fascia lata on the medial side of the femoral veins. The upper one has also been called the node of Cloquet or Rosenmüller.

Some vessels pass from the labium minus to the vestibule. From the region of the clitoris, deeper lymphatic vessels pass directly to the deep femoral nodes, or to the external iliac nodes. The distal vaginal wall, the proximal two-thirds of the urethra, and the body of the clitoris drain to a deep set of nodes. These deep nodes consist of the deep inguinal nodes and the medial group of the external iliac, obturator, and hypogastric nodes. Theoretically, lesions arising in or involving the glans clitoris or urethra can spread to the pelvic nodes directly without passing inguinal nodes. Nevertheless, iliac involvement without metastasis to the groin is seen extremely seldom (PEREZ and GRIGSBY 1992; DUBESHTER et al. 1993).

Vulvar cancer can be localized at the labia majora, the labia minora, the clitoris, and the perineum. In some cases the vagina may be involved simultaneously. These cases should be classified as vulvar carcinoma in general. Further classification problems may occur in cases with involvement of the urethra. All cases of squamous differentiation and urethral involvement should be classified as vulvar cancer. A classification may be impossible in advanced perineal cancers with involvement of the anal ring and the vulva.

The most common sites of invasive carcinoma are the labia majora and minora (70%). In 10%–15% the clitoris and in 4%–5% the area of the perineum and fourchette are the primary location. The most common mode of spread is to the superficial inguinal lymph nodes. Cases with involvement of deep femoral nodes and free superficial inguinal nodes are reported very seldom (HACKER et al. 1984; PARKER et al. 1975). The probability of spread depends on the diameter of the lesion, its depth of infiltration, its localization, and the histological grading. Most of the involved lymph nodes are localized in the ipsilateral groin. The frequency of contralateral metastasis is lower in patients with well-lateralized tumors and higher in those with lesions characterized by a larger diameter, deeper invasion, or higher grading.

Left untreated, vulvar cancer shows infiltration of adjacent organs, vagina, urethra, anus, bladder, pubic bone, mons pubis, and the structures of the pelvic floor. Cases with groin node metastasis have a 40% likelihood of involvement of pelvic nodes. Further spread and distant metastasis seldom occur because most of the women die of sequelae of local progression into the pelvis.

5.3 Diagnostic Workup and Staging

The preoperative staging should include the following procedures: Physical examination with inspection of the vulva, the anal area, the perineum, the vagina, and the cervix. Careful palpation of groin nodes has to be done for clinical nodal staging. A pelvic examination should be performed. Involvement of the urinary tract is ruled out by cystoscopy and intravenous urography. Proctosigmoidoscopy should be performed when a tumor is located near to the perineum and there is involvement of the vagina. Lymphography is seldom used in the staging of vulvar carcinoma; it is, however, of great value in the detection of small metastases in the inguinal and external iliac nodes. While computed tomography (CT) is of limited value in the staging of vulvar carcinoma, magnetic resonance imaging (MRI) is helpful to demonstrate the extent of the primary. Staging is completed by blood count, blood chemistry, and chest radiographs.

The rules for clinical staging (Table 5.1) were established at the meeting of the FIGO Committee on Gynecologic Oncology in October 1988 (PETTERSSON 1991). For the TNM classification according the UICC, see Tables 5.2 and 5.3. The staging of the American Joint Committee (AJC) is identical. The correlation of the FIGO and TNM classifications is shown in Table 5.4.

It is of doubtful value to compare clinical and surgical staging. In clinical stage FIGO I (T1N0M0), 14% of patients show lymph node involvement (HOPKINS et al. 1991). These cases will be restaged to FIGO III (unilateral) or IV (bilateral lymph node involvement). About 23% of clinical stage II (T2N0M0) patients have lymph node involvement (HOPKINS et al. 1991) on histological examination and will be regrouped into surgical stage FIGO III or

Table 5.1. Clinical staging of vulvar cancer according to FIGO (1988)

Stage 0	Carcinoma in situ
Stage Ia	A single lesion measuring 2 cm or less in diameter and with a depth of invasion of 1 mm or less
Stage Ib	Tumor confined to the vulva, 2 cm or less in diameter, without suspicious groin nodes
Stage II	Tumor confined to the vulva, exceeding 2 cm in diameter, without suspicious groin nodes
Stage III	Extension beyond the vulva, without suspicious groin nodes, or lesions of any size with suspicious groin nodes
Stage IVa	Bilateral positive groin nodes, regardless of extent of the primary
Stage IVb	Evidence of distant metastases, including to the pelvic lymph nodes

Table 5.2. T-staging (primary tumor) according to the AJC and UICC

Tis	Preinvasive carcinoma
T1	Tumor confined to the vulva and/or perineum - 2 cm or less in greatest dimension
T2	Tumor confined to the vulva and/or perineum - more than 2 cm in greatest dimension
T3	Tumor of any size with adjacent spread to the urethra and/or vagina and/or anus
T4	Tumor of any size infiltrating the bladder mucosa and/or the rectal mucosa including the upper part of the urethral mucosa and/or fixed to the bone

Table 5.3. N- and M-staging according to the AJC and UICC

N:	Regional lymph nodes
N0	No nodes palpable
N1	Unilateral regional lymph node metastasis
N2	Bilateral regional lymph node metastasis
M:	Distant metastasis
M0	No clinical metastasis
M1	Distant metastasis, including pelvic lymph node metastasis

Table 5.4. Clinical stages: correlation of the FIGO and UICC/AJC classifications

Stage	TNM
0	Tis
I	T1N0M0
II	T2N0M0
III	T3N0M0
	T1/2/3N1M0
IVa	TxN2M0
	T4NxM0
IVb	TxNxM1

Table 5.5. Stage distribution

	Source			
	21st Annual Report	Ann Arbor[a]	Munich[b]	GOG 36[c]
Stage I	29.3%	37%	23%	25%
Stage II	30.3%	26%	25%	34%
Stage III	29.5%	29%	33%	31%
Stage IV	10.5%	8%	19%	5%
No. of cases	2912	172	115	608

[a] Hopkins et al. 1991; Pettersson 1991.
[b] Lochmüller 1986.
[c] Sevin and Homesley 1986.

IV. Thus the results of surgically staged cases will be better than those of clinically staged cases in groups I and II.

In Table 5.5 the stage distribution is demonstrated. The 21st Annual Report contains the largest number of patients. Two-thirds of the patients are without clinical evidence of lymph node metastasis.

5.4 Histopathological Classification and Grading

Preinvasive forms of vulvar malignancy are called VIN (see Sect. 6.1 in Chap. 6). Of the invasive lesions, 90% are squamous cell carcinomas. The clinical appearance is that of an ulcerated endophytic lesion in one-third of cases, and an exophytic nodular growth in the others. Most of the tumors grow slowly and are better differentiated than those seen in the cervix. Histologically, 90% of the squamous cell tumors are well differentiated; only 5%–10% are anaplastic varieties. The latter have a higher probability of node involvement. In well-differentiated invasive squamous cell carcinomas, a large amount of keratin is seen at the surface and in tongues and inlays within the tumor. In moderately differentiated tumors, keratinization and pearl formation are less marked. Cells have a moderate amount of cytoplasm and are rounder. Nuclear and cellular pleomorphism are not marked. In contrast, poorly differentiated squamous cell carcinomas have a conspicuous pleomorphism; keratinization and pearl formation are absent (Ng 1991).

Verrucous and basal cell carcinomas are rare variants of squamous cell lesions with a different behavior (Sect. 6.2 in Chap. 6). Tumors playing adenoid differentiation can be metastatic or derive from the Bartholin's gland (see Sect. 6.3 in Chap. 6). Melanoma of the vulva is more common than that of other parts of the skin (see Sect. 6.4 in Chap. 6).

A pathological report should include the following important information for the physician:

- Tumor type, invasiveness
- Grading, differentiation
- Largest diameter
- Thickness, depth of invasion
- Involvement of borders
- Number of groin nodes
- Number of involved nodes
- Extranodal infiltration of the groin

Microinvasive carcinomas invade less than 5 mm of the basal membrane and have a maximum diameter of 20 mm. This subgroup of women has a very low risk of nodal involvement.

5.5 Prognostic Factors

In patients with tumors, favorable prognosis can be defined as the probability of survival or as the probability of not developing a local recurrence. Survival is governed not only by the tumor. Because vulvar cancer is primarily a disease of very old women, natural causes of death play a major role. According to the Hamburg Statistical Yearbook, a 70-year-old women has an 83% probability of surviving 5 years without tumor; this decreases to 56% at the age of 80 years, and 38% at 85 years. Old age and polypathia play an important role in the choice of treatment. Of the patients seen by LOCHMÜLLER (1983), 85% were aged over 60 years, and 80% had cardiovascular diseases demanding treatment. In such cases the physician will perform less radical surgery and will not use radiotherapy. During and after treatment, patients with polypathia have a greater chance of developing complications, e.g., wound breakdown, thrombosis, pneumonia.

In contrast, local recurrence is influenced by the following factors only: extent of the disease, biological features of the tumor, and local treatment. In a multivariate analysis, HEAPS et al. (1990) analyzed 135 cases for variables predicting local recurrence. The most significant factor was stage, followed by involvement of margin of resection: local recurrence occurred in the vicinity of the closest surgical margin in all of the cases. Depth of invasion and tumor thickness also reflected the extent of the disease. Factors numbered five to eight were histological ones: growth pattern, vascular invasion, amount of keratin, and mitotic activity. The minor influence of these histological factor is due to the fact that 90% of tumors are well differentiated, and small undifferentiated tumors are rare. A similar analysis performed by MALFETANO et al. (1985) revealed that tumor stage, tumor diameter, and depth of invasion were significantly related to improved survival.

A multivariate analysis of histological features revealed vascular involvement to be the most important factor (GOMEZ RUEDA et al. 1994). The importance of lymph vascular space involvement was stressed by PALADINI (1994), who found a correlation with survival. In addition, extranodular spread of tumor cells in the groin had a negative influence on prognosis.

Tumor markers are of limited value in vulvar cancer. Because most of the lesions are squamous cell carcinomas (SCC), antigen levels were examined by ROSE et al. (1992). In primary disease only 15% of the women showed elevated SCC antigen levels. In positive cases a decrease was seen after effective therapy. Local recurrence was associated with a very slight increase in SCC antigen levels in about half of the cases. A marked increase was seen in one case of distant metastasis.

5.6 General Management

Surgery and radiotherapy are the main therapeutic approaches for the management of vulvar cancer. Systemic chemotherapy has never played a major role in the primary treatment of this disease. Radical vulvectomy with bilateral lymphadenectomy was established as the major treatment approach for resectable vulvar cancer for many decades. Some centers, however, preferred other modalities:

- Primary irradiation (FRISCHBIER et a. 1985)
- Electroresection of the vulva and radiotherapy of the groin (LOCHMÜLLER 1986; Table 5.6)
- Vulvar electroresection, coagulation, and groin radiotherapy (KUCERA and WEGHAUPT 1988)
- Less radical surgery in early stages (HACKER and VAN DER VELDEN 1993)

Experience with these approaches is discussed later in separate sections. Modern therapeutic concepts demand a treatment optimized for individual patients. The choice of treatment has to take several aims into account:

1. To achieve
   a) Local control
   b) Regional control
   c) Systemic control
2. To minimize posttherapeutic complications
3. To optimize quality of life

Local control can be achieved by surgery and/or radiotherapy. There is a trend to extend surgery to elderly women and those with polypathia because perioperative management has been improved in recent decades. However, radical surgery is a mutilating procedure, and a high rate of posttherapeutic complications has to be tolerated (CAVANAGH et al.

1990; KNAPSTEIN et al. 1991). The risk of wound breakdown are lowered by electroresection of the vulva (KUCERA and WEGHAUPT 1988; LOCHMÜLLER 1986) or application of musculocutaneous flaps (KNAPSTEIN et al. 1991). As an alternative to the en bloc dissection, a separate groin incision can be performed to reduce postoperative morbidity (HACKER et al. 1981). A reduction of local control caused by the skin bridge left between the vulva and the groin has not been ruled out, however. Radical surgery is limited by the general condition of elderly patients and by advanced T-stages (>T2). There is a trend to reduce operative radicality (RUTLEDGE et al. 1991; DISAIA 1991; MALFETANO et al. 1985; BURRELL 1988; DISAIA et al. 1979), made possible by the detection of a greater number of cases at the early stage. In early cases, vulvar surgery can be restricted to hemivulvectomy or wide excision, thereby reducing disfiguration. Unfortunately, only a few cases are diagnosed early enough for limited surgery.

Primary radiotherapy of the vulva is not limited by age and T-stage. The outer female genitalia can fully be conserved. A disadvantage is moist desquamation, which demands intensive care for many weeks during and after irradiation. Another disadvantage is a certain number of vulvar indurations as a late effect of irradiation. A combination of wide excision and irradiation with limited doses may achieve good control and a good cosmetic result, but data about this strategy are not available.

Regional control can be achieved by groin lymph node dissection or radiotherapy. Surgery has the advantage of histologically confirmed nodal staging. In cases of extranodal infiltration and involvement of large arteries and veins, surgery cannot prevent recurrence. On the other hand, groin node dissection in stage I vulvar cancer with a minimal depth of invasion is under much debate. In laterally sited carcinoma of stage I, contralateral lymph node metastasis is extremely rare. In well-lateralized lesions without ipsilateral groin metastasis, the probability of contralateral node involvement is less than 1% (HACKER 1991). In spite of this, bilateral groin dissection is recommended because a contralateral groin recurrence is fatal in a curable carcinoma. Unilateral groin dissection should be restricted to controlled studies.

Radiotherapy of the groin is well tolerated even in bad general conditions. Effectiveness of irradiation is limited in cases of large lymph node metastases and radioresistant tumors.

Systemic disease is very rare in vulvar cancer, and one should rule out a different tumor type, e.g., amelanotic melanoma. Chemotherapy is of very limited effect in the presence of distant metastasis. Application of bleomycin and platinum derivatives is further limited by the general condition of elderly patients with vulvar cancer.

In FIGO stage III, different criteria govern the choice of therapy. In cases of unilateral lymph node involvement, radical vulvectomy with bilateral groin dissection is recommended. The distal urethra can be resected without loss of continence. However, most of these patients are not suitable for extended radical surgery. On the other hand, radiation therapy can achieve 5-year survival rates of 39% in stage III vulvar cancer (SCHREER et al. 1991).

In stage IV patients the probability of 5-year survival is 11% only (PETTERSSON 1991). A complete resection of the tumor requires extended radical procedures which most patients who are elderly and suffer from polypathia will not tolerate. Even in incurable patients, radiotherapy of the local process is indicated for palliation to improve the quality of life and avoid social isolation caused by a necrotized tumor with an intolerable smell.

5.7 Radical Surgery in Primary and Recurrent Cancer

W. WEIKEL and P.G. KNAPSTEIN

5.7.1 Introduction

The epidemiology of vulvar carcinoma casts light on several important factors that need to be taken into account when devising an operative therapy for this disease: While, among genital carcinomas, the incidence has remained constant at 4%, the proportion of premenopausal patients affected by early invasive carcinomas or VIN is rising. This can be attributed, on the one hand, to a higher incidence of viral diseases (GROSS 1986) and, on the other hand, to the greater attention paid to this potential tumor site during routine preventive examinations.

For such patients, the current surgical approach is to achieve the maximum possible retention of the affected organ and its functions, not least because of psycho-oncological considerations based on an integral, holistic view of the clinical picture presented by a patient (DISAIA et al. 1979; IVERSEN et al. 1981; HACKER et al. 1984a). As classical radical vulvar operations result in massive functional loss, more restricted operative procedures (wide local excision, partial vulvectomy) are now employed when possible. Additionally, when the disease indications necessitate extensive operative intervention, it is increasingly common for plastic/reconstructive surgery to be performed. However, the choice of a less radical operative approach must be based on the precise delineation of patients according to known risk factors.

Alongside such cases, there still remains the clinical picture of a tumor at an advanced stage of development, this being encountered primarily among older women. In this situation, radical vulvectomy continues to be the accepted approach (Cavanagh et al. 1990), although the problem of internal polypathia often raises the question of the feasibility of an operative intervention. In such cases of advanced disease, operability can also be improved by the application of plastic/reconstructive surgical measures as well as recent developments in perioperative management. The same applies to relapse surgery, which, as a result, is performed more frequently nowadays, in some cases even on the basis of palliative indications.

5.7.2 Risk Factors

In the assessment of the risks presented by a vulvar carcinoma, the most important data in the clinical examination are those relating to the topography of the tumor.

The required morphological data comprise the following:

1. Precise ascertainment of the tumor size, particularly the depth of invasion
2. Histological grading of the tumor, in which both the invasion pattern and the lymphocytic demarcation are taken into account or are evaluated separately
3. Information relating to any invasion of lymphatic or blood vessels
4. Assessment of the region surrounding the tumor with respect to VIN or primary multicentricity

5.7.3 Microcarcinoma/Stage I Cancer

Franklin and Rutledge (1971) first defined an early invasive vulvar carcinoma as one having a diameter of less than 2 cm and a depth of invasion of no more than 5 mm. More recently, the more stringent definition devised by the ISSVD has suggested that cases with the same diameter (i.e., <2 cm) and a depth of invasion not exceeding 1 mm should be classified as being at stage Ia (Kneale 1984).

5.7.4 Surgical Techniques for Primary Cancer

5.7.4.1 Wide Local Excision

Wide local excision represents the least extensive operative intervention in the vulva; to guard against recurrence, tissue located 2 cm to the side of the affected site and to a depth of 1 cm should be regarded as the minimum excision zone.

5.7.4.2 Modified Radical (Partial) Vulvectomy

Various operative procedures are distinguished on the basis of topographical considerations (Burrell et al. 1988):

1. Anterior bilateral modified radical vulvectomy (resection of the clitoris and preservation of the posterior commissure)
2. Posterior bilateral modified radical vulvectomy (preservation of the clitoris and resection of the posterior commissure)
3. Lateral or hemivulvectomy (with preservation of the clitoris)
4. Medial bilateral modified radical vulvectomy or central vulvectomy (preservation of a large part of the labia majora, but resection of the clitoris)

For all such excisions, the depth of the level of excision extends as far as the fascia of the urogenital diaphragm, which is co-planar with the fascia lata and the fascia localized over the pubic symphysis (Hacker 1991).

5.7.4.3 Simple or Skinning Vulvectomy

Simple or skinning vulvectomy involves complete peritomy of the vulva, with only the skin and the adjoining subcutaneous adipose tissue being removed. In general, the indications for this operation are rarely encountered, as it fails to provide the depth of intervention necessary to guard against recurrence in the case of an invasive carcinoma. In the event of preinvasive alterations, other methods (e.g., laser vaporization) offering markedly better cosmetic results are now available (Bornstein and Kaufmann 1988).

5.7.4.4
Radical Vulvectomy

After the publication of the studies of Taussig (1940) and Way (1960), radical vulvectomy came to be regarded as the standard surgical therapy for patients with vulvar carcinoma. Nowadays, it is still the therapy of choice for most T2 lesions. For T3 tumors, this operation can be extended, according to the involvement of the urethra, vagina, perineum, or anus. When the urethra is affected, it is possible to perform a resection as far as the lower half (Monaghan 1991). Depending on the degree of involvement, invasion of the anus should lead one to consider an anovulvectomy or a posterior exenteration (Grimshaw et al. 1991).

Basically, radical operative procedures for the vulva can be performed using two different types of incision:

1. The "butterfly" (or trapezoid) incision (Fig. 5.1) involving the removal of the inguinal lymph nodes and the vulva en bloc, with the incision starting at the superior iliac crest and extending to a midpoint far down the symphysis pubis; this is followed by an incision from the anterior superior iliac spine extending in a curve toward the groin fold to a point 4 cm below the pubic tubercle. The peritomy around the vulva takes an elliptical form, extending as far as the perineum (Monaghan 1991). The level of resection extends to the depth of the fascia. Using this excision shape, there is substantial skin loss, especially over the symphysis, so that it is usually impossible to achieve a tension-free primary wound closure.
2. Separate incisions for groin node dissection and radical vulvectomy (three-in-one or triple incision) (Fig. 5.2). In this procedure, the skin of the inguinal region and mons pubis is preserved. The peritomy of the vulva begins on the mons pubis.

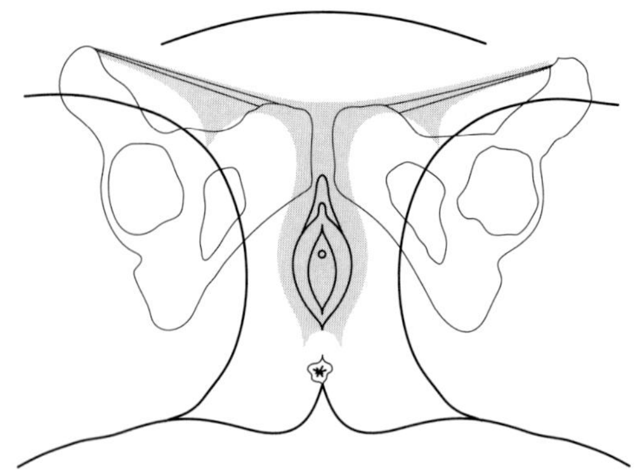

Fig. 5.1. En bloc or butterfly radical vulvectomy

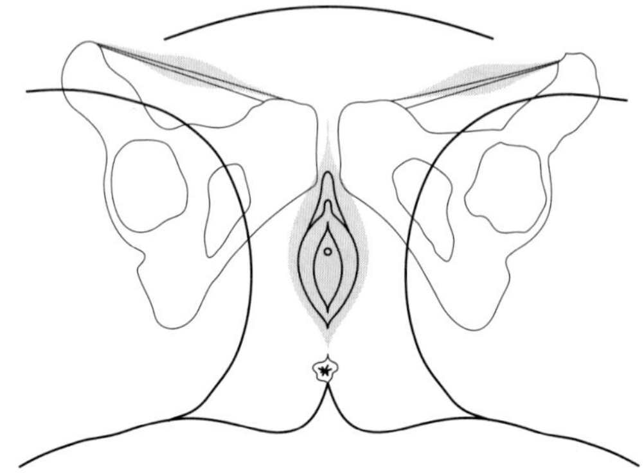

Fig. 5.2. Radical vulvectomy using the three-in-one technique

5.7.4.5
Groin Dissection

Only in 50%–75% of cases does the clinical assessment of the node status of a vulvar carcinoma prove to be accurate (Homesley et al. 1986; Podratz et al. 1982). The histopathological features of a tumor would appear to represent important indicators of lymph node metastasis. In a study of microinvasive carcinomas (tumor thickness, <5 mm) performed by the Gynecologic Oncology Group (GOG), Sedlis et al. (1987) found that the factors tumor thickness, tumor grading, lymphangiosis, clinical assessment of the inguinal region, and tumor localization were correlated with the probability of metastatic spread. In this large patient group ($n = 272$), it is especially worthy of note that 20% of the early invasive tumors exhibited lymph node involvement. For stage I tumors with favorable supplementary criteria, the recommended approach is to reduce the radicality of the lymphadenectomy by means of semilateral, surface removal (Di Re et al. 1991).

The GOG study of more advanced tumors (Homesley et al. 1993) – exhibiting metastasis in

41% of all cases – was able to confirm the relevance of all of the above-mentioned criteria with the exception of tumor localization, while additionally showing that increased patient age was correlated with the likelihood of metastatic spread.

Opinions differ with respect to the lymphatic drainage resulting from a tumor localized in the clitoris region. PLENTL and FRIEDMAN (1971) described a direct route of lymphatic drainage into the iliac lymph nodes, whereas more recent studies have been unable to confirm this finding (IVERSEN and AAS 1983). The latest GOG investigation has also demonstrated that a medial tumor site can no longer be regarded as a significant factor in the prognosis of vulvar carcinomas (HOMESLEY et al. 1993).

In the case of an advanced primary tumor, the deep inguinofemoral group of lymph nodes (CLOQUET/ROSENMÜLLER) located below the fascia lata should be removed. Whereas a frequently applied method is to split the fascia (SCHMIDT-MATTHIESEN and MICHEL 1991), preliminary reports have described a modification that preserves the fascia (MICHELETTI et al. 1990). There is general agreement that, whenever possible, the internal saphenous vein should be preserved.

An iliac lymphadenectomy would appear to be justified only in the event of involvement of the inguinal lymph nodes (FRANKLIN and RUTLEDGE 1971; CURRY et al. 1980); this can be performed extraperitoneally after transection of the inguinal ligament. However, some studies have indicated that radiotherapy of the iliac lymph nodes following radical vulvectomy and inguinal lymphadenectomy produces more favorable results than the removal of these lymph nodes (HOMESLEY et al. 1986). Studies of large patient groups have shown that lymphatic edema is a complication in 9% of patients who have undergone an inguinal lymphadenectomy (CAVANAGH et al. 1990).

5.7.4.6
Pelvic Exenteration

The surgical treatment of advanced tumors exhibiting involvement of the intestinal or bladder mucosa (T4) requires a pelvic exenteration in addition to radical vulvectomy. A distinction is made between, on the one hand, complete exenteration and, on the other hand, an anterior exenteration with cystectomy or a posterior exenteration including the removal of the anus and a part of the sigmoid colon. In addition, this operation involves the removal of the inner genitalia. To allow defecation, it is necessary to perform a colostomy, while the maintenance of urinary function requires either a urinary conduit or a continent urinary pouch (THUROFF et al. 1986). To cover the pelvic floor and the extensive skin defects, it is necessary to apply plastic surgery procedures involving appropriate skin flap grafting.

These operations require a thorough preoperative examination of a patient with respect to distant metastasis and involve difficult and complicated perioperative management such as can only be provided in specialized clinics. Studies on large patient groups have indicated a survival rate of more than 40% over a long observation period (CAVANAGH and SHEPHERD 1982; WEIKEL et al. 1991). However, owing to the considerable efforts involved in an operation of such scope, trials of primary radiotherapy or combined surgery and radiotherapy have been conducted (BORONOW 1982).

5.7.5
Surgical Techniques for Recurrent Disease

Studies of vulvar carcinomas over a long follow-up period have revealed a relapse rate (or tumor persistence) of 26% (PODRATZ et al. 1982), with the incidence of local recurrence (18%) being three times higher than that of a relapse at all other localizations (groin, pelvis, distant metastasis).

5.7.5.1
Local Recurrence

In the event of local recurrence, the operative therapy corresponds to that used to deal with a primary tumor; thus, depending on the tumor spread, it can range from a local excision in sano to complete pelvic exenteration. When there is a relapse, a difference as compared to primary therapy is that there is frequently a lack of healthy tissue to provide plastic covering of resulting skin defects: consequently, in cases of major relapses plastic surgery grafting is necessary.

5.7.5.2
Regional (Groin/Pelvis) Recurrence

Relapses in the groin are often very complicated from the point of view of surgery and are not infrequently linked with tumor generalization. In such cases, lobar grafting is an essential component of the surgical therapy. In a far from insignificant number of cases, recurrence in the pelvis can be treated by exenteration combined with radiotherapy (Hockel and Knapstein 1992). Should a supralevatorial exenteration be under consideration, the possibility of reconstructing the vagina also needs to be given due attention.

5.7.5.3 Reconstructive Procedures

One of the principal difficulties arising from radical operations on the vulva is the achievement of a tension-free closure of the wound. This problem is further exacerbated in the event of an underlying internal illness (such as arteriosclerosis or diabetes) or, in recurrent tumors, of previous radiotherapy, so that disorders of the wound-healing process have been found in up to 50% of cases in some patient groups. Surgical reconstruction involving the introduction of healthy tissue into the site of the defect offers the best and, in a great many cases, the only viable solution to such wound-healing problems. The principles underlying such operations are shown in Figs. 5.3–5.8, while the technical details can be found in a recent publication by Knapstein and co-workers (Knapstein et al. 1991).

When it is desirable to cover large skin defects over the entire vulva or to create a new perineum or a neovagina after exenteration, a myocutaneous graft may be indicated. This method utilizes not only skin and subcutaneous adipose tissue but also the underlying muscle and its substantial blood supply. Although several techniques employing various muscle groups have been devised, our experience indicates that the three myocutaneous grafts discussed below are the most suitable for vulvar surgery.

Musculus Gluteus Maximus Graft. The gluteus maximus graft (Figs. 5.3, 5.4) can be used as a skin-island flap or as a transposition flap, although it should be pointed out that the former has proved to be the safer method with respect to minimizing partial necrosis. This procedure is primarily used to cover defects in the region of the posterior vulva, the perineum, or the sacrum.

Musculus Rectus Abdominis Graft. The rectus abdominis island graft (Figs. 5.5, 5.6) is mainly employed to cover defects in the anterior vulva and

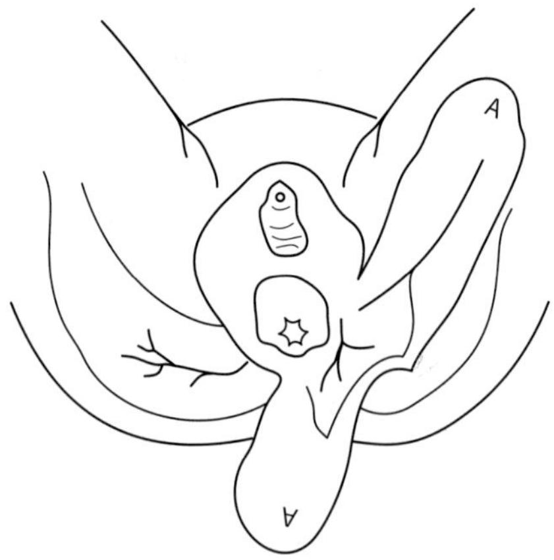

Fig. 5.3. Musculus gluteus maximus graft: The skin flap on the left side is circumcised and mobilized from the underlying tissue. The supplying inferior gluteal artery is identified. The letter *A* indicates the tip of the flap and the donor site

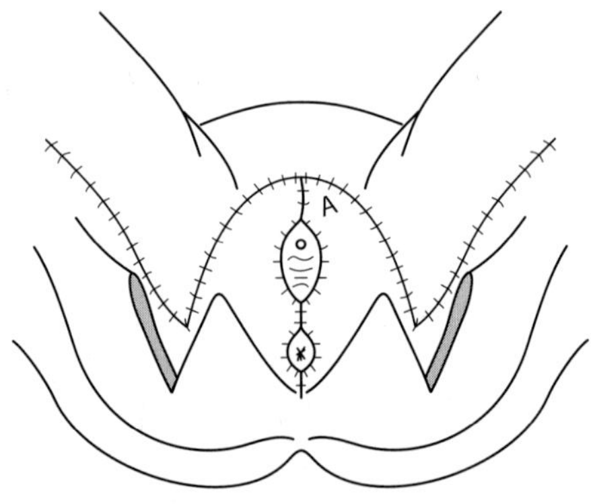

Fig. 5.4. Musculus gluteus maximus graft: Bilateral myocutaneous grafts are united and the skin edges are approximated to the skin of the mons pubis and the remaining vagina. The donor sites can be closed primarily. The letter *A* indicates the tip of the flap

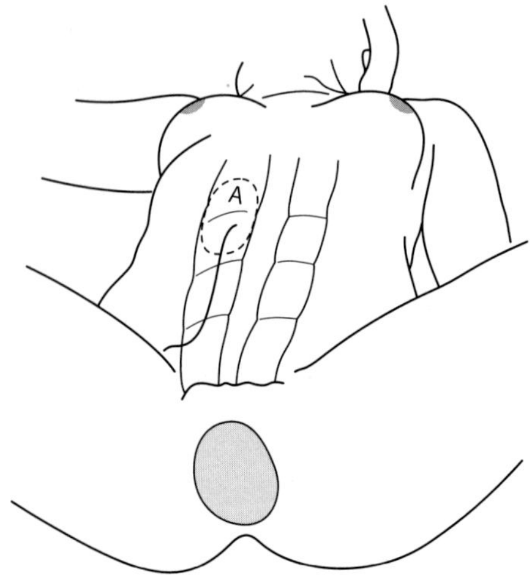

Fig. 5.5. Musculus rectus abdominis graft: An island flap from the right muscle supported by the epigastric artery is demonstrated

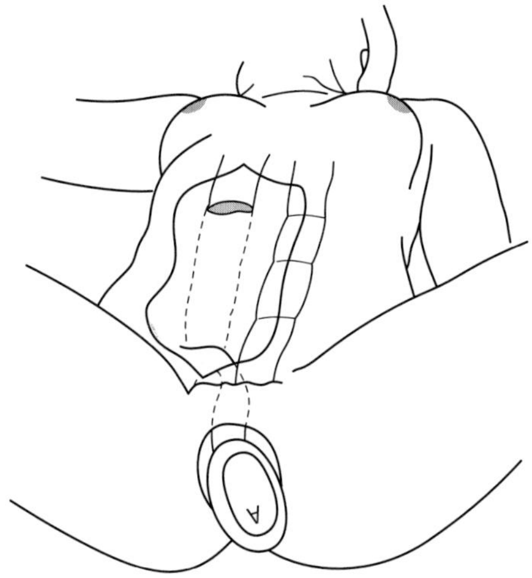

Fig. 5.6. Musculus rectus abdominis graft: The mobilized graft is brought through a subcutaneous tunnel to cover the defect

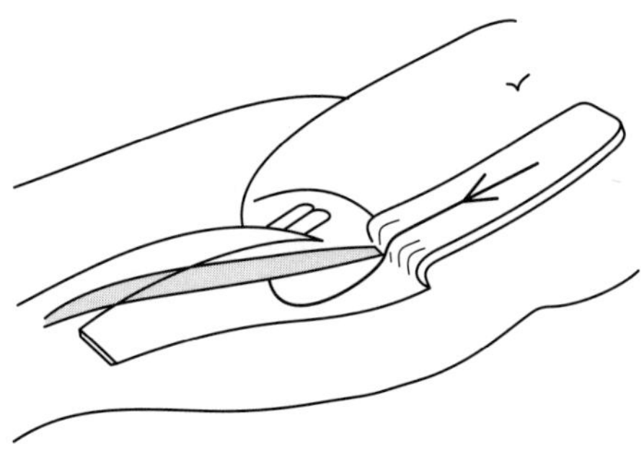

Fig. 5.7. Musculus tensor fasciae latae graft: The circumcised and elevated skin flap remains adjacent to the mobilized fascia lata with its blood support from the lateral femoral circumflex artery

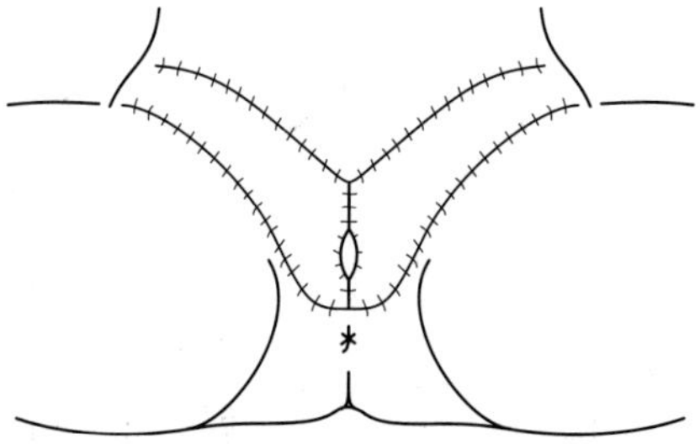

Fig. 5.8. Musculus tensor fasciae latae graft: In order to reconstruct the mons pubis and the introitus of the vagina, both flaps are sutured medially

groin regions; however, without skin, it can be used for intra-abdominal grafting, e.g., for the isolation of radiation tubes. One of the advantages of such grafts is that they frequently remain intact for relapse therapy when radiotherapy has been performed previously.

Musculus Tensor Fasciae Latae Graft. The indication for the use of a tensor fasciae latae graft (Figs. 5.7, 5.8) mainly arises from the need to cover defects in the groin region and vulva resulting from a radical operation on the vulva producing predominantly anterior defects.

5.8 Vulvectomy and Postoperative Irradiation

Some centers perform radical vulvectomy with bilateral inguinal node removal and select certain patients for postoperative irradiation. In Beijing in China, Zhang (1992) treated 76 women with advanced vulvar carcinomas of stages III and IV. A combination of radiotherapy with radical vulvectomy and inguinal lymphadenectomy gave the best results. A 5-year survival rate of 47% in stage III and 33% in stage IV cases was reported.

While radical vulvectomy with bilateral inguinal node removal itself is a mutilating and poorly tolerated procedure, the combination with extensive radiotherapy cannot be employed as a routine procedure. In some advanced cases this combination may be the only chance of achieving local control; a greater number of patients, however, do not require extensive radiotherapy. Histological workup of the vulvar resection should determine the site of the closest margin (Heaps et al. 1990): in most cases, local recurrence takes place at the site of the closest margin. Other cases may require radiation therapy of certain nodes only. The GOG 37 study tested the value of radiotherapy in cases with histologically proven groin node metastasis. On a random basis, patients received radiotherapy of the pelvis or a pelvic lymph node dissection. There was a clear advantage of radiotherapy, which increased with the number of involved nodes and the presence of palpable lymph node metastases (see Sect. 5.16).

Elderly patients with a poor general condition may not be suitable for radical surgery. Restriction of surgery to vulvectomy can reduce the duration of surgery. Irradiation of the groin nodes leads to satisfactory locoregional control.

5.9 Electroresection and Postoperative Irradiation (Munich Method)

Experiences with postoperative irradiation of the vulva were reported by LOCHMÜLLER (1986) from Munich. The surgical treatment employed was electroresection of the vulva including the introitus vaginae and clitoris. No suturing of the resection field was performed. Radiotherapy was started before the resection area had been closed, on the 4th to 5th postoperative day. In this way, radiation-induced desquamation could be avoided. Radiotherapy of the resection area was performed with 10-MeV electrons to a total dose of 40 Gy. Inguinal and lower iliac nodes were irradiated with telecobalt using a total dose of 40 Gy at the level of the nodes. From 1968 to 1978, 225 women were admitted to the First Department of Gynecology of the University Hospital in Munich, 115 of whom had a follow-up of more than 5 years. The stage distribution (Table 5.6). shows that more than half of the women had advanced (stage III and IV) tumors. Seventy-three percent of the patients with stage I disease survived 5 years, as did 55% with stage II, 29% with stage III, and 18% with stage IV (Table 5.6). Radical surgery yields better results in early stages; for advanced cases, however, electroresection and radiotherapy show good results.

Table 5.6. Results of electroresection and radiotherapy (Munich Method, LOCHMÜLLER 1983)

Stage	No.	5-year crude survival	
		n	%
I	26	19	73
II	29	16	55
III	38	11	29
IV	22	4	18

5.10 Electroresection, Coagulation, and Groin Radiotherapy (Viennese Method)

K. KUCERA

5.10.1 Introduction

In the early part of this century, inadequate dissection of the primary tumor and regional lymph nodes in patients with cancer of the vulva resulted in a 5-year survival rate of only 25%. After the middle of the century en bloc radical vulvectomy with bilateral groin dissection was the treatment of choice for all patients with operable vulvar cancer. The more aggressive surgical approach improved survival but postoperative morbidity was high. During the past decade, however, significant changes have occurred in the management of vulvar cancer:

1. Vulvar conservation for patients with small unifocal lesions and an otherwise normal vulva (DISAIA et al. 1979; IVERSEN et al. 1981; HACKER et al. 1983, 1984b; BURKE et al. 1990)
2. Elimination of routine inguinal lymphadenectomy (GREEN 1978; BENEDET et al. 1979; CURRY et al. 1980; HACKER et al. 1984b; CAVANAGH et al. 1986)
3. Omission of groin dissection for patients with stage I tumors and less than 1 mm of stromal invasion (IVERSEN et al. 1981; HACKER et al. 1983)
4. Omission of contralateral groin dissection in patients with lateral lesions and negative ipsilateral nodes (HACKER et al. 1983; FIGGE et al. 1985)
5. Use of separate incisions for groin dissections (HACKER et al. 1981)
6. Use of preoperative radiation therapy to obviate the need for exenteration in patients with advanced disease (BORONOW 1973, 1982; HACKER et al. 1984a)
7. Use of postoperative irradiation to decrease the incidence of groin recurrence in patients with multiple positive groin nodes (HOMESLEY et al. 1986).

For more than 40 years, we have adopted in Vienna a standard treatment for vulvar cancer consisting of electrosurgical vulvectomy with groin radiotherapy as a possible alternative to groin dissection. Our experience with this unchanged therapeutic method over four decades probably gives us one of the largest volumes of material covering a uniform treatment of carcinoma of the vulva. The Viennese management of vulvar cancer is of increasing interest because of a significant trend towards more conservative treatment methods. Modern treatment for vulvar cancer requires careful consideration of the most appropriate surgical procedure for the vulva and the groin and the appropriate integration of surgery and radiation therapy.

5.10.2
Methods

5.10.2.1
Electrosurgical Vulvectomy

The operation is carried out under general anesthesia. The instrument used is a flat electrode (hot knife) shaped like a ski which can cut like a scalpel and also coagulate. An incision is made in a curving line beginning 4 cm above the clitoris on the mons veneris and moving laterally to the labiocrural folds and to the anal region. The internal incision proceeds from the symphysis via the clitoris to a point close to the uretra, passes this laterally, and finally follows the border of the hymen. The depth of the incision is chosen so that the suprapubic and sublabial fatty tissue is removed to a minimal depth of 2 cm in the healthy tissue. Special care must be taken that the hot knife is moved at a suitably slow rate so that the blood vessels can be coagulated simultaneously with the incision. The entire vulva, including the tumor, is removed without any loss of blood and within a few minutes. After electroresection the remaining fatty tissue, which has already been coagulated superficially, is again coagulated with the hot knife, so that finally the entire base of the vulva is covered with a dark crust. Suturing or ligature of individual vessels is as a rule not necessary and all hemostasis is achieved by electrocoagulation.

After 4 weeks the open coagulation wound is completely cleaned and shows superficial granulation. Between 6 and 8 weeks after surgery the wound is covered by a new epidermis. This seems to be a long recuperation time but the patient can leave the hospital 3 weeks after the operation. The cosmetic effect is usually excellent and chronic edema of the lower extremities is very rare (the incidence is less than 4% after groin irradiation). The duration of the operation is only 10–20 min, and appropriate pre- and postoperative internal medical treatment leads to very good tolerance.

5.10.2.2
Groin Radiotherapy

The reason for the low primary mortality (in the last 10 years, zero) and the good tolerance of our method is that general operative removal of inguinal lymph nodes is not carried out. These nodes are definitively irradiated, radiotherapy being commenced on day 12 after surgery. A surface dose of 60 Gy is applied to the inguinal fields on both sides in an area of 6 × 16 cm, resulting in a 45 Gy focal lymph node dose at depth. Both areas are irradiated with 3 Gy so that the total dose is achieved in 20 days. The irradiated inguinal fields include not only the lymph nodes with an appropriate safety margin but also the entire area of skin up to the limit of the vulvar resection.

It is to be expressly pointed out that in our approach the radiation treatment is exclusively confined to the inguinal fields and that the tumor field proper, the vulva, does not receive any supplementary irradiation.

In the years until 1972 we used high voltage x-rays; later cobalt-60 irradiation was performed.

5.10.3
Results of Treatment

In the years 1952–1988 we employed electrosurgical vulvectomy with groin radiotherapy in a total of 837 patients with vulvar cancer. Mean age at diagnosis was 69.9 years. Follow-up information was available for all but five patients (0.6%). Ninety patients have died from causes other than vulvar cancer. The remaining 739 patients have a minimum postoperative follow-up of 5 years.

The uncorrected 5-year survival of the 837 patients with squamous vulvar cancer was 60.6% (507/837). The corrected 5-year figures (excluding deaths from causes other than vulvar cancer and those lost to follow-up) were as follows: In FIGO stage I, 183 (85.5%) out of 214 patients survived 5 years; in stage II the figure was 134 (77.9%) out of 172, in stage III, 177 (65.3%) out of 271, and in stage IV, 13 (15.3%) out of 85. Of this total of 742 patients with vulvar cancer, 507 (68.3%) survived more than 5 years after electroresection of the vulva and groin radiotherapy (Table 5.7).

Table 5.7. Carcinoma of the vulva (1952–1988): results of vulvar electroresection and groin radiotherapy (Viennese management)

FIGO stage	No.	5-year survival	
		n	%
I	214	183	85.5
II	172	134	77.9
III	271	177	65.3
IV	85	13	15.3
Total	742	507	68.3

5.10.4 Discussion

It appears to be difficult to compare results in cases of vulvar carcinoma treated according to various therapeutic measures, as results depend primarily on the extent of the cancer and its individual characteristics and only secondarily on the type of therapy. The achievements of conventional radical vulvectomy and bilateral inguinal node dissection have been extensively documented in the literature (Morley 1976; Iversen et al. 1981; Hacker et al. 1981; Podratz et al. 1982; Homesley et al. 1993). The overall 5-year survival rate following this procedure for vulvar cancer is approximately 65% (Thomas et al. 1991).

Survival and cure rates for patients with negative nodes have been excellent, ranging from 70% to 90%. The outcome for those with involved nodes is substantially worse, with 5-year survival rates ranging from 25% to 41% (Morley 1976; Hacker et al. 1981, 1983; Podratz et al. 1982). Survival of patients with involved pelvic nodes is extremely rare (Podratz et al. 1982). With electroresection of the vulva and groin radiotherapy we were able to cure 507 (68.3%) out of 742 patients with invasive squamous cell carcinoma of the vulva. It is beyond any doubt that our long-established method of treatment of vulvar cancer achieves results as good as those of other methods.

Morbidity rates following conventional radical vulvectomy and bilateral inguinal node dissection are substantial. The most commonly reported complication is that of wound breakdown, which occurs in up to 85% of patients (Podratz et al. 1982); 30%–70% of patients have chronic edema of the legs, and genital prolapse and vaginal stricture occur in 15%–20% of patients (Hacker et al. 1981; Podratz et al. 1982). All these complications are extremely rare in patients treated with electrosurgical vulvectomy and groin radiotherapy.

In a more detailed study we were able to show that 43% of the patients with clinical involvement of the inguinal nodes were successfully treated by groin radiotherapy (Kucera and Weghaupt 1988). The breakdown of clinical stage III cases according to the TNM system showed a 5-year survival of 48% although lymph nodes were palpable in 87% of these cases.

We believe in groin irradiation as an alternative to groin dissection, though we would prefer groin dissection on principle if it could be proved that considerably more than 50% of the patients with cancerous infiltration of the inguinal lymph nodes could thereby be cured. If that were the case, it would seem to us justifiable to accept the substantially higher rate of complications encountered when groin dissection is performed.

The main objection that can be raised against our method is that histological lymph node diagnosis is not available. However, to date it has not been proved beyond doubt whether the significance of lymphadenectomy is diagnostic or therapeutic.

Leg edema remains one of the long-term problems with the surgical treatment of inguinal lymph nodes. A possible alternative to groin dissection for patients with vulvar cancer is groin irradiation. Although the GOG prematurely closed the study in which patients with N0 or N1 groin nodes were randomized between groin dissection and groin radiotherapy because of an increased recurrence rate in the irradiated nodes, the GOG reported the results of another study that randomized patients with positive groin nodes between ipsilateral pelvic node dissection and bilateral groin and pelvic irradiation (Homesley et al. 1993). There was a significant survival advantage at 2 years (68% vs 54%) for the group receiving radiation therapy, as a result of a significantly decreased incidence of groin recurrence in the irradiated group (5% vs 24%).

Our long-established method is in agreement with the changing concepts in the management of vulvar cancer, and alternatives to routine groin node dissection should continue to be studied.

5.11 Primary Irradiation

I. Schreer

5.11.1 Introduction

In the gynecological literature, radiation therapy of carcinoma of the vulva is declared to be worthless. Since most skin cancers can be treated with radiation therapy very successfully, it is hard to understand why carcinoma of the vulva is said to be radioresistant. To sterilize a squamous cell carcinoma it is necessary to apply sufficient dose. Poor results obtained by Scandinavian centers (Frankendahl 1972; Bäckström 1972; Helgason et al. 1972; Jeppesen et al. 1972; Simonsen 1984) were probably derived from orthovoltage therapy and low doses. Since the introduction of megavoltage therapy, many reports with good results from small numbers of patients with advanced vulvar cancers have been published (Hacker et al. 1984; Jafari and Magalotti 1981; Pirtoli and Rottoli 1982; Perez et al. 1993). Furthermore, modern radiotherapy is able to cure lymph node metastases of the head and neck as well as breast cancer, so locoregional control of vulvar cancer should be a resolvable problem.

As an argument against radiotherapy, a high rate of severe complications is mentioned. The vulva is a radiosensitive organ, partly due to the great number of blood vessels. Thus, the radiation doses that are well tolerated are rather low. Therefore, many therapists think that it is impossible to apply radiation doses large enough to destroy a tumor.

In our experience moist desquamation is not avoidable during therapy, but with good care it is a transient complaint. Severe late complications are seldom, and the rate is comparable with that following radical surgery. Radical surgery in the treatment of carcinoma of the vulva is a very mutilating procedure. Labia majora and minora are removed. Lymph node resection of the groin impairs the drainage of the legs. Other disadvantages that must be considered are large scars in the lower abdomen or myocutaneous flaps from the upper leg, which have to be tolerated. In contrast, radiation therapy entails conservation of the outer female genitalia.

Even in centers which prefer radical vulvectomy, there will be a lot of women who cannot be treated surgically. Many patients have disease incompatible with an operation lasting several hours. Some tumors may not be resectable because they are fixed to the pubic bone. Furthermore, the number of patients who will not tolerate the removal of their entire external genitalia will increase; an analogous development led to the breast-conserving concept in breast cancer.

Early results on definite radiation of vulvar carcinoma using electrons to irradiate vulvar carcinoma were reported by Kepp et al. (1951). This paper describes the first cures of invasive vulvar carcinoma using fast electrons of 4 MeV. A reprint of the illustration published by Kepp et al. (Fig. 5.9) shows a tumor of the right labia minora before and after therapy with a single dose of 2000 r at the surface. At the Women's Hospital of the University of Göttingen from 1963 to 1967, Frischkorn (1969) treated 137 patients with high-energy electrons. The 5-year survival rate of the patients was 32%.

Similar poor results were obtained by Scandinavian centers (Frankendahl et al. 1973; Helgason et al. 1972; Jeppesen et al. 1972; Simonsen 1984). Radiation was performed with different equipment (orthovoltage and megavoltage) and low doses. Their conclusion that radiation is worthless was based upon inadequate methods.

In Stockholm, Pirtoli and Rottoli (1982) treated 19 patients with vulvar cancer using electrons. The dose was 45–58 Gy to the primary lesion. Of these women, 42% survived 5 years.

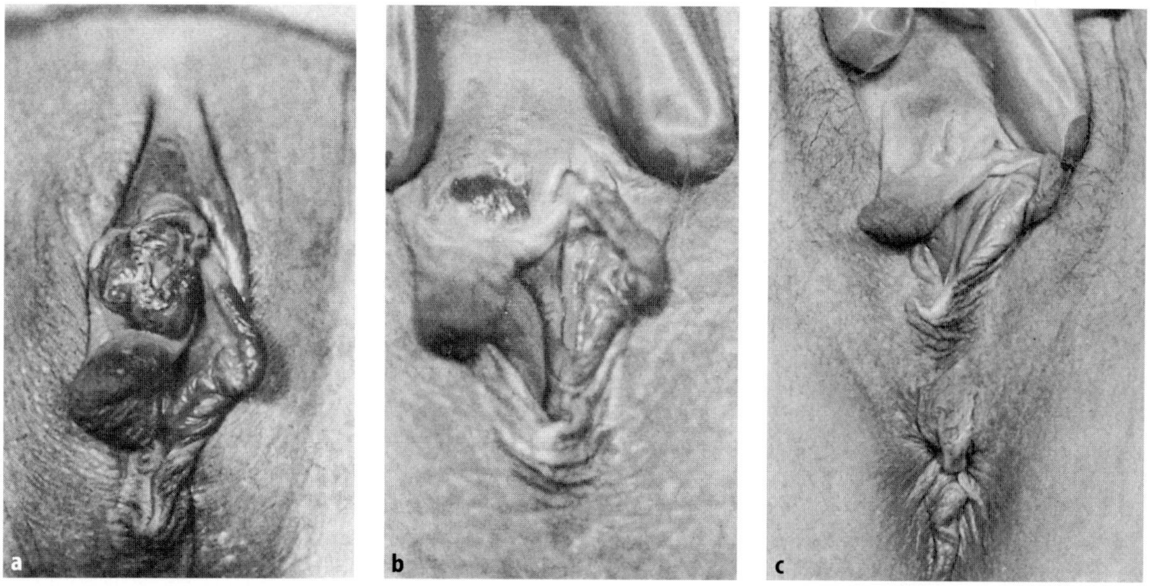

Fig. 5.9 a–c. Illustrations of one case from the first series of cases cured by radiation therapy with electrons. **a** Before irradiation: tumor of the right labia minora. **b** Appearance 44 days after therapy with 2000 r electrons of 4 MeV. **c** Appearance 137 days after primary irradiation. (From Kepp et al. 1951)

5.11.2 Radiation Treatment at the Department of Gynecological Radiology, Women's University Hospital, Hamburg

From 1956 to 1983 the primary therapy of vulvar carcinoma was irradiation. Electron therapy was introduced in the Department of Gynecology at the University of Hamburg by Schubert in 1956 and was continued by Thomsen in 1965 (Frischbier et al. 1985).

Radiation therapy was the primary treatment for all operable and inoperable carcinomas of the vulva. No radical vulvectomy was carried out. Malignancy was ensured by excisional biopsy. Partial or complete simple vulvectomy was performed in 24 patients. In all, 530 patients were treated with the same regimen (Schreer et al. 1991). The whole vulva was irradiated with electrons of 9–18 MeV supplied by an 18-MeV betatron. The energy of the electrons was modified according to tumor size and depth of infiltration. The radiation field included the whole vulva covering at least 2 cm unaffected tissue around the tumor. Care was taken that no gap occurred between the cranial border of the vulvar field and the caudal border of the groin fields. Initially, the vulva was irradiated with single doses of 3 Gy five times a week. Later, the single dose was reduced to 2 Gy in order to reduce late radiation side-effects. Total dose was 45–60 Gy (maximum).

The groin was irradiated with a combination of 18-MeV electrons and telecobalt. This mixture allows the delivery of a sufficient dose to the superficial as well as to the deep femoroinguinal nodes. Initially, the single dose was 3 Gy. Later, the single dose was reduced to 2 Gy five times a week, achieving maximum doses of 50–60 Gy, with 45 Gy at about 3 cm depth. In the presence of palpable, suspicious lymph nodes (N2, N3), lymphography was performed to demonstrate iliac nodes. In the event of suspicious findings in the iliac lymph nodes, radiation was extended to the pelvic wall by application of dorsal fields or rotating fields. A maximum dose of 60 Gy was delivered to suspicious iliac nodes.

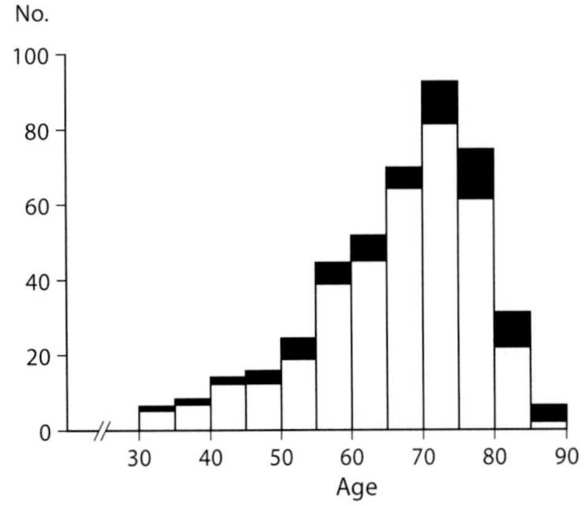

Fig. 5.10. Age distribution of patients treated by radiation. *Black areas* patients treated between 1979 and 1983. Note the increase in mean age by 5 years

Table 5.8. Patient distribution by T stage of squamous carcinoma of the vulva

Stage	No.		
Tx	29		
T1	135	T1 + T2	T1–T4
T2	193	328	417
T3	82	T3 + T4	
T4	7	89	
Total	446		

Radiotherapy of vulvar carcinoma was generally performed under inpatient conditions. During irradiation of the vulva, moist desquamative epidermatitis normally occurs in the fourth week of treatment. To complete the therapy with a sufficient dose, optimal care of the irradiated skin areas is necessary. All irritations of the vulva have to be minimized. Local treatment consists of application of ointment-containing pieces of cloth. Powder was applied onto groin fields.

Of 530 women treated, 513 had invasive squamous carcinoma, eight malignant melanoma, three sarcoma, and six noninvasive neoplasia. In 12 women, treatment was rejected or stopped before reaching 45 Gy because of poor general status. Some 46 patients were lost to follow-up. In 29 patients, the primary was removed elsewhere, so staging was impossible (Tx). The following discussion is restricted to the remaining 446 patients.

The age distribution (Fig. 5.10) demonstrates a predominance in the seventh and eighth decades. The clinical stages are shown in Tables 5.8–5.10. There were 30.3% of patients with stage T1 disease, 43.3% with stage T2, 18.4% with stage T3, and 1.6% with stage T4. The clinical nodal stage was distributed equally: 49.3% of patients had N0 or N1 disease, and 50.7%, N2 or N3 disease. The TNM classification demonstrated a significant dominance of T1 and T2 over T3 and T4 tumors. Most of the patients with T2 disease had lymph node metastases, so they had to be grouped in stage III.

5.11.2.1
Results

The 5-year survival rate was 60% for patients with T1 and 40% for those with T2 disease (Table 5.11). Survival dropped to 30.5% for patients with T3 disease. None of seven women with T4 tumors were cured. Survival also depended on lymph node status (53% of the patients with N0 or N1 disease survived, versus 37.3% with N2 or N3 disease; see Table 5.12). Among patients with T1/2N0/1 disease, 63.1% were alive after 5 years, as were 38.3% of those with T3/4N2/3 disease.

Age is an important factor for the treatment result (Table 5.13). The best results were seen in patients under 60 years of age. With advancing age, mortality increased in patients with stage I and stage II disease as well as in those with stage III and IV disease. Of all patients with squamous carcinoma, 43.8% survived 5 years. A melanoma of the vulva (see Sect. 6.4 in Chap. 6 for more details) was seen in eight patients. Three of eight women with a melanoma were alive after 5 years.

Table 5.9. Patient distribution by N stage of squamous carcinoma of the vulva

	T1, T2	T3, T4	Tx	Total (%)
N0, N1	187	16	17	220 (49.3%)
N2, N3	141	73	12	226 (50.7%)

Table 5.10. Patient distribution by T and N stage

	N0, N1	N2, N3	Nx	Total (%)
Tx	15	12	2	29 (6.5%)
T1	102	33		135 (30.3%)
T2	85	108		193 (43.3%)
T3	16	66		82 (18.4%)
T4	0	7		7 (1.6%)
Total	218	226	2	446

Table 5.11. Survival by T stage

	N0, N1	N2, N3	Total
T1	60.8%	57.6%	60%
T2	47.1%	35.2%	40%
T3	37.5%	28.8%	30.5%
T4			0%

5.11.2.2
Side-effects

Irradiation of the vulva with high-energy electrons has early and late effects. All patients suffer from a moist desquamation during therapy which heals within 2–3 weeks under good nursing care and optimal hygiene of the perineal region. Figure 5.11 shows an 80-year-old women with a carcinoma of the clitoris treated with 55 Gy electrons of 9 MeV (single dose 2.5 Gy) 3 weeks after therapy. Moist desquamation and swelling of the labia are still present. Four months later (Fig. 5.12), pubic hair has regrown and

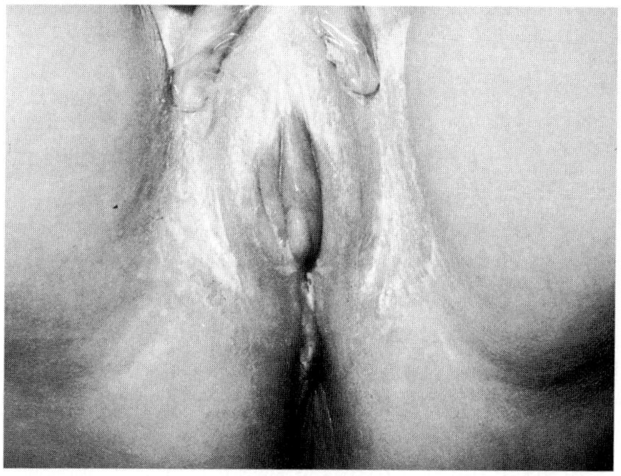

Fig. 5.11. An 80-year-old woman with a carcinoma of the clitoris treated with 55 Gy electrons of 9 MeV (single dose 2.5 Gy) 3 weeks after therapy. Moist desquamation and swelling of the labia are still present

Table 5.12. Survival by N stage

	T1, T2	T3, T4	Total
N0, N1	63.1%	37.5%	53%
N2, N3	46.1%	38.3%	37.3%

Table 5.13. Five-year survival rate in patients with vulvar carcinoma by clinical stage

Age	Stage		Total
	I, II	III, IV	
<39	83.3%	57.0%	69.2%
40–49	84.6%	64.3%	74.1%
50–59	67.7%	63.3%	65.6%
60–69	57.4%	41.1%	49.1%
70–79	37.5%	25.8%	30.2%
80+	7.7%	25.0%	16.0%
Total	52.6%	39.2%	43.8%

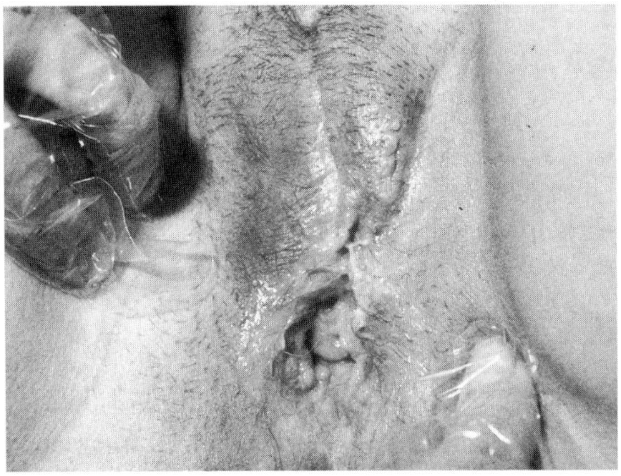

Fig. 5.12. Same patient as in Fig. 5.12, 4 months later. Pubic hair has regrown and the labia have recovered from the radiation damage

the labia have recovered from the radiation damage. Late side-effects are depigmentation, depilation, skin atrophy, and subcutaneous fibrosis.

Severe complications, e.g., ulcer or abscess, were seen in 42 patients (10.9%). Six patients developed radionecrosis of the pubic bone. Two patients suffered stenosis of the urethra. In three women a colpostomy was necessary because of rectal stenosis. Severe complications were more common in patients with stage III and IV disease (12.2%) than in those with stage I and II disease (9.2%).

Some 120 women without recurrence underwent a gynecological examination in our department. Nine presented with severe complications, such as deep ulcers, abscess, necrosis, stenosis, or radionecrosis. In seven of them a biopsy had been carried out to exclude recurrence. Therefore, we conclude that biopsy should be avoided after radiotherapy of the vulva. The follow-up should be done by a physician very familiar with radiation-induced changes of the vulva.

5.11.2.3
Treatment of Recurrences

Many physicians look upon recurrence as a fatal situation. But treatment of recurrences following primary irradiation of vulvar carcinoma is of substantial benefit. In our department 41 women with recurrence of vulvar carcinoma were treated by secondary radical vulvectomy (Frischbier and Wenn 1985). In 20 (48.8%) of these patients, recurrence occurred following a stage III primary. The size of the recurrence was 1–3 cm in 74.7%. Vulvectomy was performed by electroresection. If resection was maintained outside the radiation field, wound healing presented no problem. The survival rate was 36.6% after 3 years and 19.5% after 5 years. Results depended on the size of the recurrence.

5.11.3
Conclusions

Primary irradiation alone is not the first choice in the treatment of vulvar carcinoma. The results of radiation are comparable with radical surgery only in patients with advanced disease. There is an indication for irradiation in local inoperable lesions and patients with a poor general status precluding radical surgery.

If the tumor is fixed to the pubic bone, there is little chance of obtaining regional control by radical surgery. Electroresection with coagulation may cure some cases but runs the risk of osteonecrosis induced by heat and infection.

In cases of urethral involvement a deeper resection is necessary, with the possibility of incontinence. Using radiation treatment, patients remain continent. Shrinkage of the urethra after irradiation may occur in some cases.

Vulvar carcinoma with extensive involvement of the perineum or anus is seldom controlled by radical surgery. Radiation treatment is a good alternative in these patients. It must be said that patients receiving radiotherapy to the anus have complained of problems with defecation during therapy and need more nursing care.

Some patients, especially younger women, refuse the mutilating operation to the outer genitalia, but radiation-induced side-effects will affect the sexual life of these patients as well. A satisfying approach for the treatment of vulvar carcinoma in young patients is still lacking.

5.12
Technique of Radiation Therapy

The first cures of vulvar carcinoma by primary irradiation were made possible by the development of accelerators (Kepp et al. 1951). The technique of vulvar irradiation employed a direct field with an angulation of 50–70°. Electron irradiation had the advantage of a sufficient dose at the surface of the tumor; on the other hand, moist desquamation was induced very early. Radiation of the groin nodes was

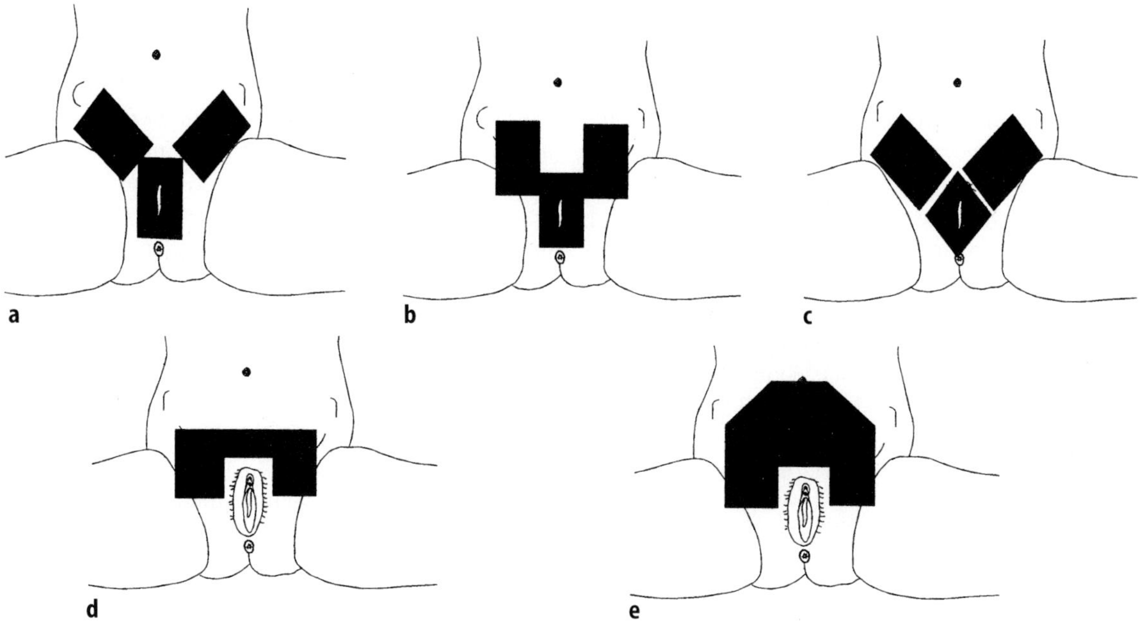

a b c d e

Fig. 5.13 a–e. Technique of vulvar irradiation. **a** Hamburg I: direct electron beam to the vulva. Oblique groin fields. **b** Hamburg II: groin fields parallel to the vulvar field. **c** Vahrson: Rotated vulvar field. Groin field oblique, parallel to the vulva field borders. **d** Lower abdominal fields with lower central shielding. **e** Lower abdominal field including the common iliac nodes

performed using oblique fields (Fig. 5.13a). Involvement of iliac nodes was not taken into account while using this technique. A disadvantage of oblique fields was the inadequate adaptation to the vulvar field. This problem was solved by the introduction of groin fields parallel to the vulvar fields (Fig. 5.13b). The external iliac nodes can be irradiated, too, by extending the groin field cranially. In Gießen (Germany), VAHRSON (1995, personal communication) used a special technique with a rotation of the vulvar field. An oblique groin field can be easily adapted to the vulvar field (Fig. 5.13c).

Some centers prefer opposing fields with a central shielding for the vulvar field (Fig. 5.13d). The same technique was applied to irradiate node-positive cases after radical vulvectomy. Recurrences were seen in 63% of advanced cases, 76% of them being central recurrences under the shielding block (DUSENBERG et al. 1994). On the other hand, radiation therapy performed after radical vulvectomy without shielding the vulva often induces wound breakdown. In advanced cases it is necessary to reach the common iliac nodes, too (Fig. 5.13e).

Control of iliac nodes is a major problem in the treatment of vulvar carcinoma. A mixture of electrons and photons is usually applied to deposit sufficient doses to the groin nodes and reduce the dose to the femoral neck. The depth of the inguinal nodes was calculated to be 3 cm. However, recent research has shown that only 18% of patients have nodes at that depth (MCCALL et al. 1995); rather, the median is 5–6 cm. Individual therapy planning and modification of the beam quality are recommended to obtain optimal results.

5.13 Further Modalities in Primary Treatment

In addition to the concepts of management of vulvar carcinomas discussed above, there are some strategies which are aimed to solve problems for subgroups of patients:

1. For early-stage tumors
   - Wide excision and radiotherapy
2. For advanced cases
   - Extended radical surgery
   - Irradiation followed by radical surgery
   - Chemotherapy
   - Combination of chemotherapy and radical surgery
   - Combination of radiotherapy and chemotherapy

PEREZ et al. (1993) compared 13 patients who underwent radical surgery and radiotherapy with 13 who had a wide excision and radiotherapy. In T1/2 cases there was no difference in the local recurrence rate. These data are not sufficent for a general recommendation, and randomized trials will have to be performed to establish a vulva-conserving therapy similar to the successful breast-conserving therapy.

In patients with locally advanced tumors, good local control is not achieved by radical vulvectomy alone. CAVANAGH et al. (1982, 1986, 1990) reported good results of pelvic exenteration in selected patients with advanced tumors. Tumor control was excellent: half of the patients survived 5 years. However, extended radical surgery can be performed in selected cases only and requires a team of specialist surgeons.

Radical surgery after irradiation is an uncommon modality but it was successfully applied in advanced cases of vulvar carcinoma by BORONOW (1991). One approach is to extend the radicality of surgery, but this causes very mutilating procedures. BORONOW (1973) began treatment with radiotherapy. After reduction of the tumor volume, vulvectomy was performed. Of 48 cases treated, 37 were primary vulvar tumors and 11 were recurrences. Of the primary cases, 43 were stage III or IV. Radiotherapy was a combination of external beam and intracavitary treatment in 26 cases, intravaginal brachytherapy alone in 13 cases, and external beam therapy alone in nine cases. When both external beam therapy and intracavitary therapy were employed, the maximum dose to the vaginal surface ranged from 63.5 to 146 Gy (median 83.25 Gy). In spite of the great number of advanced cases, 42.5% of the patients showed no viable residual cancer at vulvectomy. Analysis of results showed excellent 5-year survival rates of 75.6% for primary cases and 62.6% for recurrent cases. In a number of cases, major complications such as fistulas, stenosis of the urethra and vagina, and major necrosis of bone and introitus occurred. These complications have to be considered in relation to the mutilation caused by extended radical surgery such as exenteration. This mode of treatment has not been adopted by many institutions.

HACKER et al. (1984) delivered 33–54 Gy by external beam irradiation preoperatively and performed radical vulvectomy with groin dissection. Tumor control without major complications was achieved in 62% of cases.

The role of systemic therapy in the management of cancer of the vulva is not well defined (THIGPEN 1991). For a long time squamous cell tumors were considered to be resistant to chemotherapy. The introduction of platinum derivatives and bleomycin led to a certain success, e.g., in head and neck tumors. Unfortunately, vulvar tumors are slow-growing neoplasms with a high grade of keratinization. As the following results demonstrate, response to chemotherapy is comparatively rare. Forty-two patients with advanced vulvar cancer were treated with cisplatin, bleomycin, and methotrexate by BENEDETTI-PANICI et al. (1993). Only 10% had a partial response of the primary, while 67% had a partial or complete response of the inguinal nodes. With additional radical surgery a 3-year survival of only 24% was registered. The high percentage of response of inguinal nodes has not been confirmed by other investigators.

Chemotherapy may play a certain role in combination with surgery and/or radiotherapy. BEREK et al. (1991) treated 12 patients with a combination of cisplatin and 5-fluorouracil (5-FU). Additional surgery was applied in four women. Chemotherapy was used as a sensitizer for concurrent radiotherapy. Ten patients were alive with a median follow-up of 37 months. Combined radiotherapy and chemotherapy was tested for the treatment of locoregionally advanced vulvar cancer by KOH et al. (1993) from the University of Washington (Seattle). Seven patients had FIGO stage III, ten had stage IV, and three had recurrent disease; all were unsuitable for radical surgery. The radiation dose was 30–54 Gy, and in gross tumors, 34–70 Gy. Concurrent chemotherapy was 5-FU in 15 cases and cisplatin in five. The disease-specific 5-year survival rate was 49%.

Recently, multimodal therapy combining radiotherapy with chemotherapy has been tested in order to reduce the radiation dose and thereby avoid moist desquamation of the vulva. It is recommended that this should be done in controlled studies only! In our institution, some women with advanced recurrences were admitted in whom a small curable primary had been treated by narrow excision, chemotherapy, and external beam radiotherapy (30 Gy to the vulva and the nodes). None of them survived. WAHLEN et al. (1995) report 19 cases treated with chemotherapy and irradiation with 45–50 Gy. Complete response was obtained in ten patients; however, the number of cases is too small to draw conclusions.

On the basis of the present data and personal experience, one may expect chemotherapy to have a future in three indications:

1. In undifferentiated advanced cases
2. As a radiosensitizer in combination with irradiation
3. In cases of distant visceral metastasis

Poorest results have been seen in (a) recurrences in an irradiated field, and (b) primary chemotherapy of advanced cases not suitable for surgery.

5.14 Five-Year Results and Complications

The 5-year crude survival of 2912 cases of the 21st Annual Report (PETTERSSON 1991) was as follows: FIGO I, 71.9%; II, 54.3%; III, 36.6%; IV, 21.0%. Some authors report better results in stages I and II. HOPKINS et al. (1991) from the University of Michigan observed a 5-year survival rate of 94% in stage I and 91% in stage II. The presence of inguinal lymph node metastasis is of the greatest prognostic significance. Among 106 patients seen at the University Clinic of Oklahoma, those who were node-positive had a 5-year survival of 38%, as compared with 87% for patients without positive nodes (SHANBOUR 1992). Prognosis is affected by the site of nodal involvement. In a collection of studies presented by WURM and ROTH (1993), patients with groin node metastasis had a 5-year survival of 52%, as compared with 18% in patients with iliac node involvement.

AYHAN et al. (1993) performed a multivariate analysis of risk factors. Depth of invasion was the most significant factor, followed by grade and stage. The value of prognostic factors may depend on the stage of the disease. HOPKINS et al. (1991) found that in stage I/II, survival was significantly influenced by tumor grade, while in stage III/IV tumor size and number of positive nodes governed the prognosis. The prognostic importance of clinical and histological parameters has been described in Sect. 5.5.

The pattern of complications depends on the therapy. After radical surgery, wound breakdown (SAROSI et al. 1994: 59%), necrosis of flaps, leg edema, thromboembolism, and pneumonia are of greatest importance. The high rate of wound breakdown can be lowered by flap techniques (see Sect. 5.7). Some authors report more groin complications than vulvar complications. BURKE et al. (1995) observed vulvar complications in 8% of cases and groin complications in 11% perioperatively. Delayed groin complications were seen in 29%. Radiotherapy of the vulva can result in induration and vaginal stenosis. Necrosis of the public bone is a rare but poorly tolerated complication of electron arc therapy. After complications and recurrences in the vulvar region, social integration is often impaired by the bad smell. Radiotherapy of inguinal nodes can lead to leg edema. Unfortunately, many elderly women have preexisting edema, postthrombotic syndromes, and crural ulcers. Any impairment reduces the mobility of these women. Radiotherapy of the groin can lead to femoral neck fracture: GRIGSBY et al. (1995) saw a rate of 11% at 5 years and 15% at 10 years, but did not mention the risk of femoral neck fracture for healthy women of the same age. They found a correlation with dose, cigarette use, and preexisting osteoporosis.

5.15 Use of Interstitial Brachytherapy in the Management of Progression and Recurrences

H. JACOBS

The different treatment policies employed for cancer of the vulva have been described in the foregoing sections. There are situations where radiation therapy, and especially interstitial brachytherapy, plays a major role: in advanced disease stages and in recurrences this treatment may be successful (JACOBS 1983, 1988; JACOBS et al. 1984).

5.15.1 Patients and Methods

From 1982 through the end of 1992, 41 patients with far advanced cancers of the vulva and recurrences were treated with radiation therapy for locoregional disease at the Radiation Oncology Department in Saarbrücken. All of them were treated with interstitial brachytherapy. The mean age of the patients was 74 years, with a range of 50–84 years. They all had squamous cell carcinoma of various differentiation, most being nonkeratinizing epidermoid cell tumors (3 well differentiated, 27 moderately differentiated, 11 undifferentiated).

Of 22 patients with primary tumors with clinical stage T3N0–2, 16 were treated with radiation therapy alone after biopsy and six were treated with local (wide) excision of the primary and radiation therapy (interstitial brachytherapy).

Of the 19 patients with recurrences, 12 had been treated initially with radical vulvectomy only (with or without inguinal lymph node dissection) and seven with vulvectomy and external beam radiation.

The treatment modalities have to take into consideration: (a) the extent of the primary and its relation to the urethra and vagina, (b) the pretreatment, and (c) the general condition of the patients.

5.15.2 Treatment Technique

For advanced cancers our strategy is to treat with external beam radiation using standard portals which include the primary and the inguinal and lower iliac lymph nodes. Patients were treated in a supine position with megavoltage photons (mostly with 18 MV) over parallel opposed fields. Until 1986, cobalt-60 radiation was given over unequally loaded fields.

In several cases additional doses were delivered to the primary or to lymph nodes using fast electrons of 9 and 12 MeV. The daily fractions ranged from 1.8 to 2.5 Gy, with four or five fractions being given weekly. The tumor doses ranged from 46 to 56 Gy.

Interstitial brachytherapy using a high-dose-rate technique was administered following this external beam radiotherapy. The procedure was performed under general or spinal anesthesia, took about 30–60 min, and was well tolerated by the patients. Two different modalities were used:

1. Temporary implants with parallel stainless steel needles fixed in special templates were used for one or two fractions. The single dose ranged from 8 to 10 Gy given to a reference isodose covering the target volume. The mean total dose ranged from 16 to 20 Gy (Fig. 5.14).
2. Temporary implants with flexible catheters allowed a more conventional fractionation schedule, i.e., single doses of 2 or 3 Gy to a total dose of 20–30 Gy in most cases, and of 35 and 45 Gy in one case each. During the Past 5 years the daily dose was given in two fractions with an interval of 6 h. This schedule is now preferred (Figs. 5.15–5.17).

5.15.3 Results

Of the 16 patients with *primary tumors treated with radiation therapy alone after biopsy*, eight developed a complete remission; two of them subsequently had a local failure after 8 and 14 months and one had a lymph node relapse. Five of the 16 patients had only a partial remission and three patients showed no or only a slight response. The conventional fractionation schedule yielded better results and produced less side-effects than the treatment with higher single doses of HDR brachytherapy. Two patients developed long-lasting ulcerations and fibrosis. Telangiectasia was seen in all cases as a result of the high "physically calculated" total dose between 66 and 78 Gy.

Of the six patients with *primary tumors treated with wide excision and an interstitial "boost" only to the tumor bed*, two developed local failure and died of progression after 7 and 13 months. In three cases the interstitial brachytherapy was given as single doses of 10 Gy three times at intervals of 7 days, and in the other three cases in a fractionated regimen with daily doses of 2 Gy up to 28, 30, and 36 Gy over 3 weeks. In spite of the patients' age and clinical status, these procedures were very well tolerated.

In the group of patients with *recurrences* the pretreatment was an important prognostic factor. Patients who had not previously been irradiated showed better results, and the localization of the recurrence seemed to be important too.

Of the 12 previously nonirradiated patients, five showed a complete remission with a mean duration of 34 months. In four out of these five patients the site of the failure was the vulvovaginal region. In those cases where the failure was located in the region of the vulva, only partial remissions lasting a few months were achieved.

The control of relapse after previous surgery and radiation of the primary was very poor. The treatment was then performed as interstitial brachytherapy with the aim of palliation in order to influence pain and hemorrhage. The treatment was given in single doses of 15–20 Gy once to three times according to the results and the clinical status during the follow-up.

5.15.4 Conclusions

Interstitial brachytherapy is well suited for the treatment of advanced tumor stages, tumor progression,

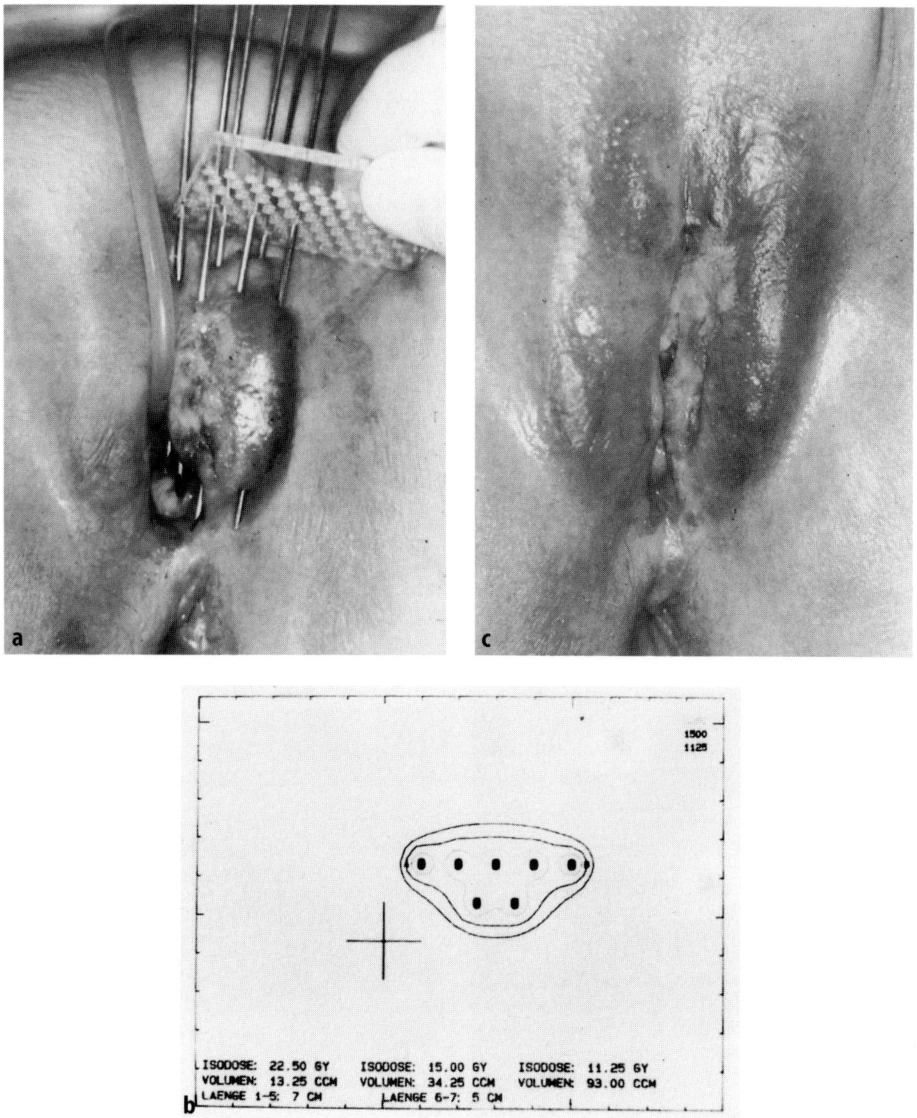

Fig. 5.14. **a** A two-plane implant performed to treat a local recurrence with palliative intention. In this case interstitial HDR brachytherapy was given in three sessions with single doses of 15 Gy (volume 34 ml), the second and third fractions being given after intervals of 10 and 12 days. **b** The dose distribution in the same patient. **c** The situation 8 months after completion of the irradiation with HDR brachytherapy; 2 months later the patient developed a new local "in-field" relapse

and recurrences because of the good dose distribution that may be achieved by using special templates and flexible catheters which allow individual tailoring with respect to the tumor and the surrounding tissues (Jacobs 1990, 1992, 1993). Brachytherapy should be used in combination with external beam radiation for the treatment of these usually inoperable large tumor masses. We prefer to use it following the external beam therapy as part of a shrinking field technique, the volume being adapted during the therapy. This can be adequately performed using modern planning systems. When the intent is curative, the interstitial HDR technique should be used in a conventional fractionation schedule with single doses of 3–5 Gy, whenever possible delivering two fractions a day with a 6-h interval between them. The interstitial HDR technique is also justified in the palliative situation, using higher single doses.

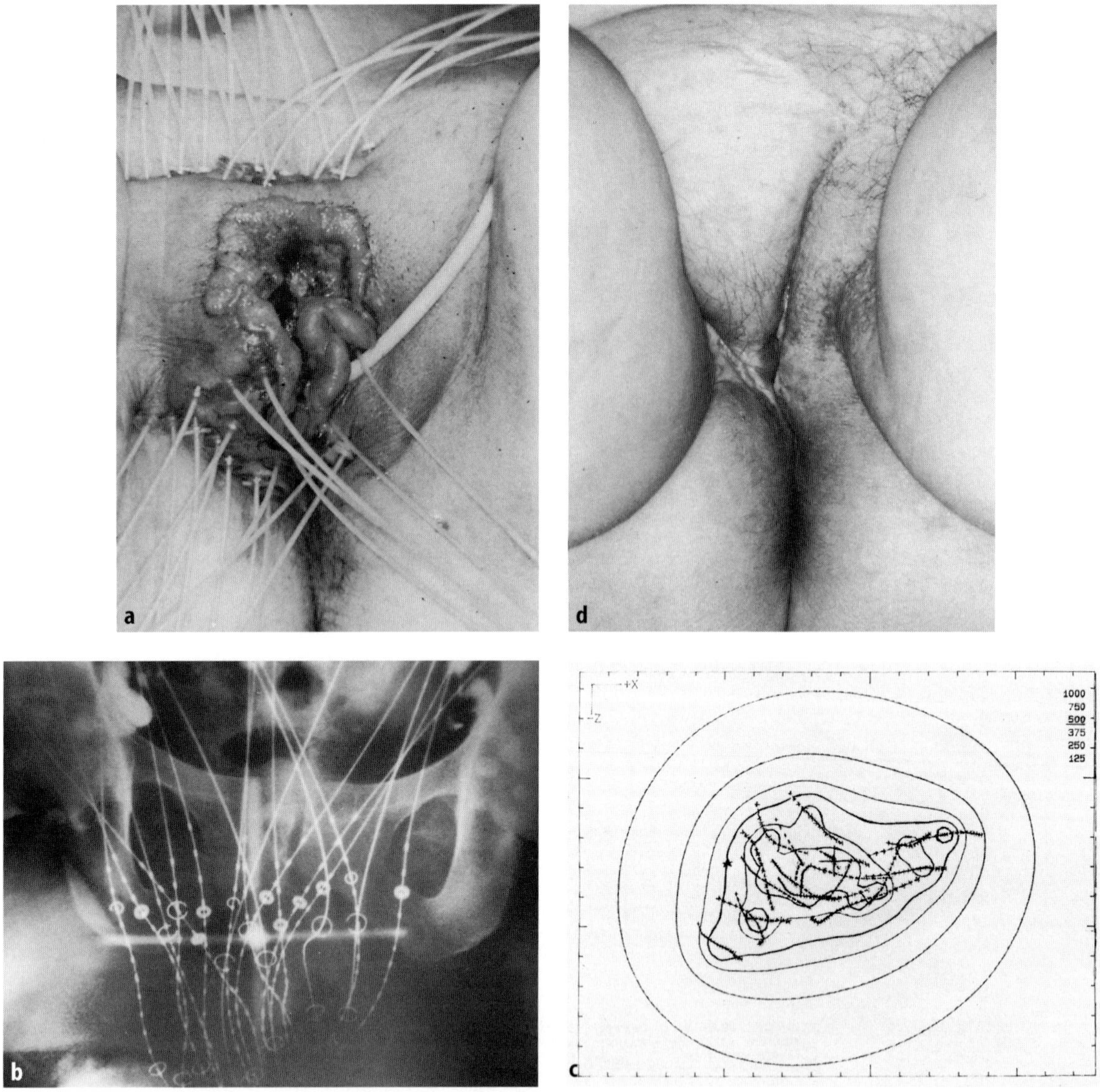

Fig. 5.15. **a** Example of interstitial brachytherapy with flexible catheters in a far-advanced vulvar cancer (T3/4). A three-plane implant was "tailored" according to the tumor extent. **b** Anterior/posterior x-ray check film showing 18 dummy wires in the flexible catheters of the implant. **c** The isodose distribution of this implant with 18 catheters. The "reference isodose" (500) encompasses the target volume. In this case the dose prescription was 2 and 3 Gy/day with an interval of 6 h between doses. The total dose was 35 Gy, given over a period of 17 days, followed by external beam radiation with 34 Gy in conventional fractions (18 MV photons). **d** The situation 56 months after completion of the combined radical irradiation with telangiectasia and local fibrosis but with excellent function of the urethra and bladder. (Twenty-one months after therapy a persistent ulcer in the right upper vulvar area was excised)

5.16 Follow-up Examinations

Many studies of vulvar carcinomas suffer from a lack of follow-up data. Because vulvar cancer is a disease of old and very old women, many patients do not consult the physician who performed primary therapy. The early detection of local recurrence is most important, and gynecological investigation consequently should be performed quarterly for at least 5 years. While the prognosis is bad in cases of groin recurrence, secondary infiltration of the vulva can be cured by surgery or radiotherapy. In addition some women may still have precursors of squamous cell cancer, which can develop to invasive cancer. Such precursors should be removed by excision or laser coagulation.

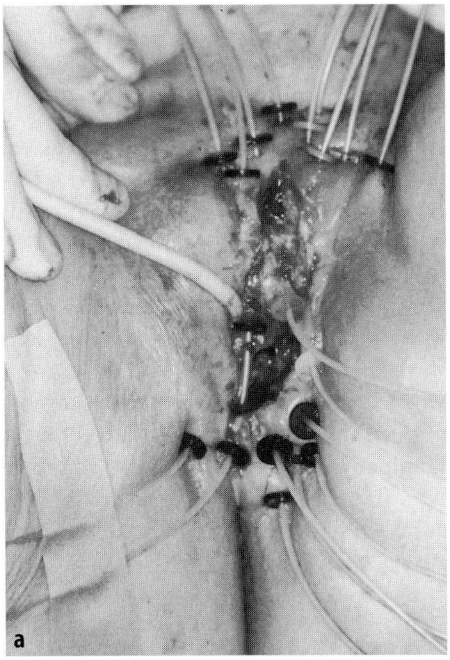

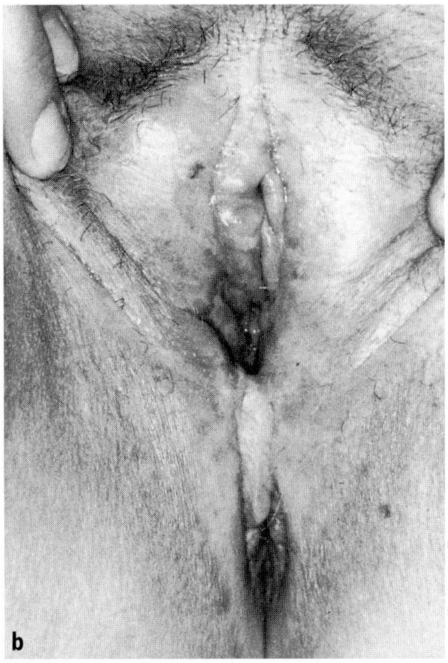

Fig. 5.16. a An interstitial implant with flexible catheters in a T2 tumor (recurrence after vulvectomy in a 74-year-old woman following external beam irradiation with 42 Gy. The implant encompasses the whole palpable mass with a "safety" margin. The additional total dose was 22 Gy with HDR brachytherapy, applied in daily doses of 4 Gy (2 Gy twice a day) 4 times a week over a total period of 8 days (last fraction 2 Gy only). **b** The situation 34 months after the irradiation with a good cosmetic and functional result

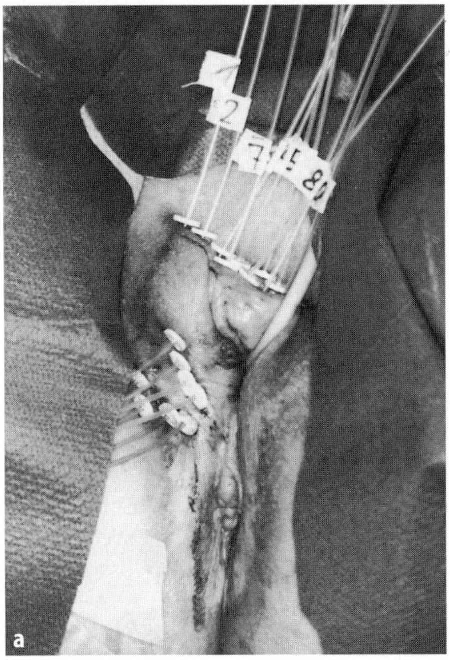

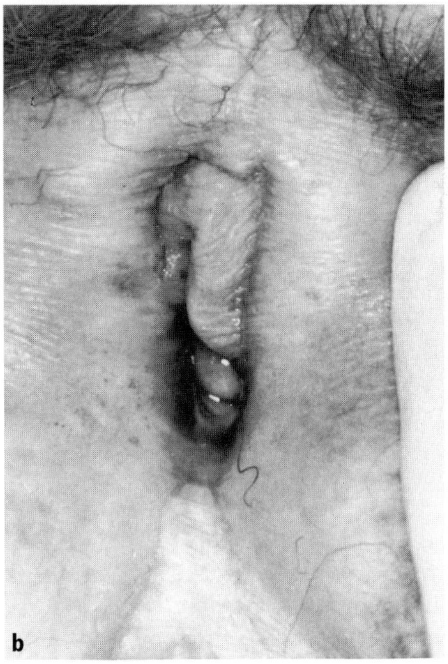

Fig. 5.17. a A two-plane implant for treatment of a vulvar cancer in a 76-year-old woman (T2). This tumor was irradiated only using interstitial HDR brachytherapy: 39 Gy (in daily fractions of 3 Gy over 3 weeks) to the reference isodose encompassing a relatively small volume of 32 ml. **b** The result 16 months after the completion of irradiation

5.17 Clinical Trials and Outlook

Much of our better knowledge of vulvar cancer has derived from GOG studies. The Gynecologic Oncology Group (GOG) was founded by the National Cancer Institute of the United States in 1970. The GOG protocols 36 and 37 deal with vulvar carcinoma. The GOG protocol 36 was entitled "Surgical-pathologic study of women with squamous cell carcinoma of the vulva" (HOMESLEY and SEVIN 1991). From 1971 to 1984, 588 patients underwent radical vulvectomy and bilateral groin dissection. Patients with nonresectable tumors and inadequate treatment were excluded. Thus, most of the patients presented with FIGO clinical stage I or II disease. The relationship between vulvar tumor and nodal involvement was defined very clearly. The probability of inguinal lymph node metastasis increased with tumor size, depth of invasion, and histological grade. Further significant predictors for groin node metastasis were capillary-like space involvement and a clitoral or perineal location. Clinically suspicious nodes were involved in 59% of the cases, but 17% of women without palpable groin nodes also had metastases.

A second study was initiated to determine whether adjunctive radiation therapy could improve survival (HOMESLEY and SEVIN 1991). In spite of the fact that radiation therapy of vulvar cancer has not been used widely in the United States, cases with groin node metastasis were entered in GOG protocol 37. This protocol was entitled "Randomized study of radiation therapy versus pelvic node resection for patients with invasive squamous cell carcinomas of the vulva having positive groin nodes." This is at present the most important study with regard to definition of the importance of radiotherapy of lymph nodes in vulvar cancer. On a random basis, patients were treated with either radiotherapy of the pelvis or a pelvic lymph node dissection. Radiotherapy included both groins and all nodes from the foramina obturatoria up to the L5-S1 interspace. The total dose was 45–50 Gy in the midplane of the pelvis. The vulvar region was not irradiated. In the other arm an epsilateral pelvic lymph node dissection was performed in cases of unilateral node involvement and a bilateral dissection when both groin nodes contained metastases. One hundred and fourteen randomized patients were analyzed for survival and failure pattern. At 2 years survival was 75% in the radiation group and 56% in the pelvic lymph mode dissection group. Survival benefit increased with the number of involved nodes and the presence of palpable node metastasis. The most common site of recurrence was the vulvar region (not irradiated) in both treatment arms. Groin failure was less frequent in the radiation group than in the extended radical surgery group. The GOG study showed that pelvic lymph node metastasis plays a major role if three or more groin nodes are involved by the tumor (CURRY et al. 1980; HOMESLEY et al. 1986). Irradiation of the pelvic nodes improved survival in patients with three of more positive groin nodes. Because pelvic metastasis does not occur on the contralateral side, when contralateral groin nodes are negative, adjuvant radiotherapy can be restricted to the ipsilateral hemipelvis. The percentage of side-effects was similar in both groups. As regards mild leg edema, more cases were found in the radiotherapy group (19% vs 11%).

SEHMAN et al. (1992) reported the first results of a GOG study on early stage I carcinomas. Between 1983 and 1989, 155 women entered the study and underwent a modified radical hemivulvectomy and ipsilateral inguinal lymphadenectomy. Patients eligible for the study were those with lesions up to 20 mm in diameter and with a thickness of 5 mm or less, without suspicious groin nodes. Results were compared with previous experiences. Vulvar recurrences were frequently salvaged by further surgery (eight of ten cases). The decision to leave the femoral nodes behind probably caused a significant increase in groin recurrence. It may be concluded that reduction of radical surgery is successful if there is careful selection of cases, appropriate investigation of specimens, and careful follow-up. The control of lymph nodes is of greater importance, because groin recurrences led to death due to cancer in five of seven cases.

A current GOG study is testing the substitution of groin dissection by radiation therapy (DUBESHTER et al. 1993). At present no results are available. Omitting groin dissection reduces the duration of surgery and the postoperative morbidity; thus it is suitable for elderly patients with multiple medical problems. Side-effects of radiotherapy are rare if the vulva is not irradiated and no groin dissection is performed (HOMESLEY et al. 1986).

Further GOG studies are addressing the modalities of groin node control, advanced cases, and melanoma of the vulva. At present detailed data are not available.

References

Ayhan A, Tuncer R, Tuncer ZS, Yuecel I, Zeyneloglu HG, Kuecuekali T, Develioglu O (1993) Risk factors for groin node metastasis in squamous carcinoma of the vulva: a multivariate analysis of 39 cases. Eur J Obstet Gynecol Reprod Biol 48:33–36

Bäckström A, Edsmyr F, Wicklund H (1972) Radiotherapy of carcinoma of the vulva. Acta Obstet Gynecol Scand 51:109

Benedet JL, Turko M, Fairey RN, et al. (1979) Squamous carcinoma of the vulva. Results of treatment. Am J Obstet Gynecol 134:201

Benedetti-Panici P, Greggi S, Scambia G, Salerno G, Mancuso S (1993) Cisplatin (P), bleomycin (B), and methotrexate (M) preoperative chemotherapy in locally advanced vulvar carcinoma. Gynecol Oncol 50:49–53

Berek JS, Heaps JM, Fu YS, Juillard GJ, Hacker NF (1991) Concurrent cisplatin and 5-fluorouracil chemotherapy and radiation therapy for advanced-stage squamous carcinoma of the vulva. Gynecol Oncol 42:197–201

Boiti Trotti A, Tseroni V, Rovea P, Nastasi U, Fracchia F (1991) II ruolo della radioterapia nel trattamento del tumore della vulva. (The role of radiotherapy in the treatment of vulvar tumors.) Minerva Ginecol 43:381–384

Bornstein J, Kaufmann RH (1988) Combination of surgical excision and CO_2 laser vaporization for multifocal vulvar intraepithelial neoplasia. Am J Obstet Gynecol 158:459

Boronow RC (1973) Therapeutic alternative to primary exenteration for advanced vulvo-vaginal cancer. Gynecol Oncol 1:223

Boronow RC (1982) Combined therapy as an alternative to exenteration for locally advanced vulvo-vaginal cancer: rationale and results. Cancer 49:1085

Boronow RC (1991) Combined radiation and surgery for locally advanced cancer of the vulva. In: Knappstein PG, di Re F, DiSaia PJ, Haller U, Sevin Bu (eds) Malignancies of the vulva. Thieme, Stuttgart, pp 133–142

Burke TW, Stringer CA, Gershenson DM, et al. (1990) Radical wide excision and selective inguinal node dissection for squamous cell carcinoma of the vulva. Gynecol Oncol 38:328

Burke TW, Levenback C, Colemann RL, Morris M, Silva EG, Gershenson DM (1995) Surgical therapy of T1 and T2 vulvar carcinoma: further experience with radical wide excision and selective inguinal lymphadenectomy. Gynecol Oncol 57:215–220

Burrell MO, Franklin EW, Campion MF, et al. (1988) The modified radical vulvectomy with groin node dissection: an eight year experience. Am J Obstet Gynecol 159:715

Cavanagh D, Shepherd JH (1982) The place of pelvic exenteration in the primary management of advanced carcinoma of the vulva. Gynecol Oncol 13:318

Cavanagh D, Roberts WS, Bryson SCP, et al. (1986) Changing trends in the surgical treatment of invasive carcinoma of the vulva. Gynecol Oncol 38:164

Cavanagh D, Fiorica JV, Hoffman MS, et al. (1990) Invasive carcinoma of the vulva. Changing trends in surgical management. Am J Obstet Gynecol 163:1007

Chamlian DL, Taylor HB (1972) Primary carcinoma of Bartholin's gland. Obstet Gynecol 39:489

Chalubinski K, Breitenecker G, Tatra G (1992) Maligne Lymphome an Vulva und Vagina. (Malignant lymphomas of the vulva and vagina) Geburtshilfe Frauenheilkd 52:630–631

Collins CG, Ramon-Lopez JJ, Lee FYL (1987) Intraepithelial carcinoma of the vulva. Am J Obstet Gynecol 108:1187

Craighead PS, du Toit PF (1993) Endodermal sinus tumour of the vulva: an interesting clinico-pathological problem. Eur J Surg Oncol 19:203–205

Crun CP, Liskow A, Petras P, Keng WC, Frick HC (1984) Vulvar intraepithelial neoplasia (severe atypia and carcinoma in situ). Cancer 54:1429–1434

Curry SL, Wharton JT, Rutledge F (1980) Positive lymph nodes in vulva squamous carcinoma. Gynecol Oncol 9:36

Di Re F, Fontanelli R, Raspagliesi F, et al. (1991) Lymph node involvement in vulvar carcinoma. In: Knapstein PG, Di Re F, Disaia PJ, Haller U, Sevin BU (eds) Malignancies of the vulva. Thieme, Stuttgart, p 86

DiSaia PJ (1991) Conservative treatment of microcarcinomas. In: Knappstein PG, di Re F, DiSaia PJ, Haller U, Sevin BU (eds) Malignancies of the vulva. Thieme, Stuttgart, pp 73–79

DiSaia P, Rich WM (1981) Surgical approach to multifocal carcinoma in situ of the vulva. Am J Obstet Gynecol 140:136–145

DiSaia PJ, Creasman WT, Rich WH (1979) An alternative approach to early cancer of the vulva. Am J Obstet Gynecol 133:825

DuBeshter B, Angel C, Lin J, Poulter CA (1993) Gynecologic tumors. In: Rubin Ph (ed) Clinical oncology, 7th edn. Saunders, Philadelphia, pp 363–418

Dusenberg KE, Carlson JW, LaPorte RM, et al. (1994) Radical vulvectomy with postoperative irradiation for vulvar cancer: therapeutic implications of a central block. Int J Radiat Oncol Biol Phys 29:989–998

Elchalal U, Dgani R, Zosmer A, Levi E, Rakovsky E, Lifschitz-Mercer B (1991) Malignant fibrous histiocytoma of the vagina and vulva successfully treated by combined chemotherapy and radiotherapy. Gynecol Oncol 42:91–93

Feuer GA, Shevchuk M, Calanog A (1989) Vulvar Paget's disease: the need to exclude an invasive lesion. Gynecol Oncol 38:81–89

Figge CD, Tamimi HK, Greer BE (1985) Lymphatic spread in carcinoma of the vulva. Am J Obstet Gynecol 152:387

Frankendahl B, Larrson LG, Westling P (1973) Carcinoma of the vulva. Acta Radiol 12:165

Franklin EW, Rutledge FD (1971) Prognostic factors in epidermoid carcinoma of the vulva. Obstet Gynecol 37:892

Friedrich EG, Wilkinson EJ (1982) The vulva. In: Blaustein A (ed) Pathology of the female genital tract. Springer, Berlin Heidelberg New York, pp 13–58

Friedrich EG, Wilkinson EJ, Fu YS (1980) Carcinoma in situ of the vulva: a continuing challenge. Am J Obstet Gynecol 136:880

Frischbier HJ, Wenn K (1985) Behandlungsergebnisse durch sekundäre Vulvektomie nach Elektronenbestrahlung eines Vulvakarzinoms. Geburtshilfe Frauenheilkd 45:494–496

Frischbier HJ, Thomsen K, Schmermund HJ, Oberheuser F, Höhne G, Lohbeck HU (1985) Die Strahlenbehandlung des Vulvakarzinoms. Geburtshilfe Frauenheilkd 45:1–5

Frischkorn R (1969) Bestrahlung der Vulva-Carcinome mit schnellen Elektronen. Geburtshilfe Frauenheilkd 29:1016

Goldberg LH, Rubin HA (1989) Management of basal cell carcinoma. Which option is best? Postgrad Med 85:57–63

Gomez Rueda N, Vighi S, Garcia A, Cardinal L, Belardi MG, di Paola G (1994) Histologic predictive factors. Therapeutic impact in vulvar cancer. J Reprod Med 39:71–76

Green TH Jr (1978) Carcinoma of the vulva. A reassessment. Obstet Gynecol 52:462

Grigsby PW, Roberts HL, Perez CA (1995) Femoral neck fracture following groin irradiation. Int J Radiat Oncol Biol Phys 32:63–67

Grimshaw RN, Ghazal Asward S, Monaghan JM (1991) The role of anovulvectomy in locally advanced carcinoma of the vulva. Int J Gynecol Cancer 1:15

Gross H (1986) Virusinfektionen der Vulva. In: Zander J, Baltzer J (eds) Erkrankungen der Vulva. Urban & Schwarzenberg, München, p 16

Haberthür F, Almendral AC, Ritter B (1993) Therapy of vulvar carcinoma. Eur J Gynaecol Oncol XIV:218–227

Hacker NF (1991) Management of stage I vulvar cancer. In: Knappstein PG, di Re F, DiSaia PJ, Haller U, Sevin Bu (eds) Malignancies of the vulva. Thieme, Stuttgart, p 80

Hacker NF, Van der Velden J (1993) Conservative management of early vulvar cancer. Cancer 71:1673–1677

Hacker NF, Leuchter RS, BEREK JS, et al. (1981) Radical vulvectomy and bilateral lymphadenectomy through separate groin incision. Obstet Gynecol 58:574–579

Hacker NF, Berek JS, Lagasse LD, et al. (1983) Management of regional lymph nodes and their prognostic influence in vulvar cancer. Obstet Gynecol 61:408

Hacker NF, Berek JS, Lagasse LD, et al. (1984a) Individualisation of treatment for stage I squamous cell vulvar carcinoma. Obstet Gynecol 63:155

Hacker NF, Berek JS, Juillard GJF, Lagasse LD (1984b) Preoperative radiation therapy for locally advanced cancer. Cancer 54:2056

Heaps JM, Fu YS, Montz FJ, Hacker NF, Berek JS (1990) Surgical-pathologic variables predictive of local recurrence in squamous cell carcinoma of the vulva. Gynecol Oncol 38:309–314

Heine O, Vahrson H (1987) Das primäre Karzinom der Bartholinischen Drüse. Geburtshilfe Frauenheilkd 47:35–40

Helgason NM, Hass AC, Latourette HB (1972) Radiotherapy in carcinoma of the vulva. Cancer 30:997

Henson D, Tarone R (1977) An epidemiologic study of cancer of the cervix, vagina, and vulva based on the Third National Cancer Survey in the United States. Am J Obstet Gynecol 129:525

Höckel M, Knapstein PG (1992) The combined operative and radiotherapeutic treatment (CORT) of recurrent tumors infiltrating the pelvic wall: first experience with 18 patients. Gynecol Oncol 46:20

Homesley BU, Homesley HD (1986) Das Vulvakarzinom. Gynäkologe 19:109–115

Homesley HD, Bundy BN, Sedlis A, Adcock L (1986) Radiation therapy versus pelvic node resection for carcinoma of the vulva with positive groin nodes. Obstet Gynecol 68: 733

Homesley HD, Sevin BU (1991) Treatment of vulvar cancer: the gynecology oncology group experience. In: Knapstein PG, di Re F, DiSaia PJ, Haller U, Sevin BU (eds) Malignancies of the vulva. Thieme, Stuttgart, pp 119–123

Homesley HD, Bundy BN, Sedlis A, Yordan E, Berek JS, Jahsan A, Mortel R (1993) Prognostic factors for groin metastasis in squamous cell carcinoma of the vulva (a GOG study) Gynecol Oncol 49:279

Hopkins MP, Reid GC, Vettrano I, Morley GM (1991) Squamous cell carcinoma of the vulva: prognostic factors influencing survival. Gynecol Oncol 43:113–117

Iversen T, Aas M (1983) Lymph drainage of the vulva. Gynecol Oncol 16:179

Iversen T, Aalders J, Christensen A, Kolstad P (1980) Squamous cell carcinoma of the vulva: a review of 424 patients, 1956–1974. Gynecol Oncol 9:271

Iversen T, Abeler V, Aalders J (1981) Individualized treatment of stage I carcinoma of the vulva. Obstet Gynecol 57:85

Jacobs H (1983) Erste Erfahrungen mit der interstitiellen Radio-Curie-Therapie. Saarländ Ärztebl II:725–730

Jacobs H (1988) Experiences with interstitial HDR afterloading therapy in genital and breast cancer. In: Vahrson H, Raute G (eds) Afterloading in the treatment of cancer of the uterus, breast, and rectum. Urban and Schwarzenberg, München, pp 258–262

Jacobs H (1990) Interstitielle Brachytherapie beim Vaginal- und Vulvakarzinom. In: Baier K, Herbolsheimer M, Sauer O (eds) Interdisziplinäre Behandlungsformen beim Mammakarzinom und bei gynäkologischen Malignomen. Bonitas-Bauer, Würzburg pp 140–150

Jacobs H (1992) Interstitial brachytherapy for advanced cancer of the vulva – a case report. Activity 6:37

Jacobs H (1993) Interstitial brachytherapy in the treatment of gynaecological tumours. In: Fietkau R, Mould RF (eds) Brachytherapy. State of the art in Germany. Nucletron International, Veenenclaal, Netherlonds, pp 192–197

Jacobs H et al. (1984) Interstitelle Brachytherapie – erste Erfahrungen mit 192-Iridium in der Kurzzeittherapie. Strahlenther Oncol 160:8–14

Jafari K, Magalotti M (1981) Radiation therapy in carcinoma of the vulva. Cancer 47:686

Jeppesen JT, Sell A, Skjöldborg H (1972) Treatment of cancer of the vulva. Acta Obstet Gynecol Scand 51:101

Kepp RK, Paul W, Schmermund HJ, Schubert G (1951) Neue Methoden in der Bekämpfung der Vulvakarzinome. Geburtshilfe Frauenheilkd 11:298–312

Knapstein P, Sevin BU, Friedberg V (1991) Reconstructive surgery in gynecology. Thieme, Stuttgart

Kneale BL (1984) Microinvasive cancer of the vulva: report of the International Society for the Study of Vulvar Disease Task Force. Proceedings of the 7th Word Congress of the ISSVD. J Reprod Med 29:454

Koh WJ, Wallace HJ III, Greer BE, et al. (1993) Combined radiotherapy and chemotherapy in the management of local-regionally advanced vulvar cancer. Int J Radiat Oncol Biol Phys 26:809–816

Kucera H, Weghaupt K (1988) The electrosurgical operation of vulvar carcinoma with postoperative irradiation of inguinal lymph nodes. Gynecol Oncol 29:158

Lee WR, McCollough WM, Mendenhall WM, Marcus RB Jr, Parsons JT, Million RR (1993) Elective inguinal lymph node irradiation for pelvic carcinomas. The University of Florida experience. Cancer 72:2058–2065

Levitan Z, Kaplan AL, Kaufman RH (1992) Advanced squamous cell cercinoma of the vulva after treatment for verrucous carcinoma. A case report. J Reprod Med 37:889–892

Lochmüller H (1983) Zur Strahlentherapie bei der Behandlung des Vulvakarzinoms. Radiologe 23:24–28

Lochmüller H (1986) Radiologische Behandlungsmethoden des Vulvakarzinoms (Münchner Methode). In: Zander J, Baltzer J (eds) Erkrankungen der Vulva. Urban & Schwarzenberg, München, pp 168–173

Mack T, Casagrande JT (1981) Epidemiology of gynecologic cancer. II. Endometrium, ovary, vagina, vulva. In: Coppleson M (ed) Gynecologic oncology: fundamental principles and clinical practice. Churchill Livingstone, New York, pp 28–30

Malfetano JH, Piver S, Tsukada Y, Reese P (1985) Univariate and multivariate analyse of 5-year survival, recurrence, and inguinal node metastases in stage I and II vulvar carcinoma.

McCall AR, Olson MC, Potkul RK (1995) The variation of inguinal lymph node depth in adult women and its importance in planning elective irradiation for vulvar cancer. Cancer 75:2286–2288

Micheletti L, Borgno B, Barbero M, et al. (1990) Deep femoral lymphadenectomy with preservation of the fascia lata: pre-

liminary report on 42 invasive vulvar carcinomas. J Reprod Med 35:1130
Monaghan JM (1991) Radical surgery of cancer of the vulva: the Gateshead experience 1974–1989. In: Knapstein PG, di Re F, DiSaia PJ, Haller U, Sevin BU (eds) Malignancies of the vulva. Thieme, Stuttgart, p 124
Morley GW (1976) Infiltrative carcinoma of the vulva: results of surgical treatment. Am J Obstet Gynecol 124:874
Ng ABP (1991) Histopathology of premalignant and malignant tumors of the vulva. In: Knapstein PG, di Re F, DiSaia PJ, Haller U, Sevin BU (eds) Malignancies of the vulva. Thiems, Stuttgart, pp 1–24
Paladini D, Cross P, Lopes A, Monaghan JM (1994) Prognostic significance of lymph node variables in squamous cell carcinoma of the vulva. Cancer 74:2491–2496
Parker RT, Duncan I, Rampose J, et al. (1975) Operative management of early invasive epidermoid carcinoma of the vulva. Am J Obstet Gynecol 123:349
Perez CA, Grigsby PW (1992) Vulva. In: Perez CA, Brady LW (eds) Principles and practice of radiation oncology. Lippincott, Philadelphia, pp 1273–1289
Perez CA, Grigsby PW, Galakatos A, Swanson R, Camel HM, Kao MS, Lockett MA (1993) Radiation therapy in management of carcinoma of the vulva with emphasis on conservation therapy. Cancer 71:3707–3716
Pettersson F (1991) Annual report on the results of treatment in gynecologic cancer. Int J Gynecol Obstet 36 (Suppl):1–315
Phillips GL, Bundy BN, Okagaki T, Kucera PR, Stehman FB (1994) Malignant melanoma of the vulva treated by radical hemivulvectomy. A prospective study of the Gynecologic Oncology Group. Cancer 73:2626–2632
Pirtoli L, Rottoli ML (1982) Results of radiation therapy for vulvar carcinoma. Acta Radiol 21:45
Plentl AA, Friedman EA (1971) Lymphatic system of the female genitalia. Saunders, Philadelphia
Podratz KC, Symmonds RE, Taylor WF (1982) Carcinoma of the vulva: analysis of treatment failures. Am J Obstet Gynecol 143:340
Reagan JW, Ng ABP (1988) Vaginal and vulvar disease. In: Wied GL, Keebler CM, Kossl ••, Reagan JW (eds) Compendium on diagnostic cytology. Chicago, p 71
Rose PG, Tak WK, Reale FR, Hunter RE (1991) Adenoid cystic carcinoma of the vulva: a radiosensitive tumor. Gynecol Oncol 43:81–83
Rose PG, Nelson BE, Fournier L, Hunter RE (1992) Serum squamous cell carcinoma antigen levels in invasive squamous vulvar cancer. J Surg Oncol 50:183–186
Rutledge FN, Mitshell MF, Munsell MF, Atkinson EN, Bass S, McGuffee V, Silva E (1991) Prognostic indicators for invasive carcinoma of the vulva. Gynecol Oncol 42:239–244
Sarosi Z, Boessze P, Danczig A, Ringwald G (1994) Complications of radical vulvectomy and adjacent lymphadenectomy based on 58% cases of vulvar cancer. Orv Hetil 135:743–746
Schmidt W, Schmid H, Villena-Heinsen C, Kuehn W, Jochum-Merger N, von Fournier D (1992) Behandlungsergebnisse beim Vulvakarzinom von 1970 bis 1990. (Results of treatment in vulvar cancer from 1970 to 1990.) Geburtshilfe Frauenheilkd 52:749–757
Schmidt-Matthiesen H, Michel RT (1991) Operationen an Vulva und Vagina. In: Zander J, Graeff H (eds) Gynäkologische Operationen. Springer, Berlin Heidelberg New York
Schreer I, Bahnsen J, Frischbier HJ (1991) Radiotherapy of vulvar carcinoma. In: Knapstein PG, di Re F, DiSaia PJ, Haller U, Sevin BU (eds) Malignancies of the vulva. Thieme, Stuttgart, pp 143–152
Schueller EF (1965) Basal cell cancer of the vulva. Am J Obstet Gynecol 93:199–208
Sedlis A, Homesley HD, Bundy BN, et al. (1987) Positive groin nodes in superficial squamous cell vulvar carcinoma. Am J Obstet Gynecol 156:1159
Sehman FB, Bundy BN, Dvoretsky PM, Creaseman WT (1992) Early stage I carcinoma of the vulva treated with ipsilateral superficial inguinal lymphadenectomy and modified radical hemivulvectomy: a prospective study of the Gynecologic Oncology Group. Obstet Gynecol 79:490–497
Shanbour KA, Mannel RS, Morris PC, Yadack A, Walker JL (1992) Comparison of clinical versus surgical staging systems in vulvar cancer. Obstet Gynecol 80:927–930
Simonsen E (1984) Invasive squamous cell carcinoma of the vulva. Ann Chir Gynaecol 73:331–338
Stening M (1980) Cancer and related lesions of the vulva. MTP Press, Lancaster, England
Sutton GP, Stehman FB, Ehrlich CE, Roman A (1987) Human papillomavirus deoxyribonucleic acid in lesions of the female genital tract: evidence for type 6/11 in squamous carcinoma of the vulvar. Obstet Gynecol 70:564
Taussig FJ (1940) Carcinoma of the vulva. An analysis of 155 cases. Am J Obstet Gynecol 40:764
Thigpen JT (1991) Systemic therapy in the management of cancer of the vulva. In: Knapstein PG, di Re F, DiSaia PJ, Haller U, Sevin Bu (eds) Malignancies of the vulva. Thieme, Stuttgart, pp 153–157
Thomas GM, Dembo AJ, Bryson CP, Osborne R, DePetrillo AD (1991) Changing concepts in the management of vulvar carcinoma. Gynecol Oncol 42:9
Thüroff JW, Alken P, Riedmiller H, et al. (1986) The Mainz pouch (mixed augmentation ileum and cecum) for bladder augmentation and continent diversion. J Urol 136:17
Tilmans AS, Sutton GP, Look KY, Stehman FB, Ehrlich CE, Hornback NB (1992) Recurrent Squamous carcinoma of the vulva. Am J Obstet Gynecol 167:1383–1389
Wahlen SA, Slater JD, Wagner RJ, Wang WA, Keeney ED, Hocko JM, King A, Slater JM (1995) Concurrent radiation therapy and chemotherapy in the treatment of primary squamous cell carcinoma of the vulva. Cancer 75:2289–2294
Way S (1960) Carcinoma of the vulva. Am J Obstet Gynecol 79:692
Weikel W, Güldütuna S, Knapstein PG, et al. (1991) Die hintere Exenteration mit plastischer Wiederherstellung beim fortgeschrittenen Vulvakarzinom. Geburtshilfe Frauenheilkd 51:814
Wurm R, Roth SL (1993) Das Vulvakarzinom. In: Roth SL, Böttcher HD (eds) Gynäkologische Strahlentherapie. Enke Verlag, Stuttgart
Young JL, Percy CL, Asire AS (1981) Surveillance, epidemiology and end results: incidence and mortality data, 1973–1977. Monogr Natl Cancer Inst 57:982
Zhang WH (1992) Combination of radiotherapy and surgery for advanced cancer of the vulva. Chinese J Oncol 14:375–378

6 Special Malignancies of the Vulva

J. BAHNSEN and H.J. FRISCHBIER

CONTENTS

6.1 Vulvar Intraepithelial Neoplasia, Bowen's Disease, and Paget's Disease

Preinvasive forms of vulvar malignancy are called vulvar intraepithelial neoplasia (VIN). About 20% of VIN appear hyperpigmented (FRIEDRICH and WILKINSON 1982). In the United States approximately 2500 new cases of VIN are diagnosed annually (YOUNG et al. 1981; CRUN et al. 1984). Ten percent of cases of vulvar carcinoma in situ progress to invasive vulvar carcinoma. The median age for carcinoma in situ is 44 years (COLLINS et al. 1987). Given that the median age for invasive vulvar cancer is more than two decades higher, it may be concluded that progression requires a long time. About 20% of patients with VIN have foci of occult early invasion that usually measure less than 1 mm. Sometimes VIN are present in the surrounding tissue of invasive lesions. About a quarter of the patients have an associated noncontiguous malignancy, e.g., cervical cancer, breast cancer, basal cell tumors, or ovarian neoplasms (FEUER et al. 1989).

For the majority of lesions wide local excision is curative. Because groin nodes are never involved, lymphadenectomy is not necessary (FRIEDRICH et al. 1980). Laser surgery can be used to remove VIN successfully (BORNSTEIN and KAUFMANN 1988). However, prior to therapy multiple biopsies, especially of irregular raised foci, have to be performed in order to exclude early invasion. Local treatment with 5-fluorouracil is not recommended as a method of achieving definitive cure as 40% of VIN persist or recur.

In multifocal VIN total excision may include most of the vulva (DISAIA and RICH 1981). To avoid total vulvectomy in a multifocal VIN, a "skinning" vulvectomy with skin grafting can be performed.

Four forms of VIN can be recognized:

1. Bowen's disease
2. Erythroplasia of Queyrat
3. Carcinoma simplex
4. Paget's disease of the vulva

Bowen's disease of the vulva is a form of intraepithelial carcinoma. Typically there is a whitish discoloration and shrinkage of the vulva. Histologically the epithelium is atypical: there is total loss of the normal stratification, with hyperkeratosis, parakeratosis, acanthosis, and thickening.

Vulvar erythroplasia of Queyrat is a variant of Bowen's disease. Hyperkeratosis and parakeratosis are not prominent. The atypical epithelium lacks maturation and stratification. No invasion is present.

In Paget's disease the epidermis contains distinctive clear cells, so-called Paget's cells, which are large and rounded or oval in shape. Nests of large pale Paget's cells are seen at the tips of the rete ridges, and single cells infiltrate upward in the epithelium. Paget's cells can be easily differentiated from surrounding keratinocytes. There is little or no alteration of the maturation. Twenty percent of patients have an associated underlying adenocarcinoma.

The gross appearance of Paget's disease is an erythematous, thickened, and irregular lesion. Usually it shows an area which is uniformly reddened, sharply demarcated, slightly elevated, edematous, and somewhat indurated.

Paget's disease of the vulva should be treated with wide local excision. There is an increased risk of

J. BAHNSEN, MD, PhD, Professor, Abteilung für Gynäkologische Radiologie, Frauenklinik, Universitätskrankenhaus Eppendorf, Martinistraße 52, D-20251 Hamburg, Germany
H.J. FRISCHBIER, MD, PhD, Professor, Klövensteenweg 64, D-22559 Hamburg-Rissen, Germany

other synchronous malignancies, and careful follow-up is necessary because recurrence is frequent.

6.2 Verrucous Carcinoma

Verrucous carcinoma of the vulva is a rare variant of squamous cell carcinoma. Clinically, the lesion mimics condylomata acuminata. The association of these tumors with condylomata acuminata is supported by the identification of human papilloma virus DNA in the neoplasm. Large tumors are called Buschke-Löwenstein tumors. Histologically they are well-differentiated carcinomas with prominent acanthosis and parakeratosis. The dermal papillae have a chronic inflammatory cell infiltrate. Keratin inclusions are not present. Cellular atypia is seen, especially at the base of the rete ridges. Growth is locally destructive; metastasis, however, is extremely rare.

Radiotherapy is contraindicated in verrucous carcinoma because some cases show a more aggressive behavior afterwards.

6.3 Primary Cancer of Bartholin's Gland

Tumors of Bartholin's gland are rare. About 1% of all vulvar carcinomas derive from this gland (Heine and Vahrson 1987). To distinguish a cancer of Bartholin's gland from other vulvar tumors, certain criteria should be fulfilled (Chamlian and Taylor 1972):

1. Histological differentiation compatible with Bartholin's gland
2. Location at the posterior part of the labia majora
3. Connection with ducts of the gland
4. Normal overlying skin

Tumors of Bartholin's gland include adenocarcinoma, adenoacanthoma, squamous cell carcinoma, and adenoid cystic carcinoma, the most frequent of which is adenocarcinoma. The periodic acid-schiff reaction is positive for the presence of mucopolysaccharides. Adenoacanthomas look like adenocarcinomas containing areas of distinct neoplastic squamous metaplasia. Squamous cell carcinomas arise from the duct of the gland. Because the histological appearance is similar to that of squamous cell carcinomas of other parts of the vulva, the above-mentioned criteria must be employed to diagnose a primary growth in Bartholin's gland. Occasionally there is fixation at the pubic bone.

Adenoid cystic carcinoma is formed by islands of relatively small cells with central areas of microcystic formation. There is a tendency for early vascular invasion by this tumor.

Adenocarcinoma and adenoid cystic carcinoma of the vulva occasionally derive from the glandulae vestibulares minores. Due to the rarity of tumors of Bartholin's gland, reports about treatment are anecdotal. The therapeutic approach is similar to that in the usual form of vulvar cancer. In many cases radical surgery is limited by fixation at the pubic bone. Radiation therapy has to include deep structures of the pelvic floor.

6.4 Melanoma

The vulva constitutes only 1% of the total skin surface, yet more than 5% of all melanomas in the female arise in this organ. Vulvar melanomas are four times more common in Caucasian women. Compared with squamous cell carcinoma, melanoma of the vulva presents at a significantly younger age. Of 112 cases cited in the 21st Annual Report, the mean age was 46 years in stage 0, 51 in stage I, 62.4 in stage II, 70.76 in stage III, and 63.7 in stage IV (Pettersson 1991). The preferred sites of growth are the clitoris and the labia minora.

The three major forms are lentigo maligna melanoma, superficial spreading melanoma, and nodular melanoma. Lentigo maligna melanoma presents as a flat freckled lesion, often with a speckled appearance; usually it remains superficial. The most common melanoma on the vulva is the superficial spreading one. Nodular melanoma is a raised tumor with an irregular surface; it carries a bad prognosis.

The stage distribution shows more stage I cases (44.7%, Pettersson 1991). The stage-dependent survival is lower compared with squamous cell carcinoma (e.g., stage I: 65.5% vs 71.7%).

The prognosis of vulvar melanoma correlates with the tumor thickness, which can be measured by the Clark or Breslow classification. As the prognosis for patients with groin node involvement is fatal, radical vulvectomy can be reduced to wide local excision. Radiotherapy is of very limited value: The radiation dose required to destroy melanoma exceeds the tolerance of the vulva in general. Nevertheless, three of eight women with melanoma of the vulva who received primary irradiation survived 5 years (see Sect. 5.11).

In 1983 the Gynecologic Oncology Group started a study of vulvar melanoma (Phillips et al. 1994). Modified radical vulvectomy was employed as minimal therapy. Groin dissection was optional. From 1983 to 1990 83 cases were entered in the study. Multivariant analysis revealed two independent factors that were indicative of groin metastasis: angiosis carcinomatosa and a central location. It was concluded that the biological behavior of vulvar melanoma is similar to that of other nongenital melanomas.

6.5 Other Special Malignancies

Adenoid cystic carcinoma of the vulva is a highly radiosensitive tumor. Adjuvant radiotherapy should be considered as a part of the primary therapy (Rose et al. 1991).

Basal cell carcinoma is the most common malignant skin cancer; however, involvement of the vulva is rare. About 2%–3% of all vulvar neoplasms are basal cell carcinomas (Schueller 1965). Metastasis is extremely rare. Most cases can be cured by wide local excision: only some large and invasive lesions may require radical surgery. Little information is available on the use of radiotherapy in the treatment of basal cell tumors of the vulva. The cure rate of basal cell carcinoma of the skin is 94%–98% (Goldberg and Rubin 1989).

The most frequent *sarcoma* of the vulva is the leiomyosarcoma. Other forms are neurofibrosarcoma, rhabdomyosarcoma, fibrosarcoma, and angiosarcoma. Wide local excision is recommended as initial treatment; however, no controlled trials are available on this topic.

References

Bornstein J, Kaufmann RH (1988) Combination of surgical excision and CO2 laser vaporization for multifocal vulvar intraepithelial neoplasia. Am J Gynecol 158:459

Chamlian DL, Taylor HB (1972) Primary carcinoma of Bartholin's gland. Obstet Gynecol 39:489

Collins CG, Ramon-Lopez JJ, Lee FYL (1987) Intraepithelial carcinoma of the vulva. Am J Obstet Gynecol 108:1187

Crun CP, Liskow A, Petras P, Keng WC, Frick HC (1984) Vulvar intraepithelial neoplasia (severe atypia and carcinoma in situ). Cancer 54:1429–1434

DiSaia P, Rich WM (1981) Surgical approach to multifocal carcinoma in situ of the vulva. Am J Obstet Gynecol 140:136–145

Feuer GA, Shevchuk M, Calanog A (1989) Vulvar Paget's disease: the need to exclude an invasive lesion. Gynecol Oncol 38:81–89

Friedrich EG, Wilkinson EJ (1982) The vulva. In: Blaustein A (ed) Pathology of the female genital tract. Springer, Berlin Heidelberg New York, pp 13–58

Friedrich EG, Wilkinson EJ, Fu YS (1980) Carcinoma in situ of the vulva: a continuing challenge. Am J Obstet Gynecol 136:880

Goldberg LH, Rubin HA (1989) Management of basal cell carcinoma. Which option is best? Postgrad Med 85:57–63

Heine O, Vahrson H (1987) Das primäre Karzinom der Bartholinischen Druse. Geburtshilfe Frauenheilkd 47:35–40

Pettersson F (1991) Annual report on the results of treatment in gynecologic cancer. Int J Gynecol Obstet 36 (Suppl):1–315

Phillips GL, Bundy BN, Okagaki T, Kucera PR, Stehman FB (1994) Malignant melanoma of the vulva treated by radical hemivulvectomy. A prospective study of the Gynecologic Oncology Group. Cancer 73:2626–2632

Rose PG, Tak WK, Reale FR, Hunter RE (1991) Adenoid cystic carcinoma of the vulva: a radiosensitive tumor. Gynecol Oncol 43:81–83

Schueller EF (1965) Basal cell cancer of the vulva. Am J Obstet Gynecol 93:199–208

Young JL, Percy CL, Asire AS (1981) Surveillance, epidemiology and end results: incidence and mortality data, 1973–1977. Monogr Natl Cancer Inst 57:982

7 Cancer of the Vagina

C.A. PEREZ

CONTENTS

C.A. PEREZ, MD, Director, Radiation Oncology Center, Mallinckrodt Institute of Radiology, Washington University Medical Center, 4511 Forest Park, Suite 200, St. Louis, MO 63108, USA

7.1 Epidemiology and Risk Factors

Primary malignant tumors of the vagina arise in this organ; there should be documentation that the lesion does not involve the cervix or vulva. It is a rare tumor, representing 1%–2% of all gynecologic malignancies (DAW 1971; HERBST et al. 1970; ROBBOY et al. 1975). Most vaginal neoplasms (more than 80%) are metastatic, involving the vagina by direct extension or by lymphatic or hematogenous routes (HILLBORNE and FU 1987).

The majority of primary vaginal cancers are squamous cell in origin. A review by HERBST et al. (1970) showed that half of the patients (47.1%) with epidermoid carcinoma were 60 years of age or older, with a peak incidence in the 50- to 70-year-old age group and a mean age of 60–65 years. No apparent etiology or associated factors predisposing a patient to this malignancy were identified.

BRINTON et al. (1990), in a study of 41 women with carcinoma in situ or invasive carcinoma of the vagina and 97 community control patients, identified low socioeconomic level, history of genital warts, vaginal discharge or irritation, a previous abnormal Papanicolaou smear, early hysterectomy, and, less significantly, vaginal trauma as potential risk factors.

Irradiation was suggested as a possible cause of primary squamous cell carcinoma of the vagina (WAY 1948). In a report of 43 patients, five of whom presented with invasive carcinoma of the vagina 7 or more years after radiation therapy for invasive carcinoma of the cervix, PRIDE et al. (1979) suggested, without statistical basis, that these lesions may have been irradiation induced. BOICE et al. (1988) reported a greater risk of developing vaginal cancer in a survey of 150000 women treated in 20 worldwide oncology clinics. A 14-fold risk was observed in women irradiated under the age of 45 years, and a dose-response relationship was found to be significant. However, an analysis of 1200 patients treated with radiation therapy over a period of 20 years at our institution showed no increase in the incidence of pelvic second neoplasias (Lee et al. 1982).

In 1971 increased incidence of clear cell adenocarcinoma of the vagina in young women was found to be associated with administration of diethylstilbestrol (DES) to the mother during pregnancy (Herbst et al. 1971). The incidence of clear cell adenocarcinoma in women prenatally exposed to DES is estimated to be between 0.14 and 1.4 per 1000 (Herbst 1988; Melnick et al. 1987).

In a recent update by Herbst and Anderson (1990), it was noted that in 1990 there were 547 cases of clear cell adenocarcinoma of the vagina and cervix recorded in the Registry for Research on Hormonal Transplacental Carcinogenesis. As summarized by Hicks and Piver (1992), the most recent findings of the Registry were: (1) 60% of registered patients had been exposed to DES or similar synthetic estrogens in utero, (2) 60% of the registered lesions were vaginal and 40% were cervical primary tumors, (3) cervical tumors were located primarily in the exocervix and vaginal lesions mainly in the upper third of the anterior vaginal wall, (4) ages at diagnosis ranged from 7 to 34 years (median, 19 years), and (5) risk of developing adenocarcinoma of the cervix or vagina in the exposed female population from birth to 34 years of age was approximately 1 case per 1000 women. This implies that these tumors are extremely rare among DES-exposed females and that DES is not a complete carcinogen. About 90% of patients were reported to have early-stage adenocarcinoma (I and II) at the time of diagnosis.

Horwitz et al. (1988) noted that the incidence of DES-induced carcinoma of the vagina and cervix increased up to 1979 and decreased slightly from 1980 to 1982; therefore continued surveillance of patients exposed to DES is critical. Median age at tumor diagnosis was 19 years (Herbst et al. 1971; Melnick et al. 1987). Herbst et al. (1971) observed a close correlation between the annual incidence of clear cell adenocarcinoma of the vagina and cervix and the estimated use of DES for pregnancy support in the United States. An association was found between the risk of developing vaginal cancer and the time of first exposure to DES; the risk was greatest for those exposed during the first 16 weeks in utero and declined for those whose exposure began in the 17th week or later (Perez et al. 1992).

Bornstein et al. (1988) reported an incidence of cervical and vaginal intraepithelial neoplasia in DES-exposed donors twice as high as in unexposed women. This was also associated with a higher incidence of herpes simplex virus and human papillomavirus infections. Their speculation that DES has a role in the development of squamous genital neoplasias in women has been demonstrated experimentally in mice (Forsberg 1975).

7.2 Topographic Anatomy and Patterns of Spread

7.2.1 Anatomy

The vagina is a muscular, dilatable tube, averaging 7.5 cm in length, that extends from the uterus to the vulva. It is located posterior to the base of the bladder and urethra and anterior to the rectum. The upper quarter of the posterior wall is separated from the rectum by a reflection of peritoneum called the pouch of Douglas. At its uppermost extent the vaginal wall meets the uterine cervix, attaching at a higher point on the posterior wall than on the anterior wall. The circular groove formed at the juncture of the vagina and the cervix is called the fornix.

The vaginal wall is composed of three layers: the mucosa, the muscularis, and the adventitia. The inner mucosal layer is formed by a thick, nonkeratinizing, stratified, squamous epithelium overlying a basement membrane containing many papillae. The epithelium normally contains no glands but is lubricated by mucous secretions originating in the cervix. The mucosa forms many transverse folds called rugae. The epithelium changes little in response to the reproductive cycle. The muscularis layer is composed of smooth muscle fibers arranged circularly on the inner portion and longitudinally on the thicker outer portion. A vaginal sphincter is formed by skeletal muscle at the introitus. The adventitia is a thin, outer connective tissue layer that merges with that of adjacent organs.

The lymphatic drainage of the vagina consists of an extensive intercommunicating network. The lymphatics in the upper portion of the vagina drain primarily via the lymphatics of the cervix, whereas those in the lowest portion of the vagina drain either cephalad to cervical lymphatics or follow drainage patterns of the vulva into femoral and inguinal nodes. The anterior vaginal wall usually drains into the deep pelvic nodes, including the interiliac and parametrial nodes.

7.2.2 Patterns of Spread

Vaginal cancers occur most commonly on the posterior wall of the upper third of the vagina. In an extensive review of the literature, PLENTL and FRIEDMAN (1971) found that 51.7% of primary vaginal cancers occurred in the upper third of the vagina and 57.6% on the posterior wall.

Tumors originating in the vagina may spread along the vaginal wall to involve the cervix or vulva. However, if biopsies of the cervix or the vulva are positive at the time of initial diagnosis, the tumor cannot be considered a primary vaginal lesion. Because of the absence of anatomic barriers, vaginal tumors readily extend into surrounding tissues. Lesions in the anterior vaginal wall may involve the vesicovaginal septum; those in the posterior wall may displace the vaginal mucosa and may eventually invade the rectovaginal septum. Vaginal cancer may invade the paracolpal and parametrial tissues, extending to the pelvic walls and even the uterosacral ligaments.

The incidence of positive pelvic nodes at diagnosis varies with the stage and location of the primary tumor. Because the lymphatic system of the vagina is so complex, any of the nodal groups may be involved regardless of the location of the lesion (PLENTL and FRIEDMAN 1971). Involvement of inguinal nodes is most common when the lesion is located in the lower third of the vagina. The reported incidence of clinically positive inguinal nodes at diagnosis ranges from 5.3% to 33%, depending on the proximal or distal location of the tumor in the vagina (BROWN et al. 1971; PEREZ et al. 1988; PLENTL and FRIEDMAN 1971; STOCK et al. 1992; WHELTON and KOTTMEIER 1962).

After treatment, a few local failures (5%–10%) are noted in patients with stage 0 disease without pelvic recurrences or distant metastases. In patients with stage I disease, the frequency of pelvic recurrences is 10%–20%. A similar incidence of distant metastases is reported. In stage II disease, in which there is more paravaginal or parametrial infiltration, the pelvic recurrence rate increases to 35%, and distant metastases are more common (22%) (Table 7.1). In patients with stage III disease, the incidence of local recurrence varies between 25% and 37%, and distant metastases have been reported in approximately 25% of patients. In patients with stage IV disease,

Table 7.1. Carcinoma of the vagina: outcome of stage I and II disease treated with radiation therapy alone. (Modified from PEREZ et al. 1983)

Investigator	No. of patients (stage)	Survival	No. of recurrences (%)		
			Pelvis	Pelvis + distant metastases	Distant metastases
Stage I					
BROWN et al. (1971)	21	85%[a]	1 (4.8)		1 (4.8)
DANCUART et al. (1988)	71		15 (21)	2 (2.8)	2 (2.8)
DELCLOS (1984)	27	63%[b]	4 (14.8)[c]		2 (7.4)
MARCUS et al. (1978)	6	80%	0	0	0
PEREZ et al. (1988)	50	75%	4 (8)	3 (6)	5 (10)
Total[d]	175		20 (11)	5 (3)	10 (6)
Stage II					
BROWN et al. (1971)	25	76%[a]	2 (8)	2 (8)[e]	1 (4)[e]
DANCUART et al. (1988)	42		7 (16.7)		2 (4.8)
DELCLOS (1984)	47	55%[b]	8 (17)[c]		3 (6.4)
MARCUS et al. (1978)	10	50%[b]	1 (10)		2 (20)
PEREZ et al. (1988)	49 (IIA)	55%	10 (20.4)	9 (18.4)	6 (12.2)
	26 (IIB)	43%	5 (19.2)	7 (26.9)	5 (19.2)
Total[d]	199		25 (12.5)	18 (9)	19 (9.5)

[a] Determinate, 5 years.
[b] Absolute, 5 years, no evidence of disease.
[c] Value is combined total of recurrences in pelvis and pelvis plus distant metastases in study by DELCLOS (1984).
[d] Excluding DELCLOS (1984).
[e] One patient had inguinal node metastasis.

Table 7.2. Carcinoma of the vagina: outcome of stage III and IV disease treated with radiation therapy alone. (Modified from Perez et al. 1983)

Investigator	No. of patients	Survival	No. of recurrences (%)		
			Pelvis	Pelvis + distant metastasis	Distant metastasis
Stage III					
Brown et al. (1971)	16	40%[a]	4 (25)	0	1 (6.3)
Dancuart et al. (1988)	42		10 (24)		5 (12)
Delclos (1984)	27	37%[b]	10 (37)[c]		0
Marcus et al. (1978)	3	100%[b]	0	0	0
Perez et al. (1988)	16	32%	0	6 (37.5)	4 (25)
Total[d]	104		14 (13.4)	6 (6)	10 (9.6)
Stage IV					
Brown et al. (1971)	13	0	5 (38.5)	2 (15.4)	1 (7.7)
Dancuart et al. (1988)	11		3 (27)	1 (9)	1 (9)
Delclos (1984)	6	0	3 (50)[c]		1 (16.7)
Marcus et al. (1978)	3	50%[b]	1 (33.3)	0	0
Perez et al. (1988)	8	10%	2 (25)	4 (50)	0
Total[d]	41		11 (29)	7 (17)	3 (7.3)

[a] Determinate, 5 years.
[b] Absolute, 5 years, no evidence of disease.
[c] Value is combined total of recurrences in pelvis and pelvis plus distant metastases in study by Delclos (1984).
[d] Excluding Delclos (1984).

there is a high incidence of pelvic failure (58%) and distant metastases (about 30%) (Table 7.2).

Tarraza et al. (1991) noted that upper (distal) vagina lesions more commonly recurred locally, whereas lower (proximal) lesions were associated with pelvic side wall and distant recurrence. Most of these patients had locally extensive tumors.

In squamous cell carcinoma of the vagina, metastases to the lungs or supraclavicular nodes may occur in patients with more advanced disease. However, Robboy et al. (1974) reported that metastases to the lungs or supraclavicular lymph nodes represented 35% of the recurrences in young women with clear cell adenocarcinoma, a proportion much greater than that found with squamous cell carcinoma of the cervix or vagina.

7.3 Clinical Presentation

Abnormal vaginal bleeding is the most common presenting symptom of primary vaginal tumors (50%–75% of patients) (Herbst et al. 1971; Livingstone 1950; Rutledge 1967; Underwood and Smith 1971). It may occur as dysfunctional bleeding or postcoital spotting. Vaginal discharge is also common. Less frequent presenting complaints are dysuria and pelvic pain, which occur with more advanced disease.

7.4 Diagnostic Workup and Staging

Following a complete history and physical examination, speculum examination and palpation of the vagina are essential in the diagnostic workup. The speculum must be rotated as it is withdrawn so that anterior/posterior wall lesions, which may occur, are not overlooked. Bimanual pelvic and rectal examinations are integral elements in the clinical evaluation of these patients.

Exfoliative cytology studies may detect early squamous cell lesions of the vagina, but this is not true for clear cell adenocarcinomas, which often start out as submucosal lesions (Barber and Sommers 1974). Biopsies are frequently obtained at the time of initial examination. Schiller's test (with Lugol's solution) and colposcopy are useful for directed biopsies in abnormal sites in the vagina. A metastatic evaluation including cytoscopy and proctosigmoidoscopy should be performed on patients with pathologically confirmed invasive vaginal carcinoma.

In addition to a chest x-ray, intravenous pyelography and when indicated barium enema or air contrast, computed tomography, and magnetic resonance imaging have been increasingly used in the evaluation of patients with tumors of the vagina (HRICAK et al. 1988; TOGASHI et al. 1986). CHANG et al. (1988) reported the results of pelvic magnetic resonance imaging in 87 women: 51 with normal vagina, 2 with benign cysts, and 34 with vaginal carcinoma (8 primary, 22 metastatic, and 8 recurrent).

Table 7.3. Clinical staging of malignant tumors of the vagina. (From PEREZ et al. 1992)

AJC[a]	FIGO[b]	
Tx		Primary tumor cannot be assessed
Tis	0	Carcinoma in situ (intraepithelial)
T1	I	Confined to vaginal mucosa
T2	II	Submucosal infiltration into parametrium, not extending to pelvic wall
	IIA[c]	Subvaginal infiltration, not into parametrium
	IIB[c]	Parametrial infiltration, not extending to pelvic wall
T3	III	Tumor extending to pelvic wall
T4	IV	Tumor extension to bladder or rectum or metastasis outside true pelvis

[a] American Joint Committee.
[b] International Federation of Gynecology and Obstetrics.
[c] Proposed subdivision for stage II lesions (PEREZ et al. 1973).

These findings were correlated with surgical-pathologic findings; the positive predictive value of the test for primary and metastatic tumors was 84% and the negative predictive value 97%. The accuracy of magnetic resonance imaging in detection of recurrent vaginal carcinoma was 82%, compared with clinical or surgical findings. The lesions are better seen on T2 predominant images using transverse planes 5 mm thick. The authors stated that this examination could effectively differentiate between fibrotic tissue and grossly recurrent tumor, findings reported by others (EBNER et al. 1988; GLAZER et al. 1985). Bone scan is indicated only in patients with stage III or IV disease, or if symptoms warrant it.

Staging should be performed jointly by the gynecologic and radiation oncologists with the patient under general anesthesia. At that time additional biopsy specimens of the vagina should be taken at various sites to determine the limits of abnormal vaginal mucosa. Multiple biopsies of the cervix are necessary to rule out a cervical primary tumor. If there is a concomitant malignant lesion of the same histology in the cervix or if biopsies demonstrate a similar tumor, the lesion must be classified as a primary cervical carcinoma and staged accordingly. According to SEDLIS and ROBBOY (1987), a vaginal neo-

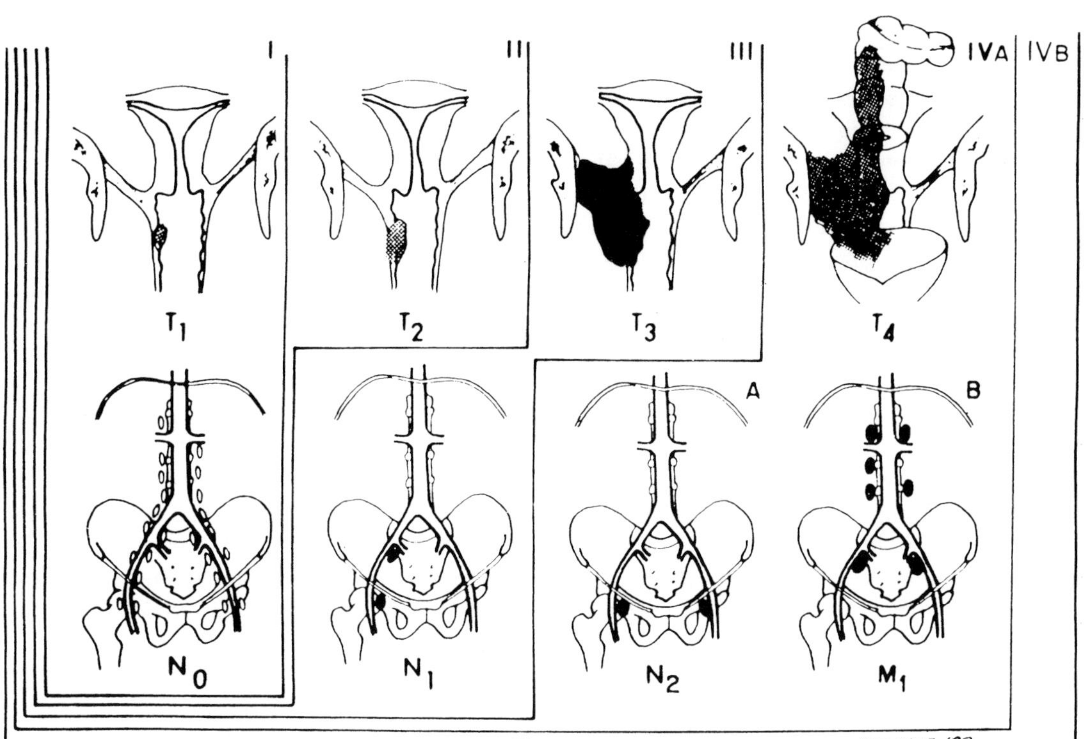

Fig. 7.1. Clinical staging in carcinoma of vagina, FIGO system. (Modified from RUBIN 1983)

plasm may be considered primary if there is neither cervical nor vulvar cancer at the time of diagnosis or for 10 years before diagnosis.

Patients are staged using the International Federation of Gynecology and Obstetrics (FIGO) or American Joint Committee (AJC) staging system (Table 7.3 and Fig. 7.1). Carcinomas in situ are superficial tumors that have not penetrated the basement membrane of the mucosal layer. They tend to be multicentric. Stage I lesions, although confined to the mucosa, may spread to involve more than one vaginal wall. We proposed that FIGO stage II be subdivided into IIA (subvaginal infiltration only) and IIB (parametrial extension) because of the larger volume and more aggressive behavior of tumors with parametrial involvement (Perez et al. 1973).

7.5 Histopathologic Classification

7.5.1 Epithelial Neoplasms

Squamous cell carcinoma has well-known histologic characteristics. It may be very difficult or impossible to distinguish between a primary vaginal squamous lesion and a recurrence of cervical or vulvar cancer. Extension to the vagina from tumors in either of these sites exceeds the frequency of primary vaginal squamous cell carcinoma. Further, squamous neoplasms may involve multiple different sites in the lower female genital tract (Choo and Morley 1980; Friedrich et al. 1980). Rarely squamous carcinomas have prominent spindle cell features (Steeper et al. 1983). A grade is assigned based on a combination of cytologic and histologic features, but correlation between grade and survival has not been established (Cavanaugh et al. 1980; Perez et al. 1992, 1974).

Verrucous carcinoma is a variant of well-differentiated squamous cell carcinoma that occasionally occurs in the vagina, presenting as a relatively large, well-circumscribed, soft cauliflower-like mass (Faaborg et al. 1979; Kraus and Perez-Mesa 1966; Powell et al. 1978; Ramzy et al. 1976; Vayrynen et al. 1981). Microscopically, the tumor exhibits a papillary growth pattern with marked hyperkeratosis and broad, bulbous pegs of acanthotic epithelium that push into the underlying stroma. Cytologic features of malignancy are lacking. Because of its well-differentiated character, the microscopic diagnosis of verrucous carcinoma may be difficult, especially if the biopsy is superficial. Verrucous carcinoma rarely, if ever, metastasizes (Perez et al. 1992).

Small cell carcinoma may occur in the vagina, either in pure form or associated with squamous or glandular elements. A high proportion will show ultrastructural or immunohistochemical evidence of neuroendocrine differentiation (Fukushima et al. 1986; Ulich et al. 1986).

Primary adenocarcinoma of the vagina is rare and occurs predominantly in postmenopausal women.

Malignant melanoma is the second most common cancer of the vagina, representing 2.8%–5% of all vaginal neoplasms (Chung et al. 1980; Iverson and Robins 1980; Norris and Taylor 1966). Melanoma is most frequent in the lower third of the vagina (Chung et al. 1980) and varies considerably in size, color, and growth pattern (Morrow and DiSaia 1976; Ragni and Tobon 1974). The tumor may be composed of spindled, epithelioid, or small lymphocyte-like cells, and the cells may or may not be pigmented. Poorly differentiated lesions are difficult to distinguish from sarcomas or squamous cell carcinomas but may be identified by their distinctive ultrastructural features or immunoperoxidase staining pattern (Berman et al. 1981). Tumor depth invasion according to the method of Breslow should be assessed since it is the best predictor of survival (Bonner et al. 1988; Iverson and Robins 1980).

7.5.2 Mesenchymal Tumors

Smooth muscle tumors, although rare, are the most common benign and malignant mesenchymal tumors in adult women (Davos and Abell 1976; Peters et al. 1985b). They are usually submucosal. The gross appearance varies greatly depending on cellularity, type and extent of degenerative change, and amount of necrosis and hemorrhage (Tavassoli and Norris 1979; Tobon et al. 1973). Microscopically, smooth muscle tumors are composed of interlacing bundles of spindle-shaped cells with blunt-ended nuclei and fibrillar cytoplasm. An epithelioid pattern and extensive myxoid change have been reported in a few vaginal smooth muscle tumors (Chen et al. 1980; Tavassoli and Norris 1979).

The behavior of some smooth muscle tumors may be difficult to predict based on histologic appearance. Important prognostic factors include status of the tumor border (infiltrative versus circumscribed), mitotic rate, and degree of cytologic atypicality.

Tavassoli and Norris (1979) concluded that smooth muscle tumors with five or more mitoses/ten high-power fields, significant cellular atypia, diameter of 3 cm or more, and infiltrating margins are at risk to recur or metastasize.

Embryonal rhabdomyosarcoma, botryoid variant, is the most common malignant tumor of the vagina in pediatric patients (90% occur in children under 5 years of age) (Copeland et al. 1985; Davos and Abell 1976). Rhabdomyosarcomas have a characteristic gross appearance consisting of multiple gray-red, translucent, grapelike masses that fill and protrude from the vagina. Microscopically there is a continuous zone of condensed round or spindle cells immediately beneath the intact vaginal epithelium. Elsewhere, the tumor is composed of small dark cells sparsely distributed in a myxoid stroma; some cells may show intensely eosinophilic cytoplasm with cross-striations (Perez et al. 1992).

Other *primary sarcomas* involving the vagina include endometrial stromal sarcoma (Berkowitz et al. 1978; Granai et al. 1984; Ulbright and Kraus 1981), alveolar soft part sarcoma (Chapman et al. 1984; Kasai et al. 1980), malignant fibrous histiocytoma (Webb et al. 1974), synovial-like sarcoma, malignant mixed tumor (Okagaki et al. 1976; Shevchuk et al. 1978), angiosarcoma (Antonioli and Burke 1975; Prempree et al. 1983), and hemangiopericytoma (Buscema et al. 1985; Hiura and Nagai 1985).

Malignant lymphoma may be localized to the female genital tract or be part of a widespread process (Chorlton et al. 1974; Harris and Scully 1984). Vaginal bleeding is the chief complaint in 65% of patients, with dyspareunia and vaginal discharge being less frequent symptoms (Perren et al. 1992; Prévot et al. 1992). In 20 patients with primary Hodgkin's disease of the vagina, 13 had localized mass or nodular elevated tumors, and diffuse involvement was rare; 12 of the tumors were stage IE or 2IIE (Prévot et al. 1992). Most primary malignant lymphomas involving the vagina are of the diffuse large cell type, but nodular lymphomas also occur. The histologic diagnosis depends on the identification of monomorphous, cytologically atypical, mitotically active lymphoid cells deeply penetrating the stroma. Characteristically, the mucosa is intact. Marker studies are useful in distinguishing difficult or equivocal cases from lymphoma-like lesions. Leukemic infiltration, especially granulocytic sarcoma, can be impossible to distinguish from malignant lymphoma. A chloroacetate esterase stain is helpful in some cases.

7.5.3 Vaginal Adenosis and Clear Cell Carcinoma

As noted by Gersell in a chapter by Perez et al. (1992), vaginal adenosis is a condition in which müllerian-type glandular epithelium is present after vaginal development is complete. A great deal of attention has been focused on this lesion since its discovery in women exposed to diethylstilbestrol (DES) in utero. It is important to emphasize that while adenosis is the most common histologic abnormality in women exposed to DES in utero, it is not strictly confined to this population (Kurman and Scully 1974; Robboy et al. 1986; Sandberg 1968; Sandberg et al. 1965).

In the DES cohort, adenosis most commonly involves the anterior wall and upper third of the vagina, but may also extend into the middle and lower thirds. The classical gross appearance of adenosis is red, velvety grapelike clusters in the vagina. The process may involve the surface epithelium and/or glands in the superficial stroma (Antonioli and Burke 1975; Robboy et al. 1979, 1977b; Sandberg et al. 1965). Microscopically, the glandular epithelium may be composed of any of the müllerian epithelial cell types. Endocervical-type mucous cells are the most common; surface adenosis is composed almost exclusively of this cell type. The glands within the lamina propria may be lined by endometrial or tubal type epithelium as well (Antonioli and Burke 1975; Hart et al. 1976).

The glandular epithelium involutes via progressive squamous metaplasia (Antonioli and Burke 1975; Hart et al. 1976). Ultimately all the glandular tissue may be replaced, leaving stromal nodules or pegs of squamous epithelium containing small mucin droplets as the only residuum of the glandular elements (Robboy et al. 1977b). The gradual evolution of glandular to squamous epithelium has been documented by sequential cytology and biopsy studies (Burke et al. 1981; Ng et al. 1975; Noller et al. 1983; O'Brien et al. 1979; Robboy et al. 1981). Other gross cervicovaginal changes associated with DES exposure and adenosis include cervical ectropion and the cervicovaginal hood and its variants (Perez et al. 1992).

Both the gross and the microscopic appearance of adenosis may be altered by any process that involves native endocervical or transition zone epithelium such as microglandular hyperplasia (Robboy and Welch 1977) or CIN (Fowler et al. 1981; Mattingly and Stafl 1976; Robboy et al. 1978; Robboy et al. 1984; Stafl and Mattingly 1974).

Whether immature squamous metaplasia in adenosis is associated with an increased risk of dysplasia or squamous cell carcinoma is a controversial issue (Robboy et al. 1977A).

Diethylstilbestrol-associated clear cell carcinomas have a predilection for the exocervix and upper third of the vagina. Robboy et al. (1982) emphasized that clear cell adenocarcinomas (CCAs) are frequently located at or near the lower margin of the zone of glandular tissue in the cervix or vagina. The tumors vary greatly in size; most are exophytic and superficially invasive (Herbst et al. 1974). Microscopically they exhibit three basic histologic patterns: tubulocystic (most common), papillary, and solid. The tumor cells are either cuboidal or columnar with clear cytoplasm and a distinct cell membrane or hobnail type with large atypical protruding nuclei rimmed by a small amount of cytoplasm. Glycogen is abundant (Herbst et al. 1974). Adenosis is associated with 97% of vaginal and 52% of cervical CCAs.

The major determinant of outcome in CCA is stage, but some pathologic features are statistically associated with better outcome including a tubulocystic growth pattern, size less than $3\,cm^2$, and less than 3 mm of stromal invasion (Herbst et al. 1974). Almost all CCAs are discovered at the time of initial examination, but a few tumors have been detected among women under surveillance for adenosis (Kaufman et al. 1982).

7.6 Prognostic Factors

The most significant factor is clinical stage of the disease, which reflects the depth of penetration into the vaginal wall or surrounding tissues (Perez et al. 1983). Age of the patient, extent of mucosal involvement, gross appearance of the lesion, and degree of differentiation and keratinization have not been identified as reliable prognostic factors (Perez et al. 1974, 1983).

Livingstone (1950) reported that lesions located in the upper vagina had a better prognosis, but other authors found no correlation between primary tumor location and treatment results (Frick et al. 1968; Perez et al. 1988; Rutledge 1967; Whelton and Kottmeier 1962).

Overexpression of HER-2/*neu* oncogenes in squamous cancer of the lower genital tract is a rare event that may be associated with aggressive biologic behavior (Berchuck et al. 1990).

Patients with nonepithelial tumors (sarcoma, melanoma) have a poor prognosis with a high incidence of local failure and distant metastasis.

7.7 General Management

The preferred treatment for most carcinomas of the vagina is radiation therapy. Some authors advocate surgery (Underwood and Smith 1971), but, in general, this approach is not favored because of the excellent tumor control and good functional results obtained with adequate irradiation. Surgical procedures may be reserved for early-stage (0, I) squamous cell carcinoma, nonepithelial tumors, stage I clear cell adenocarcinomas in young women (Hoskins et al. 1989; Webb et al. 1974), and treatment of irradiation failures.

7.7.1 Surgery

Several considerations may favor treating selected patients with surgery, particularly those with localized intraepithelial disease, young patients in whom there is a desire for preservation of ovarian function, and patients with verrucous carcinoma (Powell et al. 1978). Several authors have recommended partial or total vaginectomy for patients with in situ and superficially invasive tumors (Curtis et al. 1992; Hoffman et al. 1992; Lindeque 1987). Laser vaporization has been used with a reported 50%–100% success rate. Hoffman et al. (1992) warn that laser vaporization should not be performed unless the full extent of the abnormal vaginal epithelium can be visualized, there is no suspicion of an invasive process, and there is no gross fibrosis or distortion of the posthysterectomy vaginal cuff.

In patients with stage I invasive tumors in the middle or upper third of the vagina, surgical treatment consists of a radical hysterovaginectomy and pelvic lymph node dissection. Lindeque (1987) pointed out that most tumors require removal of the full length of the vagina, although in localized lesions a partial colpectomy may be performed. Anterior vaginal lesions may be difficult to excise with an adequate margin of healthy tissue without injury to the urethra or bladder, and in posterior lesions, special attention should be given to the anterior rectal wall. For lesions in the lower third of the vagina that may encroach on the vulva, radical vulvovaginectomy and bilateral groin lymph node dissection is the procedure of choice (LINDEQUE 1987). Direct primary closure of the surgical wound may be obtained by mobilization of lateral skin and by using simple ligatures, in an attempt to decrease tension on the wound edges (LAMONT 1984). Repair of the surgical defect can also be accomplished with myocutaneous flaps (MAGRINA and MASTERSON 1981). A few authors have suggested pelvic exenteration for more extensive lesions, but radiation therapy is the method of choice. For further details, readers are referred to surgically oriented writings (LINDEQUE 1987; PEREZ et al. 1992).

7.7.2 Irradiation

Management of patients with carcinoma of the vagina is complex, and individualized radiation therapy techniques are mandatory (CHAU 1963). PEREZ et al. (1977) reported a correlation between doses of irradiation and probability of local tumor control for various stages of vaginal carcinoma. Paravaginal and parametrial interstitial implants are both frequently used if residual tumor is present after the planned external and intracavitary therapy is completed (CHAU 1963; LAUFE and BERNSTEIN 1971; MACNAUGHT et al. 1986; PUTHAWALA et al. 1983).

A combination of irradiation and surgery has been suggested to improve therapeutic results (BORONOW et al. 1987), although more complications may be seen from combined therapy.

7.7.3 Carcinoma in Situ

Carcinoma in situ of the vagina is most often managed by either surgical excision or laser vaporization. The advantage of surgical excision is that it allows histologic review of all lesions that have been removed, making it possible to rule out invasive carcinoma (PEREZ et al. 1992). Whether laser vaporization or surgical excision is used, it is sufficient to excise only the abnormal areas after they have been visualized and identified by colposcopy. It is often helpful to use Lugol's staining of the vagina to define abnormal areas. When the stain is used for identification of abnormal areas, it is important to correlate these findings with the colposcopic findings (PEREZ et al. 1992).

On rare occasions many multifocal lesions are identified, and total vaginectomy may be necessary, with reconstruction of the vagina using a split-thickness skin graft. However, irradiation should be considered as an alternative treatment method; an intracavitary application delivering 6500–8000 cGy to the involved vaginal mucosa is adequate to control most in situ lesions. Higher doses may cause significant vaginal fibrosis and stenosis. Because vaginal carcinoma tends to be multicentric, the entire vaginal mucosa is usually treated to a dose of 5000–6000 cGy. An adequate dose distribution can be obtained using a cylinder or a vaginal applicator with as large a diameter as possible. Depending on the length of the vagina, two to four radioactive sources (1.5–2 cm in length) may be necessary.

Topical chemotherapy with 5-fluorouracil (5-FU) cream can also be used to treat vaginal carcinoma in situ (TOWNSEND 1981; WOODRUFF et al. 1975); the cream must be applied nightly, and it is necessary to use a tampon to prevent the medication from leaking out onto the vulva, where it can cause intense irritation. TOWNSEND (1981) recommends 5 g of 5-FU cream intravaginally each night for 5 days with repetition of the course every 6–12 weeks until eradication of the lesions is documented. When 5-FU cream is used, the vulva should be protected with petroleum jelly to prevent irritation.

7.7.4 Stage I

Stage I carcinoma of the vagina is usually managed by radiation therapy. These invasive lesions are 0.5–1 cm thick and may involve one or more vaginal walls. Superficial tumors may be treated with only an intracavitary cylinder covering the entire vagina (6000–6500 cGy mucosal dose) and an additional 2000–3000 cGy mucosal dose only to the tumor area. If the lesion is thicker and localized to one wall, a single plane implant may be used with an intracavitary cylinder to increase the depth dose and limit excessive irradiation to the vaginal mucosa. A dose of 6000–6500 cGy is delivered to the entire vaginal mucosa and an additional 1500 cGy calculated 0.5 cm beyond the plane of the implant to the gross tumor with the involved vaginal mucosa receiving an estimated 8000–10 000 cGy (Fig. 7.2).

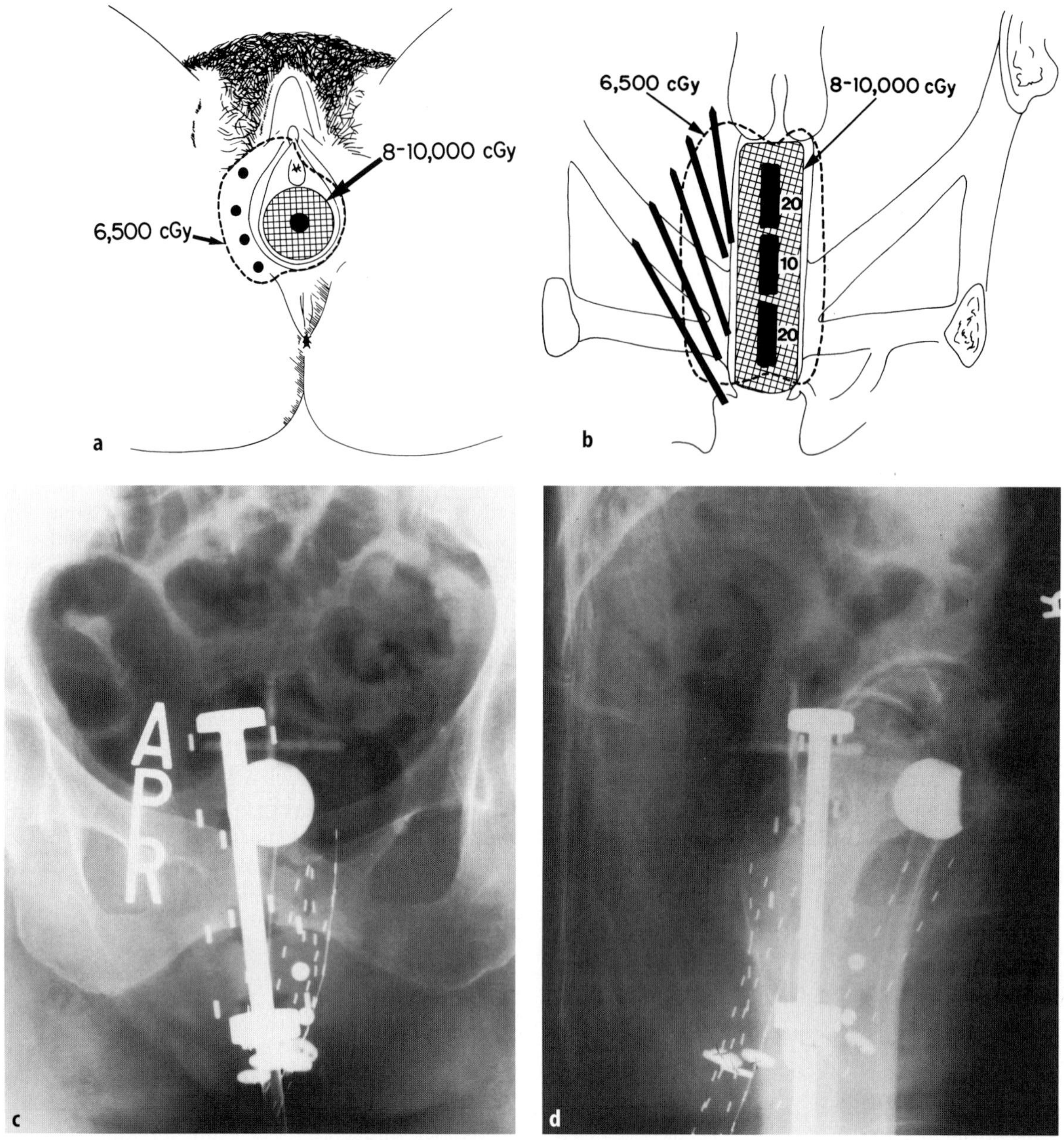

Fig. 7.2. a,b Diagrams showing the placement of an interstitial plane implant and intracavitary insertion for treatment of stage I carcinoma of the vagina (modified from Perez et al. 1977). **c** AP and **d** lateral radiographs of actual single plane implant with ^{137}Cs needles and intracavitary insertion with Delclos applicator

Use of external beam irradiation in stage I disease should be reserved for aggressive lesions (more invasive, infiltrating, or poorly differentiated) to supplement intracavitary and interstitial therapy. The whole pelvis is treated with 1000 or 2000 cGy; additional parametrial dose should be delivered with a midline (5 HVL) block to give a total of 4500–5000 cGy to the parametria. Brachytherapy doses should be adjusted accordingly.

7.7.5 Stage IIA

Patients with stage IIA tumors have more advanced paravaginal disease without extensive parametrial infiltration. They should be treated with a greater external radiation dose: 2000 cGy to the whole pelvis and an additional parametrial dose with a midline block (5 HVL) for a total of 4500–5000 cGy. A combination of intracavitary and interstitial therapy may be used to deliver a minimum of 5000–6000 cGy 0.5 cm beyond the deep margin of the tumor (in addition to the whole pelvis dose). Double-plane implants may be necessary because of extensive tumor volume. Total tumor dose should be 6500–7000 cGy.

7.7.6 Stage IIB, Stage III, and Stage IV

For advanced tumors, 4000 cGy whole pelvis and 5500–6000 cGy total parametrial doses (with midline shielding) have been given in combination with interstitial and intracavitary insertions to deliver a total tumor dose of 7500–8000 cGy to the vaginal tumor and 6500 cGy to parametrial and paravaginal extensions. An interstitial implant boost of 2000–2500 cGy is sometimes given to patients with extensive parametrial infiltration.

Boronow et al. (1987) proposed an alternative to exenterative procedures for locally advanced vulvovaginal carcinoma, using radiation therapy to treat the pelvic (internal genital) disease and a radical vulvectomy with bilateral inguinal node dissection to treat the external genital tumor. External irradiation to the pelvis and inguinal nodes consisted of 4500–5000 cGy, combined with intracavitary insertions to deliver maximum doses of 8000–8500 cGy to the vaginal mucosa with both modalities.

7.7.7 Small Cell Carcinoma

Small cell carcinoma containing neuroendocrine elements is rarely found in the female genital tract, including the vagina. As in small cell carcinoma of the lung, these tumors have a great propensity for distant dissemination, and they can be rapidly fatal (Hopkins et al. 1989). Reasonable local control has been obtained with surgical resection or radiation therapy combined with adjuvant chemotherapy. Usual drugs used are cyclophosphamide, doxorubicin (Adriamycin), and vincristine (CAV), with administration of 12 cycles, some prior to initiation of radiation therapy. Doses of irradiation are similar to those administered for squamous cell carcinoma. Of ten patients treated at our instiution with this approach, only one has survived for more than 5 years.

7.7.8 Clear Cell Adenocarcinoma

Surgery for stage I clear cell adenocarcinoma may have the advantage of ovarian preservation and better vaginal function following skin graft. However, this requires removal of most of the vagina and reconstructive procedures. The surgical procedure may involve radical pelvic surgery such as hysterectomy with pelvic lymphadenectomy, total vaginectomy, and replacement of the vagina with split-thickness skin graft (Hicks and Piver 1992). The vagina is dissected first before the abdominal procedure; a radical hysterectomy and lymph node dissection are necessary to encompass the area from the parametria and paracolpium to the side walls of the pelvis. Periaortic nodes should be sampled before the procedure to determine presence of lymphatic dissemination. Senekjian et al. (1987) reported on 176 patients treated with radical therapy and 43 with local therapy for stage I vaginal clear cell adenocarcinoma. Less extensive procedures comprising wide local excision combined with radiation therapy showed similar results, leading the authors to conclude that the combination of wide local excision with preservation of vaginal function and fertility, retroperitoneal pelvic lymphadenectomy to rule out lymph node metastasis, and subsequent local irradiation is effective treatment for tumors smaller than 2 cm. Because the tumor often spreads subepithelially, it is important that the surgeon obtain frozen section biopsies of the distal margins of resection to determine the lower margins of the surgical resection. However, Fletcher (1980a) and Wharton et al. (1975) advocate intracavitary or transvaginal irradiation alone for treatment of small tumors; this approach yields excellent tumor control with a functional vagina and preservation of ovarian function.

For more extensive lesions, external radiation therapy is essential. Techniques are similar to those described above.

7.7.9 Nonepithelial Tumors

Rhabdomyosarcoma of the vagina is generally treated with a combination of surgical resection, irradiation, and systemic chemotherapy (Piver et al. 1973). This multidisciplinary approach became the main modality of treatment in the 1970s. The Intergroup Rhabdomyosarcoma Study Group carried out numerous clinical trials, establishing the combination of vincristine, dactinomycin, and cyclophosphamide (VAC) given for 1 or 2 years as effective adjuvant therapy after surgery for stage I disease, with or without irradiation. With highly effective systemic chemotherapy and irradiation, radical surgery including pelvic exenteration can be avoided in many patients. After complete resection, irradiation of the entire pelvis is not required, thus avoiding its adverse effects. Flamant et al. (1990) reported that 15 of 17 girls with rhabdomyosarcoma of the vagina or vulva were cured after treatment with local incision, interstitial or intracavitary brachytherapy, and 18 months of alternating VAC and vincristine and doxorubicin. Twelve patients were studied for long-term sequelae: 11 had normal puberty, two had a total of three healthy children, 11 had normal menses, and ten had normal menarche.

Melanoma and leiomyosarcoma are treated primarily with radical surgical resection (vaginectomy, hysterectomy, and pelvic lymphadenectomy) (Bonner et al. 1988). Vaginal melanomas are aggressive and, according to some authors, are less suitable for radical excision (Harwood and Cummings 1982; Levitan et al. 1989).

Radical surgery, including vaginectomy, Wertheim hysterectomy and vaginectomy, or pelvic exenteration, has been used for the treatment of localized malignant lymphomas of the vagina. Satisfactory results with a combination of external irradiation and intravaginal brachytherapy combined with chemotherapy have been reported. Most often used chemotherapy is cyclophosphamide, doxorubicin, vincristine, and prednisone (CHOP) or bleomycin and CHOP (BACOP), usually six cycles. Prévot et al. (1992) felt that radical surgery should be avoided in relatively young women (49 years, mean age) and preference should be given to partial surgery combined with radiation therapy and multiagent chemotherapy. Similar treatment recommendations were made by Perren et al. (1992) for stage IE and nonbulky tumors of low and intermediate grade. They noted that many women with this tumor were likely to be sexually active, and some may wish to remain fertile, in which case combination chemotherapy as the sole modality is preferred, even for patients with localized disease.

Patients with endodermal sinus tumor of the vagina are preferentially treated with surgery and chemotherapy, since this lesion often occurs in young women and preservation of ovarian function is desired. Brachytherapy may occasionally be used, and in one instance, preservation of hormonal function and subsequent pregnancy were reported (Aartsen et al. 1993).

7.7.10 Vaginal Recurrences

Vaginal carcinoma can frequently be effectively treated with surgery after radiation therapy local failure. The surgical procedure may range from a wide local excision or partial vaginectomy to a posterior or total pelvic exenteration. Meticulous and regular follow-up examinations are important to detect the recurrence early (Perez et al. 1992).

7.8 Radiation Therapy Techniques

Irradiation treatment guidelines for vaginal carcinoma are outlined in Table 7.4.

7.8.1 External Irradiation

External irradiation should be administered using AP:PA pelvic portals that encompass the entire vagina down to the introitus and the pelvic lymph nodes to the proximal common iliac chain. Portals of 15 × 15 cm or 15 × 18 cm at the skin (16.5 × 16.5 cm or 16.5 × 21 cm at the isocenter) are usually adequate. The distal margin of the tumor should be identified with a radiopaque marker or bead when simulation radiographs are taken. In tumors involving the middle or lower third of the vagina, the inguinal and adjacent femoral lymph nodes should be electively treated (4500–5000 cGy), which requires a modification of the standard portals (Fig. 7.3a). For patients with clinically palpable nodes, additional doses of 1500 cGy (calculated at 4–5 cm) are necessary with reducing portals (Fig. 7.3b). These doses can be achieved by using unequal loadings (2AP to 1PA) with 10- to 18-MV photons, in which case a 2-cm bolus should be used when palpable lymph nodes are present. Alternatively, equal loading with photons may be used to deliver 4500–5000 cGy to the pelvic and inguinal nodes. If necessary, reduced AP portals are used to deliver a boost dose to the inguinal nodes with ^{60}Co or electrons (12–16 MeV). Special attention is needed to avoid areas of overlap (Fig. 7.3b). A combination of 6-MV x-rays on the AP portal and 18-MV photons on the PA portal will yield

Table 7.4. Carcinoma of the vagina: treatment guidelines at Mallinckrodt Institute of Radiology. (From PEREZ 1992)

FIGO stage	External radiation therapy		Brachytherapy	Total tumor dose (cGy)
	Whole pelvis	Parametrial (midline block)		
0			Intracavitary: 6500–8000 cGy SD to tumor; 6000 cGy to entire vagina	6500–8000
I Superficial			Intracavitary: 6500–8000 cGy SD to entire vagina	6500–8000
0.5 cm thick			Intracavitary/interstitial: 6500 cGy at 0.5 cm (mucosa, 10 000 cGy)	6500–7000
IIA	2000	3000	Intracavitary/interstitial: 5000–6000 cGy TD	7000–7500
IIB	2000	3000	Intracavitary/interstitial: 6500–7000 cGy TD	7500
III, IV	4000	1000[a]	Intracavitary: 5000–6000 cGy Interstitial: 2000–3000 cGy boost to parametrium	8000

Distal vagina lesions: inguinal lymph nodes receive 5000 cGy (at 3 cm). Interstitial doses are usually calculated 0.5 cm from plane of implant.
SD, surface dose; TD, tumor dose.
[a] Additional 1000-cGy boost to parametrium.

a higher dose to the inguinal nodes in relation to the midplane tumor dose. After a specified tumor dose is delivered to the whole pelvis (2000–4000 cGy, depending on extent of tumor), a midline rectangular or wedge block is interposed, and additional irradiation is given to the parametrial tissues.

The use of an anterior transmission block for irradiation of the inguinal lymph nodes in conjunction with the pelvic tissues has been described (DIGEL et al. 1989).

7.8.2 Brachytherapy

Intracavitary therapy is carried out using vaginal cylinders such as the Burnett, Bloedorn, Delclos, or MIRALVA applicators. Domed cylinders may be used for homogeneous irradiation of the vaginal cuff. DELCLOS (1984) recommends that a short cesium source be used at the top to obtain a uniform dose around the dome, since a lower dose is noted at the end of the linear cesium sources. SHARMA and BHANDARE (1991) described an ellipsoid design for the dome of Delclos applicators to obtain a more homogeneous dose. The largest possible diameter should be used to improve the ratio of mucosa to tumor dose (FLETCHER 1980a). The Bloedorn applicator consisted of a device incorporating the configuration of vaginal colpostats and a vaginal cylinder; although extensively used, it was never described in detail (DELCLOS 1984). Afterloading vaginal cylinders have been designed using a central hollow metallic cylinder, in which the sources are placed, and plastic "jackets" of varying diameter and 2.5 cm in length, which are inserted over the cylinder. In some instances the cylinders have lead shielding to protect portions of the vagina. In general, the vulva is sutured with silk or chromic catgut for the duration of the implant.

When the lesion is in the upper third, the upper vagina can be treated with the same intracavitary arrangement used for carcinoma of the uterine cervix, including an intrauterine tandem and vaginal colpostats. The middle and distal vagina are treated with a subsequent insertion of a vaginal cylinder. If the entire dose has been delivered to the upper vagina, a blank source can be used in the cylinder. Otherwise, a lower intensity source can be inserted to deliver the desired dose. Alternatively, the insertion can be condensed in one procedure using the MIRALVA (Mallinckrodt Institute of Radiology afterloading vaginal applicator) (PEREZ et al. 1990), which incorporates two ovoid sources and a central tandem that can be used to treat the entire vagina (alone or in combination with the uterine cervix). The vaginal cylinder or uterine tandem never carries an active source at the level of the ovoids to prevent excessive doses to the bladder or the rectum. The applicator has vaginal apex caps and additional cylinder sleeves that allow for increased diameters. A tandem in the uterus can be used when clinically indicated, with standard loadings, depending on the depth of the uterus (Fig. 7.4). When the tandem and vaginal cylinder are used, the strength of the sources in the ovoids should be 15 mg Ra eq.

When any type of vaginal applicator is used, it is important to determine the surface dose in addition to the tumor dose. Tables have been generated for ^{137}Cs sources (FLETCHER 1980b; SHARMA et

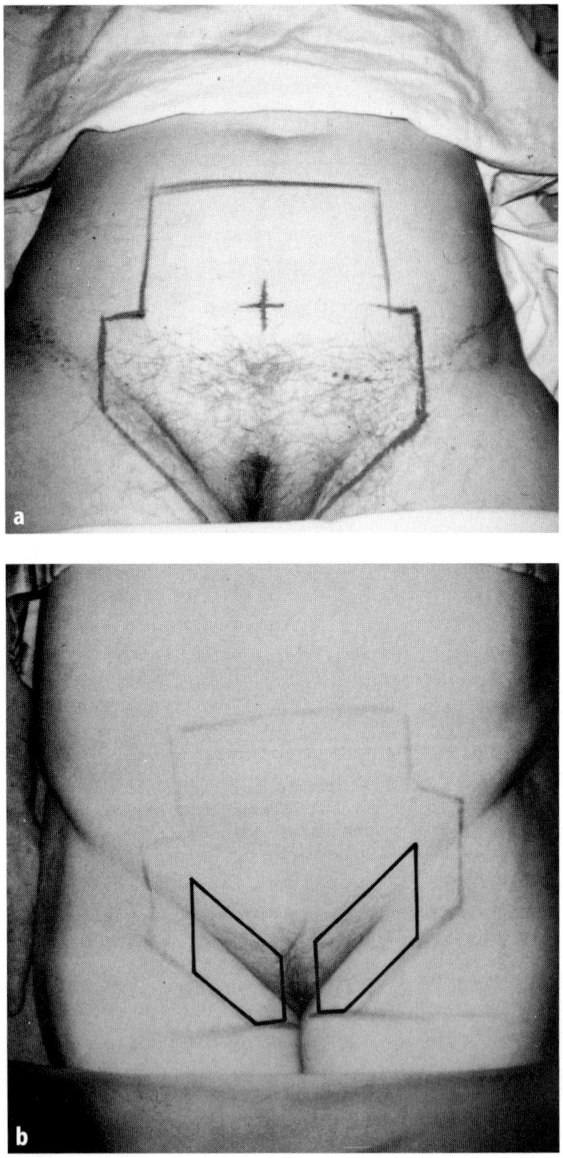

Fig. 7.3. **a** Example of portal used to treat the whole pelvis and the inguinal lymph nodes in carcinoma of the vagina. **b** Variation of treatment portals, with small fields to boost the inguinal lymph node dose with ^{60}Co or electrons (12–16 MeV). Overlap of this field should be carefully avoided. (From Perez 1992)

al. 1979). Vaginal molds for individualized intracavitary applications have been described (Bertoni et al. 1983).

Muench and Nath (1992) described a shielded vaginal applicator used with encapsulated americium (^{241}Am) and recently published careful dosimetry studies. A few patients with recurrent pelvic, including vaginal, tumors have been treated with this applicator with significant reduction of bladder and rectal doses because of the profound effect of the shielding on the 60 keV emitted by the isotope. The half-value layer of ^{241}Am is only 0.125 mm of lead (compared with 6 mm for ^{137}Cs photons).

Interstitial therapy with ^{137}Cs, ^{226}Ra needles, or afterloading ^{192}Ir needles has been employed. Depending on the extent and thickness of tumor, single-plane, double-plane, or volume implants should be planned. ^{252}Cf has been used in a few patients (Shpikalov and Atkochyus 1989).

7.8.3 High-Dose-Rate Brachytherapy

High-dose remote afterloading applicators are increasingly used in the treatment of cancer, particularly in gynecologic malignancies. The International Commission of Radiation Units and Measures (ICRU) defines high-dose-rate (HDR) brachytherapy as exceeding 1200 cGy/h. Nanavati et al. (1993) reported on 13 patients with primary vaginal carcinoma treated with this modality in combination with external irradiation. Median tumor diameter was 4 cm. Five tumors were stage I, four were IIA, and four were IIB. External irradiation consisted of 4500 cGy to the pelvis in 180-cGy daily fractions, five fractions per week, with anterior/posterior and lateral opposed fields, using 10- or 18-MV photons. Brachytherapy was administered with a Microselectron HDR unit, 10 Ci ^{192}Ir source, and a 3-cm-diameter vaginal applicator (including intrauterine tandem when an intact uterus was present). Initially, doses ranged from 2000 to 2800 cGy in three or four weekly fractions of 700 cGy. Because of decreased complications with increased fractionation, the dose prescription was changed to 2000 cGy in four 500-cGy fractions. With a median follow-up of 2.6 years, local control was achieved in 12 patients (92%), and 11 (85%) are alive and disease free. There was no significant acute or chronic intestinal or urinary tract grade 3 or 4 toxicity. Moderate to severe vaginal stenosis occurred in six patients (46%), more frequently in those who were not sexually active and refused vaginal dilation. One patient developed a partial small bowel obstruction during the external irradiation that was resolved with conservative therapy.

Stock et al. (1992) described results in 15 patients with carcinoma of the vagina treated with HDR brachytherapy; dose per treatment ranged from 300 to 800 cGy with median dose of 700 cGy, for a total dose of 2100 cGy. The median interval between fractions was 2 weeks. Brachytherapy was combined

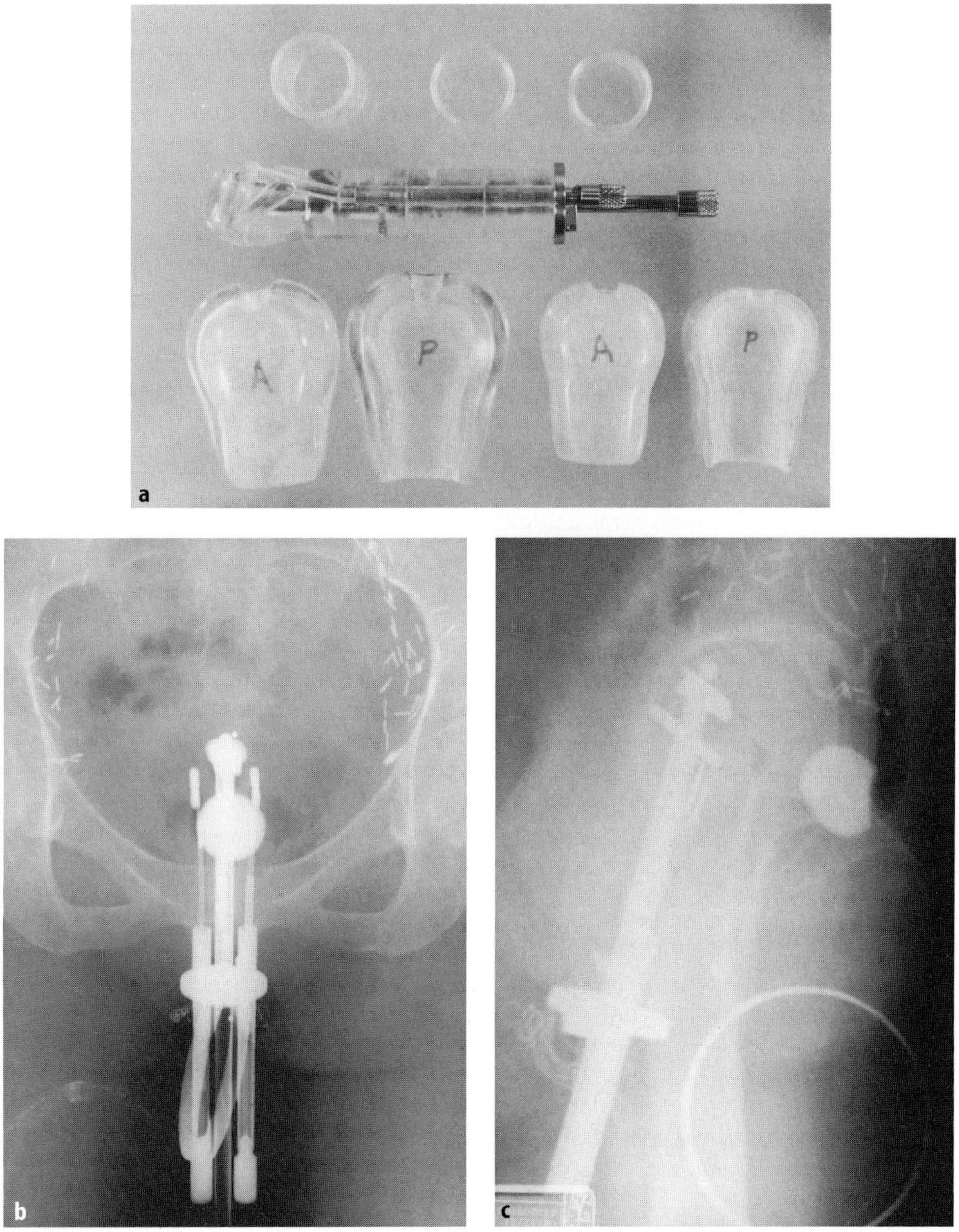

Fig. 7.4. a Mallinckrodt Insitute of Radiology afterloading vaginal applicator (MIRALVA) used for vaginal or uterovaginal applications. **b,c** Radiographs of MIRALVA applicator in place for irradiation of postradical hysterectomy vaginal cuff. (From PEREZ 1992)

with external irradiation (300–6300 cGy with a median dose of 4200 cGy, 180–236 cGy per fraction). The median total tumor dose from both components was 6300 cGy. Five-year actuarial survival was 50% in the brachytherapy compared with 9% in the external beam alone patients ($P < 0.001$), although a larger percentage of stage IV lesions occurred in the external beam alone group (36% vs 5% in the brachytherapy group). Local tumor control was 50% for stage I, 47% for stage II, and 40% for stage III. Survival closely paralleled tumor control. There was no significant difference in outcome in the two brachytherapy groups. The morbidity of therapy was reported for all 49 patients, including those treated with low dose rate, but no comment was made comparing the low- and high-dose-rate groups.

7.9 Role of Chemotherapy

As noted by McGuire in a chapter by PEREZ et al. (1992), drugs evaluated in phase II for squamous cancer of the vagina include cisplatin, etoposide, mitoxantrone, doxorubicin, lomustine, and semustine. Only doxorubicin has significant activity in squamous cancer of the vagina although the numbers of patients in each study are small. Table 7.5 summarizes the data of single-agent activity in squamous carcinomas of the vagina (PEREZ et al. 1992).

All combinations contain cisplatin, suggesting that there may be some activity of this drug in squamous vaginal cancer although the larger phase II study concluded there was minimal activity (THIGPEN et al. 1986a). Most patients in the phase II study had received prior radiation therapy, which may have abrogated the response rate. Table 7.6 summarizes the published literature regarding combination therapy in squamous vaginal cancer.

Several reports have used chemotherapy concomitant with radiation therapy in patients with locally advanced disease, making it difficult to assess the effects of chemotherapy on the disease.

PATTON et al. (1991) reported on 46 patients with advanced squamous carcinoma of the cervix and vagina treated with pelvic intra-arterial chemotherapy perfusion (mitomycin C, bleomycin, and cisplatin) and intravenous vincristine. After completion of a minimum of one and a maximum of three cycles of chemotherapy, patients were reevaluated for radiation therapy, which was administered to 41 patients (usually doses of 4000–7000 cGy to the pelvis but in seven patients, 5000–6000 cGy). Brachytherapy was administered to 28 patients (median dose, 4608 mgh). Response to initial chemotherapy was complete in 11 patients (24%) and partial in 24 (52%). Complications of chemotherapy included three treatment-related deaths, interstitial pneumonitis secondary to bleomycin in two patients, severe neutropenia in two patients, and one

Table 7.5. Single-agent cytotoxics in squamous vaginal cancer. (From PEREZ et al. 1992)

Drug response	Dose and schedule	Patients treated	Complete response	Partial
Etoposide[a]	100 mg/m² days 1, 3, 5 q 4 weeks	16	0	0
Mitoxantrone[b]	12 mg/m² q 3 weeks	9	0	0
Cisplatin[c]	50 mg/m² q 3 weeks	16	1	0
Lomustine[d]	100 mg/m² q 6 weeks	3	0	0
Semustine[d]	150 mg/m² q 6 weeks	2	0	0
Doxorubicin[e]	90 mg/m² q 3 weeks	7	1	1[f]

[a] SLAYTON et al. (1987).
[b] MUSS et al. (1989).
[c] THIGPEN et al. (1986a).
[d] OMURA et al. (1978).
[e] PIVER et al. (1978).
[f] Patient treated with doxorubicin combined with Cytoxan and 5-fluorouracil.

Table 7.6. Combination regimens in squamous vaginal cancer. (From PEREZ et al. 1992)

Regimen response	Dose and schedule	Patients treated	Complete response	Partial
Bleomycin Vincristine Mitomycin C Cisplatin[a]	15 mg/m² days 1, 2, 3 1.4 mg/m² day 3 10 mg/m² day 3 60 mg/m² day 3 Cycle q 4 weeks	2	0	1
Cisplatin Dichloromethotrexate[b]	Not given	3	2	0
Bleomycin Methotrexate Cisplatin[c]	10 mg days 1, 8, 15 40 mg/m² days 1, 15 50 mg/m² day 4 Cycle q 3 weeks	1	1	0

[a] BELINSON et al. (1985).
[b] PETERS et al. (1985a).
[c] KATIB et al. (1985).

instance each of cerebral vascular accident, congestive heart failure, pulmonary embolus, and severe thrombocytopenia. Complications after radiation therapy included one enterovesical fistula, four cases of severe radiation enteritis, and one contracted bladder with urinary insufficiency. Five-year survival was 30%, and median survival was 18 months.

There are no published data regarding cytotoxic therapy for the extremely rare primary adenocarcinoma arising in the vagina. FOWLER et al. (1979) described one complete response and one partial response lasting 13 and 10 months, respectively, after treatment with pulse melphalan, 1 mg/kg over 5 days each month. ROBBOY et al. (1974) described 13 cases of vaginal and cervical clear cell carcinoma treated with various drugs used singly or in combination suggesting activity with 5-fluorouracil and vinblastine although details of neither the responses nor their durations are well described.

BRAND et al. (1989) reported on chemotherapy and/or immunotherapy in six patients with recurrence after primary therapy. The results were uniformly poor, as has been seen in cutaneous melanoma. Thus no standard chemotherapy can be recommended at this time for mucosal melanomas of the vagina.

Recent data suggest that both cisplatin and ifosfamide are active against mixed mesodermal tumors arising from the uterus (SUTTON et al. 1989; THIGPEN et al. 1986b), while doxorubicin remains the standard therapy for treatment of leiomyosarcoma (MUSS et al. 1985); however, there is no information on efficacy in similar vaginal tumors.

Embryonal rhabdomyosarcoma (sarcoma botryoides) requires a multidisciplinary approach that frequently includes combination chemotherapy, radiation therapy, and surgical resection (COPELAND et al. 1985; PIVER and ROSE 1988). HAYS et al. (1985) reported a good outcome with multimodality therapy (one tumor-related death in 24 cases) in children under the age of 4 years. In their study therapy in 24 vaginal primaries consisted of VAC combination therapy in all patients before or after surgery (six patients had no surgery, and 14 had preoperative chemotherapy until maximum tumor response was seen). Only eight patients were treated with radiation therapy. Of note, 20 of the patients in this series had avanced disease at presentation and were managed without exenterative surgery with excellent results. Thus current therapy for embryonal rhabdomyosarcoma should still be individualized, but excellent results in locally advanced disease can be attained with preoperative VAC followed by nonexenterative surgery in most cases. Radiation therapy can probably be reserved for patients with positive surgical margins.

7.10 Other Therapeutic Approaches

RYAN et al. (1992) described a vaginal applicator with a central obturator and an acrylic template for placement of microwave antennae and thermometry probes for administration of brachytherapy and hyperthermia. At the time of publication the applicator had been used in three patients with satisfactory results. Future modifications of the applicator will incorporate air cooling of antennas to further smooth the temperature distribution.

7.11 Results of Therapy

Following adequate therapy, the survival rates of patients with carcinoma of the vagina are comparable to those reported for carcinoma of the cervix, which range from 20% to 80% at 5 years, depending on stage of the disease (Table 7.7) (BENEDET et al. 1983; BROWN et al. 1971; GALLUP et al. 1987; KUCERA et al.

Table 7.7. Pooled survival data of 12 studies using low-dose-rate brachytherapy for stage I and II vaginal cancer. (From NANAVATI et al. 1993)

	Survival, stage I	Survival, stage II	Overall complications (%)
NORI et al. (1983)	10/14	4/6	
PUTHAWALA et al. (1983)	1/1	12/16	22
CHU and BEECHINOR (1984)	7/8	8/19	20
GALLUP et al. (1988)	1/1	6/11	33
PEREZ et al. (1988)	37/50	38/75	12
MANETTA et al. (1988)	5/6	9/15	21
SPIRTOS et al. (1989)	17/18	4/5	17
MANETTA et al. (1990)	6/9	6/15	34
KUCERA and VAVRA (1991)	13/16	4/5	
DAVIS et al. (1991)	9/14	4/9	
REDDY et al. (1991)	12/15	16/22	18
STOCK et al. (1992)	2/6	13/27	22
Total	120/158 (76%)	124/225 (55%)	12–34
Total for stage I and II combined		244/383 (64%)	

1985; Manetta et al. 1988; Perez et al. 1977; Prempree and Amornmarn 1985; Reddy et al. 1987; Rubin et al. 1985; Shimm and Ropar 1986; Spirtos et al. 1989; Whelton and Kottmeier 1962). Perez et al. (1988) noted a somewhat higher incidence of pelvic failures in patients with carcinoma of the vagina treated with irradiation in comparison with 1054 patients with invasive cervical carcinoma, although the differences were not statistically significant.

Results after surgical treatment are more sparse than with radiation therapy. Woodman et al. (1988) treated 11 patients with intraepithelial neoplasia following hysterectomy for cervical carcinoma in situ with tumor control in all patients. Nine of ten patients questioned continued to enjoy satisfactory sexual intercourse after treatment. Lee and Symmonds (1976) described 66 patients previously treated for in situ carcinoma of the cervix who were subsequently treated for primary carcinoma in situ of the vagina with wide local excision, partial vaginectomy, or total vaginectomy. They stated that 58 patients (88%) were alive and disease free at the time of the report; six others had died of intercurrent disease without recurrent carcinoma. One patient had recurrent carcinoma of the vagina, resulting in death. These results are not superior to those reported with irradiation alone, and the authors made no statement about the status of the vaginal mucosa and functional results. Audet-LaPointe et al. (1990) reported 70.5% tumor control in 34 patients with vaginal intraepithelial neoplasia treated with CO_2 laser therapy. Curtis et al. (1992) reported that 10 of 12 women (83%) with intraepithelial neoplasia showed no evidence of recurrence after partial colpectomy. One patient complained of dyspareunia, vaginal shortening, and stress incontinence treated with vaginoplasty.

Davis et al. (1991) treated 52 patients with stage I or II carcinoma of the vagina with surgery alone and 14 with surgery plus irradiation. Pelvic and para-aortic lymph nodes were assessed in 17 patients. Only one patient of 17 (6%) with stage I tumor had positive pelvic nodes as opposed to 8 of 31 patients (26%) with stage II disease. One patient with stage II disease had para-aortic lymph node involvement. Surgery was based on tumor volume and ability to obtain clear pathologic margins (partial vaginectomy in six patients, radical hysterectomy plus vaginectomy in 25 patients, and exenteration in 21 patients). One patient had preoperative irradiation; 13 had adjuvant postoperative irradiation, and 23 additional patients were treated with irradiation alone. Median follow-up was 5.4 years for patients with stage I and 3.2 years for those with stage II. The central and regional failure rate for stage I was 11% and 5% and for stage II, 9% and 7%, respectively. Distant metastases developed in 5% of the patients with stage I and 22% of those with stage II. Survival was comparable for patients with squamous cell carcinoma, clear cell carcinoma, and adenocarcinoma. Five-year survival without disease was comparable for the three modalities (Fig. 7.5).

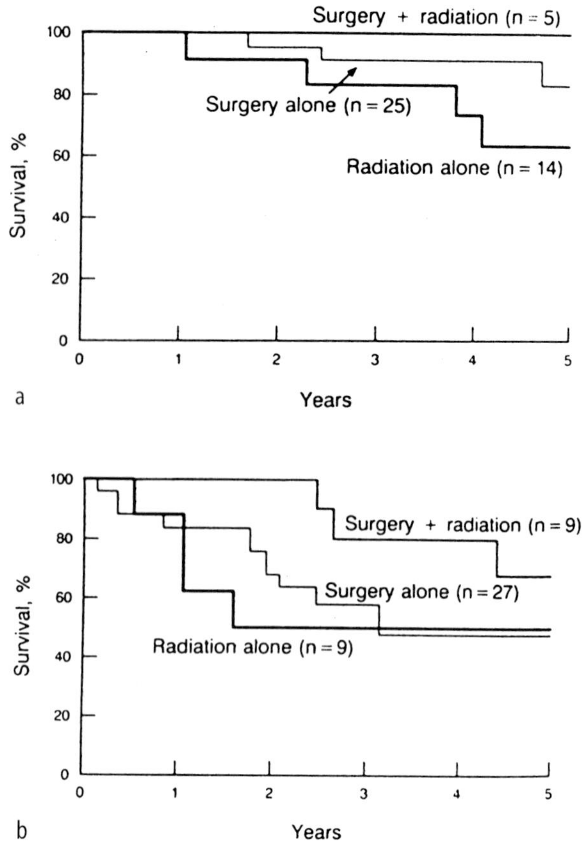

Fig. 7.5 a,b. Survival correlated with treatment modality. **a** Stage I disease ($P = 0.89$). One patient was lost to follow-up. **b** Stage II disease ($P = 0.64$). (From Davis et al. 1991)

Hoffman et al. (1992) described results in 32 women, 31 having had previous hysterectomy, who were treated for carcinoma in situ or occult, superficially invasive carcinoma of the vagina with upper vaginectomy. Fourteen patients had undergone previous treatment for vaginal intraepithelial neoplasia. Nine had invasive cancer on final pathologic examination. Among the remaining 23 patients, recurrence of vaginal neoplasia developed in four (17%) after surgical treatment, with a mean time to recurrence of 78 weeks. Nineteen patients were alive with no evidence of recurrent tumor at a mean follow-up interval of 152 weeks. Of 15 patients treated with upper vaginectomy and no history of radiation therapy, five had vagina adequate for intercourse.

RUTLEDGE (1967) reported a 35% 5-year survival rate in 70 patients with invasive vaginal carcinoma (including advanced stages) treated with irradiation; some patients died of intercurrent disease. BROWN et al. (1971) and PEREZ and CAMEL (1982) reported 80%–90% tumor control and survival rates in patients with carcinoma in situ and stage I invasive carcinoma. These authors cautioned against overly aggressive therapy in these early lesions because of the possibility of producing mucosal injury and interference with sexual function. BROWN et al. (1971) noted no new cases of in situ or invasive carcinoma developing after radiation therapy for carcinoma in situ or early invasive carcinoma of the vagina.

PEREZ et al. (1988) noted that 15 of 16 patients (93%) with stage 0 carcinoma of the vagina treated with irradiation had control of the tumor 5 years after treatment. In stage I the pelvic tumor control was 86% (43 of 50 patients). In patients with more advanced tumors the pelvic control decreased significantly (40%–50%, depending on tumor extent and techniques used). Similar results were reported by PREMPREE and AMORNMARN (1985) in 88 patients.

PEREZ and CAMEL (1982) reported that in carcinoma in situ and stage I vaginal carcinoma treated with brachytherapy, tumor control in the pelvis was the same with or without external beam irradiation. However, better tumor control (65%) was observed in stage II and III with the addition of external irradiation in comparison with brachytherapy only (40%). Likewise, MACNAUGHT et al. (1986), in an analysis of 78 cases of primary vaginal carcinoma, 61 of which were squamous cell carcinoma, reported better tumor control and survival with combination external beam and interstitial treatment compared with brachytherapy alone, despite the staging distribution being in favor of the patients treated with brachytherapy only. In stage III and stage IVA vaginal carcinoma irradiation has resulted in only 25%–50% pelvic tumor control; therefore higher doses with a greater contribution from the external irradiation are being used.

PREMPREE and AMORNMARN (1985) and PUTHAWALA et al. (1983) described tumor control rates in the pelvis ranging from 65% to 80% with a combination of external irradiation and, when appropriate, paravaginal or parametrial interstitial implant, in addition to intracavitary brachytherapy.

DANCUART et al. (1988), in 167 patients with primary squamous cell carcinoma of the vagina treated with irradiation alone at M.D. Anderson Hospital, reported central failure rates of 18% in 71 patients with stage I disease, 14% in 42 patients with stage II, 24% in 38 patients with stage III, and 30% in 11 patients with stage IVA disease. A few pelvic or central failures combined with distant metastases were noted in each stage. There was no significant difference in the failure rate when brachytherapy or external irradiation or combination of both was used. These authors postulated that since the incidence of pelvic failures was low there is no need to irradiate the whole pelvis in these patients. They advocated the treatment of subclinical disease in the inguinal lymph nodes with 4000 or 5000 cGy. In our experience, however, the incidence of pelvic failures in stages IIA and IIB is relatively high, and we do recommend whole pelvis and parametrial irradiation.

KUCERA and VAVRA (1991) reported on 434 patients treated with irradiation for invasive vaginal carcinoma, with more details for 110 treated in more recent years. Intracavitary radium was the standard primary treatment, to deliver 6000–9000 cGy to the tumor and 3000 cGy to the surrounding vagina. In more advanced lesions external irradiation (5600 cGy to the lateral pelvic wall) was delivered. Five-year survival in shown in Table 7.8. Five-year survival was higher in patients with tumors in the upper third (21 of 35, 60%) than in those with tumors in the middle or lower third (19 of 51, 37.5%) or involving the whole vagina (5 of 24, 20.8%).

LEUNG and SEXTON (1993) treated 103 patients with radiation therapy consisting of brachytherapy alone, external beam irradiation alone (38 patients), or a combination of the two. Doses ranged from 3000 to 7000 cGy before 1985 and 5000 to 6300 cGy thereafter. Local relapse-free survival for patients in all stages was 60%. Results were better after 1965, although the difference did not reach statistical significance. The inguinal lymph nodes were not routinely irradiated unless involved at presentation. Only one

Table 7.8. Carcinoma of the vagina: 5-year survival of 434 patients treated between 1952 and 1984. (From KUCERA and VAVRA 1991)

Stage	Number	5-year survival
I	73	56 (76.7%)
II	110	49 (44.5%)
III	174	54 (31.0%)
IV	77	14 (18.2%)
Total	434	173 (39.9%)

patient presented with inguinal disease; three other cases developed following treatment of the primary tumor. Overall incidence of distant metastases was 21% (18 of 84). Survival for the entire population was 58% at 5 years and 42% at 10 years, with better results for patients receiving external beam irradiation.

As with tumors at other sites, it is important to achieve a homogeneous dose distribution throughout the target volume. PEREZ et al. (1977) reviewed distribution of the radiation dose and found that in several patients whose tumors recurred, distribution had been suboptimal (nonhomogeneous) because of inadequate placement of the needles, lack of an intravaginal cylinder, or treatment to a volume smaller than the tumor.

BORONOW et al. (1987) advocated a combination of surgery and irradiation for the treatment of patients with advanced vulvovaginal cancer. Practically all of the 37 patients they treated with this technique had advanced primary tumors of the vulva. The 5-year survival rate for the primary cases was 75.6%. For the patients with recurrent disease the 5-year survival rate was 62.6%. In the majority of the patients (94.8%) the bladder and rectum were preserved.

HOPKINS et al. (1989) reported on three patients with small cell tumors containing neuroendocrine granules treated with a combination of irradiation and chemotherapy. As in the lung counterpart, local tumor control was good, but distant metastasis to the brain, bones, and other organs was frequent.

7.11.1 Patients with a History of Previously Treated Uterine Tumors

Several authors have described the appearance of vaginal carcinoma after successful treatment of primary carcinoma of the cervix (CHOO and ANDERSON 1982; KANBOUR et al. 1974; STUART et al. 1981).

PEREZ and co-workers reported that patients with carcinoma of the vagina who had a history of previously treated primary carcinoma of the cervix or the endometrium (irradiation, hysterectomy, or combination of both) and received treatment over 5 years before the diagnosis of vaginal carcinoma had survival and tumor control rates equal to patients with de novo primary vaginal carcinoma (PEREZ and CAMEL 1982; PEREZ et al. 1988). The possibility of the vaginal lesion being a local recurrence or metastasis was considered unlikely, since 95% of the recurrences following treatment of primary carcinoma of the cervix or the endometrium occur within 5 years after therapy. It is concluded that these lesions are most likely second primaries that should be treated with definitive radiation therapy and a curative aim.

7.11.2 Clear Cell Adenocarcinoma

FLETCHER (1980a) reported that 17 of 19 young women with clear cell adenocarcinoma treated with irradiation (two combined with surgery) were alive and tumor free (one had recurrence of an extensive lesion, and one patient died of pulmonary emboli after removal of radium needles). Fifteen patients were followed up for more than 2 years.

SENEKJIAN et al. (1987) noted 92% and 88% 5- and 10-year survival rates in 43 patients with stage I clear cell vaginal carcinoma treated with local therapy (vaginectomy, local excision alone or combined with irradiation), which was comparable with the results in 126 patients treated with vaginectomy and radical hysterectomy. However, at 10 years the actuarial recurrence rate for the local excision subgroup was 45% in comparison to only 13% for the patients treated with more radical surgery. Patients who received local irradiation (with or without excision) had a recurrence rate of 27%. Recurrences were more frequently noted in patients with tumors larger than 2 cm, with invasion of 3 mm or more, and with a predominant histologic pattern other than tubulocystic. Pelvic lymph node metastases were noted at death in 12% of the patients.

SENEKJIAN et al. (1988) also reported the results in 76 patients with stage II clear cell adenocarcinomas of the vagina, which were subdivided into three substages according to the classification proposed by PEREZ et al. (1973). Twenty-two of the patients were treated with surgery alone (vaginectomy with radical hysterectomy in 13 patients and vaginectomy with total or partial pelvic exenteration in nine); radiation therapy alone was used in 38 patients, and a combination of vaginectomy, radical hysterectomy, and external irradiation or other treatment approaches was used in 12 patients. The 5-year survival rate was approximately 80% and the 10-year survival rate 65% without significant differences among the three treatment modalities (Fig. 7.6).

SENEKJIAN et al. (1989) reported on 21 of 527 patients, most of whom had stage II or III clear cell

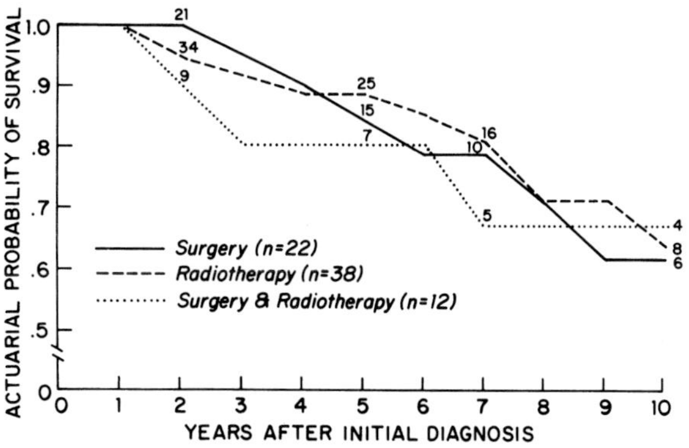

Fig. 7.6. Survival for stage II vaginal clear cell carcinoma by treatment modality. (From SENEKJIAN et al. 1988)

adenocarcinoma of the cervix and vagina and were treated with pelvic exenteration (in ten cases combined with irradiation). Eleven patients survived tumor free from 0.2 to 12.9 years. Of nine patients with stage II vaginal clear cell adenocarcinoma, 89% survived 5 years and 84% survived 10 years.

7.11.3 Squamous Cell Carcinoma of the Neovagina

Nine cases of squamous cell carcinoma in a neovagina created to treat vaginal agenesis have been reported. Three of the tumors were adenocarcinoma associated with the use of small or large bowel for vaginal reconstruction. Four patients were treated by primary surgery and apparently have not developed a recurrence (two radical vaginectomies and two exenterations). Three of four previously reported patients were primarily treated with radiation therapy, although unfortunately a high failure rate has been noted (HOPKINS and MORLEY 1987). BALTZER and ZANDER (1989) also favor surgical treatment of these tumors.

7.11.4 Nonepithelial Tumors

Conventional therapy has been anterior exenteration with urinary diversion (ureteroileostomy or ureterosigmoidostomy), occasionally with resection of the colon including colostomy. This approach was found to be relatively ineffective except in patients with small tumors and carried a high complication rate (HILGERS 1975; MAHESH KUMAR et al. 1976). DANIEL et al. (1959) reported only two survivors among 13 children with vaginal rhabdomyosarcoma. DAVOS and ABELL (1976) described no survivors among five patients treated with surgery or radiation therapy. HELDERS et al. (1972) reported ten cases from the Mayo Clinic and reviewed 49 cases previously reported, showing that only nine (18%) had been cured, primarily after surgery alone. Treatment consisted of hysterectomy and total vaginectomy. Combination of several modalities has significantly improved the treatment results of these patients (FRIEDMAN et al. 1986; GHAVIMI et al. 1975; HOLTON et al. 1973; KILMAN et al. 1973; PRATT et al. 1972). KILMAN et al (1973) noted that with a combination of surgery, irradiation, and chemotherapy only 4 of 38 patients (11%) died during the first year of therapy, and 29 (76%) were alive at the end of 5 years. GROSFELD et al. (1972) reported 6 of 13 (46%) patients with pelvic rhabdomyosarcoma surviving after combined therapy. PIVER et al. (1973) reported three patients with vulvovaginal rhabdomyosarcoma who survived without disease after aggressive treatment with surgery, irradiation, and triple chemotherapy (vincristine, dactinomycin, and cyclophosphamide). The use of less radical surgical operations, with removal of gross tumor but conserving normal anatomy if feasible, was suggested by KILMAN et al. (1973), avoiding the need for cystectomy, urinary diversion, and rectal resection.

The combination of irradiation and chemotherapy with conservation surgery has been shown to improve tumor control while decreasing morbidity. Permanent local tumor control with cytotoxic drugs alone has been shown to be less than 15% (GHAVIMI et al. 1984).

RANEY et al. (1990) reported on patients treated in the Second Intergroup Rhabdomyosarcoma Study, including 20 patients with vaginal primary lesions. Patients were treated with vincristine, dactinomycin, and cyclophosphimide (VAC) for two courses and then reassessed with biopsies; patients showing less than 50% tumor reversal had limited surgical excision of the tumor. Patients showing a complete response received two additional courses of chemotherapy followed by wide local excision of the tumor. Patients were randomized to continue chemotherapy or a combination of irradiation and chemotherapy for a total of 2 years. If the tumor exhibited no response, patients were treated with more extensive surgery followed by radiation therapy and additional chemotherapy. Initially a radiation dose of 2500 cGy was recommended, but because of poor response the dose was increased to 4000–4500 cGy in 4–5 weeks. Disease-free survival in the entire group of patients in this protocol was 52% at 3 years, with 85% survival for those with vaginal primary tumors.

PETERS et al. (1985a) reported a 36% 5-year survival rate in nine patients with one leiomyosarcoma and a 17% rate in seven patients with mixed müllerian tumors of the vagina after various forms of therapy, including pelvic irradiation. Three of four patients who underwent exenteration were alive and tumor free for 84–161 months. These results underscore the importance of local therapy, since in all 14 treatment failures, the tumor first recurred within the pelvis, and in seven of the 14 this location was the only site of recurrence.

Results of treatment of vaginal melanoma are poor. Recent review of the literature shows a 5-year survival rate of 8.4% (Table 7.9); there is a high incidence of distant metastases, possibly because only 5% of the patients had lesions less than 2 mm thick (CHUNG et al. 1980). REID et al. (1989) abstracted data for meta-analysis of 129 patients reported in the literature, including 15 treated at their institution. Tumors occurred most frequently in the lower third of the vagina (34%), with the anterior one-third (38%) being the most common area. Patients were treated with wide local excision or partial vaginectomy (24 patients), radical surgery (31), radiation therapy (26), or combinations thereof (13 patients). There was no significant difference in survival when correlated with therapeutic modality (Fig. 7.7). Local recurrence developed in 40.7% of patients, regional failures in 19.7%, and distant metastases in 35%.

Irradiation may have a role in the primary management of vaginal melanomas, although follow-up is short (BONNER et al. 1988; CHUNG et al. 1980; HARWOOD and CUMMINGS 1982; SON 1980). In a review of the literature MORROW and DISAIA (1976) found reports of one patient surviving 5 years following radiation therapy, none of ten surviving following local excision (with or without irradiation), and 3 of 19 surviving after radical exenterative surgery. HARWOOD and CUMMINGS (1982) described a complete response in four patients with vaginal melanoma treated with irradiation, although two subsequently relapsed. HARRISON et al. (1987) reported one of three patients with vaginal melanoma treated with irradiation surviving 7.5 years; the other two died with distant metastases but had the local tumor controlled.

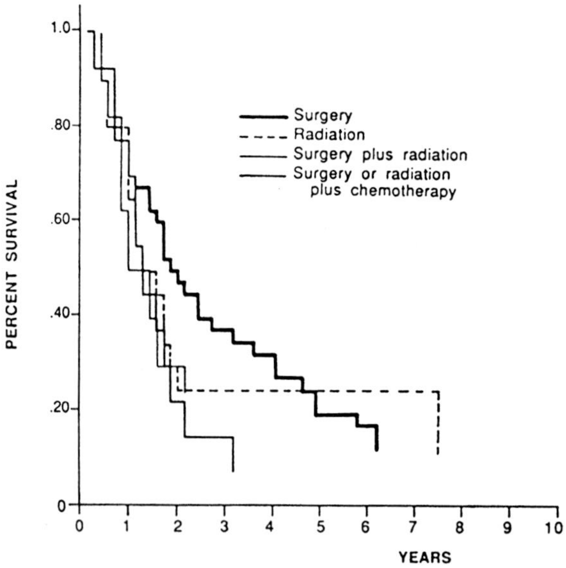

Fig. 7.7. Percent survival of vaginal melanoma by treatment regimens of surgery ($n = 55$), irradiation ($n = 26$), surgery plus irradiation ($n = 11$), and surgery or irradiation with adjunctive chemotherapy ($n = 13$) ($P = 0.47$). (From REID et al. 1989)

Table 7.9. Survival correlated with treatment modality in vaginal melanoma. (From LEVITAN et al. 1989)

Method of treatment	Survival [no. (%)]	
	2 years	5 years
Wide local excision	4/16 (25)	1/15 (6.6)
Wide excision plus irradiation	1/5 (20)	0/5
Wide excision plus node dissection	2/7 (28.6)	1/7 (14.3)
Radiation therapy	3/22 (13.6)	2/21 (9.5)
Radical surgery	15/38 (39.5)	3/35 (8.6)
Total	25/88 (28.4)	7/83 (8.4)

BONNER et al. (1988) reported on ten patients with malignant melanoma: three were treated with conservative surgery, six had radical surgery, and no further procedures were performed on one with metastatic disease. Two patients survived for more than 5 years, one for 38 months, and one for 29 months. Two patients, one treated initially with a wide local excision and the other with anterior pelvic exenteration, were alive several months after retreatment of a recurrence with high-fraction irradiation. In five of the six patients treated with radical surgery, four developed locoregional lymph node failure as the first site of recurrence (one patient had inadequate information regarding site of first relapse); all of the patients managed with local excision developed locoregional recurrent tumor, prompting the authors to conclude that locoregional control of vaginal melanoma is difficult to achieve with surgery alone.

ROGO et al. (1991) reported on 22 cases of vulvovaginal melanoma treated with conservation surgery or irradiation or both. Eight patients (36%) were alive 5 years and four 10 years after treatment. Eleven patients had stage I, six had stage II, three had stage III, and two had stage IV tumors. Inguinal lymph node recurrences and distant metastases were the most common sites of failure. Results were comparable to those obtained with radical surgery.

7.12 Sequelae of Treatment

The most common complications following surgery are wound infection and secondary bleeding. Surgery-associated urinary fistulae were reported in 2 of 19 patients by BELL and BERMAN (1982). Pulmonary embolus, occasionally fatal, may be noted. LINDEQUE and MONAGHAN (to be published) have found no surgical fatalities, emboli, or fistulae in 23 patients treated surgically for vaginal carcinoma. A possible disadvantage to extensive vaginal surgery is loss of vagina, which may be prevented by adequate vaginal reconstruction, using vulvovaginoplasty or myocutaneous flap. Vaginal reconstructive surgery, other than primary skin graft, is usually not performed at the time of initial operation but as a subsequent separate procedure (LINDEQUE 1987).

PEREZ et al. (1988) reported grade 2–3 complications in about 5% of patients treated for stage 0 and stage I lesions and in about 15% of patients with stage II lesions. No complications were reported in stage III and stage IV disease, probably because the patients died shortly after treatment. The most common major complications were proctitis (two), rectovesicovaginal fistulae (three), and vesicovaginal fistulae (two). The most common minor complications were fibrosis of the vagina and small areas of mucosal necrosis, which were noted in about 10% of patients.

HINTZ et al. (1980) analyzed 16 patients with cancer of the vagina locally controlled for a minimum of 18 months and indicated that doses of irradiation greater than 9800 cGy to the lower vaginal mucosa (both external and brachytherapy contributions) will result in a higher incidence of complications. The posterior wall of the vagina appears more sensitive to irradiation, as does the distal vaginal mucosa. In contrast, the upper vagina (vault) tolerated doses in the range of 14000 cGy. HINTZ et al. (1980) advocated dose rates of less than 80 cGy an hour. These authors cautioned against placing radioactive needles on the surface of the vaginal cylinder because this may increase the frequency of vaginal necrosis.

7.13 Follow-up Examinations

Careful follow-up after initial treatment by the gynecologic and radiation oncologists is critical to facilitate early detection of tumor recurrences and assess sequelae of therapy and quality of life of the patient. We see our patients every 3 months during the first year, every 6 months during the second and third years, every 6 months during the fourth and fifth years, and annually thereafter.

7.14 Summary and Outlook

There are two major difficulties in the management of vaginal carcinoma. First, irradiation alone has not provided adequate results in stage III and stage IV disease. Pelvic failures and distant metastases occur in half of the patients with advanced disease. The second problem is that the results of therapy for patients with nonepithelial tumors (sarcomas, melanomas) are poor.

Carcinoma in situ of the vagina should preferentially be treated with intracavitary irradiation to the entire vaginal mucosa. Superficial stage I carcinomas can be treated with an intracavitary cylinder to the entire vagina. A single-plane implant may be added for thicker lesions confined to one vaginal wall. Supplemental external irradiation should be used only for aggressive stage I lesions.

Stage IIA carcinoma patients should receive 2000–4000 cGy to the whole pelvis and 5000–6000 cGy total dose to the lateral pelvic wall. Interstitial and intracavitary therapy should supplement external beam irradiation.

Stage IIB to stage IV carcinoma patients have received higher doses to the whole pelvis and lateral parametrium. Improvements in therapeutic techniques are necessary, including combinations of irradiation and surgery.

Clear cell adenocarcinoma stage I disease may be treated with surgery or intracavitary or transvaginal irradiation. Irradiation is necessary for large lesions.

Melanomas and leiomyosarcomas are surgically treated. Rhabdomyosarcoma is treated with surgical resection, irradiation, and chemotherapy.

The use of hypoxic sensitizers to enhance the effects of irradiation in large tumors is under investigation (WASSERMAN et al. 1980). Effective chemotherapeutic agents to treat systemic disease are necessary, especially in patients with advanced disease who have a high incidence of distant metastasis.

References

Aartsen EJ, Delemarre JFM, Gerretsen G (1993) Endodermal sinus tumor of the vagina: radiation therapy and progeny. Obstet Gynecol 81:893–895

Antonioli DA, Burke L (1975) Vaginal adenosis: analysis of 325 biopsy specimens from 100 patients. Am J Clin Pathol 64:625–638

Antonioli DA, Rosen S, Burke L, Donahue V (1979) Glandular dysplasia in diethylstilbestrol-associated vaginal adenosis. Am J Clin Pathol 71:715–721

Audet-LaPointe P, Body G, Vauclair R, Drouin P, Ayoub J (1990) Vaginal intraepithelial neoplasia. Gynecol Oncol 36:232–239

Baltzer J, Zander J (1989) Primary squamous cell carcinoma of the neovagina. Gynecol Oncol 35:99–103

Barber HRK, Sommers SC (1974) Vaginal adenosis, dysplasia, and clear cell adenocarcinoma after diethylstilbestrol treatment in pregnancy. Obstet Gynecol 43:645–652

Belinson JL, Stewart JA, Richards AL, McClure M (1985) Bleomycin, vincristine, mitomycin-C, and cisplatin in the management of gynecological squamous cell cancer. Gynecol Oncol 20:387–393

Bell HG, Berman ML (1982) Management of primary vaginal carcinoma. Gynecol Oncol 14:154–163

Benedet JL, Murphy KJ, Fairey RN, Boyes DA (1983) Primary invasive carcinoma of the vagina. Obstet Gynecol 62:715–719

Berchuck A, Rodriguez G, Kamel A, Soper JT, Clarke-Pearson DL, Bast RC Jr (1990) Expression of epidermal growth factor receptor and HER-2/*neu* in normal and neoplastic cervix, vulva, and vagina. Obstet Gynecol 76:381–387

Berkowitz RS, Ehrmann RL, Knapp RC (1978) Endometrial stromal sarcoma arising from vaginal endometriosis. Obstet Gynecol 51:34S–37S

Berman ML, Tobon H, Surti U (1981) Primary malignant melanoma of the vagina: clinical, light, and electron microscopic observations. Am J Obstet Gynecol 139:963

Bertoni F, Bertoni G, Bignardi M (1983) Vaginal molds for intracavitary curietherapy: a new method of preparation. Int J Radiat Oncol Biol Phys 9:1579–1582

Boice JD Jr, Engholm G, Kleinerman RA, et al. (1988) Radiation dose and second cancer risk in patients treated for cancer of the cervix. Radiat Res 116:3–55

Bonner JA, Perez-Tamayo C, Reid GC, Roberts JA, Morley GW (1988) The management of vaginal melanoma. Cancer 62:2066–2072

Bornstein J, Adam E, Adler-Storthz K, Kaufman RH (1988) Development of cervical and vaginal squamous cell neoplasia as a late consequence of in utero exposure to diethylstilbestrol. Obstet Gynecol Surv 43:15–21

Boronow RC, Hickman BT, Reagan MT, Smith RA, Steadham RE (1987) Combined therapy as an alternative to exenteration for locally advanced vulvovaginal cancer. II. Results, complications, and dosimetric and surgical considerations. Am J Clin Oncol 10:171–181

Brand E, Fu YS, Lagasse LD, Berek JS (1989) Vulvovaginal melanoma: report of seven cases and literature review. Gynecol Oncol 33:54–60

Brinton LA, Nasca PC, Mallin K, et al. (1990) Case-control study of in situ and invasive carcinoma of the vagina. Gynecol Oncol 38:49–54

Brown GR, Fletcher GH, Rutledge FN (1971) Irradiation of "in situ" and invasive squamous cell carcinomas of the vagina. Cancer 28:1278–1283

Burke L, Antonioli D, Friedman EA (1981) Evolution of diethylstilbestrol-associated genital tract lesions. Obstet Gynecol 57:79–84

Buscema J, Rosenshein NB, Taqi F, Woodruff JD (1985) Vaginal hemangiopericytoma: a histopathologic and ultrastructural evaluation. Obstet Gynecol 66:82S

Cavanaugh D, Praphat H, Ruffolo EH (1980) Cancer of the vagina. Obstet Gynecol Ann 9:311–325

Chang YCF, Hricak H, Thurnher S, Lacey CG (1988) Vagina: evaluation with MR imaging. II. Neoplasms. Radiology 169:175–179

Chapman GW, Genda J, Williams T (1984) Alveolar soft-part sarcoma of the vagina. Gynecol Oncol 18:125

Chau PM (1963) Radiotherapeutic management of malignant tumors of the vagina. Am J Roentgenol Radium Ther Nucl Med 89:502–523

Chen KTK, Hafez GR, Gilbert EF (1980) Myxoid variant of epithelioid smooth muscle tumor. Am J Clin Pathol 74:350–353

Choo YC, Anderson DG (1982) Neoplasms of the vagina following cervical carcinoma. Gynecol Oncol 14:125–132

Choo YC, Morley GW (1980) Multiple primary neoplasms of the anogenital region. Obstet Gynecol 56:365–369

Chorlton I, Karnei RF, King FM, Norris HJ (1974) Primary malignant reticuloendothelial disease involving the vagina, cervix, and corpus uteri. Obstet Gynecol 44:735–748

Chu AM, Beechinor R (1984) Survival and recurrence patterns in the radiation treatment of carcinoma of the vagina. Gynecol Oncol 19:298

Chung AF, Casey MJ, Flannery JT, Woodruff JM, Lewis JL Jr (1980) Malignant melanoma of the vagina: report of 19 cases. Obstet Gynecol 55:720–727

Copeland LJ, Gershenson DM, Saul PB, Sneige N, Stringer CA, Edwards CL (1985) Sarcoma botryoides of the female genital tract. Obstet Gynecol 66:262–266

Curtis P, Shepherd JH, Lowe DG, Jobling T (1992) The role of partial colpectomy in the management of persistent vaginal neoplasia after primary treatment. Br J Obstet Gynaecol 99:587–589

Dancuart F, Delclos L, Wharton JT, Silva EG (1988) Primary squamous cell carcinoma of the vagina treated by radiotherapy: a failures analysis – the M.D. Anderson Hospital experience 1955–1982. Int J Radiat Oncol Biol Phys 14:745–749

Daniel WW, Koss LG, Brunschwig A (1959) Sarcoma botryoides of the vagina. Cancer 12:74

Davis KP, Stanhope CR, Garton GR, Arkinson EJ, O'Brien PC (1991) Invasive vaginal carcinoma: analysis of early-stage disease. Gynecol Oncol 42:131–136

Davos I, Abell MR (1976) Sarcoma of the vagina. Obstet Gynecol 4:342–350

Daw E (1971) Primary carcinoma of the vagina. J Obstet Gynecol Br Commonw 78:853

Delclos L (1984) Gynecologic cancers: pelvic examination and treatment planning. In: Levitt SH, Tapley N (eds) Technological basis of radiation therapy: practical clinical applications. Lea & Febiger, Philadelphia, pp 193–227

Digel CA, Lastner GMF, Zinreich ES (1989) The use of transmission block in the radiation therapy portal for treatment of the inguinal nodes in late stage pelvic malignancies. Radiol Technol 53:227–232

Ebner F, Kressel HY, Mintz MC, et al. (1988) Tumor recurrence versus fibrosis in the female pelvis: differentiation with MR at 1.5 T. Radiology 166:333–340

Faaborg LL, Smith ML, Newland JR (1979) Uterine cervical and vaginal verrucous squamous cell carcinoma. Gynecol Oncol 8:104–109

Flamant F, Gerbaulet A, Nihoul-Fekete C, Valteau-Couanet D, Chassagne D, Lemerle J (1990) Long-term sequelae of conservative treatment by surgery, brachytherapy, and chemotherapy for vulval and vaginal rhabdomyosarcoma in children. J Clin Oncol 8:1847–1853

Fletcher GH (1980a) Tumors of the vagina and female urethra. In: Fletcher GH (ed) Textbook of radiotherapy, 3rd edn. Lea & Febiger, Philadelphia, pp 821–824

Fletcher GH (1980b) Squamous cell carcinoma of the uterine cervix. In: Fletcher GH (ed) Textbook of radiotherapy, 3rd edn. Lea & Febiger, Philadelphia, pp 720–773

Forsberg JG (1975) Late effects in the vaginal and cervical epithelia after injections of diethylstibestrol into neonatal mice. Am J Obstet Gynecol 121:101

Fowler WC, Brantley JC, Edelman DA (1979) Clear cell adenocarcinoma of the genital tract. South Med J 72:15–16

Fowler WC, Schmidt G, Edelman DA, Kaufman DG, Fenoglio CM (1981) Risks of cervical intraepithelial neoplasia among DES-exposed women. Obstet Gynecol 58:720–724

Frick HC II, Jacox HW, Taylor HC Jr (1968) Primary carcinoma of the vagina. Am J Obstet Gynecol 101:695

Friedman M, Peretz BA, Nissenbaum M, Paldi E (1986) Modern treatment of vaginal embryonal rhabdomyosarcoma. Obstet Gynecol Surv 41:614–618

Friedrich EG, Wilkinson EJ, Sui YS (1980) Carcinoma in situ of the vulva: a continuing challenge. Am J Obstet Gynecol 136:830

Fukushima M, Twiggs LB, Okagaki T (1986) Mixed intestinal adenocarcinoma-argentaffin carcinoma of the vagina. Gynecol Oncol 23:387

Gallup DG, Talledo E, Shah KJ, Hayes C (1987) Invasive squamous cell carcinoma of the vagina: a 14-year study. Obstet Gynecol 69:782–785

Ghavimi F, Exelby PR, D'Angio GJ, et al. (1975) Multidisciplinary treatment of embryonal rhabdomyosarcoma in children. Cancer 35:677–686

Ghavimi F, Herr H, Jereb B, Exelby PR (1984) Treatment of genitourinary rhabdomyosarcoma in children. J Urol 132:313–319

Glazer HS, Lee JKT, Levitt RG, et al. (1985) Radiation fibrosis: differentiation from recurrent tumor by MR imaging. Radiology 156:721–726

Granai CO, Walters MD, Safaii H, Jelen I, Madoc-Jones H, Moukhtar M (1984) Malignant transformation of vaginal endometriosis. Obstet Gynecol 64:592–595

Grosfeld JL, Smith JP, Clatworthy W (1972) Pelvic rhabdomyosarcoma in infants and children. J Urol 107:673–675

Harris NL, Scully RE (1984) Malignant lymphoma and granulocytic sarcoma of the uterus and vagina. Cancer 53:2530

Harrison LB, Fogel TD, Peschel RE (1987) Primary vaginal cancer and vaginal melanoma: a review of therapy with external beam radiation and a simple intracavitary brachytherapy system. Endocurietherapy/Hyperthermia Oncol 3:67–72

Hart WR, Townsend DE, Aldrich JO, Henderson BE, Roy M, Benton B (1976) Histopathologic spectrum of vaginal adenosis and related changes in stilbestrol-exposed females. Cancer 37:763

Harwood AR, Cummings BJ (1982) Radiotherapy for mucosal melanomas. Int J Radiat Oncol Biol Phys 8:1121

Hays DM, Shimada H, Raney RB, Tefft M, Newton W, Christ WM, Lawrence W, Ragab A, Maurer HM (1985) Sarcomas of the vagina and uterus: the Intergroup Rhabdomyosarcoma Study. J Pediatr Surg 20:718–724

Helders RD, Malkasian GD, Soule EH (1972) Embryonal rhabdomyosarcoma of the vagina. Am J Obstet Gynecol 107:484–502

Herbst AL (1981) Clear cell adenocarcinoma and the current status of DES-exposed females. Cancer 48:484

Herbst AL (1988) The effects in the human of diethylstilbestrol (DES) use during pregnancy. In: Miller RW, Takamatsu NO, Miya HI, Gan K (eds) Unusual occurrences as clues to cancer etiology. Taylor & Francis, Tokyo, pp 67–75

Herbst AL, Anderson D (1990) Clear cell adenocarcinoma of the vagina and cervix secondary to intrauterine exposure to diethylstilbestrol. Semin Surg Oncol 6:343–346

Herbst AL, Scully RE (1970) Adenocarcinoma of the vagina in adolescence: a report of 7 cases including 6 clear-cell carcinomas (so-called mesonephromas). Cancer 25:745

Herbst AL, Green TH Jr, Ulfelder H (1970) Primary carcinoma of the vagina. Am J Obstet Gynecol 106:210–218

Herbst AL, Ulfelder H, Poskanzer DC (1971) Adenocarcinoma of the vagina: association of maternal stilbestrol therapy with tumor appearance in young women. N Engl J Med 284:878–881

Herbst AL, Robboy SJ, Scully RE, Poskanzer DC (1974) Clear-cell adenocarcinoma of the vagina and cervix in girls: Analysis of 170 Registry cases. Am J Obstet Gynecol 119:713–724

Hicks ML, Piver MS (1992) Conservative surgery plus adjuvant therapy for vulvovaginal rhabdomyosarcoma, diethylstilbestrol clear cell adenocarcinoma of the vagina, and unilateral germ cell tumors of the ovary. Obstet Gynecol Clin North Am 19:219–233

Hilborne LH, Fu YS (1987) Intraepithelial, invasive and metastatic neoplasms of the vagina. In: Wilkinson EJ (ed) Pathology of the vulva and vagina. Churchill Livingstone, New York, p 184

Hilgers RD (1975) Pelvic exenteration for vaginal embryonal rhabdomyosarcoma: a review. Obstet Gynecol 45:175–180

Hintz GL, Kagan AR, Chan P, Gilbert HA, Nussbaum H, Rao AR, Wollin M (1980) Radiation tolerance of the vaginal mucosa. Int J Radiat Oncol Biol Phys 6:711–716

Hiura M, Nagai N (1985) Vaginal hemangiopericytoma: a light microscopic and ultrastructural study. Gynecol Oncol 21:376

Hoffman MS, DeCesare SL, Roberts WS, Fiorica JV, Finan MA, Cavanagh D (1992) Upper vaginectomy for in situ and occult, superficially invasive carcinoma of the vagina. Am J Obstet Gynecol 166:30–33

Holton CP, Chapman KE, Lackey RW, Hatch EI, Baum ES, Favara BE (1973) Extended combination therapy of childhood rhabdomyosarcoma. Cancer 32:1310–1316

Hopkins MP, Morley GW (1987) Squamous cell carcinoma of the neovagina. Obstet Gynecol 69:525–527

Hopkins MP, Kumar NB, Lichter AS, Peters WA III, Morley GW (1989) Small cell carcinoma of the vagina with neuroendocrine features: a report of three cases. J Reprod Med 34:486–491

Horwitz RI, Viscoli CM, Merino M, Brennan TA, Flannery JT, Robboy SJ (1988) Clear cell adenocarcinoma of the vagina and cervix: incidence, undetected disease, and diethylstilbestrol. J Clin Epidemiol 41:593–597

Hoskins WJ, Perez C, Young RC (1989) Gynecologic tumors. In: DeVita VT Jr, Hellman S, Rosenberg SA (eds) Cancer: principles and practice of oncology, 3rd edn. Lippincott, Philadelphia, pp 1099–1161

Hricak H, Lacey CG, Sandles LG, Chang YC, Winkler ML, Stern JL (1988) Invasive cervical carcinoma: comparison of MR imaging and surgical findings. Radiology 166:623–631

Iverson K, Robins RE (1980) Mucosal malignant melanomas. Am J Surg 139:660

Kanbour AI, Klionsky B, Murphy AL (1974) Carcinoma of the vagina following cervical cancer. Cancer 34:1838

Kasai K, Yoshida Y, Okumura M (1980) Alveolar soft part sarcoma in the vagina: clinical features and morphology. Gynecol Oncol 9:227

Katib S, Kuten A, Steiner M, Yudelev M, Robinson E (1985) The effectiveness of multidrug treatment by bleomycin, methotrexate, and cisplatin in advanced vaginal carcinoma. Gynecol Oncol 21:101–102

Kaufman RH, Korhonen MO, Strama T, Adam E, Kaplan A (1982) Development of clear cell adenocarcinoma in DES-exposed offspring under observation. Obstet Gynecol 59:68S–72S

Kilman JM, Clatworthy HW Jr, Newton WA Jr, et al. (1973) Reasonable surgery for rhabdomyosarcoma: a study of 67 cases. Ann Surg 178:346–351

Kraus FT, Perez-Mesa C (1966) Verrucous carcinoma: cervical and pathologic study of 105 cases involving oral cavity, larynx and genitalia. Cancer 19:27

Kucera H, Vavra N (1991) Radiation management of primary carcinoma of the vagina: clinical and histopathological variables associated with survival. Gynecol Oncol 40:12–16

Kucera H, Langer M, Smekal G, Weghaupt K (1985) Radiotherapy of primary carcinoma of the vagina: management and results of different therapy schemes. Gynecol Oncol 21:87–93

Kurman RJ, Scully RE (1974) The incidence and histogenesis of vaginal adenosis: an autopsy study. Hum Pathol 5: 265

Lamont A (1984) Wondgenesing en wondhegting (wound healing and suturing). South African J Cont Med Ed 2:95–99

Laufe LE, Bernstein ED (1971) Primary malignant melanoma of the vagina. Obstet Gynecol 37:148–154

Lee JY, Perez CA, Ettinger N, Fineberg BB (1982) The risk of second primaries subsequent to irradiation for cervix cancer. Int J Radiat Oncol Biol Phys 8:207–211

Lee RA, Symmonds RE (1976) Recurrent carcinoma in situ of the vagina in patients previously treated for in situ carcinoma of the cervix. Obstet Gynecol 48:61–64

Leung S, Sexton M (1993) Radical radiation therapy for carcinoma of the vagina: impact of treatment modalities on outcome: Peter MacCallum Cancer Institute experience 1970–1990. Int J Radiat Oncol Biol Phys 25:413–418

Levitan Z, Gordon AN, Kaplan AL, Kaufman RH (1989) Primary malignant melanoma of the vagina: report of four cases and review of the literature. Gynecol Oncol 33:85–90

Lindeque BG (1987) The role of surgery in the management of carcinoma of the vagina. Baillieres Clin Obstet Gynaecol 1:319–329

Lindeque BG, Monaghan JM (to be published) The role of surgery in the management of primary vaginal cancer. J Obstet Gynecol

Livingstone RC (1950) Primary carcinoma of the vagina. Thomas, Springfield, ILL

MacNaught R, Symmonds RP, Hole D, Watson ER (1986) Improved control of primary vaginal tumors by combined external beam and interstitial radiotherapy. Clin Radiol 37:29–32

Magrina JF, Masterson BJ (1981) Vaginal reconstruction in gynecologic oncology: a review of techniques. Obstet Gynecol Surv 36:1–10

Mahesh Kumar APM, Wrenn EL Jr, Fleming ID, Omar Hustu H, Pratt CB (1976) Combined therapy to prevent complete pelvic exenteration for rhabdomyosarcoma of the vagina or uterus. Cancer 37:118–122

Manetta A, Pinto JL, Larson JE, Stevens CW Jr, Pinto JS, Podczaski ES (1988) Primary invasive carcinoma of the vagina. Obstet Gynecol 72:77–81

Manetta A, Gutrecht EL, Berman ML, DiSaia PJ (1990) Primary invasive carcinoma of the vagina. Obstet Gynecol 76:639–642

Marcus RB, Million RR, Daly JW (1978) Carcinoma of the vagina. Cancer 42:2507–2512

Mattingly RF, Stafl A (1976) Cancer risk in diethylstilbestrol-exposed offspring. Am J Obstet Gynecol 126:543

Melnick S, Cole P, Anderson D, Herbst A (1987) Rates and risks of diethylstilbestrol-related clear-cell adenocarcinoma of the vagina and cervix: an update. N Engl J Med 316:514–516

Morrow CP, DiSaia PJ (1976) Malignant melanoma of the female genitalia: a clinical analysis. Obstet Gynecol Surv 31:233

Muench PJ, Nath R (1992) Dose distributions produced by shielded applicators using ^{241}Am for intracavitary irradiation of tumors in the vagina. Med Phys 19:1299–1306

Muss HB, Bundy BN, DiSaia PJ, Homesley HD, Fowler WC Jr, Creasman W, Yordan E (1985) Treatment of recurrent or advanced uterine sarcoma: a randomized trial of doxorubicin versus doxorubicin and cyclophosphamide. Cancer 55:1648–1653

Muss HB, Bundy BN, Christopherson WA (1989) Mitoxantrone in the treatment of advanced vulvar and vaginal carcinoma. Am J Clin Oncol 12:142–144

Nanavati PJ, Fanning J, Hilgers RD, Hallstrom J, Crawford D (1993) High-dose-rate brachytherapy in primary stage I and II vaginal cancer. Gynecol Oncol 51:67–71

Ng AB, Reagan JW, Hawliczek S, Wentz WB (1975) Cellular detection of vaginal adenosis. Obstet Gynecol 46:323–328

Noller KL, Townsend DE, Kaufman RH, et al. (1983) Maturation of vaginal and cervical epithelium in women exposed in utero to diethylstilbestrol (DESAD Project). Am J Obstet Gynecol 146:279–285

Nori D, Hilaris BS, Stanimir G, Lewis JL Jr (1983) Radiation therapy of primary vaginal carcinoma. Int J Radiat Oncol Biol Phys 9:1471

Norris HJ, Taylor HB (1966) Melanomas of the vagina. Am J Clin Pathol 46:420–426

O'Brien PC, Noller KL, Robboy SJ, Barnes AB, Kaufman RH, Tilley BC, Townsend DE (1979) Vaginal epithelial changes in young women enrolled in the national cooperative diethylstilbestrol adenosis (DESAD) project. Obstet Gynecol 53:300–308

Okagaki T, Ishida T, Hilgers RD (1976) A malignant tumor of the vagina resembling synovial sarcoma: a light and electron microscopic study. Cancer 37:2306

Omura GA, Shingleton HM, Creasman WT, Blessing JA, Boronow RC (1978) Chemotherapy of gynecologic cancer with nitosoureas: a randomized trial of CCNU and methyl-

CCNU in cancer of the cervix, corpus, vagina, and vulva. Cancer Treat Rep 62:833–835
Patton TJ, Kavahagh JJ, Delclos L, et al. (1991) Five-year survival in patients given intra-arterial chemotherapy prior to radiotherapy for advanced squamous carcinoma of the cervix and vagina. Gynecol Oncol 42:54–59
Perez CA (1992) Vagina. In: Perez CA, Brady LW (eds) Principles and practice of radiation oncology, 2nd edn. Lippincott, Philadelphia, pp 1258–1272
Perez CA, Camel HM (1982) Long-term follow-up in radiation therapy of carcinoma of the vagina. Cancer 49:1308–1315
Perez CA, Madoc-Jones H (1987) Carcinoma of the vagina. In: Perez CA, Brady LW (eds) Principles and practice of radiation oncology. Lippincott, Philadelphia, pp 1023–1035
Perez CA, Arneson AN, Galakatos A, Samath HK (1973) Malignant tumors of the vagina. Cancer 31:36–44
Perez CA, Arneson AN, Dehner LP, Galakatos A (1974) Radiation therapy in carcinoma of the vagina. Obstet Gynecol 44:862–872
Perez CA, Korba A, Sharma S (1977) Dosimetric considerations in irradiation of carcinoma of the vagina. Int J Radiat Oncol Biol Phys 2:639–649
Perez CA, Bedwinek JM, Breaux SR (1983) Patterns of failure after treatment of gynecologic tumors. Cancer Treat Symp 2:217
Perez CA, Camel HM, Galakatos AE, Grigsby PW, Kuske RR, Buchsbaum G, Hederman MA (1988) Definitive irradiation in carcinoma of the vagina: long-term evaluation of results. Int J Radiat Oncol Biol Phys 15:1283–1290
Perez CA, Slessinger E, Grigsby PW (1990) Design of an afterloading vaginal applicator (MIRALVA). Int J Radiat Oncol Biol Phys 18:1503
Perez CA, Gersell DJ, Hoskins WJ, McGuire WP (1992) Vagina. In: Hoskins WJ, Perez CA, Young RC (eds) Principles and practice of gynecologic oncology. Lippincott, Philadephia, pp 567–590
Perren T, Farrant M, McCarthy K, Harper P, Wiltshaw E (1992) Lymphomas of the cervix and upper vagina: a report of five cases and a review of the literature. Gynecol Oncol 44:87–95
Peters WA III, Juman NB, Morley GW (1985a) Carcinoma of the vagina: factors influencing outcome. Cancer 55:892–897
Peters WA III, Kumar NB, Andersen WA, Morley GW (1985b) Primary sarcoma of the adult vagina: a clinicopathologic study. Obstet Gynecol 65:699–704
Piver MS, Rose PG (1988) Long-term follow-up and complications of infants with vulvovaginal embryonal rhabdomyosarcoma treated with surgery, radiation therapy, and chemotherapy Obstet Gynecol 71:435–437
Piver MS, Barlow JJ, Wang JJ, Shah NK (1973) Combined radical surgery, radiation therapy and chemotherapy in infants with vulvo-vaginal embryonal rhabdomyosarcoma. Obstet Gynecol 42:522–526
Piver MS, Barlow JJ, Xynos FP (1978) Adriamycin alone or in combination in 100 patients with carcinoma of the cervix or vagina. Am J Obstet Gynecol 131:311–313
Plentl AA, Friedman EA (1971) Lymphatic system of the female genitalia: the morphologic basis of oncologic diagnosis and therapy. Saunders, Philadelphia, pp 51–74
Powell JL, Franklin EW III, Nickerson JF, Burrell MO (1978) Verrucous carcinoma of the female genital tract. Gynecol Oncol 6:565–573
Pratt CB, Husto HO, Fleming ID, Pinkel D (1972) Combination treatment of childhood rhabdomyosarcoma with surgery, radiotherapy, and combination chemotherapy. Cancer Res 32:606–610
Prempree T, Amornmarn R (1985) Radiation treatment of primary carcinoma of the vagina: patterns of failure after definitive therapy. Acta Radiol Oncol 24:51–56
Prempree T, Tang C-K, Hatef A, Forster S (1983) Angiosarcoma of the vagina: a clinicopathologic report. A reappraisal of radiation treatment of angiosarcomas of the female genital tract. Cancer 51:618–622
Prévot S, Hugol D, Audouin J, Diebold J, Truc JB, Decroix Y, Poitout P (1992) Primary non-Hodgkin's malignant lymphoma of the vagina: report on three cases and review of the literature. Pathol Res Pract 188:78–85
Pride GL, Schultz AE, Chuprevich TW, Buchler D (1979) Primary invasive squamous carcinoma of the vagina. Obstet Gynecol 53:218–225
Puthawala A, Syed AMN, Nalick R, McNamara C, DiSaia PJ (1983) Integrated external and interstitial radiation therapy for primary carcinoma of the vagina. Obstet Gynecol 62:367–372
Ragni MV, Tobon H (1974) Primary malignant melanoma of the vagina and vulva. Obstet Gynecol 43:658–664
Ramzy I, Smont MS, Collins JA (1976) Verrucous carcinoma of the vagina. Am J Clin Pathol 65:644
Raney RB Jr, Gehan EA, Hays DM, Tefft M, Newton WA Jr, Haeberlen V, Maurer HM (1990) Primary chemotherapy with or without radiation therapy and/or surgery for children with localized sarcoma of the bladder, prostate, vagina, uterus, and cervix: a comparison of the results in Intergroup Rhabdomyosarcoma Studies I and II. Cancer 66:2072–2081
Reddy S, Lee MS, Graham JE, et al. (1987) Radiation therapy in primary carcinoma of the vagina. Gynecol Oncol 26:19–24
Reddy S, Saxena VS, Reddy S, et al. (1991) Results of radiotherapeutic management of primary carcinoma of the vagina. Int J Radiat Oncol Biol Phys 21:1041
Reid GC, Schmidt RW, Roberts JA, Hopkins MP, Barrett RJ, Morley GW (1989) Primary melanoma of the vagina: a clinicopathologic analysis. Obstet Gynecol 74:190–199
Robboy SJ, Welch WR (1977) Microglandular hyperplasia in vaginal adenosis associated with oral contraceptives and prenatal diethylstilbestrol exposure. Obstet Gynecol 49:430
Robboy SJ, Herbst AL, Scully RE (1974) Clear cell adenocarcinoma of the vagina and cervix in young females: analysis of 37 tumors that persisted or recurred after primary therapy. Cancer 34:606–614
Robboy SJ, Scully RE, Herbst AL (1975) Pathology of vaginal and cervical abnormalities associated with prenatal exposure to diethylstilbesterol. J Reprod Med 15:13
Robboy SJ, Prat J, Welch WR (1977a) Squamous cell neoplasia controversy in the female exposed to diethylstilbestrol. Hum Pathol 8:483
Robboy SJ, Scully RE, Welch WR, Herbst AL (1977b) Intrauterine diethylstilbestrol exposure and its consequences: pathologic characteristics of vaginal adenosis, clear cell adenocarcinoma, and related lesions. Arch Pathol Lab Med 101:1
Robboy SJ, Keh PC, Nickerson RJ, et al. (1978) Squamous cell dysplasia and carcinoma in situ of the cervix and vagina after prenatal exposure to diethylstilbestrol. Obstet Gynecol 51:528–535
Robboy SJ, Kaufman RH, Prat J, et al. (1979) Pathologic findings in young women enrolled in the national cooperative diethylstilbestrol adenosis (DESAD) project. Obstet Gynecol 53:309–317

Robboy SJ, Szyfelbein WM, Goellner JR, et al. (1981) Dysplasia and cytologic findings in 4589 young women enrolled in diethylstilbestrol-adenosis (DESAD) project. Am J Obstet Gynecol 140:579–586

Robboy SJ, Welch WR, Young RH, Truslow GY, Herbst AL, Scully RE (1982) Topographic relation of cervical ectropion and vaginal adenosis to clear cell adenocarcinoma. Obstet Gynecol 60:546

Robboy SJ, Hill EC, Sandberg EC, Czernobilsky B (1986) Vaginal adenosis in women born prior to the diethylstilbestrol era. Hum Pathol 17:488–492

Robboy SJ, Noller KL, O'Brien P, et al. (1984) Increased incidence of cervical and vaginal dysplasia in 3980 diethylstilbestrol-exposed young women: experience of the National Collaborative Diethylstilbestrol Adenosis Project. JAMA 252:2959

Rogo KO, Andersson R, Edbom G, Stendahl U (1991) Conservative surgery for vulvovaginal melanoma. Eur J Gynaecol Oncol 12:113–119

Rubin P (1983) Clinical oncology: a multidisciplinary approach, 6th edn. American Cancer Society, Atlanta

Rubin SC, Young J, Mikuta JJ (1985) Squamous carcinoma of the vagina: treatment, complications, and long-term follow-up. Gynecol Oncol 20:346–353

Rutledge F (1967) Cancer of the vagina. Am J Obstet Gynecol 97:635–655

Ryan TP, Taylor JH, Coughlin CT (1992) Interstitial microwave hyperthermia and brachytherapy for malignancies of the vulva and vagina. I. Design and testing of a modified intracavitary obturator. Int J Radiat Oncol Biol Phys 23:189–199

Sandberg EC (1968) The incidence and distribution of occult vaginal adenosis. Am J Obstet Gynecol 101:322

Sandberg EC, Danielson RW, Cauwet RW, et al. (1965) Adenosis vaginae. Am J Obstet Gynecol 93:209

Sedlis A, Robboy SJ (1987) Disease of the vagina. In: Kurman RJ (ed) Blaustein's pathology of the female genital tract. Springer, Berlin Heidelberg New York, p 113

Senekjian EK, Frey KW, Anderson D, Herbst AL (1987) Local therapy in stage I clear cell adenocarcinoma of the vagina. Cancer 60:1319–1324

Senekjian EK, Frey KW, Stone C, Herbst AL (1988) An evaluation of stage II vaginal clear cell adenocarcinoma according to substages. Gynecol Oncol 31:56–64

Senekjian EK, Frey K, Herbst AL (1989) Pelvic exenteration in clear cell adenocarcinoma of the vagina and cervix. Gynecol Oncol 34:413–416

Sharma SC, Bhandare N (1991) A new design of Delclos dome cylinders using standard Cs-137 sources. Int J Radiat Oncol Biol Phys 21:511–514

Sharma SC, Gerbi B, Madoc-Jones H (1979) Dose rates for brachytherapy applicators using ^{137}Cs sources. Int J Radiat Oncol Biol Phys 5:1893

Shevchuk M, Fenoglio CM, Lattes R, et al. (1978) Malignant mixed tumor of the vagina probably arising in mesonephric rests. Cancer 42:214

Shimm DS, Ropar M (1986) Radiation therapy of carcinoma of the vagina. Acta Obstet Gynecol Scand 65:449–452

Shpikalov VL, Atkochyus VB (1989) Interstitial radiotherapy of malignant tumors of the vagina. Neoplasma 36:729–737

Slayton RE, Blessing JA, Beecham J, et al. (1987) Phase II trial of etoposide in the management of advanced or recurrent squamous carcinoma of the vulva and carcinoma of the vagina: a Gynecologic Oncology Group Study. Cancer Treat Rep 71:869–870

Son YH (1980) Primary mucosal malignant melanoma: appraisal of role of radiation therapy. Acta Radiol Oncol 19:177

Spirtos NM, Doshi BP, Kapp DS, Teng N (1989) Radiation therapy for primary squamous cell carcinoma of the vagina: Stanford University experience. Gynecol Oncol 35:20–26

Stafl A, Mattingly RF (1974) Vaginal adenosis : a precancerous lesion? Am J Obstet Gynecol 120:666

Steeper TA, Piscioli F, Rosai J (1983) Squamous cell carcinoma with sarcoma-like stroma of the female genital tract. Cancer 52:890

Stock RG, Mychalczak B, Armstrong JG, Curtin JP, Harrison LB (1992) The importance of brachytherapy technique in the management of primary carcinoma of the vagina. Int J Radiat Oncol Biol Phys 24:747–753

Stuart GC, Allen HH, Anderson RJ (1981) Squamous cell carcinoma of the vagina following hysterectomy. Am J Obstet Gynecol 139:311–315

Sutton GP, Blessing JA, Rosenshein N, Photopulos G, DiSaia PJ (1989) Phase II trial of ifosfamide and mesna in mixed mesodermal tumors of the uterus (a Gynecologic Oncology Group study). Am J Obstet Gynecol 161:309–312

Tarraza MH Jr, Muntz H, Decain M, Granai OC, Fuller A Jr (1991) Patterns of recurrence of primary carcinoma of the vagina. Eur J Gynaecol Oncol 12:89–92

Tavassoli FA, Norris HJ (1979) Smooth muscle tumors of the vagina. Obstet Gynecol 53:689–693

Thigpen JT, Blessing JA, Homesley HD, Berek JS, Creasman WT (1986a) Phase II trial of cisplatin in advanced or recurrent cancer of the vagina: a Gynecologic Oncology Group Study. Gynecol Oncol 23:101–104

Thigpen JT, Blessing JA, Orr JW, DiSaia PJ (1986b) Phase II trial of cisplatin in the treatment of patients with advanced or recurrent mixed mesoderma sarcomas of the uterus: a Gynecologic Oncology Group Study. Cancer Treat Rep 70:271–274

Tobon H, Murphy AI, Salazar H (1973) Primary leiomyosarcoma of the vagina: light and electron microscopic observation. Cancer 32:450

Togashi K, Nishimura K, Itoh K, et al. (1986) Uterine cervical cancer: assessment with high-field MR imaging. Radiology 160:431–435

Townsend DE (1981) Intraepithelial neoplasia of the vagina. In: Coppleson M (ed) Gynecologic oncology: fundamental principles and clinical practice. Churchill Livingstone, New York, pp 339–344

Ulbright TM, Kraus FT (1981) Endometrial stromal tumors of extra-uterine tissue. Am J Clin Pathol 76:371

Ulich TR, Liao S-Y, Layfield L, Romansky S, Cheng L, Lwein KT (1986) Endocrine and tumor differentiation markers in poorly differentiated small-cell carcinoids of the cervix and vagina. Arch Pathol Lab Med 110:1054–1057

Underwood RB, Smith RT (1971) Carcinoma of the vagina. JAMA 217:46–52

Vayrynen M, Romppanen T, Koskela E, Castren O, Syrjanen K (1981) Verrucous squamous cell carcinoma of the female genital tract: report of three cases and survey of the literature. Int J Gynaecol Obstet 19:351–356

Wasserman TH, Stetz J, Phillips TL (1980) Clinical trials of misonidazole in the United States. In: Brady LW (ed) Radiation sensitizers: their use in the clinical management of cancer. Masson, New York, pp 387–396

Way S (1948) Primary carcinoma of the vagina. J Obstet Gynaecol Br Emp 55:739

Webb MJ, Symmonds RE, Weiland LH (1974) Malignant fibrous histiocytoma of vagina. Am J Obstet Gynecol 119:190

Wharton JT, Rutledge FN, Gallagher HS, Fletcher G (1975) Treatment of clear cell adenocarcinoma in young females. Obstet Gynecol 43:365–368

Whelton J, Kottmeier HL (1962) Primary carcinoma of the vagina. Acta Obstet Gynecol Scand 41:22–40

Woodman CB, Mould JJ, Jordan JA (1988) Radiotherapy in the management of vaginal intraepithelial neoplasia after hysterectomy. Br J Obstet Gynaecol 95:976–979

Woodruff JD, Parmley TH, Julian CG (1975) Topical 5-fluorouracil in the treatment of vaginal carcinoma in situ. Gynecol Oncol 3:124

8 Cancer of the Female Urethra

B. Micaily and M.F. Dzeda

CONTENTS

8.1 Epidemiology

Carcinoma of the female urethra is uncommon, with approximately 1500 cases reported in the literature (Grigsby 1992). It represents 0.02% of all cancers found in women and less than 0.1% of all gynecologic malignancies (Johnson and O'Connell 1983; Weghaupt et al. 1984). The peak incidence occurs in the fifth and sixth decades, although cases have been reported in children as young as 4 years and women in their ninth decade (Hopkins and Grabstald 1986). This cancer appears to be more common in white women (85%) than black women (12%) (Hopkins and Grabstald 1986).

The causes for female urethral cancer remain unclear. Various factors such as chronic urethral irritation, caruncle, polyps, viral infections, fibrosis, coitus, and parturition have been suggested as causative agents, but there has been no substantiating evidence (Narayan and Konety 1992).

B. Micaily, MD, Department of Radiation Oncology, Allegheny University Hahnemann, Broad and Vine, Mail Stop 200, Philadelphia, PA 19102-1192, USA
M.F. Dzeda, MD, Department of Radiation Oncology, Allegheny University Hahnemann, Broad and Vine, Mail Stop 200, Philadelphia, PA 19102-1192, USA

8.2 Anatomy and Pattern of Spread

The female urethra is 3–4 cm long and is arbitrarily divided into proximal and distal sections (Leeson et al. 1988). It extends from the urinary bladder, passes through the urogenital diaphragm, and terminates at the vestibule, forming the urethral meatus (Figs. 8.1, 8.2). Most of the urethra remains buried in the anterior wall of the vagina.

The urethra is surrounded by a layer of longitudinal smooth muscle which is continuous with the detrusor muscle of the bladder. The proximal end of the muscular wall forms the internal sphincter. The voluntary urethral sphincter is located at the level of the urogenital diaphragm. The lamina propria comprises the middle layer and contains loose fibroconnective tissue as well as numerous venous plexuses similar to the cavernous tissue of the male. The inner epithelial surface contains several histologies. The proximal third is lined with transitional epithelium which merges internally with the bladder. The distal two-thirds is composed of nonkeratinizing stratified squamous epithelium with patches of psuedostratified columnar epithelium that continues externally onto the vulva. The distal urethra additionally contains small mucous recesses and the periurethral Skene's glands. These glands are concentrated in the region of the meatus but extend along the entire urethra and are lined by psuedostratified and stratified columnar epithelium.

The lymphatics of the distal urethra, like those of the vulva, drain into the superficial and deep inguinal lymph nodes. The drainage of the proximal urethra is mainly to the obturator, internal and external iliac, and presacral lymph nodes.

Tumors originating from the distal urethra can resemble a urethral caruncle or present as a papillary growth protruding from the meatus (Hopkins and

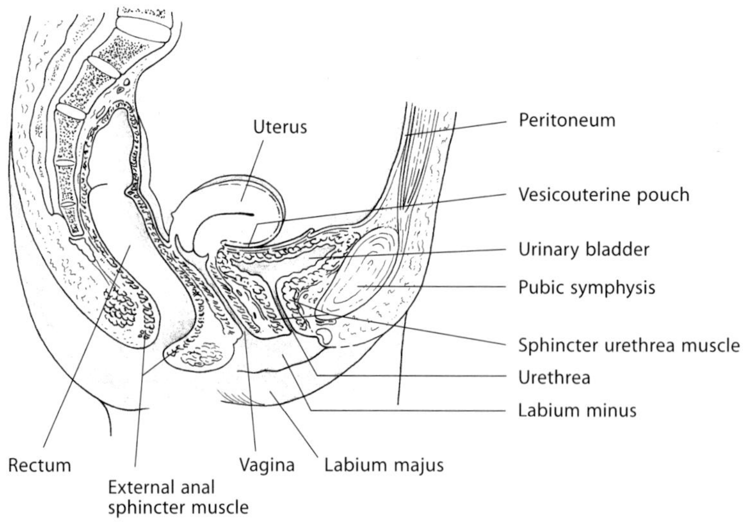

Fig. 8.1. Sagittal section of female pelvis at mid-plane

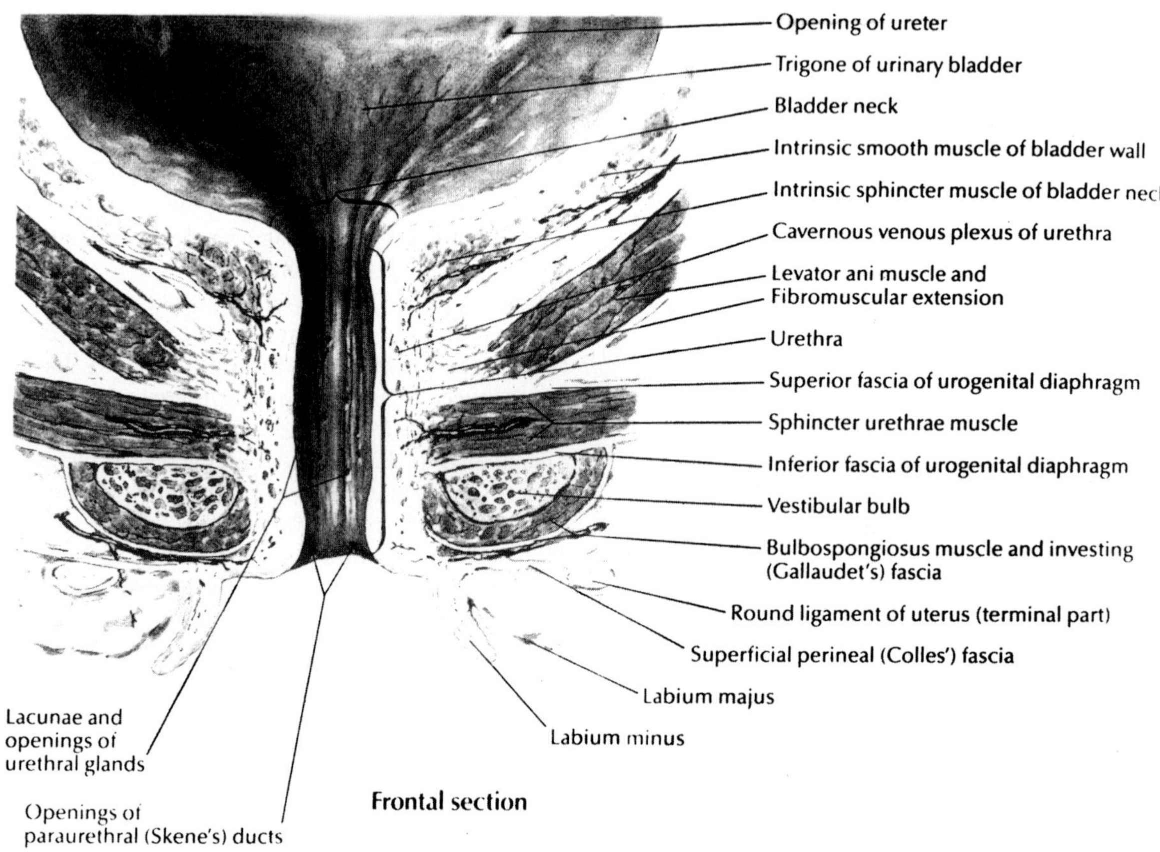

Fig. 8.2. Anatomy of female pelvis. Coronal section at the plane of the urethra

Grabstald 1986). These lesions may be detected at an earlier stage because of their tendency to bleed and superficial location (Antoniades 1969). As these tumors progress, they may enlarge, ulcerate, and extend to the perineum (Peterson et al. 1973).

In more advanced stages, malignancies of the proximal urethra can erode into the vaginal vault, extend downward to involve the entire urethra, and infiltrate the urinary bladder (FORMAN and LICHTER 1992). Tumors are confined to the distal urethra in approximately 30%–40% of cases (GRABSTALD 1973; JOHNSON and O'CONNELL 1983).

Regional lymph node spread is uncommon in early tumors of the urethral meatus, but in more advanced stages, clinically positive nodes at presentation are found in approximately 30% of patients (ANTONIADES 1969; CHU 1973; DESAI et al. 1973; GRABSTALD et al. 1966; SAILER et al. 1988; WEGHAUPT et al. 1984). The majority of these will represent metastatic disease rather than infection. In a report from Memorial Sloan-Kettering Cancer Center, 25 of 79 patients demonstrated clinically positive nodes during the course of their disease (GRABSTALD et al. 1966). Pathologic examination was performed in 24 of 25 patients, with confirmation of cancer in 22. Of 26 patients who underwent pelvic node sampling, 13 were found to have lymph node metastases.

Distant metastases at presentation was found in 5 of 79 patients and developed in an additional six patients in the same study from MSKCC (GRABSTALD et al. 1966). The most common sites were lung, bone, brain, and liver. Distant spread was found to be more common in adenocarcinoma and did not seem to correlate with lymphatic involvement.

8.3 Symptoms

Due to the nonspecific nature of symptoms, the average time between onset and diagnosis is usually 5–6 months (HOPKINS and GRABSTALD 1986). A summary of presenting symptoms from three institutions is given in Table 8.1 (BRACKEN et al. 1976; GRABSTALD et al. 1966; PETERSON et al. 1973). The most common symptom is bleeding, occurring in more than half of the patients. Other common complaints are urinary frequency, dysuria, and the development of a urethral mass. less frequently encountered are perineal pain, dyspareunia, and incontinence. Some patients present with advanced disease, including urethrovaginal and vesicovaginal fistulas as well as inguinal lymphandenopathy.

Table 8.1. Presenting symptoms in 209 women from three institutions. (BRACKEN et al. 1976; GRABSTALD et al. 1966; PETERSON et al. 1973)

Symptom	Percent
Bleeding	55
Urinary frequency	42
Dysuria	41
Urethral mass	30
Perineal pain	16
Incontinence	7
Dyspareunia	6

8.4 Diagnostic Workup

A thorough history and physical examination should be performed, with attention to the groin and lower extremities to assess regional lymph node status. A bimanual pelvic examination under general anesthesia is done at the time of cystourethroscopy to evaluate the extent of local involvement. Urine cytology can be obtained, but definitive pathologic diagnosis is best documented by biopsy of the primary tumor.

Routine laboratory studies include a complete blood count, blood chemistry, and urinalysis. Radiographic studies should consist of a chest x-ray as well as computed tomography of the abdomen and pelvis. Magnetic resonance imaging appears to be superior in assessing lymph node status and local disease in the pelvis and is valuable as a complementary study (Fig. 8.3). In asymptomatic patients with early stage disease, the yield in obtaining a bone scan is

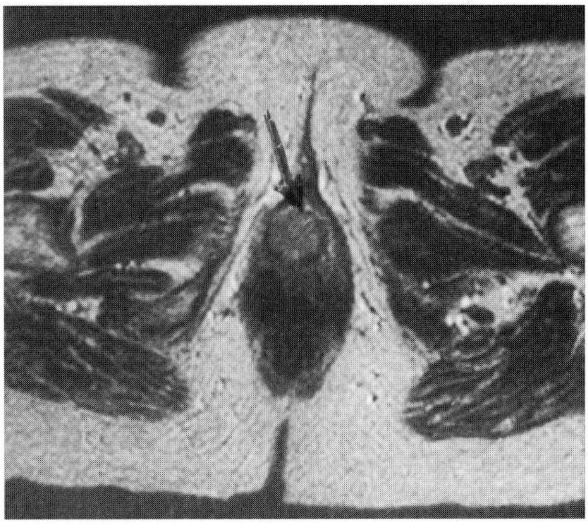

Fig. 8.3. Magnetic resonance image of the female pelvis. Cross-sectional view at the urethral meatus, in a patient with distal urethral squamous cell carcinoma. Note periurethral and anterior vaginal wall extension of the tumor (*solid arrow*)

extremely small and can be omitted. Additional studies that should be considered as optional are intravenous pyelography and lymphangiography.

8.5 Staging

There have been several attempts to formulate a universally accepted staging system for carcinoma of the female urethra. The two most frequently used systems are the Grabstald staging system based on pathological criteria and the Prempree modification of Taggart and associates, which is clinically based (Tables 8.2, 8.3) (GRABSTALD et al. 1966; PREMPREE et al. 1984). Most authors use the Prempree modification, since this system distinguishes distal one-half from entire urethral involvement, reflecting the treatment and prognosis of female urethral cancer. The American Joint Committee on Cancer TNM staging system is shown in Table 8.4 (BEAHRS et al. 1992).

Table 8.2. Grabstald staging system for carcinoma of the female urethra. (GRABSTALD et al. 1966)

Stage 0	In situ (limited to mucosa)
Stage A	Submucosal (not beyond submucosa)
Stage B	Muscular (infiltrating periurethral muscle)
Stage C	Periurethral
C1	Infiltrating muscular wall of vagina
C2	Infiltrating muscular wall of vagina with invasion of vaginal mucosa
C3	Infiltrating other adjacent structures such as bladder, labia, or clitoris
Stage D	Metastasis
D1	Inguinal lymph nodes
D2	Pelvic lymph nodes below aortic bifurcation
D3	Lymph nodes above aortic bifurcation
D4	Distant

Table 8.3. Prempree modification for staging of carcinoma of the female urethra. (PREMPREE et al. 1984)

Stage I	Disease limited to the distal one-half of the urethra
Stage II	Disease involving the entire urethra, with extension to the periurethral tissues, but not involving the vulva or bladder neck
Stage III	
A	Disease involving the urethra and vulva
B	Disease invading vaginal mucosa
C	Disease involving the urethra and bladder neck
Stage IV	
A	Disease invading parametrium or paracolpium
B	Metastases
1	Inguinal lymph nodes
2	Pelvic nodes
3	Para-aortic
4	Distant

8.6 Pathology

Tumors tend to be low grade when the anterior urethra is involved (GRABSTALD 1973). Squamous cell carcinoma is the most frequent histology in female urethral cancer, accounting for 70% of all cases. Transitional cell carcinoma is found in 15% and adenocarcinoma in approximately 10% of cases (MEIS et al. 1987; SAILER et al. 1988). A predilection for adenocarcinoma has been described in black women (MEIS et al. 1987). Melanoma is found in 3% and usually arises from the distal urethra (SAILER et al. 1988). Although rare, the female urethra is the most common site of origin of primary melanoma of the genitourinary tract (LEVINE 1980). Less common histologies include lymphoma, anaplastic tumors, and leiomyosarcomas (MOSTOFI et al. 1992; SAILER et al. 1988). Metastases to the urethra have been

Table 8.4. TNM classification for carcinoma of the urethra. (BEAHRS et al. 1992)

Primary tumor (T)	
TX	Primary tumor cannot be assessed
T0	No evidence of primary tumor
Tis	Carcinoma in situ
Ta	Noninvasive papillary, polypoid, or verrucous carcinoma
T1	Tumor invades subepithelial connective tissue
T2	Tumor invades the periurethral muscle
T3	Tumor invades the anterior vagina or bladder neck
T4	Tumor invades other adjacent organs
Regional lymph nodes (N)	
NX	Regional lymph nodes cannot be assessed
N0	No regional lymph node metastasis
N1	Metastasis in a single lymph node, 2 cm or less in greatest dimension
N2	Metastasis in a single lymph node, more than 2 cm but not more than 5 cm in greatest dimension; or multiple lymph nodes, none more than 5 cm in greatest dimension
N3	Metastasis in a lymph node more than 5 cm in greatest dimension
Distant metastasis (M)	
MX	Presence of distant metastasis cannot be assessed
M0	No distant metastasis
M1	Distant metastasis

reported for ovarian carcinomas, uterine carcinomas and choriocarcinomas, lung cancers, and lymphomas (Mostofi et al. 1992).

8.7 Prognostic Factors

The two most significant factors affecting prognosis in female urethral cancer are overall TNM staging and location. Small tumor size and distal location were found to be favorable prognostic factors. Grigsby and associates reported a 5-year progression-free survival of 81%, 37%, and 7% for patients with lesions less than 2 cm, 2–4 cm, and greater than 4 cm, respectively (Grigsby and Corn 1992). Bracken and associates noted a similar correlation between tumor size and survival (Bracken et al. 1976). They observed 5-year survival rates of 60%, 46%, and 13% in patients with tumors less than 2 cm, between 2 and 4 cm, and 5 cm or greater, respectively. Women with early meatal tumors had an excellent outlook, achieving nearly a 90% 5-year survival rate (Antoniades 1969; Hopkins and Grabstald 1986). Involvement of the entire urethra, fixed lesions, infiltration of adjacent structures, and lymph node metastasis are poor prognostic variables (Garden et al. 1993).

Histologic subtype has not been found to be a statistically significant prognostic factor in most studies (Antoniades 1969; Bracken et al. 1976; Garden et al. 1993). One exception is primary melanoma, which does signify a poor prognosis (Hopkins and Grabstald 1986).

8.8 Surgery

Tumors located in the distal third of the urethra which are superficial and limited to the mucosa (Tis, T1) can be treated surgically by laser surgery, local excision, or transurethral resection. Lesions invading the periurethral musculature (T2) may be managed utilizing partial urethrectomy, if clear margins are possible. Up to two-thirds of the distal urethra can be resected without causing urinary incontinence (Grabstald 1982).

Tumors involving the proximal or entire urethra often extend into adjacent structures and metastasize to the inguinal and pelvic lymph nodes. Standard surgical management involves cystourethrectomy (anterior exenteration) and pelvic lymph node dissection. In some cases, the entire vagina must be resected and vaginal reconstruction is performed using gracilis myocutaneous flaps. When the tumor involves the inferior pelvic rami or symphsis public, the en bloc resection includes the pubic rami to ensure an adequate surgical margin (Klein et al. 1983).

8.9 Treatment of Lymph Nodes

When inguinal lymph nodes are clinically involved, lymphadenectomy or irradiation is recommended. When the nodes are clinically negative, prophylactic lymphadenectomy has not been proven to be superior to therapeutic node dissection (Levine 1980). However, several investigators have recommended prophylactic inguinal node irradiation (Foens et al. 1991; Garden et al. 1993; Hahn et al. 1991). Foens et al. (1991) found a significantly higher inguinal failure rate in patients not receiving inguinal treatment (52%) than in those who received treatment to the inguinal nodes (10%), which corresponded to a superior 5-year survival (60% vs 18%).

8.10 Radiation Therapy

Early stage lesions of the urethral meatus are usually treated with interstitial brachytherapy. More bulky and invasive lesions of the anterior urethra are managed with branchytherapy in combination with external beam irradiation. In very advanced tumors of the posterior or entire urethra, preoperative irradiation followed by exenterative surgery has given the best results.

For localized disease or early meatal tumors with minimal invasion, interstitial brachytherapy is the treatment of choice. This technique features afterloading catheters utilizing iridium-192 to form a volume implant, usually arranged in a circular pattern around the urethral orifice, with the actual placement of catheters dependent on the tumor volume (Fig. 8.4). The treatment volume is defined through the use of MRI imaging and clinical evaluation. Pretreatment planning is then performed in conjunction with the physicist to determine the number of strands, the number of seeds, and the activity per seed to best encompass the specified target volume.

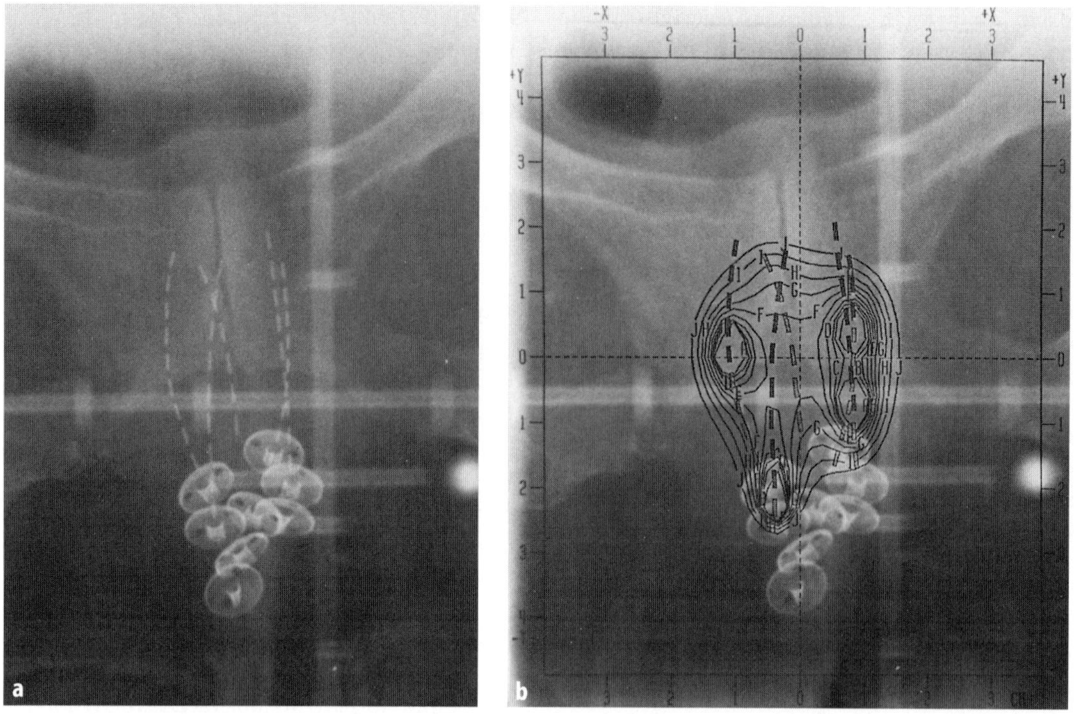

Fig. 8.4. **a** Anteroposterior view of interstitial urethral implant with iridium-192 seeds, using the afterloading technique. Forty-two seeds were used, with a seed activity of 0.48 mg radium equivalent per seed. **b** Overlay of isodose distribution on the above radio-graph; G line represents 90 cGy/h

The patient, under spinal or general anesthesia, is placed in the lithotomy position. A Foley catheter is inserted into the bladder and the balloon inflated. The actual length of the urethra can be determined by deflating the balloon after grasping the distal end of the catheter and measuring the length between the finger and the balloon. The Foley catheter is used as the central source of the implant. Other sources are positioned by using stainless steel trocars spaced 1 cm apart, guided either by a template or free-hand. Blind-end plastic catheters are threaded into the trocars, and a metal stylet is used to keep the catheters in place as the trocars and removed. Metal buttons are placed over the catheter and crimped while the stylet remains in position. The stylet is then removed and the buttons sutured. When the catheters are secured, the iridium-192 strands are placed into the catheters and fastened. After verification of source placement by x-ray, a dose of 6000–7000 cGy is delivered at 60–120 cGy per hour to the periphery of the implant volume when the implant is to be used alone.

For large, bulky tumors with extension to the urinary bladder or involvement of the vagina, labia, or entire urethra, an implant alone will not be sufficient to control disease. For these patients, external beam irradiation is followed by interstitial brachytherapy. The whole pelvis is treated to 4500–5000 cGy in 4–5 weeks by external beam irradiation for control of subclinical disease. The four-field pelvic technique is preferred, which allows for field shaping and treatment to the potential areas of disease while reducing the treatment side-effects (Fig. 8.5). The portals should cover the inguinal, external iliac, and internal iliac lymph nodes. If the inguinal nodes are involved, they are boosted to a total of 6000–6500 cGy with appropriate beam energy and quality. Alternatively, the patient can be treated through anterior and posterior fields if the energy of the beam is at least 10 MV, but this does not permit shielding of sensitive structures, such as the posterior wall of the rectum. After a several-week break, an additional 2000–3500 cGy is delivered by the interstitial implant for a tumor does of 7000–8000 cGy.

Care should be taken while delivering external beam irradiation to the perineum in patients with extensive disease. Confluent moist desquamation may develop and interfere with the completion of treatment. This may be prevented by eliminating the

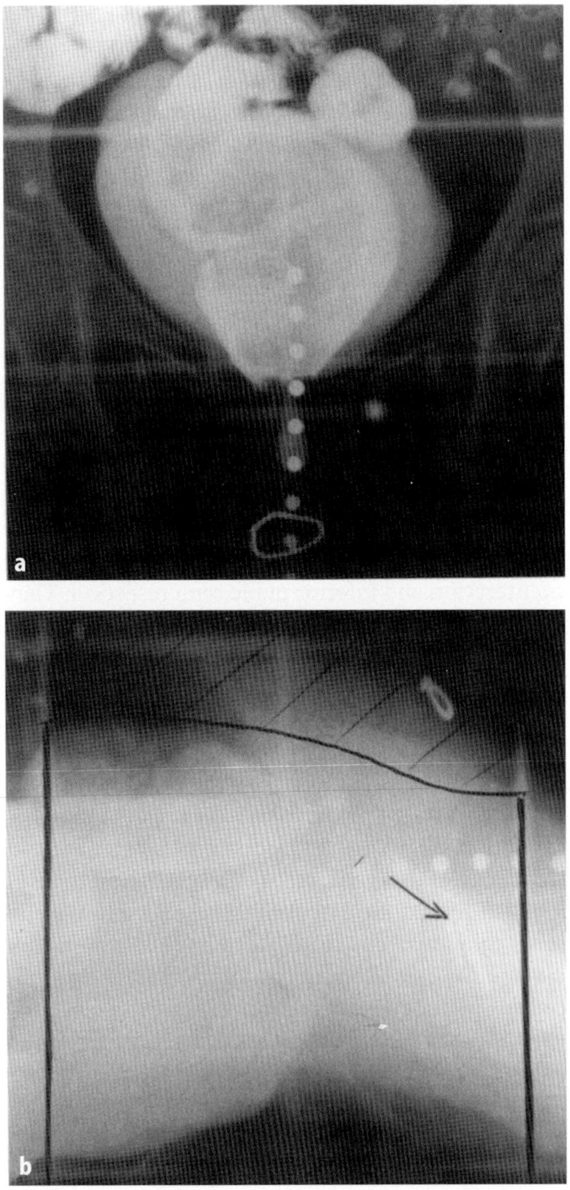

Fig. 8.5. **a** Anterior simulation and **b** right lateral simulation films of a four-field pelvis technique for urethral cancer. The patient is prone on a wedge-shaped sponge with the bladder and rectum filled with contrast. Note displacement of small bowel loops outside the radiotherapy field. Markers on the urethral meatus and anus are shown on the lateral simulation films. Note the inclusion of inguinal nodes on both anterior and lateral fields and sparing of the posterior rectal wall as well as the anus on lateral fields

differences in tissue thickness of the perineum by either using bolus or tissue compensators. In some patients, we have found it useful to treat with the legs closed to homogenize the does when the perineum is splayed.

8.11 Results of Therapy

8.11.1 Surgery

Early meatal cancers of the female urethra can be cured by surgery alone. Grabstald et al. (1966) cured five of seven patients after partial urethrectomy. The remaining two patients developed both local and distant metastases at 6 and 20 months. Peterson and colleagues reported on two patients with squamous cell carcinoma of the anterior urethra who were successfully treated with surgical excision (Peterson et al. 1973). They additionally reported on a patient with adenocarcinoma of the anterior urethra treated with local excision. Four years later she developed local and inguinal node recurrence and was cured with salvage irradiation.

Grabstald et al. (1966) have reported their results on 15 patients with advanced disease treated by anterior or total exenteration. At 5 years, there were three survivors. Bracken et al. (1976) performed radical surgery in seven patients and had follow-up in six patients. Four failed locally, with one of these salvaged by external beam irradiation for a perineal recurrence.

8.11.2 Radiation Therapy

Radiation therapy alone has been successful for tumors of the urethral meatus or distal urethra. Early meatal tumors have cure rates from 70% to 90% (Antoniades 1969; Prempree et al. 1984; Taggart et al. 1972). Antoniades (1969) reported 100% 5-year survival in eight patients with meatal tumors, seven of whom were treated with interstitial implant alone. Prempree et al. (1984) treated three patients with lesions confined to the anterior urethra with interstitial brachytherapy, reporting 100% local control and 5-year survival. They additionally reported on four patients with lesions limited to the entire urethra treated with external beam or external beam plus interstitial irradiation, achieving local control and 5-year survival in two of the four patients. Chu (1973) reported 5-year NED survival in 7 of 11 patients (64%) with distal lesions treated by interstitial brachytherapy alone or combined with external beam irradiation. Weghaupt et al. (1984) achieved

71% 5-year survival in 42 patients with tumors of the anterior urethra managed with intracavitary and external beam irradiation (WEGHAUPT et al. 1984). Forty percent of the patients had clinically positive lymph nodes, and if these were larger than 2 cm, they were dissected midway through the external beam treatments.

Tumors of the proximal and entire urethra are a therapeutic challenge. ANTONIADES (1969) reported a poor prognosis in 4 of 11 patients (36%) alive at 5 years utilizing brachytherapy and external beam irradiation. BRACKEN et al. (1976) treated 44 patients, reporting 25% 5-year survival for stage C and 20% for stage D lesions. PREMPREE et al. (1984) treated seven patients, five with irradiation alone and two preoperatively. Four of five had had no evidence of disease (NED) at 5 years, one had NED at 2 years, and one died of intercurrent disease. WEGHAUPT et al. (1984) reported 50% 5-year survival in 20 patients with posterior or entire urethral involvement treated as previously described for anterior urethral cases. KLEIN et al. (1983) reported on five females receiving preoperative irradiation followed by anterior exenteration and inferior pubic rami resection. They had a 40% 5-year survival rate. Tables 5 and 6 list the treatment results.

Table 8.5. Summary of results for low stage female urethral carcinoma

Reference	No. of pts.	Treatment	5-year survival
GRABSTALD et al. (1966)	26	R	3/13 (23%)
		S	8/10 (80%)
		R+S	2/3 (67%)
BRACKEN et al. (1976)	30	R (19)	(40%–45%)[a]
		S (3)	
		R+S (8)	
TAGGART et al. (1972)	15	R	8/15 (53%)[b]
ANTONIADES (1969)	9	R	8/9 (89%)
CHU (1973)	11	R	7/11 (64%)
PREMPREE et al. (1984)	7	R	5/7 (71%)
WEGHAUPT et al. (1984)	42	R	30/42 (71%)
DESAI et al. (1973)	10	R	4/10 (40%)
POINTON and POOLE-WILSON (1968)	26	R	20/26 (77%)[c]

R, radiation therapy; S, surgery; R+S, radiation therapy plus surgery.
[a] Estimated from survival curve.
[b] Two-year NED survival.
[c] Three-year survival.

Table 8.6. Summary of results for advanced stage female urethral carcinoma

Reference	No. of pts.	Treatment	5-year survival
GRABSTALD et al. (1966)	48	R	1/14 (17%)
		S	3/17 (18%)
		R+S	5/17 (29%)
BRACKEN et al. (1976)	44	R (35)	(20%–25%)[a]
		S (8)	
		R+S (1)	
TAGGART et al. (1972)	22	R (18)	4/22 (18%)[b]
		S (4)	
ANTONIADES (1969)	11	R	4/11 (36%)
CHU (1973)	8	R	0/8 (0%)
PREMPREE et al. (1984)	7	R (5)	
		R+S (2)	4/5 (80%)[c]
WEGHAUPT et al. (1984)	20	R	10/20 (50%)
DESAI et al. (1973)	6	R	1/6 (17%)
POINTON and POOLE-WILSON (1968)	52	R	22/52 (42%)[d]

R, Radiation therapy; S, surgery; R + S, radiation therapy plus surgery.
[a] Estimated from survival curve.
[b] Two-year NED survival.
[c] One additional patient, NED at 2 years.
[d] Three-year survival.

8.12 Complications

Complications following radiation therapy vary in frequency and severity according to the method of irradiation and the extent of disease. Urethral strictures may develop, requiring dilatation or urinary diversion. Less commonly encountered complications include local necrosis, vaginal stenosis, urinary incontinence, cystitis, osteomyelitis, radiation enteritis, and small bowel obstruction. Fistula formation is a severe complication which may be inevitable when there is local tumor extension into adjacent organs with ensuring necrosis of tumor. Most institutions report a complication rate of 12%–30% (ANTONIADES 1969; CHU 1973; FOENS et al. 1991; GRIGSBY and CORN 1992; PREMPREE et al. 1984; TAGGART et al. 1972). GARDEN et al. (1993) have updated their results at MDAH and report 49% complications in 27 of 55 patients achieving local control. However, in patients treated since 1980, they have observed only 27% complications and none were scored as severe. They explain this improvement by the treatment of multiple fields each day and use of the shrinking-field technique.

Aggressive surgical approaches such as anterior exenteration and inferior pubic rami resection have resulted in complications including rectovaginal fistula, perineal herniation, small bowel fistula, pelvic abscess, and fracture of the superior pubic rami

(KLEIN et al. 1983; NARAYAN and KONETY 1992). This is in addition to the permanent ostomies necessitated by the surgical procedure.

8.13 Chemotherapy

Due to poor local control and treatment-related complications in patients with advanced stage carcinoma of the female urethra, several investigators have attempted combined-modality approaches utilizing concomitant chemotherapy and irradiation. Two institutions have published case reports of patients with advanced squamous cell carcinoma of the female urethra utilizing concomitant 5-fluorouracil, mitomycin-C, and external beam irradiation as used in anal cancer with impressive early results (JOHNSON et al. 1989; SHAH et al. 1985). Another area of interest is neoadjuvant M-VAC (methotrexate, vinblastine, doxorubicin, and cisplatin) for transitional cell carcinoma of the female urethra, which has been successful in bladder cancer (SCHER et al. 1988).

References

Antoniades J (1969) Radiation therapy in carcinoma of the female urethra. Cancer 24:70

Beahrs OH, Henson DE, Hutter RVP, Kennedy BJ (eds) (1992) American Joint Committee on Cancer, manual for staging of cancer, 4th edn. Lippincott, Philadelphia

Bracken RB, Johnson DE, Miller LS, et al. (1976) Primary carcinoma of the female urethra. J Urol 116:188

Chu AM (1973) Female urethral carcinoma. Radiology 107: 627

Delclos L (1982) Carcinoma of the female urethra. In: Johnson DE, Boileau MA (eds) Genitourinary tumors. Grune & Stratton, New York, p 275

Desai S, Libertino JA, Zinman L (1973) Primary carcinoma of the female urethra. J Urol 110:693

Foens CS, Hussey DH, Staples JJ, et al. (1991) A comparison of the roles of surgery and radiation therapy in the management of carcinoma of the female urethra. Int J Radiat Oncol Biol Phys 21:961

Forman JD, Lichter AS (1992) The role of radiation therapy in the management of carcinoma of the male and female urethra. Urol Clin North Am 19:383

Garden AS, Zagars GK, Delclos L (1993) Primary carcinoma of the female urethra. Results of radiation therapy. Cancer 71:3102

Grabstald H (1973) Tumors of the urethra in men and women. Cancer 32:1236

Grabstald H (1982) Commentary: urethral cancer. In: Johnson DE, Boileau MA (eds) Genitourinary tumors. Grune & Stratton, New York, p 287

Grabstald H, Hilaris B, Henschke U, et al. (1966) Cancer of the female urethra. JAMA 197:835

Grigsby PW (1992) Female urethra. In: Perez CA, Brady LW (eds) Principles and practice of radiation oncology, 2nd edn. Lippincott, Philadelphia, p 1059

Grigsby PW, Corn BW (1992) Localized urethral tumors in women: indications for conservative versus exenterative therapies. J Urol 147:1516

Hahn P, Krepart C, Malaker K (1991) Carcinoma of female urethra. Urology 37:106

Hopkins SC, Grabstald H (1986) Benign and malignant tumors of the male and female urethra. In: Walsh PC, Gittes RF, Perlmutter AD, Stamey TA (eds) Campbell's urology, 5th edn. Saunders, Philadelphia, p 1441

Johnson DE, O'Connell JR (1983) Primary carcinoma of the female urethra. Urology 21:42

Johnson DW, Kessler JF, Ferrigni RG, Anderson JD (1989) Low dose combined chemotherapy/radiotherapy in the management of locally advanced urethral squamous cell carcinoma. J Urol 141:615

Klein FA, Whitmore WF, Herr HW, et al. (1983) Inferior pubic rami resection with en bloc radical excision for invasive proximal urethral carcinoma. Cancer 51:1238

Leeson TS, Leeson CR, Paparo AA (1988) Text/atlas of histology. Saunders, Philadelphia, p 566

Levine RL (1980) Urethral cancer. Cancer 45:1965

Meis JM, Ayala AG, Johnson DE (1987) Adenocarcinoma of the urethra in women: a clinicopathologic study. Cancer 60:1038

Mostofi FK, Davis CJ, Sesterhenn IA (1992) Carcinoma of the male and female urethra. Urol Clin North Am 19:347

Narayan P, Konety B (1992) Surgical treatment of female urethral carcinoma. Urol Clin North Am 19:373

Peterson DT, Dockerty MB, Utz DC, et al. (1973) The peril of primary carcinoma of the urethra in women. J Urol 110:72

Pointon RCS, Poole-Wilson DS (1968) Primary carcinoma of the urethra. Br J Urol 40:682

Prempree T, Amornmarn R, patanaphan V (1984) Radiation therapy in primary carcinoma of the female urethra. II. An update on results. Cancer 54:729

Sailer SL, Shipley WU, Wang CC (1988) Carcinoma of the female urethra: a review of results with radiation therapy. J Urol 140:1

Scher HI, Yagoda A, Herr HW, et al. (1988) Neoadjuvant M-VAC (methotrexate, vinblastine, doxorubicin and cispatin) for extravesical urinary tract tumors. J Urol 139:475

Shah AB, Kalra JK, Silber L, et al. (1985) Squamous cell cancer of the female urethra. Urology 25:284

Taggart CG, Castro JR, Rutledge FN (1972) Carcinoma of the female urethra. AJR 114:145

Weghaupt K, Gerstner GJ, Kucera H (1984) Radiation therapy for primary carcinoma of the female urethra: a survey over 25 years. Gynecol Oncol 17:58

9 Cancer of the Cervix

K. MORITA

CONTENTS

9.1 Epidemiology and Risk Factors

In general, cancer incidence is reported in cases per 100000 population per year. The cumulative incidence for cervical cancer varies from 4.2 in Israel to 48.9 in Goiania (Brazil), where cervical cancer is the most common malignancy in women. This disease is most common in Latin America and Africa, and is less frequent in Jewish and European women. Circumcision of Jewish and Moslem men has in the past

K. MORITA, MD, Director, Aichi Cancer Center Hospital, 1-1 Kanokoden, Chikusa-ku, 464 Nagoya, Japan

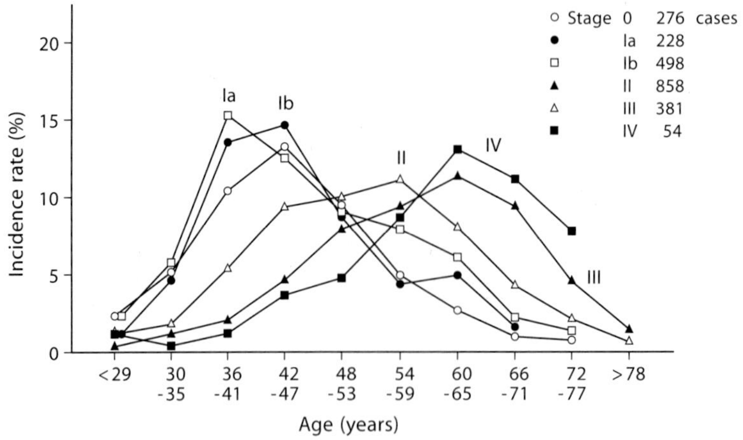

Fig. 9.1. Age distribution in each clinical stage. (SEKIBA 1981)

Table 9.1. Risk factors for invasive cervical cancer. (PETERS et al. 1986)

	Relative risk
Coitus before age 15	16.1
≥3 sexual partners	3.5
Genital warts (≥2 episodes)	5.0
Cigarette smoking (≥4 years)	4.0

been postulated to reduce cervical cancer; however, decreased incidence of cervical carcinoma has not been observed among the partners of non-Jewish circumcised men. Therefore, it is presumed that Jewish women have a genetic resistance to tumor of the cervix (ABOU-DAOUD 1967).

The peak age incidence for carcinoma of the cervix is between 45 and 55 years. The peak incidence for carcinoma in situ lies between the ages of 25 and 40 years (BARBER 1982), while for invasive carcinoma the highest incidence occurs between about 40 and 50 years in stage Ib, and at more than 50 years in stages IIb–IVa (SEKIBA 1981) (Fig. 9.1).

Risk factors for invasive cervical carcinoma are listed in Table 9.1 (PETERS et al. 1986). Cervical carcinoma is more frequent in women of low socioeconomic status, women who begin sexual intercourse at a young age, women with a large number of sexual partners such as prostitutes, and women who become pregnant at a young age (KESSLER 1976; CHAMBERLAIN 1981). Conversely, the low frequency of cancer of the cervix in nulliparous women has long been acknowledged. Tobacco smoking has also been reported to be an independent risk factor for invasive cervical carcinoma (TREVATHAN et al. 1983) or perhaps a co-factor in this disease (BRINTON et al. 1986).

In animal experiments the administration of hormonal chemicals can promote cervical carcinoma (HERBST et al. 1979; BOYCE et al. 1972), but there is no evidence to support a relationship between the use of hormonal compounds and cervical dysplasia.

The human papilloma virus (HPV), especially of types 16 and 18 (HPV-16/18), is suspected to be a factor in the genesis of cervical carcinoma (BEAUDENON et al. 1986), and studies indicate that almost 50% of intraepithelial neoplasias show evidence of HPV infection (ZUR HAUSEN et al. 1974). Although the exact mechanism for the development of cervical carcinoma has not yet been explained, HPV infection appears to play an important role in the transformation process (VAN DEN BRULE et al. 1989; CRUM and LEVINE 1984), and the presence of HPV-16/18 DNA in cells of the cervix is associated with an increased risk for cervical carcinoma (risk factor = 2.1–9.1) (REEVES et al. 1989).

The finding of higher antibody titers against herpesvirus type 2 (HSV-2) in cervical carcinoma patients than in controls suggests a cause and effect relation. RAPP et al. (1974) reported that HSV-2 virus probably plays a role in the genesis of cervical carcinoma; however, a direct etiologic role has not been established. Although it is now considered that HSV-2 virus is not important in the development of cervical carcinoma, infection with either of these viruses (HPV-16/18 or HSV-2) is associated with a significantly higher risk for cervical neoplasia.

Micronutrient deficiency, including folic acid and vitamin A deficiencies, has been suggested to affect the invasive progression of intraepithelial disease (carcinoma in situ) (BUTTERWORTH et al. 1982; LA VECCHIA et al. 1984).

9.2 Topographic Anatomy and Patterns of Spread

9.2.1 Anatomy

The uterus is located in the middle of the true pelvis, behind the urinary bladder and in front of the rectum. The fallopian tubes enter the uterus in the lateral portions (Figs. 9.2, 9.3). The uterus is divided into the fundus, corpus, and cervix. The cervix is separated from the corpus by the internal uterine orifice and is divided into two regions. A supravaginal portion above the ring of attachment contains the endocervical canal, and a vaginal portion projects into the vault. The cervix has a central orifice (external os) which is a transverse opening with an anterior and a posterior lip. The vaginal wall forms a circular cul-de-sac around the cervix. The anterior fornix forms a shallow fold, and the posterior fornix is the deepest. The cervix is covered by a stratified squamous epithelium that is continuous with the vaginal epithelium. At the external orifice this changes abruptly into a more rugous columnar epithelium.

The uterus is suspended in a midpelvic portion by anterior, posterior, and posterolateral ligaments. The anterior vesicouterine tissues pass from the lateral aspects of the uterus to the lateral aspects of the bladder and then to the pubis. The posterior uterosacral ligaments pass posteriorly, lateral to the rectum, to the os sacrum. The cardinal ligaments sweep from the pelvic wall to the lateral aspects of the cervix. These ligaments represent the pathways of major uterine and vaginal arteries, veins, and lymphatics, and at the same time form the usual pathways of direct tumor invasion.

The uterus is highly vulnerable to compression by parametrial invasion of tumor, because the ureters pass anteroinferiorly and medially through the parametrium to the bladder and are only 1.5 cm lateral to the cervix (Figs. 9.4, 9.5). The most common site of obstruction in cervical cancer is the ureterovesical junction or the distal third of the ureter.

The main artery supplying the uterus is the uterine artery, which originates from the internal iliac (hypogastric) artery. The uterine artery enters the uterine cervix through the lower margin of the broad ligament, which arches over the ureter about 2 cm from the uterus (Figs. 9.4, 9.5).

The cervix has a rich lymphatic network. At the lateral aspects of the cervix these lymphatics form three major collecting trunks. The superior channels follow the path of the uterine artery laterally through the broad ligament to the node near the junction of internal iliac (hypogastric) and external iliac arteries (=interiliac lymph nodes – the uppermost component of the internal iliac nodes). The middle lymphatics drain into the obturator lymph nodes. The channels originating from the most inferior aspect of the cervix drain toward the posterior pelvic wall to

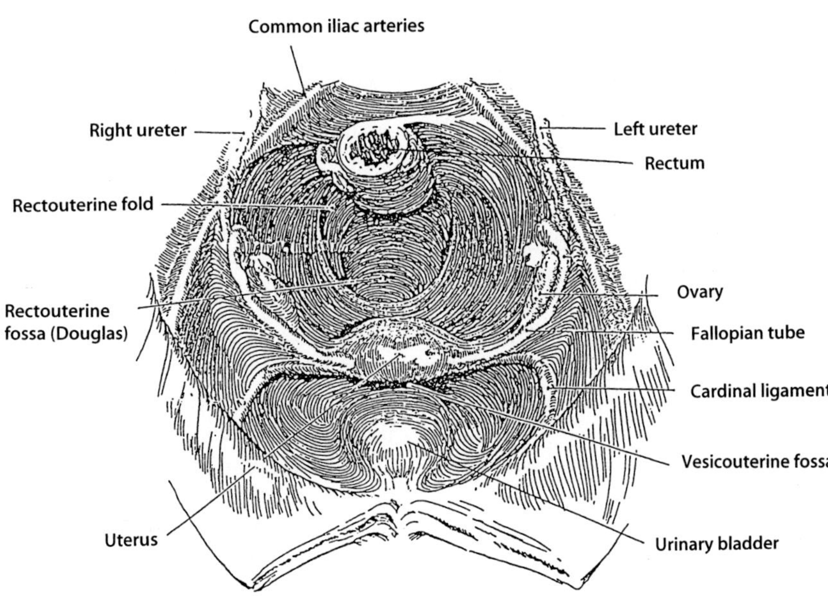

Fig. 9.2. Anatomy of the pelvis observed from above

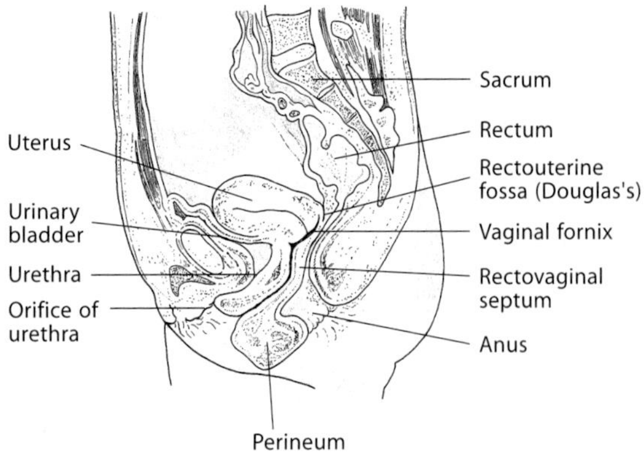

Fig. 9.3. Anatomy of the pelvis observed on a sagittal view

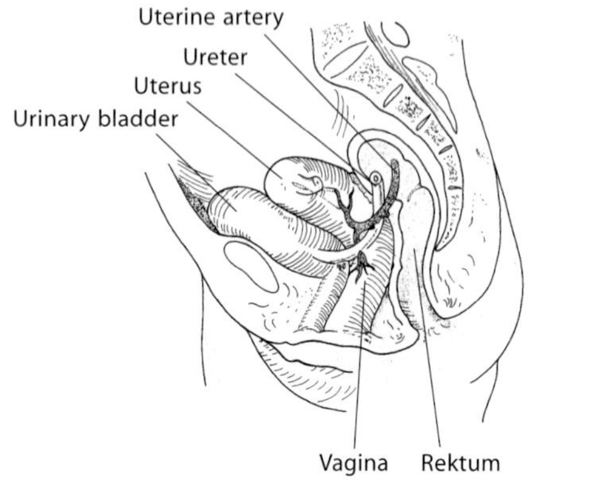

Fig. 9.5. Position of the uterine artery and ureter observed on a sagittal view

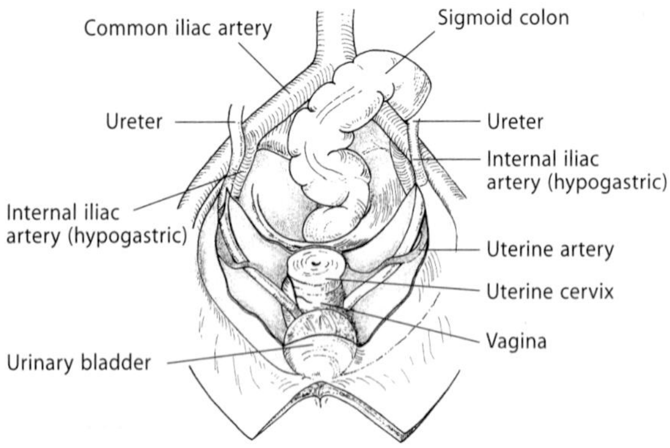

Fig. 9.4. Position of the pelvic arteries and ureters observed from above

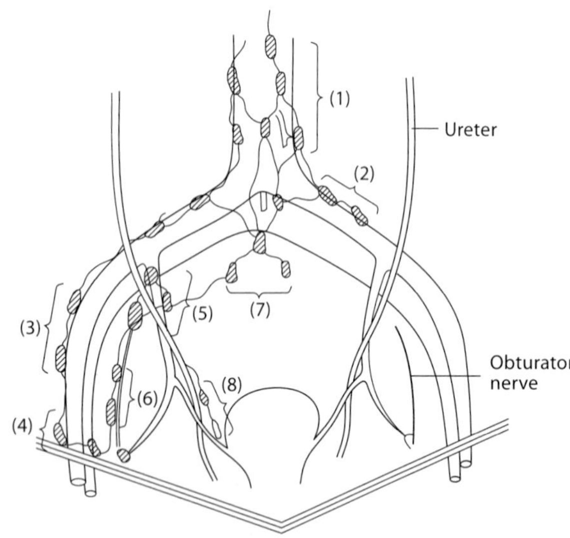

Fig. 9.6. Lymphatic drainage of the uterus. *1*, Para-aortic lymph nodes; *2*, common iliac lymph nodes; *3*, external iliac lymph nodes (a group of six to eight nodes that tend to be uniformly larger than the nodes of the other iliac groups); *4*, suprainguinal lymph nodes; *5*, internal iliac (hypogastric) lymph nodes; *6*, obturator lymph nodes (surrounding the obturator vessels and nerves); *7*, sacral lymph nodes; *8*, parametrial lymph nodes (traversing the parametria) and paracervical or ureteral lymph nodes (located above the uterine artery where it crosses the ureter)

the internal iliac (hypogastric) lymph nodes. The interiliac, obturator, external iliac, and internal iliac (hypogastric) nodes drain into the common iliac and para-aortic lymph nodes. Lymph channels from the posterior aspects of the cervix drain through the uterosacral ligament to sacral and superior rectal lymph nodes. These drain to common iliac and para-aortic lymph nodes. A few lymph nodes are occasionally found in the tissue immediately surrounding the cervix (=parametrial and paracervical lymph nodes), but these have not been given much consideration in the treatment of cancer of the cervix. The anatomic location of pelvic lymph nodes is demonstrated in Fig. 9.6.

9.2.2 Patterns of Spread

Squamous cell carcinoma of the uterine cervix usually arises from the squamocolumnar junction of the cervix, which moves from the outer surface of the portio vaginalis in young women to the inner cervical canal in old women, and is preceded by cervical dysplasia and carcinoma in situ. Although it is certain that dysplasia or carcinoma in situ proceeds to invasive cancer, less agreement exists about the time scale of progression. Most investigators accept the figure of more than 10 years, as reported by Patton and others (Patton 1969; Barron and Richart

1968, 1970). Invasive carcinoma occurs when the malignant epithelial cells break through the basement membrane and enter the stroma.

9.2.2.1 Direct Invasion

Cervical carcinoma may spread by direct extension into the paracervical tissue, the vagina, or the endometrium.

Lateral Spread to the Paracervical Tissues. The anterior, posterior, and posterolateral ligaments and their associated connective tissues form the parametrium and represent the pathway of major uterine vessels and lymphatics. At the same time the parametrial tissues form the usual pathways of tumor infiltration and metastasis. Parametrial extension is very important from both a prognostic and a therapeutic viewpoint. In advanced stages parametrial infiltration ultimately reaches to the structure of the lateral pelvic wall. This pattern of spread often causes ureteral obstruction and progressive loss of renal function. Continued local growth also progressively involves the bladder anteriorly or the rectum posteriorly.

Inferior Spread to the Vagina. Inferiorly, cervical cancer spreads by direct invasion into the upper vaginal wall. Microscopic extension usually occurs beyond visible or palpable disease. There is further spread into the lower vagina from which metastases to the inguinal lymph nodes can occur.

Superior Spread to the Endometrium. Extension of the cancer into the lower uterine segment may occur. Such extension is difficult to ascertain clinically, and its presence or absence is not a criterion for staging. However, those having extension of the cancer into the endometrium have a worse prognosis, presumably because such extension is associated with an increased incidence of distant metastasis (Perez et al. 1981) (see Table 9.18).

Table 9.2. Pelvic lymph node metastases in carcinoma of the uterine cervix

Reporters	Year	Stage I	Stage II	Stage III
Morton et al.	1964	9/38 (23.7)%	10/42 (23.8%)	
Liu and Meigs	1955	42/231 (18.2%)	76/190 (40.0%)	
Christensen et al.	1964	29/167 (17.4%)	27/104 (26.0%)	
Parker et al.	1967	15/95 (16.0%)	7/16 (44.0%)	
Gray et al.	1958	5/44 (11.4%)	6/17 (35.3%)	
Masubuchi et al.[a]	1954	5/62 (8.0%)	13/59 (22.0%)	9/29 (31.0%)
Tachibana et al.[a]	1960	12/102 (11.8%)	98/413 (23.8%)	6/12 (50.0%)
Ogino et al.[a]	1953	18/81 (22.2%)	89/300 (29.7%)	38/70 (54.3%)
Shiiki et al.[a]	1956	17/55 (30.9%)	35/104 (33.7%)	
Mori et al.[a]	1953	5/27 (18.5%)	39/113 (34.0%)	45/64 (70.3%)
Inoue et al.	1984	105/484 (21.7%)	160/391 (40.9%)	
Total		262/1386 (18.9%)	560/1749 (32.0%)	98/175 (56.0%)

[a]These data were accumulated by Nishimura (1965).

Table 9.3. Frequency of para-aortic lymph node metastases

Reporters	Year	Stage Ib	Stage IIa	Stage IIb	Stage III	Stage IV
Sudarsanam et al.	1978	11/155 (7%)	3/21 (14%)	4/22 (18%)	5/19 (26%)	0/3
Nelson et al.	1977		2/16 (13%)	7/47 (15%)	15/39 (38%)	
Piver et al.	1977			6/46 (13%)	18/49 (36%)	4/7 (57%)
Wharton et al.	1977	0/21	0/10	10/47 (21%)	14/42 (33%)	
Lagasse et al.	1980	8/143 (5%)	4/22 (18%)	19/58 (33%)	19/64 (31%)	1/4
Buchsbaum	1979	4/16	0/4	1/15	34/104 (33%)	4/10 (40%)
Averette et al.	1975	3/40 (8%)	2/9 (22%)	2/9 (22%)	2/20 (10%)	1/2
Delgado et al.	1977	0/18		8/18 (44%)	5/13 (36%)	
Hughes et al.	1980	6/140 (4%)	3/35 (8%)	11/45 (24%)	23/96 (40%)	10/23 (43%)
Total		32/533 (6%)	14/117 (12%)	69/307 (22%)	135/446 (30%)	20/49 (41%)

9.2.2.2
Lymphatic Spread

Metastases usually occur by way of the lymphatics, although blood-borne metastases do occur. The obturator, internal iliac (hypogastric), and external iliac lymph nodes are frequently involved. According to Plentyl and Friedman (1971), the anatomic distribution of nodal metastases in 700 patients with cervical cancer was as follows: external iliac 23%, obturator 19%, internal iliac 17%, and common iliac 12%. An additional 21% of patients had metastatic involvement of parametrial or paracervical lymph nodes. The incidence of metastases to pelvic lymph nodes according to clinical stage is summarized in Table 9.2. By averaging a large number of reports, the frequency of involvement of pelvic lymph nodes from stage I through stage III is about 19%, 32%, and 56%, respectively. Table 9.3 shows the distribution of para-aortic lymph nodes metastases according to clinical stage, as reported by various researchers.

9.2.2.3
Hematogenous Spread

Spread by hematogenous dissemination is relatively unusual in the early stages of cervical cancer, but the risk increases with more advanced stages. Metastases to the lungs, kidneys, and skeleton occur via the systemic circulation, while metastases to the liver probably occur by way of the vaginal plexus and port acaval anastomosis. Carlson et al. (1987) reported distant metastases in 4.7% of stage Ib, 9.2% of stage IIa, 16.2% of stage IIb, 19.8% of stage III, and 24% of stage IV patients.

9.3
Diagnostic Workup and Staging

9.3.1
Diagnostic Workup

Every patient with carcinoma of the cervix should be jointly evaluated and staged by the radiation oncologist and the gynecologist. An outline of the diagnostic workup for carcinoma of the cervix is presented in Table 9.4.

In order to decide on the clinical staging, the following examinations are permissible: physical examination (palpation and inspection), Papanicolaou (Pap) test, colposcopy, endocervical curettage, hysteroscopy, cystoscopy, proctoscopy, intravenous urography, and x-ray examination of the lungs and skeleton. Suspected bladder or rectal involvement should be confirmed by biopsy. The findings of optional examinations such as lymphangiography, angiography, laparoscopy, computed tomography, and magnetic resonance imaging of the pelvis and abdomen should not form the basis for deciding on the clinical staging by FIGO, because generally these modalities are not yet available.

For many years, Pap smears have been performed at the time of routine pelvic examination for early detection of preinvasive cervical carcinoma. The purpose of periodic cytologic screening with the Pap smear is to prevent the development of invasive cervical cancer. This system divides exfoliated cells into five groups or classes. Because different laboratories often used to modify the system and report the re-

Table 9.4. Diagnostic workup for carcinoma of the uterine cervix

Standard diagnostic procedures
Physical examination by vaginal inspection and vaginal and rectal palpation (under anesthesia, preferably)
Cytological examination: punch biopsy or pap smears
Intravenous pyelography
Laboratory studies
- Complete blood cell count
- Blood chemistry, including tumor markers
- Urinalysis

Chest radiography

Procedures ordered for particular stages
Dilatation and curettage (cytologic smears by Papanicolaou)
Colposcopy (early stages)
Barium enema examination (stage IIb, III, IVa)
Rectosigmoidscopy including biopsy (stage IIb, III, IVa)
Cystoscopy including biopsy (stage IIb, III, IVa)

Procedures ordered when needed in individual cases
Computed tomography of the pelvic and abdominal region
Lymphography
Magnetic resonance imaging (MRI) of pelvic region
Sonogram of the liver
Bone scan (if positive, skeletal survey)

Table 9.5. Nomenclature in cervical cytology

Pap smear	WHO system
Class I	Normal
Class II	Atypical
Class III	Dysplasia
	Mild
	Moderate
	Severe
Class IV	Carcinoma in situ
Class V	Invasive squamous cell carcinoma
	Adenocarcinoma

sults of Pap tests differently, in 1973 the World Health Organization established guidelines regarding the terminology for reporting Pap tests: normal, atypical, dysplasia, carcinoma in situ, invasive squamous cell carcinoma, and adenocarcinoma (Table 9.5). One of the most important steps that can be taken to minimize false-negatives is to perform a proper smear of the cervix. To obtain an optimal Pap smear, the transformation zone must be sampled. Currently colposcopy is a recommended method for evaluating an abnormal Pap smear.

Any grossly visible cervical lesion should be biopsied. Pap smears and colposcopic examination are not substitutes for cervical biopsy. The inflammation that accompanies many cervical carcinomas can be misleading on the colposcopic examination and the Pap smear, resulting in a false evaluation.

Intravenous urography should be routinely performed because ureteral obstruction remains a major prognostic factor in cervical cancer. Patients with ureteral obstruction are considered to have stage IIIb disease due to the marked invasion of the parametrium. Approximately 4% of patients with stage Ib or II disease are reclassified to a higher stage because of the finding of ureteral obstruction (Table 9.6).

Cystoscopy and rectosigmoidoscopy should be performed in all patients with late stage IIb, III, or IVa disease (van Nagell et al. 1975; Shingleton et al. 1971; Lindell and Anderson 1987) (Table 9.7). In about 20% of stage IIIb patients, positive biopsies are obtained from the vesical membrane.

Recently squamous cell carcinoma (SCC) antigen levels have been widely used for cervical squamous

Table 9.6. Ureteral obstruction related to clinical stage in cervical cancer. (van Nagell et al. 1983)

Stage prior to IVP	No. of patients	Ureteral obstruction
I	716	15 (2.1%)
II	780	48 (6.2%)
III	427	138 (32.3%)
IV	227	101 (44.5%)

IVP, intravenous pyelography.

Table 9.7. Cystoscopic findings in patients with cervical cancer

Stage prior to cystoscopy	No. of patients	Bullous edema	Invasive cancer (positive biopsies)	Vesicovaginal fistula
I	517	3 (0.6%)	0	0
II	562	10 (1.8%)	0	0
III	331	27 (8.1%)	64 (19.3%)	0
IV	162	2 (1.4%)	33 (20.4%)	5 (3.1%)
Total	1572	42	97	5

Summation from three reports (Shingleton et al. 1971; van Nagell et al. 1975; Lindell and Anderson 1987).

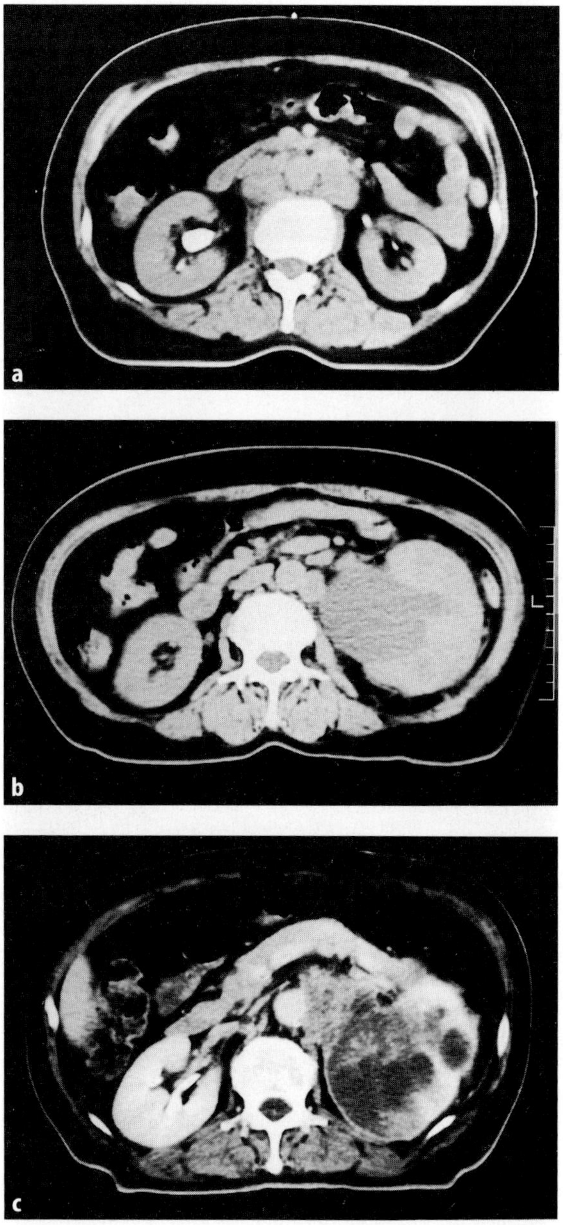

Fig. 9.7a–c. CT findings in respect of para-aortic lymph node metastases. **a** Multiple para-aortic lymph node metastases. **b** Left ureteral obstruction and hydronephrosis due to para-aortic lymph node metastases. **c** Loss of renal function and cystic changes of the left kidney due to long-term ureteral obstruction. A metastatic lesion of para-aortic lymph node is invading the wall of the abdominal aorta

Table 9.8. CT scan in the evaluation of para-aortic nodes

Reporters	Year	No. of cases	FIGO stage	Sensitivity (%)	Specificity (%)	Accuracy (%)
Kilcheski et al.	1981	36	I–IV, rec			80
Brenner et al.	1982	42	I–IV, rec	77	86	83
Bandy et al.	1985	44	I–IV, rec	75	91	86
Camilien et al.	1986	61	I–IV	67	100	98

rec, recurrent.

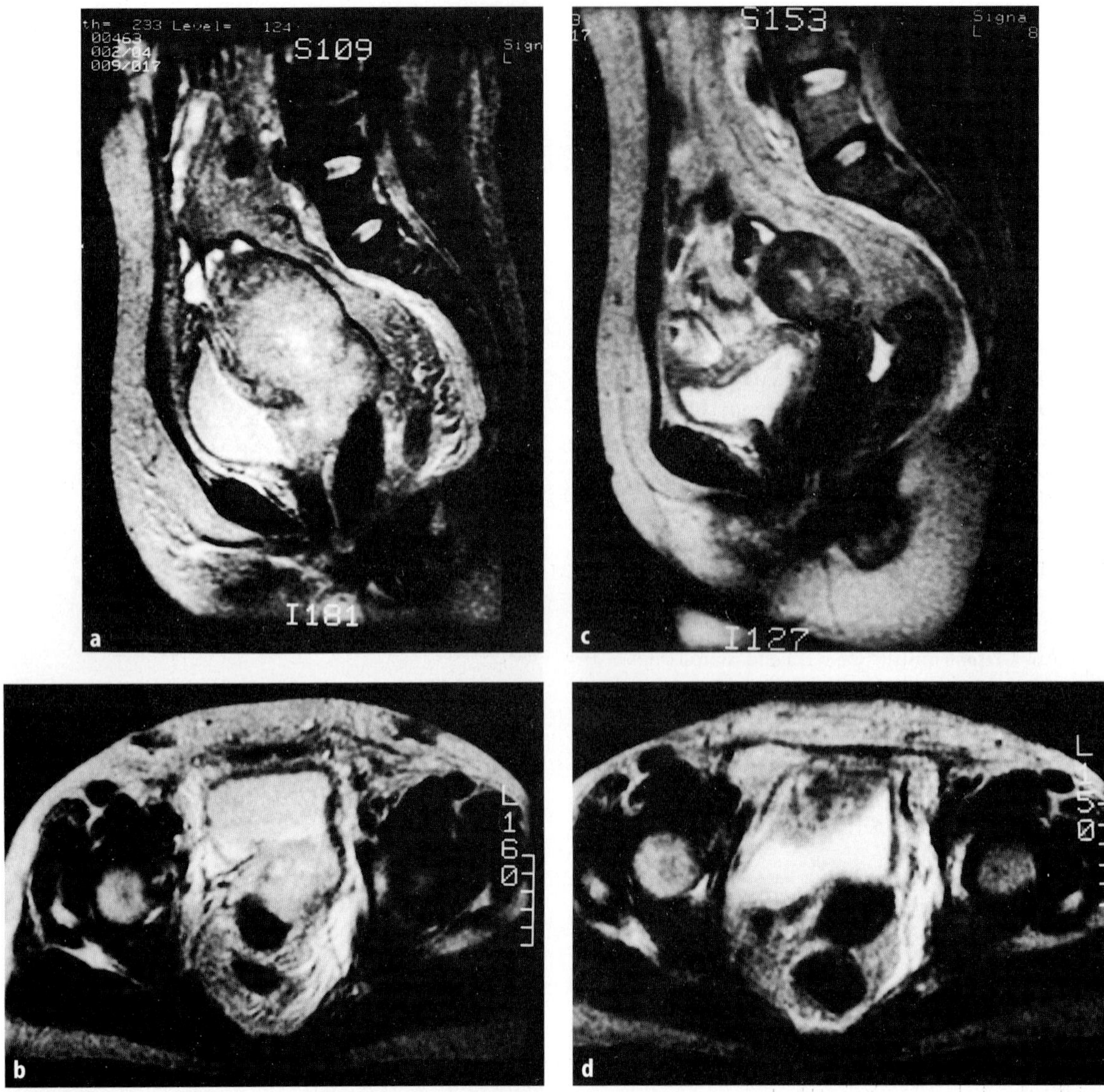

Fig. 9.8 a–d. MRI findings before and after radiation therapy for cervical cancer. **a,b** Before treatment: Cervical tumor invades the uterine body. The left posterior wall of the urinary bladder is under pressure due to the cervical tumor, but cystoscopically mucosal tumor invasion was not observed (stage IIIB; T2-weighted images). **c,d** After treatment: The tumor shadow has disappeared completely

carcinoma. The titer value correlates with stage, tumor volume, and prognosis (Maiman et al. 1989; Patner and Mann 1989). In advanced stages, abnormal serum values are found in more than 70% of patients (Maruo et al. 1985; Senekjian et al. 1987; Holloway et al. 1989). Carcinoembryonic antigen (CEA) has also been used to monitor the response to therapy and for the follow-up of cervical carcinoma (Kjorstad and Orjasaester 1982; TeVelde et al. 1982). The titer correlates with tumor volume. An elevated SCC or CEA level after treatment may precede the clinical diagnosis of recurrence.

Until recently, bilateral pedal lymphangiography was widely used. The specificity of the lymphangiogram is very high (more than 90%) (Heller et al. 1990; Kolstad 1983; Fletcher and Rutledge 1972; Horiot et al. 1988), but the sensitivity for the detection of metastases remains low because not all the lymph nodes can be visualized [e.g., obturator or internal iliac (hypogastric) nodes cannot be seen] and also small metastatic lesions cannot be adequately detected. Moreover, lymphangiography is a fairly difficult and expensive study; at present, many institutions use the study sparingly in cervical cancer.

Among cross-sectional imaging techniques, ultrasonography currently does not play a major role in cancer staging. Morphologic features of the tumor and depth of invasion are important prognostic factors, as are tumor size and lymph node metastases (see Table 9.13).

Computed tomography (CT) is not used for the evaluation of either tumor size or depth of stromal invasion (Kim et al. 1990; Camilien et al. 1988; Parker et al. 1990) because the major limitation in CT evaluation of carcinoma of the cervix lies in difficulty of direct tumor visualization. The reported overall accuracy of CT with respect to parametrial invasion is about 60%. Overstaging of the local tumor extent is a common problem when using CT. With regard to the delectability of pelvic lymph node metastases, the specificity of CT scan is very high [75% of enlarged pelvic lymph nodes on CT scans were found by Vercamer et al. (1987) to contain metastases, while 97% of the patients with negative nodes on CT scan were pathologically negative]. However, histologically positive pelvic nodes are often missed on CT scan (low sensitivity). Therefore, at present no reliable evaluation supports either the accuracy of this procedure or its value in staging or therapeutic decisions.

Computed tomography have proved more valuable for evaluation of para-aortic lymph nodes metastases than for evaluation of the pelvic region (Camilien et al. 1988; Kilcheski et al. 1981; Brenner et al. 1982; Bandy et al. 1985) (Table 9.8, Fig. 9.7). It is highly desirable for abnormal or suspicious lymph node radiographic findings to be confirmed by surgical procedures or CT-guided thin-needle aspiration biopsies.

Magnetic resonance imaging (MRI) may be helpful for assessment of the cervical localization of the primary tumor and its extracervical extension (Angel et al. 1987; Janus et al. 1989; Lien et al. 1991) (Fig. 9.8). Tumor location, tumor diameter, depth of cervical stromal invasion, and extension of tumor to the uterine corpus are accurately demonstrated on T2-weighted images, the tumor being distinguished from the low-signal intensity cervix and parametrium. MRI is also valuable in ruling out parametrial, pelvic side wall, vaginal, vesical, or rectal involvement. The use of Gd-DTPA does not increase the diagnostic accuracy of MRI for tumor depiction. Improvements in MRI technology now permit noninvasive evaluation of tumor size and depth of penetration. As a result, MRI can facilitate the choice of treatment option and thus affect patient prognosis. In the near future, modern imaging techniques such as MRI and PET may be applied routinely to decide on staging or the choice of therapeutic methods.

9.3.2 Staging

The classification of the International Federation of Gynecology and Obstetrics (FIGO), which has undergone periodic modifications since 1937, is still widely used. In 1985, the Oncology Committee of FIGO made changes in the FIGO classification of cervical carcinoma, which were published in 1987 (Table 9.9). The changes in the new classification were limited to stage Ia, and their impact is not clear. The Society of Gynecologic Oncologists (SGO) in the United States officially opposed the new FIGO staging classification and recommended that the definition of stage Ia carcinoma be "less than 3 mm of invasion with no lymphovascular invasion." In order to decide on the FIGO clinical staging of cervical cancer it is necessary to use physical examinations (i.e., inspection, vaginal and rectal palpation, and biopsy), laboratory studies, and radiographic evaluation as outlined previously (Table 9.9). The clinical staging must be concluded before the treatment is initiated. The official stage of the patient for the purpose of reporting treatment results may not be altered after the surgical procedure.

The TNM Committee of the Union International Contre le Cancer (UICC) has also promulgated its recommendations for the classification of gynecological tumors since 1966. In the UICC classification adopted in 1987, cases with regional lymph node metastases are classified as stage IIIb regardless of the T category (Table 9). Various imaging techniques, including lymphangiography, CT, and MRI, may be used in order to assess the N and M categories.

Table 9.9. Staging of carcinoma of the uterine cervix

UICC categories (1987)	FIGO stages (1988)	
T: Primary tumor		
TX		Primary tumor cannot be assessed
T0		No evidence of primary tumor
Tis	0	Carcinoma in situ, intraepithelial carcinoma (cases of stage 0 should not be included in any therapeutic statistics for invasive carcinoma)
T1	I	Carcinoma strictly confined to the cervix (extension to corpus should be disregarded)
T1a	IA	Preclinical carcinoma of the cervix, diagnosed by microscopy only
T1a1	IA1	Minimal microscopic stromal invasion
T1a2	IA2	Lesions detected microscopically that can be measured. The upper limits of the measurement should not show a depth of invasion of more than 5 mm taken from the base of the epithelium, either surface or glandular, from which it originates; and a second dimension, the horizontal spread, must not exceed 7 mm
T1b	IB	Lesions of greater dimensions than T1a2, whether seen clinically or not
T2	II	Carcinoma invades beyond the uterus but not to the pelvic wall or to lower third of the vagina
T2a	IIA	Without parametrial invasion
T2b	IIB	With parametrial invasion
T3	III	Carcinoma extends to the pelvic wall and/or involves the lower third of the vagina and/or causes hydronephrosis or nonfunctioning kidney
T3a	IIIA	Tumor involves the lower third of the vagina; no extension to the pelvic wall
T3b	IIIB	Tumor extends to the pelvic wall and/or causes hydronephrosis or nonfunctioning kidney
T4	IVA	Tumor invades the mucosa of the bladder or rectum and/or extends beyond the true pelvis. (Presence of bullous edema is not sufficient evidence to classify a tumor as T4.)
N: Regional lymph nodes		
Regional lymph nodes include paracervical, parametrial, hypogastric (obturator), common iliac, internal and external iliac, presacral and sacral nodes		
NX		Regional lymph nodes cannot be assessed
N0		No regional lymph node metastasis
N1		Regional lymph node metastasis
M: Distant metastasis		
MX		Presence of distant metastasis cannot be assessed
M0		No distant metastasis
M1	IVB	Distant metastasis

N.B. Stage grouping in UICC classification:

Stage 0	T1s	N0	M0	M0
Stage IA	T1a	N0	M0	M0
Stage IB	T1b	N0	M0	M0
Stage IIA	T2a	N0	M0	M0
Stage IIB	T2b	N0	M0	M1
Stage IIIA	T3a	N0		
Stage IIIB	T1–3a	N1		
	T3b	Any N		
Stage IVA	T4	Any N		
Stage IVB	Any T	Any N		

9.4 Histopathologic Findings

The WHO pathological classification of cervical carcinoma is shown in Table 9.10.

9.4.1 Squamous Cell Carcinoma

The majority of carcinomas of the cervix are squamous cell carcinomas. Squamous cell carcinoma of the cervix typically arises at the active squamocolumnar junction from a preexisting dysplastic lesion, although some dysplasia may remain stationary. Once the basement membrane has been breached and stromal invasion occurs, the process is generally regarded as irreversible. Microinvasive carcinoma is now considered an important form of cervical carcinoma. Generally a depth of 3–5 mm from the epithelial stromal junction is considered to be the limit of microinvasion. Progression from mild dysplasia to invasive cancer takes several years, but wide variations exist.

The first growth pattern is exophytic (polypoid), arising from the ectocervix. The exophytic growth of an endocervical lesion may be toward the canal lumen, which would expand the cervix. The second basic growth pattern is infiltrative, which becomes ulcerative if necrosis occurs. An infiltrative lesion of the ectocervix is more likely to involve the vaginal fornices and upper vagina, whereas an endocervical infiltrating lesion often invades the corpus and lateral parametria. The infiltrative and endocervical types are more likely to produce lymphatic metastases than is the exophytic type.

Table 9.10. WHO classification of pathology for carcinoma of the uterine cervix

Squamous cell carcinoma
Dysplasia (mild, moderate, and severe)
Carcinoma in situ
Squamous cell carcinoma
Keratinizing
Large cell nonkeratinizing
Small cell nonkeratinizing
Adenocarcinoma
Adenocarcinoma, endocervical type
Endometrioid adenocarcinoma
Clear cell (mesonephroid) adenocarcinoma
Adenoid cystic carcinoma
Adenosquamous carcinoma
Undifferentiated carcinoma

Most squamous cell carcinomas of the cervix show some evidence of epithelioid differentiation. In only 5% of cases is the keratinizing type seen. The nonkeratinizing type is divided into two groups; large cell type and small cell type. The large cell type is the most common. Wentz and Reagan (1959) speculated from animal experiments that the keratinizing type develops on the ectocervix, the large cell nonkeratinizing type arises from the transformation zone, and the small cell nonkeratinizing type arises from the endocervix. The histologic grading of the large cell type is of little prognostic value. Stage for stage, patients with the large cell nonkeratinizing type have a better prognosis than do those with the keratinizing type, when treated with irradiation. With radical surgery no such prognositc difference is noted (van Nagell et al. 1977; Randall et al. 1988). Therefore, the poorer survival of patients with the keratinizing type appears to be related to the intrinsic radiation resistance of this type.

Small cell carcinomas consist almost entirely of round, oval, or fusiform elements in which the nucleus is set in a scanty cytoplasm and the mitotic rate is high. This small cell variant is considered a highly malignant carcinoma by many authors (van Nagell et al. 1988). Among patients with negative pelvic nodes, Inoue (1984) noted a substantially reduced 5-year survival rate for the small cell nonkeratinizing type in comparison with large cell nonkeratinizing and large cell keratinizing lesions. The prognosis in small cell carcinoma is poor regardless of the therapeutic method employed, probably due to their tendency to display vascular invasion and give rise to extrapelvic metastases.

9.4.2 Adenocarcinoma

The WHO has adopted a classification of cervical adenocarcinoma that includes four subtypes: endocervical, endometrial, clear cell (mesonephric), and adenoid cystic. The relative frequency of these types, and of adenosquamous carcinoma, is demonstrated in Table 9.11. Pure adenocarcinoma of the cervix accounts for 5%–20% of all cervical carcinomas in various series, and the incidence may be increasing. The origin of cervical adenocarcinomas is usually considered to be more endocervical or higher in the canal than for squamous lesions. Endocervical and endometrial curettage is essential in evaluating these cases, if the results of

Table 9.11. Frequencies of various histologic types in cervical adenocarcinoma

Cell type	Percent of all cases
Endocervical	47%–69%
Endometrioid	1%–17%
Clear cell	0%–13%
Adenoid cystic	0%–3%
Adenosquamous	8%–25%

gross colposcopic and cytologic examinations are negative.

Endocervical and endometrial adenocarcinomas often resemble each other closely. When an adenocarcinoma extends to involve both the endometrium and the endocervix, the identification of a cervical adenocarcinoma cannot be accomplished except by examination of the complete uterus. The behavior of such carcinomas of the uterine body and the cervix resembles that of a cervical squamous cell carcinoma.

The prognosis of cervical adenocarcinoma is significantly worse than that of epidermoid carcinoma (Pettersson 1988). This difference in prognosis may be attributable to the growth patterns of these tumors and their intrinsic properties. Characteristically, adenocarcinomas grow endophytically and expand into the lower uterine body. As a result, the tumor volume is much larger and the stromal invasion is also deeper than would be appreciated on clinical examination. In general, the extent of differentiation reflects the degree of malignancy inasmuch as the more undifferentiated variants proliferate and infiltrate more rapidly and metastasize early (Berek et al. 1985; Hopkins et al. 1988). The incidence of pelvic lymph node metastases and the recurrence rate of poorly differentiated adenocarcinomas are much higher than in the case of poorly differentiated squamous cell carcinomas. Cure in patients with lymph node metastases appears to be unusual.

9.4.3 Endometrioid Carcinoma

The endometrioid pattern of cervical adenocarcinoma is uncommon and is usually diagnosed only when benign squamous elements are present (adenoacanthoma). Some authors regard adenosquamous cancer as a variant of this group.

9.4.4 Clear Cell (Mesonephroid) Adenocarcinoma

When the mesonephric duct, which sometimes penetrates the uterus at about the level of the internal os in the fetus, persists in adults, the remnants are found dispersed as isolated tubules lined by a single layer of cuboidal, clear, nonmucinous epithelium in which the cell borders are blurred and the nuclei are round or oval. Rarely, cervical mesonephroid adenocarcinomas arise from these mesonephric remnants. Their occurrence is associated with in utero exposure to diethylstilbestrol (DES) during the first trimester of pregnancy (Melnick et al. 1987). Histologically, these tumors are characterized by clear cells in hobnail, solid, or tubulocystic patterns. Tumor cells contain glycogen but no mucin. They are usually well differentiated.

9.4.5 Adenoid Cystic Carcinoma (Cylindroma)

Adenoid cystic carcinoma is characterized histologically by small basal cells with hyperchromatic nuclei surrounding the central area of amorphous material. In general, these tumors have a high mitotic rate and exhibit high vascularity. Overall survival rate may be poorer than for pure squamous cell carcinoma, and lung metastases are common.

9.4.6 Adenosquamous Carcinoma

Adenosquamous cell carcinomas of the cervix represent 2%–5% of all cervical carcinomas (Regan et al. 1973). The simultaneous presence of an epidermoid carcinoma and an adenocarcinoma has been observed on a number of occasions and may be responsible for "mixed" tumors consisting of squamous and glandular elements derived from two distant sources. There are, however, instances of adenosquamous carcinoma and mucoepidermoid carcinoma of the cervix that have originated from a single source. Tamimi and Figgi (1982) re-ported that survival was poorer in patients with cervical adenosquamous carcinoma than in those with pure adenocarcinoma. However, no statistically significant difference in prognosis between adenosquamous carcinomas and pure adenocarcinomas was found when other prognostically significant variables were controlled (RANDALL et al. 1988; KILGORE et al. 1988).

A rare histologic variant of cervical adenosquamous carcinoma is the glassy cell carcinoma initially described by GLUCKMAN and CHERRY in 1956. These tumors are poorly differentiated and biologically aggressive, with a tendency to develop extrapelvic metastases.

9.5 Prognostic Factors

The prognosis of cervical cancer depends on various factors such as the histologic type of the tumor, its size (transverse diameter), the depth of stromal invasion, and the presence of lymph node metastases. Therefore, the FIGO stage of the disease is no longer the exclusive parameter used in selecting the treatment strategy.

9.5.1 Age

Cervical carcinoma is relatively rare in women under 20 years of age, and most cases occurring before that age have been adenocarcinoma. Some investigators (RUTLEDGE et al. 1992; GYNNING et al. 1983) have demonstrated that the stage-corrected survival for women under 40 years is worse than that for older women, while others (KJORSTAD 1977; BALTZER et al. 1982; CARMICHAEL et al. 1986) have reported that there is no difference. MEANWELL et al. (1988) reported that survival for younger women (usually under 40 years) is actually better than that for older women: older women are more likely to have complicating medical factors that may prevent definitive treatment.

9.5.2 Other Host-Related Factors

Several researchers reported that anemia, a high neutrophile count, an increased number of pregnancies, high oral temperatures over 100°F (VAN HERIK 1965; KAPP and LAWRENCE 1984), and arterial hypertension (JENKINS and STRYKER 1968) are associated with lower disease-free survival. A greater incidence of pelvic recurrence and lower survival are observed in patients with anemia (hemoglobin below 10–11 g/dl.) (BUSH et al. 1978). Pregnancy may have an adverse effect on survival.

9.5.3 Stage

The more advanced a cancer is before treatment, the poorer the prognosis. Reports from several medical centers around the world make it clear that a stepwise decrease in survival from stage I through stage IV is universally observed (Jpn. Soc. Obstet. Gynecol. 1990) (Table 9.12). Figure 9.9 shows the 5-year survival by stage reported from 44 clinics contributing to volumes 12–21 of the Annual Reports on the Results of Treatment in Gynecological Cancer published by FIGO. The average survival by stage has remained almost constant from 1950 to 1981. The data from volumes 21 and 22 are actuarial survival data and, therefore, not comparable with the previous data. The 5-year survival rates for stage I cases improved from 75% to 85% and those for stage II from 53% to 66%. For stage III the change was from 26% to 39% and for stage IV from 6% to 11%.

9.5.4 Tumor Size

Especially in stage Ib, interest has focused on the relationship of lesion size to prognosis, because the frequency of regional lymph node metastases correlates with the tumor size (Table 9.13). In patients with bulky tumors there is a higher incidence of lymphatic metastases and lower survival. MORITA (1994, unpublished) has demonstrated the relationship

Table 9.12. Five-year survival in the different stages in 105 institutions in Japan. (Jpn Soc Obstet Gynecol 1990)

Stage	No. of patients	5-year cumulative survival rate
Ia	954	92.3%
Ib	1168	84.0%
IIa	282	68.8%
IIb	1212	65.6%
IIIa	39	53.8%
IIIb	982	41.4%
IVa	132	18.2%
IVb	87	4.6%
Total	4856	68.1%

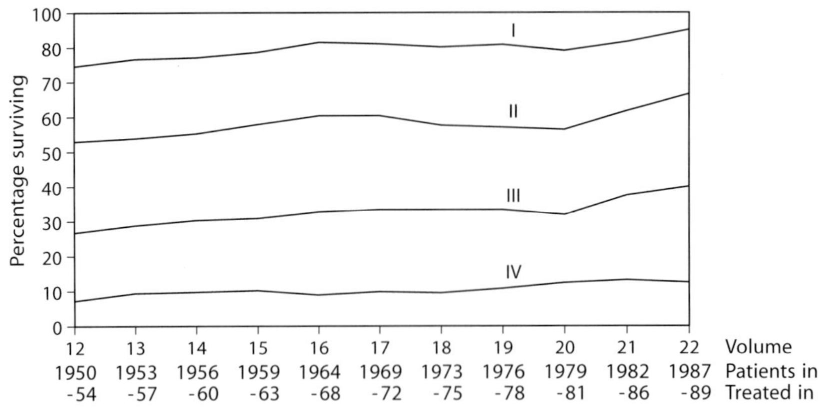

Fig. 9.9. Five-year survival rates by stage and period of treatment in patients with carcinoma of the cervix (Annual Report on the Results of Treatment in Gynecological Cancer, volume 22, International Federation of Gynecology and Obstetrics, Stockholm, 1995). Data for the last two volumes are given as corrected actuarial survival, and for the previous volumes as crude direct 5-year survival

Table 9.13. Influence of tumor size on pelvic lymph node metastasis and survival rate

Authors	Year	Tumor size	Indicator and results	
Delgado et al.	1990	Occult ca.	3-year disease-free survival	94.6%
		3 cm or less		85.5%
		Greater than 3 cm		68.4%
Chung et al.	1981	4 cm or less	Pelvic node metastatic rate	20%
		Greater than 4 cm		59%
Lange	1960	Less than 1 cm	Pelvic node metastatic rate	11%
		1–3 cm		25%
		Greater than 3 cm		47%
Piver and Chung	1975	3 cm or less	Pelvic node metastatic rate	21%
		Greater than 3 cm		40%

Table 9.14. Tumor size and site of relapse. (Morita K 1994, unpublished data)

Stage and tumor size	No. of cases	Local control rate	Region of first relapse			
			Portio	Vagina	Parametrium Pelvic lymphnodes	Extrapelvic region
IB ≤4 cm	87	98.8% (86/87)	1 (1%)	0	0	3 (3%)
>4 cm	25	88.0% (22/25)	1 (4%)	0	2 (8%)	2 (8%)
IIA ≤4 cm	70	97.1% (68/70)	1 (1%)	1 (1%)	0	5 (7%)
>4 cm	30	90.0% (27/30)	1 (3%)	1 (3%)	1 (3%)	5 (17%)
IIB ≤4 cm	39	89.7% (35/39)	3 (8%)	1 (3%)	0	3 (8%)
>4 cm	36	88.9% (32/36)	2 (6%)	1 (3%)	1 (3%)	5 (14%)
>4 cm[a]	31	77.4% (24/31)	3 (9%)	0	4 (13%)	10 (31%)

[a] High degree of parametrial invasion.

between tumor size by stage and the frequency of local/regional recurrence and extrapelvic metastases (Table 9.14). Failures in pelvis and extrapelvic metastasis increase with the size of cervical tumor and the degree of parametrial invasion.

9.5.5 Depth of Invasion

The frequency of lymph node metastases in a large number of patients with early invasive cervical carcinoma treated by radical hysterectomy is shown in Table 9.15. No lymph node metastases were found among patients with stromal invasion of 3 mm or less. In contrast, approximately 9% of patients with tumors demonstrating stromal invasion of 3.1–5 mm had lymph node metastases.

In invasive carcinoma of the cervix, the depth of invasion is also related to the rate of nodal metastases and prognosis. The combination of the data of Boyce et al. (1984) and those of Gauthier et al. (1985) shows that the rates of pelvic node metastases for lesions measuring 5 mm or less, 6–10 mm, 11–15 mm, and greater than 15 mm in thickness are 2.5%, 4%, 26%, and 44%, respectively. Inoue (1984) has also observed a higher incidence of metastatic lymph nodes in the presence of deep stromal invasion. These patients had a lower 5-year survival. The depth of invasion was evaluated by Inoue as a prognostic factor in 628 patients after radical hysterectomy for stage IB–IIB cervical carcinoma. Pelvic lymph node metastases showed significant increases with tumor invasion deeper than 5, 10, and 30 mm (Table 9.16).

Table 9.15. Frequency of lymph node metastases related to stromal invasion in patients with stage IA cervical cancer. (van Nagell et al. 1993)

Depth of stromal invasion	No. of cases	No. of patients with with positive nodes
≤1.0 mm	162	0%
1.1–3.0 mm	407	0%
3.1–5.0 mm	124	9%

Table 9.16. Nodal metastases relating to the maximum depth of tumor invasion. (Inoue 1984)

Depth of tumor invasion	No. of patients	Parametrial Extension	Nodal metastases (%)
0–4.9 mm	97	0 (0.0%)	1 (1.0%)
5–9.9 mm	153	5 (3.3%)	19 (12.4%)
10–14.9 mm	169	29 (17.2%)	44 (26.0%)
15–29.9 mm	183	63 (34.4%)	63 (34.4%)
30–•• mm	26	15 (57.7%)	16 (61.5%)
Total	628	112 (17.8%)	143 (22.8%)

9.5.6 Invasion of the Lymphovascular Space

Invasion of the lymphovascular space influences the survival rate and the frequency of pelvic lymph node metastases (Crissman et al. 1985; Delgado et al. 1990) (Table 9.17). Baltzer et al. (1982) reported that 70% of patients with microscopic evidence of blood vessel invasion died compared with 30% of those with lymph channel invasion. Thus the significance of the former may differ substantially from that of the latter.

9.5.7 Endometrial Stromal Invasion

The present clinical stage classification disregards tumor extension into the corpus because its diagnosis is usually difficult clinically. However, Perez et al. (1981) reported that endometrial stromal invasion does influence the prognosis (Table 9.18). Transvaginal ultrasonography and MRI make it possible to detect the endometrial stromal invasion precisely.

9.5.8 Histopathologic Variables

In squamous cell carcinoma, Inoue (1984) noted a substantially reduced 5-year survival rate for the small cell type in comparison with the large cell nonkeratinizing type among patients with negative

Table 9.17. Influence of invasion of the lymphovascular space (LVSI) in stage Ib cervical cancer on pelvic lymph node metastasis and survival

Source	LVSI negative			LVSI positive		
	No.	Percent survival	Percent pelvic node metastasis	No.	Percent survival	Percent pelvic node metastasis
Boyce et al. (1984)	94	97	6	41	71	32
Crissman et al. (1985)	40	85	8	30	64	17
Delgado et al. (1990)	360	90	8	276	78	25
Total	494	91	8	347	76	25

Table 9.18. Prognostic significance of endometrial extension from carcinoma of the uterine cervix. (Perez et al. 1981)

Stage	Endometrial invasion and 3-year survival rate		
	Positive D&C	Admixture of normal endometrium and cervical ca. (contamination)	Negative D&C
IB	22/31 (71%)	46/53 (88%)	105/116 (91%)
IIA	10/17 (59%)	12/13 (92%)	26/34 (76%)
IIB	24/50 (48%)	13/16 (81%)	37/47 (79%)
III	9/30 (30%)	5/11 (45%)	9/21 (43%)

D&C, dilatation and curettage.

Table 9.19. Corrected 5-year survival rates among patients with cervical cancer, in relation to the cell type. (Inoue 1984)

Cell type	Pelvic lymph node metastasis		Total
	Positive	Negative	
Large cell nonkeratinizing	320/335 (95.5%)*	59/93 (63.4%)	379/428 (88.6%)
Keratinizing	67/68 (99.9%)**	17/20 (85.0%)	84/88 (95.5%)
Small cell nonkeratinizing	16/20 (80.0%)***	3/5 (60.0%)	19/25 (76.0%)
Adenocarcinoma	39/42 (92.9%)	4/11 (36.4%)	43/53 (81.1%)
Total	442/465 (95.1%)	83/129 (64.3%)	524/594 (88.2%)

Significant differences between * and ** ($P < 0.05$) and * and *** ($P < 0.005$).

Table 9.20. Frequency of pelvic lymph node metastases and survival in early-stage squamous cell carcinoma of the cervix

Reporters	Negative nodes		Positive nodes	
	No.	Percent survival	No.	Percent survival
Larson et al. (1987)	164	92	30	67
Monaghan et al. (1990)	392	91	102	50
Soisson et al. (1990)	271	90	49	67
Delgado et al. (1990)	545	86	100	83[a]
Kamura et al. (1992)	281	91	64	63

[a] Excluded patients with grossly positive pelvic lymph nodes.

Table 9.21. Five-year survival rates and number of positive nodes in relation to clinical stage. (Inoue 1984)

No. of positive nodes	5-year survival rates (%)		
	Ib cases	IIa cases	IIb cases
0 (N0)	348/379 (92)*1	68/74 (92)	139/167 (83)*2
1 (N1)	43/47 (91)*3	6/10 (60)	31/41 (75)
2 or 3 (N2)	22/31 (71)*4	5/8 (63)	24/41 (56)
4–18 (N4)	8/16 (50)	1/1 (-)	10/28 (36)
Unresectable	5/11 (45)	1/3 (33)	2/18 (10)

Significant differences between *1 and *2 ($P < 0.05$) and *3 and *4 ($P < 0.05$).

pelvic nodes (Table 9.19). Generally speaking, every type of adenocarcinoma of the cervix has a poorer prognosis than does squamous carcinoma.

9.5.9 Regional Lymph Node Metastasis

The risk of lymph node metastasis is related to histologic type and grade, stage, presence of parametrial infiltration, lesion size, depth of penetration into the cervical wall, and invasion of the lymphatic space. The existence of lymph node metastasis has a powerful effect on the patient's prognosis (Larson et al. 1987; Monaghan et al. 1990; Soisson et al. 1990; Kamura et al. 1992). The survival rates of patients with negative and patients with positive nodes average 91% and 56%, respectively (Table 9.20). Involvement of the common iliac nodes carries a much worse prognosis.

The number of nodes involved also influences the survival rate. From the collected data, patients with one to three nodal metastases without parametrial invasion have a 72% 5-year survival rate, compared with a rate of 40% in patients with more than three involved nodes (Inoue et al. 1984; Inoue and Morita 1990) (Table 9.21).

9.6 Treatment Policy

9.6.1 Squamous Cell Carcinoma

9.6.1.1 Preinvasive and Microinvasive Carcinoma

The primary method of therapy for preinvasive (stage 0) and microinvasive (stage Ia1 and Ia2) carcinoma of the cervix is surgery.

Carcinoma In Situ. Although the definitive therapy for grade 3 (severe dysplasia and carcinoma in situ) cervical intraepithelial neoplasia (CIN) is conization of the cervix, selected patients can be managed by outpatient therapy with cryotherapy or laser ablation. A new technique for the diagnosis and therapy of preinvasive lesions of the cervix employs a thin wire loop electrode to excise the lesions and the transformation zone. In the past, abdominal or vaginal hysterectomy was the treatment for CIN-3. However, based on current evidence, this treatment choice is no longer justified.

Stage Ia. Stage Ia1 microinvasive carcinoma is so small that it cannot be measured. A simple hysterectomy might be considered the standard therapy for the healthy patient who does not desire further childbearing. But nearly half of women with microinvasive carcinoma of the cervix are younger than 40 years and many of these women desire future fertility. Women who desire to preserve fertility or who are poor surgical risks can be managed by conization and followed closely (every 3 months for the first 2 years).

The proper management of stage Ia2 cervical carcinoma is less clear. Simple hysterectomy or modified radical hysterectomy can be chosen. Three series in the literature report only two recurrences among 178 patients who were treated by simple hysterectomy with 3 mm or less invasion (Yajima and Noda 1979; Larsson et al. 1983; van Nagell et al. 1983). When the depth of penetration of the stroma by tumor is more than 3 mm, pelvic lymphadenectomy combined with radical hysterectomy is the preferred treatment (Fennell 1978; Nelson et al. 1975; Seski et al. 1977). With every treatment method the tumor control is close to 100%. Radiation therapy is also entirely suitable for cases that are considered to be medically inoperable. In stage Ia1 cases, only intracavitary irradiation should be chosen.

9.6.1.2 Stage Ib and IIa Cervical Carcinoma

Stage Ib and IIa cervical carcinoma can be managed equally well by radical hysterectomy and pelvic lymphadenectomy or definitive irradiation. There has often been disagreement between those who advocate radical surgery and those who support irradiation for the treatment of carcinoma of the cervix in stage Ib and IIa. A direct comparison of the results obtained with these modalities is extremely difficult because there is a definite selection of patients. Surgery and radiation therapy are complementary rather than competitive methods of treatment, and optimal results cannot be obtained with either modality alone. Patients should be treated with close communication between the gynecologist and the radiation oncologist, and an integrated team approach should be vigorously pursued. The preference for one procedure over the other depends on the institution, the gynecological and radiation oncolgical staff, the general condition of the patient, and the characteristics of the lesion.

An operation has usually been preferred by young women because of the desire to preserve ovarian function and the possibility of a more pliable vagina following surgery. Radiation therapy is generally chosen for older women, especially in the presence of some medical problems. Sometimes the presence of a conical vagina in older patients militates against successful intacavitary radiation therapy.

Thinness is desirable in patients undergoing hysterectomy because it makes surgery easier. Radiation injury is more common in the thin patient than in the obese patient.

Tumor configuration is also an important factor during treatment planning. Barrel-shaped endocervical tumors in stage Ib have a higher incidence of local recurrence (Durrance 1969) because of their extension beyond the curative isodose of radiation. O'Quinn et al. (1980) reported that such tumors often contain areas of poorly perfused hypoxic tumor cells that are resistant to radiation therapy. Radical hysterectomy or extrafascial hysterectomy following radiation therapy is better than radiotherapy alone. GALLION et al. (1985) reported a reduction in the recurrence rate among patients with bulky tumors (more than 4 cm in diameter) from 47% to 16% with the addition of extrafascial hysterectomy.

Cell type is important in determining the optimal treatment method for each patient. Patients with keratinizing squamous cell cancers have a worse prognosis than do those with large cell nonkeratinizing cancers when treated with irradiation (VAN NAGELL et al. 1977; RANDALL et al. 1988). No such prognostic difference is observed when radical surgery is employed. The poorer survival of patients with keratinizing tumors appears to be related to the intrinsic resistance of these tumors to radiation. The prognosis in small cell cancers is poor regardless of the therapeutic method employed, because of their propensity for vascular invasion and extrapelvic metastases. Radiotherapy combined with multiagent chemotherapy following guidelines for the management of small cell carcinoma of the lung is recommended (VAN NAGELL et al. 1988).

9.6.1.3
Stage IIb, III, and IVa Cervical Carcinoma

The treatment for cervical carcinoma more advanced than stage IIa is irradiation. According to the summarized results from 14 institutions in Germany and Austria, the 5-year survival rate in stage II cases is inversely proportional to the frequency of surgical treatment (Table 9.22). In stage IIb, practically all patients are treated with irradiation alone, and the 5-year survival rate is 60%–65%. Occasionally, a conservative hysterectomy is performed after high-dose preoperative irradiation in patients with a barrel-shaped cervix and limited medial parametrial infiltration.

Table 9.22. Relationship between 5-year survival and frequency of surgical treatment in carcinoma of the uterine cervix (stage II)

Frequency of surgical treatment	No. of institutes	No. of patients	5-year survival
In 1982 (Annual Report No. 18)			
0.4%–6.4%	5	651	63.1%
11.5%–35.7%	4	513	58.7%
54.5%–81.8%	4	273	54.2%
In 1985 (Annual Report No. 19)			
2.8%–11.4%	5	505	56.2%
20.8%–37.9%	5	477	53.7%
45.5%–60.6%	4	186	50.0%

Summarized results from 14 institutes in Austria and Germany.

In stage IIIb, the 5-year survival rate ranges from 25% to 50%. This variation may be related to the socioeconomic status of the patients, the extent of the disease, the techniques of irradiation, and the doses delivered to the parametria.

Isolated cases of stage IVa cervical carcinoma with involvement of the bladder or rectum without pelvic side wall involvement can be treated by pelvic extenteration, but the best choice of therapy is primary irradiation. Interstitial parametrial implants have rarely been used to supplement standard external and intracavitary techniques. If brachytherapy procedures cannot be performed for medical reasons or because of an unusual anatomic configuration of the pelvis or the tumor, higher doses of external irradiation alone may be used. A higher incidence of central-pelvic recurrences is observed among patients treated with external beam alone than among patients receiving brachytherapy in addition to external beam irradiation. In stage IIIb–IVb there is a need for prospective multi-institutional trials to determine the efficacy of adjuvant chemotherapy.

9.6.2
Adenocarcinoma

9.6.2.1
Adenocarcinoma In Situ

Adenocarcinomas of the cervix appear to be increasing in frequency relative to squamous cancers (TAMIMI and FIGGE 1982; BEREK et al. 1985). The average age at diagnosis is about 10 years less than that of women with invasive adenocarcinoma. Usually simple hysterectomy is the treatment of choice. For young women who desire to retain childbearing ability, cone biopsy may be recommended if the margins are clear and the patient agrees to close follow-up.

9.6.2.2
Invasive Adenocarcinoma

Although cervical adenocarcinomas have been reported to have a poorer prognosis than squamous cell cancers of a similar stage (PETTERSSON 1988), this difference in survival may be attributable to the growth patterns of these tumors. Characteristically, adenocarcinomas grow endophytically and often invade the cervical stroma. Therefore, the tumor volume of adenocarcinomas is much larger than would be appreciated on clinical examination. Recently, MRI of the pelvis has enabled more accurate definition of the depth of stromal invasion and the total volume of these lesions. When these findings match those of squamous cell carcinomas, the survival is similar for both types (Shingleton et al. 1981; Rutledge et al. 1968; Weiner and Wizenberg 1975).

There is considerable disagreement in the literature regarding the optimal therapy for invasive adenocarcinoma of the cervix because combined surgical treatment and radiation therapy does not improve survival substantially compared with radical hysterectomy or radiation therapy alone. From several reports, the average 5-year survival for adenocarcinoma of the cervix is 75% for stage I and 50% for stage II disease.

At present, the recommended treatment for stage I and IIa disease is radical hysterectomy and pelvic node dissection. Adjuvant whole-pelvis irradiation should be added in those cases with lymph node metastases, lymphovascular space invasion, grade 3 histology, or lesions greater than 3 cm in diameter. Removal of the ovaries is indicated for endometrioid and for poorly differentiated adenocarcinomas based on the risk of a second primary or metastatic involvement. When radiation therapy is chosen for such early cases, adjuvant simple hysterectomy after irradiation is recommended.

In the case of stage IIb disease, radiation therapy is chosen. If the parametrial invasion disappears after treatment, simple hysterectomy is recommended. The prognosis for more advanced cases seems to be especially poor in spite of intensive radiation therapy.

9.6.3 Cervical Cancer in Pregnancy

Carcinoma of the cervix coincident with pregnancy is relatively rare, occurring in 0.4%–1.01% of pregnancies (Greer et al. 1989; Jolles 1988). Optimal treatment for pregnant patients with cervical cancer depends on the stage of disease and the trimester at the time of diagnosis. A histologic specimen should be obtained using directed biopsies, because the reported risk for abortion after first trimester conization is 15%–33% (Moore et al. 1966; Averette et al. 1970) and conization during the pregnancy is often associated with severe hemorrhage.

Patients with microinvasive carcinoma (less than 3 mm stromal invasion without lymphovascular space invasion) can continue the pregnancy while undergoing observation with repeat cytology and colposcopy to assess tumor growth. Vaginal or abdominal hysterectomy should be performed 2–3 months post partum.

For invasive cervical carcinoma in stage Ib and IIa it is recommended that radical surgery be performed as soon as possible. If cervical cancer is diagnosed late in the second trimester, it may be possible to delay surgery for a short time until the fetal lungs have matured. The surgical procedure of choice is cesarean section followed by radical hysterectomy and pelvic lymhadenectomy. Vaginal delivery is contraindicated, because of the increased risk of hemorrhage and infection.

Radiation therapy is the therapeutic method of choice in pregnant patients with stage IIb–IVa cervical cancer. In the first trimester radiation therapy should be started immediately and will often induce spontaneous abortion. When advanced stage disease is diagnosed in the second trimester, hysterectomy should be performed prior to radiation, because fetal tissues are less sensitive to radiation and treatment-abortion is often delayed. If advanced stage cervical cancer is diagnosed during the third trimester, cesarean section should be performed as soon as fetal lung maturity is established, with radiation therapy initiated shortly thereafter. Available data suggest that survival rates in the pregnant and nonpregnant patients are statistically similar (Hacker et al. 1982).

9.6.4 Carcinoma of the Cervical Stump

Subtotal hysterectomy, a relatively popular procedure for benign conditions of the uterus in past years, is rarely performed today. Malignant transformation occurs in the residual cervical stump following subtotal hysterectomy with the same frequency as in the intact uterus. The natural history and patterns of spread of carcinoma of the cervical stump are similar to those of cervical carcnoma in the intact uterus. Individualized management should take into account the altered anatomy as well as the volume and stage of tumor.

Surgery for stage Ib or IIa tumors is rendered somewhat more difficult by the presence of postoperative adhesions in the pelvis. When irradiation is administered, the lack of a uterine cavity makes intracavitary radiotherapy more difficult. If possible, at least one source should be inserted into the remaining cervical canal. It is important to deliver more whole-pelvis irradiation. Occasionally, transvaginal irradiation may be used to boost the dose delivered to central disease in the stump. If bulky disease is present in the cervix, parametrium, or vagina, interstitial brachytherapy is also advisable.

Patients with carcinoma of the cervical stump have a similar survival rate to those with cervical carcinoma of the intact uterus (Table 9.23). The difficulty of irradiating stump cancer substantially increases the late complication rate (MILLER et al. 1984). This is undoubtedly due to the emphasis on external radiation in the face of a greater likelihood of adhesions of the bladder, sigmoid colon, and small bowel to the stump after supracervical hysterectomy.

9.6.5 Brachytherapy

Optimal radiotherapy of invasive carcinoma of the cervix consists in a combination of external whole-pelvis irradiation and intracavitary brachytherapy. External irradiation delivers a substantial dose to all pelvic structures, including the upper vagina, the cervix and body of the uterus, the fallopian tubes and ovaries, the parametria, and the pelvic lymph nodes. Intracavitary irradiation gives its highest dose to the upper portion of the vagina, the cervix, body of the uterus, and the paracervical area. Brachytherapy is essential to the successful treatment of cervical cancer by radiation therapy. Because of the rapid dose fall-off, brachytherapy can deliver a high dose to the primary lesion of the uterine cervix, and at the same time can protect the adjacent normal organs such as the rectosigmoid, the bladder, and the small bowel. However, as the only modality used for treating pelvic lymph nodes, it is inadequate.

Based on clinical experience, different systems of intracavitary therapy have been presented for the treatment of ervical carcinoma. Originally, three basic systems were developed: the Stockholm system, the Paris system, and the Manchester system. Most of the systems used throughout the world are derived from these three basic systems. The differences are largely in the number and duration of applications, and the placement of sources.

9.6.5.1 Type of Radioactive Material

Radium, cobalt, cesium, and iridium are the most frequently used radioactive substances. Radium is less often used nowadays because of the potential for leaks of radon gas and shielding problems. Rather, cesium has become the most popular isotope because of its low cost, long half-life (30 years), ease of shielding, and ease of safe encapsulation. Three to four tubular sources in a tandem arrangement are placed in a metal tube in the uterine canal, and two tubular sources are placed into ovoids in the vaginal colpostats. The active length and actual length of each source is about 15 mm and 20 mm, respectively. Usually each source contains 10, 15, or 20 mg of radium or radium-equivalent millicuries of radioactive cesium.

In spite of its relatively short half-life, since the 1970s cobalt (1–4 Ci) has been widely used in Japan as a source for remote afterloading systems with a high dose rate because of its high specific radioactivity. Recently, the remote afterloading system using a radioactive iridium point source has been applied not only for intracavitary insertion in cases of cervical cancer but also for intracavitary or interstitial radiotherapy for various malignancies (Table 9.24).

Table 9.23. Five-year survival rate following radiation for carcinoma of the cervical stump

Stage	No. of cases	5-year survival rate
I	181	86%
II	192	72%
III	110	47%
IV	35	26%

Summation from the results of IGBOELE et al. (1983), MILLER et al. (1984), NASS et al. (1978), OATS (1976), PREMPREE et al. (1979).

Table 9.24. Radium and its substitutes used for cervical cancer

	Half-life	Energy of γ-ray (MeV)	Half-value layer (cmPb)
^{226}Ra	1600 years	0.047–2.45	1.3
^{60}Co	5.26 years	1.17, 1.33	1.2
^{137}Cs	30 years	0.662	0.65
^{192}Ir	74.2 days	0.136–1.07	0.3

9.6.5.2
Applications

More than 100 different types of applicators have been developed for intracavitary brachytherapy of cervical cancer. At present, the most frequently used applicator in the United States is the Fletcher and Suit type (Suit and Fletcher 1963), while the TAO type (Tazaki et al. 1965) is that most often employed in Japan. Both types are modifications of the Manchester system. For intracavitary brachytherapy for cervical cancer, both the tandem and the colpostat are almost always applied to deliver the dose to the lesion as homogeneously as possible. A narrow vaginal vault may, however, prevent use of the colpostat. In some institutes a long linear source extending the whole length of the uterine canal and the upper vagina is always employed without the use of the colpostat. It must be noted that the tandem alone provides a poor dose distribution, especially when used for the treatment of bulky cervical tumors.

9.6.5.3
Dose Rate

In intracavitary brachytherapy for carcinoma of the uterine cervix using a low dose rate, the usual source arrangement delivers 40–60 cGy per hour at the paracervical point (point A). Dose rates exceeding 70–80 cGy per hour result in a higher percentage of complications without any advantage for treatment of the cervical cancer, if the same fractionation schedule is used (Pierquin et al. 1989).

Low-dose-rate intracavitary radiation therapy has some disadvantages: (a) exposure of the medical staff is unavoidable; (b) the physical and psychological burden for patients is large due to the long treatment time; (c) it is difficult to maintain the precise position of applicators during treatment. In 1960 Henschke and co-workers presented a remote afterloading technique with a low dose rate. Radiation exposure of medical staff was markedly reduced but the disadvantages of conventional brachytherapy were not completely solved, because of the long treatment time. High-dose-rate remote afterloading intracavitary radiation therapy was de-

Table 9.25. High-dose-rate (HDR) brachytherapy regimens

Authors	XRT dose (Gy)	HDR fractionation			
		HDR dose/Fr (Gy)	No.	Frequency	HDR timing
Utely et al. (1984)	50	8–10	5	Twice weekly	Concurrent
Teshima et al. (1988)	42–60	7.5	3–6	Weekly	Concurrent
Joslin (1989)	24	10	4	Weekly	Concurrent
Chen et al. (1991)	44–58	5–8.5	3	Twice weekly	After XRT
Roman et al. (1991)	30–64	8–10	1–3	Weekly	Concurrent
Arai et al. (1992)	45–65	5–6	4–5	Weekly	Concurrent
Kataoka et al. (1992)	30–60	6–7.5	4–5	Weekly	After XRT

Fr, fraction.

Table 9.26. Treatment protocol for cervical cancer. (Arai et al. 1984)

Size of tumor	External irradiation		Intracavitary irradiation	
	WP (Gy)	CS (Gy)	High DR (Gy/Fr)	Low DR (Gy/Fr)
IB	0	45	29/5	50/5
II				
Small	0	50	29/5	50/5
Large	20	30	23/4	40/3
III				
Small	20–30	20–30	23/4	40/3
Large	30–40	15–25	15/3–24/4	25/2–40/3
IVA	40–50	10–25	15/3–20/4	25/2–33/3

WP, whole-pelvis field; CS, pelvis field with central shielding; DR, dose rate; Fr, fraction.

Table 9.27. Comparison of intracavitary irradiation. (ARAI et al. 1979)

	Direct insertion of radioactive sources with low dose rate	Afterloading technique with low dose rate	Remote Afterloading technique with high dose rate
Sources	Ra, Cs, Co	Ra, Cs, Co	Cs, Co, Ir
Exposure of medical staff	(+++)	(+)	(–)
Treatment time	24–48 h	24–48 h	10–20 min
Physical/mental burden for patient	(+++)	(+++)	(+)
Danger of urinary infection	(++)	(++)	(–)
Applicator movement during therapy	(++)–(+++)	(++)–(+++)	(–)
Need to shield ward	(+)	(+)	(–)
Biological disadvantage[a]	(–)	(–)	(+)
Cost of device	(–)	(–)	(+++)

[a] Decrease in therapeutic ratio due to dose rate effect.

Table 9.28. Policies of treatment with irradiation for carcinoma of the uterine cervix (PEREZ 1993)

Tumor stage	Tumor extent	External irradiation (Gy)[a]		Brachytherapy (2 insertions) (mgh)[b]
		Whole pelvis	Additional parametrial dose (midline shield)	
Ib (small)	Superficial ulceration Less than 2 cm in diameter or involving fewer than two quadrants		45	6500–7000
Ib (large)	Four-quadrant involvement No endocervical component or significant expansion	10	40	7000–7500
IIa	Cervix not barrel shaped	20	30	8000
Ib–IIa (bulky)[c] IIb, IIIa–b	Barrel-shaped cervix	20	30 + 10	8000
IIb, IIIb, IV	Poor pelvic anatomy Patients not readily treated with intracavitary insertions (barrel-shaped cervix not regressing, inability to locate external os)	40	20	6500

[a] 180 cGy/day, five weekly fractions, using 18-MV or higher photon beams.
[b] 60–80 cGy/h at point A. In patients over 65 years of age, or with a history of previous pelvic inflammatory disease or pelvic surgery, doses should be reduced by 10%.
[c] In stages Ib and IIa, if complete regression is not obtained, extrafascial conservative hysterectomy should be performed (reduce brachytherapy dose to 6000 mgh).

Table 9.29. Doses[a] of radiation used in the treatment of cancer of the cervix. (CROOK and ESCHE 1994)

Intracavitary brachytherapy[b]	External whole pelvis[c]	Total paracentral[b]
8000 (2 insertions)		8000
4000 (1 insertion)	4500 (150–170 cGy/fraction)	8500
3500 (1 insertion)	4950–5100 (150–170 cGy/fraction)	8500
3000 (1 insertion)	5000 split: 2500 (250 × 10) 2 weeks' rest 2500 (250 × 10)	8000
–	7000 (5000 plus reduced-field boost)	7000

[a] All doses calculated in cGy.
[b] Calculated at point A. When a tandem only is used, the dose is calculated at 2 cm lateral to its center.
[c] Central axis dose at midpelvis.

veloped by HENSCHKE et al. (1964) and O'CONNELL et al. (1967) to overcome these weak points completely. In ICRU report No. 38, "high dose rate" refers to any dose rate higher than 0.2 Gy/min. (12 Gy/h). Usually a dose rate as high as 2–5 Gy/min at point A is used. A variety of treatment schedules including high dose rates are summarized in Table 9.25. From their experience, ARAI et al. (1984) estimated the dose rate factor to be 0.55–0.60. Fifty Gy/2–3 insertions at a low dose rate (one insertion per week) give almost the equivalent effect to 29 Gy/5 insertions in 4 weeks (one insertion per week) (Table 9.26). ARAI et al. (1979) cited various advantages of intracavitary irradiation with a high dose rate compared with the conventional low-dose-rate technique (Table 9.27).

9.6.5.4 Total Brachytherapy Doses

ARAI et al. (1984), PEREZ (1993) and CROOK and ESCHE (1994) have clarified the interrelationship between external and intracavitary irradiation (Tables 9.26, 9.28, and 9.29, respectively). The total brachytherapy dose depends on the magnitude of the external dose with or without a midline shield. In general, the following basic principles apply (BRENNER and HALL 1991): (a) the relative proportion of external radiation therapy increases with increasing tumor bulk and stage; (b) exceptionally (stage IA or superficial type of stage IB, smaller than 1 cm) the intracavitary irradiation may be applied with no external beam therapy (GRIGSBY and PEREZ 1991); (c) external radiation therapy precedes intracavitary brachytherapy except for small tumors; (d) at least two intracavitary applications are more effective than one.

9.6.5.5 Timing of Brachytherapy

In early stages such as Ib and IIa, intracavitary brachytherapy can be performed before or during external radiotherapy. For advanced cancer, brachytherapy should follow external irradiation. By then, the tumor shrinkage facilitates the insertion and placement of sources. According to the size of the tumor and its extent, there should be a high degree of tailoring of techniques (timing, number of insertions, and total brachytherapy dose) to each patient's needs. Intervals of longer than 2 weeks between external irradiation and intracavitary brachytherapy should not be allowed because of the possibility of tumor regrowth and vaginal narrowness after external irradiation.

9.6.5.6 Dose Expression and Points of Calculation

The use of the term "milligram hours" alone to express the dose from a brachytherapy source when employing the original Stockholm or Paris method is no longer acceptable because it is impossible to ascertain doses in the lesion and critical organs. In the Manchester system, specific points such as points A and B were proposed to estimate the brachytherapy dose to the lesion more precisely. Formerly, point A was defined as being 2 cm lateral to the central canal of the uterus and 2 cm up from the mucous membrane of the lateral fornix, and point B was 5 cm lateral to the midline of the pelvis and 2 cm cephalad from the lateral fornix (ICRU 1985) (Fig. 9.10). In practice, on an x-ray film point A is defined as being 2 cm superior to the inferior end of the intrauterine source and 2 cm lateral from the central canal. If a radiopaque marker is clipped on the cervix at the level of the external os, then this point becomes an

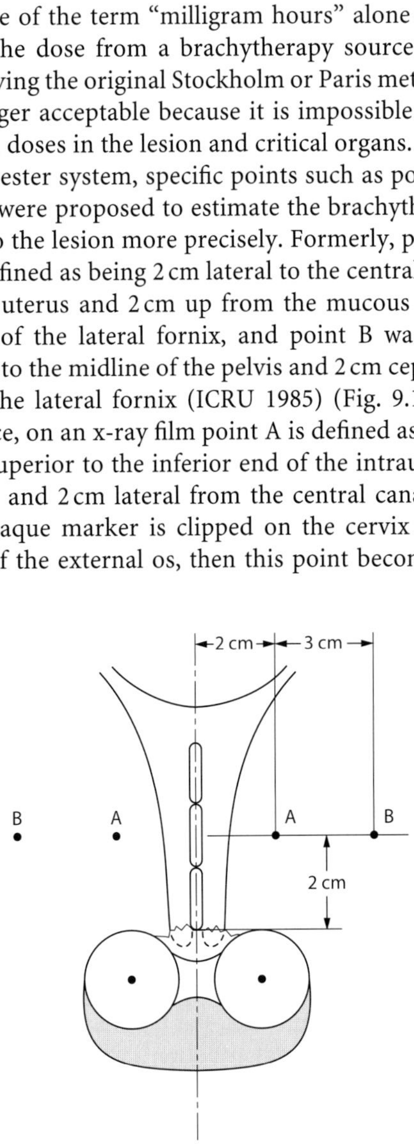

Fig. 9.10. The Manchester system. Definition of points *A* and *B*. Originally point *A* was defined as a point 2 cm lateral to the central canal of the uterus and 2 cm up from the mucous membrane of the lateral fornix, in the axis of the uterus. Point *B* was defined as being in the transverse axis through point *A*, 5 cm from the midline. In clinical practice, dose calculations are often made from radiographs and point *A* is taken 2 cm up from the flange of the intrauterine source and 2 cm lateral from the central canal, as indicated in the figure. (From ICRU Report 38, 1985)

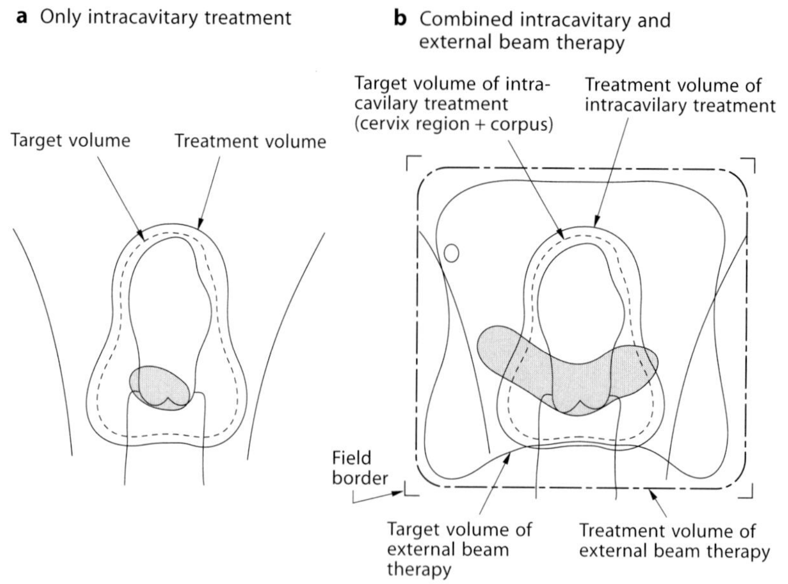

Fig. 9.11 a,b. Treatment of cervical carcinoma, stage IIb. Examples of target volume and treatment volumes. **a** Tumor volume (*hatched*): 4 × 3 × 2 cm. The almost pear-shaped target volume includes the entirety of the palpable and visible tumor as well as the whole uterus. The planned, pear-shaped treatment volume encompasses the target volume. **b** Tumor volume (*hatched*): 9 × 5 × 4 cm. The target volume for brachytherapy will only include the major parts of the tumor volume, but will include the whole uterus. To treat the rest of the tumor volume and further subclinical disease throughout the pelvis and the regional lymphatics, external beam therapy will be used, with brachytherapy as boost therapy

accurate reference point (point CO). Usually point A corresponds to the lateral border of the cervical crossing of the ureter and uterine artery and point B to the position of the distal margin of bilateral parametria or bilateral obturator lymph nodes.

In 1985, the ICRU committee provided new definitions and guidelines concerning dose and treatment volume specification for reporting intracavitary therapy in gynecology. These were required because the tremendous developments in computer technology had come to allow the easy calculation of the dose at any point or the minimum and maximum doses within a target volume for brachytherapy. With these data, it is possible to calculate the optimum doses at various locations and the optimum dose distribution in the surrounding normal tissues (Fig. 9.11).

The ICRU guidelines provided the following definitions:

1. *Target volume.* Tissues that are to be irradiated to a specified absorbed dose according to a specified time-dose pattern.
2. *Treatment volume.* The volume enclosed by a relevant isodose surface selected by the radiotherapist, and encompassing at least the target volume.
3. *Reference volume.* The volume enclosed by the reference isodose surface. The treatment dose level defining the treatment volume may be equal to or different from this reference dose level.

In order to define "the dose given to the treatment volume," the ICRU (1985) recommended that an absorbed dose level of 60 Gy might be widely accepted as the appropriate reference level for classical low-dose-rate therapy. For intracavitary therapy at medium or high dose rates, the dose level which is equivalent to 60 Gy delivered at the low dose rate has to be indicated. When intracavitary therapy is combined with external beam therapy, the isodose level to be considered is the difference between 60 Gy and the dose delivered at the same location by external beam therapy.

The reference volume is defined by means of three dimensions (Fig. 9.12). It is recommended that the dose distributions be computed in at least planes, the oblique frontal plane and the oblique sagittal plane, both of which contain the intrauterine source.

9.6.5.7 Reference Points Relative to Lymph Node Regions

Estimation of the absorbed dose at reference points relative to lymph node regions using well-defined bony structures is particularly useful when in-

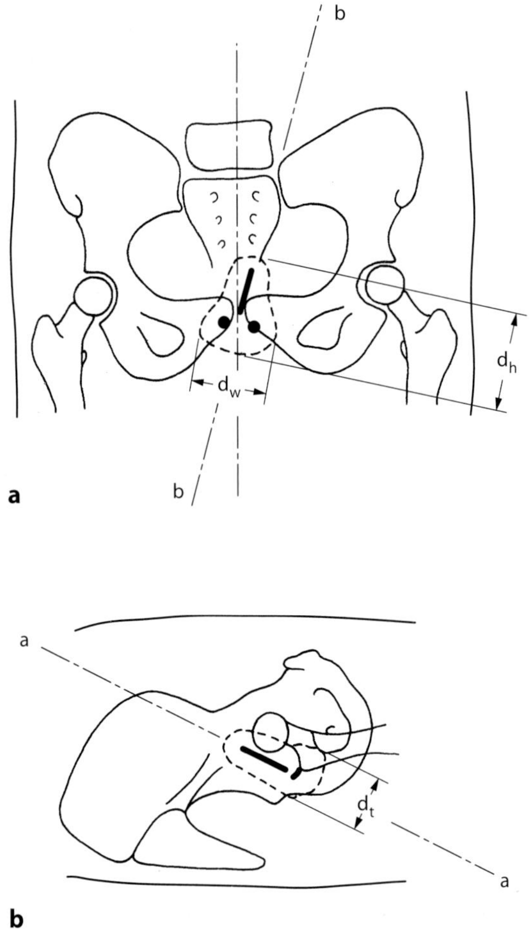

Fig. 9.12 a,b. Geometry for measurement of the size of the pear-shaped 60-Gy isodose surface (*broken line*) in a typical treatment of cervical carcinoma using one rod-shaped uterine applicator and two vaginal applicators. *Plane a* is the "oblique" frontal plane that contains the intrauterine device. *Plane b* is the "oblique" sagittal plane that contains the intrauterine device. The height (d_h) and the width (d_w) of the reference volume are measured in plane a as the maximal sizes parallel and perpendicular to the uterine applicator, respectively. The thickness (d_t) of the reference volume is measured in plane b as the maximal size perpendicular to the uterine applicator

tracavitary therapy is combined with external beam therapy. The lymphatic trapezoid proposed by FLETCHER in 1980 is used to estimate the dose to mid-external iliac lymph nodes (EXT), to the low common iliac lymph nodes (COM), and to the low para-aortic lymph nodes (PARA) (Fig. 9.13). The pelvic wall reference points presented by CHASSAGNE et al. in 1977 are intended to be representative of the absorbed dose at the distal part of the parametrium and at the obturator lymph nodes (Fig. 9.14).

9.6.5.8 Reference Points Relative to Organs at Risk

The determination of the absorbed dose to organs at risk is obviously useful in order to estimate the normal tissue tolerance limits. In 1977 CHASSAGNE and HORIOT proposed reference points for the expression of the absorbed dose to the bladder and the rectum (Fig. 9.15).

The bladder reference point is obtained as follows. A Foley catheter is used. The balloon must be filled with 7 cm^3 of radio-opaque fluid. The catheter is pulled downwards to bring the balloon against the urethra. On the lateral radiograph, the reference point is obtained on an anteroposterior line drawn through the center of the balloon. The reference point is taken on this line at the posterior surface of the balloon. On the frontal radiograph, the reference point is taken at the center of the balloon.

The rectal reference point is obtained as follows. On the lateral radiograph, an anteroposterior line is drawn from the lower end of the intrauterine source (or from the middle of the intravaginal sources). The point is located on this line 5 mm behind the posterior vaginal wall. The posterior vaginal wall is visualized, depending upon the technique, by means of an intravaginal mold or by opacification of the vaginal cavity with a radio-opaque gauze used for the packing. On the anteroposterior radiograph, this reference point is at the lower end of the intrauterine source or at the middle of the intravaginal sources.

9.6.5.9 Interstitial Implantation

Interstitial brachytherapy is sometimes used in patients with residual tumor or tumor recurrence following irradiation, in whom the usual patterns of intracavitary therapy are impossible, for boosting the dose to a vaginal nodule or to parametrium that has previously been externally irradiated. CROOK and ESCHE (1994) demonstrated that there are certain clear indications for interstitial therapy: (a) centropelvic recurrence after radical surgery, (b) distorted anatomy that prohibits an adequate intracavitary insertion, and (c) bulky parametrial side wall disease.

Interstitial implants with needles or catheters, in which the radioisotopes [usually ^{192}Ir seeds or wires for low-dose-rate irradiation and ^{192}Ir point sources (usually 8–10 Ci) for high-dose-rate irradiation] are implanted in limited tumor volumes, have a definite

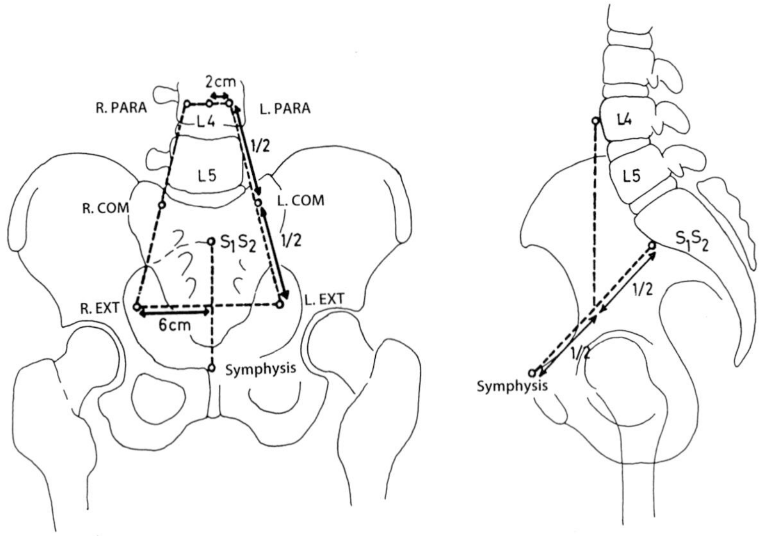

Fig. 9.13. Determination of the lymphatic trapezoid. *Left* an anteroposterior view; *right* a lateral view

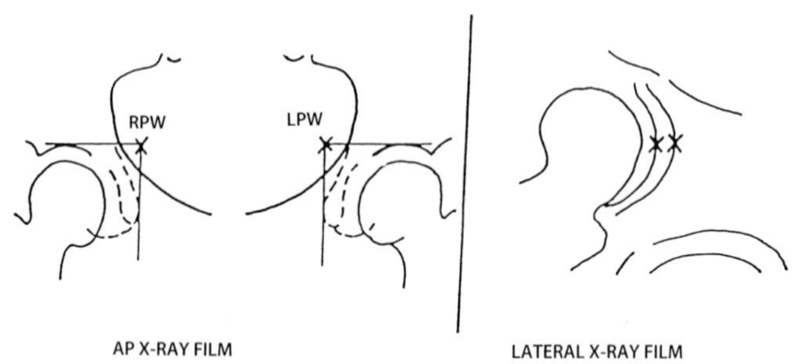

Fig. 9.14. Determination of the right (*RPW*) and left (*LPW*) pelvic wall reference points

role in the treatment of cervical cancer. However, their application requires a high level of technical skill if severe complications are to be avoided (Goddis et al. 1983; Aristizabel et al. 1987).

9.6.6 Teletherapy

Radiation therapy for invasive carcinoma of the cervix consists in a combination of external whole-pelvis irradiation and intracavitary brachytherapy with radioactive sources placed in the vagina and uterine cervix. External pelvic irradiation is administered prior to intracavitary insertion in patients with (a) bulky cervical lesions such as bulky stage Ib, stage IIb, stage IIIb or stage IVa disease, in order to improve the geometry of the intracavitary application; (b) exophytic, easily bleeding tumors; and (c) tumors with a necrotic large ulcer. In early-stage cases without a bulky lesion, the intracavitary insertion is performed before or during the external irradiation for the parametrial lymph node region, because intracavitary therapy provides the greatest benefit.

External pelvic irradiation alone is less successful, being associated with increased complications (Castro et al. 1970; Chadha 1988). Morita and coworkers (1988) compared the results in a group of patients who received external irradiation without brachytherapy and a group who received external irradiation combined with intracavitary irradiation (Table 9.30). A dose of more than 70 Gy was necessary to obtain satisfactory locoregional control. On the other hand, the greater the total dose, the higher the frequency of late complications. These findings may indicate that external radiotherapy alone should not be applied in routine practice, but rather reserved for patients unfit for brachytherapy. The dynamic conformal technique using a multileaf

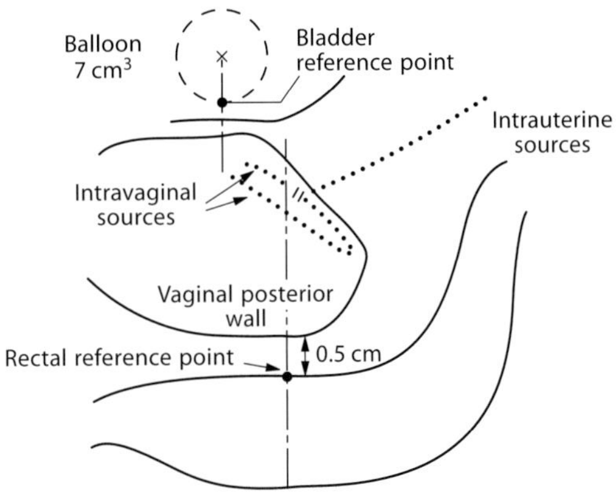

Fig. 9.15. Determination of the reference points for bladder and rectum

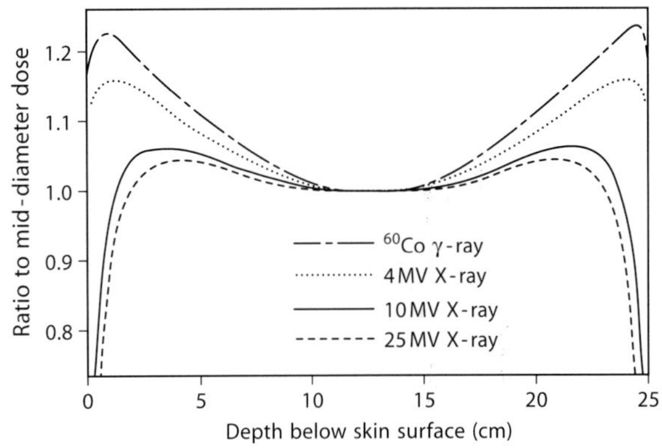

Fig. 9.16. Dose profile used in anteroposterior and posteroanterior portals with different photon energies. With photons below 10 MV, higher integral doses are delivered to the bladder and rectum (pelvic diameter =25 cm)

Table 9.30. Local control rate and late complications involving the rectum and urinary bladder in grades 2 and 3 and total dose at point A (cervical cancer in stage IB and II with external radiotherapy alone). (Morita et al. 1988)

Total dose (Gy) (point A)	No. of patients	Local control rate	Late complications in grades 2 and 3	
			Rectum	Bladder
65–69	12	58.3%	25.0%	16.7%
70–74	24	87.5%	25.0%	8.3%
75–79	38	94.8%	28.9%	10.5%
80–84	25	88.0%	60.0%	20.0%

collimator may be considered one of the most suitable external radiotherapy techniques when intracavitary radiotherapy is not possible (Morita et al. 1974).

9.6.6.1 Beam Energy

Depending on the thickness of the patient's pelvis, high-energy x-ray beams with 10 MV or higher energy produced by a linear accelerator or microtron are applied. The dose profiles for anteroposterior (AP) and posteroanterior (PA) parallel portals using different x-ray beam energies and a ^{60}Co γ-ray beam are shown in Fig. 9.16. With the ^{60}Co γ-ray beam and x-ray beams of less than 6 MV, more complicated field arrangements, e.g., the four-field pelvic box technique or biaxial pendulum irradiation, should be used in order to minimize the dose to the bladder and the rectum and to avoid subcutaneous fibrosis while delivering an adequate dose to the cervix and the parametria.

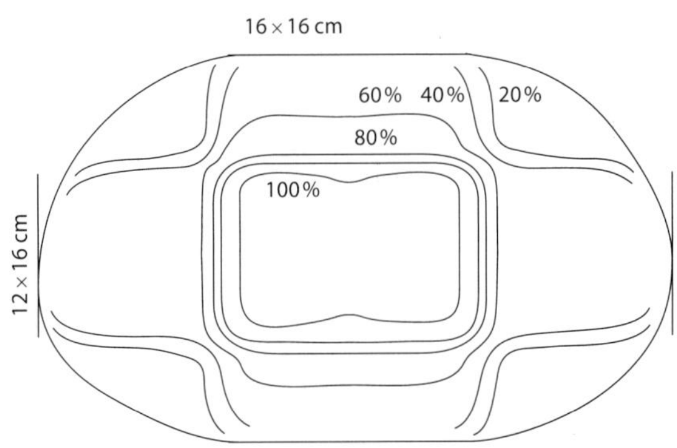

Fig. 9.17. Examples of isodose curves for "box" irradiation of the pelvis with 6-MV x-rays

9.6.6.2 Portals

Anterior and posterior fields or anterior (Fig. 9.16), posterior, and two lateral fields (so-called box technique) are most commonly employed (Fig. 9.17). The AP and PA fields extend superiorly to the top of the fifth lumbar vertebra to cover all of the common iliac nodes (Greer et al. 1990), and inferiorly to the upper half of the vagina and the foramina obturatoria (usually the lower margin of the symphysis) (Fig. 9.18). A 2-cm margin lateral to the bony pelvis is adequate as the lateral border. The usual field is about 16 × 16 cm at the midplane. When there is vaginal involvement, the entire length of the vagina should be treated down to the introitus (dashed line in Fig. 9.18). It is important to identify the distal extension of the tumor by submucosal insertion of a small silver rod or by placing a radiopaque bead on the vaginal wall. A

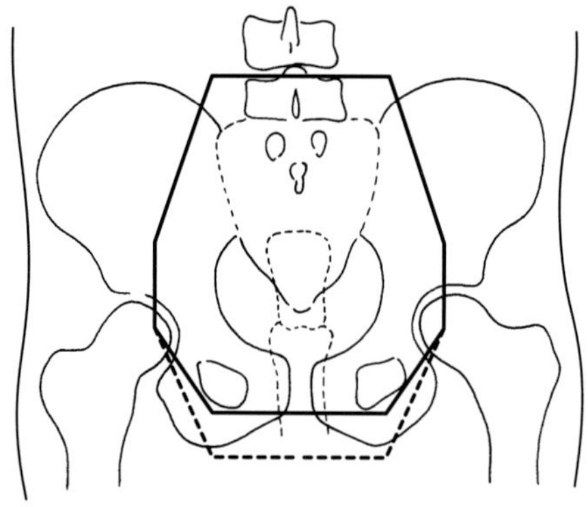

Fig. 9.18. Diagram of standard whole-pelvis portals used in external irradiation for carcinoma of the uterine cervix. If there is vaginal tumor extension, the lower margin of the field is drawn at the introitus (*dashed line*)

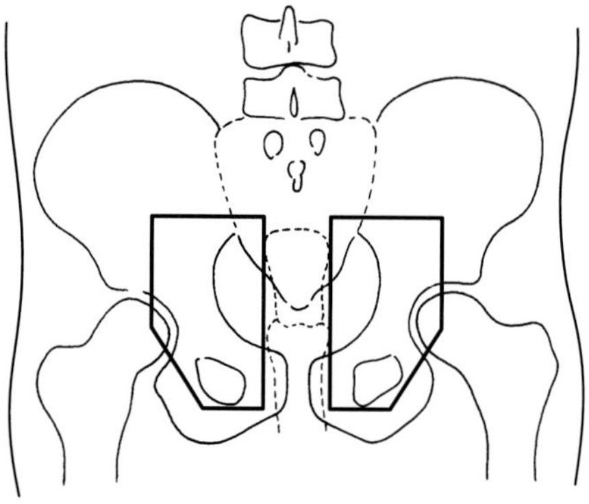

Fig. 9.20. Diagram of reduced portals used for parametrial boost in patients with stage IIB and IIIB disease after completion of whole-pelvis irradiation. If there is unilateral parametrial involvement, only half of the pelvis is treated. A rectangular block is used to shield volume treated with brachytherapy

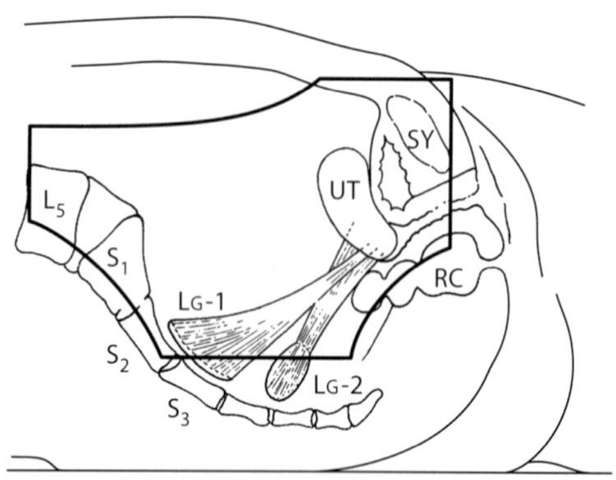

Fig. 9.19. Diagram of conformed lateral portal with the box technique for cancer of the uterine cervix. *L_5*, Fifth lumbar vertebra; *S_1–S_3*, sacral vertebrae; *LG-1*, uterosacral ligament; *LG-2*, cardinal ligament; *UT*, uterus; *SY*, symphysis; *RC*, rectum

conformal radiotherapy technique using a customized shielding block or a multileaf collimator should be used for all fields to exclude normal tissue as far as possible.

With the box technique, lateral fields are usually 10–12 × 16 cm (Fig. 9.19). The lateral fields should cover the external iliac nodes anteriorly (usually at the anterior aspect of the pubic symphysis) and the sacral nodes posteriorly (usually at the S2–3 junction). Barium in the rectum is useful for simulation of the posterior border of the lateral fields. In patients with a bulky primary lesion or uterosacral ligament involvement, the posterior border of the lateral field should be placed at the S3–4 junction.

Central shielding is usually at least five half-value layers thick. Since the pelvic geometry of the applicators changes considerably during intracavitary irradiation with a low dose rate, a simple shielding block, such as straight shields 4 cm wide at the axis of the beams, is often used. However, in the case of high-dose-rate intracavitary radiotherapy, it is preferable to shape the central shielding with "step-wedged" matching to the isodose configuration from the brachytherapy.

Patients should be treated with a full bladder to remove the small bowel from the treatment volume. The prone position is sometimes more reproducible for obese patients.

When the parametrial invasion persists after 50 Gy has been given, an additional 10 Gy in five fractions may be administered with reduced portals of 8 × 12 cm (Fig. 9.20). In stage IIIA the portals should be modified to cover the inguinal lymph nodes because of the increased probability of metastases.

Simulation films should be taken with radiopaque markers placed on the external os and at the lower end of the tumor extensions into the vagina. The bladder and rectum can be visualized with radiopaque material in the lumen. Repeated portal check films are essential for set-up verification.

Serial CT images of the pelvis facilitate the construction of the three-dimensional dose distribution to the tumor volume and normal organs at risk for radiation damage. In order to deliver the radiation dose precisely to the primary tumor and the pelvic lymph node region, Takahashi (1965) proposed the "conformation radiotherapy technique." This technique represents an improvement of the moving-field technique, and since 1972 it has been chiefly developed at the Aichi Cancer Center. A three-dimensional model of the 90% dose region and the dose distributions of two typical axial transverse planes when using the conformation technique are shown in Fig. 9.21. With two axial arc therapy using a multileaf collimator, such a sophisticated high-dose region can be achieved (MORITA et al. 1988, 1995).

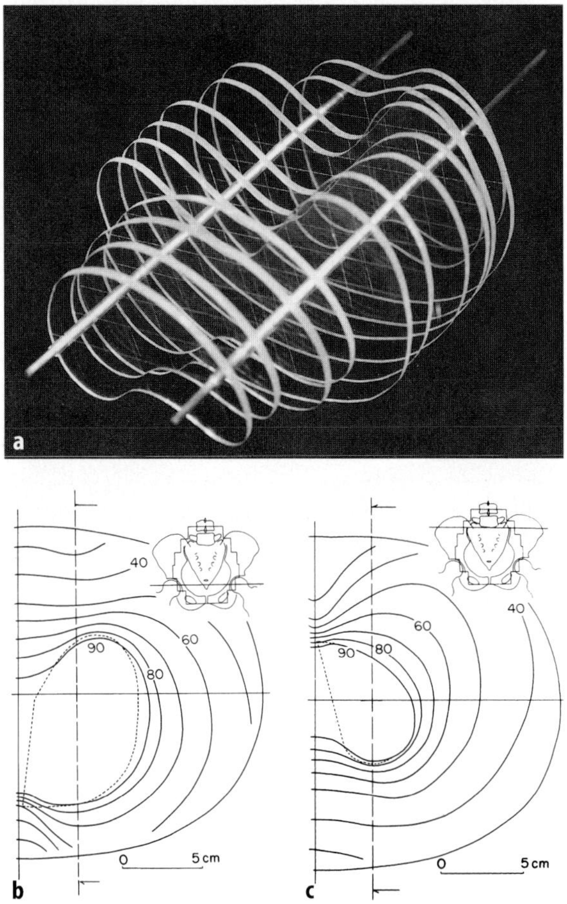

Fig. 9.21a–c. Three-dimensional model of the 90% dose region for pelvic irradiation with the dynamic conformal technique (biaxial and bisegmental) using a multileaf collimator and isodose curves in two transverse planes. (From MORITA et al. 1974)

9.6.6.3 Radiation Doses

The administered radiation doses are expressed in fraction size, number of fractions per week, and total dose.

1. *Fraction size.* Usually, five fractions of 1.8 Gy per day (total weekly dose of 9 Gy) are used. Fractions of 1.5–1.7 Gy are recommended in patients over 75 years of age because they minimize acute normal tissue reactions. All fields should be treated every day to reduce the late complications.
2. *Total dose.* The dose to the whole pelvis from external irradiation with or without an appropriate shielding block (center splitter) varies from 40 to 50 Gy according to the size of the primary tumor. In stage IIb and IIIb the local/marginal parametrial recurrence rate has been found to be reduced with doses of radiation of more than 50 Gy to the parametrium (PEREZ et al. 1983b). Dose variation in the irradiated volume should not exceed 10%.

9.6.6.4 Extended Field Radiotherapy

The tendency of cervical cancer to display stepwise lymphatic spread makes it possible to apply extended field irradiation in selected patients. The frequency of para-aortic lymph node metastases ranges from about 8% in stage Ib to 30% in stage IIIb disease (Table 9.3). If metastatic para-aortic lymph nodes are confirmed, the retroperitoneal tissue is irradiated either through a separate portal or with a so-called extended field, which includes both the para-aortic and the pelvic region.

In patients with pelvic node involvement, there is a more than 50% risk of spread to the para-aortic

Table 9.31. Five-year survival rates relating to number of positive nodes with or without postoperative extended field radiotherapy for carcinoma of the uterine cervix. (INOUE and MORITA 1995)

Treatment method and authors	No. of positive nodes			Total
	1	2 or 3	4 or more	
IB–IIB treated by radical hysterectomy	86%	68%	39%	71%
plus postoperative whole-pelvis radiotherapy	49/57	27/40	7/18	82/115
(INOUE and OKUMURA 1984)				
IB–IIB treated by radical hysterectomy	94%	73%	71%	82%
plus postoperative extended field	21/22	11/15	10/14	42/51
radiotherapy (INOUE and MORITA 1995)				

nodes (Emami et al. 1980; Ballon et al. 1981). It is difficult to decide on the indications for prophylactic extended field irradiation because treatment tolerance is often reduced as a result of the transperitoneal surgical procedure (Haie et al. 1988).

Two randomized trials comparing extended field and pelvic radiation therapy (Haie et al. 1988; Rotman et al. 1990) revealed that extended field radiotherapy with 45 Gy did succeed in eradicating para-aortic lymph node metastases and reduced the rate of subsequent distant failure. Para-aortic lymph node irradiation should only be applied in patients with early-stage disease and a high probability of pelvic control, since the severe complication rate in the extended field group is obviously higher than that in the standard whole-pelvis group. The risk-benefit ratio decreases with advancing stage because of the reduced chance of ultimate locoregional control, and the increased risk of distant metastases. Recently Inoue and Morita (1995) reported on the basis of long-term observations that the number of positive nodes seems to be the best indicator when

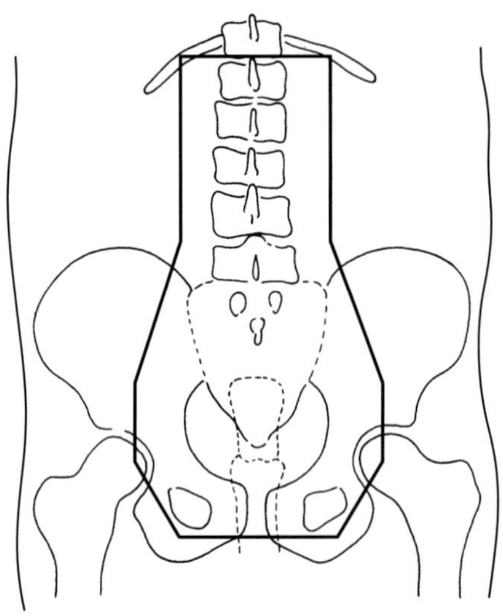

Fig. 9.22. Diagram of extended pelvic and para-aortic portal

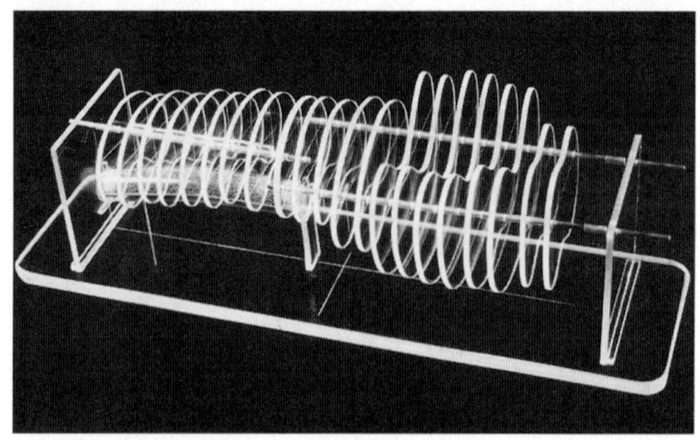

Fig. 9.24. Three-dimensional model of the 90% dose region for the pelvic and para-aortic regions with the dynamic conformal technique (biaxial and bisegmental) using a multileaf collimator and synchronous movement of the treatment couch. (Inoue and Morita 1995)

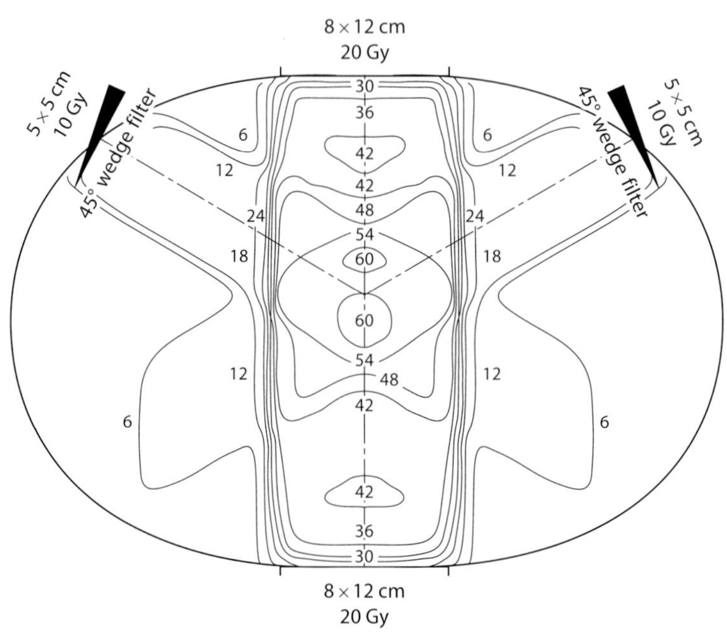

Fig. 9.23. Isodose curve of three stationary fields for the para-aortic lymph node region

deciding whether extended field radiotherapy should be given after radical hysterectomy (Table 9.31).

The fields extend up to the level of the dome of the diaphragm (usually the upper margin of T12). Most centers use an AP-PA parallel opposed pair, and usually the width is at least 8 cm (Fig. 9.22). In radiotherapy for the para-aortic lymph node region, the use of lateral or oblique portals after 30 Gy (so-called field-shrinking technique) decreases small bowel damage (Fig. 9.23). Using the two-axial dynamic conformal technique with a multileaf collimator system it is possible to obtain a high-dose region coincident with the sophisticated target region (MORITA et al. 1995) (Fig. 9.24).

Fraction size should not exceed 1.8 Gy a day. Usually a total dose of 45 Gy is administered for subclinical disease and 50 Gy for known para-aortic lymph node metastases. A dose greater than 50 Gy may be delivered without an unacceptably high risk of small bowel injury (JOLLES 1988; MUNZENRIDER et al. 1991).

9.7 Radical Surgery for Cervical Cancer

R. KREIENBERG and D. KIEBACK

Radical surgery for cervical cancer is an alternative treatment to radiation that needs to be considered when planning treatment for any given cervical cancer. In 85% of cases, cervical cancer presents as squamous cell carcinoma of the cervical surface epithelium; 5% of the cancers are adenocarcinomas arising from the cervical glands. While some authors prefer radiotherapy to surgery in cases of adenocarcinoma, up to now the general opinion is that the histologic differentiation should not be a major factor in deciding between treatment modalities. The differential indication is dependent on tumor stage and tumor size. Therefore, the surgical concepts will be presented in that order.

Additional consideration will be given to the surgical treatment of radiation failure and to the role of combined treatment with radiation and radical surgery in primary therapy and in the treatment of recurrence.

9.7.1 General Considerations

Multivariate analysis has shown that invasion, stage, presence or absence of symptoms, lymph node involvement, vascular space invasion, and grade are of prognostic significance in cervical cancer. Lymph node metastasis correlates with tumor size, tumor volume, lymphovascular space invasion, and tumor differentiation. Histology, age, parity, and menopausal status are not prognostic factors (Table 9.32, Figs. 9.25–9.29) (BURGHARDT et al. 1992; BUXTON et al. 1990; FRIEDBERG and BECK 1989; KREIENBERG et al. 1990). Recent data suggest that tumors that test positive for human papillomavirus type 18 may be

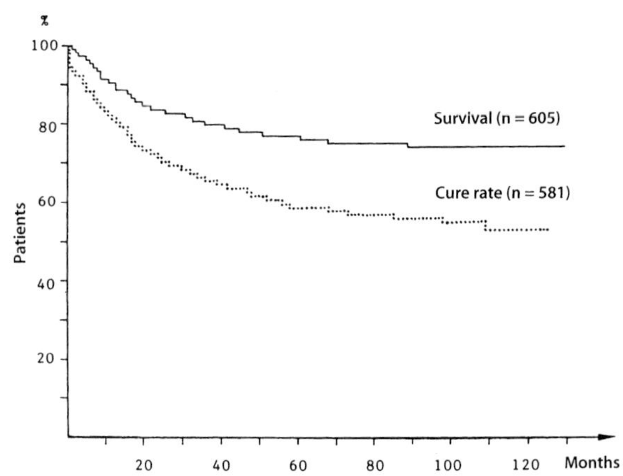

Fig. 9.25. Actuarial survival of patients with cervical cancer (Mainz 1975–1984; retrospective analysis)

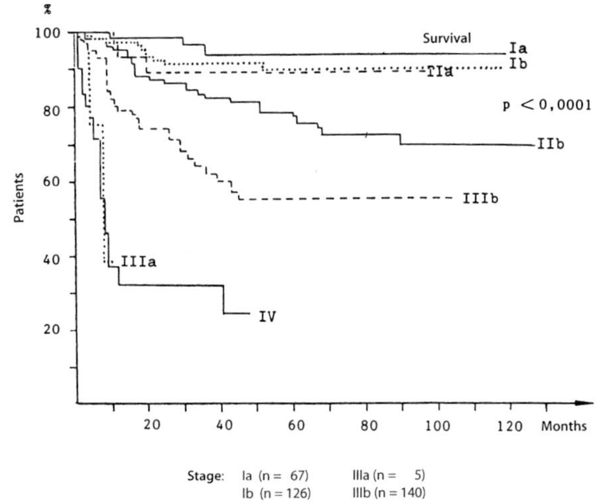

Fig. 9.26. Actuarial survival of patients with cervical cancer by tumor stage (FIGO) (Mainz 1975–1984; retrospective analysis)

Table 9.32. Factors predicting recurrence of cervical cancer. (Modified from BUXTON et al. 1990)

Variable	Classification	Recurred	χ^2	Tails	*P*
Cervical invasion	<50%	7/95	27.4	2	0.00001
	>50%	8/26			
	Entire cervix +/– parametria	10/20			
Stages	Ia	0/10	17.1	3	0.0007
	Ib occ.	5/66			
	Ib	18/59			
	IIa	2/6			
Symptoms	No	8/90	13.2	1	0.0003
	Yes	16/51			
Nodal disease	No	16/116	7.6	1	0.0058
	Yes	9/25			
Vascular invasion	No	14/103	6.7	1	0.0096
	Yes				
Grade	I	0/18	7.2	2	0.0275
	II	8/37			
	III	14/42			
Cell type	Squamous	18/112	1.593	2	0.4509
	Adenosq.	3/16			
	Adeno.	3/12			
Age	<40	16/96	0.058	1	0.8909
	>40	9/45			
Parity	0	8/36	2.04	3	0.5642
	1–2	10/48			
	3–4	5/42			
	>4	2/15			
Menopausal status	Pre	23/124	0.332	1	0.5643
	Post	2/17			

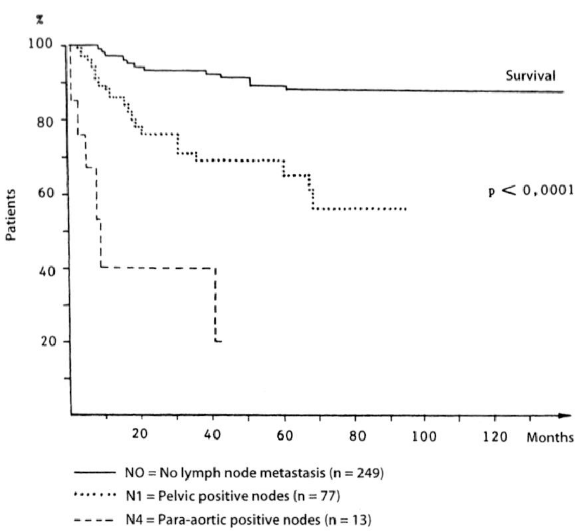

Fig. 9.27. Actuarial survival of patients with cervical cancer in relation to the location of nodal metastases (Mainz 1975–1984; retrospective analysis)

more prone to recurrence (BURNETT et al. 1992). The same may apply to tumors in patients with preoperative thrombocytosis (RODRIGUEZ et al. 1993).

Patient age and weight have been shown to have no limiting consequences for the surgical indication (LEVRANT et al. 1992). Obesity, on the other hand, may influence radiotherapy.

9.7.2 Primary Treatment

9.7.2.1 *Stage Ia*

A depth of invasion of 5 mm already bears a risk of pelvic nodal disease of 1.2% (DISAIA and CREASMAN 1989). Therefore, the Gynecologic Oncology Group has been proposing a maximum depth of invasion of 3 mm as a limit for this tumor stage, to set these small tumors with only local disease apart from larger le-

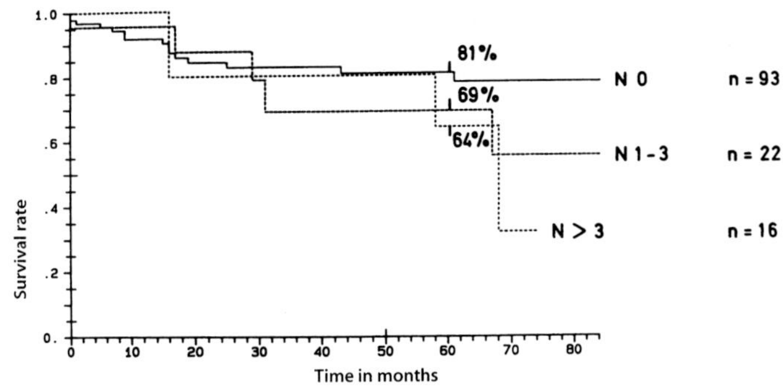

Fig. 9.28. Actuarial survival of patients with cervical cancer in relation to the number of positive lymph nodes (Mainz 1972–1986; retrospective analysis)

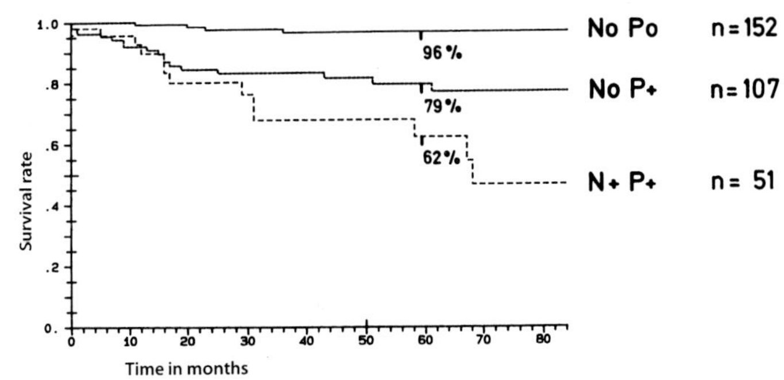

Fig. 9.29. Actuarial survival of patients with cervical cancer in relation to nodal metastasis and/or parametrial involvement (Mainz 1972–1986; retrospective analysis); N0, no nodal metastasis; N+, nodal metastasis; P0, no parametrial involvement; P+, parametrial involvement

sions with metastatic potential. The treatment of stage Ia disease consists in a cone biopsy or simple hysterectomy. Cone biopsy is considered adequate if the entire tumor is removed in the cone and the margins are free of invasive foci and of carcinoma in situ (Morris et al. 1993). All other cases should be treated by simple hysterectomy by the vaginal or abdominal route (Jones et al. 1993). Cone biopsy is preferred (assuming it is an option) in the young patient desiring more children, and hysterectomy after the completion of family planning.

9.7.2.2 Stage Ib

Tumor stage Ib comprises a wide variety of tumors from very localized processes with a depth of invasion of ≥3 mm and no palpable mass up to exophytic growths of up to 8 cm. Accurate staging can be a problem in the latter cases, as the cervix and the vaginal fornices cannot be adequately visualized and also the bimanual examination has to be performed with care so as to avoid the possibility of profuse bleeding from the tumor. For these reasons, treatment of large exophytic lesions is mostly by radiation. In addition to dosimetric considerations, starting radiotherapy by external beam treatment is especially rewarding in these cases, as many lesions "melt away" under radiation and the cervix is found to have reformed at the time of intracavitary treatment, facilitating placement of the radiation sources. It has been suggested that the differentiation between exophytic and endophytic growth patterns may identify different biologic tumor behavior, with radiation therapy being superior in exophytic lesions and surgery in endophytic tumors (Trelford et al. 1993).

As long as there is no evidence of lymphatic spread after staging of the tumor, surgery and radiation therapy can be considered equally curative in stage Ib disease. The decision on the form of treatment will depend on factors like patient operability, the desire to preserve ovarian function in the premenopausal state, and the histology of the tumor.

Table 9.33. Histologic staging versus clinical staging in cervical cancer. (Modified from TEUFEL et al. 1990)

Clinical FIGO stage	Histologic FIGO staging			
	I (%)	IIa (%)	IIb (%)	III (%)
I ($n = 237$)	69	7	9	15
IIa ($n = 15$)	13	27	20	40
IIb ($n = 92$)	27	14	31	28

In the absence of an expertly read lymphogram, the reliability of lymph node staging has to be considered very limited. The patient with a poorly differentiated lesion with lymphovascular space invasion will therefore often be referred for primary radiotherapy, while the lack of such indicators of high metastatic potential will make surgery a more attractive treatment modality (HUGHES et al. 1980).

The European treatment philosophy for cervical cancer favors the surgical approach. The main arguments are that surgical staging is by nature more accurate (Table 9.33), the lymph node status can be ascertained, and the accuracy of the prognosis is thereby enhanced (FRIEDBERG and BECK 1989).

The removal of the tumor may also be of subjective value to the patient. Whether the factors mentioned above translate into a better clinical outcome for the patient has been the subject of much controversy; however, there have been no adequate clinical trials that permit a final comparative evaluation of radiotherapy and surgery.

It should be kept in mind, that skill, availability of adequate equipment, and clinical judgement are important variables affecting the quality of radiotherapy as well as surgery. The availability of optimum treatment conditions is therefore an important additional factor in deciding on the treatment for the individual patient.

Surgical treatment consists in a radical hysterectomy (Wertheim) with removal of the uterus, the intra-abdominal part of the round ligaments, the cardinal ligaments, and the paravaginal parametria after mobilization and lateralization of the ureters, the sacrouterine ligaments, and a portion of the vagina (usually 2–3 cm infracervically). The ovaries can be preserved if no macroscopic abnormalities are present. This procedure is combined with a pelvic lymphadenectomy (Meigs). The original Meigs approach is often modified by extending the removal of the lymph nodes to include the common iliac nodes and submitting them for frozen section early in the course of the operation to assess the operability of the lesion. Frozen section evaluation of lymph nodes during surgery carries a specificity of 100% (BJORNSSON et al. 1993) but a sensitivity of only 68%. It needs to be stressed that the extent of the parametrial dissection during radical hysterectomy should be tailored to the size and aggressiveness of the tumor, as reflected by the classes of radicality described by PIVER et al. (1974b).

Surgery is considered as adequate treatment only in the absence of extensive pelvic lymph node involvement. In cases with positive high common iliac nodes, radiotherapy is the treatment of choice. In the United States, if multiple positive nodes are found during exploratory surgery, radical hysterectomy is often abandoned and radiotherapy administered postoperatively, as it still offers a chance for cure in these patients (SUTTON et al. 1993). In Europe, radical lymphadenectomy including the para-aortic nodes is frequently performed (BURGHARDT et al. 1992; FRIEDBERG and BECK 1989). Adjunctive irradiation in these cases is used less and less frequently as a variety of studies using combinations of radical surgery and radiotherapy have failed to demonstrate improved survival, but have shown a considerable increase in morbidity due to the combined approach. Adjuvant chemotherapy is still under investigation.

With these arguments in mind, in Europe tumors of ≤4 cm in diameter are generally treated by radical hysterectomy and pelvic lymphadenectomy. Some centers, mainly in the United States, reserve surgical treatment for younger women who profit from the conservation of their ovarian function.

Larger tumors of ≥4 cm in diameter, especially the intracervical barrel-shaped lesions, present a considerable problem. The isodose distribution of classical radiotherapy is poor, with a significant risk of tumor persistence or central recurrence. Radical surgery, on the other hand, while eliminating the primary tumor, is faced with a high incidence of extensive lymphatic spread in these lesions. Unfortunately, combining conventional radiation and surgery has failed to improve survival in these patients, too. Especially radiotherapy followed by hysterectomy has resulted in a prohibitive complication rate even when administering a specially designed radiation dosage, and does not improve survival (RUTLEDGE et al. 1976). Recently, pilot data have become available suggesting a place for multimodality treatment with chemoradiation and surgery in these cases (PARHAM et al. 1993).

9.7.2.3
Stages IIa/IIb/IIIa

It appears logical that surgery should also be considered a suitable treatment modality for larger lesions if lymph nodes are negative and the tumor can be completely removed. Vaginal involvement in stage IIa disease will necessitate at least partial vaginectomy, often combined with immediate elongation of the remaining vagina, i.e., by the technique of Simmons and Pratt, in order to prevent postoperative dyspareunia. In stage IIb disease the involvement of the parametria will govern the treatment decision. As long as a sufficient plane can be found laterally to completely resect the tumor, these cancers are also amenable to surgical treatment. The same is true for stage IIIa disease that warrants a total vaginectomy. Today, however, lesions of this extent are very rarely treated surgically. This policy has been evolving because the incidence of lymph node involvement increases steeply with advanced tumor stages. Radiation therapy is appropriate in these cases. With nodal involvement in the area of the common iliac vessels, radiotherapy potentially involves extended fields to the para-aortic areas. In cases with positive para-aortic nodes, extended field radiotherapy has been shown to have a favorable effect on survival (Hughes et al. 1980). Some centers also treat lymph node involvement surgically by radical lymphadenectomy, with equal success in local control. These findings may remind us that extensive nodal spread indicates systemic disease with distant metastasis as the predominant site of tumor progression. It is important to recognize these cases by very careful assessment of the nodal status, in an effort to improve our as yet insufficient arsenal of adjuvant systemic treatment options, i.e., chemotherapy.

Table 9.34. Intra- and postoperative complications of radical hysterectomy (n = 325). (Modified from Teufel et al. 1990)

Complication	No.	%
Intraoperative bleeding	3	0.9
Delayed wound healing	4	1.2
Postoperative bleeding and/or abscess	13	4.0
Lung embolism	6	1.8
Ureteral and/or bladder injury, fistulas	5	1.5
Thrombosis	6	1.8
Lymph cyst formation	13	4.0
Lymph edema	10	3.1
Injury to nerves	1	0.3
Post void residual urine volume >100 cc	10	3.1
Death	3	0.9

The key to the prognosis of cervical cancer lies in the volume of tumor present regardless of the clinical tumor stage (Baltzer et al. 1982; Burghardt et al. 1992; Lohe et al. 1978; Zander et al. 1981). Clinical examination, even in combination with diagnostic imaging techniques, is currently unable to accurately predict the extent of tumor spread found in the surgical specimen. Cut-through hysterectomies should be avoided whenever possible. Aggressive radiotherapy is required to salvage these patients, at the cost of considerable morbidity.

9.7.2.4
Stage IV

Radiotherapy is the primary treatment modality for stage IV disease.

9.7.2.5
Complications

In contrast to complications from radiotherapy, which often arise after a long latency period, surgical complications are usually acute in their occurrence and management (Table 9.34). General complications such as excessive bleeding and wound infection also occur with radical hysterectomy. The most notable specific complications of this type of surgery are injuries to the urinary tract, especially the ureters and the bladder (Methfessel et al. 1992; Kinney et al. 1992). These injuries can be classified as injuries occurring during surgery, unintentionally or with partial bladder resection, and secondary leak formation or fistulation secondary to the inflammatory tissue response in the former vicinity of the tumor or during wound healing. The former complications, if undetected during surgery, are usually symptomatic within the first 48 h postoperatively, while the latter occur after 4 days or more in the context of an otherwise uncomplicated clinical course. Many of these problems can be managed conservatively; only rarely is reoperation necessary for reversal of a fistula or even formation of a urinary conduit. Surgical bowel injury is rare and usually detected and managed during the primary procedure.

Partial denervation of the bladder may occur with extensive parametrial dissection, resulting in neurogenic bladder dysfunction sometimes requiring prolonged self-catheterization (Chen 1989; Iio et al. 1993). This type of disorder seems to respond favorably to treatment with beta-stimulants (Kinney et al.

1992). Instability of the urethra can be a problem with extensive vaginal resections (LORAN and PUSHKAR 1992). Neural disturbances of bowel function have also been described and may require specific treatment (SCHREUDER et al. 1993).

9.7.3
Treatment of Recurrent Cervical Cancer

Pelvic side wall recurrence after initial surgery or radiation carries a bad prognosis. After surgery, external beam radiotherapy is usually administered, sometimes combined with intratumoral implantation of gold seeds or iridium needles. A combination of surgical tumor reduction with afterloading therapy via intraoperatively placed tubes (CORT) has also been advocated for pelvic side wall recurrence after surgery and external beam radiotherapy (HÖCKEL et al. 1989). A definitive evaluation of this technique is not currently possible owing to a lack of controlled trials. This type of recurrent disease is a field of intense investigation of multimodality therapy involving combinations of surgery, chemotherapy, radiotherapy, and differentiating or radiosensitizing agents.

Central pelvic recurrence of cervical cancer after surgery or irradiation is best treated with pelvic exenteration, if this is possible. If surgery has been the primary treatment modality, an attempt at salvage with radiation is usually made before choosing the exenteration approach. In Europe, primary exenteration for recurrent disease without previous radiotherapy appears distinctly more popular than in the United States.

Depending on the exact location of the tumor, either removal of the bladder, vagina, uterus (if present), and surrounding tissues is performed (anterior exenteration), or removal of the rectum, vagina, uterus (if present), and surrounding tissues (posterior exenteration), or combined removal of the rectum and bladder with the vagina, uterus (if present), and surrounding tissues (total exenteration). Subgrouping of pelvic exenterations into further anatomically defined entities may be helpful in comparing operative modalities between treatment centers and in developing a more individualized treatment approach (MAGRINA 1990).

Depending on the organs removed, formation of a urinary conduit, increasingly performed as a continent conduit by techniques like the Mainz pouch (Fig. 9.30) (HOHENFELLNER 1987), and/or of an end descending colostomy becomes necessary as part

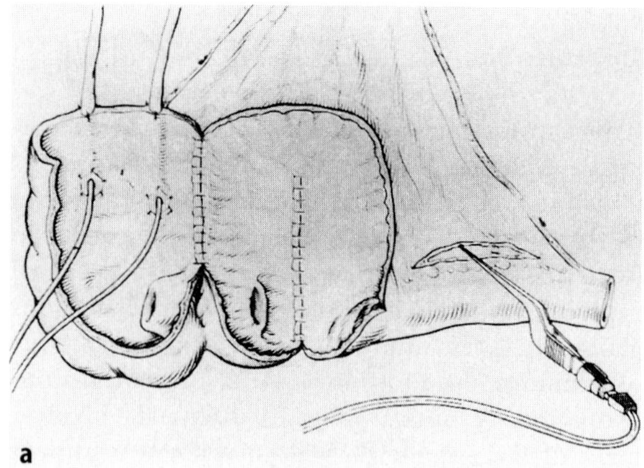

a

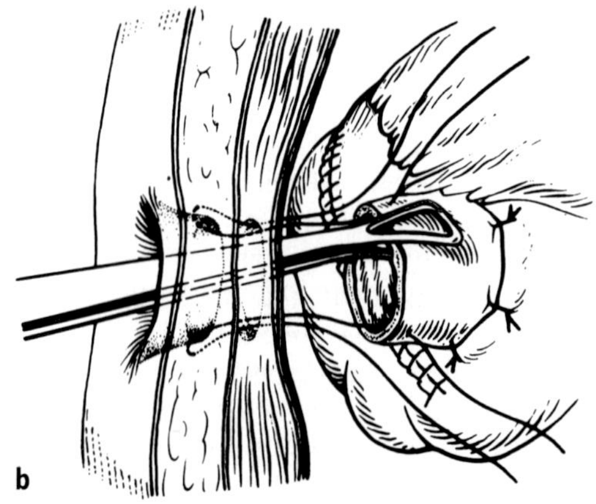

b

Fig. 9.30 a,b. Mainz pouch (FRIEDBERG and BECK 1989; HOHENFELLNER 1987). **a** Anatomic construction; **b** Transumbilical continent urinary stoma

of the above-mentioned interventions. The ileal neobladder has been used with great success in benign bladder disease. So far, however, there are no data on its application in radical surgery for malignant gynecologic tumors (HAUTMANN et al. 1988; WENDEROTH et al. 1990).

Increasingly, attempts are being made to avoid colostomy by low rectal anastomosis if the puborectal portion of the colon is not affected (Fig. 9.31) (FRIEDBERG 1988; HATCH et al. 1990). Rectal J pouch reservoir may decrease the frequency of tenesmus and defecation in low coloproctostomy (WHEELESS and HEMPLING 1989).

If desired, vaginal reconstruction can be performed simultaneously by a variety of procedures. The largest study, in respect of 440 cases, has concerned the use of two introverted m. gracilis flaps, which has the additional advantage of bringing nonirradiated well-vascularized tissue into the denuded pelvic cavity. The total complication rate of this procedure was 5.4% (RUTLEDGE et al. 1976). Al-

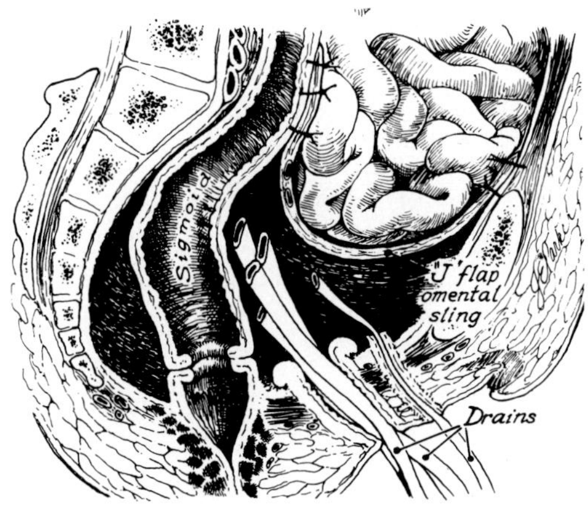

Fig. 9.31. Low rectal reanastomosis with omental flap in pelvic exenteration for recurrent cervical cancer

ternatively, tissue quality permitting, a vaginal reconstruction can be performed with a large bowel segment, i.e., from the cecum or sigmoid (PRATT 1961) or from the ascending colon. Other approaches are the adaptation of the Williams procedure (WILLIAMS 1964), the pudendal thigh fasciocutaneous flap (GLEESON et al. 1994), or the bulbocavernosus myocutaneous flap (CURRIE et al. 1993). Also, the distally based rectus abdominis flap has been reported to be suitable for this purpose (PURSELL et al. 1990). In the absence of nodal disease, the cure rate with this type of radical surgery is about 50% (RUTLEDGE 1987), contrasting markedly with a median life expectancy of only 9 months if the surgical attempt has to be abandoned after exploration. Contraindications to exenteration are lack of surgical planes, intraperitoneal tumor spread, and positive peritoneal washings. Nodal disease in the pelvic nodes decreases the benefit of the operation to a maximum of 21.9%, and disease of the common iliac or para-aortic nodes contraindicates the continuation of the exenteration (RUTLEDGE 1987). These patients do not profit significantly from surgery.

9.7.4 Future Developments

Multiple aspects of cervical cancer warrant further investigation. The areas of investigation mentioned here can only offer a rudimentary idea of promising research topics. Multimodality treatment, already generating encouraging results (PARHAM et al. 1993), will require more extensive study. The surgeon will probably have an expanded role in the development of these approaches (BALCH 1990). Tumor angiogenesis warrants further study as a prognostic factor (CHADWICK et al. 1993) and possibly as a therapeutic target. The impaired T lymphocyte function observed in cervical dysplasia (CROWLEY-NORWICK et al. 1993) and its role in the malignant transformation appears equally important. In the area of human papillomavirus research the interaction between viral proteins and the tumor suppressor gene p53 may provide insights into carcinogenesis as well as an avenue for molecular therapy.

Steroid receptors, specifically retinoic acid receptors, and their interaction with interferons are an active field of clinical investigation. Encouraging results have been reported for a combination of 13 cis-retinoic acid and interferon-α (LIPPMAN et al. 1992).

9.8 Combined Primary Radiation Procedures (Brachy- and Teletherapy)

9.8.1 Japanese Experiences with High-Dose-Rate Afterloading and Teletherapy

K. MORITA

9.8.1.1 Indications for Radiation Therapy

In Japan, radiation therapy has been used in the treatment of cervical carcinoma since the 1940s, usually for locally advanced stages such as III and IV. By contrast, the treatment of choice for patients with early stages such as IB and II is surgery. When radiation therapy is used in early-stage disease, it is usually for certain medically inoperable conditions or in patients more than 60–65 years old.

Table 9.35. Results of treatment by treatment method for carcinoma of the uterine cervix (1982–1986, 150 institutions in Japan). [From *Jpn J Obstet Gynecol* (1993) 43:324]

Stage	Radiotherapy		Surgery	
	No. of cases	No. of 5-year survivors	No. of cases	No. of 5-year survivors
IB	146	98 (67.1%)	939	778 (82.9%)
II	375	217 (57.9%)	920	645 (70.1%)
III	605	262 (43.3%)	73	35 (47.9%)
IV	94	14 (14.9%)	2	0 (0.0%)
Total	1220	591 (48.4%)	1934	1458 (75.4%)

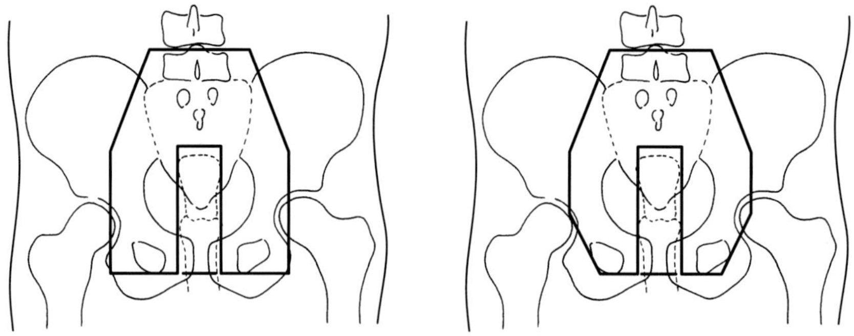

Fig. 9.32. Diagram of two standard whole-pelvis portals used in external irradiation for carcinoma of the uterine cervix

The treatment results for cervical carcinoma in Japan are shown in Table 9.35 (Jpn. Soc. Obstet. Gynecol. 1993). In stage Ib and II, the treatment results of radiation therapy in Japan have usually been 10%–15% worse than those of surgery, because of the aforementioned use of irradiation in patients who are inoperable due to old age or poor general condition.

9.8.1.2
Methods of Radiation Therapy

Radiation therapy for patients with carcinoma of the uterine cervix is essentially based on a combination of intracavitary treatment and external whole-pelvis irradiation.

External Irradiation. External whole-pelvis irradiation is usually delivered with 6- to 10-MV x-rays through 15 × 15 to 16 × 18 cm anteroposterior and posteroanterior ports (two opposing portals), because the average thickness of Japanese women is about 20 cm. For T1b and small T2 lesions, whole-pelvis irradiation using central shielding of 4 cm width at the midline is performed. In Fig. 9.32, the two shapes of central shielding used in Japan are shown. In advanced stages, such as large IIb, III, and IVa, 20–40 Gy is administered by whole-pelvis irradiation without central shielding; thereafter, central shielding is placed. The role of external radiotherapy increases and that of intracavitary irradiation decreases in advanced stages. External irradiation is usually given with doses of 180 cGy per fraction and five fractions per week. The policy regarding irradiation for carcinoma of the uterine cervix recommended by the Japanese Society of Gynecology and Obstetrics is summarized in Table 9.26 (Arai et al. 1984).

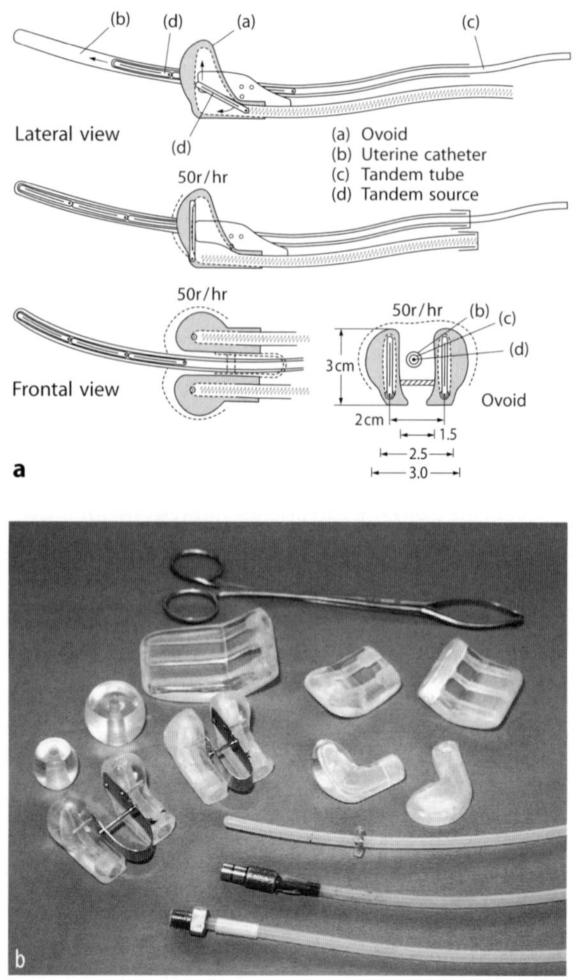

Fig. 9.33 a,b. TAO applicators for **a** LDR and **b** HDR afterloading systems

Intracavitary irradiation is usually given during the course of external irradiation. When the cervical orifice cannot be found due to the presence of a large primary lesion or adequate geometry does not exist in the pelvis due to the degree of vaginal invasion, external irradiation is delivered prior to the first application to decrease the size of the lesion and improve the relationship of the applicators to the cervix and vagina.

Intracavitary Irradiation. In 1965 Tazaki and co-workers developed a new type of afterloading applicator system (the TAO system) for cervical carcinoma, modifying the Manchester system (TAZAKI et al. 1965) (Fig. 9.33). Several sizes of ovoid applicator are available, matching the width of the vaginal vault. Mini-ovoids are also available for the narrow vaginal vault.

High-dose-rate remote afterloading intracavitary radiation therapy (HDR-RALS) was introduced in Japan by WAKABAYASHI et al. (1966). A clinical trial of HDR-RALS for patients with cervical carcinoma was initiated by Arai and co-workers in 1968. In 1979 they reported having obtained almost the same treatment results with high-dose-rate as with low-dose-rate intracavitary irradiation without a significant increase in the radiation injury of surrounding healthy tissues (ARAI et al. 1979, 1992) (Table 9.36). From their long-term clinical experience, it was confirmed that high-dose-rate therapy to a total dose of 29 Gy in five fractions, once a week, produces the same effect as low-dose-rate therapy to a total dose of 50 Gy in four fractions, once a week. The conversion factor from low dose rate to high dose rate is about 0.6 (29/50). Based on these results, guidelines on radiation therapy for cervical carcinoma were presented in 1980 to standardize the treatment schedule (Table 9.26). In 70% of the hospitals, "once a week" application is performed. However, 4 Gy/fraction and "twice a week" application is also recommended because of the biologic advantages, and a total dose of 36 Gy in nine fractions, twice a week, might give almost the same effect. The results obtained at several large hospitals in Japan using low-dose-rate and high-dose-rate intracavitary irradiation for cervical cancer are demonstrated in Table 9.37.

The main features of the remote afterloading device with a high dose rate in Japan are as follows (MORITA et al. 1988):

1. As the radiotherapy source, ^{60}Co is used in almost all hospitals (96%), because the diameter of the ^{60}Co source is smaller than that of the ^{137}Cs source. Recently, remote afterloading devices with a ^{192}Ir source have also gradually become more popular.
2. Acrylite is usually used as the material for the tandem applicator in 90% of the hospitals. When using the flexible acrylite applicator it is easy to confirm the source position using a diagnostic x-ray beam. It is sometimes difficult, however, to correct a pronounced deviation of the uterine body, and in such cases a metallic tandem applicator is also used.
3. The one-point source of type A (Table 9.38) is used for the intrauterine source. During the treatment, the one-point source is moved and stopped repeatedly, to obtain the optimal dose distribution.
4. As an ovoid, about 65% of hospitals use the "boot-styled" TAO applicator (Fig. 9.33), which resembles to the original Manchester ovoid system. The perpendicular standing position of the linear radium source is suitable for irradiating primary tumors of the portio, and for protecting the urinary bladder and the rectum from excessive exposure. Several sizes of vaginal applicator are available according to the size of the vaginal vault and the extension of the tumor.
5. As bilateral ovoid sources, two-point sources (type B) are usually used (Table 9.38). The isodose curve of a type B ^{60}Co source is almost the same as that of a tubular radium source. In 35% of hospitals, the one-point source (type A) is used for bilateral ovoid sources as well as the tandem source. Currently the straight type of ovoid appli-

Table 9.36. Comparison of local failure and late complication rates between high-dose-rate and low-dose-rate intracavitary irradiation. (ARAI et al. 1992)

Local failure rate

Stage	High-dose-rate intracav. irrad.		Low-dose-rate intracav. irrad.	
	No. of cases	Local failure rate	No. of cases	Local failure rate
I	147	5%	13	0%
II	256	14%	70	12%
III	515	24%	143	31%
IVA	74	33%	10	60%
IVB	30	43%	10	60%

Late complication rate

Organ	Late complication rate more than grade 2	
	High-dose-rate intracav. irrad.	Low-dose-rate intracav. irrad.
Rectosigmoid colon	10.6%	18.0%
Urinary bladder	6.7%	7.8%
Small intestine	2.9%	0.4%

Table 9.37. Results of radiotherapy for cervical cancer in Japan[a]

Reporter, institution	Year	No. of cases	5-year cumulative survival rate						Late complication rate more than grade 2			
			IB	II	(IIA	IIB)	III	IVA	All	Rectum	Bladder	Small intestine
Treatment with low-dose-rate intracavitary irradiation:												
Okawa et al. Tokyo W.C.H.	1987	98	82	77			53	29	12.2			
Akine et al. Nat.C.C.	1988	142	82		75	56				40	11.5	0.5
Narimatsu et al. Nat. Sapporo H.	1992	231	70	67			46	22		10	3	
Arai et al. NIRS	1992	77	83		74	47	34	29		18	8	0.4
Takekawa et al. Tokushima Univ.	1993	280	77	71	74	70	54	33	8.6			
Teshima et al. Osaka Univ.	1993	89	89	73			45			5		
Kato and Morita Aichi C.C.	1993	214	89	70	79	60	50			6.5	0.5	0
Treatment with high-dose-rate intracavitary irradiation:												
Koga et al. Miyazaki Univ.	1987	34	85	68					3.7			
Teshima et al. Osaka A.D.C.	1987	105		69			61	29		7.6	5.7	1.0
Arai et al. N.I.R.S.	1992	403	88		77	67	52	24		10.6	6.7	2.9
Kataoka et al. Ehime Univ.	1992	140	72		89	69	64	17		20.7		
Kikuchi et al. Asahikawa Univ.	1992		80	74			63					
Ito et al. Keio Univ.	1992	291	84	71			47	12		13.6	0.8	

[a] Compiled in part from proceedings of congresses held in Japan and from personal communications.

cator is usually used; this type of applicator can be easily inserted in elderly patients with a narrow vagina, but is not suitable for bulky tumors of the portio.

In the opinion of some radiation oncologists in Japan, low-dose-rate brachytherapy is more effective against local recurrence of cervical carcinoma after radical radiotherapy or adenocarcinoma of the uterine cervix than is high-dose-rate brachytherapy owing to several biologic advantages. Therefore, they emphasize that an afterloading or remote afterloading brachytherapy unit with a low dose rate should be maintained together with the high-dose-rate equipment.

9.8.1.3 Fast Neutron Therapy in Japan

In Japan fast neutron therapy for squamous cell carcinoma of the uterine cervix in stage IIIb was started in 1975 (Morita et al. 1985). The fast neutron beams used were produced by bombarding a thick beryllium target with 30-MeV deuterons delivered from the NIRS medical cyclotron. Mean energy was about 13 MeV. Patients were divided into two groups, with treatment by photons or fast neutrons. The whole pelvis was irradiated by two opposing external portals with a mixed schedule, three times weekly by photon therapy and twice weekly by neutron therapy. The dose range was 50–55 Gy per 5–5.5 weeks, with an RBE value of 3.0 for neutron therapy, i.e., 7.2 Gy per 10 fractions for neutron therapy and 25.5 Gy per 15 fractions for photon therapy. The photon radiation group was treated to the whole pelvis with two opposing portals in the dose range of 50–55 Gy per 5–5.5 weeks, 5 times weekly. All patients in both groups then underwent intracavitary irradiation by means of the remote afterloading high-dose-rate technique. The treatment was administered in two fractions with an interval of 1 week during the last 2 weeks of external irradiation, to give a dose of 11–13 Gy at point A.

Table 9.38. Types of ^{60}Co souces for HDR intracavitary irradiation. (MORITA et al. 1988)

Type of source		No. of hospitals	No. of sources		
Tandem	Ovoid		1–2	3	4–6
A	A	50 (43%)	3	45	2
A	B	58 (50%)	0	36	22
B	B	8 (7%)	1	7	0
Total		116	4 (3%)	88 (76%)	24 (21%)

Source of type A = one-point source of ^{60}Co. The source is located 3–5 mm from the top of the tube.
Source of type B = two-point source of ^{60}Co. The anterior source is located 3–5 mm from the top of the tube, and the distance between the two sources is usually 10 mm (9–11 mm). The dose distribution of the type B source, with two-point sources, is almost the same as that of the radium tube with a linear source.

The local control rate was 73% (33/45) after neutron therapy and 66% (35/53) after photon irradiation (Table 9.39). For medium-volume tumors, local control rate increased, though not statistically significantly, to 83% (19/23) for the neutron group, and was 65% (17/26) for the photon group. The 5-year survival rate was 49% in both groups. There was no significant difference in complications between the neutron therapy and the photon therapy group. About 60% of patients in both groups experienced no radiation-related complications.

These results indicate that there were no significant differences between the neutron therapy and the photon therapy group with regard to local control rate, survival rate, frequency of radiation complications, or prognostic pattern. The results were similar to those of the M.D. Anderson Hospital (MORALES et al. 1981; PETERS et al. 1979). Neutron therapy is considered to be more effective for slow-growing tumors; however, squamous cell carcinoma of the uterine cervix is characterized as a relatively rapid-growing tumor, and thus represents only a minor indication for fast neutron therapy.

9.8.2 Low-Dose-Rate Afterloading: The Manchester System

R.D. HUNTER

9.8.2.1 The Classical Manchester System

The technique for the treatment of cancer of the cervix by intracavitary therapy that eventually became known as the Manchester System had its origins in the two pioneering systems of the 1920s that were developed in Paris and Stockholm. When the Christie Hospital and the Holt Radium Institute were merged in 1932 under the leadership of Professor Ralston Paterson, a team led initially by Margaret Todd and supported by the physicist Jack Meredith concentrated on the development of a system that they felt might retain the strengths and improve on the weaknesses of the two original systems.

The first step was the development of a new style of uterine and vaginal applicator. The uterine tubes that evolved were of a soft rubber and incorporated a flange designed to lie at the external os of the cervix and to prevent the sources from slipping deep into the uterine cavity. These soft rubber tubes also allowed the sources to follow the normal anatomy of the uterine canal. Tube lengths of 6 cm, 4 cm, 3.5 cm, and 2 cm became the basis of the system, with the first two (6 and 4 cm) offering optimum system treatment and to be used if possible and the latter two (3.5

Table 9.39. Fast neutron therapy for carcinoma of the uterine cervix in stage IIIB. (MORITA et al. 1985)

	Fast neutrons		Photons	
	Large tumor volume	Medium tumor volume	Large tumor volume	Medium tumor volume
Local control rate	64% (14/22)	83% (19/23)	67% (18/27)	65% (17/26)
	73% (33/45)		66% (35/53)	
5-year cumulative survival rate	49%	49%		
Rate of distant metastases	45%	22%	26%	15%
	33%		21%	
Radiation complications				
Moderate	32% (11 cases)		33% (13 cases)	
Severe	6% (2 cases)		8% (3 cases)	

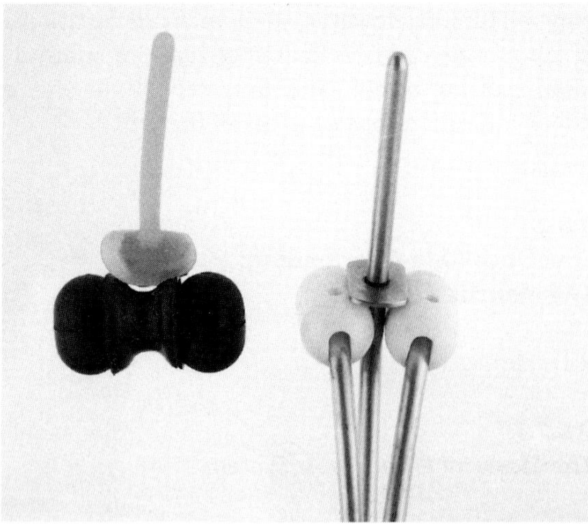

Fig. 9.34. Classical Manchester radium applicators (*left*) and the equivalent modern Manchester afterloading applicator (*right*); AP view (6 cm central tube and small ovoids)

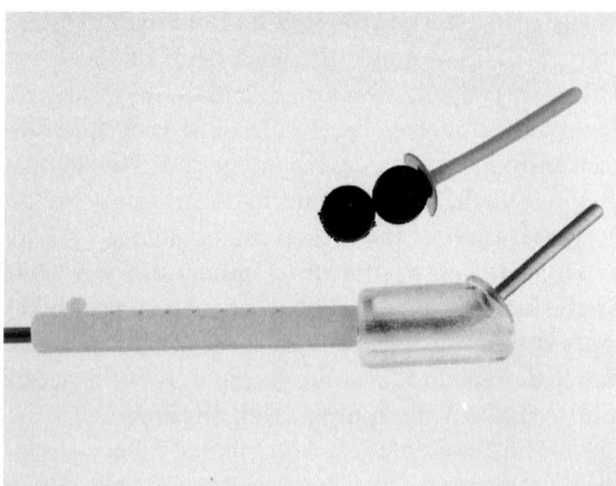

Fig. 9.35. *Above* classical Manchester applicators with small ovoids in tandem. *Below* the equivalent Manchester afterloading applicator

and 2.0) being recognised as non-standard tubes to be utilised only when the uterine canals could not accommodate one of the first two.

The vaginal applicators which developed (Fig. 9.34) were entirely novel. The corks of Paris and the silver boxes of Stockholm were discarded in favour of new firm rubber ovoids designed so that the dose distribution from the standard radium G tubes which were used in the system followed the line of the surface of the individual applicators. This resulted in an ellipsoid shape to the applicators which were known as ovoids. Three sizes were developed with diameters of 3.0, 2.5 and 2 cm based on a clinical project which measured the width of the upper vagina in a series of patients. The applicators were designed to be mounted transversely across the upper vagina and were partly stabilised by the use of a rubber washer (0.1 mm) or spacer (1.0 cm) which was placed between the ovoids and helped to stretch the sources laterally into the fornices and to fill the space available.

Table 9.40. Radium content of intrauterine tubes and ovoids and dose rate at point A

Intrauterine tube	Loaded	Dose rate (cGy/h)	
Long	15 + 10 + 10 mg	34.3	
Medium	15 + 10 mg	34.1	
Short	20 mg	27.3	
Vaginal ovoids	Loaded	Dose rate (cGy/h)	
		With spacer	With washer
Large	22.5 mg	18.3	18.9
Medium	20.0 mg	18.8	19.0
Small	17.5 mg	18.9	19.0

With satisfactory applicators the decision was made to allow the isodose distribution from the treatment to run parallel to the surface of the uterine applicator throughout its length and to create a dose distribution that threw the dose laterally at the level of the cervix and vagina while following the lines of the applicators and not throwing the dose anteriorly into the bladder or posteriorly into the rectum.

Some patients proved unsuitable for standard applicators because they had short uterine cavities, small vaginal diameters or extension of disease down the vagina. They were treated using modified applicators for the uterus or modified positioning of standard applicators, typically ovoids, placed in series or tandem down the vagina (Fig. 9.35). The use of these non-standard applicators or applications resulted in the need for alterations to the standard treatment plans to be able to accommodate the different dose distributions.

To achieve all these specifications Meredith used differential loading of the applicators with radium G tubes, the final loadings are shown in Table 9.40. The effect of these loadings was to create a system that produced a pear-shaped distribution when viewed AP and a banana-shaped distribution when viewed laterally (Fig. 9.36). Perhaps the most important feature of the system was the fact that provided standard applicators were used and positioned correctly

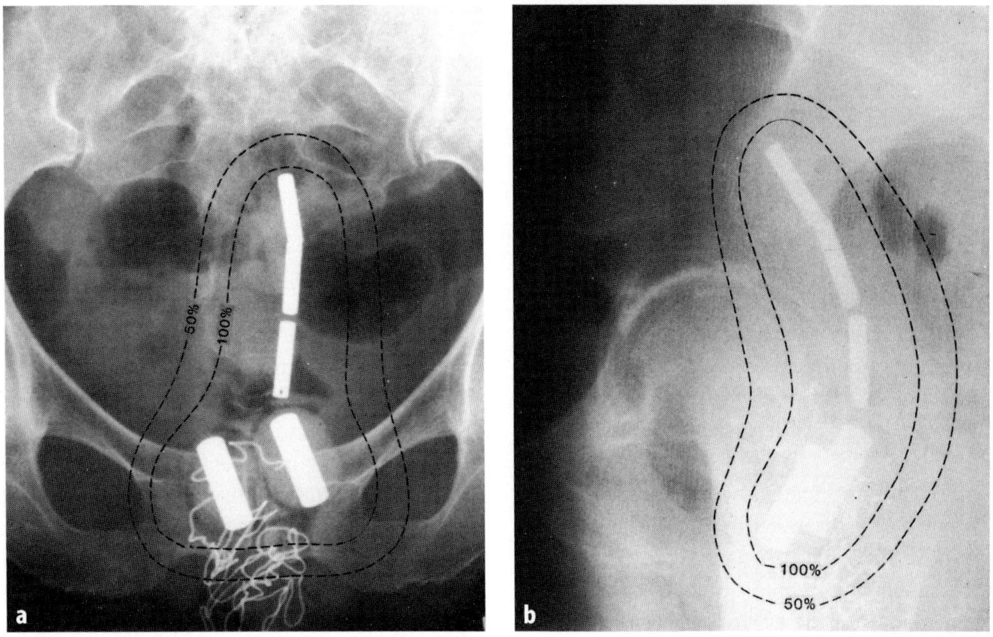

Fig. 9.36. **a** AP view of radium applicators with dose distribution superimposed. **b** Lateral view. (100% = all points receiving the same dose rate as point A.)

the dose rate at point A was the same no matter what combination was employed. The figure in ideal geometry using Meredith loading patterns was 57 Roentgen (R) per hour to the dosimetry point – point A (53 cGy per hour).

The final part of the development of the system was the introduction of the concept of point A. Prior to this time dosage for intracavitary therapy had been expressed in milligrams of radium times number of hours (mghrs). Point A emerged from a perceived need to be more precise and to try to express exposure of the tissues which were being targeted by the treatment. There was a clear understanding that this type of treatment was entirely inhomogeneous and that the exposure gradients around the sources were very steep. This was particularly true close to the sources. On the other hand, more than 3 cm from the sources the exposure being delivered was recognised to be too low to contribute in a major fashion to the control of cancer of the cervix.

The concept recognised a volume lateral to the cervix or lower uterus in which the dose was important because that was the line of spread of many of the cancers and was also the site of key tissues like the uterine artery and the ureter. Within this volume Tod and Meredith (1938) defined point A (Fig. 9.37) because they recognised the need to define a point rather than a volume in this inhomogeneous treatment. Although the anatomical and pathological factors mentioned above were important in the definition of point A, it is critical to an understanding of the Manchester System and its clinical use that it is understood that point A is an ideal geometry point and relates to optimum siting of standard applicators. The clinicians then considered that they were dealing with a standard dose distribution in relation to the applicators and a fixed dose rate to point A.

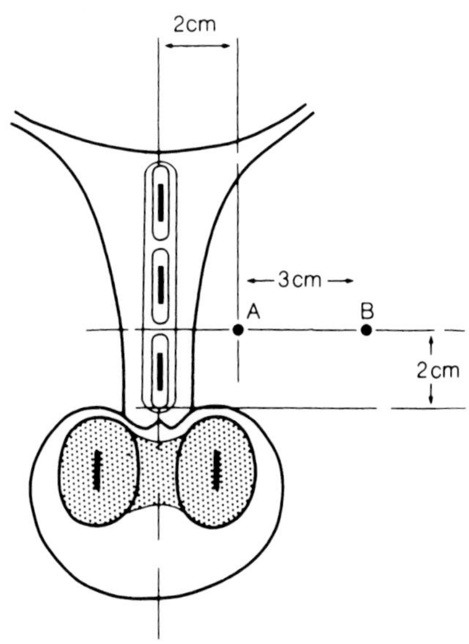

Fig. 9.37. The modern Manchester definition of point *A*

In Manchester the A point has always been used with this philosophy and this has meant that provided correctly loaded standard applicators are used, that they are positioned correctly and that the dose to the rectum as measured by rectal probe has not been more than two-thirds of the dose to point A, then a standard point A dose rate has been assumed and the treatments completed using standard times. The nett effect of these decisions is that the Manchester Cervix Radium System could be thought of and used as a time system provided all the constraints mentioned above are operating. All of the clinical work that led to the definition of the optimum schedules and doses was undertaken following this philosophy.

Technically the applicators were inserted under general anaesthetic, often with the patient in the knee-chest position. This approach gave a single operator an excellent view, made uterine cannulation simpler and made uterine perforation easier to detect. The applicators were held in position by gauze packing employing a radiopaque thread within the packing itself and this was carefully placed to maximise the distance from the vaginal sources to the anterior rectal wall before filling the rest of the vagina to the introitus.

The next phase in the introduction of the system clinically was a definition of optimum schedules. For intracavitary therapy alone and intracavitary therapy with kilovoltage x-ray therapy this work was completed in 1952 with the publication of *Studies in Optimum Dosage* (Paterson 1952). This followed a series of clinical studies in which different treatment schedules utilising different numbers of fractions, overall time and treatment times were employed and assessed. For intracavitary therapy alone the optimum schedule that emerged was 2×70 h of radium, 7–10 days apart, and this gave an exposure of 8000 R to point A. This converts to 7500 rads or cGy. The original publications of Todd suggested there was considerable normal tissue tolerance still available with the chosen schedules. For patients treated with x-ray therapy and intracavitary treatment, different studies pointed to the best results being obtained from a parameterial kilovoltage x-ray technique delivering 3000 R to point B (3 cm lateral to point A) and 1500 R to point A in 15 fractions in 21 days followed by two intracavitary applications, again at 7- to 10-day intervals, delivering a dose of 6500 R (6000 rads/cGy at point A).

The technique then proved popular internationally and many features of the Manchester approach were translated to other centres. Undoubtedly its strength was its simplicity for the operator and the physicist. It did, however, demand a high degree of operator skill and employed pre-loaded radium which ultimately became unacceptable for radiation protection reasons. Many hundreds of patients were treated utilising the system and it remains the basis of modern practice in Manchester. Utilised alone in early cancer of the cervix (small volume stage IB and IIA) it produces results that are outlined in Table 9.41. The 5-year survival for a group of patients treated between 1980 and 1988 with intracavitary therapy alone was 79%. Primary tumour control in this group was achieved with the radium alone in 96%. Surgical salvaging of primary tumour failure was unusual. Mortality was more frequently due to lateral pelvic, para-aortic and pulmonary metastatic disease. Morbidity of the same group, assessed using the modern Franco-Italian glossary, is also shown in Table 9.41. Morbidity utilising this system is located primarily at the lower urinary tract/bladder and sigmoid colon. The combined grade 2 and grade 3 complication rate utilising the system was found to be 12%. Morbidity also included early menopause in the younger patients and upper vaginal stenosis or mucosal thinning in spite of the use of post-treatment vaginal dilators and hormone replacement therapy in younger patients.

Table 9.41. Five-year results for patients with stage I and IIa disease who were treated with radical intracavitary therapy alone. Complications graded by the Franco-Italian Glossary

No. of patients	193
Primary failure	8 (4%)
Died of disease	41 (21%)
Morbidity	
G2	14 (7%)
G3	8 (4%)
G4	1 (0.5%)

9.8.2.2 The Modern Manchester System

The conversion of the classical Manchester System to the modern caesium afterloading system began in 1978 and was based on the use of the flexible LDR (low-dose-rate) Selectron system. Applicators were designed to physically mimic those of the radium system (Figs. 9.34, 9.35). Caesium pellet loading patterns were designed to reproduce the dose distributions of the Manchester System in ideal geometry. This was achieved easily by constructing sources from a mixture of active and inactive pellets, each of

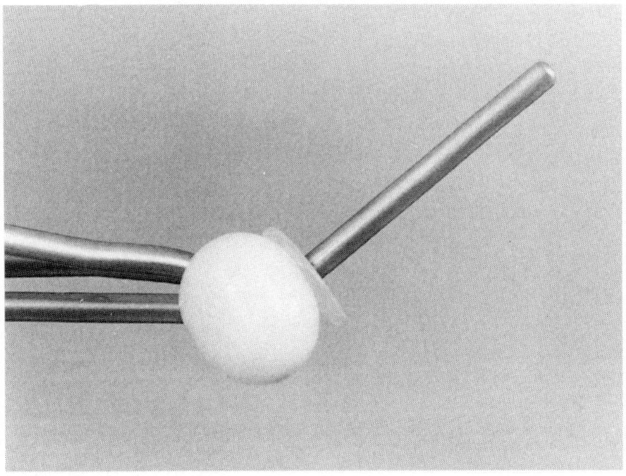

Fig. 9.38. The relationship of ovoids to central tube in the modern Manchester System

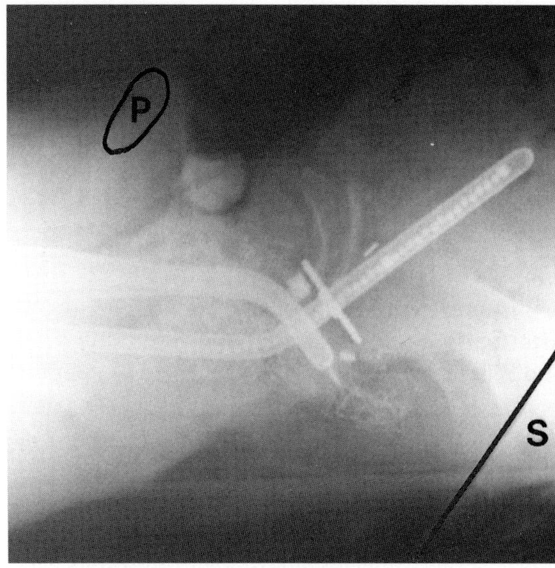

Fig. 9.39. Lateral radiograph of pelvis with modern applicators in situ. Air in the bladder allows the posterior wall to be identified

which were 2.5 mm in diameter. In practice each 5 mg of radium was replaced by an active pellet distributed evenly within the relevant portion of the applicators.

The LDR Selectron system offered a choice of pellet strength ranging from 20 to 40 mCi (60–120 µGy/h at 1 m). For a combination of patient and hospital factors the introduction of the low-dose-rate afterloading system at the Christie Hospital utilised 40-mCi pellets. During the last decade this resulted in treatments that have been delivered at between 140 and 180 cGy per hour to point A, i.e. 2.8–3.5× the dose rates of the old system. The afterloading technique was introduced in a manner that ensured that all the individual variables of this system, including patient selection, fractionation and overall time, were controlled to allow only the dose to point A to vary.

Clinical experience has confirmed that dose rate correction factors which reduce the absolute dose need to be applied when moving from the classical radium dose rates to the higher dose rates of the new system.

Modern Manchester applicators are designed of lightweight alloy and employ uterine lengths of 6 cm and 4 cm (with a fixed uterine flange) angled at 40° forward to the line of the vaginal component. This angle was chosen after studying a large series of radium insertions. The vaginal ovoids retain their classical shape except that the small ovoids have been extended posteriorly by 0.5 cm to build packing into this particular size (Fig. 9.38). The three afterloading tubes are held together by a clamp fixing the ovoid carriers to the uterine tube in a manner that ensures that the relationship of the three applicators is as close to the ideal as is physically possible. They are now typically inserted with the patient in the lithotomy position under general anaesthetic and retained using gauze in a manner similar to the radium system (Fig. 9.39). Applicators are available to accommodate unusually short uterine canals and the fixed position uterus and to allow tandem loading of the vaginal part of the uterine tube if required.

Extensive clinical experience has suggested that for intracavitary therapy alone, if all other parameters remain the same, then a dose rate correction factor downwards of 12%–20% is optimum in terms of cancer control survival and late morbidity when moving from the classical radium dose rate to the dose rate of the new system (Hunter 1991). For treatments employing intracavitary therapy with external beam therapy, the optimum dose rate correction factor lies in the range 10%–20%, depending on the balance of external beam and intracavitary therapy.

The modern afterloading system therefore maintains the strong links with the past by utilising standard applicators, standard loading patterns and, as a result, standard dose distributions and the concept and philosophy of point A. The clinical studies in the conversion to afterloading have strengthened the concept of point A by achieving statistically significant correlations between the dose to point A and the critical end points of central cancer control and morbidity. It is easy to criticise the use of such a rigid system and the use of ideal geometry point A, but the practical reality is that the system has not been surpassed since its introduction and will not be until a more accurate, practical and internationally acceptable way of expressing dose to critical tissues from an inhomogeneous system of intracavity therapy emerges.

9.8.3 Experiences with High-Dose-Rate Afterloading and Teletherapy in Germany: The Würzburg Method

M. Herbolsheimer and K. Rotte

Primary radiation therapy plays an important role in the management of cervical cancer. Compared with radical surgery it yields almost identical results even in early stages (Newton 1975; Morley and Seski 1976; Hamberger et al. 1978; Rotte 1981, 1983, 1985, 1987; Hanks et al. 1983; Haie et al. 1988; Horiot et al. 1988; Piver et al. 1988; Kim et al. 1989; Lowrey et al. 1992; Averette et al. 1993). The choice of the treatment seems to be based on local tradition and personal experience rather than on scientific data. Objective reasons for preferring surgery are the preservation of ovarian function, the opportunity to carry out pelvic and abdominal evaluation, and the assumption that surgery leaves a more functional vagina in sexually active patients. On the other hand radiation therapy avoids major intraoperative and postoperative surgical complications. Thus in early cervical cancer (stage IB and IIA) a general guideline for the treatment management cannot be recommended (Zola et al. 1989). Patients should be treated with close collaboration between the gynecologist and the radiotherapist.

9.8.3.1 Brachytherapy

According to the approach adopted at the Röntgen- und Strahlenabteilung der Universitäts-Frauenklinik Würzburg, curative radiotherapy as a primary modality has to comprise a combination of brachytherapy and external beam therapy, brachytherapy being an integral element of the whole treatment. Thus we do not consider brachytherapy only as a boost to external pelvic irradiation. Consequently we define a first-rank target volume (uterus), in which only brachytherapy is involved, and a second-rank target volume (parametria and pelvic/para-aortic lymphatics), which is covered by external beam therapy (Fig. 9.40). This separation allows us to utilize the full scope of brachytherapy with its steep dose gradient, i.e. high doses to the tumorous tissue are associated with low doses to the organs at risk. Moreover, optimization of the dose distribution is much more effective if brachytherapy is not only a boost. This approach has already been reported by Rotte (1968, 1981, 1983, 1985, 1987) and Gauwerky (1977, 1980).

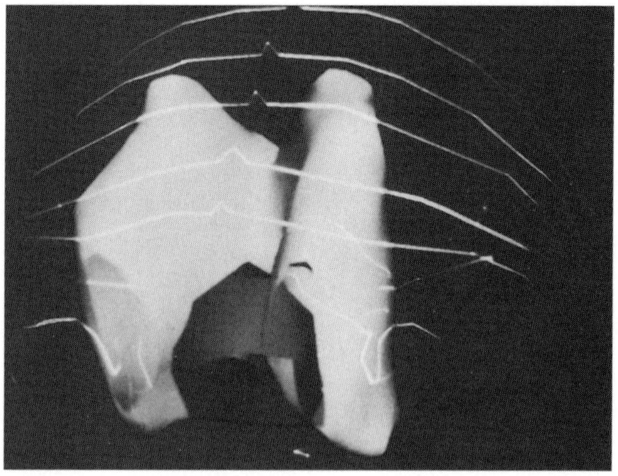

Fig. 9.40. Three-dimensional presentation of pelvic target volumes in primary irradiation of cervical cancer. The first rank volume = dark (brachytherapy) is flanked by the second rank volumes = light (external beam therapy)

According to the policy at our clinic, stage I and early stage II tumors are treated facultatively by either surgery or primary radiotherapy, depending on the individual circumstances. Together with the majority of therapists, we agree with the opinion of Fletcher (1971) that irradiation is the treatment of choice for patients with more advanced tumors. Thus stage IIB and stage III cases are irradiated primarily. In patients with stage IV tumors a palliative treatment depending on individual circumstances is chosen.

In brachytherapy we have replaced the classical radium applications continuously by a remote-controlled HDR afterloading technique since 1971. The afterloading applicator is a combination of a ring which is placed at the portio and an intracervical tube (Rotte 1975; Löffler and van der Laarse 1988). We can choose between different rings, with diameters of 26 mm, 30 mm, and 34 mm, and different tubes of variable lengths between 20 mm and 60 mm. As shown in Fig. 9.41, the tubes are angulated because of the divergence of the cervical and vaginal axes. Normally an angle of 60° between ring and tube is suitable. The diameters of the ring and tube are

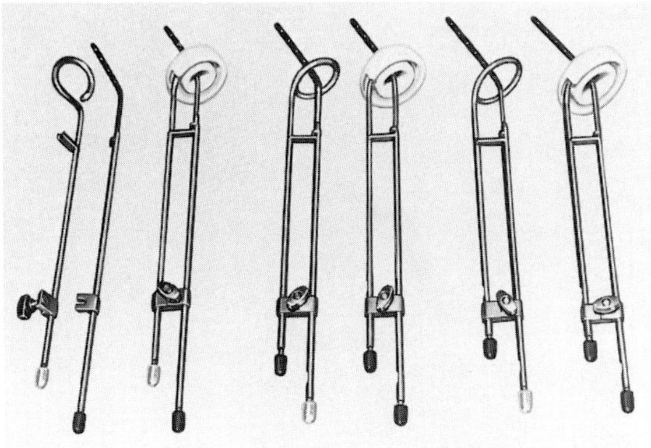

Fig. 9.41. Selection of applicator sets with different ring diameters and tube lengths. Additional plastic covers are placed over the ring

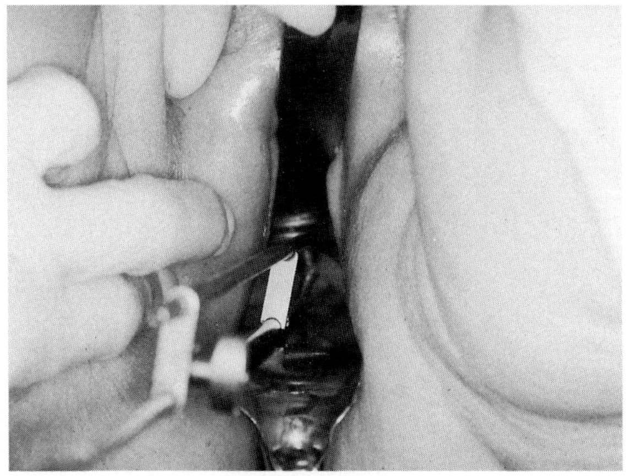

Fig. 9.42. Coupled ring and tube in situ

4 mm and 3 mm, respectively. In order to avoid direct contact between the tube and the cervical tissue, a plastic husk can be placed over the tube. Thus the outer diameter is enlarged to 6 mm. In cases with no tumorous infiltration of the portio, a plastic cover of 3 mm thickness may be placed over the ring for the same reason (Fig. 9.41). In such cases we have to be aware of the changed applicator geometry, as the distance between the ring and our reference point (Manchester point A) is enlarged. The applicator will be afterloaded later by the HDR-MicroSelectron. A ^{192}Ir source, having a diameter of 1 mm and a nominal activity of 10 Ci (370 MBq), is moved in steps of 2.5 mm.

The chosen tube should be about 10–15 mm shorter than the cavity length (in order to avoid direct contact with the fundus wall) but not shorter because the endometrial tumor spread cannot always be defined correctly. An endometrial extension considerably influences the prognosis in stages I and II (Perez et al. 1975). Therefore after cervical dilatation with Hegar's dilators (up to Hegar 7) under general anesthesia the length of the uterine cavity is measured and the tube is inserted.

The ring is correctly placed and fixed to the tube by a special coupling mechanism (Fig. 9.42). With this fixation we obtain right-angled axes of the ring and the intracervical part of the tube and a tube position exactly in the center of the ring. The procedure is supported by percutaneous ultrasound control because especially in cases showing an exophytic portio tumor the risk of inserting the tube into a via falsa is relatively high.

A measuring tube containing a fivefold semiconductor detector chain is inserted into the rectum, and a catheter with a Foley balloon filled with 7 ml contrast fluid is inserted into the bladder. A measuring tube with one semiconductor detector at its top is placed in the center of the balloon.

Finally vaginal gauze packing is applied to hold the applicator in place and to increase the distance between the applicators and the organs at risk. The gauze contains a contrast thread for its identification on the radiographs which will be taken after application. This simple procedure can facilitate the optimization of the dose distribution considerably, as will be described later.

One could argue that a dilatation to Hegar 7 requires local anesthesia, only. But if vaginal gauze packing is performed we need a totally relaxed patient in order to obtain a sufficient distance between the applicator and the organs at risk. This is especially true for the ring. Thus general anesthesia is preferred. The whole application procedure lasts about 5–10 min, so that anesthesia can be restricted to a relatively short time.

The application has to be deferred in cases of pyometra. An indwelling drainage tube is inserted for a few days and antibiotic therapy is administered.

A principal requirement for adequate brachytherapy planning is knowledge of the applicator geometry and its relationship to specific anatomic points. This means we need a reproducible source arrangement in order to achieve a suitable dose distribution. Our planning procedure is based on isocentric orthogonal radiographs of the pelvis (Fig. 9.43) which are taken at a C-bow in the application room. Roentgen catheters (dummies) are inserted into the ring and tube. Tungsten markers show the potential (standard) dwell positions on the radiographs. The patient is, of course, placed on the same table during application, roentgen examination, and

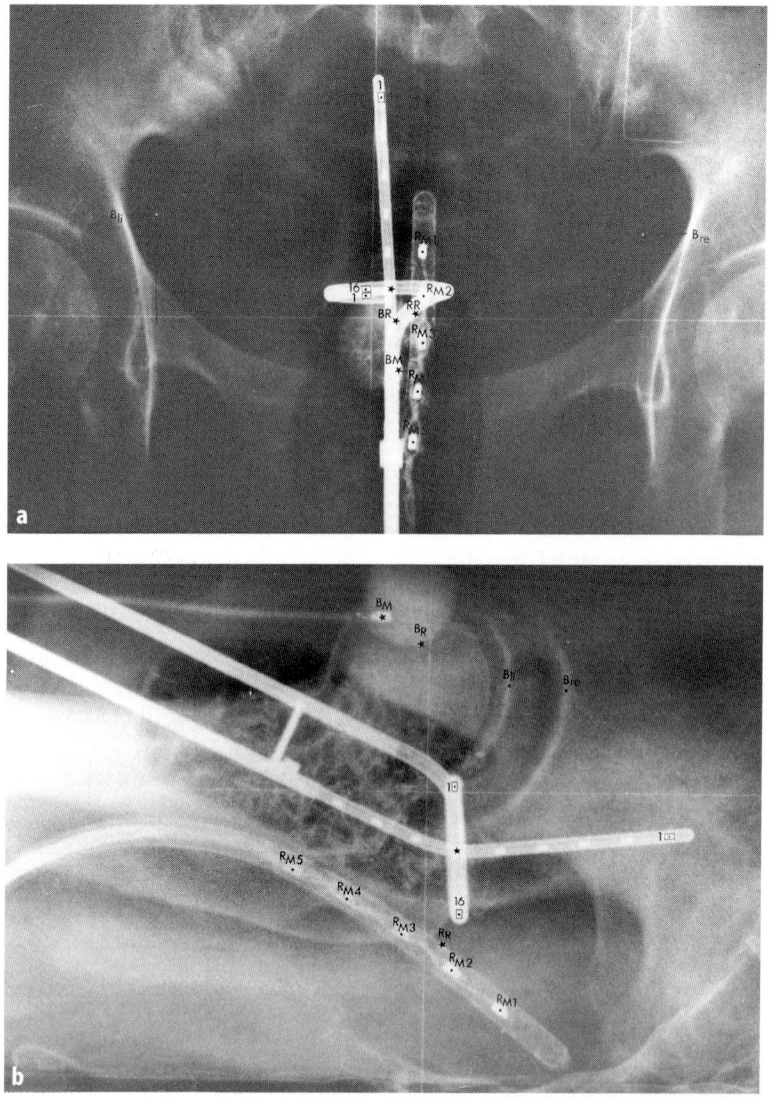

Fig. 9.43 a,b. Isocentric orthogonal radiographs of the pelvis showing the applicators and the measurement tubes in the rectum and bladder. Special points are marked for the digitizing procedure. **a** Frontal view; **b** lateral view

irradiation. The radiographs are digitized with a graphics tablet; sometimes additional isocentric stereo images can facilitate the digitizing procedure. The computer-controlled planning system calculates the dose distribution in three dimensions. This is a standard distribution belonging to a program which is stored in the computer for each applicator combination. These standard programs facilitate the planning procedure. The resulting dose distribution can be optimized easily by changing the number and/or the weight of the active source positions or by shifting these positions (Fig. 9.44). This optimization is influenced by the calculated absorbed doses to the reference points of the organs at risk (SAUER 1992). These points are determined according to the recommendation of the ICRU (1985) as is shown in Fig. 9.15. Quality assurance is achieved by comparing the calculated doses to the measurement points with the doses being measured directly. If there are differences of more than 10%, the digitizing procedure is repeated. If there are no relevant differences, the calculated doses to the reference points are reliable and confirm a correct correlation between the radiation plan and the doses which are actually delivered to these points.

As we have already pointed out elsewhere (LÖFFLER and VAN DER LAARSE 1988; HERBOLSHEIMER 1993), imaging procedures must always

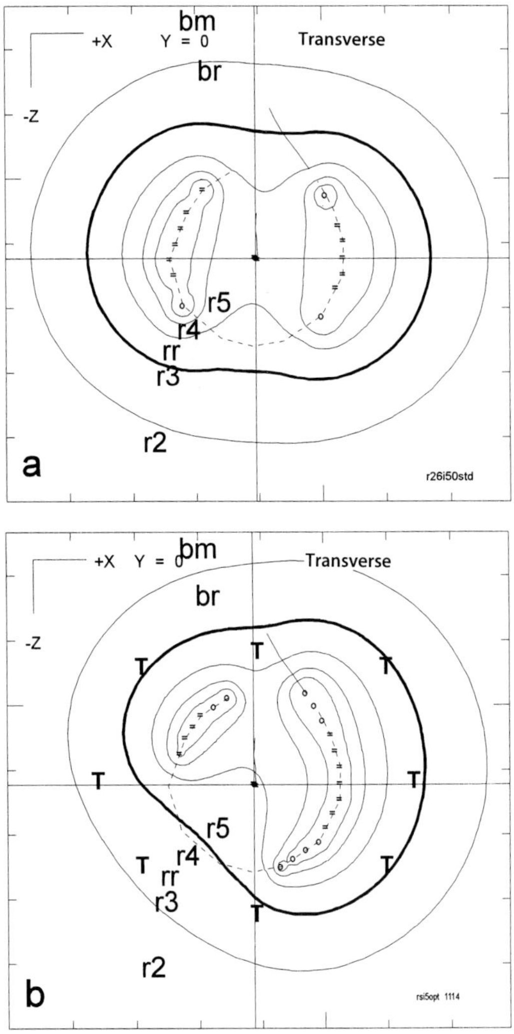

Fig. 9.44. **a** Standard isodose distribution within the ring plane. The rectum marked with the letters *rr* and *r2–r5* is shifted to the right side of the applicator and receives an overdose. The bladder points are *br* and *bm*. **b** The dwell positions and weights are calculated using mathematical optimization. The letters *T* mark the target envelope points, located according to the standard reference isodose shape. (From SAUER 1992)

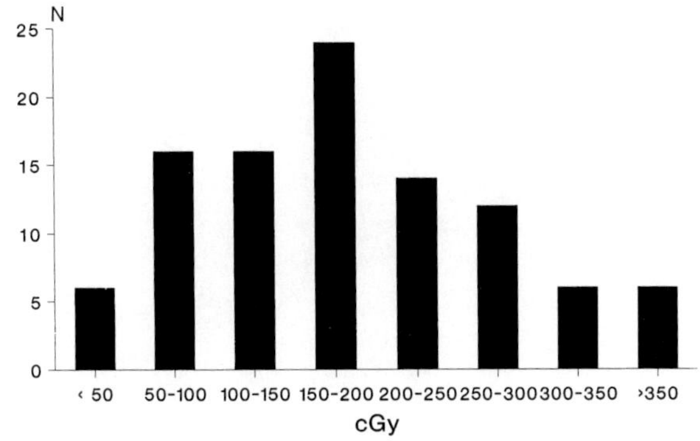

Fig. 9.45. Difference between reference (calculated) dose and dose measured (measurement point) in the bladder in patients treated with HDR afterloading (n = 100)

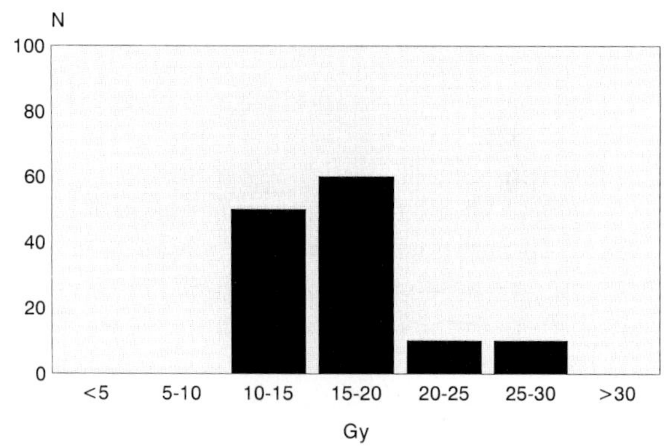

Fig. 9.46. Number of late complications related to the measured dose in patients with cervical cancer treated with radium (n = 102)

be considered as an integral element of treatment planning because they are the only way to determine reference points of the organs at risk. Only the absorbed doses to these standardized points allow comparisons of treatment regimens and they are better correlated with clinical side-effects. Dose measurements alone are no alternative because they represent unreproducible points which are not related to a dose maximum. We have confirmed this by a retrospective study of 100 applications in cervical cancer. Figure 9.45 shows the differences between the doses to the reference point and the measurement point (center of the Foley balloon) of the bladder. On average, the differences are 2 Gy per fraction (SAUER et al. 1994).

Figure 9.46 shows the number of late complications, related to the measured dose, in 102 patients treated in the radium era. Only measured values were taken to estimate the risk of side-effects. There was no correlation between the doses and the clinical signs.

In another study we reviewed the assumed mobility of the organs at risk in 103 afterloading applications in which 71 ring-tube combinations were used. In each case a second set of orthogonal images was obtained after irradiation and was digitized, too. We were able to show that the mobility of the organs at risk did lead to relevant geometric uncertainty (SAUER et al. 1994). The mean standard deviation between the two sets of dose values was 13%; from this a geometric uncertainty of about 3 mm could be estimated. Thus the study confirmed

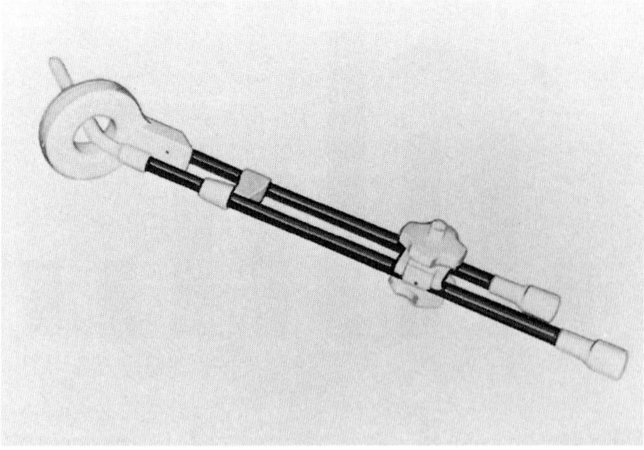

Fig. 9.47. Plastic ring-tube combination suitable for MRI. The applicator is used for planning as well as for performing intracavitary brachytherapy in cervical cancer

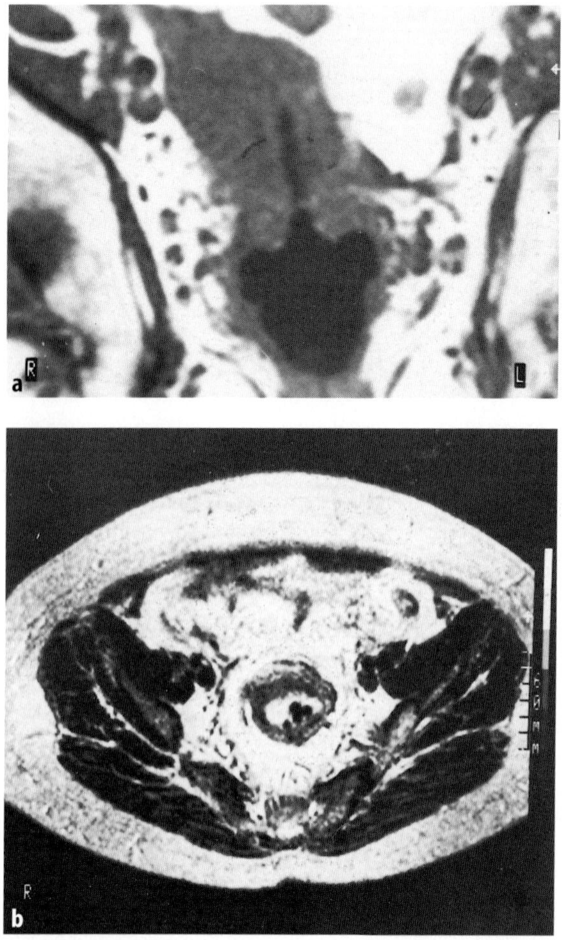

Fig. 9.48. **a** Double angulated coronal MR slice (T1-weighted SE sequence) of the pelvis showing the plastic applicator and the vaginal tamponade in situ as well as the surrounding tissue (vasa iliacae internae, plexus uteri) in cervical cancer stage IB. **b** Transverse T2-weighted SE sequence MR slice showing parametrial infiltration by a stage IIB carcinoma of the cervix. (Images printed with permission of the Institute für Röntgendiagnostik der Universität Würzburg.)

the high geometric precision of the digitized reference points.

As in cases of endometrial cancer, we ensure that the reference doses to rectum and bladder do not exceed 7 Gy per fraction, or 60 Gy within 6 weeks, including the dose contribution from the external beam therapy. Similar recommendations have been reported elsewhere (Neeff 1941; Frischkorn 1983). It is known that the cumulated doses to the rectum and bladder do not always correspond to the clinical complication rate (Esche et al. 1987) even if they are calculated precisely. But in our cases, our previously mentioned study on the accuracy of the treatment planning was confirmed by the rate of side-effects, as will be discussed later.

As with primary irradiation in endometrial cancer, we have supported our treatment planning by magnetic resonance (MR) images since the beginning of 1993. This imaging procedure provides suitable assistance in treatment planning for cervical cancer, as is well known (Hricak et al. 1988; Wijrdeman and Bakker 1988; Schmidt et al. 1991; Hawnaur et al. 1992). In order to use MRI not only as support but as an integral element in the treatment planning, we have replaced our common metallic precious steel applicators with a plastic ring-tube combination (Fig. 9.47), which is not merely a phantom for planning but a suitable applicator, i.e., exchange is not necessary after the MR examination. Of course, the applicator allows optimization of the dose distribution in the same way as conventional applicators.

We choose double-angulated MR slices parallel to the dose distribution axis which is determined by the axis of the cervical tube (Fig. 9.48). The slices have the same scale as the orthogonal exposures.

In cervical cancer, MRI plays a less important role than in the treatment planning of endometrial carcinoma. Nevertheless, it is useful to adapt the reference isodose to the course of the organs at risk. Moreover, the doses to the reference points of the organs at risk, calculated by the orthogonal exposures, can be compared with the doses to equivalent points which are calculated by digitizing the MR slices. Of course, in patients who are not fit for MR examinations, for whatever reason (e.g., claustrophobia, metal implants, pacemakers, poor general state of health), a conventional planning procedure is still performed.

We apply five fractions of 8.5 Gy, 10 days apart, to the Manchester point A. The dosage is equivalent to the former radium therapy.

9.8.3.2
Teletherapy

The brachytherapy applications are scheduled within the course of megavoltage treatment to the pelvic lymphatics, which are irradiated using 10-MeV photons from a linear accelerator. A bisegmental arc rotation with two isocenters is utilized. The planning is supported by computed tomography (CT) in several slices (Fig. 9.49). The target volumes are defined with regard to the individual anatomy and to the area irradiated by brachytherapy. Distention of the reference isodose of brachytherapy at the level of the ring would cause overlapping with the external beam portals. Thus we combine the movement of the gantry (four segments of 30°) with a fixed collimator rotation of about 12°, which results in a teletherapy dose contribution of less than 10 Gy to the reference volume of the brachytherapy. Due to the arc rotation the skin is more spared and the dose profile at the borderline of the target volumes is smoother than with shielded fixed fields. This represents a suitable adaptation to parametrial tumor distention and helps to avoid hot spots due to the assumed mobility of the uterus. On the other hand, such hot spots in a small margin may even be desirable on the side of the tumorous parametrial infiltration. In these cases the uterus is removed with the shortened parametrium and the overdosage covers mostly tumorous tissue. We have been able to show that the rate of side-effects is not enlarged under these circumstances. The lower margin of the portals is at the inferior border of the obturator foramen, and the upper margin at the L4–5 interspace.

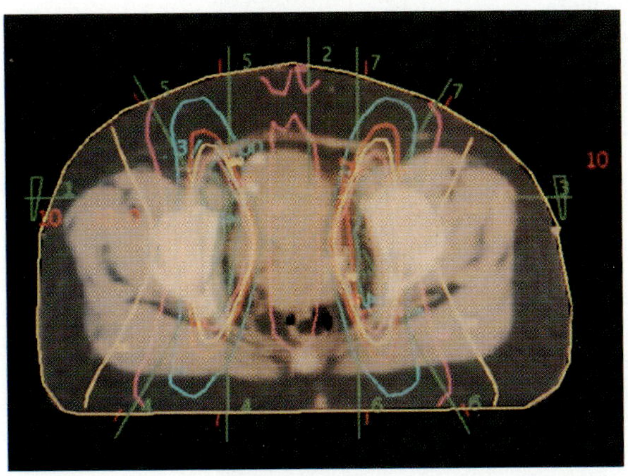

Fig. 9.49. Transverse CT slice of the pelvis. Isodose distribution of external beam therapy (biaxial bisegmental arc rotation) in the central beam plane

The arc rotation technique which we use is similar to long-established techniques employed during the telecobalt era in order to compensate skin reactions due to the relatively small build-up effect of telecobalt machines (Surmont et al. 1956; Heinzel 1961; Frischbier and Hasse 1965; Vahrson 1973).

We apply 25 fractions of 2 Gy to the maximum point. The target volume is enclosed by the 80% isodose at least. If the total treatment time is prolonged (e.g., due to intervening public holidays) the physical total dose is changed according to a modified linear quadratic concept. For this reason we developed a computer-assisted biologic treatment planning system (Baier 1987).

Irradiation of the para-aortic region is only performed in cases of histologically proven lymph node metastases or in those patients in whom CT or MRI is suggestive of para-aortic metastases. As in cases of endometrial cancer, we do not perform adjuvant treatment. From the study of Haie et al. (1988) it can be concluded that adjuvant para-aortic irradiation is of limited value. Chism et al. (1975) calculated an increase in 5-year survival of only 1% whereas considerable side-effects have to be taken into account. The assumed rate of para-aortic lymph node metastases is about 10% in stage IIa tumors and increases to about 30% in stage III tumors (Perez 1992; Roth et al. 1994); consequently most patients would be irradiated for no good reason. Only in young patients in a good general condition and patients with pelvic lymph node metastases or a stage III tumor can adjuvant para-aortic irradiation be justified. In such special high risk cases a benefit of about 10% can be assumed (Rotman et al. 1990).

The target volume is adjacent to the pelvic portals. The upper margin is at the T12-L1 interspace. Treatment planning is based on several CT slices. Fractionation and dosage are the same as to the pelvic lymphatics, which are irradiated simultaneously.

The radiation technique depends on individual circumstances (extension of the tumorous infiltration and its spatial relationship to the kidneys, craniocaudal angulation of the target volume with regard to an exposure of the spinal cord, etc.). It may involve a combination of fixed fields with or without wedge filters or arc rotation therapy. Irrespective of this, we have to deal with severe acute side-effects to the intestine, including the stomach, which are primarily due to the large treatment volume. Moreover, the prognosis following radiation therapy in patients with para-aortic metastases is poor (HAIE et al. 1988).

In this context it is worthwhile to perform a biopsy of scalene lymph nodes in high-risk cases because the rate of metastases to this area is about 20% or more (BUCHSBAUM and LIFSHITZ 1976). As the mean survival time of patients with positive scalene lymph nodes is less than 1 year (DIPAOLO et al. 1990), therapy should be only symptomatic.

9.8.3.3 Special Situations

In patients showing a *residual tumor* at the portio after intracavitary brachytherapy we apply an interstitial boost to the tumor (Fig. 9.50). We choose between a low dose rate (LDR) technique with iridium wires (similar to our boost technique in breast-conserving therapy) and a fractionated high-dose-rate (HDR) technique with a single iridium source. Therapy planning is supported by stereo or orthogonal radiographs that are digitized. The dose distribution is calculated according to the Paris System (PIERQUIN et al. 1978). The boost doses depend on the individual situation. Usually a boost of 4 times 4.3 Gy is applied by HDR afterloading (equivalent to 20 Gy by LDR afterloading).

The *interstitial version of brachytherapy* as a boost to intracavitary applications or for use in patients with recurrent tumors after irradiation is usually the sole way to apply a sufficient tumor dose without exceeding the tolerance dose of the connective tissue, including the organs at risk. Successful attempts at increasing local tumor control by means of interstitial brotherapy in gynecologic tract cancer have been reported by several authors (MARTINEZ et al. 1985; MARTINEZ 1989; SYED et al. 1986; NORI and HILARIS 1987; SYED and PUTHAWALA 1987; DONATH et al. 1992). But as already pointed out by HORIOT et al. (1989), this procedure requires some experience and one has to be aware of complications such as bleeding and inflammation.

We consider *external beam radiation after a radical Wertheim's hysterectomy* to be justified only in cases of pelvic and/or para-aortic lymph node involvement and/or if lymphangiosis carcinomatosa or infiltration of blood vessels beyond the uterus is present (ROTTE 1987). This procedure is also recommended by others (KUCERA and VAVRA 1990; PEREZ 1992; VAVRA et al. 1992). An increasing incidence of lymph node metastases from 15% (no evidence of lymphangiosis carcinomatosa or infiltration to the parametrial vessels) to almost 70% if lymph or blood vessels have been infiltrated has been reported (CHUNG et al. 1980; FULLER et al. 1982; FRIEDBERG and BECK 1989). As is well known, patients with positive lymph nodes have a considerably worse prognosis (INOUE and OKUMURA 1984). Nevertheless, there are individual constellations that restrict the indications for postoperative radiotherapy in patients with

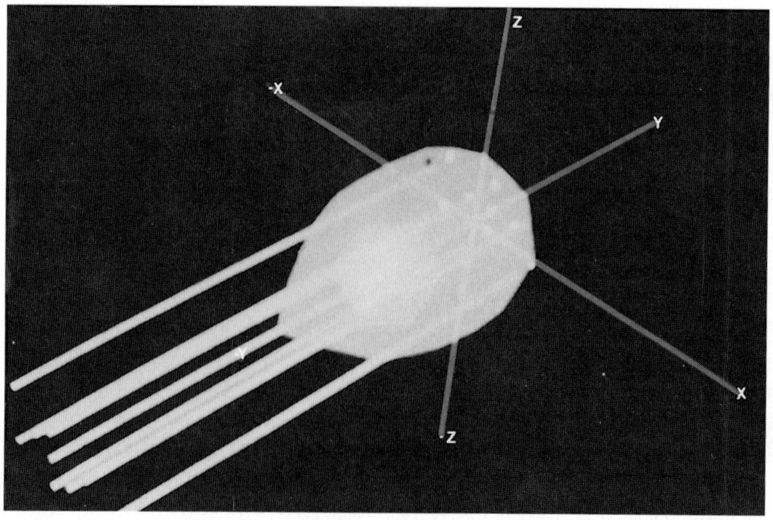

Fig. 9.50. Three-dimensional representation of the reference volume of interstitial brachytherapy to the uterine cervix

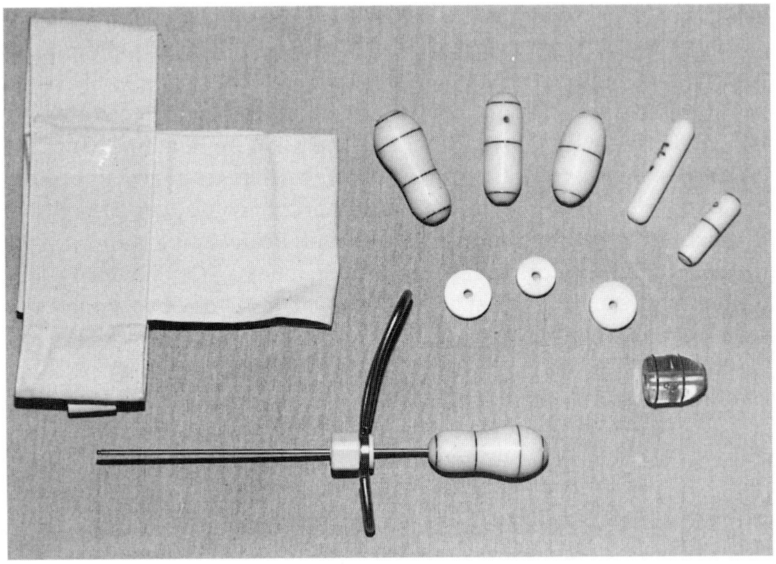

Fig. 9.51. Selection of individually manufactured plastic vaginal applicators. The rigid tube for the ^{192}Ir source is placed in the center line. The vaginal applicators are fixed with a so-called perineal bow. This bow is fixed to the patient with a special bandage. Note: The applicator is fixed to the patient using the aforementioned accessories and not fixed to the table

lymph node metastases: If radical pelvic and para-aortic lymph node dissection has been performed (e.g., more than 25 lymph nodes have been dissected) and only a few lymph nodes are involved, one has to weigh the potential benefit of irradiating the lymphatics against the increased side-effects. If surgery is incomplete, the results of postoperative radiotherapy will be worse than after a radical operation or after primary irradiation (Rotte 1987) and an increased rate of side-effects has to be expected. In such cases we apply 25 fractions of 2 Gy to the whole pelvis, normally utilizing a box technique. If necessary the para-aortic region is irradiated simultaneously, as described above. If the removed vaginal cuff is insufficient, five brachytherapy fractions of 8 Gy are delivered the applicator surface using a suitable vaginal applicator (Fig. 9.51) Care should, however, be exercised when performing vaginal insertions. Because of the surgical treatment the organs at risk may be closer to the applicator than in patients with an intact uterus. This again stresses the necessity of imaging procedures and computerized brachytherapy planning.

To avoid postoperative radiotherapy in general we advise the gynecologist to perform only an exploratory laparotomy if it becomes obvious during the operation that radical surgery will not be possible, for whatever reason. Such a patient is a candidate for primary irradiation.

We do not perform *preoperative irradiation*, though it is usual in several centers (Rampone et al. 1973; Perez et al. 1985; Calais et al. 1989; Gerbaulet et al. 1992d; Touboul et al. 1992). It may be suitable to decrease the possibility of viable tumor cells and to decrease the risk of distant tumor dissemination, and it may be justified in special cases in order to transform a primarily inoperable tumor into an operable one; however, it increases the rate of postoperative complications. Moreover there is no proof of increased survival rates following preoperative radiotherapy (Rotte 1987).

There is no general agreement as to the influence of histologic type on the prognosis, especially when the stages have been analyzed separately (Kilgore et al. 1988; Vavra et al. 1989; Eifel et al. 1990; Perez 1992). The rate of adenocarcinomas in our patient groups was about 5%. They were treated in the same way as squamous cell carcinomas, and we have seen no significant differences with regard to outcome.

The special case of a *carcinoma of the cervical stump* after subtotal hysterectomy (a relatively popular treatment modality for benign conditions of the uterus in former years) is something of a challenge for radiotherapy because it is often difficult to achieve adequate source arrangements in brachytherapy. We try, if possible, to apply a combination of a short tube and a ring. Brachytherapy is usually combined with external beam therapy of the whole pelvis.

There is controversy over how to manage so-called *bulky tumors or barrel-shaped intracervical lesions* (PEREZ et al. 1985; WHEEMS et al. 1985; HORIOT et al. 1988, 1989; BLOSS et al. 1992; COLEMAN et al. 1992; MARUYAMA et al. 1992). Our primary treatment in such special cases does not differ from the usual technique and dosage except that in selected cases we additionally give an interstitial boost to the cervix; we then use the technique described by HORIOT et al. (1989).

The management of *recurrences* is individual, depending above all on previously applied doses and on the site, shape, and distention of the tumor. Individual treatment is required in stage IV primaries, too. Our results and those reported in the literature (VAN NAGELL et al. 1979; KREBS et al. 1982; SCHULZ-WENDTLAND et al. 1991) are not satisfactory. Mostly due to synchronous or metachronous distant metastases about 80% of our patients died within the first 2 years after the diagnosis of a recurrence.

We consider general management policies not to be practicable. This is true for each kind of radiation as well as for surgical or systemic treatment forms.

9.8.3.4
Results

Our results in respect of primary irradiation are summarized in Tables 9.42–9.44 and in Fig. 9.52. The data presented in Table 9.42 concern only patients who were treated according to the approach described above. The survival and the recurrence rate do not differ considerably from the literature data (HAMBERGER et al. 1978; KUIPERS 1984; PEREZ et al. 1985; DISAIA et al. 1987; TESHIMA et al. 1987; HORIOT et al. 1988; HORIOT et al. 1989; VAHRSON and RÖMER 1988; KATAOKA et al. 1992a,b; TEUFEL et al. 1992; HAMMER et al. 1993; SMIT and SCHMITT 1993; CHATANI et al. 1994a,b). A review that we performed in 1512 patients, including some historical groups, revealed similar survival rates with ^{226}Ra and HDR afterloading treatment (Fig. 9.52), again confirming the well-known fact that HDR and LDR regimens (including radium therapy) can be considered equivalent (ROTTE 1983, 1987, 1991; KUIPERS 1984; BATES 1989; MARTH et al. 1991; ORTON et al. 1991; TESHIMA et al. 1993; ORTON and SOMNAY 1994; CHATANI et al. 1994b).

Our results in early tumor stages are comparable to those achieved with radical surgery.

Our group of patients treated by HDR afterloading showed only modest acute side-effects (mild diarrhea and/or mild cystitis). Severe late reactions did not occur; even in historical groups such reactions were seldom (ROTTE 1983), and they have been further restricted to occasional cases of transient rectal or bladder irritation following optimization of the dose distributions. No fistulas occurred in our patients. The tendency towards a reduction in side-effects is obvious from Table 9.43, where side-

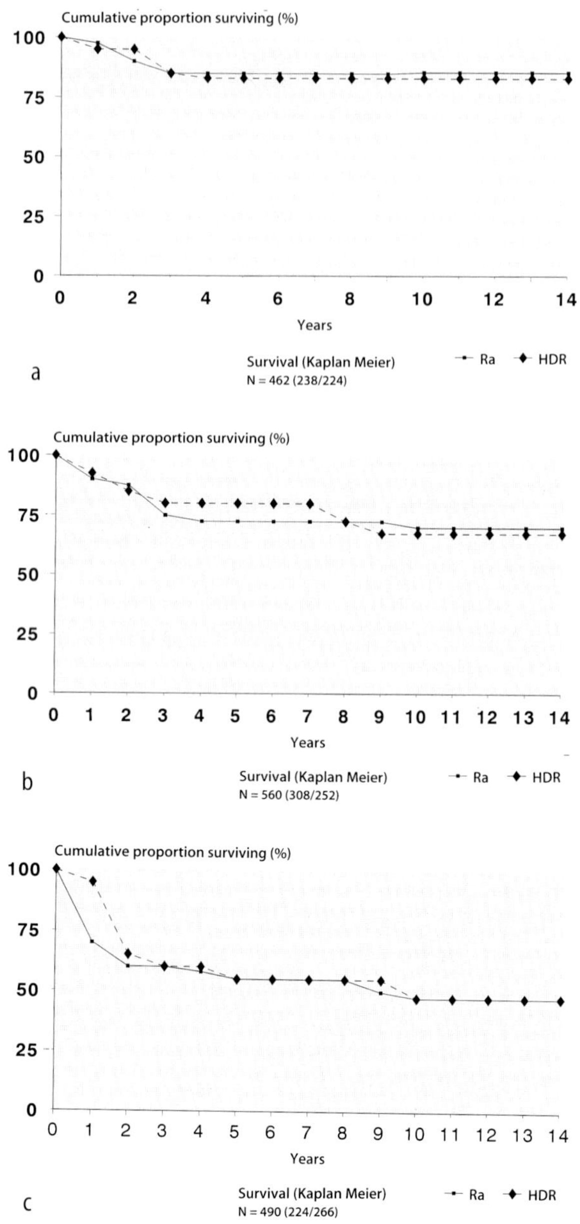

Fig. 9.52 a–c. Actuarial survival rates of primary irradiation in cervical cancer, 1973–1988; comparison of ^{226}Ra and HDR afterloading treatment. **a** Stage I; **b** stage II; **c** stage III

Table 9.42. Results achieved at the UFK Würzburg between 1984 and 1992 using primary irradiation for cervical cancer (according to the approach described in the text)

	Stage					
	IB	IIA	IIB/IIA + B	III	IV	I–IV
Pelvic recurrences	2/59 (3.4%)	2/39 (5.1%)	5/76 (6.6%)	13/68 (19.1%)	1/4	26/241 (10.8%)
Tumor progression	–	1/39 (2.6%)	4/76 (5.2%)	6/68 (8.8%)	3/4	14/241 (5/8%)
Pelvic relapses in total	2/59 (3.4%)	3/39 (7.7%)	9/76 (11.8%)	19/68 (28%)	4/4	40/241 (16.6%)
Distant metastases (+/– pelvic relapses)	3/59 (5.1%)	9/39 (23.1%)	27/76 (35.5%)	34/68 (50.0%)	4/4	77/241 (32.0%)
5-year crude survival	89%	75%		41%	–	66%

Table 9.43. Comparison of the results achieved at UFK Würzburg using ^{226}Ra and HDR afterloading for carcinoma of the cervic (n = 1512)

Complication	Complication rate (%)			
	Radium		HDR afterloading	
	1973–1979	1980–1988	1973–1979	1980–1988
Bladder ulcer	2.4	2.2	5.7	1.1
Bladder fistula	0.0	0.0	0.0	0.0
Rectal ulcer	11.6	5.8	6.9	1.4
Rectal fistula	1.2	0.2	1.5	0.0
All complications	15.3	8.3	14.1	2.5

Table 9.44. Comparison of the results achieved at UFK Würzburg with standard planning and individualized planning

Characteristic	Patient planning subgroup	
	Standard	Individualized
Total no. of cases	26	24
Recurrences[a]		
Stage I	0/6	0/2
Stages IIa/IIb	5/11	3/13
Stage III	4/9	5/9
All stages	9/26	8/24
Complications		
Bladder ulcer	3	0
Bladder fistula	0	0
Rectal ulcer	1	0
Rectal stenosis	0	0
Rectal fistula	0	0
All complications	4/26	0/24

[a] Stages cited are the FIGO stages.

effects after radium and HDR afterloading are compared: Until 1988 radium was used simultaneously with the afterloading technique, which was increasingly used after its introduction in 1973. As to the radium, we replaced "milligram-hours" by isodose distributions in 1980. This led to a considerable decrease in side-effects. During the first years of afterloading (1973–1979) the complication rate was higher than with the radium therapy that we performed after 1980, and was about as high as in the radium period up to 1979, although we had designed a fractionation protocol according to the linear-quadratic model based on the studies of Fowler and Stern (1963). This was doubtless due to the smaller therapeutic range of HDR compared with LDR irradiation (Kummermehr 1990). However, after the introduction of individualized treatment planning (afterloading period 1980–1988) the complication rate decreased below the level of both radium periods. As the total group included more than 1500 patients it was, of course, heterogeneous. In order to eliminate this disadvantage and to scrutinize the real validity of dose optimization we compared two selected groups with identical features, i.e., same stage, age, and state of health and, of course, absolutely identical teletherapy and HDR afterloading procedures. Fifty patients were analyzed under these strict conditions after a follow-up period of 3 years. The first group was treated according to standard plans, while the second underwent brachytherapy after we had optimized the dose distribution. Deliberately restricting the analysis to objective side-effects, we saw no reactions within the individually planned patient group but there were several complications in the group treated on the basis of standard plans. There was no difference between the groups with respect to the recurrence rate (Table 9.44). Though the groups are rather small (which could not be avoided, given the numerous strict inclusion criteria) we can state that the implementation of our policy to reduce the incidence of complications did not result in an increased rate of recurrences.

To summarize, one can suggest that the decreased therapeutic breadth of HDR treatment techniques can be more than compensated by a sufficiently optimized treatment planning procedure. Its accuracy is due to a reproducible geometry of the source arrangement which is guaranteed by the short treatment times.

9.8.4 The Paris Method

A. Gerbaulet, M. Maher, C. Haie-Meder, E. Lartigau, and H. Marsiglia

9.8.4.1 The Classical Paris Method

At the turn of the twentieth century, surgery alone was the treatment of choice for carcinoma of the cervix. However, following the discovery of x-rays by W. Roentgen and radium by Marie Curie, new modalities of treatment were introduced into the management of such cancers. Over the ensuing decades a great deal of progress was made, culminating in what became known as the "Paris school," led by Regaud (1929), which resulted in the establishment of rules for a method using intracavitary radium sources in continuous low-dose-rate irradiation. This method had the following characteristics:

Colpostat. This vaginal device consisted of two special types of ovoids known as "corks," which were mounted on diverging prongs, connected by a transverse metal spring. The corks could accommodate radium sources of three different sizes, and variation in the tension applied to the spring ensured that the corks were appropriately situated in each lateral fornix.

Uterine Catheter. For the uterine source, a hollow gum elastic tube was employed into which radium sources were introduced, allowing the entire uterine cavity to be irradiated. In later years, a central upper vaginal cork was sometimes added to ensure a more uniform irradiation of the cervix.

Sources. Radium was manufactured as tubes of different activities, usually 10, 20, and 30 mg.

Time-Dose Relationship. Intracavitary radium applications were performed in one, or more often in several sessions; the aim of the fractionation was to decrease the tumor volume and to ensure that the position of the radioactive material at each session was satisfactory. The irradiation was specified in milligram-hours (mgh), which was the product of the total activity of the sources and the duration of irradiation. Treatment generally fell between 4500 and 9000 mgh.

9.8.4.2 The Modern Techniques Derived from the Paris Method

Of course, the above-described classical but historical Paris method has been modified over the years. The experience of the "French school" with intracavitary radium therapy resulted in much progress, improved results, and notably a decrease in the morbidity of treatment for carcinoma of the cervix (Lamarque and Coliez 1951).

There are three techniques which have their origin in the original Paris method: the Institut Gustave-Roussy method (Chassagne et al. 1969, 1977; Gerbaulet et al. 1990a,b,c, 1992a; Pierquin et al. 1987b; Rosenwald and Dutreix 1970), the Créteil method (Pierquin and Marinello 1975; Pierquin et al. 1987b), and the R. Huguenin method (Chassagne et al. 1968; Delouche and Gest 1972; Rosenwald and Dutreix 1970). The first of these is the most frequently used and will be described in detail.

The Institut Gustave-Roussy Method

The Gustave-Roussy system has four main principles: (a) individually tailored irradiation, (b) abso-

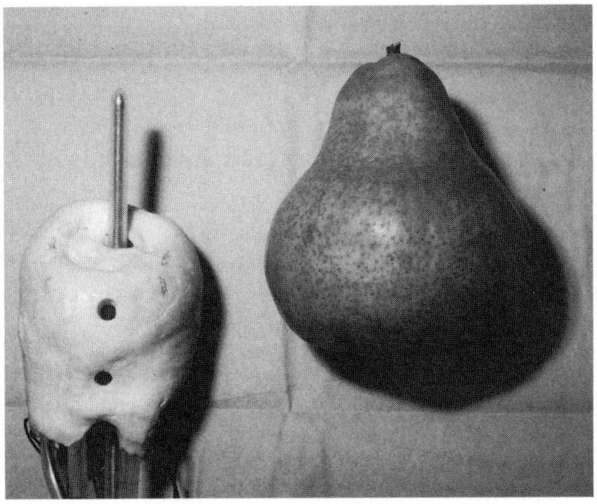

Fig. 9.53. Molded applicator with uterine catheter and pear-shaped reference volume

lute knowledge of the dose distribution within the tumor, the neighboring organs (bladder, rectum), the draining nodes, and the pelvic side walls, (c) total radiation protection for the medical staff and visiting family, and (d) good patient tolerance. This method was devised by D. CHASSAGNE and A. DUTREIX in the 1960s. Initially they tried to apply an afterloading technique using iridium wires in plastic tubes. This technique was intermediate between the classical Regaud method and our current intracavitary brachytherapy. Its major disadvantage was the inability to ensure that the sources remained in a constant position throughout the application time. As a result of this drawback a mould applicator was devised in the Institute Gustave-Roussy in 1964. Initially a vaginal mould applicator (which was in fact the first step in the development of the current individualized method) used radium tubes, but these were rapidly replaced by iridium and cesium miniaturized souces.

Moulded Applicator. To construct an individually specific moulded applicator four steps are necessary: (1) cervicovaginal impression using dental paste, (2) acrylic mould fabrication from the negative of the impression, (3) source outline and positioning of the plastic catheters within the mould, and (4) guide insertion to aid x-ray localization (CHASSAGNE and PIERQUIN 1965; CHASSAGNE and GERBAULET 1975; GERBAULET et al. 1990a, 1992b). This applicator is individually made to order for each patient, resulting in perfect adaptation to the patient's anatomic features and to the tumor topography (Fig. 9.53). In addition this technique affords reasonable comfort for the patient, and eliminates the risk of displacement of the mould device.

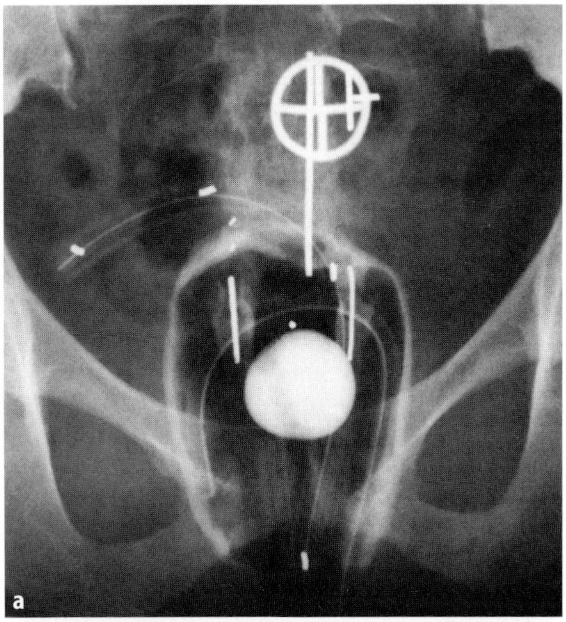

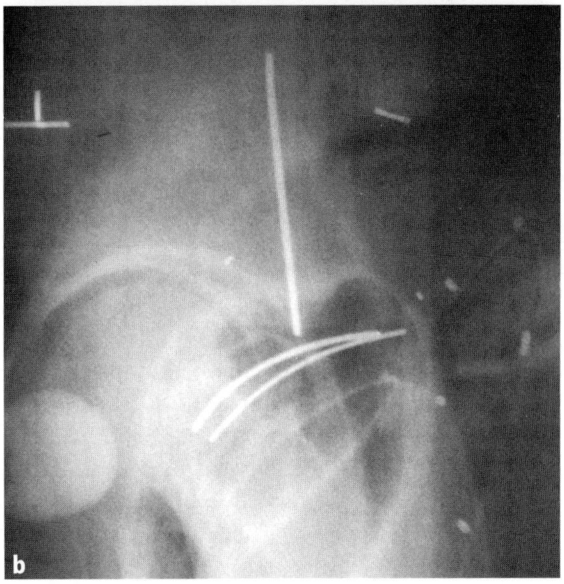

Fig. 9.54a,b. X-ray control with dummy sources: AP and lateral views

Sources. The geometry of the source placement is entirely governed by the topography of the tumor, thereby assuring maximum quality of irradiation with an optimal dose distribution. The Institut Gustave Roussy method is a low-dose-rate system and the radionuclide used is cesium-137. Sources of ten different lengths are available in increments of

8 mm from 16 to 88 mm. The choice of source length to be employed depends on the needs of each individual case (Chassagne and Gerbaulet 1975; Dutreix and Wambersie 1975; Gerbaulet et al. 1990a, 1992a,b).

The preferred position of the uterine source, which is contained in a plastic flexible catheter, is as follows: upper limit, the upper third of the uterus; lower limit, level with the vaginal sourcese (Fig. 9.54).

For the vaginal sources, the preferred positions are: parallel to each other and parallel to the face of the mould, which abuts onto the cervix while simultaneously being lateralized in front of the right and the left cervical lips. Their lengths are dictated by the topography of the tumor and the size of the cervix. The distance between the two vaginal sources is equal to the average length of both of them.

The geometric positioning of the sources is decided by the radiotherapist according to the individual anatomy of the patient and to the characteristics of the tumor.

Although, presently the Institut Gustave Roussy system utilizes a low dose rate in its gynecologic treatments, it can be adapted to a high dose rate.

Afterloader. A remote afterloader (curietron), which automatically projects cesium sources, is used to place the radioactive material in the required positions (Chassagne et al. 1968; Chassagne and Gerbaulet 1975; Gerbaulet et al. 1983, 1990c, 1992a,c). This is a bedside apparatus. It is equipped with four independent motors driving four independent cables to transfer the sources from their holding safe to the patient's moulded applicator and vice versa. Source transfer is by a pneumatic drive system which is independent for each cable and precludes the need for staff to handle the radioactive material.

A further advantage of the remote afterloading device is the ability to optimize dose distribution with the aid of computerized dosimetry data, by varying source length, source activity, and duration of treatment time attributed to each source.

The use of the moulded applicator and the curietron allows the patient to stand up daily, thereby decreasing the risk of complications associated with continuous bed rest. Interruption of treatment for nursing needs, doctors' visits and family visits is possible through the use of an automatic disconnecting system operated from outside the treatment room. When the system is disconnected the radioactive sources are pneumatically driven to the source safe in the curietron, ensuring complete radioprotection for anyone entering the treatment room. The cumulative amount of time taken up by such interuptions is automatically calculated by the curietron machine in the estimation of the total treatment time.

Dosimetry. After the moulded applicator is positioned in the vagina in the operating room, dummy sources are placed into the protruding catheters. Orthogonal x-ray localization films are then taken. These x-ray films are used to check source positioning and eventually to modify the positioning, if required, in order to optimize the dose distribution. The following day, further x-ray films are taken for dosimetric calculations. This 24-hour delay in taking the films on which dosimetry is based takes into account the overnight upward migration of the moulded applicator, which in our experience is a common phenomenon, particularly in young women with limited disease undergoing uterovaginal brachytherapy. Such movement of the mould may be due to strong uterine contractions following placement of the uterine plastic catheter.

Forecast computerized dosimetry is performed on each application. Isodose distributions are plotted in at least three planes: the oblique frontal (Fig. 9.55a) and oblique sagittal (Fig. 9.55b) planes containing the intrauterine tube, and also the lymphatic trapezoid defined by G.H. Fletcher (Bridier et al. 1981; Chassagne et al. 1969, 1977; Chassagne and Horiot 1977; Dutreix and Wambersie 1975; Duff et al. 1982; Gerbaulet et al. 1990a, 1992a,b; Prade et al. 1977; Rosenwald and Dutreix 1970).

Report 38 of the ICRU deals with the problems of dose and volume specification for reporting intracavitary therapy for cervical carcinoma. (Chassagne et al. 1977; Chassagne and Horiot 1977; Gerbaulet et al. 1992d; Icru 198•; Lambin et al. 1993). In the Institut Gustave-Roussy method, we apply the following ICRU recommendations for each case:

1. *Description of the technique.* The description includes the radionuclide, the number and length of sources used, the source specification expressed in reference air kerma rate $Gy\,h^{-1}\,m^2$ (the reference air kerma rate of a source is the kerma rate to air, in air at a reference distance of 1 m, corrected for air attenuation), the type of applicator, and a note of any shielding material employed.
2. *Total reference air kerma* is the new specification for brachytherapy applications and replaces the

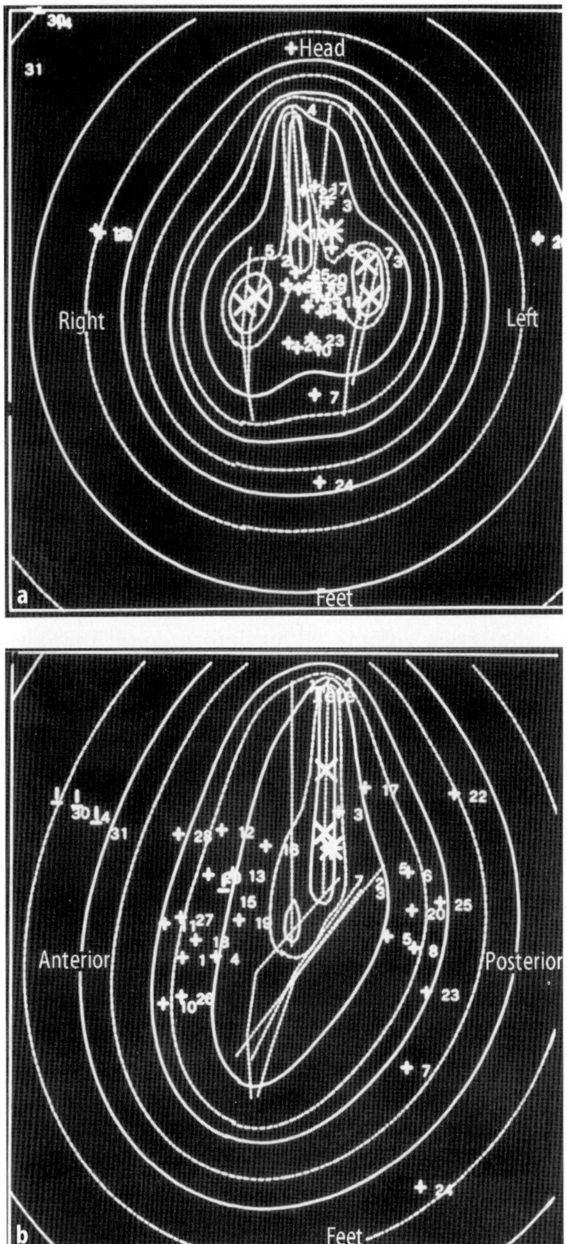

Fig. 9.55 a,b. Computerized dosimetry in two planes (**a** oblique frontal; **b** oblique sagittal): addition of two brachytherapy sessions

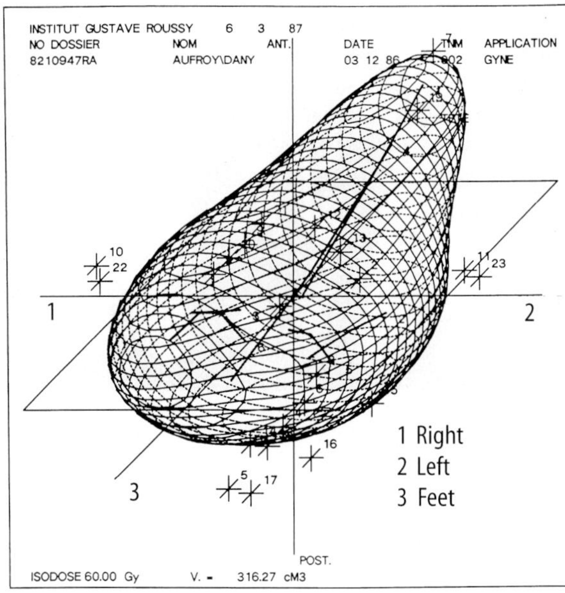

Fig. 9.56. Sixty-Gy reference volume to be reported according to the ICRU 38 recommendations

former concept of mgh. It is the sum of the products of reference air kerma rate and duration of the application for each source. This quantity is expressed in cGy m^2. It is proportional to the integral dose to the patient and can also serve as a useful index for radioprotection of staff.

3. *Reference volume* is defined as the volume enclosed by the reference isodose curve (60 Gy) (Fig. 9.56). When two or more intracavitary applications are performed, the treated volume to be considered is that resulting from all applications. When intracavitary treatment is combined with exernal beam therapy, the volume to be considered is that enveloped by the difference between 60 Gy and the dose delivered to the same volume by external beam therapy. This volume is defined by means of three dimensions representing the classical pear-shaped dose distribution. The height and the width are measured in the oblique frontal plane, and the thickness is measured in the oblique sagittal plane (Fig. 9.57).
4. *Reference points:* The following definitions apply in cases where the doses are calculated from two orthogonal radiographs, AP and lateral. The determination and specification of the absorbed dose to the organs at risk (bladder, rectum) and reference points related to bony structures are obtained and expressed as follows.
   a) Bladder reference point: Prior to placing the uterine source and vaginal mould, a Foley catheter is inserted into the bladder. The balloon is filled with 7 cc of radiopaque fluid. The catheter tube is pulled downwards to bring the balloon against the vesical urethral orifice. On the lateral radiograph, the reference point is obtained on an anterior-posterior line drawn through the balloon center and is positioned at the posterior surface of the balloon. On the

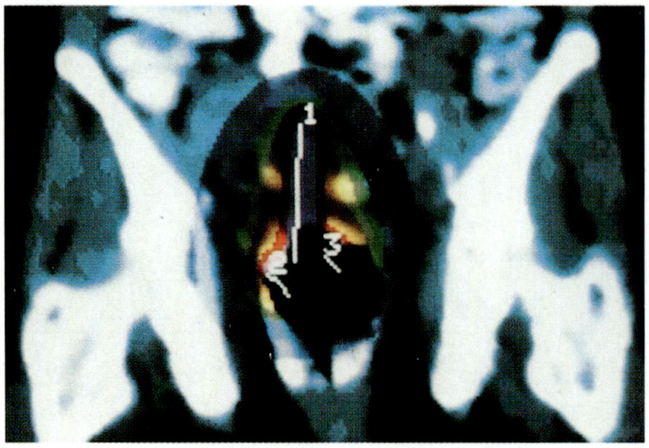

Fig. 9.57. Report of isodose distribution on a frontal scanner rebuilding

AP radiograph, the reference point is taken at the center of the balloon.

b) Rectal reference point: On the lateral radiograph, an anteroposterior line is drawn from the lower end of the intrauterine source. The reference point is located on this line 5 mm below the posterior external surface of the mould. On the AP radiograph, this reference point is at the lower end of the intrauterine source.

c) Lymphatic Fletcher trapezoid (Fig. 9.58): On the lateral film a line is drawn from the junction of S1–2 to the top of the symphysis pubis. A line is then drawn from the middle of that line to the middle of the anterior aspect of L4. A trapezoid is contructed in a plane passing through a transverse line in the pelvic brim plane and a line passing through the midpoint of the anterior aspect of the L4 body. A point 6 cm lateral to the midline at the inferior end of this figure is used to give an estimate of the dose rate to the mid-external iliac lymph nodes. At the top of the trapezoid, points 2 cm lateral to the midline at the level of L4 are used to estimate the dose to the low para-aortic area.

d) Pelvic wall reference point (D. Chassagne): This can be visualized on an AP and a lateral radiograph and related to fixed bony structures. It is intended to be representative of the absorbed dose at the distal ends of the parametria and the obturator lymph nodes. On an AP radiograph, the pelvic wall reference point is intersected by the following two lines: a horizontal line tangential to the highest point of the acetabulum, and a vertical line tangential to the inner aspect of the acetabulum. On a lateral radiograph, the highest points of the right and left acetabulum in the cranial-caudal direction are joined and the lateral projection of the pelvic wall reference point is located at the mid distance of these points.

5. *Level of dose rate (DR).* Three levels of dose rate are defined: $<2\,Gy\,h^{-1}$ (low, or LDR); $2 < 12\,Gy\,h^{-1}$ (medium, or MDR); and $>12\,Gy\,h^{-1}$ (high, or HDR). Dose rate is calculated on the reference isodose curve (60 Gy). We have limited our experience to the use of LDR. The overall treatment time should always be documented. In patients undergoing more than one application, the duration of each should be carefully recorded together with the time interval between them.

For those patients undergoing exclusive brachytherapy in either one or more applications, the total prescribed dose in our institution is 60 Gy delivered to the target volume taking into account the dose received by adjacent critical organs.

Concluding Remarks. Such a treatment scheme, based on forecast dosimetry and the combination of a remote afterloading system and mould applicator, has, in our current experience of more than 8000 cases since 1968, yielded the following results: maximum comfort for and tolerance by patients, maximum quality of treatment through prevention of source displacement, and finally optimal dose distribution within the tumor volume. By using different source lengths and treatment times for each source, a change in the dose distribution without modification of the mould or source tubes can be achieved. Such precise knowledge of dose distribution, with optimal dose to the tumor and minimal dose to critical organs, allows an increase in local control to be achieved while concurrently decreasing complication rates and providing complete radioprotection for staff (Gerbaulet et al. 1992d; Lambin et al. 1993).

THE CRETEIL METHOD

"This system is based on a principle of direct proportionality between the dimensions of uterine and the length of the vaginal sources. The system defines a reference isodose of fixed value encompassing a target volume of constant anatomic structures. The target volume always contains the same anatomic structures independent of the tumor extent" (Pierquin and Marinello 1975) (see also Chassagne and Pierquin 1965; Chassagne et al.

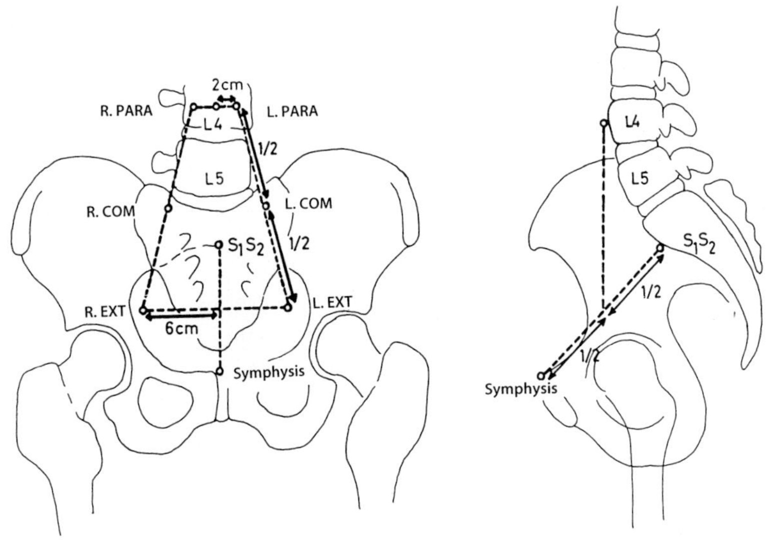

Fig. 9.58. Lymphatic trapezoid plane

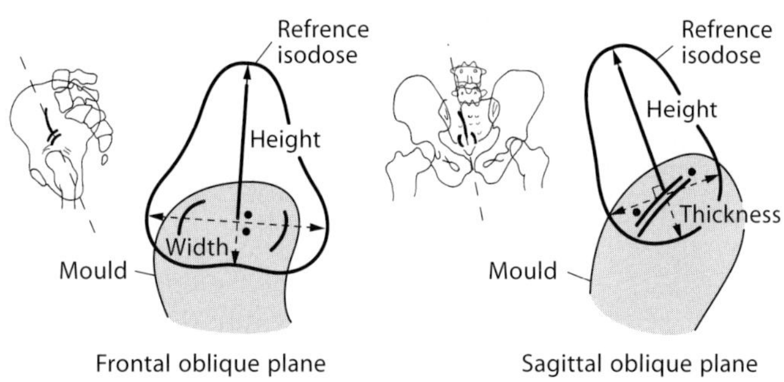

Fig. 9.59. Créteil method: reference isodose

1969; Dutreix et al. 1982; Pierquin et al. 1987b). This technique is based upon the following practical principles:

Predictive Technique. It is a predictive system adapted for each patient, using a cervicovaginal plastic mould in tandem with a semirigid uterine catheter. For the uterine loading, the upper limit of the source is 0.5 cm below uterine fundus. The lower limit of the uterine source is: (a) 0.5 cm protrusion from the cervix into the vagina if the cervix is less than 4 cm in diameter, and (b) 1.5 cm protrusion from the cervix into the vagina if the cervix is more than 4 cm in diameter.

For the cervicovaginal loading two lateral arcs on either side of the cervical mould are used. Their length is equal to 0.8 times the transverse diameter of the mould.

Sources. Iridium wires with the same uniform linear exposure rate are used for both uterine and vaginal sources.

Afterloading Procedure. In this method, the remote afterloader (projector of sources) is not employed: it is a manual afterloading technique.

Dosimetry. The usual prescribed total dose is 60 Gy calculated at the reference isodose of 4 Gy per day, assuming a linear nominal exposure rate of 1 mRhm/cm (Fig. 9.59). The treatment volume contains the cervix, the proximal parametria, and the upper third of vagina.

Time-Dose Relationship. A single uterovaginal application is the norm. All sources have equal dwell times.

THE SAINT CLOUD METHOD

An applicator system with precalculated isodoses for gynecologic curietherapy using the curietron afterloading system forms the basis of this method (CHASSAGNE et al. 1968; DELOUCHE and GEST 1972). It consists of: (a) an arrangement of single-use plastic devices with a central uterine catheter and two vaginal catheters bearing barrel-type ovoids; (b) a joining block tunneled with three holes which slides over the three catheters and rests in the vagina, maintaining the ensemble in place. Various sizes of catheters and joining blocks are available (Fig. 9.60).

Sources. The radioactive material used is cesium, as in the Institute Gustave-Roussy method. However, the position of vaginal sources is different: they are placed parallel to the long axis of the vagina, lateralized into each fornix. The same linear activity is used for uterine and vaginal sources.

Afterloader. The remote afterloader (curietron) is used, permitting automatic disconnection, as in the Institut Gustave-Roussy method.

Dosimetry. The isodoses pertaining to each application are generated by a computer and collected in a book. To determine the dose to be delivered, the isodoses are superimposed on the x-ray control films.

Time-Dose Relationship. In most cases, a single uterovaginal application is carried out. However, for large tumors, brachytherapy may be fractionated.

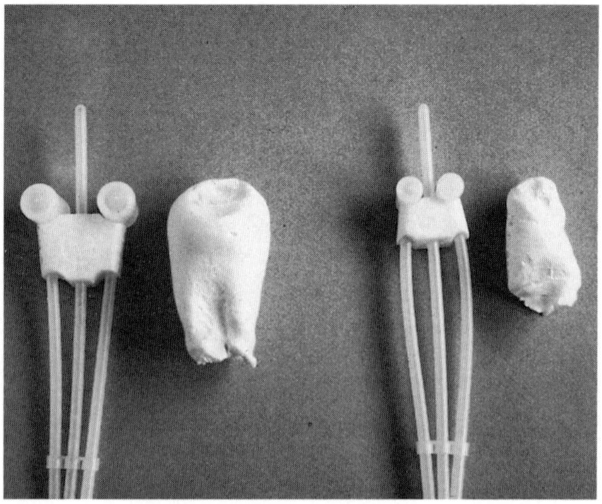

Fig. 9.60. Saint-Cloud method: applicator system

9.8.4.3
Conclusion

After many years of radium therapy for carcinoma of the cervix, satisfactory results have ensured that brachytherapy holds an important place in the treatment of these cancers. Gradual progress has ensured achievement of a radiobiological effect equivalent to that obtained with conventional radium sources, but with the additional advantages of:

1. A tailored application for each case
2. Improved treatment tolerance for the patient
3. Improved radiation protection for the staff
4. Improved precision in the knowledge of the dose distribution

The three main French methods deriving from the original Paris system differ from each other in technique and isodose selection. We have been employing the Gustave-Roussy technique for 25 years, and more than 8000 cases have been treated by this method.

In conclusion, we would like to share with the reader the assessment made by one of the innovators of the Gustave Roussy method, Daniel Chassagne, who expressed the merits of this technique as follows:

1. "From the radioprotection point of view, our goal was very quickly achieved: nobody in the staff, including ward nurses and technicians, now receive any exposure from cesium gynecologic brachytherapy.
2. For the patient, during the treatment time:
   a) Tolerance to a mechanical connection to a remote afterloader is excellent, provided that elementary precautions are taken, such as for example attaching the cables to a crib located above the patient's legs.
   b) Psychological tolerance is surprisingly good. Patients generally understand very well the purpose of this technique and are willing and cooperative. The patient no longer feels isolated and is considered as a normal patient (that is to say without any exposure risk) by the staff.
   c) Venous thrombosis occurring due to mandatory bedrest is now very rare since we allow the patient to get up twice a day for half an hour.
   d) We have not seen any adverse effects from this small interruption of irradiation, for a treatment which normally lasts 6 days.

3. Technical errors and accidents were very few (less than 1%) during the first years of use and have now completely disappeared; the benefits of this technique are obvious and outweigh the rare inconveniences.

9.8.5 Cervical Interstitial Brachytherapy

W.A. LONGTON, B. MICAILY, and L.W. BRADY

Interstitial brachytherapy for cervical cancer has been utilized for more than 70 years in one form or another. Standard intracavitary brachytherapy may not be adequate or even possible due to the distorted anatomy caused by the tumor burden (WATERMAN et al. 1947; WATERMAN and RAPHAEL 1950; ARNESON 1938; CORSCADEN et al. 1948). So perineal implants using templates should be able to overcome this problem theoretically (FEDER et al. 1978; MARTINEZ et al. 1984; SYED and FEDER 1977). Templates to guide and help direct interstitial implantation have been used since the 1950s. Recently, a variety of templates have been designed and utilized with varying degrees of tumor control and complication rates.

Pitts and Waterman compared conventional intracavitary radiation (prior to 1925) and direct transvaginal insertion of long, low-intensity radium needles (after 1925) in 110 consecutive stage III cervical cancer patients and found an increase in 5-year survival, from 14% to 31%, in favor of the interstitial implant (FEDEB et al. 1978). Even though this showed an increase in survival, interstitial radiation was seldom preferred to intracavitary radiation, primarily because of the high rate of complications.

9.8.5.1 *Interstitial Techniques and Results*

Interstitial radiotherapy using a template has been utilized since 1951, (GREEN and JENNINGS 1951). Various templates have been designed for use over the past 30 years. Three of these templates are the Syed-Neblett parametrial butterfly in 1978, MUPIT (Martinez Universal Perineal Interstitial Implant) in 1984, and the Hammersmith perineal hedgehog (see Figs. 9.62–9.64, 9.66).

In the late 1970s, a perineal template was designed using a butterfly pattern of holes where hollow guide needles are placed in the parametrial area. This is called the *Syed-Neblett template*, which consists of two superimposed lucite plates, each 1.2 cm thick, held together by screws. Holes are drilled in a butterfly pattern through both plates with a larger hole in the center (Figs. 9.61, 9.62). Between 20 and 30 needles are inserted in the perineum through the predrilled holes in the template. The template is secured to the patient's perineum with sutures. The hollow needles are afterloaded with ^{192}Ir seeds (in ribbons) with send activity equal to 0.3–0.45 mg Ra eq. Each ribbon contains five or six seeds with an overall length of 4–5 cm. Dose to the lateral

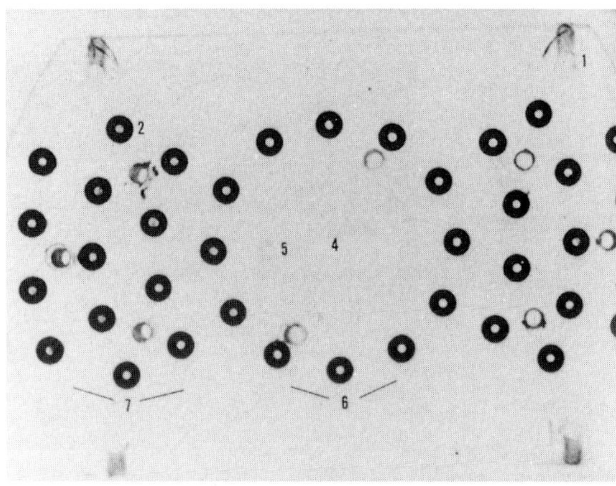

Fig. 9.61. One of two lucite plates which form the "butterfly" template. *1*, hole for suture fixation; *2*, rubber doughnut in well surrounding needle hole; *3*, hole for Allen head machine screw; *4*, opening for grooved plastic vaginal guide; *5*, special ridge for alignment of vaginal guide; *6*, paracervical ring. (From FEDEB et al. 1978)

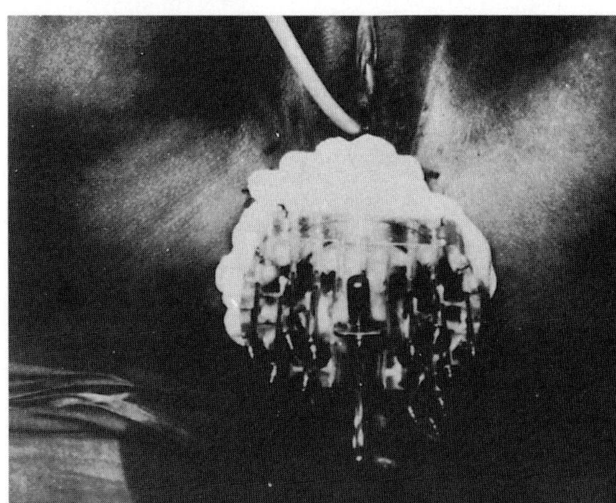

Fig. 9.62. "Transperineal butterfly" implant completed, ready for afterloading. (From FEDEB et al. 1978)

Table 9.45. Advanced carcinoma of the cervix treated by external and interstitial intracavitary applications

Endocurietherapy	Stage[a]	Patients[b]	No. of patients alive with tumor	No. of patients alive with no gross tumor[c]
Two interstitial-intracavitary applications	3	23	1	14
	4a	2	0	0
One conventional intracavitary and one interstitial-intracavitary application	3	12	2	7
	4a	1	0	0
Total		38	3	21

[a] UICC–FIGO.
[b] Absolute.
[c] Followed for 16–40 months (average 24 months).

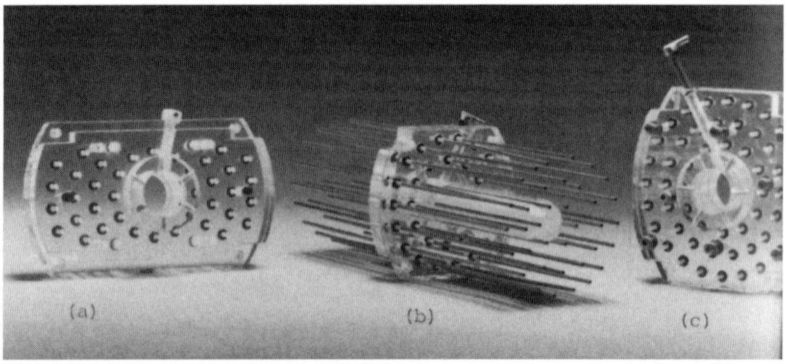

Fig. 9.63 a–c. Templates used at Hammersmith: **a** Syed-Neblett template; **b, c** Small and large Hammersmith hedgehogs. (From BRANSON et al. 1985)

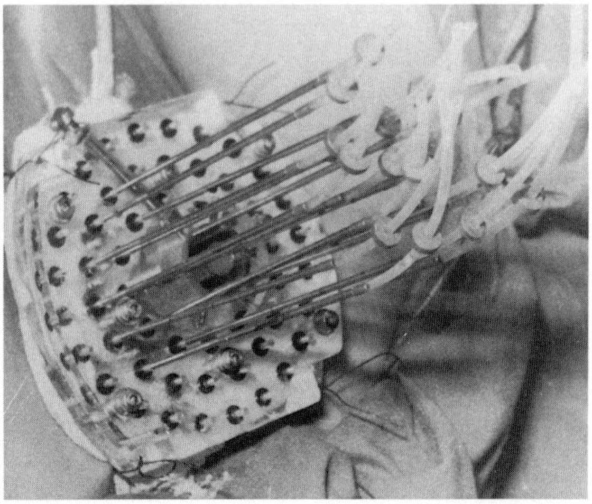

Fig. 9.64. Large Hammersmith hedgehog in position, showing needles, "outer tubing," and lead washers. (From BRANSON et al. 1985)

parametrium is 40–80 cGy/h, to the medial parametrium, 80–120 cGy/h, and to the bladder and rectum, 30–50 cGy/h. This device was used in 38 patients, all of whom received 50 Gy external beam whole-pelvic radiation. Some had two interstitial-intracavitary applications while some had one conventional intracavitary and one interstitial-intracavitary application. Follow-up in these patients was an average of 24 months. Results are shown in Table 9.45; 8% of the patients developed complications, with only one requiring surgical intervention (FEDEB et al. 1978).

BRANSON et al. (1985) reported on the difficulty of treating lesions in the lower vagina and vulva with the Syed-Neblett template and redesigned the template pattern from a butterfly to a three or four complete ring pattern (Figs. 9.63, 9.64). Using this device, they treated three cervical cancer patients and the results are listed in Table 9.46. They called these two new templates the small and large *Hammersmith Perineal Hedgehogs*. Due to the small number of pa-

Table 9.46. Results obtained by Branson et al. using interstitial implants ("Hedgehogs")

	Age	Needles	Dose (Gy)	XRT (Gy)	Follow-up (months)	Tumor response
Stage IIIB	40	28	25	50	7	Nil
Vaginal recurrence	75	18	60	50	8	Complete
Vaginal recurrence	42	15	44	50	8	Partial

Table 9.47. Method of brachytherapy in study group

FIGO stage	Total no. of patients	Brachytherapy	
		Template	Fletcher suit
IB	14	22	6
IIA	8	11	4
IIB	25	38	9
III (A + B)	26	41	11
IVA	2	4	0
Total	75	116	30

tients and short follow-up, no definitive statement could be made in regard to tumor control and chronic complications. However, the authors believed that the technique was satisfactory and the dose distribution acceptable.

Gaddis et al. (1983) reported the results in 75 treated patients using at least one perineal interstitial implantation for cervical cancer. All patients received 50 Gy external beam radiation in 5–6 weeks and then two brachytherapy procedures; at least one of these implant procedures was interstitial. Interstitial brachytherapy was used if patients presented with poor geometry, large bulky disease, or parametrial infiltration. All others received Fletcher Suit tandem and ovoid application. Brachytherapy was performed at 2-week intervals following external beam therapy. The methods of brachytherapy is listed in Table 9.47. Dosimetry plots for the implant were based on an ideal geometric model which assumes that the source guides are straight, perpendicular to the template, and placed at equal tissue depths. Median follow-up was 17 months, and showed a survival rate less than with conventional treatment programs. The frequency and location of recurrent cancer are shown in Table 9.48. Non-tumor-associated fistulas occurred in 16% of patients and nonfistula grade 3 reactions in 24% (Table 9.49). In summary, survival rates were less than with conventional treatment and the complication rates were higher.

Aristizabal et al. (1987) reported 21 consecutive patients with locally advanced invasive cervical carcinoma. Some of these patients had compromised anatomy, preventing performance of conventional intracavitary brachytherapy. Therefore, transperineal interstitial brachytherapy was substituted for intracavitary irradiation. All patients received 40–50 Gy external beam whole-pelvis irridation in 4–6 weeks followed by brachytherapy procedures at 2-week intervals. A Syed type perineal template was used. The tandem in the center was not loaded in some of the patients due to distorted anatomy secondary to tumor burden. Mean follow-up was 26 months. Local control was 100% for stages IB and IIB and 86% for stage IIIB (Table 9.50). High-grade (II and III) complication rate was 33%. The number of patients were small and the follow-up was short in this study.

Aristizabal et al. (1987) treated 43 patients with stage IIB cervical carcinoma with external beam radiation plus intracavitary brachytherapy and 45 similar patients with external beam radiation and interstitial brachytherapy. In a retrospective analysis they found the local failure rate for intracavitary therapy to be 16% and that for interstitial therapy, 17% (Fig. 9.65). The survival rate was similar for both groups. The complication rate was much higher for interstitial (22%) than for intracavitary (7%) therapy (Table 9.51). However, the numbers in each group were small, compromising the value of interpretation.

Martinez (1984) treated 37 patients with advanced or recurrent cervical carcinomas with the *MUPIT device*. The MUPIT (Martinez Universal Perineal Interstitial Template) consists of an acrylic predrilled template, cover plate, acrylic cylinders, obturators, screws, and stainless steel needles (Fig. 9.66). Three mid-template holes are present along the midline: (a) Foley catheter, (b) vaginal cylinder, and (c) rectal cylinder (Fig. 9.67, 9.68). The apparatus can be sutured to the perineum once it is in place. There are small holes in the template for trocar

Table 9.48. Frequency and location of recurrent cancer in the study group

FIGO stage	Total no. of patients	All recurrences		Recurrences in treatment field	
		No.	(%)	No.	(%)
IB	14	6	(42.7)	5	(35.7)
IIA	8	1	(12.5)	0	(0.0)
IIB	25	8	(32.0)	5	(20.0)
III (A + B)	26	16	(61.5)	12	(46.2)
IVA	2	0	(0.0)	0	(0.0)
Total	75	31	(41.3)	22	(29.3)

Table 9.49. Frequency of grade 2, grade 3, and fistulous adverse effects due to radiation

Stage	Total no. of patients	Patients with significant adverse effects	Adverse effects			
			Grade 2[a]	Grade 3[a]	Fistulas	Total
IB	14	3	2	5	2	9
IIA	8	1	3	1	0	4
IIB	25	6	5	6	6[b]	17
III	26	6	3	6	4	13
IVA	2	0	0	0	0	0
Total	75	16	13	18	12	43

[a] Includes proctosigmoiditis, cystitis, and vaginal necrosis.
[b] Six fistulas in four patients.

Table 9.50. Control of local tumor achieved by Aristizabal et al. (1987) in patients with locally advanced invasive cervical carcinoma[a]

Stage	No. of pts.	%
IB	2/2	100
IIB	3/3	100
IIIB	13/15	86
IVA	0/1	0
Total	18/21	85

[a] Mean follow-up = 26 months; four patients died of distant metastases.

Table 9.51. Complications reported by Aristizabal et al. (1987) using intracavitary and interstitial brachytherapy for stage IIB cervical carcinoma

Technique	Frequency	Grade	
		II	III
Intracavitary	3/43 (7%)	0	0
Interstitial	10/45 (22%)[a]	6	4

[a] $P = 0.044$.

placement (12.5 mm apart) (Fig. 9.69). There are two types of horizontal rows: type I = perpendicular to the template; type II = angled 13° laterally outward. The volume covered by type I alone is 4 cm on either side of the midline. If type II is added, it will extend out to 7 cm laterally (Fig. 9.70). The vaginal and rectal cylinders have intracavitary ability. The activity per seed of the central sources is one-half to one-third that at the periphery. Near the midsagittal plane, the treatment volume is reduced in the anteroposterior dimension to decrease the rectal and bladder doses. The implant dose is defined by using the cross-sectional plane at the center of the implant. In the study by Martinez the dose ranged from 35 to 37 Gy, and the dose rate was 0.75–1.1 Gy per hour. The brachytherapy radiation was given as a supplement to external beam radiation which consisted of 36 Gy to the whole pelvis in 4 weeks. After brachytherapy, a midline block was placed and the pelvic side wall was boosted to a total of 50 Gy with 180-cGy fractions. Minimum follow-up was 1 year. Seventy-eight percent of patients were followed for more than 2 years, and local control was obtained in

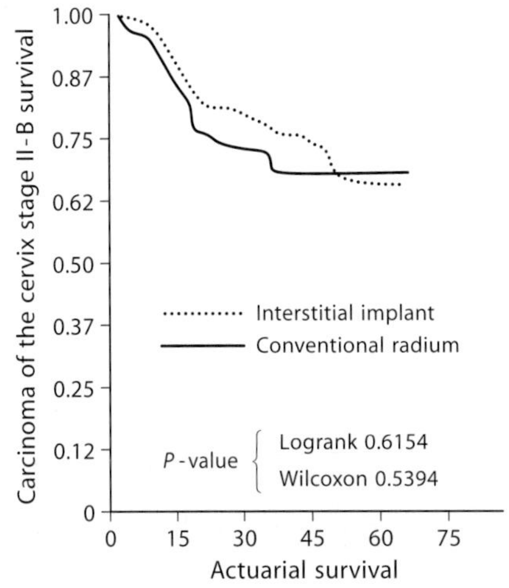

Fig. 9.65. The overall disease-free survival and the actuarial survival were similar for the intracavitary and interstitial implant groups. (From ARISTIZABAL et al. 1987)

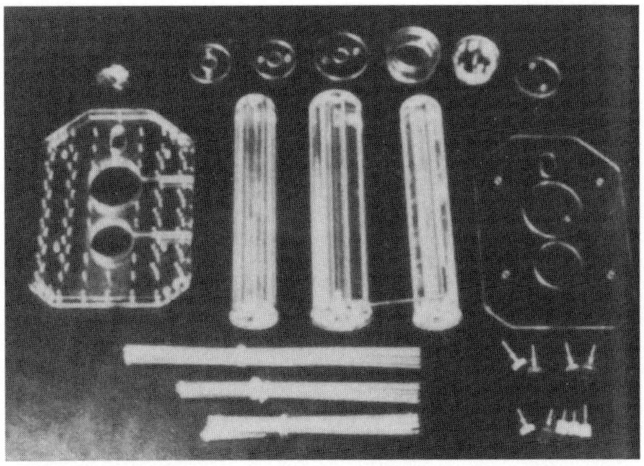

Fig. 9.66. MUPIT contains an acrylic predrilled template and cover plate, acrylic cylinders, obturators, screws, and stainless steel needles. (From MARTINEZ 1984)

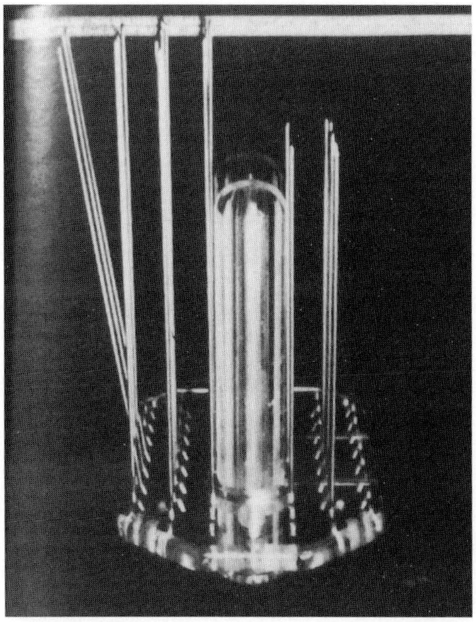

Fig. 9.67. MUPIT with two rows of straight needles on the *right* and three rows of straight needles and one row of angled needles on the *left*. Different lengths can be utilized. (From MARTINEZ 1984)

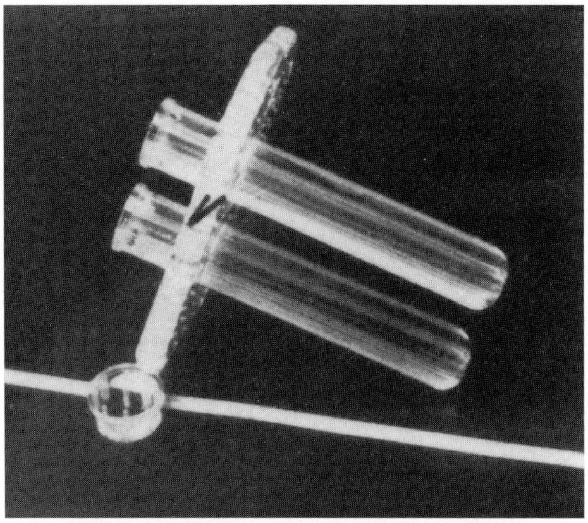

Fig. 9.68. Acrylic predrilled template attached to both the rectal and vaginal cylinders. (From MARTINEZ 1984)

31/37 patients (83%), with central failure in six (17%). The use of a central tandem is avoided if possible because it is felt that the tandem significantly disrupts the homogeneity of the dose distribution, producing a much higher central dose (increasing the rectal and bladder doses). A complication rate of 2/37 (5.4%) was noted. These results are very good compared with other published results, possibly due to decreased use of a tandem and utilization of a uniform dose without trying to create a hot spot (MARTINEZ et al. 1984; MARTINEZ 1983). (see Fig. 9.71 for intraoperative placement film.)

CHOY et al. (1994) reported a vaginal template used to treat 21 patients with cervical carcinoma with vaginal stenosis or inadvertent diagnosis after hysterectomy. Eight peripheral holes and one control hole are drilled in the template (Figs. 9.72, 9.73). The dose rate ranged from 13 to 16 Gy/day with an implant time usually of 4 days. All patients received external beam radiation at 2.5 Gy/day, four fractions/week, to a total dose of 40 Gy with a midline block at 35 Gy. Follow-up ranged from 22.7 to 54.6 months. Of the 21 patients in this study, nine (41%) had re-

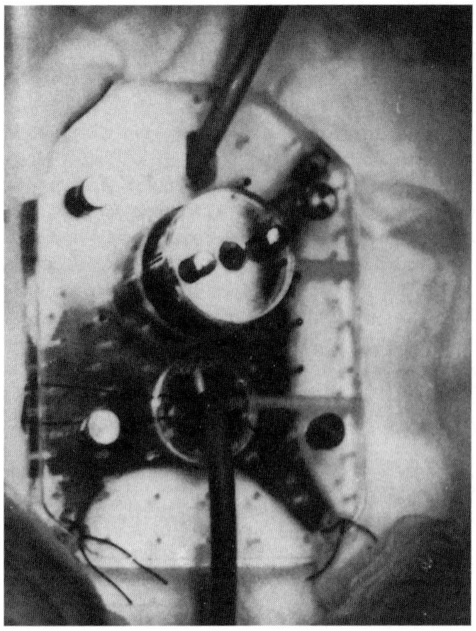

Fig. 9.69. Completed MUPIT implant in a patient with stage IIIB cancer of the cervix. (From MARTINEZ 1984)

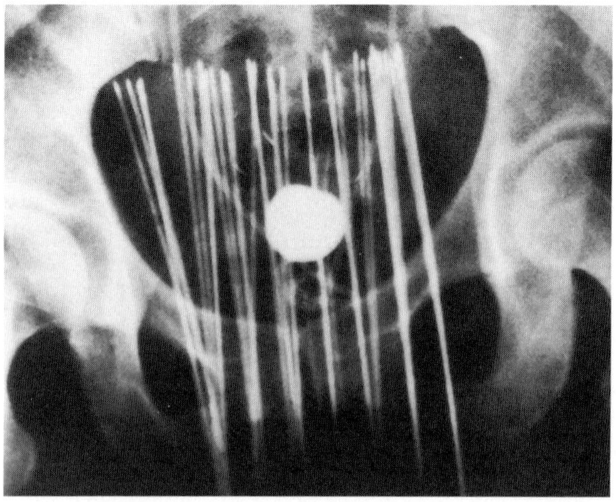

Fig. 9.70. Intraoperative radiograph in case of stage IIIB cervical carcinoma with tumor fixation to the right pelvic side wall and bilateral hydronephrosis with bilateral stent tubes. Angled needles were used on the right to cover the pelvic wall extension of the tumor. (From MARTINEZ et al. 1985)

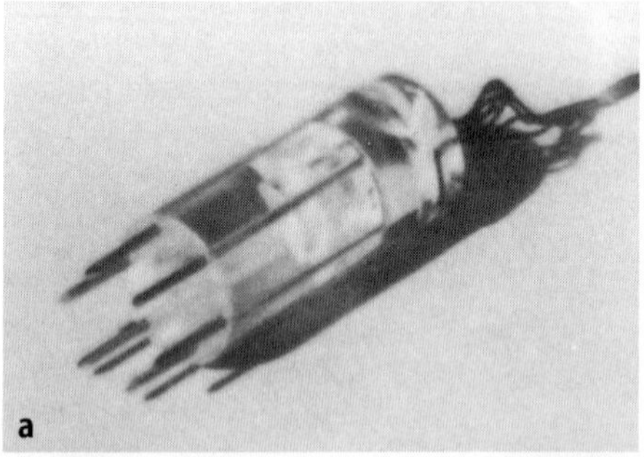

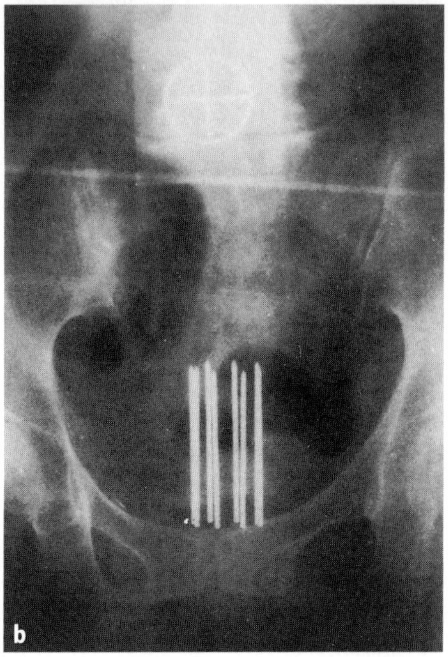

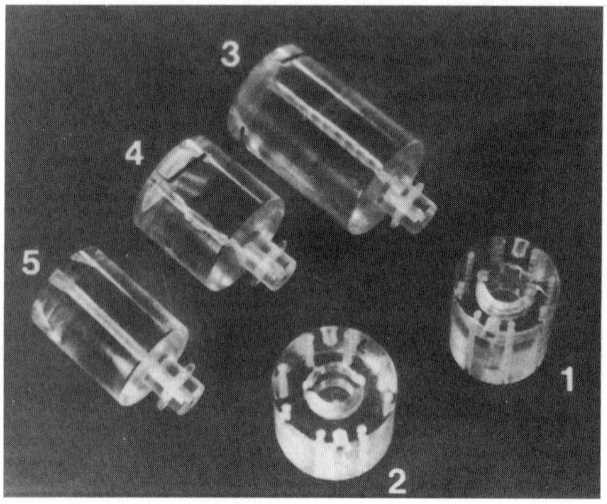

Fig. 9.71. Front (*1* and *2*) and end pieces (*3*, *4* and *5*) of different lengths and diameters. Front and end pieces of the same diameter (*1* with *5*, diameter 2 cm; *2* with *3* or *4*, diameter 2.5 cm) but of a different length can be combined for treating patients with different vaginal lengths. Note the bayonet-type of locking device. (From CHOY et al. 1994)

◀
Fig. 9.72. **a** An assembled applicator with the needles. **b** Radiographic image of an implant with template. (From CHOY et al. 1994)

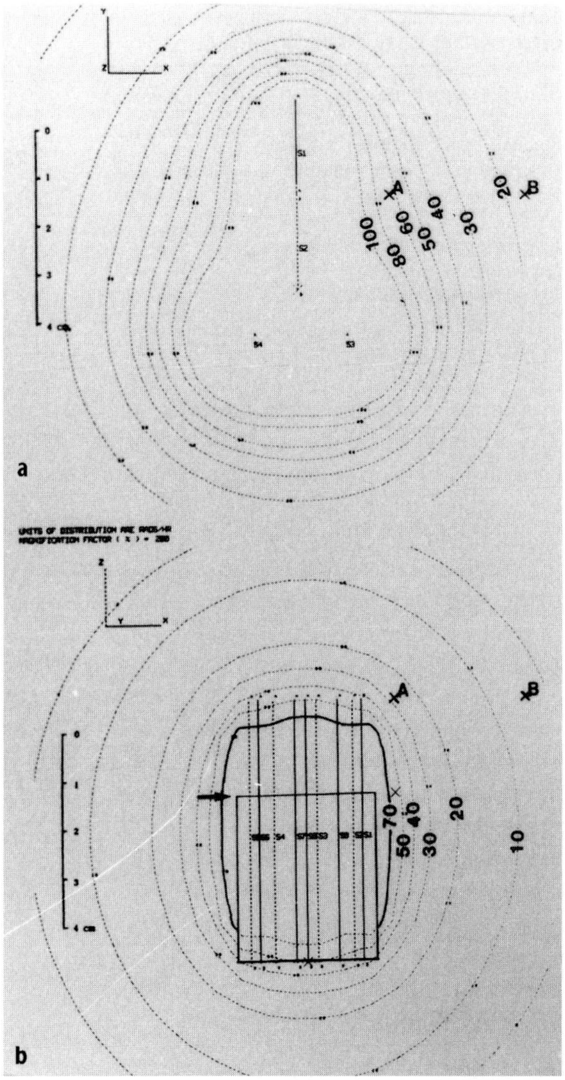

Fig. 9.73. **a** The isodose of intracavitary treatment with intrauterine tandem and vaginal ovoids; dose is prescribed at point *A*. **b** The isodose from a typical vaginal template implant. Dose is prescribed at 70 cGy/h. Dose at point *A* is 28 cGy/h; thus point *A* receives about 40% of the dose. The *arrow* marks the cranial limit of the front pieces, and the needles are protruding beyond this. (From Choy et al. 1994)

current disease. Seven of the patients had grade I (proctitis) complications. One disadvantage of this system is that the dose at point A is much lower than with conventional intracavitary therapy, i.e., 30% versus 60% when comparing isodose curves (Fig. 9.74).

Randall et al. (1993) reported four patients treated for recurrent cervical cancer with interstitial reirradiation. Two had squamous cell carcinoma, one adenosquamous carcinoma, and one

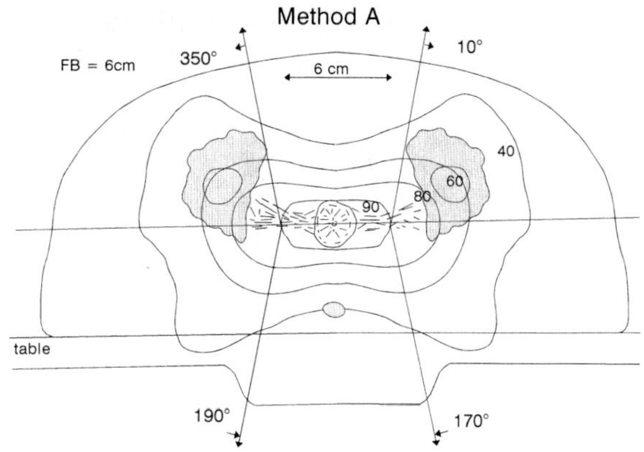

Fig. 9.74. Isodose curve of method A. Rotation radiation with two axes at a distance of 6 cm. Rotation angles are 10–170° and 190–350°. The length of the fields is fitted to the patient's size, while the width is constantly 6 cm. Note the steep decline to the bladder and rectum and the high dose at the pelvic wall

adenocarcinoma. All patients had received external beam whole-pelvic radiation. The Syed-Neblett template was used. Local control was achieved in two of the four patients (50%). Distant failures occurred in two patients (50%).

9.8.5.2 Conclusions

Brachytherapy plays an integral part in the treatment of cervical carcinoma. It is usually performed with intracavitary placement instead of interstitial. It has been shown that these two modalities can yield similar results, and since it is not always possible to use a tandem and ovoids due to vaginal stenosis or anatomic anomalies or due to tumor burden, there may be benefit from interstitial brachytherapy. Also, in patients who have received radiation therapy to the pelvic area before, there may be benefit from reirradiation using interstitial implantation. The complication rate of interstitial brachytherapy is much higher in most series, especially if a tandem is used.

The proximity of bladder and rectum to the cervix, and parametrial structures, and their relative radiosensitivity are the primary determinants of the maximum dose of radiation which can be delivered to the cervix and parametrial tissues. The dose distribution from intracavitary placement is suboptimal in cases of poor geometry and/or large tumor with significant lateral and/or anterior-posterior extension. Interstitial implantation is advantageous in these settings if dose distribution is homogeneous and excessive radiation to bladder and rectum and other vital structures can be avoided.

The advantages of interstitial brachytherapy include the following: Theoretically, the radiation dose distribution conforms to the tumor volume. An intact anatomy is not required, and the dose can be tailored to specific anatomic conditions, e.g., implantation of the pelvic side wall, recurrent tumors after hysterectomy. The technique is best used for small-volume tumors.

The disadvantages of interstitial brachytherapy are that it is an invasive procedure with potential significant short-and long-term complications. The risk increases with inexperience.

Intracavitary brachytherapy offers the following advantages: it is noninvasive, there is a uniform dose distribution, and it is ideal for small-volume centrally located tumors. It is disadvantageous when there is distorted anatomy due to tumor bulk, the patient's anatomy, or prior surgery, e.g., as in the case of recurrent tumors after radical surgery. There is also a limited dose contribution to the pelvic side wall.

From the review of current literature, it is apparent that the key elements in achieving maximum tumor control and minimum complications can be summarized as follows:

- Proper patient selection
- Proper patient preparation
- Multidisciplinary approach
- Preimplant treatment planning
- Proper integration of external radiation and interstitial dose

9.9 The Hamburg Experience with Exclusive Teletherapy

J. Bahnsen, H.J. Frischbier, and V. Stelte

Definitive irradiation of cervical cancer should consist of brachytherapy and teletherapy. Brachytherapy allows us to deliver high doses to the primary tumor without causing damage to the bladder and bowel. Additional teletherapy is necessary to destroy tumor cells distant from the primary in the pelvis. In some cases, however, brachytherapy is impossible or contraindicated (Table 9.52). There may be anatomic factors, such as stenosis of the vagina, that make the application impossible, or a multimorbid situation may preclude anesthesia. In very advanced cases the region of bulky tumor is too large to profit from brachytherapy. In the presence of involvement of bladder or rectum (stage IVA), brachytherapy is very risky because the applicator may perforate these organs and cause fistulas. Most of these cases are either so advanced or in such a bad general condition that ultraradical surgery is not possible. In such cases, many radiotherapists deliver a small dose for palliation only. In the Department of Gynecologic Radiology in Hamburg, special methods of exclusive teletherapy with curative intention have been developed and applied for 30 years (Frischbier and Hasse 1965). The additional irradiation of para-aortic nodes and the left supraclavicular fossa is described elsewhere.

Table 9.52. Indications for exclusive teletherapy because brachytherapy is impossible or inferior

Brachytherapy impossible:
Cervical canal not passable
Stenosis of the vagina
Destruction of urinary bladder
Destruction of rectum
Brachytherapy inferior:
No analgesia possible
Extremely bulky disease
"Frozen pelvis"

9.9.1 Description of the Methods

The methods have been derived from Mellor, who in 1960 reported results of radiotherapy in patients with cervical cancer treated by megavoltage therapy alone. Mellor was the first to use a biaxial rotation method for this purpose. In our institution the method was modified and standardized: The axes are placed parallel to the cervical canal at a distance of 3 cm (method A, Fig. 9.75) or 2.5 cm (method B, Fig. 9.76). Rotation angles are constantly 10–170° and 190–350°. With this technique the skin reaction is minimal, even at high doses. The length of the fields is fitted to the size of the patient. The upper margin is placed at 4–5, while the lower margin is the lower margin of the foramen obturatorium. The upper margin includes the common iliac nodes, but not the aortic nodes. The lower margin includes the nodes in the foramina obturatoria, a common site of metastasis from cervical cancer. The width of the fields is kept constant (6 cm in method A, 8 cm in method B). Computer planning of the technique re-

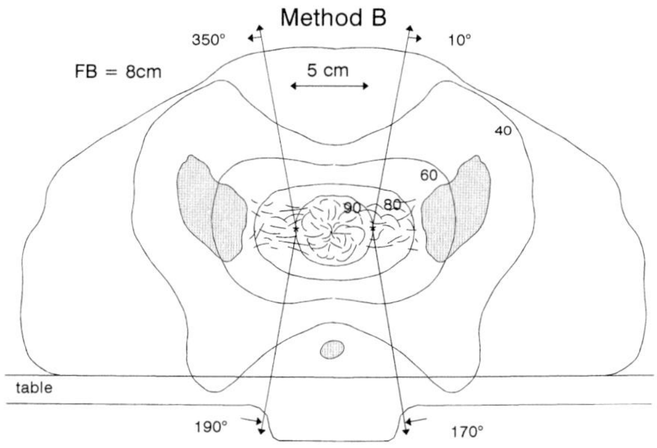

Fig. 9.75. Isodose curve of method B. There is similarity to method A (Fig. 9.76) but the distance of the axes is 5 cm and the field width is 8 cm. Note the larger high-dose area

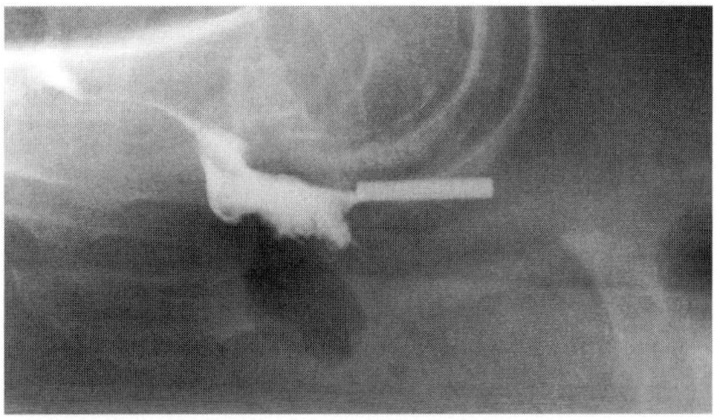

Fig. 9.76. Control of the horizontal correctness of the axes. The vagina is filled with 5 ml contrast medium. The cervical canal is exactly at the position of the axis marked by a 2 cm metal tube. The irregular shape of the vagina is caused by grossly infiltrating tumor

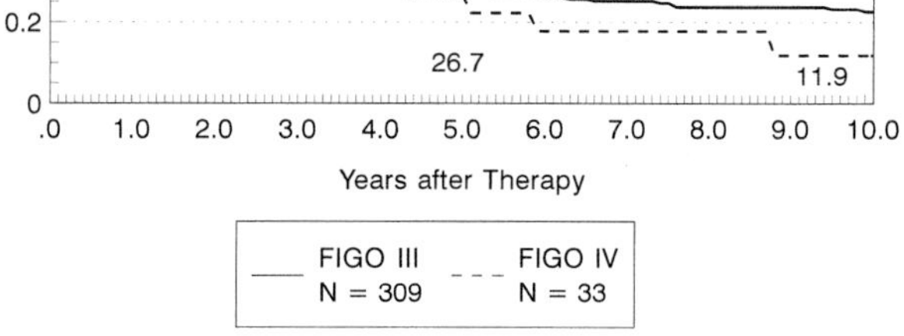

Fig. 9.77. Survival of FIGO stage III and IV patients with advanced cervical cancer not suitable for brachytherapy

sults in an isodose curve (Figs. 9.75, 9.76) with a maximum in the cervix and a high dose in the paracervical tissue. The high-dose area includes the lymph nodes at the pelvic wall. A steep decline of the dose ventral and dorsal of the cervix minimizes the doses at the bladder and rectum.

As indicated above, the method is used in two variants: method A has a smaller high-dose area and is used for tumors less than 40 mm in diameter, while method B has a larger high-dose area and allows the irradiation of larger primaries. Because the larger area of high dose in method B results in a higher frequency of acute and late side-effects, it is seldom used. After shrinking of the tumor, one should switch to method B. The method has been applied to a great number of women with constant parameters. The shape of the isodose curves is very similar in lean and adipose patients. The position of the axis is controlled after instillation of 5 ml contrast medium into the vagina (Fig. 9.77). In most of the cases it is possible to visualize the beginning of the cervical canal. It is recommended that the horizontal position of the axes be controlled every 1 or 2 weeks, and the distance of the axes twice a week. The precision of the position of the axis is very important for the success of the methods.

Initially, the dose at the axis was calculated in a midline plane. 3.5 Gy was applied daily, alternating between the right and left axes. Total dose was 80 Gy at the maximum (cervix) and 60 Gy at the pelvic wall. For radiobiologic reasons, however, the method was modified. Now a dose of 2 Gy is delivered to the maximum (1 Gy from the right and left axes daily). Upon reaching 60 Gy, the length of the field is reduced to the size of the cervical tumor. This method was developed for a ^{60}Co machine in 1965 (FRISCHBIER and HASSE 1965). For use on a linear accelerator the parameters must be modified. The radiotherapy is generally delivered under inpatient conditions because intensive supervision and care are necessary.

9.9.2 Results

Results of exclusive teletherapy in cervical cancer are rarely published (MELLOR 1960; KOECK and HILLSINGER 1971). The treatment outcome and survival rates in our patients have been reported by ULMER and FRISCHBIER (1982). The following data are the preliminary results cited in a thesis by V. Stelte. From 1965 to 1993 a total of 377 women with cervical cancer were treated by the biaxial rotation method. Their ages ranged from 27 to 90 years (median 64.8 years); 34.7% were more than 70 years of age. Of all the cases, 82.0% were FIGO stage III, and 8.8% stage IV. Most of the patients had a staging lymphography. In 26% metastasis to the aortic nodes was suspected by lymphography. Only 8.8% were grouped in stage IV, because there were major lymphographic signs of metastasis or histologically proven involvement. Twenty-seven patients were in a poor general condition, unsuitable for surgery or brachytherapy. In eight patients staging was incomplete. In 62.9% of the patients there was infiltration of both parametria, and in a further 18.5% infiltration of one parametrium. In 49 cases, infiltration of the parametria was doubtful because physical investigations were discrepant. No parametrial infiltration was present in 5.6% of the cases. Involvement of the vagina was observed in 66.8%, and in 21.8% the involvement exceeded one-third of the vagina. [In the radium era, major infiltration of the vagina was a contraindication to radium application because the tamponage would have resulted in a distance between the source and involved vagina; this would have resulted in an underdose and subsequent recurrence.] Involvement of the bladder was suspected after cystoscopy in 32 cases and histologically proven in 11 cases. Infiltration of the rectum was present in four cases. An obstruction of one or two ureters was found in 9.3%, and hydronephrosis in an additional 6.3%.

9.9.3 Follow-up

Analysis of follow-up is based on outpatient controls in our clinic and reports from other institutions. Survival status was obtained from the registration office. Of 309 FIGO III cases the 5-year survival rate (Kaplan-Meier) was 28.5% and the 10-year rate, 22.6%. The median follow-up of the survivors was 7.7 years. Of 33 cases classified as FIGO IV, 26.7% survived 5 years and 11.9% 10 years (median follow-up: 5.2 years).

9.9.4 Side-Effects

Because high doses are required to cure advanced cervical cancer, some side-effects have to be tolerated. Early side-effect are diarrhea, nausea, dysuria, and pollakiuria. During radiotherapy nearly all patients developed diarrhea. In 6.6% of the cases therapy had to be stopped owing to the poor general condition of the patient or to an acute bowel reaction. Three patients developed thrombosis, and one pulmonary embolism.

During follow-up, seven patients developed a vesicovaginal fistula and one, a vesicorectovaginal fistula. Fistulas were counted only if they were not associated with a local recurrence. An obstruction of the ureter was noted in four cases. Some women developed late bowel complications. Resection of small bowel was performed in three cases (0.8%); an artificial anus was constructed in ten cases (2.7%). Obstruction caused by tumor growth was not counted as a therapy-related complication.

9.9.5 Conclusion

The presented data show that a substantial percentage of patients with advanced cervical cancer not suitable for brachytherapy will survive after irradiation with appropriate methods and high doses. Thus low-dose radiotherapy for palliation only should be restricted to fatal cases.

9.10 Preoperative and Postoperative Radiotherapy

K. Morita

The routine combination of radiation and surgery does not improve results. However, some selected irradiated patients do benefit from postirradiation hysterectomy and at least one-quarter of patients treated initially by surgery required postoperative irradiation.

9.10.1 Preoperative Radiotherapy

There are two indications for postirradiation hysterectomy: (a) a bulky stage Ib–IIa cervical cancer and (b) a stage Ib–IIa tumor that has not regressed during radiation therapy.

The original rationale for adding surgery to irradiation was the alleged inability of irradiation to completely eradicate the tumor at bulky primary sites. Bulky endocervical lesions (5%–10% of stage Ib and II cancers) are especially prone to irradiation failure because of the large hypoxic cell population (O'QUINN et al. 1980). In addition, extension of the malignant growth into the endometrium and/or myometrium produces dosimetric problems resulting in an underdose to those areas (DURRANCE et al. 1969). After whole-pelvis irradiation with about 50 Gy, these patients undergo extrafascial hysterectomy. Gallion and co-workers (1985) reported a reduction in the recurrence rate in patients with bulky barrel-shaped stage IB tumors from 47% to 16% with the addition of extrafascial hysterectomy. Since these large-volume tumors have a high incidence of lymph node metastases, para-aortic lymph node sampling should be routinely performed at the time of surgery. Other authors have reported that radical surgery with postoperative irradiation is an equally effective method of treating bulky stage IB cervical cancer (RETTENMAIER et al. 1982).

Another indication for postirradiation extrafascial hysterectomy is the failure of a stage IB tumor to regress during radiation therapy. In 1982, HARDT and co-workers reported that patients with no palpable or visible evidence of a cervical tumor 1 month after completing radiation therapy had a 95% 5-year survival rate. In contrast, patients with obvious disease in the cervix at this time had a recurrence rate of 80%. For this reason, patients with stage Ib disease whose tumors do not respond by the time radiation therapy is completed should be considered candidates for extrafascial hysterectomy provided that there is no evidence of extracervical spread on CT scan.

9.10.2 Radiation Following Radical Hysterectomy

There are few controlled studies showing improved survival among patients who have undergone pelvic irradiation following radical surgery in the presence of positive pelvic nodes (MORROW et al. 1980; FULLER et al. 1989; KINNEY et al. 1989) (Table 9.53). In 1980, MORROW and co-workers reported the results of a randomized trial addressing the significance of postoperative irradiation. There was a trend toward improved survival with radiation, particularly in patients with more than three positive lymph nodes, although the survival rates of the irradiated and nonirradiated groups were not significantly different. In addition, the incidence of pelvic recurrences was reduced in those who received radiation.

Table 9.53. Postoperative radiotherapy for pelvic node metastasis after radical hysterectomy

Authors	Year	5-year disease-free survival (%)	
		Postoperative radiotherapy	No postoperative radiotherapy
MORROW et al.	1980	60% (30 cases)	59% (144 cases)
FULLER et al.	1982	56% (32 cases)	61% (39 cases)
KINNEY et al.	1989	63% (60 cases)	65% (60 cases)

Table 9.54. Five-year survival rates and number of positive nodes in relation to parametrial invasion. (INOUE and MORITA 1990)

No. of positive nodes	5-year survival rates	
	Stages IB and IIA	Stage IIB
0	470/508 (92%)	85/112 (76%)
1	46/51 (90%)	34/47 (72%)
2–3	32/48 (67%)	19/32 (59%)
4 or more	8/13 (62%)	11/32 (34%)
Unresectable	5/11 (45%)	3/21 (9%)

KINNEY and co-workers (1989) also evaluated the use of postoperative irradiation in a retrospective study. Although long-term survival was essentially the same in both groups, postoperative radiation therapy improved short-term survival and reduced the frequency of local recurrences.

Based on their analysis of 875 postoperatively irradiated patients, INOUE and MORITA (1990) reported that the 5-year survival rates of those patients with one positive node can be improved up to the level of those without nodal metastases by administering 45–50 Gy of postoperative irradiation. But in cases with more than two lymph node metastases after radical hysterectomy and pelvic lymphadenectomy, the 5-year survival rate decreased from 92% to 66% in stage Ib–IIa and from 75% to 47% in stage IIb (Table 9.54). In these reports the number of treated patients is too small to draw definite conclusions. A prospective multi-institutional trial is needed to evaluate the efficacy of postoperative radiation therapy in patients with histologically confirmed pelvic lymph node metastases.

At present, postoperative radiotherapy is usually performed in high-risk groups. If metastastic pelvic lymph nodes, positive parametrial invasion, or positive surgical margins are found after radical hysterectomy, postoperative irradiation is delivered. When metastatic lymph nodes or parametrial invasion is histologically confirmed, 50–60 Gy in fractions of 1.7–1.8 Gy/day is administered to the whole pelvis. Patients with positive common iliac or para-aortic node metastases, or metastases to more than three pelvic lymph nodes, should receive 45–50 Gy to the para-aortic region as well.

For patients in whom postoperative irradiation is indicated because of positive surgical margins, one may employ a combination of external irradiation consisting of 20–30 Gy to the whole pelvis and 20 Gy to the parametria with a midline block combined with an intracavitary insertion for 40–50 Gy to the vaginal epithelium with two colpostats.

In patients receiving postoperative irradiation, extreme care should be taken, especially with respect to intracavitary insertions, because the bladder and the rectosigmoid may lie closer to the radioactive source than in patients with an intact uterus. When external beam whole-pelvis irradiation is administered, the risk of small bowel complications increases because postoperative adhesions can prevent mobilization of the small bowel loops.

9.11 Chemotherapy, Radiosensitization, and Hyperthermia

9.11.1 Chemotherapy

Chemotherapy is usually chosen for patients with stage III and IV disease, for those with extrapelvic metastases, and for those with recurrent disease after surgery and irradiation, because these patients have a low chance of cure with standard treatment modalities.

9.11.1.1 Single-Agent Chemotherapy

The response of squamous cell carcinoma of the cervix to single-agent chemotherapy is summarized in Table 9.55. The principal chemotherapeutic agents that have been combined with radiation to treat cervical cancer are 5-fluorouracil (5-FU) and cisplatin. The best responses were obtained with cisplatin. Choo and co-workers (1986) randomized patients with stage IIb, IIIa, or IIIb disease to receive cisplatin plus radiation versus radiation alone. Cisplatin was given in a dose of 25 mg/m^2 intravenously on day 1 of radiation therapy and was repeated at weekly intervals during the period of irradiation. A complete response was observed in 55% of patients in the combined therapy arm as opposed to only 20% of the patients treated with radiation therapy alone. Although the exact mechanism of the combined effect is unknown, available evidence suggests that cisplatin inhibits the repair of radiation damage in mammalian cells. In these reports the usual dose of cisplatin was 50 mg/m^2 every 3 weeks. At present, several cisplatin analogs such as carboplatin (CBDCA) are used instead of cisplatin because of their reduced nephrotoxicity. In most studies the response of cervical cancer to cisplatin has been short-lived (3–6 months).

9.11.1.2 Combination Chemotherapy

Data on the efficacy of combination chemotherapy in the treatment of squamous cell carcinoma of the cervix are presented in Table 9.56. Although the response rates using combination regimens appear to exceed those achieved with single agents, their toxicity is also substantial. Therefore, none of these combinations is definitely superior to single-agent cisplatin in terms of duration of response or survival, particularly in patients with recurrent disease after primary therapy. Large prospective randomized trials are necessary to compare the various regimens.

9.11.1.3 Intra-arterial Chemotherapy

The location of cervical carcinoma has provided a rationale for the trial of regional perfusion of chemotherapy using intra-arterial infusion. Unfortunately, responses have been uncommon and of short duration. Complication rates have also been significant. A few studies have reported (Ohta 1978; Carlson et al. 1981; Kavanagh et al. 1982) a reduction in complications and some responses. Randomized comparisons will be required to establish any benefits of intra-arterial infusions.

Table 9.55. Response of squamous cell carcinoma of the uterine cervix to single-agent chemotherapy

Drugs	Reporter(s)	Year	No. of patients	Overall response[a]
Alkylating agents				
Cyclophosphamide	Smith et al.	1967	91	20% (0%)
	Perez et al.	1985	228	14%
Chlorambucil	Moore et al.	1968	26	27% (4%)
	Perez et al.	1985	44	25%
Antimetabolites				
5-Fluorouracil	Malkasian et al.	1964	22	23% (0%)
	Perez et al.	1985	348	20%
Methotrexate	Perez et al.	1985	77	16%
Mitotic inhibitor				
Vincristine	Perez et al.	1985	44	23%
Antitumor antibiotics				
Doxorubicin	Slavik	1975	20	15% (0%)
	Cavins and Geisler	1978	18	39% (6%)
	Perez et al.	1985	78	10%
Bleomycin	Mathe	1970	18	33% (5%)
	Krakoff	1977	32	31% (6%)
	Perez et al.	1985	172	10%
Other agents				
Cisplatin	Thigpen et al.	1981	34	39% (9%)
	Perez et al.	1985	52	40%
	Potter et al.	1989	68	40% (16%)
Carboplatin	McGuire et al.	1989	175	15% (8%)
Iproplatin	McGuire et al.	1989	177	11% (4%)
Hexamethylmelamine	Perez et al.	1985	49	22%
	Stolinsky and Bateman	1973	21	38% (0%)
CCNU or methyl-CCNU	Perez et al.	1985	120	4%

[a] Complete response rate is shown in parentheses.

Table 9.56. Response of squamous cell carcinoma of the uterine cervix to combination chemotherapy

Regimen	Reporter(s)	Year	No. of patients	Overall response[a]
Bleomycin, methotrexate	Piel et al.	1973	8	62% (37%)
	Conroy et al.	1976	20	60% (0%)
Bleomycin, mitomycin C	Greenberg et al.	1982	18	11% (0%)
	Perez et al.	1985	33	36% (15%)
Bleomycin, mitomycin C, vincristine	Baker et al.	1973	50	60% (16%)
	Perez et al.	1985	91	51% (15%)
Doxorubicin, bleomycin	Barlow et al.	1973	25	13% (0%)
Doxorubicin, methyl-CCNU	Day et al.	1978	31	45% (29%)
Doxorubicin, methotrexate	Perez et al.	1985	59	66% (22%)
Cisplatin, doxorubicin	Perez et al.	1985	19	31 (10%)
	Trope et al.	1986	31	17% (7%)
Cisplatin, bleomycin, mitomycin C, vincristine	Perez et al.	1985	14	43% (29%)
	Alberts et al.	1987	54	22% (7%)
	Giannone et al.	1987	16	44% (13%)
Cisplatin, bleomycin, ifosfamide	Buxton et al.	1989	49	69% (20%)
Cisplatin, bleomycin, velban	Perez et al.	1985	33	66% (18%)
Cisplatin, bleomycin, vincristine, methotrexate	Perez et al.	1985	15	66% (20%)
Carboplatin, bleomycin, vincristine, methotrexate	Rustin and Newlands	1988	19	26% (0%)

[a] Complete response rate in parentheses.

9.11.2 Combined Chemotherapy and Radiotherapy

9.11.2.1 Chemotherapy as a Radiosensitizer

Several studies on the use of chemotherapeutic agents as radiosensitizers for cervical carcinoma have been reported. PIVER and co-workers (1974a) reported that in stage IIb–IIIb patients with cervical carcinoma a significant improvement in the 2-year survival rate was achieved in the stage IIb group receiving irradiation and hydroxyurea (74%) in comparison with the control IIb group treated with irradiation and a placebo (44%); this was also true for stage IIIb patients (52% compared with 33%). Increased toxicity was, however, observed in the hydroxyurea group. HRESHCYSHYN and co-workers (1979) reported almost the same results among patients with stage IIIb and IV patients; the complete response rate was 68% for the hydroxyurea-treated group and 49% for the placebo group ($P < 0.05$). Recently, the radiosensitizing effect of small doses of doxorubicin and cisplatin has been compared with that of hydroxyurea. BANJAMAN and co-workers (1979) found that the radiosensitizing effect of doxorubicin was superior to that of hydroxyurea. Cisplatin has also been shown to be a radiation sensitizer, at least for hypoxic cells (RUNOWICZ et al. 1989; WONG et al. 1989; SKOV and MACPHAIL 1991). Although the exact mechanism of radiation potentiation by cisplatin is unknown, available evidence suggests that cisplatin inhibits the repair of radiation damage in mammalian cells (COUGHLIN and RICHMOND 1989).

9.11.2.2 Concurrent Use of Chemotherapy

In 1984 CUMMINGS and co-workers reported on the combined effect of 5-FU and radiation therapy. In order to achieve such a combined effect, tumor cells must be exposed to 5-FU for at least 24 h after radiation therapy has begun. The higher the concentration of drug per given period, the more likely the tumor will respond. For locally advanced or recurrent cervical cancer, radiation therapy combined with chemotherapy using cisplatin or cisplatin and 5-FU has been tried recently in many institutions. Whether these combined treatment regimens can provide a significant improvement in long-term survival remains unclear, although several trials reported encouraging results (KUSKE et al. 1989; CHOO et al. 1986; MONYAK et al. 1988; WONG et al. 1989).

9.11.3 Hyperbaric Oxygen

Clinical evaluation of radiation therapy under hyperbaric oxygen in the treatment of cervical carcinoma has provided discrepant results. In a randomized clinical trial of 320 patients with stage III–IVa disease treated at four institutions, WATSON and co-workers (1978) reported 5-year survival rates of 33% in the group treated with hyperbaric oxygen and radiotherapy and 27% in the control group treated in air ($P = 0.08$). The local recurrence rate was 33% for the 161 patients treated with oxygen and 53% for the 159 patients treated in air ($P = 0.001$). Morbidity among the patients treated with hyperbaric oxygen was greater than among those treated in air. The difference was particularly striking for complications of the bowel (13 vs 2 severe complications). On the other hand, FLETCHER and co-workers (1977) demonstrated no significant benefit in survival or tumor control among patients in whom hyperbaric oxygen was used. The morbidity was again greater in patients treated with hyperbaric oxygen than in the control group. In these trials an increased incidence of distant metastasis was not observed following hyperbaric oxygen.

9.11.4 Hypoxic Cell Radiosensitizers

Among the hypoxic cell radiosensitizers, misonidazole has been the most investigated drug. In a randomized study of 331 patients with stage IIb, III, or IVa cervical carcinoma treated with misonidazole or a placebo and irradiation. OVEGAARD and co-workers (1989) found no significant difference in local control (50% vs 54%) or disease-free survival (47% vs 46%). But patients with hemoglobin levels below 7 g/100 mL. had significantly lower local tumor control (24% vs 47%). The results reported by LEIBEL and the RTOG group (1987) are similar to those reported by OVERGAARD and co-workers.

9.11.5 Hyperthermia and Irradiation

Many biologic findings reveal that hyperthermia in combined with radiation is of potential benefit for cancer therapy. Hyperthermia has been clinically applied mainly for superficial tumors by using microwave or ultrasound, and the reported results of treatment regimens combining hyperthermia and radiation are very encouraging. However, studies evaluating hyperthermia in the treatment of carcinoma of the uterine cervix have been sparse because of thermal limitations in attempting to deliver adequate heat to the pelvis (HIRAOKA et al. 1987; SEKIBA et al. 1993).

From 1983 through 1985 seven patients with locally advanced stage IIIb or IVa disease and large pelvic lymph node metastases were treated by external radiotherapy combined with hyperthermia, using an 8-MHz radiofrequency capacitive heating device. External irradiation was given at a rate of 1.8 Gy five times a week to a total dose of 50–55 Gy. In five cases intracavitary irradiation (22–29 Gy/2 insertions/10 days) was performed after external radiotherapy. Hyperthermia was incorporated into the external radiotherapy (2 times/week, 5–8 times in total). Temperature measurements were usually performed by thin Teflon-coated microthermocouples which were inserted in the cervical tumors, the rectum, and the urinary bladder. Six months after combined treatment the huge primary tumors and regional lymph node metastases had disappeared completely in three cases (Fig. 9.78) (FUWA et al. 1987). Thermal response was strongly related to a minimum tumor temperature of more than 42°C. Hyperthermia for deep-seated cervical tumors has two disadvantages: (a) the frequency of hyperthermia to more than 42°C decreased greatly when the thickness of the subcutaneous fat layer exceeded 15 mm; (b) it is often difficult to achieve a whole tumor volume temperature of more than 42°C.

SHARMA and co-workers (1989) reported a 70% disease-free survival rate at 18 months in 20 patients with stage IIb or III carcinoma of the uterine cervix treated with a combination of irradiation and hyperthermia (13.5 MHz, 42°–43°C, 30 min before irradiation), compared with a 50% disease-free survival rate among 22 patients treated with irradiation alone. Radiotherapy combined with local or regional hyperthermia can be recommended chiefly for advanced IIIb and IVa cases with huge primary tumors or large pelvic metastases, when the body of the patient is sufficiently thin.

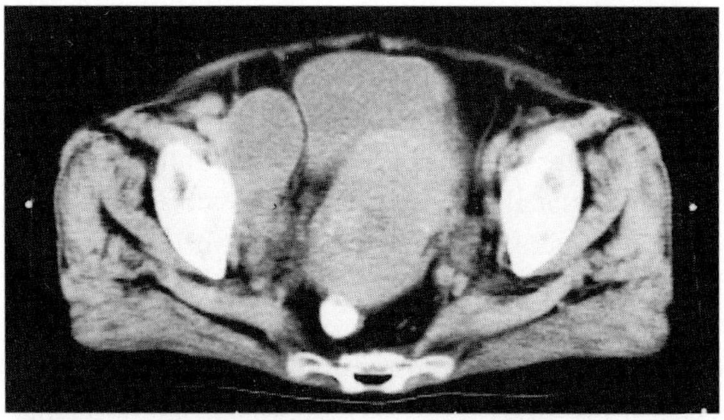

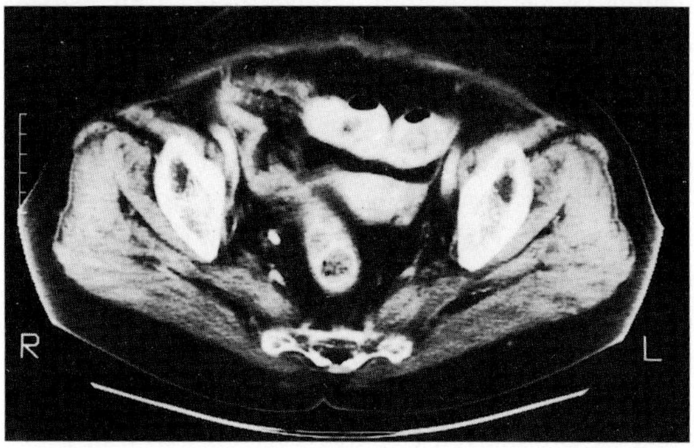

Fig. 9.78. Results of radiation therapy combined with regional hyperthermia with RF wave for cervical cancer in stage IIIB with large pelvic node metastases

9.12 Treatment Results and Complications

9.12.1 Treatment Results

The summarized 5-year survival rates by FIGO stage following radiation therapy for cancer of the cervix are shown in Table 9.57. The average survival by stage 57 remained almost constant from 1950 to 1980 (PETTERSSON 1988). Treatment results often vary significantly from one institution to another (Tables 9.12, 9.35, 9.37, 9.42). In general, survival rates are

Table 9.57. Five-year survival rate of patients with cervical cancer according to stage. (PETTERSSON 1988)

Stage	No. of patients	5-year survival
I	10933	79.4%
II	12561	58.2%
III	9139	31.4%
IV	1461	8.4%

Table 9.58. Five-year survival after extended field radiation for cervical carcinoma with para-aortic nodal metastases

Authors	Year	No. of patients	Radiation dose (Gy)	5-year survival	Incidence of severe complications
Hughes et al.	1980	38	45–51	30%	
Piver et al.	1981	21	60	10%	62%
		10	44–50	43%	10%
Tewfik et al.	1982	23	50–55	22%	35%
Potish	1983	81	43.5–50.75	40%	2%
Rubin et al.	1984	14	40–50	43%	36%
Nori et al.	1985	27	50–52	30%	
Gaspar et al.	1989	18	40–60	17%	
Lovecchio et al.	1989	36	45	50%	
Podczaski	1990	35	42.5–51	39%	9%

Table 9.59. Failures in the pelvis after radiation therapy for cervical cancer by stage

Author(s)	Stage	No. of patients	Failure in pelvis
Marcial[a]	I	439	3%
	IIA	329	15%
	IIB	549	21%
	IIIA	235	31%
	IIIB	156	53%
	IVA	22	68%
Perez et al.	I	1801	8%
	IIA	1962	17%
	IIB	2233	25%
	III	1660	36%
	IV	171	65%

[a] Summarized data from three institutes.

highest in centers where there is a standardized evaluation system and multidisciplinary consultation, allowing therapy to be individualized. The average results in the United States reported in the Pattern of Care Study (Coia et al. 1990) and in Japan (Table 9.35) (Jap. Soc. Obstet. Gynecol. 1993) are inferior to those reported by large centers with more experience. Failure analysis and diffusion of the optimal treatment techniques by stage are essential to improve the average results.

Survival rates for cervical cancer patients with para-aortic lymph node metastases treated by extended field radiation are summarized in Table 9.58. Five-year survival rates range from 17% to 50% (mean = 35%).

Control rates in the pelvis by stage are shown in Table 9.59. In stages I and II, the local control rate reaches more than 80%. By contrast, in stages III and IV the local control rate is about 60% and 30%, respectively. Perez and co-workers (1983a) reported that local/regional parametrial recurrences correlate with dose to the lateral parametrium in patients with various stages of cervical cancer. In stages II and III better tumor control is obtained with higher doses of radiation. The pattern of failure by stage after radiotherapy was reported by Perez et al. (1986) (Table 9.60). Unsurprisingly, the more advanced the stage, the more frequent is distant metastasis with or without local failure.

9.12.2 Complications Related to Radiation

Complications of radiation are generally divided into acute (during or immediately after therapy) and late (more than 6 months after therapy). Acute complications are often easily reparable but the late injuries are usually irreparable, because they are often caused by arteriocapillary fibrosis in vasculoconnective tissues (Rubin et al. 1984).

The radiation tolerance of an organ or tissue is defined as the dose required to produce a given risk of severe complications (Rubin 1990) (Table 9.61). A hollow viscus such as the bowel needs only a focal overdose to become nonfunctional because of a stricture or fistula, whereas a parenchymal organ like the liver and lung may need to sustain a large area of damage to cause loss of function.

It is clear that the cure rate does rise as the dose increases up to the tolerance levels of the surrounding normal tissues. Beyond this level little increase in control rate can be expected, but a serious increase in the incidence of late complications occurs.

The complications after radiation therapy for cervical carcinoma depend not only on the total dose, the volume of the high dose region, the fractionation schedule, the dose rate of the intracavitary irradiation, and the energy of the external radiation, but

Table 9.60. Site of failure after radiation therapy for cervical cancer. (PEREZ et al. 1986)

Stage	No. of patients	Local[a]	Sites of recurrence		
			Pelvic	Pelvic + DM	DM only
IB	312	7 (2.2%)	0	16 (5.1%)	25 (8.0%)
IIA	98	5 (5.1%)	1 (1.0%)	7 (7.1%)	16 (16.3%)
IIB	276	13 (4.7%)	16 (5.8%)	17 (6.2%)	44 (15.9%)
III	237	31 (13.1%)	22 (9.3%)	34 (14.3%)	42 (17.7%)
IV	18	9 (50.0%)	1 (5.6%)	4 (22.2%)	3 (16.7%)

DM, Distant metastases.
[a] Includes local only; local and parametrial; local, parametrial, and distant metastases; and local and distant metastases.

Table 9.61. Normal tissue tolerance. (RUBIN and CASARETT 1968)

Organ	Injury	Volume	TD5/5	T50/5
Intestine	Ulcer, perforation,	400 cm^2	45 Gy	55 Gy
	hemorrhage	100 cm^2	50 Gy	65 Gy
Rectum	Ulcer, stricture	75 cm^2	60 Gy	75 Gy
Bladder	Contracture	Whole	60 Gy	80 Gy
Ureter	Stricture	5–10 cm	75 Gy	100 Gy
Uterus	Ulcer, necrosis	Whole	>100 Gy	>200 Gy
Vagina	Ulcer, fistula	Whole	90 Gy	>100 Gy

TD5/5: the dose that produces a 5% incidence of a specified complication within 5 years of treatment.
TD50/5: the dose that produces a 50% incidence of a specified complication within 5 years of treatment.

also to a lesser degree on other factors such as age, other medical problems (e.g., diabetes, vascular disease), previous pelvic surgery, race, and the socioeconomic level of the patient. In order to achieve satisfactory treatment results, a certain percentage of radiation-induced complications is unavoidable. The more advanced the stage, the greater the dose and the larger the portals necessary for disease eradication. With advanced disease, higher risks of injury are therefore anticipated and justified. The rate of major late complications of radiation therapy for stage Ib and IIa carcinoma of the cervix ranges from 3% to 5%, and for stage IIb and III disease, from 10% to 15%. The generally acceptable level of radiation-induced complications may be 5%–10%.

In the past, Kottmeier's grading system for late complications of the rectum, sigmoid, and urinary bladder was usually used (KOTTMEIER 1964):

Grade 1: Complications signifying transient injury requiring no or minimal medical care
Grade 2: Complications requiring continuous conservative treatment for more than 6 months
Grade 3: Complications requiring surgical treatment
Grade 4: Death resulting directly or indirectly from complications

Recently, the acute and late effects scoring system for normal tissues after irradiation developed by RTOG/EORTC has often been used to compare the treatment results of each institution (Table 9.62). In 1995 these two large organizations, RTOG and EORTC, presented the new late effect normal tissue (LENT) scoring system (RUBIN et al. 1995) (Table 9.63). There is general agreement that LENT toxicity should include five grades. Grade 0 indicates no toxicities and grade 4 indicates fatality or loss of an organ and structure. In order to evaluate the late radiation effects, LENT scores/scales are divided into four major categories: subjective (symptoms), objective (signs), management, and analytic (SOMA). In the near future, the validity of the new LENT scoring system will be evaluated by various group studies.

The dose distribution, dose rate, and the fractionation are different in external pelvic irradiation and transvaginal irradiation. Also, there are important differences in radiation tolerance among various brachytherapy techniques due to the differences in source distribution and dose rate. Simple addition of the doses received at points (for example, point A or point B) in the parametrium from intracavitary sources and from external pelvic irradiation may give equal sums, but may produce different reactions. In spite of its weak points, simple addition of the doses at point A is now widely used. In 1985 the ICRU (International Committee on Radiation Units and Measurements) produced guidelines for the reporting of rectal and bladder complications.

Radiation-induced complications at various locations are discussed below:

Table 9.62. Acute and late radiation morbidity scoring systems

	0	Grade I	Grade II	Grade III	Grade IV
Acute radiation morbidity scoring criteria (RTOG)					
Lower GI, including pelvis	No change	Increased frequency or change in quality of bowel habits not requiring medication; rectal discomfort not requiring analgesics	Diarrhea requiring parasympatholytic drugs (e.g., diphenoxylate); mucous discharge not necessitating sanitary pads; rectal or abdominal pain requiring analgesics	Diarrhea requiring parenteral support; severe mucous or blood discharge necessitating sanitary pads; abdominal distention (flat plate radiograph demonstrates distended bowel loops)	Acute or subacute obstruction, fistula or perforation; GI bleeding requiring transfusion; abdominal pain or tenesmus requiring tube decompression or bowel diversion
Genitourinary	No change	Frequency of urination or nocturia twice pretreatment habit, dysuria, urgency not requiring medication	Frequency of urination or nocturia less frequent than every hour; dysuria, urgency, bladder spasm requiring local anesthetic (e.g., phenazopyridine)	Frequency with urgency and nocturia hourly or more frequently, dysuria, pelvis pain or bladder spasm requiring regular, frequent narcotic; gross hematuria with or without clot passage	Hematuria requiring transfusion; acute bladder obstruction not secondary to clot passage; ulceration or necrosis
Late radiation morbidity scoring scheme (RTOG/EORTC)					
Small/large intestine	None	Mild diarrhea; mild cramping; bowel movement 5 times daily; slight rectal discharge or bleeding	Moderate diarrhea and colic; bowel movement >5 times daily; excessive rectal mucus or intermittent bleeding	Obstruction or bleeding requiring surgery	Necrosis, perforation, fistula
Bladder	None	Slight epithelial atrophy; mild telangiectasia (microscopic hematuria	Moderate frequency; generalized telangiectasia; intermittent macroscopic hematuria	Severe frequency and dysuria; severe generalized telangiectasia (often; with petechiae); frequent hematuria reduction in bladder capacity (<150 cc)	Necrosis; contracted bladder capacity (<100 cc); severe hemorrhagic cystitis

9.12.2.1 Skin

With megavoltage irradiation with more than 10 MV x-rays, acute skin reactions are modest, usually consisting of slight erythema and transient epilation. When ^{60}Co γ-rays or less than 6 MV x-rays are used, subcutaneous fibrosis is sometimes observed in advanced-stage patients due to the high dose of external radiation.

9.12.2.2 Uterine Cervix and Corpus

The cervix and corpus of the uterus can tolerate high doses of radiation. Doses of more than 100 Gy in about 2 weeks are routinely tolerated. Asymptomatic pseudomembranous inflammation of the portio and vagina occurs following the intracavitary treatment. The epithelia of the uterus and vagina have a remarkable ability to recover from radiation injury and the smooth muscle and stroma of the uterus seem little affected by such a high dose. After radiation therapy the uterus shows strong radiation-induced atrophic and fibrotic changes. These changes pass unnoticed in the uterus, because the uterus is not called on to function after radiation therapy.

9.12.2.3 Vagina

Postirradiation ulcers of the portio or the vaginal vault develop 6–12 months after treatment. They rarely develop unless the original cervical cancer was

Table 9.63. New SOMA-LENT scoring system for late radiation effects in normal tissues, proposed by RTOG/EORTC in 1995

Small intestine/colon

	Grade 1	Grade 2	Grade 3	Grade 4	SCORING
Subjective					
Stool frequency	2–4 per day	5–8 per day	>8 per day	Refractory diarrhea	— <u>Instructions</u> Score the 13
Stool consistency	Bulky	Loose	Mucous, dark, watery		— SOM parameters — with 1–4
Pain	Occasional and minimal	Intermittent and tolerable	Persistent and intense	Refractory/rebound	
Constipation	3–4 per week	Only 2 per week	Only 1 per week	No stool in 10 days	—
Objective					
Melena	Occult/occasional	Intermittent and tolerable, normal hemoglobin	Persistent, 10%–20% decrease in hemoglobin	Refractory or frank blood, >20% decrease in hemoglobin	— (Score = 0 if there are no toxicities)
Weight loss from time of treatment	≥5%–10%	>10%–20%	>20%–30%	>30%	— Total the scores and
Stricture	$>\frac{2}{3}$ normal diameter with dilatation	$\frac{1}{3}$–$\frac{2}{3}$ normal diameter with dilatation	$<\frac{1}{3}$ normal diameter	Complete obstruction	— divide by 13
Ulceration	Superficial ≤1 cm^2	Superficial > 1 cm^2	Deep ulcer	Perforation, fistulas	—
Management					
Pain	Occasional nonnarcotic	Regular nonnarcotic	Regular narcotic	Surgical intervention	— LENT score:
Stool consistency/frequency	Diet modification antidiarrheal	Regular use of nonnarcotic	Continuous use of narcotic antidiarrheal		—
Bleeding	Iron therapy	Occasional transfusion	Frequent transfusions	Surgical intervention	— ———
Stricture	Occasional diet adaptation	Diet adaptation required	Medical intervention, NG suction	Surgical intervention	—
Ulceration			Medical intervention	Surgical intervention	—

Analytic		
CT	Assessment of wall thickness, sinus, and fistula formation	Y/N Date:
MRI	Assessment of wall thickness, sinus, and fistula formation	Y/N Date:
Absorption studies	Assessment of protein and fat absorption and metabolic balance	Y/N Date:
Barium radiograph	Assessment of lumen and peristalsis	Y/N Date:

Rectum

	Grade 1	Grade 2	Grade 3	Grade 4	SCORING
Subjective					
Tenesmus	Occasional urgency	Intermittent urgency	Persistent urgency	Refractory	— <u>Instructions</u> Score the 14
Mucosal loss	Occasional	Intermittent	Persistent	Refractory	— SOM parameters
Sphincter control	Occasional	Intermittent	Persistent	Refractory	— with 1–4
Stool frequency	2–4 per day	4–8 per day	>8 per day	Uncontrolled diarrhea	—
Pain	Occasional and minimal	Intermittent and tolerable	Persistent and intense	Refractory and excruciating	—
Objective					
Bleeding	Occult	Occasionally > 2/week	Persistent/daily	Gross hemorrhage	— (Score = 0 if there are no
Ulceration	Superficial ≤ 1 cm^2	Superficial > 1 cm^2	Deep ulcer	Perforation, fistulas	— toxicities)
Stricture	$>\frac{2}{3}$ normal diameter with dilatation	$\frac{1}{3}$–$\frac{2}{3}$ normal diameter with dilatation	$<\frac{1}{3}$ normal diameter	Complete obstruction	
Management					
Tenesmus and stool frequency	Occasional, ≤2 antidiarrheals/week	Regular, >2 antidiarrheals/week	Multiple, >2 antidiarrheals/day	Surgical intervention/permanent colostomy	— Total the scores and divide by 11
Pain	Occasional nonnarcotic	Regular nonnarcotic	Regular narcotic	Surgical intervention	—
Bleeding	Stool softener, iron therapy	Occasional transfusion	Frequent transfusions	Surgical intervention/permanent colostomy	—
Ulceration	Diet modification, stool softener	Occasional steroids	Steroids per enema, hyperbaric oxygen	Surgical intervention/permanent colostomy	— — LENT score:
Stricture	Diet modification	Occasional dilatation	Regular dilatation	Surgical intervention/permanent colostomy	— ———
Sphincter control	Occasional use of incontinence pads	Intermittent use of incontinence pads	Persistent use of incontinence pads	Surgical intervention/permanent colostomy	——

Table 9.63 *(continued)*

Rectum

	Grade 1	Grade 2	Grade 3	Grade 4	
Analytic					
Barium enema	Assessment of lumen and peristalsis				Y/N Date:
Proctoscopy	Assessment of lumen and mucosal surface				Y/N Date:
CT	Assessment of wall thickness, sinus, and fistula formation				Y/N Date:
MRI	Assessment of wall thickness, sinus, and fistula formation				Y/N Date:
Anal manometry	Assessment rectal compliance				Y/N Date:
Ultrasound	Assessment of wall thickness, sinus, and fistula formation				Y/N Date:

Bladder/urethra

	Grade 1	Grade 2	Grade 3	Grade 4	SCORING
Subjective					
Dysuria	Occasional and minimal	Intermittent and tolerable	Persistent and intense	Refractory and excruciating	— Instructions Score the 14
Frequency	3–4 h intervals	2–3 h intervals	1–2 h intervals	Hourly	— SOM parameters
Hematuria	Occasional	Intermittent	Persistent with clot	Refractory	— with 1–4
Incontinence	<Weekly episodes	<Daily episodes	≤2 pads/undergarments/ day	Refractory	
Decreased stream	Occasionally weak	Intermittent	Persistent but incomplete obstruction	Complete obstruction	—
Objective					
Hematuria	Microscopic, normal hemoglobin hemoglobin	Intermittent macroscopic, <10% decrease in	Persistent macroscopic, 10%–20% decrease in hemoglobin	Refractory, >20% decrease in hemoglobin	— (Score = 0 if there are no toxicities)
Endoscopy	Patchy atrophy or telangiectasia without bleeding	Confluent atrophy or telangiectasia with gross bleeding	Ulcerations into muscle	Perforation, fistula	— Total the scores and divide by 14
Maximum volume	>300–400 cc	>200–300 cc	>100–200 cc	≤100 cc	—
Residual volume	25 cc	>25–100 cc	>100 cc		—
Management					
Dysuria	Occasional nonnarcotic	Regular nonnarcotic	Regular narcotic	Surgical intervention	— LENT score:
Frequency	Alkalization	Occasional antispasmodic	Regular narcotic	Cystectomy	—
Hematuria/ telangiectasia	Iron therapy	Occasional transfusion or single cauterization	Frequent transfusion or coagulation	Surgical intervention	— ______
Incontinence	Occasional use of incontinence pads	Intermittent use of incontinence pads	Regular use of pad of self-catheterization	Permanent catheter	—
Decreased stream		<Once-a-day self-catheterization	Dilatation, >once-a-day self-catheterization	Permanent catheter, surgical intervention	—
Analytic					
Cystography	Assessment of mucosal surface				Y/N Date:
Volumetric analysis	Assessment of bladder capacity in milliliters				Y/N Date:
Contrast radiography	Assessment for ulcers, capacity, and contractility				Y/N Date:
Ultrasound	Assessment of wall thickness, sinus, and fistula formation				Y/N Date:
Electromyography	Assessment of sphincter activity using intraluminal pressure transducer, contraction pressure, and volume curves				Y/N Date:

S, Subjective; O, objective; M, management; A, analytic.

advanced, with extensive local ulceration. These ulcers are slow-healing and are difficult to distinguish from persistent cancer. One factor which may be related to the incidence of such ulceration is malpositioning of the intracavitary sources. Conservative management consisting of simple cleaning, good nutrition, and broad-spectrum antibiotics usually suffices.

Vaginal stenosis has been observed in approximately 70% of patients (Abitbol et al. 1974). This complication can be minimized by continuing sexual activity or by using a vaginal dilator immediately after radiation therapy.

9.12.2.4
Sigmoid and Rectum

The sigmoid and rectum are more susceptible to radiation injury than other pelvic organs. This susceptibility has been a major factor in determining which of the many techniques is preferable.

Acute Reactions. Acute radiation proctosigmoiditis (diarrhea with abdominal pain and occasional nausea) usually occurs in the 3rd week of external irradiation. Symptoms of the early reaction are diarrhea, tenesmus, and occasional minor hemorrhage, because the irradiation produces a loss of bowel epithelium. These symptoms usually appear near the end of the external whole-pelvis irradiation or within a few days after brachytherapy. The daily dose has an influence on the reaction. With less than 1.6 Gy daily fractions these acute reactions are less frequent than with the usual 1.8- to 2.0-Gy dose. Several days to a couple of weeks after irradiation, bowel habits return to normal. The relationship of the late reaction to the early reaction is not clear. Severe early reactions are not always followed by late reactions (RUBIN 1984).

Late Reactions. The late rectosigmoidal reaction is one of the most frequent complications after radiation therapy for cervical cancer. With usual treatment, the frequency of late injury of the rectosigmoid region is about 10%–15% in grade 2 of Kottmeier's grading and less than 5% in grade 3. Symptoms are diarrhea, tenesmus, bleeding, and a burning sensation in the rectum. Late rectal reactions may be divided into localized lesions of the anterior wall of the rectum caused by the vaginal brachytherapy and more diffuse changes involving that segment of rectum and sigmoid treated by the external pelvic irradiation. The apparent threshold of complications is a combined external and brachytherapy dose of 70–75 Gy (PEREZ et al. 1984; POURQUIER et al. 1985). Damage manifests from 6 months to 5 years or longer after treatment, with a median latent interval of 19 months (CROOK et al. 1987). The shorter the latent interval, the more severe is the degree of injury; this is especially true if the latent interval is less than 12 months.

An excessive rectal dose from intracavitary brachytherapy is usually caused by inadequate packing that separates the vaginal sources from the rectovaginal septum, a uterine retroflexion, an unusually long uterine tandem filling an enlarged uterine canal, excessive doses from vaginal sources, a narrowed vagina, misplacement of a vaginal source into the posterior fornix, or the slipping of the uterine tandem into the vagina. In intracavitary brachytherapy careful radioactive source placement and vaginal packing and roentgenologic confirmation of the source position are important.

Late rectal ulceration (a grade 2 complication) generally heals with conservative management. Rectovaginal fistulas, repeated severe hemorrhage, and rectal narrowing are unusual and are considered surgical problems. The less frequent large bowel reaction from high-dose external pelvic irradiation appears as a fibrous narrowing of the bowel lumen of the rectum or rectosigmoid. Symptoms consist in alternating diarrhea and constipation and blood and mucus in the stool. Barium enema reveals a narrowed segment with rigid walls. Sometimes colostomy is necessary.

9.12.2.5
Urinary Bladder

From clinical experiences it may be concluded that the limit of tolerance for the urinary bladder is somewhat higher than that for the rectosigmoid. Acute cystitis is uncommon either with external irradiation or following intracavitary applications. This complication is best treated by bladder irrigation and antibiotics.

Large hematuria from ulceration of the urinary bladder sometimes occurs in the vicinity of a brachytherapy applicator. Fibrotic contracture of the bladder is rare unless the whole bladder receives more than 60 Gy. Late urinary injury occurs in 0.5%–2% of patients and has a longer latent period than for the rectosigmoid, appearing at a median of 28 months.

9.12.2.6
Ureter

The ureter runs in the parametrium a scant 1.5 cm from the lateral vaginal fornix. High doses are routinely delivered to this portion of the ureter. The tolerance of the ureter appears high, given that late ureteral complications are rarely observed. SLATER and FLETCHER (1971) reported 134 patients with ureteral obstruction out of 1416 irradiated patients with normal pretreatment pyelograms. In 108 of these instances active pelvic recurrence was present near the ureter. Only five the remaining 26 patients had ureteral obstruction resulting from radiation-induced periureteral fibrosis. Therefore, late ureteral obstruction is usually indicative of disease recurrence in the parametrium.

9.12.2.7 Small Bowel

Late small bowel complications (bleeding, obstruction, necrosis, severe malabsorption) is seen in 1%–3% of patients (Haie et al. 1988; Rotman et al. 1990). In whole-pelvis irradiation, only a limited portion of the small bowel is included. The small bowel is the most sensitive portion of the gastrointestinal tract, but the normal motility of the small bowel usually prevents the administration of excessive doses to any one segment. In patients with previous pelvic surgery or pelvic inflammatory disease, the incidence of small bowel injury after radiation therapy increases sharply. The maximal tolerance dose in such instances might be estimated to be about 40 Gy. The clinical picture is usually that of progressive and recurrent intestinal obstruction. Surgical relief of this obstruction is generally required. When lymph node metastases are identified in the para-aortic region, longer segments of the small bowel must be irradiated. Doses of about 50 Gy in 5 or more weeks delivered to the para-aortic nodes are associated with serious subsequent small bowel damage in 10% of patients. In order to control the para-aortic lymph node metastases by irradiation, doses of about 50 Gy in 5.5–6 weeks should be given. In such instances, serious subsequent small bowel damage occurs in more than 10% of patients.

9.13 Follow-up Examinations

The diagnosis of persistent or recurrent carcinoma of the cervix after radiotherapy may be difficult. The suspected tumor must be distinguished from a slowly regressing neoplasm, and from postirradiation fibrosis. Even positive biopsy results during the first few months after irradiation must be critically evaluated to rule out confusion with a slowly regressing lesion.

Because the majority of recurrences appear within the first 2 years following treatment, follow-up visits should be most frequent during that time (Van Nagell et al. 1979; Fuller et al. 1989). Patients should be examined at least every 2–3 months after treatment for 2 years and every 6 months thereafter. The interval can be significantly prolonged after 5 years, because of the very low incidence of recurrence. At each visit, physical examination includes careful assessment of the supraclavicular and inguinal nodes for metastases as well as abdominal and transvaginal and transrectal pelvic examination. Vagina and cervix should be inspected and cervical cytologic specimens should be obtained. Because of the difficulty in discriminating between a cytologically positive beginning recurrence and "normal" irradiated senile atrophic colpitis, a histologic specimen should be obtained in any doubtful case. In addition, an annual chest x-ray and intravenous pyelography should be performed to rule out pulmonary metastases and occult recurrence in the pelvis.

Periodic transvaginal ultrasonography and pelvic and abdominal CT scan may be helpful in monitoring patients for recurrence. Serial serum SCC, CEA, and/or CA-125 antigen measurements are required in monitoring for recurrence, as continuously elevating SCC values indicate a recurrence some months prior to clinical examination.

9.14 Management of Progression and Recurrences

Although patients who fail after initial treatment have a poor prognosis, though some patients with limited pelvic disease and particularly with central recurrences can be salvaged by additional aggressive therapy. About 15%–20% of radiation therapy failures present with an isolated pelvic recurrence.

9.14.1 Locoregional Recurrences

9.14.1.1 Locoregional Recurrences After Definitive Irradiation

After full irradiation of the initial carcinoma, the salvage therapy of choice is usually surgery. Pelvic exenteration is indicated for biopsy-proven mobile centropelvic recurrence after failure of radiation therapy, without clinically evident distant metastases or side wall disease.

The overall 5-year survival rate after partial or complete pelvic exenteration has been about 15%–20%. Recent treatment results show almost 30% improvement over previous results due to selection of optimal cases and various technical developments (PENALVER et al. 1989; HATCH et al. 1990; MORLEY et al. 1989) (Table 9.64).

In order to control small central recurrences of the cervical region, brachytherapy alone is sometimes successfully administered.

Generally, reirradiation of persistent or recurrent carcinoma of the cervix initially managed with irradiation gives a low yield and a high complication rate. The techniques used in the initial treatment (especially the total dose and treatment volume) and the period between the two treatments must be taken into account. For inoperable cases, 40–45 Gy (1.8 Gy/fraction) of external irradiation to limited volumes is usually given, preferentially with multiple portals or a moving beam. Some patients are treated with interstitial irradiation by means of either removable low-dose-rate afterloading ^{192}Ir sources or permanent ^{125}I seeds which are implanted intraoperatively at the time of exploratory laparotomy.

In some patients combined use may be made of weekly regional hyperthermia. PRASAVINICHAI and co-workers (1978) reported a 17.6% 5-year survival rate for 51 patients with recurrent tumors limited to the pelvis who were treated with irradiation alone (31 patients), pelvic exenteration (10) or a combination of exploratory laparotomy, debulking, and irradiation (10).

9.14.1.2 Locoregional Recurrences After Previous Surgery

Intrapelvic recurrences after surgical procedures can be more easily treated with irradiation. When a small recurrence is seen at the vaginal stump, a combination of whole-pelvis irradiation and intracavitary therapy is recommended. Usually whole-pelvis irradiation to a total dose of 40 Gy, depending on tumor volume, and an additional parametrial dose with midline shielding, for a total of 50–60 Gy, should be administered. Intracavitary irradiation is less effective because only intravaginal sources can be used. Intracavitary irradiation of 20–30 Gy at point A is delivered during or after external irradiation. The results of salvage radiotherapy are summarized in Table 9.65.

Table 9.64. Operative mortality and 5-year survival after pelvic exenteration for radiation therapy failures

Authors	Year	No. of patients	Operative mortality	5-year survival
BRICKER	1970	207	7.7%	35%
KETCHAM et al.	1970	162	7.4%	38%
SYMMONDS et al.	1975	198	8.1%	33%
RUTLEDGE et al.	1977	296	13.5%	37%
AVERETTE et al.	1984	92	23.9%	37%
KRAYBILL et al.	1988	99	14.1%	45%
LAWHEAD et al.	1989	65	9.2%	23%
SHINGLETON et al.	1989	143	6.3%	50%
MORLEY et al.	1989	100	2.0%	61%

Table 9.65. Radiation therapy after surgical failure for carcinoma of the uterine cervix

Reporter	Year	No. of patients	Pelvic control	5-year survival
HOGAN et al.	1982	24	38%	22%
THOMAS et al.	1987	17	47%	47%
JOBSEN et al.	1989	18	61%	44%
POTTER et al.	1990	28	–	30%

For paravaginal or parametrial recurrences, interstitial irradiation with a dose of 20–30 Gy is sometimes given.

9.14.2 Extrapelvic Recurrences

Chemotherapy is frequently administered alone, and occasionally combined with surgery or irradiation. Multiple cytotoxic agent combinations are employed, usually cisplatin (50–75 mg/m^2) and 5-FU (700–1000 mg/m^2). For para-aortic, mediastinal, or supraclavicular lymph node metastases, 45–50 Gy in 5 weeks is palliatively administered. For hepatic metastases, selective intrahepatic arterial infusion using 5-FU is sometimes tried. Surgical treatment is to be preferred for solitary or a few hematogenous pulmonary metastases, if it is feasible.

9.15 Future Prospects

It is clear that carcinoma of the cervix offers the best opportunity for prevention among all forms of cancer. Prevention may be achieved through avoidance of sexually transmitted diseases, maintenance of a lean body mass, avoidance of high-fat diets, or hormonal means. The Papanicolaou smear (Pap test) has proved to be an effective tool for screening the population and reducing the risk of cancer through early detection of its precursor lesions, particularly in low socioeconomic populations.

Using radiotherapy, permanent tumor control in the pelvis can be achieved in about 95% of patients with stage I disease, and about 80% of those with stage II disease. The routine combination of radiation and surgery is not justified. For patients with stage Ib or IIa cervical cancer, the identification of high-risk subgroups for distant metastasis may allow early use of adjuvant chemotherapy with further improvements in survival. Appropriate selection of chemotherapeutic agents is very important. Various kinds of combination chemotherapy including cisplatin are often used. Preliminary results in respect of adjuvant chemotherapy should be followed with larger, prospective randomized studies.

Tumor control rates decrease with advancing disease, being slightly over 30% in patients who have stage IIIb disease with a large tumor more than 4 cm in diameter. Current research into radiotherapy for these advanced cervical cancer includes different fractionation schedules, hyperthermia, heavy-ion therapy, and the combination of irradiation and chemotherapy.

Heavy ion therapy using carbon ions for locally advanced cervical cancer has been tried at NIRS in Japan since June 1994. In March 1996 the primary response to carbon-ion therapy was evaluated in three patients with cervical cancer of stage IIIb or IVa. The response rate achieved was impressive, since a complete response was obtained in every case. The clinical study is continuing so that efficacy can be better defined.

The combination of locoregional hyperthermia and chemotherapeutic agents such as cisplatin seems to be effective in patients with irresectable local recurrence of cervical cancer in a previously irradiated region.

In patients with advanced cervical cancer, it is important to identify optimal combinations of radiotherapy and chemotherapy not only to enhance the chance of eliminating the tumor in the irradiated volume, but also to reduce metastases outside the irradiated volume.

References

Abitbol M, Davenport JH (1974) The irradiated vagina. Obstet Gynecol 44:249–254

Abou-Daoud KT (1967) Epidemiology of carcinoma of the cervix uteri in Lebanese Christians and Moslems. Cancer 20:1706–1714

Alberts DS, Kronmal R, Baker LH, et al. (1987) Phase II randomized trial of cisplatin chemotherapy regimens in the treatment of recurrent or metastatic squamous cell cancer of the cervix. A Southwest Oncology Group study. J Clin Oncol 5:1791–1798

Anderson Cancer Center between 1965 and 1985. (1990) Cancer 65:2507–2514

Angel C, Beecham JB, Rubens DJ, et al. (1987) Magnetic resonance imaging and pathologic correlation in stage IB cervix cancers. Gynecol Oncol 27:357–365

Annual report of Japanese Society of Obstetrics & Gynecology. (1993) Jpn J Soc Obstet Gynecol 43:1324–1329

Arai T, Morita S, Iinuma T (1979) Radiotherapy for cancer of the uterine cervix using HDR remote afterloading system. Determination of the optimal fractionation. Clin Cancer Treat (Jpn) 25:605–612

Arai T, Akanuma A, Ikeda M, et al. (1984) Standardization of radiotherapy for carcinoma of the uterine cervix. Clin Oncol (Jpn) 30:496–500

Arai T, Nakano T, Morita S, et al. (1992) High-dose rate remote afterloading intracavitary radiation therapy for cancer of the uterine cervix. A 20 year experience. Cancer 69:175–180

Aristizabal SA, Woolfit B, Valencia A, et al. (1987) Interstitial parametrial implant in carcinoma of the cervix stage IIB. Int J Radiat Oncol Biol Phys 13:445–450

Arneson AM (1938) Use of interstitial radiation in the treatment of cancer of the cervix. Radiology 30:167–180

Averette HE, Nasser N, Yankow SL (1970) Cervical conization in pregnancy. Am J Obstet Gynecol 106:543–550

Averette HE, Ford JJ, Dudan RC, et al. (1975) Staging of cervical cancer. Clin Obstet Gynecol 18:215–232

Averette HE, Nelson JH, Ng AG, et al. (1976) Diagnosis and management of microinvasive (stage IA) carcinoma of the uterine cervix. Cancer 38:414–420

Averette HE, Lichtinger M, Sevin BU, et al. (1984) Pelvic exenteration: a 15-year experience in a general metropolitan hospital. Am J Obstet Gynecol 150:179–186

Averette HE, Nguyen HN, Donato DM, et al. (1993) A 25-year prospective experience with the Miami technique. Cancer 71:1422–1437

Baier K (1987) Ein biologisches Planungssystem fur die routinemässige klinische Strahlentherapie. Roentgen-Berichte 16:180–191

Baker LH, Opipari M, Wilson H (1973) Mitomycin C, vincristine and bleomycin therapy for advanced cervical cancer. Obstet Gynecol 52:146–152

Balch CM (1990) The surgeon's expanding role in cancer care. Cancer 65:604–609

Ballon SC, Berman ML, Lagasse LD, et al. (1981) Survival after extraperitoneal pelvic and paraaortic lymphadenectomy and radiation therapy in cervical carcinoma. Obstet Gynecol 57:90–95

Baltzer J, Lohe KJ, Köpcke W, et al. (1982) Histologic criteria for the prognosis in patients with operated squamous cell carcinoma of the cervix. Gynecol Oncol 13:184

Bandy LC, Clarke PD, Silverman PM, et al. (1985) Computed tomography in evaluation of extrapelvic lymphadenopathy in carcinoma of the cervix. Obstet Gynecol 65:73–76

Banjamin I, Xynos FP, Rana MW (1979) Effects of adriamycin and hydroxyurea on human squamous cell carcinoma of cervix transplanted into nude mice. Fed Proc 28:1319–1324
Barber HRK (1982) Incidence, prevalence and median survival rates of gynecologic cancer. Modern concepts of gynecologic oncology. John Wright PSG, Boston, pp 1–19
Barlow J, Piver M, Chuang J (1973) Adriamycin and bleomycin alone and in combination in gynecologic cancers. Cancer 32:735–740
Barron BA, Richart RM (1968) A statistical model of the natural history of cervical carcinoma based on a prospective study of 557 cases. JNCI 41:1343–1353
Barron BA, Richart RM (1970) A statistical model of the natural history of cervical carcinoma. II. Estimates of the transition time from dysplasia to carcinoma in situ. JNCI 45:1025–1028
Bates T (1989) Historical review and critical evaluation of different techniques of intracavitary brachytherapy for carcinoma of the cervix from the clinical standpoint. In: Rotte K, Kiffer J (eds) Changes in brachytherapy. Wachholz, Nürnberg, pp 29–33
Beaudenon S, Kremsdorf D, Croissant O, et al. (1986) A novel type of human papillomavirus associated with genital neoplasias. Nature 321:246–249
Berek JS, Hacker NF, Fu YS, et al. (1985) Adenocarcinoma of the uterine cervix: histologic variables associated with lymph node metastasis and survival. Obstet Gynecol 65:46–57
Bjornsson M, et al. (1993) Accuracy of frozen section for lymph node metastasis in patients undergoing radical hysterectomy for carcinoma of the cervix. 24th Annual Meeting of the Society of Gynecologic Oncologists. Abstract No. 56
Bloss JD, Berman ML, Mukhererhee J, et al. (1992) Bulky stage IB cervical carcinoma managed by primary radical hysterectomy followed by tailored radiotherapy. Gynecol Oncol 47:21–27
Boyce JG, Lu T, Nelson JJ, et al. (1972) Cervical carcinoma and oral contraception. Obstet Gynecol 40:139–146
Boyce JG, Fruchter RG, Nicastri AD, et al. (1984) Vascular invasion in stage I carcinoma of the cervix. Cancer 53:1175–1181
Branson MR, et al. (1985) A device for interstitial therapy of low pelvis tumors. The Hammersmith Perineal Hedgehog. Br J Radiol 58:537–542
Brenner DE, Whitley NO (1983) Computed tomography in invasive carcinoma of the cervix: an appraisal. Obstet Gynecol 62:218–224
Brenner DE, Whitley NO, Prempree T, et al. (1982) An evaluation of the computed tomographic scanner for the staging of carcinoma of the cervix. Cancer 50:2322–2328
Brenner DJ, Hall EJ (1991) Fractionated high dose rate versus low dose rate regimens for intracavitary brachytherapy of the cervix. I. General considerations based on radiobiology. Br J Radiol 64:133–141
Bricker EM (1970) Pelvic exenteration. In: Advances in Surgery, vol 4. Chicago Year Book, Chicago
Bridier A, Dutreix A, Gerbaulet A, et al. (1981) Calcul previsionnel des dimensions des isodoses en curietherapie gynecologique. J Eur Radiother 23:139–156
Brinton L, Haenszel W, Stolley P, et al. (1986) Cigarette smoking and invasive cervical cancer. JAMA 255:3265–3268
Buchsbaum HJ (1979) Extrapelvic lymph node metastases in cervical carcinoma. Am J Obstet Gynecol 133:814–824
Buchsbaum HJ, Lifshitz S (1976) The role of scalene lymph node biopsy in advanced carcinoma of the cervix uteri. Surg Gynecol Obstet 143:246–248
Burghardt E, Pickel H (1978) Local spread and lymph node involvement in cervical cancer. Obstet Gynecol 52:138–148
Burghardt E, Baltzer J, Tulusan AH, et al. (1992) Result of surgical treatment of 1028 cervical cancers studied with volumetry. Cancer 70:648–655
Burnett AF, Barnes JC, Johnson JC, et al. (1992) Prognostic significance of polymerase chain reaction detected human papillomavirus of tumors and lymph nodes in surgery treated stage IB cervical cancer. Gynecol Oncol 47:343–347
Bush RS, Jenkins RD, Allt WE, et al. (1978) Definitive evidence for hypoxic cells influencing cure in cancer therapy. Br J Cancer 37:302–306
Butterworth CE, Hatch KD, Gore H, et al. (1982) Improvement in cervical dysplasia associated with folic acid therapy in users of oral contraceptives. Am J Clin Nutr 39:73–81
Buxton EJ, Meanwell CA, Hilton C, et al. (1989) Combination bleomycin, ifosfamide, and cisplatin chemotherapy in cervical cancer. J Natl Cancer Inst 81:359–367
Buxton EJ, Saunders N, Blackledge GRP, et al. (1990) Prognosefaktoren beim operativ behandelten Zervixkarzinom. In: Teufel G, Pfleiderer A, Ladner HA (eds) Therapie des Zervixkarzinoms. Springer, Berlin Heidelberg New York, pp 78–85
Calais G, Le Floch O, Chauvert B, et al. (1989) Carcinoma of the uterine cervix stage Ib and early stage II. Prognostic value of the histological tumour regression after initial brachytherapy. Int J Radiat Oncol Biol Phys 17:1231–1235
Camilien L, Gordon D, Fruchter RG, et al. (1988) Predictive value of computerized tomography in the presurgical evaluation of primary carcinoma of the cervix. Gynecol Oncol 30:209–215
Carlson JJ, Freedman RS, Wallace S, et al. (1981) Intraarterial cis-platinum in the management of squamous cell carcinoma of the uterine cervix. Gynecol Oncol 12:92–98
Carlson V, Delclos L, Fletcher GH (1987) Distant metastases in squamous-cell carcinoma of the uterine cervix. Radiology 88:961–969
Carmichael JA, Clarke DH, Moher D, et al. (1986) Cervical carcinoma in women aged 34 and younger. Am J Obstet Gynecol 154:264–275
Castro JR, Issa P, Fletcher GH (1970) Carcinoma of the cervix treated by external irradiation alone. Radiology 95:163–166
Cavins JA, Geisler HE (1978) Treatment of advanced unresectable cervical carcinoma already subjected to complete irradiation therapy. Gynecol Oncol 6:256–263
Chadha M (1988) Stage IIb carcinoma of the cevix managed with radiation therapy: an analysis of prognostic factors. Endocurietherapy Hyperthermia Oncol 4:219–228
Chadwick D, Steinhoff M, Calabresi P, et al. (1993) Tumor angiogenesis as a prognostic factor in cervical carcinoma (abstract). 24th Annual Meeting of the Society of Gynecologic Oncologists
Chamberlain G (1981) Etiology of gynecological cancer. J R Soc Med 74:246–254
Chassagne D, Pierquin B (1965) La plesiocurietherapie cancer du vagin par moulage plastique avec iridium 192. Preparation non radio-active. J Radiol 46:89–93
Chassagne D, Gerbaulet A (1975) Remote after-loading with conventional sources. In: Hilaris BS (ed) After-loading – 20 years of experience 1955–1975. Memorial Sloan-Kettering Cancer Center, New York, pp 195–200
Chassagne D, Horiot JC (1977) Propositions pour une definition commune des points de reference en curietherapie gynecologique. J Radiol 58:371–378
Chassagne D, Delouche G, Rocoplan JA, et al. (1968) Description et premiers essais du Curietron (projecteur polyvalent

de sources radio-actives permettant une protection complete en curietherapie gynecologique. J Radiol 50:910–913
Chassagne D, Attia AB, Pierquin B (1969) Description d'un programme de calcul des doses sur ordinateur en curietherapie gynecologique. Ses applications cliniques. J Radiol 50:906–911
Chassagne D, Gerbaulet A, Dutreix A, et al. (1977) Utilisation pratique de la dosimetrie par ordinateur en curietherapie gynecologique. J Radiol 58:387–393
Chatani M, Matayoshi Y, Masaki N, et al. (1994a) Long term follow-up results of high-dose rate remote afterloading intracavitary radiation therapy for carcinoma of the uterine cervix. Strahlenther Onkol 170:269–276
Chatani M, Matayoshi Y, Masaki N, et al. (1994b) A prospective randomized study concerning the point A dose in high-dose rate intracavitary therapy for carcinoma of the uterine cervix. Strahlenther Onkol 170:636–642
Chen DX (1989) Urinary complications following radical hysterectomy for 621 patients with cancer of uterine cervix. Chung Hua Chung Liu Tsa Chih 11:67–70
Chen MS, Lin FJ, Hong CH, et al. (1991) High dose-rate afterloading technique in the radiation treatment of uterine cervical cancer: 339 cases and 9 years experience in Taiwan. Int J Radiat Oncol Biol Phys 20:915–919
Chism SE, Park RC, Keys HM (1975) Prospects for para-aortic irradiation in treatment of cancer of the cervix. Cancer 35:1505–1509
Choo YC, Choy TK, Wong LC (1986) Potentiation of radiotherapy by cis-dichlorodiammine platinum (II) in advanced cervical carcinoma. Gynecol Oncol 23:94–100
Choy D, Wong LC, Sham J (1994) Vaginal template for cervical carcinoma with vaginal stenosis or inadvertent diagnosis after hysterectomy. Int J Radiat Oncol Biol Phys 28:457–462
Christensen A, Lange P, Neilsen E (1964) Surgery and radiotherapy for invasive cancer of the cervix: surgical treatment. Acta Obstet Gynecol 43:59–68
Chung CK, Nahas WA, Stryker JA, et al. (1980) Analysis of factors contributing to treatment failures in stage IB and IIA carcinoma of the cervix. Am J Obstet Gynecol 138:550–556
Chung CK, Nahhas WA, Zaino R, et al. (1981) Histologic grade and lymph node metastasis in squamous cell carcinoma of the cervix. Gynecol Oncol 12:348–356
Coia L, Won M, Lanciano R, et al. (1990) The patterns of care outcome study for cancer of the uterine cervix. Cancer 66:2451–2456
Coleman DL, Gallup DG, Wolcott HD, et al. (1992) Patterns of failure of bulky-barrel carcinomas of the cervix. Am J Obstet Gynecol 166:916–920
Conroy J, Lewis G, Brady L (1976) Low dose bleomycin and methotrexate in cervical cancer. Cancer 37:550–558
Corscaden JA, Gusberg SB, Donlan CP (1948) Precision dosage in interstitial irradiation of cancer of the cervix uteri. Am J Roentgenol 60:522–534
Coughlin CT, Richmond RC (1989) Biological and clinical development of cisplatin combined with radiation: concepts, utility, projections for new trials and the emergence of carboplatin. Semin Oncol 16:31–39
Crissman JD, Makuch R, Budharja M (1985) Histopathologic grading of squamous cell carcinoma of the uterine cervix. Cancer 55:1590–1598
Crook JM, Esche BA (1994) The uterine cervix. In: Cox JD (ed) Radiation oncology, 7th edn. Mosby, St. Louis, Chap. 26
Crook JM, Esche BA, Chaaplain G, et al. (1987) Dose-volume analysis and the prevention of radiation sequelae in cervical cancer. Radiother Oncol 8:321–332
Crowley-Norwick P, Edwards R, Kuykendall K, et al. (1993) Helper/inducer T lymphocytes and natural killer cells are depleted in cervical dysplasia. 24th Annual Meeting of the Society of Gynecologic Oncologists. Abstract No. 48
Crum CP, Levine RU (1984) Human papillomavirus infection and cervical neoplasia. New perspectives. Int J Gynecol Pathol 3:376–388
Cummings B, Keane T, Thomas G, et al. (1984) Results and toxicity of the treatment of anal canal carcinoma by radiation therapy or radiation therapy and chemotherapy. Cancer 54:2062–2065
Currie J, Abbas F, Fields A, et al. (1993) The versatility of the bulbocavernosus myocutaneous flap in vaginal reconstruction. 24th Annual Meeting of the Society of Gynecologic Oncologists. Abstract No. 60
Day T, Wharton J, Gottlieb JA, et al. (1978) Chemotherapy for squamous carcinoma of the cervix: doxorubicin-methyl CCNU. Am J Obstet Gynecol 132:545–551
Deckers PJ, Ketcham AS, Sugarbaker EV, et al. (1971) Pelvic exenteration for primary carcinoma of the uterine cervix. Obstet Gynecol 37:647–652
Delgado G, Chun B, Caglar H, et al. (1977) Para-aortic lymphadenectomy in gynecologic malignancies confined to the pelvis. Obstet Gynecol 50:418–423
Delgado G, Bundy B, Zaino R, et al. (1990) Prospective surgical pathological study of disease-free interval in patients with stage IB squamous cell carcinoma of the cervix: a Gynecologic Oncology Group study. Gynecol Oncol 38: 352–358
Delouche G, Gest J (1972) Un nouveau modele d'applicateur a isodoses precalculees pur la curietherapie gynecologique par cutietron. J Radiol 53:227–232
DiPaolo M, Tulusan AH, Breuel C, et al. (1990) Der Stellenwert der Skanenusbiopsie im Therapieplan des fortgeschrittenen Kollumkarzinoms. Geburtshilfe Frauenheilkd 50:310–313
DiSaia PJ, Creasman WT (1989) Clinical gynecologic oncology, 3rd edn. Mosby, St. Louis, p 72
DiSaia PJ, Bundy B, Curry SL (1987) Phase III study on the treatment of women with cervical cancer stage IIB, IIIB, and IVA (confined to the pelvis and/or paraaortic nodes) with radiotherapy alone versus radiotherapy plus immunotherapy with i.v.C. parvum: a GOG study. Gynecol Oncol 26:386–397
Donath D, Clark B, Kaufmann C, et al. (1992) HDR interstitial brachytherapy of lower gynaecological tract cancer. In: Mould RF (ed) International brachytherapy. Nucletron International, Veenendaal, pp 219–225
Durrance FY (1969) Radiotherapy following simple hysterectomy in patients with stage I and II carcinoma of the cervix. Am J Roentgenol 106:165–174
Dutreix A, Wambersie A (1975) Specification of gamma-ray brachytherapy sources. Br J Radiol 48:1034
Dutreix A, Marinello G, Wambersie A (1982) Dosimetrie en curietherapie. Masson, Paris, pp 163–190
Eifel PJ, Morris M, Oswald MJ, et al. (1990) Adenocarcinoma of the uterine cervix: prognosis and patterns of failure in 367 cases treated at the M.D. Anderson Cancer Center between 1965 and 1985. Cancer 65:2507–2514
Emami B, Watring WG, Tak W, et al. (1980) Para-aortic lymph node radiation in advanced cervical cancer. Int J Radiat Oncol Biol Phys 6:1237–1241
Engelshoven JMA, Van Versteege CWM, Ruys JHJ, et al. (1984) Computed tomography in staging untreated patients with cervical cancer. Gynecol Obstet Invest 18:289–295

Esche BA, Crook JM, Isturiz J, Horiot J-C (1987) Reference volume, milligram-hours and external irradiation for the Fletcher applicator. Radiother Oncol 9:255–261
Feder BH, Syed AMN, Neblett D (1978) Treatment of extensive carcinoma of the cervix with the transperitoneal butterfly. A preliminary report on the revival of Waterman's approach. Int J Radiat Oncol Biol Phys 4:735–742
Fennell RH (1978) Microinvasive carcinoma of the uterine cerix. Obstet Gynecol Surg 33:406–444
Fletcher GH (1971) Cancer of the uterine cervix: Janeway lecture. Am J Roentgenol Rad Ther Nucl Med 111:225–242
Fletcher GH (1980) Textbook of radiotherapy, 3rd edn. Lea & Febiger, Philadelphia, pp 720–769
Fletcher GH, Rutledge FN (1972) Extended field technique in the management of the cancers of the uterine cervix. Am J Roentgenol 114:116–122
Fletcher GH, Lindberg RD, Carerao JB, et al. (1977) Hyperbaric oxygen as a radiotherapeutic adjuvant in advanced cancer of the uterine cervix: preliminary results of a randomized trial. Cancer 39:617–623
Fouchee JH, Greiss FC, Loch FR (1969) Stage IA squamous cell carcinoma of the uterine cervix. Am J Obstet Gynecol 105:46–54
Fowler JF, Stern BE (1963) Dose-time relationships in radiotherapy and the validity of cell survival curve models. Br J Radiol 36:163–173
Friedberg V (1988) Möglichkeiten der Funktionserhaltung bei erweiterten gynäkologischen Tumoroperationen. Gynäkologe 21:315–318
Friedberg V, Beck T (1989) Ergebnisse operativer Therapie des Zervixkarzinoms im Stadium IIb. Geburtsh Frauenheilkd 49:782–786
Frischbier H-J, Hasse J (1965) Die biaxiale Telekobalt-Pendelbestrahlung des Kollumkarzinoms. Strahlentherapie 140:32–36
Frischkorn R (1983) Die Strahlentherapie des Endometriumkarzinoms. Gynäkologe 16:104–113
Fuller AF Jr, Elliott N, Kosloff C, et al. (1982) Lymph node metastases from carcinoma of the cervix, stages IB and IIA: implications for prognosis and treatment. Gynecol Oncol 13:165–174
Fuller AT, Elliott N, Kosloff C, et al. (1989) Determinants of increased risk for recurrence in patients undergoing radical hysterectomy for stage IB and IIA carcinoma of the cervix. Gynecol Oncol 33:34–39
Fuwa N, Morita K, Kimura C (1987) Experience of radiotherapy combined with local hyperthermia using 8MHz RF capacitive heating for advanced cervical cancer. Jpn J Clin Oncol 33:799–806
Gaddis O, Morrow CP, Klement V, et al. (1983) Treatment for cervical carcinoma employing a template for transperitoneal interstitial Ir192 brachytherapy, Int J Radiat Oncol Biol Phys 9:819–827
Gallion HH, van Nagell JR Jr, Donaldson ES, et al. (1985) Combined radiation therapy and extrafascial hysterectomy in the treatment of stage IB barrel-shaped cervical cancer. Cancer 56:262–265
Gaspar LE, Cheung AY, Allen H (1989) Cervical carcinoma: treatment results and complications of extended-field irradiation. Radiology 172:271–277
Gauthier P, Gore I, Shingleton HM, et al. (1985) Identification of histopathologic risk groups in stage IB squamous cell carcinoma of the cervix. Obstet Gynecol 66:569–580
Gauwerky F (1977) Kurzzeit-Afterloading-Curietherapie gynakologischer Karzinome. Technik und Problematik. Strahlenther 153:793–801
Gauwerky F (1980) Weibliche Genitalorgane. In: Scherer E (ed) Strahlentherapie. Radiologische Onkologie, 2nd edn. Springer, Berlin Heidelberg New York, pp 661–722
Gerbaulet A, Michel G, Haddad E, et al. (1983) Surgical management and integrated therapies in cervical cancer. Eur J Gynecol Oncol 1:74–80
Gerbaulet A, Vuong T, Haie C, et al. (1990a) Endocavitary brachytherapy in cervical carcinoma. In: The cervix and lower female genital tract. Societa Milanesa di studi gineclogici, Milano 8:235–242
Gerbaulet A, Haie C, Chassagne D (1990b) Role de la curietherapie dans le traitement des cancers gynecologiques. Bull Cancer Radiother 77:245–250
Gerbaulet A, Haie C, Michel G, et al. (1990c) Cervix radiosurgical treatment in early invasive carcinoma according to prognostic factors. Experience of the Gustav-Roussy Institute. In: The cervix and lower female genital tract. Societa Milanesa di studi Ginecologica, Milano 8:111–116
Gerbaulet A, Haie-Meder H, Delapierre M, et al. (1992a) Curietherapie des cancers du col uterin. Method de l'lnstitut Gustave-Roussy. Bull Cancer Radiother 79:107–117
Gerbaulet A, Horiot JC, Dutreix A (1992b) Cancers de l'uterus. In: Le Bourgeois J-P, Chavaudra J, Eschwege F (eds) Radiotherapie oncologique. Hermann, Paris, pp 269–281
Gerbaulet A, Horiot JC, Dutreix A (1992c) Cancers gynecologiques: generalites sur la radiotherapie des cancers gynecologiques. In: Le Bourgeois J-P, Chavaudra J, Eschwege F (eds) Radiotherapie oncologique. Hermann, Paris, pp 253–268
Gerbaulet A, Kunkler I, Kerr GR, et al. (1992d) Combined radiotherapy and surgery: local control and complications in early carcinoma of the uterine cervix – the Villejuif experience 1975–1984. Radiother Oncol 23:66–73
Giannone L, Brenner DE, Jones HW, et al. (1987) Combination chemotherapy for patients with advanced carcinoma of the cervix: trial of mitomycin-c, vincristine, bleomycin, and cisplatin. Gynecol Oncol 26:178–187
Gleeson N, Baile W, Roberts WS, et al. (1994) Pudendal thigh fasciocutaneous flap for vaginal reconstruction in gynecologic cancer patients. Gynecol Oncol 54:269–274
Gluckman A, Cherry C (1956) Incidence, histology and response to radiation of mixed carcinoma (adenoacanthomas) of the uterine cervix. Cancer 9:971–978
Goddis O, Morrow CP, Klement V, et al. (1983) Treatment for cervical carcinoma employing a template for transperineal interstitial Ir-192 brachytherapy. Int J Radiat Oncol Biol Phys 9:819–827
Gray MJ, Gusberg SB, Guttman R (1958) Pelvic lymph node dissection following radiotherapy. Am J Obstet Gynecol 76:629–636
Green JA, Jennings WA (1951) New techniques in radium and radon therapy. J Facult Radiol 2:206–223
Greenberg BR, Hanningan J, Gerretson L (1982) Sequential combination of bleomycin and mitomycin in advanced cervical cancer: an American experience. A Northern California Oncology Group Study. Cancer Treat Rep 66:163–168
Greer BE, Easterling TR, McLennan DA, et al. (1989) Fetal and maternal considerations in the management of stage IB cervical cancer during pregnancy. Gynecol Oncol 34:61–65
Greer BE, Koh WJ, Figge DC, et al. (1990) Gynecologic radiotherapy fields defined by intraoperative measurements. Gynecol Oncol 38:421–424

Grigsby PW, Perez CA (1991) Radiotherapy alone for medically inoperable carcinoma of the cervix: stage Ia and carcinoma in situ. Int J Radiat Oncol Biol Phys 21:375–378

Grumbine FC, Rosenhein NB, Zerhouni EA, et al. (1981) Abdominopelvic computed tomography in the preoperative evaluation of early cervical carcinoma. Gynecol Oncol 12:286–290

Gynning I, Johnsson JE, Alm P, et al. (1983) Age and prognosis in stage IB squamous cell carcinoma of the uterine cervix. Gynecol Oncol 15:18–28

Hacker NF, Berek JS, Lagasse LD, et al. (1982) Carcinoma of the cervix in pregnancy. Obstet Gynecol 58:735–739

Hahn GM (1975) Radiotherapy and chemotherapy: some parallels and differences. Radiology 114:203–211

Haie C, Pejovic MH, Gerbaulet A, et al. (1988) Is prophylactic para-aortic irradiation worthwhile in the treatment of advanced cervical carcinoma? Results of a controlled clinical trial of the EORTC radiotherapy group. Radiother Oncol 11:101–112

Hamberger AD, Fletcher GH, Wharton JT (1978) Results of treatment of early stage I carcinoma of the uterine cervix with intracavitary radium alone. Cancer 41:980–985

Hammer J, Zoidl JP, Altendorfer C, et al. (1993) Combined external and high-dose rate intracavitary radiotherapy in the primary treatment of cancer of the uterine cervix. Radiother Oncol 27:66–68

Hanks GE, Herring DF, Kramer S (1983) Patterns of care outcome studies: results of the national practice in carcinoma of the cervix. Cancer 51:959–967

Hardt N, van Nagell JR Jr, Hanson MB, et al. (1982) Radiation-induced tumor regression as a prognostic factor in patients with invasive cervical cancer. Cancer 49:35–43

Hatch KD, Gelder MS, Soong SJ, et al. (1990) Pelvic exenteration with low rectal anastomosis: survival, complications and prognostic factors. Gynecol Oncol 38:462–467

Hautmann RE, Egghart G, Frohneberg D, et al. (1988) The ileal neobladder. J Urol 139:39–45

Hawnaur JM, Johnson RJ, Hunter RD, et al. (1992) The value of magnetic resonance imaging in assessment of carcinoma of the cervix and its response to radiotherapy. Clin Oncol 4:11–17

Heinzel F (1961) Über die Notwendigkeit der Rotationsbestrahlung in der Telekobalttherapie. Strahlentherapie 116:180–187

Heller PB, Malento JH, Bundy BN, et al. (1990) Clinical pathologic study of stage IIB, III and IVA carcinoma of the cervix: extended diagnostic evaluation for paraaortic node metastasis – a Gynecologic Oncology Group study. Gynecol Oncol 38:425–430

Henschke UK, Hilaris BS, Mahan GD (1960) "Afterloading" applicator for radiation therapy of carcinoma of the uterus. Radiology 74:834–839

Henschke UK, Hilaris BS, Mahan GD (1964) Intracavitary radiation therapy of cancer of the uterine cervix by remote afterloading with cycling sources. Am J Roentgenol 96:45–56

Herbolsheimer M (1993) Is individual treatment planning in gynaecological brachytherapy necessary? In: Mould RF, Muller R-P (eds) Brachytherapy in Germany. Nucletron International, Veenendaal, pp 145–155

Herbst AL, Cole P, Norusis MJ, et al. (1979) Epidemiologic aspects and factors related to survival in 384 registry cases of clear cell adenocarcinoma of the vagina and cervix. Am J Obstet Gynecol 135:876–886

Hiraoka M, Jo G, Akuta K, et al. (1987) Radiofrequency capacitive hyperthermia for deep-seated tumors. I. Studies on thermometry. Cancer 60:121–127

Höckel M, Kutzner J, Bauer H, et al. (1989) Eine neue experimentelle Methode zur Behandlung von Beckenwandrezidiven gynakologischer Malignome. Geburtshilfe Frauenheilkd 49:1–5

Hohenfellner R (1987) Mainz-Pouch mit umbilicalem Stoma. Akt Urol 18:1–4

Hogan WM, Littman P, Griner L, et al. (1982) Results of radiation therapy given after radical hysterectomy. Cancer 49:1278–1285

Holloway R, To A, Moradi M, et al. (1989) Monitoring the course of cervical carcinoma with the squamous cell carcinoma serum radioimmunoassay. Obstet Gynecol 74:944–949

Hopkins MP, Schmidt RW, Roberts JA, et al. (1988) The prognosis and treatment of stage I adenocarcinoma of the cervix. Obstet Gynecol 72:915–922

Horiot JC, Pigneux J, Pourquier H, et al. (1988) Radiotherapy alone in carcinoma of the intact uterine cervix according to G.H. Fletcher guidelines: a French cooperative study of 1383 cases. Int J Radiat Oncol Biol Phys 14:605–611

Horiot JC, Pourquier H, Schraub S, et al. (1989) Current status of the management of cancer of the cervix in daily practice and in clinical research. In: Mould RF (ed) Brachytherapy 2. Nucletron International, Leersum, pp 199–214

Hreshchyshyn MM, Aron BS, Boronow RC, et al. (1979) Hydroxyurea or placebo combined with radiation to treat stages IIIB and IV cervical cancer combined to the pelvis. Int J Radiat Oncol Biol Phys 5:317–322

Hricak H, Lacey CG, Chang YC, et al. (1988) Invasive cervical carcinoma: comparison of MR imaging and surgical findings. Radiology 166:623–631

Hughes RR, Brewington KC, Hanjani P, et al. (1980) Extended irradiation for cervical cancer based on surgical staging. Gynecol Oncol 19:153

Hunter RD (1991) Female genital tract. In: Ponton R (ed) The radiotherapy of malignant disease. Springer, Berlin Heidelberg New York, pp 279–308

ICRU (1985) Dose and volume specification for reporting intracavitary therapy in gynecology, ICRU Report 38 (International Commission on Radiation Units and Measurements, Bethesda, Maryland)

Igboeli P, Kapp DS, Lawrence R, et al. (1983) Carcinoma of the cervical stump: comparison of radiation therapy factors, survival and patterns of failure with carcinoma of the intact uterus. Int J Radiat Oncol Biol Phys 9:153-159

Iio S, Yoshioka S, Nishio S, et al. (1993) Urodynamic evaluation for bladder dysfunction after radical hysterectomy. Jpn J Urol 84:535–540

Inoue T (1984) Prognostic significance of the depth of invasion relating to nodal metastases, parametrial extension, and cell types. A study of 628 cases with stage IB, IIA, and IIB cervical carcinoma. Cancer 54:3035–3042

Inoue T, Morita K (1990) The prognostic significance of number of positive nodes in cervical carcinoma stages IB, IIA, and IIB. Cancer 65:1923–1927

Inoue T, Morita K (1995) Long-term observation of patients treated by postoperative extended-field irradiation for nodal metastases from cervical carcinoma stages IB, IIA, and IIB. Gynecol Oncol 58:4–10

Inoue T, Okumura M (1984) Prognostic significance of parametrial extension in patients with cervical carcinoma stages IB, IIA and IIB: a study of 628 cases treated by

radical hysterectomy and lymphadenectomy with or without postoperative irradiation. Cancer 54:3035–3042
Inoue T, Chihara T, Morita K (1984) The prognostic significance of the size of the largest nodes in metastatic carcinoma from the uterine cervix. Gynecol Oncol 19:187–198
Janus CL, Mendelson DS, Moore S, et al. (1989) Staging of cervical carcinoma: accuracy of magnetic resonance imaging and computed tomography. Clin Imaging 13:114–116
Jenkins RD, Stryker JA (1968) The influence of the blood pressure on survival in cancer of the cervix. Br J Radiol 41:913–920
Jobsen JJ, Leer JW, Cleton FJ, et al. (1989) Treatment of locoregional recurrence of carcinoma of the cervix by radiotherapy after primary surgery. Gynecol Oncol 33:368–371
Jolles CJ, Freedman RS, Hamberger AD, et al. (1986) Complications of extended-field therapy for cervical carcinoma without prior surgery. Int J Radiat Oncol Biol Phys 12:179–183
Jolles LJ (1988) Gynecologic cancer associated with pregnancy. Semin Oncol 6:417–424
Jones WB, Lewis JL, Rubin SC, et al. (1993) Early invasive carcinoma of the cervix. Gynecol Oncol 51:26–32
Joslin CAF (1989) High-activity source afterloading in gynecological cancer and its future prospects. ECHO 5:69–81
Jpn. Soc. Obstet. Gynecol. (1987) The general rules of uterine cervical cancer. Kanehara, pp 1–88
Jpn. Soc. Obstet. Gynecol. (1990) The 29th annual report on the treatment results of the cervical cancer. Jpn J Obstet Gynecol 40:299–309
Jpn. Soc. Obstet. Gynecol. (1993) The 30th annual report on the treatment results of the cervical cancer. Jpn J Obstet Gynecol 45:275–314
Kamura T, Tsukamoto N, Tsuruchi N, et al. (1992) Multivariate analysis of the histopathologic prognostic factors of cervical cancer in patients undergoing radical hysterectomy. Cancer 69:181–193
Kapp DS, Lawrence R (1984) Temperature elevation during brachytherapy for carcinoma of the uterine cervix: adverse effect on survival and enhancement of distant metastasis. Int J Radiat Oncol Biol Phys 10:2281–2292
Kataoka M, Kawamura M, Hamamoto K, et al. (1992a) Results of the combination of external beam and high-dose rate intracavitary irradiation for patients with cervical carcinoma. Gynecol Oncol 44:48–52
Kataoka M, Kawamura M, Nisiyama Y (1992b) Patterns of failure and survival in locally advanced carcinoma of the uterine cervix treated with high-dose rate intracavitary irradiation system. Int J Radiat Oncol Biol Phys 22:31–35
Kavanagh JJ, Rutledge F, Wharton JT, et al. (1982) Palliation of advanced recurrent pelvic malignancies by selective intra-arterial combination chemotherapy. Proc Am Soc Clin Oncol 1:109–116
Kessler II (1976) Human cervical cancer as a venereal disease. Cancer Res 36:783–788
Ketcham AS, Deckers PJ, Sugarbaker EV, et al. (1970) Pelvic exenteration for carcinoma of the uterine cervix. Cancer 26:513–519
Kiffer J (ed) Changes in brachytherapy. Wachholz, Nürnberg, pp 154–163
Kilcheski TS, Arger PH, Mulhern CJ, et al. (1981) Role of computed tomography in the presurgical evaluation of carcinoma of the cervix. J Comput Assist Tomogr 5:378–383
Kilgore LC, Soong S-J, Gore H, et al. (1988) Analysis of prognostic features in adenocarcinoma of the cervix. Gynecol Oncol 31:137–148
Kim RY, Trotti A, Wu CJ, et al. (1989) Radiation alone in the treatment of cancer of the uterine cervix: analysis of pelvic failure dose response relationship. Int J Radiat Oncol Biol Phys 17:973–978
Kim SH, Choi BI, Lee HP, et al. (1990) Uterine cervical carcinoma: comparison of CT and MR findings. Radiology 175:45–51
Kinney WK, Alvarez RD, Reid GC, et al. (1989) Value of adjuvant whole-pelvis irradiation after Wertheim hysterectomy for early-stage squamous carcinoma of the cervix with pelvic nodal metastasis: a matched-control study. Gynecol Oncol 34:258–265
Kinney WK, Egorshin EV, Ballard DJ, et al. (1992) Urodynamic study on urinary disturbance after therapy of uterine cancer. Jpn J Gynecol Obstet 44:440–446
Kjorstad KE (1977) Carcinoma of the cervix in the young patient. Obstet Gynecol 50:28–36
Kjorstad KE, Orjasaester H (1982) The prognostic value of CEA determinations in the plasma of patients with squamous cell cancer of the cervix. Cancer 50:283–286
Koeck G, Hillsinger WR (1971) Dosage tolerance of pelvic structures with cobalt 60 rotation radiation therapy. Am J Roentgenol 111:260–266
Kolstad P (1983) Recent clinical developments in gynecologic oncology. Raven Press, New York
Kottmeier HL (1964) Complications following radiation therapy in carcinoma of the cervix. Am J Obstet Gynecol 88:854–866
Krakoff IH (1977) Clinical, pharmacologic, and therapeutic studies of bleomycin given by continuous infusion. Cancer 40:2027–2032
Kraybill WG, Lopez M, Bricker EM (1988) Total pelvic exentration as a therapeutic option in advanced malignant disease of the pelvis. Surg Gynecol Obstet 166:259–267
Krebs HB, Helmkamp BF, Sevin BU, et al. (1982) Recurrent cancer of the cervix following hysterectomy and pelvic node dissection. Obstet Gynecol 59:422–427
Kreienberg R, Ebert J, Beck T, et al. (1990) Die Therapie des Zervixkarzinoms an der Univ. Frauenklinik Mainz. In: Teufel G, Pfleiderer A, Ladner HA (eds) Die Therapie des Zer. Vix Karzinoms. Springer, Berlin Heidelberg New York, pp 134–146
Kucera H, Vavra N (1990) Ein Risiko-Score für das operierte Zervixkarzinom im Stadium Ib und seine Bedeutung für die postoperative Bestrahlung. Wien klin Wochenschr 15:432–437
Kuipers T (1984) High dose-rate intracavitary irradiation: results of treatment. In: Mould RF (ed) Brachytherapy 1984. Nucletron International, Leersum, pp 169–175
Kummermehr J (1990) Strahlenbiologische Überlegungen zum Einfluss der Dosisleistung in der Brachytherapie. In: Baier K, Herbolsheimer M, Sauer O (eds) Interdisziplinäre Behandlungsformen beim Mammakarzinom und bei gynäkologischen Malignomen. Bonitas-Bauer, Würzburg, pp 29–54
Kuske RR, Perez CA, Grigsby PN, et al. (1989) Phase I/II study of definitive radiotherapy and chemotherapy (cisplatin and 5-fluorouracil) for advanced or recurrent gynecologic malignancies. Am J Clin Oncol 12:467–473
Lagasse LD, Creasman WT, Shingleton HM, et al. (1980) Results and complications of operative staging in cervical cancer: experience of the Gynecologic Oncology Group. Gynecol Oncol 9:90–98

Lamarque P, Coliez R (1951) Les cancers des organes genitaux de la femme. In: Delherm L (ed) Electroradiotherapie. Masson, Paris, pp 2549–2573

Lambin P, Gerbaulet A, Kramar A, et al. (1993) Phase III trial comparing two low dose rates in brachytherapy of cervix carcinoma: report at two years. Int J Radiat Oncol Biol Phys 25:405–412

Lange P (1960) Clinical and histological studies on cervical carcinoma: precancerous, early metastases and tubular structures in the lymph nodes. Acta Pathol Microbiol Scand 50(Suppl 143):9–28

Larsh DM, Stringer CA, Copeland LJ, et al. (1987) Stage IB cervical carcinoma treated with radical hysterectomy and pelvic lymphadenectomy: role of adjuvant radiotherapy. Obstet Gynecol 69:378–390

Larson D, Stringer CA, Copeland LJ, et al. (1987) Stage Ib cervical carcinoma treated with radical hysterectomy and pelvic lymphadenectomy: role of adjuvant radiotherapy. Obstet Gynecol 69:378–381

Larsson G, Alm P, Gullberg B, et al. (1983) Prognostic factors in early invasive carcinoma of the uterine cervix: a clinical, histopathologic, and statistical analysis of 343 cases. Am J Obstet Gynecol 146:145–152

La Vecchia C, Franceschi S, DeCarli A, et al. (1984) Dietary vitamin A and the risk of invasive cervical cancer. Int J Cancer 34:319–326

Lawhead RJ, Clark DG, Smith DH, et al. (1989) Pelvic exenteration for recurrent or persistent gynecologic malignancies: a 10-year review of the Memorial Sloan Kettering Cancer Center experience (1972–1981). Gynecol Oncol 33:279–282

Leibel S, Bauer M, Wasserman T, et al. (1987) Radiotherapy with or without misonidazole for patients with stage IIIB or stage IVA squamous cell carcinoma of the uterine cervix: preliminary report of a Radiation Therapy Oncology Group randomized trial. Int J Radiat Oncol Biol Phys 48:571–576

Leman MH, Benson WL, Kurman RJ, et al. (1976) Microinvasive carcinoma of the cervix. Obstet Gynecol 48:571–576

Levrant SG, Fruchter RG, Maiman M (1992) Radical hysterectomy for cervical cancer: morbidity and survival in relation to weight and age. Gynecol Oncol 45:317–322

Lien HH, Blomlie V, Kjerstad K, et al. (1991) Clinical stage I carcinoma of the cervix: value of MR in determining degree of invasiveness. Am J Roentgenol 156:1191–1194

Lindell LK, Anderson B (1987) Routine pretreatment evaluation of patients with gynecologic cancer. Obstet Gynecol 69:242–248

Lippman SM, Kavanagh JJ, Parades-Espinoza M (1992) 13-cis retinoic acid plus interferon 2 alpha. Highly active systemic therapy for squamous cell carcinoma of the cervix. J Natl Cancer Inst 84:241–245

Liu W, Meigs JU (1955) Radical hysterectomy and pelvic lymphadenectomy. A review of 473 cases including 244 for primary invasive carcinoma of the cervix. Am J Obstet Gynecol 69:1–32

Löffler E, van der Laarse R (1988) Technique and individual afterloading treatment planning simulating classic Stockholm brachytherapy for cervix cancer. In: Vahrson H, Rauthe G (eds) High-dose rate afterloading in the treatment of cancer of the uterus, breast and rectum. Strahlenther Onkol 82(Suppl):83–89

Lohe KJ, Burghardt E, Hillemanns HG, et al. (1978) Early squamous cell carcinoma of the uterine cervix. II. Clinical results of a cooperative study in the management of 419 patients with early stromal invasion and microcarcinoma. Gynecol Oncol 6:31–38

Loran OB, Pushkar DU (1992) Urethral instability after radical hysterectomy. J Urol (Paris) 98:210–212

Lovecchio JL, Averette HE, Donato D, et al. (1989) Five-year survival of patients with periaortic nodal metastases in clinical stage IB and IIA cervical carcinoma. Gynecol Oncol 34:43–51

Lowrey GC, Mendenhall WM, Million RR (1992) Stage IB or IIA-B of the intact uterine cervix treated with irradiation: a multivariate analysis. Int J Radiat Oncol Biol Phys 24:205–210

Magrina JF (1990) Types of pelvic exenterations: a reappraisal. Gynecol Oncol 37:363–366

Maiman M, Feurer G, Boyce J (1989) Value of squamous cell carcinoma antigen levels in invasive cervical carcinoma. Gynecol Oncol 32:96–104

Malkasian GS, Decker D, Muney E (1964) Preliminary observations of carcinoma of the cervix treated with 5-fluorouracil. Am J Obstet Gynecol 88:82–89

Marcial VA (1977) Carcinoma of the cervix: present status and future. Cancer 39:945–958

Marcial VA, Bosch A (1970) Radiation induced tumor regression in carcinoma of the uterine cervix. Prognostic significance. Am J Roentgenol 108:113–122

Marth C, Lang T, Koza A, et al. (1991) Vergleich der konventionellen Radium mit einer High-dose-rate-Afterloading-Brachytherapie beim Zervixkarzinom. Geburtshilfe Frauenheilkd 51:100–105

Martinez A (1984) A multiple site perineal applicator (MUPIT) for treatment of prostatic anorectal and gynecologic malignancies. Int J Radiat Oncol Biol Phys 10:297–305

Martinez A (1989) Interstitial and external beam therapy for the treatment of locally advanced cancers of the female genital tract. In: Rotte K, Kiffer J (eds) Changes in brachytherapy. Wachholz, Nürnberg, pp 154–163

Martinez A, Edmundson GK, Cox RS, et al. (1985) Combination of external beam irradiation and multiple-site perineal applicator (Mulpit) for treatment of locally advanced or recurrent prostatic, anorectal and gynecologic malignancies. Int J Radiat Oncol Biol Phys 11:391–398

Maruo T, Shibata K, Kimura A, et al. (1985) Tumor-associated antigen, TA-4, in the monitoring of the effects of therapy for squamous cell carinoma of the uterine cervix: serial determinations and tissue localization. Cancer 56:302–308

Maruyama Y, van Nagell JRV, Powell D, et al. (1992) Predictive value of specimen histology after preoperative radiotherapy in the treatment of bulky/barrel carcinoma of the cervix. Am J Clin Oncol 15:150–156

Mathe G (1970) Study of the clinical efficacy of bleomycin in human cancer. BMJ 2:243–249

McGuire WP, Arseneau J, Blessing JA, et al. (1989) A randomized comparative trial of carboplatin and iproplatin in advanced squamous carcinoma of the uterine cervix: a Gynecologic Oncology Group study. J Clin Oncol 7:1462–1469

Meanwell CA, Kelly KA, Wilson S, et al. (1988) Young age as a prognostic factor in cervical cancer: analysis of population based data from 10,002 cases. BMJ 296:386–392

Mellor HM (1960) Carcinoma of the cervix uteri treated by supervoltage only. Br J Radiol 33:20–25

Melnick S, Cole P, Anderson D (1987) Rates and risks of diethylstibesterol-related clear cell adenocarcinoma of the vagina and cervix. N Engl J Med 316:514–518

Methfessel HD, Retzke U, Methfessel G (1992) Urinary fistula after radical hysterectomy with lymph node excision. Geburtshilfe Frauenheilkd 52:88–91

Miller BE, Copeland LJ, Hamberger AD, et al. (1984) Carcinoma of the cervical stump. Gynecol Oncol 18:100–108

Monaghan JM, Ireland D, Mor-Yosef S, et al. (1990) Role of centralization of surgery in stage IB carcinoma of the cervix: a review of 498 cases. Gynecol Oncol 37:206–218

Monyak DJ, Twiggs LB, Potish RA, et al. (1988) Tolerance and preliminary results of simultaneous therapy with radiation and cisplatin for advanced cervical cancer. NCI Monogr 6:369–373

Moore JG, Wells RG, Morton DG (1966) Management of superficial cervical cancer in pregnancy. Obstet Gynecol 27:307–314

Moore G, Bross I, Austman R (1968) Effects of chlorambucil in 374 patients with advanced cancer. Cancer Chemother Rep 52:661–664

Morales P, Hussey DH, Maor MH, et al. (1981) Preliminary report of the M.D. Anderson Hospital randomized trial of neutron and photon irradiation for locally advanced carcinoma of the uterine cervix. Int J Radiat Oncol Biol Phys 7:1533–1540

Morita K (1988) Conformation radiotherapy computerized systemization of radiotherapy from CT/MRI to linear accelerator. In: Kärcher KH (ed) Progress in radiotherapy IV. Monduzzi Editore, Bologna, pp 1–5

Morita K, Uchiyama Y (1988) Present status of brachytherapy, especially HDR afterloading in Japan. In: Vahrson H, Rauthe G (eds) High dose rate afterloading in the treatment of cancer of the uterus, breast and rectum. Urban & Schwarzenberg, München, pp 16–21

Morita K, Kimura C, Takahashi K, et al. (1974) Verbesserung der Dosisverteilung bei der Konformationsbestrahlung des Kollumkarzinoms. Strahlentherapie 147:487–497

Morita K, Fuwa N, Kato E, et al. (1988) Results of conformation radiotherapy for carcinoma of the uterine cervix. External radiotherapy alone vs combined intracavitary and external radiotherapy. Endocurietherapy/Hyperthermia Oncology 4:137–148

Morita K, Uchiyama Y, Kato E (1995) Conformation radiotherapy: Japanese experiences. In: Kogelnik E (ed) Proceedings of 5th International Meeting on Progress in Radio-Oncology. Monduzzi Editore, Bologna, pp 333–338

Morita S, Arai T, Nakano T, et al. (1985) Clinical experience of fast neutron therapy for carcinoma of the uterine cervix. Int J Radiat Oncol Biol Phys 11:1439–1445

Morley GW, Seski JC (1976) Radical pelvic surgery versus radiation therapy for stage I carcinoma of the cervix (exclusive of microinvasion). Am J Obstet Gynecol 126:785–796

Morley GW, Hopkins MP, Lindenauer SM, et al. (1989) Pelvic exenteration, University of Michigan: 100 patients at 5 years. Obstet Gynecol 74:934–942

Morris M, Mitchell MF, Silva E, et al. (1993) Cervical conization as definitive therapy for early invasive squamous carcinoma of the cervix. Gynecol Oncol 51:193–196

Morrow CP, Shingleton HM, Averette HE, et al. (1980) Is pelvic radiation beneficial in the postoperative management of stage IB squamous cell carcinoma of the cervix with pelvic node metastasis treated by radical hysterectomy and pelvic lymphadenectomy? A report from the Presidential panel at the 1979 Annual Meeting of the Society of Gynecologic Oncologists. Gynecol Oncol 10:105–110

Morton DG, Lagasse LD, Moore JG, et al. (1964) Pelvic lymphadenectomy following radiation in cervical carcinoma. Am J Obstet Gynecol 88:932–940

Munzenrider JE, Doppke DP, Brown AP, et al. (1991) Three dimensional treatment planning for para-aortic node irradiation in patients with cervical cancer. Int J Radiat Oncol Biol Phys 21:229–242

Nass JM, Brady LW, Glassburn JR, et al. (1978) The radiotherapeutic management of carcinoma of the cervical stump. Int J Radiat Oncol Biol Phys 4:279–281

Neeff TC (1941) Die Bestimmung der Radium-Toleranzdosen auf Grund der Nebenwirkungen an der Harnblase bei der Strahlenbehandlung des Gebärmutterkrebses. Strahlentherapie 70:11–22

Nelson JH, Averette HE, Richart RM (1975) Detection, diagnostic evaluation and treatment of dysplasia and early carcinoma of the cervix. Cancer 25:134–135

Nelson JH Jr, Boyce J, Macasaet M, et al. (1977) Incidence, significance and follow-up of para-aortic lymph node metastases in late invasive carcinoma of the cervix. Am J Obstet Gynecol 128:336–340

Newton M (1975) Radical hysterectomy or radiotherapy for stage I cervical cancer. Am J Obstet Gynecol 123:535–542

Nishimura T (1965) Pelvic lymph node metastases in carcinoma of the uterine cervix. J Clin Obstet Gynecol (Jpn) 11:135–142

Nori D, Hilaris BS (1987) Role of interstitial implantation in gynecological cancer. In: Nori D, Hilaris BS (eds) Radiation therapy of gynecological cancer. Liss, New York, pp 283–296

Nori D, Valentine E, Hilaris BS (1985) The role of paraaortic node irradiation in the treatment of cancer of the cervix. Int J Radiat Oncol Biol Phys 11:1469–1475

O'Connell D, Joslin CA, Howard N, et al. (1967) Treatment of uterine carcinoma using the Cathetron. Br J Radiol 40:882–892

O'Quinn AG, Fletcher GH, Wharton JT (1980) Guidelines for conservative hysterectomy after irradiation. Gynecol Oncol 9:68–70

Oats JJN (1976) Carcinoma of the cervical stump. Br J Obstet Gynecol 83:896–899

Ohta A (1978) Basic and clinical studies on the simultaneous combination treatment of cervical cancer (especially advanced cases) with a carcinostatic agent and radiation. J Tokyo Med Coll 36:529–537

Orton CG, Somnay A (1994) Results of an international review on patterns care in cancer of the cervix. In: Mould RF, Battermann JJ, Martinez AA, Speiser BL (eds) Brachytherapy from radium to optimization. Nucletron International, Veenendaal, pp 49–54

Orton CG, Seyedsadr M, Somnay A (1991) Comparison of high and low dose rate remote afterloading for cervix cancer and the importance of fractionation. Int J Radiat Oncol Biol Phys 21:1425–1434

Overgaard J, Bentzen SM, Kolstad P, et al. (1989) Misonidazole combined with radiotherapy in the treatment of carcinoma of the uterine cervix. Int J Radiat Oncol Biol Phys 16:1069–1072

Parham G, Syed S, Savage E (1993) Concurrent chemoradiation followed by modified abdominal hysterectomy, pelvic and retroperitoneal para-aortic lymphadenectomy: effective multimodality treatment for advanced bulky cervical cancer. 24th Annual Meeting of the Society of Gynecologic Oncologists. Abstract No. 58

Parker LA, McPhail AH, Yankaskas BC, et al. (1990) Computed tomography in the evaluation of clinical stage IB carcinoma of the cervix. Gynecol Oncol 37:332–334

Parker RT, Wilbanks GD, Yowell RK, et al. (1967) Radical hysterectomy with and without preoperative radiotherapy for cervical cancer. Am J Obstet Gynecol 99:933–943

Paterson R (1952) Studies in optimum dosage. Br J Radiol 25:505–516
Patner B, Mann WJ (1989) Does preoperative serum squamous cell carcinoma (SCC) antigen level predict occult extracervical disease in patients with stage IB invasive squamous cell carcinoma of the cervix? Gynecol Oncol 32:95–103
Patton SF (1969) Diagnostic cytology of the uterine cervix. Williams & Wilkins, Baltimore
Penalver MA, Bejany DE, Averette HE, et al. (1989) Continent urinary diversion in gynecologic oncology. Gynecol Oncol 34:274–280
Perez CA (1992) Uterine cervix. In: Perez CA, Brady LW (eds) Principles and practice of radiation oncology, 2nd edn. Lippincott, Philadelphia, pp 1143–1202
Perez CA (1993) Carcinoma of the cervix. In: Devita JT, Hellman S, Rosenberg SA (eds) Cancer. Principles and practice of oncology, 4th edn. J.B. Lippincott, Philadelphia, pp 1168–1195
Perez CA, Kao MS, et al. (1985) Radiation therapy alone or combined with surgery in the treatment of barrel-shaped carcinoma of the uterine cervix (stages IB, IIA, IIB). Int J Radiat Oncol Biol Phys 11:1903–1909
Perez CA, Zivnuska F, Askin F, et al. (1975) Prognostic significance of endometrial extension from primary carcinoma of the uterine cervix. Cancer 35:1493–1504
Perez CA, Camel HM, Askin F, et al. (1981) Endometrial extension of carcinoma of the cervix. A prognostic factor that may modify staging. Cancer 48:170–180
Perez CA, Bedwinek JM, Breaux SR (1983a) Patterns of failure after treatment of gynecologic tumors. Cancer Treat Symp 2:217–231
Perez CA, Breaux S, Madc-Jones H, et al. (1983b) Radiation therapy alone in the treatment of carcinoma of uterine cervix. I. Analysis of tumor recurrence. Cancer 51:1393–1402
Perez CA, Breaus S, Bedwinek JM, et al. (1984) Radiation therapy alone in the treatment of carcinoma of the uterine cervix. II. Analysis of complications. Cancer 54:235–246
Perez CA, Camel HM, Walz BJ, et al. (1986) Radiation therapy alone in the treatment of carcinoma of the uterine cervix: a 20-year experience. Gynecol Oncol 23:127–134
Peters LJ, Hussey DH, Fletcher GH, et al. (1979) Second preliminary report of the M.D. Anderson study of neutron therapy for locally advanced gynecological tumors. In: Barendsen GW, Broerse JJ, Breur K (eds) High-LET radiations in clinical radiotherapy. Oxford University Press, Oxford
Peters RK, Thomas D, Hagan DG, et al. (1986) Risk factors for invasive cervical cancer among Latinas and non-Latinas in Los Angeles County. J Natl Cancer Inst 7:1063–1069
Pettersson F (1988) Annual report on the results of treatment in gynecological cancer. International Federation of Gynecology and Obstetrics, FIGO, Stockholm, vol 20
Pettersson F (1995) Annual report on the results of treatment in gynecological cancer. International Federation of Gynecology and Obstetrics, FIGO, Stockholm, vol 22
Piel I, Slaton R, Perlia CP (1973) Combination chemotherapy with bleomycin and disseminated cervical carcinoma: a preliminary study. Gynecol Oncol 1:184–189
Pierquin B, Marinello G (1975) Plesiocurietherapie des cancers du col de l'uterus. La methode de Creteil. J Eur Radiother 2:231–245
Pierquin B, Dutreix A, Paine CH, Chassagne D, Marinello G, Ash D (1978) The Paris system in interstitial radiation therapy. Acta Radiol Oncol 17:33
Pierquin B, Gauwerky F, Luin B, et al. (1987a) The Paris system in interstitial radiation therapy. Acta Radiol Oncol 17:33–41
Pierquin B, Wilson JF, Chassagne D (1987b) Cervix. In: Modern brachytherapy. Masson, New York, pp 175–203
Pierquin B, Mazeron JJ, Grimard L, et al. (1989) Normal tissue tolerance in brachytherapy. Front Radiat Ther Oncol 23:194–201
Piver MS, Barlow JJ (1977) High dose irradiation to biopsy confirmed aortic node metastases from carcinoma of the uterine cervix. Cancer 39:1243–1246
Piver MS, Chung WS (1975) Prognostic significance of cervical lesion size and pelvic node metastases in cervical carcinoma. Obstet Gynecol 46:507–512
Piver MS, Barlow JJ, Vongtama V, et al. (1974a) Hydroxyurea and radiation therapy in advanced cervical cancer. Am J Obstet Gynecol 20:969–972
Piver MS, Rutledge FN, Smith JP (1974b) Five classes of extended hysterectomy for women with cervical cancer. Obstet Gynecol 44:265–272
Piver MS, Barlow JJ, Krisnamsetty R (1981) Five-year survival in patients with biopsy confirmed aortic node metastasis from cervical carcinoma. Am J Obstet Gynecol 139:575–582
Piver MS, Marchetti DL, Patton T, et al. (1988) Radical hysterectomy and pelvic lymphadenectomy versus radiation therapy for small (less than or equal 3 cm) stage IB cervical carcinoma. Am J Clin Oncol 11:21–24
Plentl AA, Friedman EA (1971) Lymphatic system of the female genitalia. Saunders, Philadelphia
Podczaski E, Stryker JA, Kaminski P, et al. (1990) Extended-field radiation therapy for carcinoma of the cervix. Cancer 66:251–258
Potish R, Adcock L, Jones TJ, et al. (1983) The morbidity and utility of peraortic radiotherapy in cervical carcinoma. Gynecol Oncol 15:1–9
Potter ME, Hatch KD, Potter MY, et al. (1989) Factors affecting the response of recurrent squamous cell carcinoma of the cervix to cisplatin. Cancer 63:1283–1287
Potter ME, Alverez RD, Gay FL, et al. (1990) Optimal therapy for pelvic recurrence after radical hysterectomy for early-stage cervical cancer. Gynecol Oncol 37:74–77
Pourquier H, Dubois JB, Delard R (1985) Cancer of the uterine cervix. Dosimetric guidelines for prevention of late rectal and rectosigmoid complications as a result of radiotherapeutic treatment. Int J Radiat Oncol Biol Phys 8:1887–1895
Prade M, Gerbaulet A, Charpenier P, et al. (1977) Confrontation histologie-dosimetrie apres curietherapie et chirurgie dans les cancers du col stades I et II. J Radiol 5:375–380
Prasasvinichai S, Glassburn JR, Brady LW, et al. (1978) Treatment of recurrent carcinoma of the cervix. Int J Radiat Oncol Biol Phys 4:957–961
Pratt JH (1961) Sigmoidovaginostomy: a new method of obtaining satisfactory vaginal depth. Am J Obstet Gynecol 81:535–545
Prempree T, Patanaphan V, Scott RM (1979) Radiation management of carcinoma of the cervical stump. Cancer 43:1262–1273
Pursell SH, Day TG Jr, Tobin GR (1990) Distally based rectus abdominis flap for reconstruction in radical gynecologic procedures. Gynecol Oncol 37:234–238
Rampone JF, Klem V, Kolstad P (1973) Combined treatment of stage IB carcinoma of the cervix. Obstet Gynecol 41:163–167
Randall ME (1993) Interstitial reirradiation for recurrent gynecologic malignancies: results and analysis of prognostic factors. Gynecol Oncol 48:23–31

Randall ME, Constable WC, Hahn SS, et al. (1988) Results of radiotherapeutic management of carcinoma of the cervix with emphasis on the influence of histologic classification. Cancer 62:48–59

Rapp F, Duff R (1974) Oncogenic conversion of normal cells by inactivated herpes simplex virus. Cancer 34:1353–1366

Reeves WC, Brinton LA, Garcia M, et al. (1989) Human papillomavirus infection and cervical cancer in Latin America. N Engl J Med 320:1437–1443

Regan JW, Ng ABP (1973) The cellular manifestations of uterine carcinomas. In: Norris HJ, Hertig AT, Abell MR (eds) The uterus. Williams & Wilkins, Baltimore

Regaud C (1929) Radiotherapy of carcinoma of the cervix uteri. Paris method. Am J Roentgenol 21:392–404

Rettenmaier MA, Casanova DM, Micha JP, et al. (1982) Radical hysterectomy and tailored postoperative radiation therapy in the management of bulky stage IB cervical cancer. Cancer 63:2220–2224

Roche WD, Norris HJ (1975) Microinvasive carcinoma of the cervix: the significance of lymphatic invasion and confluent patterns of stromal growth. Cancer 36:180–187

Rodriguez GC, Clarke-Pearson DL, Soper JT, et al. (1993) The negative prognostic implications of thrombocytosis in women with stage IB cervix cancer. Gynecol Oncol 83:445–448

Roman TN, Souhami L, Freeman CR, et al. (1991) High doserate afterloading intracavitary therapy in carcinoma of the cervix. Int J Radiat Oncol Biol Phys 20:921–926

Rosenwald J-C, Dutreix A (1970) Etude d'un programme sur ordinateur pour le calcul des doses en curietherapie gynecologique. J Radiol 51:651–654

Roth SL, Nitz U, Mosny D (1994) Der Wert der adjuvanten Strahlen- oder Chemotherapie nach primar operativer Therapie eines Zervixkarzinoms. Gynäkologe 27:89–98

Rotman M, Choi K, Guse C, et al. (1990) Prophylactic irradiation of the paraaortic lymphnode chain in stage IIB and bulky stage IB carcinoma of the cervix, initial treatment results of RTOG 79-20. Int J Radiat Oncol Biol Phys 19:513–521

Rotte K (1968) Ulkus und Fistel als Komplikationen an Blase und Rektum bei der Strahlenbehandlung des Kollumkarzinoms. Zentralbl Gynäkol 90:1149–1159

Rotte K (1975) Übersicht über die Afterloadingverfahren in der gynakologischen Strahlentherapie. Strahlentherapie 150:237–242

Rotte K (1981) Ferngesteuerte Afterloadingverfahren. In: Wannenmacher M, Schreiber HW, Gauwerky F, et al. (eds) Kombinierte chirurgische und radiologische Therapie maligner Tumoren. Urban & Schwarzenberg, München, pp 313–319

Rotte K (1983) Das ferngesteuerte Nachladeverfahren (remote-controlled afterloading) für die intrakavitare Kontakttherapie (Brachytherapie) gynäkologischer Karzinome. Radiologe 23:20–23

Rotte K (1985) Klinische Ergebnisse der Afterloading-Kurzzeittherapie im Vergleich zur Radiumtherapie. Strahlentherapie 161:323–328

Rotte K (1987) Die Bedeuting der Strahlentheapie fur die Behandlung des Kollumkarzinoms. Gynäkol Rundsch 27:1–10

Rotte K (1991) Comparison between high dose rate afterloading and conventional radium therapy. In: Sauer R (ed) Interventional radiation therapy. Springer, Berlin Heidelberg New York, pp 311–315

Rubin P (1984) The Franz Buschke Lecture: late effects of chemotherapy and radiation therapy: a new hypothesis. Int J Radiat Oncol Biol Phys 10:5–34

Rubin P (1990) Law and order of radiation sensitivity. Absolute versus relative. In: Vaeth JL, Meyer JL (eds) Radiation tolerance of normal tissue Front Radiat Ther Oncol 23:7–39

Rubin P, Casarett GW (1968) Clinical radiation pathology, vols I and II. Saunders, Philadelphia

Rubin P, Constine LS, Fajardo LF, et al. (1995) Overview of late effects normal tissues (LENT) scoring system. Radiother Oncol 35:9–60

Rubin SC, Brookland R, Mikuta JJ, et al. (1984) Long-term survival following extended field radiotherapy. Gynecol Oncol 18:213–221

Runowicz CD, Wadler S, Rodriguez-Rodriguez L, et al. (1989) Concomitant cisplatin and radiotherapy in locally advanced cervical carcinoma. Gynecol Oncol 34:395–401

Rustin GJS, Newlands ES (1988) Phase I–II study of carboplatin, vincristine, methotrexate, and bleomycin (COMB) in carcinoma of the cervix. Br J Cancer 58:818–824

Rutledge FN (1987) Pelvic exenteration: an update of the U.T.M.D. Anderson Hospital experience and review of the literature. In: Gynecologic cancer: diagnosis and treatment strategies. 29

Rutledge FN, Gutierrez AG, Fletcher GH (1968) Management of stage I and II adenocarcinomas of the uterine cervix on the intact uterus. Am J Roentgenol 102:161–168

Rutledge FN, Galakatos AE, Wharton JT, et al. (1975) Adenocarcinoma of the uterine cervix. Am J Obstet Gynecol 122:236–242

Rutledge FN, Wharton JT, Fletcher GH (1976) Clinical studies with adjunctive surgery and irradiation therapy in the treatment of carcinoma of the cervix. Cancer 38:596–602

Rutledge FN, Smith JP, Wharton JT, et al. (1977) Pelvic exenteration: analysis of 196 patients. Am J Obstet Gynecol 129:881–887

Rutledge FN, Mitchell JF, Munsell J (1992) Youth as a prognostic factor in carcinoma of the cervix: a matched analysis. Gynecol Oncol 44:123–135

Sauer OA (1992) Individual dose distribution optimization with the ring applicator for HDR cervical cancer brachytherapy. In: 7th International Brachytherapy Working Conference Baltimore, Washington. Nucletron, Veenendaal, pp 203–207

Sauer OA, Gotz-Gersitz U, Gullenstein M-L, et al. (1994) Precision of the dose calculated for bladder and rectum in HDR gynecological brachytherapy. Endocurie Hypertherm Oncol 10:79–82

Schmidt BF, Hirnle P, Kaulich TW, et al. (1991) Wert der Kernspintomographie zur Planung der HDR-Afterloading-Brachytherapie bei Zervixkarzinmomen. Fortschr Röntgenstr 155:109–116

Schreuder HW, Vierhout ME, Veen HF (1993) Disabling constipation following Wertheim's radical hysterectomy. Ned Tijdschr Geneeskd 137:1059–1062

Schulz-Wendtland R, Bauer M, Teufel G, et al. (1991) Zervixkarzinomrezidive und ihre Behandlung an der Universitats-Frauenklinik Freiburg in den Jahren 1976 bis 1985. Strahlenther Onkol 167:82–88

Sekiba K (1981) Early diagnosis of the cervical cancer. Sougou Rinshou 33:131–135

Sekiba K, Hasegawa T, Kobayashi Y (1993) Hyperthermic treatment for gynecological malignancies. In: Matsuda T (ed) Cancer treatment by hyperthermia, radiation and drugs. Taylor & Francis, London, pp 261–270

Senekjian EK, Young JM, Weiser P, et al. (1987) An evaluation of squamous cell carcinoma antigen in patients with cervical squamous cell carcinoma. Am J Obstet Gynecol 157:433–440

Seski JC, Abel MR, Morley GW (1977) Microinvasive squamous carcinoma of the cervix: definition, histologic analysis, late results of treatment. Obstet Gynecol 50:410–417

Sharma S, Patel FD, Sandhu APS, et al. (1989) A prospective randomized study of local hyperthermia as a supplement and radiosensitizer in the treatment of carcinoma of the cervix with radiotherapy. Endocurie Hypertherm Oncol 5:151–160

Shingleton HM, Fowler JR, Koch GG (1971) Pretreatment evaluation in cervical cancer. Am J Obstet Gynecol 110:385–390

Shingleton HM, Gore H, Bradley DH, et al. (1981) Adenocarcinoma of the cervix. I. Clinical evaluation and pathologic features. Am J Obstet Gynecol 139:799–806

Shingleton HM, Song SJ, Gelder MS, et al. (1989) Clinical and histopathologic factors predicting recurrence and survival after pelvic exenteration for cancer of the cervix. Obstet Gynecol 73:1027–1034

Silvio A, Aristizabal MD, Surwit EA (1983) Treatment of advanced cancer of the cervix with transperitoneal insterstitial irradiation. Int J Radiat Oncol Biol Phys 9:1013–1017

Simon NL, Gore H, Shingleton HM, et al. (1986) Study of superficially invasive carcinoma of the cervix. Obstet Gynecol 68:19–26

Skov K, MacPhail S (1991) Interaction of platinum drugs with clinically relevant x-ray doses in mammalian cells: a comparison of cisplatin, carboplatin, iproplatin, and tetraplatin. Int J Radiat Oncol Biol Phys 20:221–225

Slater JM, Fletcher GH (1971) Ureteral strictures after radiotherapy for carcinoma of the uterine cervix. Am J Roentgenol 111:269–281

Slavik M (1975) Adriamycin activity in genitourinary and gynecologic malignancies. Cancer Chemother Rep 6:297–306

Smit BJ, Schmitt G (1993) High-dose rate (HDR) Afterloading Therapie in Kombination mit perkutaner Therapie beim inoperablen Zervixkarzinom. In: Roth L, Böttcher HD (eds) Gynäkologische Strahlentherapie. Enke, Stuttgart, pp 38–47

Smith JP, Rutledge F, Burns B, et al. (1967) Systemic chemotherapy for carcinoma of the cervix. Am J Obstet Gynecol 97:800–809

Soisson AP, Soper JT, Clarke-Pearson DL, et al. (1990) Adjuvant radiotherapy following radical hysterectomy for patients with stage IB and IIA cervical cancer. Gynecol Oncol 37:390–398

Stolinsky D, Bateman J (1973) Further experience with hexamethyl-melamine in the treatment of carcinoma of the cervix. Cancer Chemother Rep 57:497–503

Sudarsanam A, Charyulu K, Belinson J, et al. (1978) Influence of exploratory celiotomy on the management of carcinoma of the cervix: a preliminary report. Cancer 41:1049–1053

Suit HE, Fletcher GH (1963) Modification of Fletcher ovoid system for afterloading using standard-sized radium tubes. Radiology 81:126–134

Surmont J, Guy E, Fajbisowicz S, et al. (1956) Possibilites de coodination correcte de la curie et de la roentgentheraie dans le traitement du cancer du col. J Radiol 37:252–259

Sutton G, Bundy B, Delgado G, et al. (1993) Evaluation of pelvic radiotherapy following radical hysterectomy in patients with clinical stage Ib squamous carcinoma of the cervix: a study of the gynecologic oncology group. 24th Annual Meeting of the Society of Gynecologic Onocologists. Abstract No. 19

Syed AM, Feder BH (1977) Technique of afterloading interstitial implants. Radiol Clin North Am 46:458–475

Syed AMN, Puthawala AA (1987) Interstitial-intracavitary Syed-Neblett applicator in the treatment of carcinoma of the cervix. In: Nori D, Hilaris BS (eds) Radiation therapy of gynecologial cancer. Liss, New York, pp 297–307

Syed AMN, Puthawala AA, Neblett D, et al. (1986) Transperitoneal interstitial intracavitary "Syed-Neblett" applicator in the treatment of carcinoma of the uterine cervix. Endocurie Hypertherm Oncol 2:1–13

Symmonds RE, Pratt JH, Webb MJ (1975) Exentrative operations: experience with 198 patients. Am J Obstet Gynecol 121:907–916

Takahashi S (1965) Conformation radiotherapy: rotation techniques as applied to radiography and radiotherapy of cancer. Acta Radiol 242 (Suppl):1–142

Taki I, Sugimori H, Matsuyama T, et al. (1979) The treatment of microinvasive carcinoma. Obstet Gynecol Surv 34:839–845

Tamimi HK, Figge DC (1982) Adenocarcinoma of the uterine cervix. Gynecol Oncol 13:335–342

Tazaki E, Arai T, Oryu S (1965) TAO-type afterloading device for the cervical cancer. Jpn J Clin Rad 10:768–775

Terris M, Wilson F, Nelson JJ (1973) Relation of circumcision to cancer of the cervix. Am J Obstet Gynecol 117:1056–1066

Teshima T, Chatani M, Hata K, et al. (1987) High-dose rate intracavitary therapy for carcinoma of the uterine cervix: general findings of survival and complication. Int J Radiat Oncol Biol Phys 13:1035–1041

Teshima T, Chatani M, Hata K, et al. (1988) High dose-rate intracavitary therapy for carcinoma of the uterine cervix: II. Risk factors for rectal complication. Int J Radiat Oncol Biol Phys 14:281–286

Teshima T, Inoue T, Ikeda H, et al. (1993) High-dose rate and low-dose rate intracavitary therapy for carcinoma of the uterine cervix: Cancer 72:2409–2414

Teufel F, Nestle U, Senst A, et al. (1990) Ist die Radikaloperation im Stadium IIb zu rechtfertigen? In: Teufel G, Pfleiderer A, Ladner HA (eds) Therpie des Zerviskarzinoms. Springer, Berlin Heidelberg New York, pp 153–171

Teufel G, Ladner H-A, Pfleiderer A (1992) Therapie des Zervixkarzinoms in der Frauenklinik Freiburg 1975–1986. In: Ladner H-A, Pfleiderer A, Profous CZ (eds) Gynäkologische Radiologie. Springer, Berlin Heidelberg New York, pp 47–67

TeVelde ER, Persijn JP, Ballieux RE, et al. (1982) Carcinoembryonic antigen serum levels in patients with squamous cell carcinoma of the uterine cervix: clinical significance. Cancer 49:1866–1869

Tewfik HH, Buchsbaum HJ, Latourette HB, et al. (1982) Paraaortic lymph node irradiation in carcinoma of the cervix after exploratory laparotomy and biopsy proven positive aortic nodes. Int J Radiat Oncol Biol Phys 8:13–21

Thigpen T, Shingleton H, Homesley H, et al. (1981) Cisplatinum in treatment of advanced or recurrent squamous cell carcinoma of the cervix: a phase II study of the Gynecologic Oncology Group. Cancer 48:889–894

Thomas GM, Dembo AJ, Black B, et al. (1987) Concurrent radiation and chemotherapy for carcinoma of the cervix recurrent after radical surgery. Gynecol Oncol 27:254–260

Tod M, Meredith WJ (1938) A dosage system for use in the treatment of cancer of the uterine cervix. Br J Radiol 11:809–824

Touboul E, Lefranc JP, Blondon J, et al. (1992) Preoperative radiation therapy and surgery in the treatment of "bulky" squamous cell carcinoma of the uterine cervix (stage IB, IIA and IIB operable tumours). Radiother Oncol 24: 32–40

Trelford J, Tsodikov A, Yakolev A (1993) Exophytic or endophytic stage I squamous carcinoma of the cervix - is there a difference in survival by therapy? 24th Annual Meeting of the Society of Gynecologic Oncologists. Abstract No. 54
Trevathan E, Layde P, Webster LA, et al. (1983) Cigarette smoking and dysplasia and carcinoma in situ of the uterine cervix. JAMA 250:499–503
Trope C, Horvath G, Haadem K, et al. (1986) Doxorubicin-cisplatin combination chemotherapy for recurrent carcinoma of the cervix. Cancer Treat Rep 70:1325–1330
Tsukamoto N, Kaku T, Matsukuma K, et al. (1989) The problem of stage Ia (FIGO 1985) carcinoma of the uterine cervix. Gynecol Oncol 34:1–9
Ulmer HU, Frischbier H-J (1982) Die ausschliessliche percutane Strahlenbehandlung fortgeschrittener Kollumkarzinome. Geburtshilfe Frauenheilkd 42:243–344
Utley JF, von Essen CF, Horn RA, et al. (1984) High dose-rate afterloading brachytherapy in carcinoma of the uterine cervix. Int J Radiat Oncol Biol Phys 10:2259–2263
Vahrson H (1973) Die biaxiale bisegmentale Telekobaltpendelbestrahlung in der Therapie des Kollumkarzinom. Habilitationsschrift, Univ. Giessen
Vahrson H, Römer G (1988) 5-year results with HDR afterloading in cervix cancer: dependence on fractionation and dose. In: Vahrson H, Rauthe G (eds) High dose rate afterloading in the treatment of cancer of the uterus, breast and rectum Strahlenther Onkol 82 (Suppl):139–146
van den Brule AJ, Claas EC, Du MM, et al. (1989) Use of anticontamination primers in the polymerase chain reaction for the detection of human papilloma virus genotypes in cervical scrapes and biopsies. J Med Virol 29:20–27
Van Herik M (1965) Fever as a complication of radiation therapy for carcinoma of the cervix. Am J Roentgenol 93:104–109
van Nagell JR Jr, Sprague AD, Roddick JW (1975) The effect of intravenous pyelography and cystoscopy on the staging of cervical cancer. Gynecol Oncol 3:87–93
van Nagell JR Jr, Donaldson ES, Parker JC, et al. (1977) The prognostic significance of cell type and lesion size in patients with cervical cancer treated by radical surgery. Gynecol Oncol 5:142–149
van Nagell JR Jr, Rayburn W, Donaldson ES, et al. (1979) Therapeutic implications of patterns of recurrence in cervical cancer. Cancer 44:2354–2359
van Nagell JR Jr, Greenwell N, Power DE, et al. (1983) Microinvasive carcinoma of the cervix. Am J Obstet Gynecol 145:981–995
van Nagell JR Jr, Powell DE, Gallion HH, et al. (1988) Small cell carcinoma of the uterine cervix. Cancer 62:1586–1598
van Nagell JR Jr, Higgins RV, Powell DE (1993) Invasive cervical cancer. In: Knapp RC, Berkowitz RS (eds) Gynecologic oncology. McGraw-Hill, New York, pp 192–221
Vavra N, Sevelda P, Barrada M, et al. (1989) Die Bedeutung der primären Bestrahlung des invasiven Adenokarzinoms der Cervix uteri. Geburtshilfe Frauenheilkd 49:793–796
Vavra N, Sevelda P, Seifert M (1992) Zum Wert der adjuvanten Bestrahlung bei Lymphgefässeinbrüchen bei Patientinnen mit einem Zervixkarzinom in histopathologischen Stadium Ib und negativen Lympknoten. Strahlenther Onkol 168:524–527
Vercamer R, Janssens J, Usewils R, et al. (1987) Computed tomography and lymphography in the presurgical staging of early carcinoma of the uterine cervix. Cancer 60:1745–1750
Wakabayashi M, Irie G, Sugahara T, et al. (1966) Remote afterloading device for cancer of the uterine cervix. Jpn J Clin Radiol 11:678–684
Waterman GW, Raphael SI (1950) Treatment of cancer of the cervix by radium and deep X-rays. N Engl J Med 242:689–691
Waterman GW, DiLeone R, Tracy E (1947) The use of long interstitial radium needles in the treatment of cancer of the cervix. Am J Roentgenol 57:671–678
Watson ER, Halnan KE, Dische S, et al. (1978) Hyperbaric oxygen and radiotherapy: a Medical Research Council trial in carcinoma of the cervix. Br J Radiol 51:879–887
Weiner S, Wizenberg MJ (1975) Treatment of primary adenocarcinoma of the cervix. Cancer 35:1514–1519
Wenderoth UK, Bachor R, Egghart G, et al. (1990) The ileal neobladder: experience and results of more than 100 consecutive cases. J Urol 143:492–497
Wentz WB, Reagan JW (1959) Survival in cervical cancer with respect to cell type. Cancer 12:384–396
Wharton JT, Jones H, Day TJ, et al. (1977) Preirradiation celiotomy and extended field irradiation for invasive carcinoma of the cervix. Obstet Gynecol 49:333–338
Wheeless CR, Hempling RE (1989) Rectal J-pouch reservoir to decrease the frequency of tenesmus and defection in low coloproctostomy. Gynecol Oncol 35:136–138
Wheems D, Mendenhall W, Bova F (1985) Carcinoma of the intact uterine cervix, stage IB-IIA-B, >6 cm in diameter: irradiation alone versus preoperative irradiation and surgery. Int J Radiat Oncol Biol Phys 11:1911–1914
Wiggings DL, Granai CO, Steinhoff MM, et al. (1995) Tumor angiogenesis as a prognostic factor in cervical carcinoma. Gynecol Oncol 56:353–356
Wijredman HK, Bakker CJ (1988) Multiple slice MR imaging as an aid in radiotherapy of carcinoma of the cervix uteri. A case report. Strahlenther Onkol 164:44–47
Williams EA (1964) Congenital absence of the vagina: a simple operation for its relief. J Obstet Gynecol Br Comm 24:511–512
Wong LC, Choo YLC, Choy D, et al. (1989) Long-term follow-up of potentiation of radiotherapy by cis-platinum in advanced cervical cancer. Gynecol Oncol 35:159–163
Yajima A, Noda K (1979) The results of treatment of microinvasive carcinoma (stage IA) of the uterine cervix by means of simple and extended hysterectomy. Am J Obstet Gynecol 135:685–693
Zander J, Baltzer J, Lohe KJ, et al. (1981) Carcinoma of the cervix: an attempt to individualize treatment. Results of a 20-year cooperative study. Am J Obstet Gynecol 13:752–759
Zola P, Volpe T, Castelli G (1989) Is the published literature a reliable guide for deciding alternative treatments for patients with early cervical cancer? Int J Radiat Oncol Biol Phys 16:785–787
zur Hausen H, Meihof W, Scheiber W, et al. (1974) Attempts to detect virus-specific DNA in human tumors. I. Nucleic aid hybridizations with complementary RNA of human wart virus. Int J Cancer 13:650–659

10 Cancer of the Endometrium

M. Herbolsheimer and K. Rotte

CONTENTS

10.1 Epidemiology and Risk Factors

The incidence of endometrial cancer is extremely heterogeneous, displaying geographic as well as ethnic differences. One can estimate that the median incidence in Western industrial countries is about 25 cases per 100 000 women (Kolles et al. 1989), whereas less than 2 cases per 100 000 women are reported in the statistics of certain regions in India and Japan, for example (Waterhouse et al. 1977). Even with regard purely to the United States there are remarkable regional differences: one can find data showing the incidence to range from less than 20 (Connecticut) to more than 40 cases (California) per 100 000 women (Demopoulos 1977; Waterhouse et al. 1977).

Everywhere, however, the incidence is rising (Cramer et al. 1974; Boronow 1976; Mestwerdt and Kranzfelder 1980; Kucera and Vavra 1991). Besides this absolute increase there is a relative one in comparison with cervical cancer: Before 1920 the ratio was still 1:17 (Rabe 1990), but it has changed continuously in favor of endometrial cancer (Rotte 1975; Baltzer and Maassen 1991) and at present this tumor is regarded as the most common malignancy of the female genital tract (Nori et al. 1987; Kolles et al. 1989; Kucera and Vavra 1991). Gusberg (1988) values the current ratio at 3:1.

One reason for this significant tendency is obviously the increasing frequency of prophylactic cancer examinations that lead to earlier detection of cervical cancer. Another reason could be the higher life expectancy of the population. The median age of patients with endometrial carcinoma is more than 60 years (Fig. 10.1): only 5% occur in women younger than 40 (Gallup and Stock 1984), whereas about 75% occur at or beyond the sixth decade (Rabe 1990; Ratanatharathorn and Powers 1990; Petterson 1991), and so the group at risk is increasing.

There are a number of possible risk factors:

1. Long-term effects of estrogen due to, for example, early menarche and late menopause (Creasman and Weed 1981), exogenous estrogen exposure (Brinton et al. 1992), obesity, which leads to in-

M. Herbolsheimer, MD, Akademischer Oberrat, Röntgen- und Strahlenabteilung, Universitäts-Frauenklinik, Josef-Schneider-Straße 4, D-97080 Würzburg, Germany. *Present address*: Institut für Radiologie, Klinikum Fulda, Pacelliallee 4, D-36043 Fulda, Germany

K. Rotte, MD, Professor (em.), Röntgen- und Strahlenabteilung, Universitäts-Frauenklinik, Josef-Schneider-Straße 4, D-97080 Würzburg, Germany

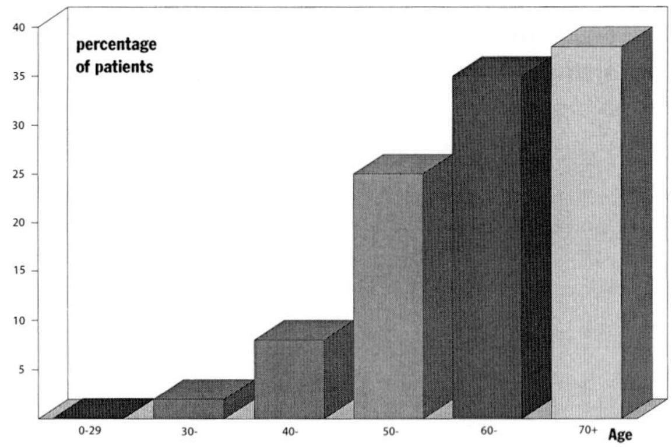

Fig. 10.1. Age distribution of patients with carcinoma of the corpus uteri. (According to the Annual Report vol. 21, 1991)

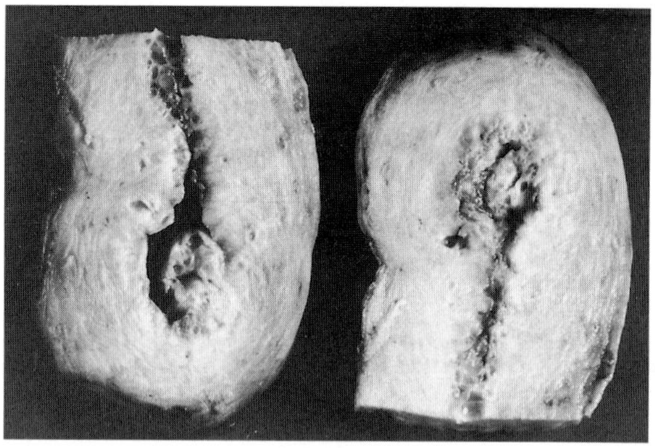

Fig. 10.2. Uterine preparation showing exophytic endometrial cancer

creased estrogen synthesis in the fatty tissue (Rotte 1975; Schindler 1977), or, in younger women, long-term treatment with ovulation inhibitors (Silverberg et al. 1977). In general, unopposed estrogen is a risk factor (Smith et al. 1975; Gusberg 1976; Davies et al. 1981; Persson et al. 1989).

2. Polycystic ovarian disease and estrogen-secreting ovarian tumors (McDonald et al. 1977).
3. Different endocrine-metabolic disorders, especially in combination with typical symptoms such as diabetes mellitus, hypertension, obesity, or nulliparity (Vahrson 1970; Brinton et al. 1992).
4. The positive association with colon and ovarian cancers (Leung and DePetrillo 1993) and breast cancer in patient histories is obviously due to hormonal stimulus (Cook 1966; MacMahon and Austin 1969; Herbolsheimer et al. 1987). Schünemann and Jourdain (1989) found syntropy in 7% of cases.

It is apparent that an excess of estrogen is common to all risk factors.

10.2 Topographic Anatomy and Patterns of Spread

The local origin of the tumor is the fundus uteri and the cornu uteri in about 80% of cases. The tumor growth is either exophytic or endophytic. Well-differentiated tumors often display exophytic growth and slight myometrial infiltration (Willgeroth 1994). The exophytic spread turns towards the uterine cavity, which may be expanded by tumor masses (Fig. 10.2). The growth may further extend downwards to the cervical tract. Endophytic tumors invade the myometrium, and in advanced cases may reach the peritoneal covering with subsequent ascites. Consequently peritoneal seeding is more common with endometrial carcinoma than with cervical cancer. Another reason for peritoneal seeding is the tendency of endometrial malignancies to seed transtubally (Glassburn et al. 1992). Spread per continuitatem to the fallopian tube and the ovaries is also known. The ovaries are involved in about 5%–10% of cases (Berman et al. 1980).

Lymphatic spread depends on the site of the tumor and its growth direction. It usually follows the route of the lymphatics of the mesosalpinx or along the iliac vessels. There may also be invasion of the nodes of the obturator fossa or along the ligamentum teres uteri, or of the inguinal lymph nodes (Fig. 10.3). There is a clear relationship between stage, myometrial infiltration, grading, and classification of the tumor (Morrow et al. 1973; Creasman et al. 1976; Aalders et al. 1980; Thigpen et al. 1986). If there is a combination of an undifferentiated tumor and deep myometrial infiltration, the risk of positive lymph nodes is higher than 30% (Kucera et al. 1989). As a consequence of this the 5-year survival rate is considerably reduced (Jones 1975; Kucera et al. 1990b; Lanciano et al. 1993).

Remote metastases occur relatively late but more often than with cervical carcinoma because of the good vasculature in the corpus uteri. The organs of predilection are the lungs, liver, and skeletal system (Salazar et al. 1977). The incidence of lung and liver metastases is somewhat more than 5%, while bone metastases occur in about 3% of cases (Plentl and Friedman 1971).

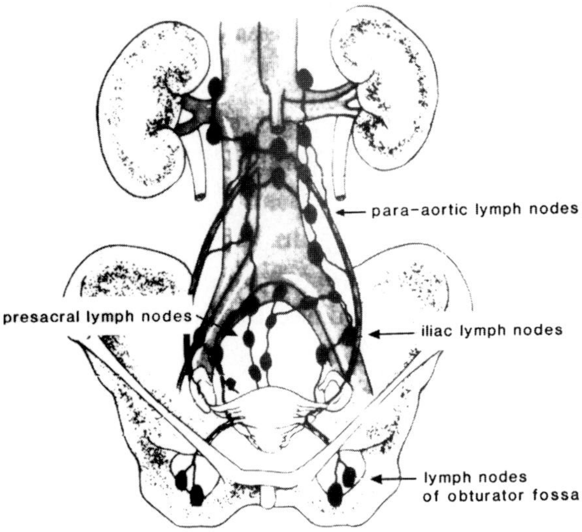

Fig. 10.3. Schematic diagram of regional lymphatic vessels and lymph nodes of the corpus uteri. (Modified from KNÖRR et al. 1989)

10.3 Diagnostic Workup and Staging

Each case of postmenopausal vaginal discharge or bleeding and each instance of irregular bleeding, whatever the age of the patient, is suspicious of endometrial carcinoma, though this symptom can have several other causes, such as endometritis, different forms of polyps or estrogen-secreting ovarian tumors. It has to be considered that about 20% of patients with postmenopausal bleeding will have a genital tract malignancy, and within this group endometrial cancer is the most frequent. When bleeding is present in women older than 80 years, the rate of endometrial carcinoma increases to 60% (MORROW and TOWNSEND 1987).

Pyometra and hematometra may be seen in patients with stenosis of the cervical canal. These findings in a postmenopausal woman should suggest endometrial cancer (DEVITA et al. 1993).

In the above cases it is obligatory to perform a fractionated curettage of the cervix and the uterine cavity. This should be done under general anesthesia so that simultaneous clinical examination of the pelvic organs can be performed while the patient is relaxed. Moreover, in patients with a clinically manifest tumor, relaxation is a precondition for accurate tumor staging. If bleeding recurs, the curettage should be repeated, for only one examination does not guarantee absolute security (BUTLER 1976). In some cases it is probably wise to perform a hysteroscopy, despite the disadvantage of risk of tumor cell spread to the peritoneal cavity through the fallopian tubes.

Rectoscopy and cystoscopy are well-established procedures for the confirmation or exclusion of stage IV tumors (see Tables 10.1a and 10.1b). Moreover, they should be performed to obtain information on other lesions (e.g., inflammation, ulcers) relevant to therapeutic strategies.

Table 10.1a. Clinical staging of endometrial carcinoma (according to the FIGO and TNM systems)

FIGO		TNM
O	Preinvasive carcinoma (carcinoma in situ)	Tis
I	Limited to corpus uteri	T1
Ia	Uterine tube length ≤8 cm	T1a
Ib	Uterine tube length >8 cm	T1b
II	Encroachment to cervix uteri	T2
III	Extension to pelvic structures outside the uterus	T3
IV	Infiltration of bladder and/or rectum and/or extension outside the pelvis	T4/M1
IVa	Infiltration of mucosa of bladder and/or rectum	T4
IVb	Remote metastases	M1

Table 10.1b. Histopathological staging of endometrial carcinoma [according to the new versions of FIGO (1989) and the TNM system (1987)]

FIGO		TNM
O	Preinvasive carcinoma (carcinoma in situ)	Tis
Ia	Limited to endometrium	T1a
Ib	Myometrial infiltration ≤1/2 of thickness of endometrium	T1b
Ic	Myometrial infiltration >1/2 of thickness of endometrium	T1b
IIa	Encroachment to endocervical glandular tissue	T2
IIb	Cervical stroma invasion	T2
IIIa	Infiltration of serosa and/or adnexa and/or positive peritoneal cytology	T3
IIIb	Vaginal metastases	T3
IIIc	Metastases to pelvic and/or para-aortic lymph nodes	T3
IVa	Infiltration of mucosa of bladder and/or rectum	T4
IVb	Remote metastases including intra-abdominal and/or inguinal lymph nodes	M1

In contrast to several authors (ENGLMEIER et al. 1985; CACCIATORE et al. 1989; BRANDNER et al. 1991) who report reliable imaging of the uterus by vaginal or intrauterine ultrasonography, we consider such ultrasound procedures to be useful staging examinations only when there are more advanced alterations of the uterus, such as extensive tumor infiltration of the myometrium with a thickened uterine wall or an expanded uterine cavity. Nevertheless, ultrasonography is, of course, a very suitable diagnostic method for the detection of liver metastases, and is indeed the most commonly used procedure for this purpose.

The indication for conventional roentgenological imaging is usually restricted to the search for remote metastases of the lung or skeletal system in patients at risk and to investigation of the intestine (e.g., barium enema) and urinary tract. The same holds true for bone scintigraphy (GLASSBURN et al. 1992). Some authors (ANDERSON et al. 1976; ROTH et al. 1985) perform hysterography for imaging of the uterine cavity. Computed tomography (CT) has no value in providing detailed findings, though GLASSBURN et al. (1992) recommend CT for the detection of the depth of myometrial invasion and as a screening method in patients with advanced tumor stages. CT screening for para-aortic lymph node metastases may be of use as a suitable replacement for lymphangiography. The results of our CT examinations with regard to brachytherapy planning were disappointing.

By contrast, magnetic resonance imaging is of proven diagnostic value (HRICAK et al. 1986, 1991; LUKAS et al. 1986) and has also become part of radiotherapy planning and therapeutic monitoring for several tumor entities (GLATSEIN et al. 1985; FISCHER et al. 1994). According to the extent of myometrial invasion, relatively high sensitivity and specificity are reported using contrast-enhanced imaging (BELLONI et al. 1990; SIRONI et al. 1992). Increased spatial resolution has been achieved by using an endorectal coil (BONER et al. 1994), and shorter acquisition times by the use of turbo-spin echo sequences (HEUCK et al. 1994). Such technical improvements can help to facilitate the determination of the target volumes.

Finally, the cytologic examination of endometrial cells for early tumor detection should be mentioned. However, unlike in the case of cervical cancer, the reliability is only about 50% (GLASSBURN et al. 1992), and the different procedures are afflicted with technical problems because they represent invasive procedures (BALTZER and LOHE 1986). This also holds true for morphological studies of cells or tissue specimens (MESTWERDT and KRANZFELDER 1983). Consequently these procedures cannot be recommended as screening methods and should be restricted to risk groups, such as patients with diabetes mellitus, hypertension, and obesity or postmenopausal women treated with estrogen for a long time (IVERSEN and SEGADAL 1985, BALTZER and LOHE 1986). According to ANTUNES et al. (1979), risk in the latter patients is increased by up to a factor of 8. Special aspects of peritoneal cytology are discussed later in Section 10.5.

Laboratory studies (complete blood count, blood chemistry, urinalysis, liver function tests) should be done routinely.

Staging is based on the classification schemes of the International Federation of Gynecology and Obstetrics (FIGO) and the International Union against Cancer (UICC). In the past, the prognostic value of staging was limited because more than 70% of the patients were assigned to stage I (BORONOW 1969; PETTERSON 1991; CREASMAN 1992; GLASSBURN et al. 1992), and the differentiation into stages Ia and Ib (Table 10.1a), which was based on a uterine tube length of ≤8 cm or >8 cm, had for some time been considered insufficient (AALDERS et al. 1980; BARAM et al. 1985; HORDING and HANSEN 1985). Therefore in 1988 FIGO accepted modifications in regard to the depth of myometrial infiltration in stage I and to local tumor spread in stages II and III (Table 10.1b). This histopathological classification guarantees a more adequate staging (LANCIANO et al. 1993) but has the disadvantage that a comparison of operative and radiotherapeutic results is not possible. It was proposed bearing in mind that only a minority of the patients are treated by primary radiotherapy; such patients are still to be classified according to the old scheme. This special aspect will be discussed in detail in Sect. 10.11.

10.4 Histopathological Classification and Grading

Atypical adenomatous hyperplasia of the endometrium counts as precancerosis (PARK et al. 1992). The term "adenomatous hyperplasia" was introduced by GUSBERG (1947). The atypical type is characterized by a diffuse adenomatous proliferation with an increasing depletion of stroma. It leads to adenocarcinoma in situ showing an even more pronounced polymorphism of cell nuclei. Atypical

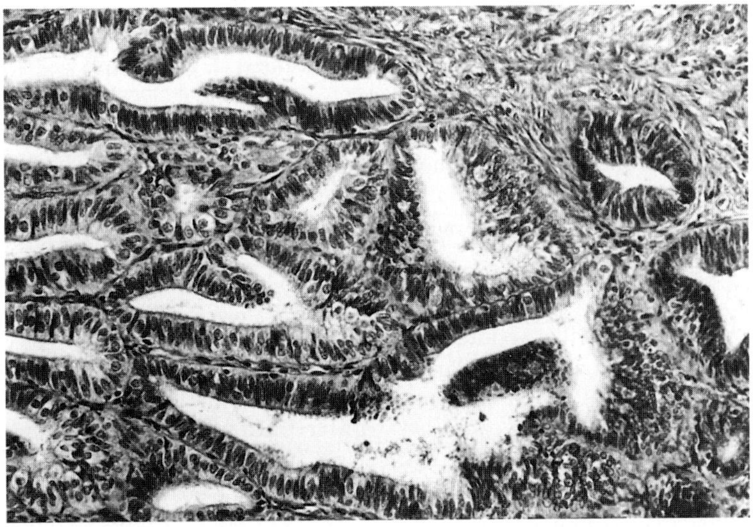

Fig. 10.4. Endometrioid adenocarcinoma infiltrating the myometrium. (Courtesy of the Labor für Gynäkopathologie, Universitäts-Frauenklinik Würzburg.) H&E

adenomatous hyperplasia and endometrial cancer can develop concomitantly. Invasive cancer associated with hyperplasia is often progesterone receptor positive and better differentiated (AYHAN et al. 1991).

MECKE et al. (1994) found an endometrial carcinoma in 16% of their group of 73 patients showing adenomatous hyperplasia of any grade. If only grade 3 adenomatous hyperplasia (which represents the atypical type) was considered, the rate rose to 57%. According to PARK et al. (1992), atypical adenomatous hyperplasia progresses to cancer in about 30% of cases. The common treatment for adenomatous hyperplasia is simple hysterectomy or, depending on individual circumstances, the application of gestagens (LINDAHL and WILLEN 1991).

The most common type of invasive uterine tumor is endometrioid adenocarcinoma (Fig. 10.4), with an incidence of about 60%. In contrast to other types (Table 10.2), such as adenosquamous carcinoma, clear cell carcinoma, squamous cell carcinoma, serous carcinoma, and, of course, the unclassifiable (undifferentiated) neoplasms and the different forms of sarcoma, it carries a favorable prognosis (HENDRIKSON et al. 1982; CHRISTOPHERSON et al. 1982; MORROW and TOWNSEND 1987; CREASMAN et al. 1987; ROSENBERG et al. 1989a; WILSON et al. 1990; GREVEN et al. 1993; WILLIAMS et al. 1994).

Mixtures of pure endometrioid carcinomas and the secretory forms are not infrequent (LEE and BELINSON 1991; WILLIAMS et al. 1994). WILLIAMS et al. (1994) pointed out that the prognostic features of these mixed tumors are related to the predominance of the different components. In their study the behavior of a mixed serous and endometrioid carcinoma containing more than 50% serous differentiation was similar to that of pure serous tumors. Carcinomas with a serous component of less than 25% could not be distinguished clinically and prognostically from pure endometrioid carcinomas. Mixed forms containing 25%–50% serous features could only be suggested to carry an increased risk. Papillary carcinomas are related to a significantly higher risk of recurrences in comparison to other histological types (MANDELL et al. 1985b; VAVRA et al. 1993).

Histopathological grading according to the amount of tubular and solid structures is shown in Table 10.3. Up to 5% of instances of a nonsquamous

Table 10.2. Subtypes of invasive endometrial carcinoma

Anglo-American nomenclature	German synonyms
Endometrioid adenocarcinoma	Endometrioides Adenokarzinom
Secretory	Sekretorisch
Papillary	Glandulär, glandulär-papillär
Ciliated cell	Solide
Adenosquamous	Adenosquamös
Adenoacanthoma	Adenokankroid
Mucinous carcinoma	Muzinöses Adenokarzinom
Clear cell carcinoma	Klarzelliges Karzinom
Serous (papillary) carcinoma	Serös-papilläres Karzinom
Squamous cell carcinoma	Plattenepithelkarzinom

Table 10.3. Histopathological grading according to FIGO

G1	Well-differentiated adenocarcinoma without solid areas
G2	Moderately differentiated adenocarcinoma with partly solid areas
G3	Predominantly solid or entirely undifferentiated carcinoma

or nonmorular solid growth pattern are related to G1, more than 50% to G3, and the rest to G2. Notable nuclear atypia inappropriate for the architectural grade results in a higher grouping, i.e., G1 or G2 tumors are classified as G2 or G3 tumors. Nuclear grading takes precedence in serous, squamous cell, or clear cell adenocarcinomas. Adenocarcinomas with squamous differentiation are graded according to the nuclear grade of the glandular component (PETTERSON 1991).

Remaining uterine body malignancies are accounted for by the different forms of sarcoma, lymphomas, mixed müllerian tumours (*Müller'sche Mischtumoren*), and distant metastases, mostly from breast and gastrointestinal tract cancer (KUMAR and HART 1982). Sarcoma accounts for about 5% of all malignancies of the corpus uteri (KEMPSON and BARI 1970; SALAZAR et al. 1978a). The most common type is leiomyosarcoma, followed by carcinosarcoma and other mixed mesodermal forms. Different types of sarcoma are sometimes seen about 10–20 years after radiation treatment (WILLIAMSON and CHRISTOPHERSON 1972). The poor prognosis of sarcomas is due to the early infiltration of vessels followed by remote metastases in the lungs and liver (FLEMING et al. 1984). The incidence of pelvic lymph involvement is also high, with estimates ranging from 25% to 50% at time of presentation (GLASSBURN et al. 1992).

The mixed müllerian tumor, which occurs in about 3%–5% of uterine malignancies, has a worse prognosis than endometrial carcinoma (MARTH et al. 1990), but it has similar prognostic parameters. Only parity is an exception, for it seems to have a beneficial influence selectively on mixed müllerian tumors, whatever the latency from the last birth. This is unique in oncology.

Myometrial penetration and consequently the infiltration of lymph nodes are two of the generic prognosticators in endometrial carcinoma. Their incidence is related to the degree of tumor differentiation (CREASMAN et al. 1976, 1987; AALDERS et al. 1984a,b; STOKES et al. 1986: THIPGEN et al. 1986; GRIGSBY et al. 1987).

In an analysis by CREASMAN et al. (1987), only about 1% of tumors restricted to the endometrium

Table 10.4. Correlation between grading and lymph node metastases in endometrial carcinoma. (According to CREASMAN et al. 1976)

Grading	Lymph node metastases (%)	
	Pelvic	Para-aortic
I	3	1
II	10	4
III	36	28

showed pelvic lymph node metastases. This rate increased to 25% in cases showing infiltration of the outer third of the myometrium. The incidence of para-aortic lymph node involvement rose from about 1% to nearly 20%.

PLENTL and FRIEDMAN (1971) found that decreased survival was directly related to depth of myometrial infiltration and histological differentiation. In a retrospective review of 262 surgically staged endometrial malignancies by KADAR et al. (1992b), tumor stage, myometrial infiltration, grading, cervical stromal penetration, vascular space involvement, and age were found to be prognostic factors for survival. CREASMAN et al. (1976, 1987) observed a clear positive correlation between grading and lymph node infiltration (Table 10.4). They observed a similar correlation regarding myometrial infiltration and the risk of involved lymph nodes. They calculated this risk to be 4% when only the inner third of the myometrium was infiltrated, but 30% when there was an infiltration of the outer third. Similar results have been reported by KUCERA et al. (1989), as mentioned in Sect. 10.2.

There is a clear relationship between lymph node infiltration rate and survival (JONES 1975; LANCIANO et al. 1993). The 5-year survival rate is about 80% if the tumor is limited to the corpus uteri, but less than 50% in cases of lymph node involvement (KUCERA 1993). Moreover, undifferentiated tumors show a higher frequency of lymphangiosis carcinomatosa (KUCERA 1993). Generally speaking, the greater the depth of myometrial infiltration and the less the tumor differentiation (these two factors are correlated), the greater is the likelihood of extrauterine spread and/or lymph node metastases.

10.5 Other Prognostic Factors: Tumor Markers and Estrogen/Progesterone Receptors

There is no general agreement as to the prognostic significance of carcinoembryonic antigen (CEA).

KJORSTADT and ÖRJASETER (1977) saw increased CEA levels in less than 40% of women with endometrial cancer. On the other hand, the marker seems to have a high prognostic value in cases that show no decrease in the level of CEA after treatment (VAN NAGELL et al. 1977). Serum CA-125 is elevated in some cases (NILOFF et al. 1984). DUK et al. (1986) and GLASSBURN et al. (1992) report that the marker has been found to be elevated especially in patients with clinically advanced or recurrent tumors. Although it is more often present in ovarian cancer (DUK et al. 1986), CA-125 thus seems to be useful for the detection of tumor progression and recurrence. The tumor-associated antigen CA 15-3, which plays a role in the follow-up of breast cancer, sometimes shows an increased level in gynecological tumors. CROMBACH et al. (1986) report pathological serum concentrations in 27% of their patients. Despite the aforementioned findings, in general there are no tumor markers specific for endometrial carcinoma.

Cytoplasmic estrogen and progesterone receptor status appears to be an important prognostic factor (EHRLICH et al. 1988; CREASMAN 1992). Patients with receptor-positive lesions have a significantly better disease-free survival than those with receptor-negative lesions. This is not surprising because a positive correlation has been reported between hormone receptor concentration and the degree of tumor differentiation (JÄNNE et al. 1979; MCCARTY et al. 1979). Analyses showed that the presence of either estrogen receptors or progesterone receptors, as well as the presence of both receptor types, was significantly associated with histological differentiation (CREASMAN et al. 1985).

Hormone response depends on the receptor status. Receptor-negative patients are normally hormone-resistant (BENRAAD et al. 1980; CREASMAN et al. 1980; DEPPE 1990). The estrogen receptor is more frequently present than the progesterone receptor, but the latter seems to be more significant for the prediction of the response to hormones (KUCERA 1993). KLEINE (1984) reported that in 63% of his patients with an endometrial carcinoma, the tumor tissue contained both receptor types, while in 10% only estrogen and in 6% only progesterone receptors were present.

Carcinomas with high progesterone receptor levels have a significantly better prognosis in all stages than those with low levels or absence of progesterone receptors. Multivariate comparisons suggest that the prognostic significance of a progesterone receptor level of more than 50 fmol is greater than that of histopathological grading, estrogen receptor status, and age (PFLEIDERER et al. 1989). Particularly patients with advanced tumor stages who respond to hormone therapy have a considerably longer mean survival time than nonresponders (REIFENSTEIN 1971; KUCERA 1993). However, there is a well-known discrepancy between the presence of female sex steroid receptors and the response to hormones. KOHORN (1976) and KAUPPILA (1984) reported that only one-third of unselected patients with advanced or recurrent tumors responded to progestin, for instance. This may be due to the fact that the examined specimens can contain receptor-positive normal tissue surrounding a receptor-negative tumor, which leads to a wrong positive analysis (STECK et al. 1991). Another reason for the discrepancy between the receptor level and the response to hormones is the heterogeneous differentiation of a tumor population (MORTEL et al. 1984). Only one-third of endometrial cancers with development of metastases and recurrences are progesterone receptor-positive (KLEINE et al. 1990).

As it is known that estriol administration can increase the level of both receptor types (JÄNNE et al. 1979; POLLOW et al. 1986), it has been proposed that tamoxifen should be administered for a short time before progesterone acetate (GURPIDE 1981; CARLSON et al. 1984).

In this context it should be mentioned that the presence of 17β-hydroxysteroid dehydrogenase in receptor-positive cells may help to predict hormone dependency (NEUMANNOVA et al. 1985; MÄENTAUSTA et al. 1992). However, at present this is not of clinical relevance. The same holds true with regard to oncogenes. The overexpression of the growth receptor protein HER-2/*neu* or of different mutations of p53, a nuclear protein playing an important role in the regulation of the cell cycle, is suggested to have a certain significance in gynecological tumors (BERCHUCK et al. 1991; BOSARI et al. 1993). BERCHUCK et al. (1991) reported a positive correlation between a high expression or overexpression of HER-2/*neu* and the rate of relapses and mortality. Cathepsin-D should also be mentioned (NAZEER et al. 1992) as a possible prognosticator.

The role of epidermal growth factor and its relationship to other prognosticators is not yet evident (BAUKNECHT et al. 1989; BERCHUCK et al. 1989). The content of desoxyribonucleic acid (DNA) and DNA ploidy are considered to have a strong correlation with tumor differentiation and consequently with patient prognosis (AMBROS and KURMAN 1992; GRIMM et al. 1992). The rate of recurrences is correlated with the amount of tetra- or aneuploid cells (BRITTON et al. 1989; LINDAHL et al. 1989). In several studies an increased recurrence rate has been found to be correlated with aneuploidy, increasing percentage of S-phase fraction, DNA index, and proliferative index (Iversen et al. 1988; Britton et al. 1989; Rosenberg et al. 1989b; Lindahl and Gullberg 1991; Takahashi et al. 1991; Podratz et al. 1993).

Kühn et al. (1989) showed that adenocarcinomas were much more diploid and had a lower S-phase fraction than mixed müllerian tumors and clear cell carcinomas. A clear correlation between these factors and conventional prognostic parameters such as stage, myometrial infiltration, grading, and hormone receptors has been shown. Thus, DNA-aneuploid tumors with a high S-phase fraction were related to a decreased survival rate. Kühn et al. suggested DNA index and S-phase fraction to be superior to grading in terms of prognostic significance. Their findings resemble the results of Rosenberg et al. (1989b), who found about 85% of papillary serous carcinomas to be aneuploid whereas most endometrioid carcinomas were diploid. According to these authors the duration of the S-phase should also be taken into account as another prognosticator.

In a multivariate analysis it was found that malignant peritoneal cytology was an independent and important prognostic factor (Creasman et al. 1987), whereas other investigators (Milosevic et al. 1992; Leung and DePetrillo 1993) consider peritoneal cytology not to be an independent prognosticator but a surrogate for other prognostic factors. A study by Kadar et al. (1992a) showed that positive cytology had a significant adverse effect on survival only if there was tumor spread outside the uterus, whereas Harouny et al. (1988) reported a correlation between disease-free survival and negative cytology even in stage I tumors. Overall, the value of peritoneal cytology is thus controversial (Lurain 1992).

There is no general agreement as to the prognostic value of the patient's age, either. Clinical studies in radiotherapy show heterogeneous results as to the survival rates in different age groups (Sturm 1977; Rustowski and Kupsc 1982; Greer and Hamberger 1983; Aalders et al. 1984a; Huguenin et al. 1992; Kadar et al. 1992b). Our own historical patient group (Sturm 1977) showed no influence of age on survival; similarly, Rustowski and Kupsc (1982) studied corrected survival and found that there was not a statistically significant relationship with age.

Over the past several years it has increasingly been considered likely that there are different types of endometrial cancer (Lee and Scully 1989; Pfleiderer 1991). The first type, carrying a good prognosis, is characterized by clinical symptoms such as diabetes mellitus, obesity, hypertension, infertility (or at least low parity), and late menopause, as well as by advanced patient age. It shows an estrogen anamnesis, is related to adenomatous hyperplasia, and is characterized by high progesterone and estrogen levels. Normally there is a stage I tumor and no deep myometrial infiltration.

The second type is the exact opposite to the first as regards the typical risk factors, the receptor status, and the depth of infiltration. There is no estrogen anamnesis and no hyperplastic origin. Most tumors are of stage III and belong to the group of unfavorable histopathological subtypes (secretory carcinomas). Thus there tends to be early metastatic spread to the regional lymph nodes. For these reasons the prognosis is poor, as reflected in a significantly lower 5-year survival rate in comparison to the first type (Wilson et al. 1990).

It is difficult to ascertain exactly the prognostic significance of the various risk factors, but overall it can be stated that the most important tumor-related prognosticators are the degree of myometrial infiltration, the presence of vascular space invasion, the tumor grade and histological type, and, of course, the stage (Lewis et al. 1970; Plentl and Friedman 1971; Boronow et al. 1984; DiSaia et al. 1985; Hanson et al. 1985; Creasman et al. 1987; Morrow et al. 1991; Kadar et al. 1992b). The probability of disease recurrence depends primarily on the number of these tumor-related risk factors (Kadar et al. 1992b).

10.6 General Management: Surgery or Primary Irradiation?

Review of the current literature concerning this question reveals almost general agreement that the cornerstone of curative treatment for endometrial carcinoma is abdominal hysterectomy and bilateral oophorectomy and – in accordance with the individual risk – facultative lymphadenectomy. Only patients who are not fit for surgery should be treated by primary radiation therapy (Pfleiderer 1991; Frischkorn 1983; Kucera 1993).

Surgery is suggested to be the more effective treatment in stages I and II in terms of the 5-year survival rates achieved. According to other authors (Lochmüller 1978; Vahrson 1991) and to our historical patient group (Rotte 1975), the difference is about 15% (85% vs 70%). Moreover, the histological

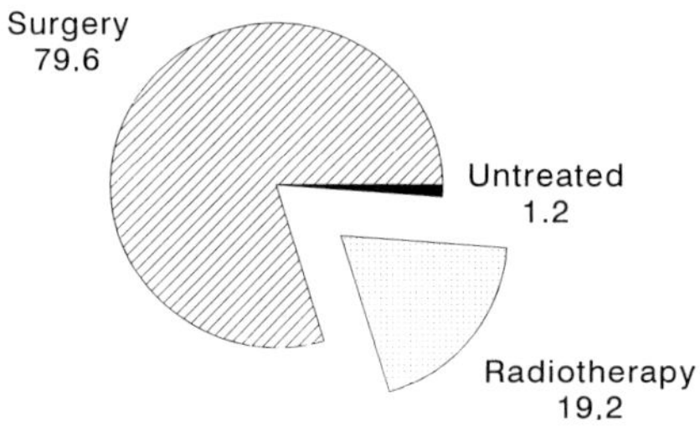

Fig. 10.5. Frequency with which surgery and radiotherapy were used for the treatment of carcinoma of the corpus uteri at UFK Würzburg, 1972–1993 ($n = 2042$)

findings are more reliable indicators of the real stage, and so they play an important role in the decision whether to employ adjuvant therapy. It must not be forgotten, however, that patients who undergo primary irradiation in general represent a negative selection, and it is not yet proven that the advantages of surgical staging result in clear advantages for patients (Vahrson 1991). In stage III disease, primary radiation therapy should generally be preferred (Frischkorn 1983; Morrow and Townsend 1987; Baltzer and Maassen 1991).

Of course, nobody denies that radiotherapy as a primary modality is an alternative to surgery in certain cases such as typical patients with clinical risk factors, especially if these are combined with cardiac complications and high age, whatever the tumor stage. But in nearly all publications considering the optimal form of therapy from a gynecological point of view one finds the conviction that surgery (alone or followed by adjuvant radiotherapy) should be employed when a curative indication exists. Consequently, representative results of primary radiotherapy are not generally available. Of course, this is also true of the Universitäts-Frauenklinik Würzburg, though about 20% of our inpatients with endometrial cancer are irradiated primarily (Fig. 10.5).

Nevertheless, before answering the question as to whether surgery or radiotherapy is appropriate, it is worthwhile to consider the reasons for the poorer results of irradiation. Analysis of common applicator techniques, of imaging, and of planning procedures shows that most treatment concepts have not met the state of the art presently achievable. Consequently, it can be suggested that the dose distribution has not been sufficiently adapted to the individual target volume. Especially in treatment protocols using brachytherapy only as a boost to percutaneous irradiation of the whole pelvis, the possibilities of optimization of the dose distribution have not been exhausted. It should be stressed that the neglect of optimization can lead to both worse results and more severe side-effects. These aspects will be discussed in Sects. 10.7 and 10.11 and then we shall deal again with the question of the relative merits of surgery and radiotherapy.

10.7 Primary Irradiation

10.7.1 Brachytherapy

In cases in which the intent is curative, radiotherapy as a primary modality has to involve a combination of brachytherapy and megavoltage external beam treatment. For adequate brachytherapy, there are three general requirements:

1. A spatial dose distribution that is adapted to the individual anatomical situation.
2. A practicable technique with regard to radiation protection and reproducible source positions.
3. A temporal dose distribution that is short enough to avoid clinical complications without reducing therapeutic breadth.

This list of principal requirements can be completed by several special requirements, as is shown in Table 10.5. It is well known that in former times the problem of satisfying all of these requirements could not be solved. An overview of the historical development of brachytherapy has been presented by Mould (1993).

The classic radium methods such as the Paris technique (Regaud 1922), the Manchester system (Paterson and Parker 1934), and the method of Fletcher (1962) were above all protocols for cervical carcinoma with a low degree of individualization. The Stockholm technique (Heyman 1935) using more flexible applicator forms is the basis of the classic packing of the uterine cavity with radium sources (Heyman et al. 1941). It allowed the dose distribution to be adapted to the varying cavity

Table 10.5. Requirements for optimal brachytherapy

Individual dose distribution
Practicable technique
Total radiation protection
Reproducible source positions
Constant geometry of implants
Short treatment time
Great therapeutic breadth

forms and sizes in an almost optimal way, especially in patients with an exophytic tumor. Additionally, a more uniform dose distribution was delivered to the entire myometrium (RUTLEDGE and DELCLOS 1980). However, as a radium therapy this technique did not permit sufficient radiation protection. Also, owing to the long treatment times, the immobilized patients developed clinical complications. Venous thrombosis was the most frequent among these, occurring especially when there was accompanying hypertension, obesity, and diabetes mellitus. This complication occurred in our department, for example, in 7% of cases (ROTTE 1990).

Packing techniques using cobalt-60 pellets were reported by MORTON et al. (1953) and HENDRICKS et al. (1955). These manual procedures had the same disadvantages as classical packing with regard to radiation protection and clinical complications. MÜLLER (1951) inserted a balloon into the uterine cavity which was filled with liquid radionuclides (normally cobalt-60). This procedure had to be abandoned because of the risk of contamination.

SIMON and SILVERSTONE (1976) developed a modified Heyman packing technique using hollow capsules that were afterloaded by cesium-137 sources. The staff exposure was considerably reduced in comparison to radium applications and therefore accuracy in the placement of the capsules was enhanced. But the negative clinical consequences of a relatively long treatment time could not yet be avoided, and this manual technique guaranteed only restricted radiation protection. It should be mentioned that initial attempts to avoid radiation exposure were made in Sweden in the 1960s using remote afterloading machines and radium sources (WALSTAM 1962). In general, the first remote afterloading techniques operated at low dose rates, whatever the nuclide chosen. Only when fractionated high-dose-rate (HDR) afterloading techniques were introduced was total radiation protection achieved. Moreover, short treatment times avoided clinical complications and resulted in reproducible source positions. But what about the requirement for an individual dose distribution?

High-dose-rate afterloading has been in use for about 30 years for irradiation of endometrial carcinoma. Its development is associated with the name of ULRICH HENSCHKE (JOSLIN 1989): in the early 1960s, Henschke presented important guidelines for the remote HDR treatment of gynecological tumors (HENSCHKE et al. 1963, 1966). In the following years and decades a variety of brachytherapy techniques for uterine cancer were proposed (SUIT et al. 1963; JOSLIN et al. 1967; LIVERSAGE et al. 1967; ROTTE et al. 1973; VON ESSEN et al. 1974; BUSCH et al. 1977; GLASER et al. 1977; SNELLING 1977; DELCLOS et al. 1980; BAUER et al. 1981; BJÖRNSSON and SORBE 1982; NORI et al. 1982; KUMAR and GOOD 1985; RIIPPA et al. 1985; KAUPPILA et al. 1987; PIERQUIN et al. 1987; RAUTHE et al. 1988; LUNDBERG et al. 1989; KUCERA et al. 1990b; JOSLIN 1991; LADNER 1992; ROSE et al. 1993; TESHIMA et al. 1993; PERNOT et al. 1994). The proposals considered:

1. The shape and the flexibility of applicators. These included single intrauterine probes with ovoids (tandem and colpostats with or without a connection), semiflexible intrauterine probes, intrauterine capsules with flexible tubes, or double-rod-shaped intrauterine probes (Fig. 10.6), which we used in our historical patient group (ROTTE 1985, 1988). It must be mentioned that many of the rigid applicators were initially designed for cervical cancer but were also used in endometrial carcinoma.
2. The choice of nuclide: usually cobalt-60, cesium-137, or iridium-192.
3. The spatial arrangement of sources: a unique oscillating source, a unique source moving in steps, a so-called train of differently weighted pellets, or a train containing active sources and spacers.

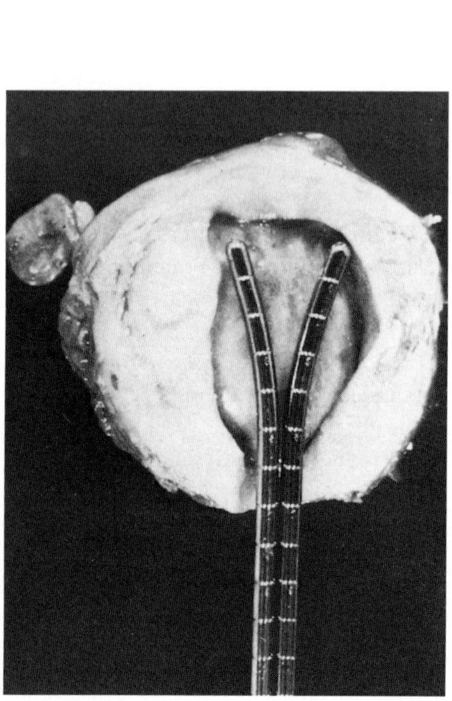

Fig. 10.6. Frontal view of a uterine preparation with a double-rod-shaped applicator for endometrial cancer in situ. (From ROTH et al. 1985)

4. The reference dose rate according to the International Commission on Radiation Units (1985): low-dose-rate (LDR) treatment with less than 2 Gy/h, medium-dose-rate (MDR) treatment with 2–12 Gy/h, or HDR treatment with more than 12 Gy/h.

Each treatment protocol entails an interplay of these four elements, which results in various combinations. The question of the most suitable combination is difficult to answer, but it is worthwhile to discuss the special aspects of each point listed above after the presentation of our treatment technique.

Optimal brachytherapy in primary irradiation of endometrial carcinoma that meets the already formulated requirements with regard to spatial and temporal dose distribution and radiation protection should combine selectively the advantages of classic packing with those of remote HDR afterloading. A precondition for this is the use of sufficiently small sources and computerized treatment planning. Since 1988 such a treatment modality, modified HDR packing, has been employed at the Universitäts-Frauenklinik Würzburg. The afterloading machine (MicroSelectron HDR) with its small iridium-192 source, having a diameter of 1 mm, allows us to pack the uterine cavity with a maximum of 18 hollow plastic capsules, the capsule diameters available being 8, 6, 5, and 4 mm (Fig. 10.7). The nominal activity of the source is 10 Ci (370 GBq).

After cervical dilation with Hegar's dilators under general anesthesia, the capsules are inserted (Fig. 10.8). Each capsule contains a semirigid Roentgen catheter (dummy) to facilitate the correct placement of the applicators. The procedure is supported by percutaneous ultrasound control, because in endometrial malignancies there is a relatively high risk of perforation. The number of capsules depends, of course, on the size of the uterine cavity; normally six to ten applicators are required to pack the uterus adequately, though in one case we had to insert 16 capsules. In order to obtain an optimal distribution we ensure that additional capsules are placed in the cervix to cover the lower uterine segment and the cervical tract. We insert these additional capsules in each patient irrespective of the tumor stage. A measuring tube containing a fivefold semiconductor detector chain is inserted in the rectum, and another containing one semiconductor detector in the center of a Foley balloon is inserted in the bladder.

Finally, vaginal gauze packing is applied to hold the applicator tubes in place and to increase the distance between applicators and organs at risk. This is a general requirement because each kind of dose optimization would have a considerably decreased effectiveness without this simple manipulation.

Insertion of the applicators has to be deferred in cases of pyometra, which is usually due to obstruction of the cervical canal by endocervical growth of the tumor. In such patients an indwelling drainage tube is inserted for a few days and antibiotic therapy administered. One has to beware of rupture of the cervix, which may be caused by the dilation up to Hegar 12, necessitated by the amount of applicators being inserted. This risk has been already pointed out by Rutledge and Delclos (1980).

The whole procedure lasts about 7–12 min (except for cases where additional fractionated curettage is performed to establish or correct the stage). Thus anesthesia is restricted to this relatively short time.

After insertion of the applicators, isocentric orthogonal radiographs of the pelvis are taken to show the relationship of the position of the capsules to the organs at risk and to bony structures (Fig. 10.9). Tungsten markers of the dummies show the potential dwell positions on the orthogonal radiographs.

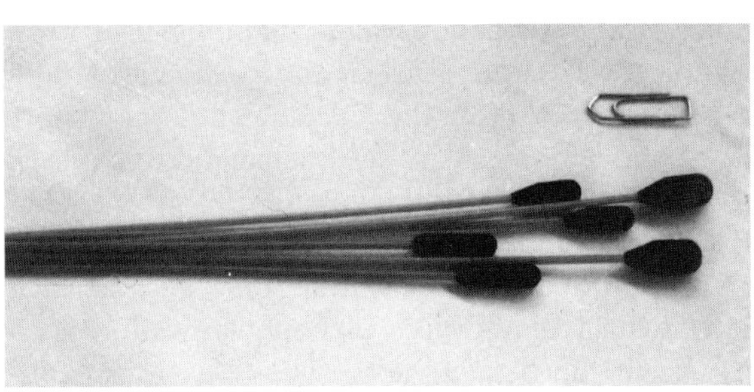

Fig. 10.7. Heyman capsules of different sites for use in remote-controlled afterloading of endometrial cancer (the paper clip illustrates the dimensions of the applicators)

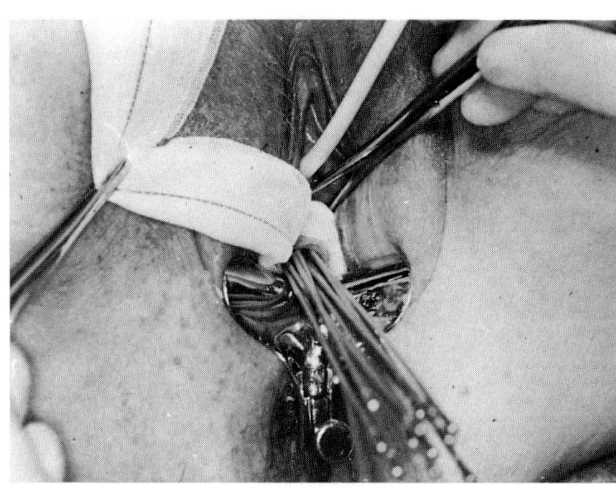

Fig. 10.8. Heyman capsules in situ after application

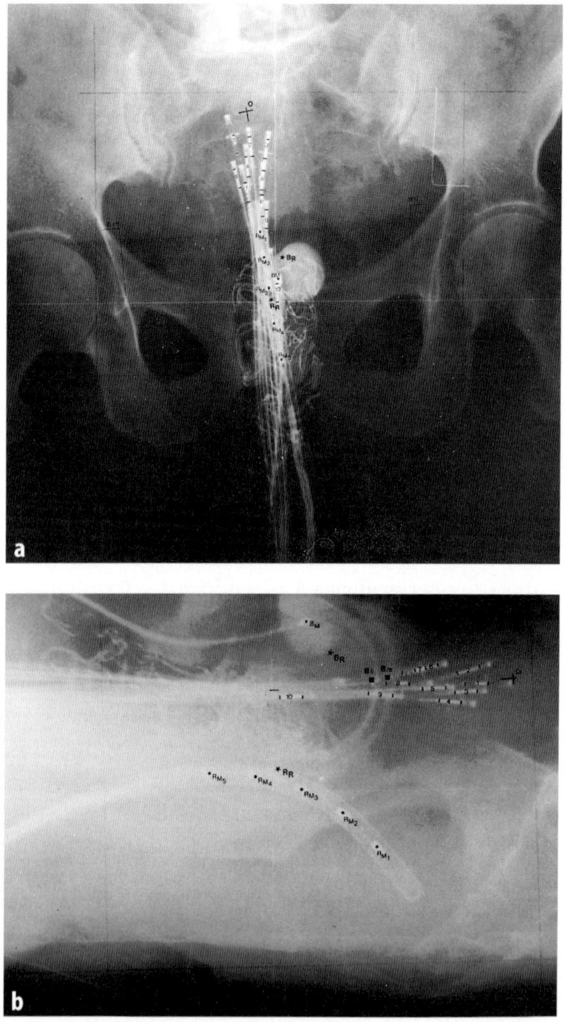

Fig. 10.9 a,b. Orthogonal radiographs of modified Heyman packing showing the applicator bundle and the measurement probes. a Frontal view; b lateral view

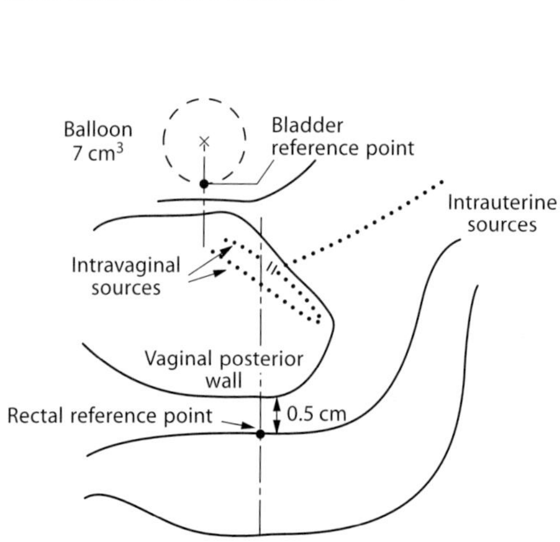

Fig. 10.10. Schematic drawing illustrating the determination of the reference points for the bladder and rectum. (From ICRU report 38)

Of course, the patients is positioned on the same table during insertion of the applicators, x-ray examination, and irradiation. By digitizing the radiographs with a graphics tablet and using a computer-controlled planning system, an individual dose distribution in three dimensions is produced. In some cases isocentric stereo images can facilitate the digitizing procedure. The calculated doses to the measurement points in the rectum and bladder are compared with those measured directly by rectum and bladder probes. If there are no relevant differences, the calculated doses at the reference points of organs at risk (Fig. 10.10) – as recommended in the ICRU report 38 (1985) – are reliable and confirm a correct correlation between the radiation plan and the doses actually delivered. We have accepted differences of up to 10%–15% in our intracavitary brachytherapy in general because to date such differences have not shown a negative influence on the rate of clinical side-effects. Greater deviations require the digitizing procedure to be repeated. If the differences remain, they are normally due to the fact that the patient has moved between the anteroposterior and the lateral exposure; new radiographs are then necessary. Detailed technical aspects have already been discussed elsewhere (Rotte 1990, 1992; Herbolsheimer 1989; Herbolsheimer et al. 1988, 1991, 1992).

It is of interest to know whether such differences in doses are due to the well-known mobility of the organs at risk, especially of the rectum, or to the reconstruction procedure. Thus we investigated 103 brachytherapy applications in patients with gynecological cancer, in whom 32 Heyman packing applications were performed. This study was also designed to examine the geometrical precision of the reference points which are constructed using the orthogonal radiographs. Therefore we repeated the reconstruction of the applicator and the measurement probes using a second set of orthogonal images acquired after the irradiation. The values were compared with those of the original treatment planning: The mean standard deviation between the two sets of dose values was 13%. From this a geometrical uncertainty of about 3 mm can be estimated (Sauer et al. 1994), which is due to the mobility of the organs at risk. The second set of radiographs was taken about 1 h after the first one. Within this interval each intracavitary application, planning procedure, and treatment can be completed. Thus the results confirm that the mobility of the organs at risk has relatively little influence on the accuracy of our treatment planning.

In order to facilitate the planning procedure, a standard program is stored in the computer. Optimization according to the individual case can be performed by changing the time weights of the different capsules. This weighting is possible since we use dummies with a binary code in order to distinguish the capsules from each other. This method of optimization requires imaging of the outer shape of the uterus. As already pointed out by others (HRICAK et al. 1986, 1991; PFÄNDNER et al. 1993), magnetic resonance imaging (MRI) is a suitable procedure to achieve this aim. Since the beginning of 1993 we have been using MRI for our treatment planning (Fig. 10.11). In order to integrate the images into the brachytherapy planning procedure we choose double-angulated slices parallel to the dose distribution axis that is determined by the course of the uterine axis. The slices must have the same scale as the orthogonal exposures, of course. In accordance with the images, the reference isodose combines several reference points determined individually on the uterine surface. MRI plays an important role in cases where tumoral infiltration has produced an irregular shape of the myometrium and it also helps to avoid excessive doses to every point of the organs at risk. This is especially true of segments of the small bowel which may be adherent to the uterine surface.

As already mentioned, we have been performing this planning procedure only since the beginning of 1993. Up to that date and in cases that are not suitable for MRI (e.g., because of metal implants, a pacemaker, claustrophobia, advanced age, and/or poor general state of health), conventional planning was

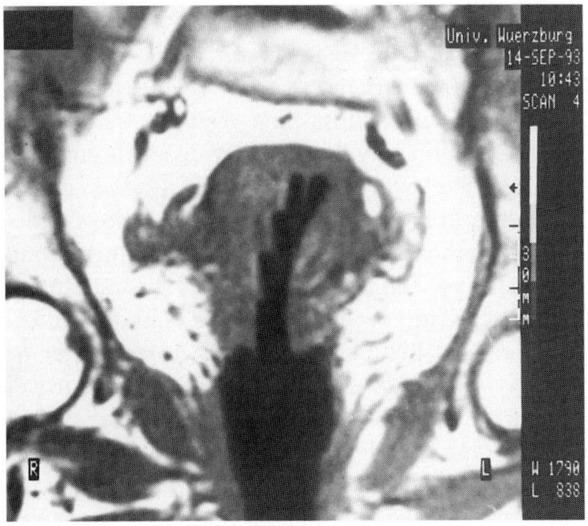

Fig. 10.11. T1-weighted double-angulated MR slice showing packing capsules in the uterine cavity

or is performed. This means that a standard reference point indicated as point MY (= abbreviation of "myometrium") is chosen. MY is comparable with the Manchester point A in irradiation of cervical cancer. MY is situated 2 cm below and lateral to the top of the dose distribution axis, i.e., the axis of the uterine cavity. The reference volume related to MY is, of course, only an approximation to the serosa of the uterus.

In each case of Heyman packing we apply five fractions of 10 Gy, 10 days apart, to the reference isodose. External beam therapy is performed simultaneously (see Sect. 10.7.2). We ensure that the reference doses to the rectum and bladder do not exceed 7 Gy per afterloading fraction, or 60 Gy within 6 weeks, including the contribution of teletherapy. Similar recommendations have been made by others (FRISCHKORN 1983). Because of the relatively great distance from the applicators in Heyman packing, the average range is 3–5 Gy per fraction.

We would suggest that our generally low rate of side-effects (see Sect. 10.11) is partly an effect of the dose calculation for the critical tissues, though some investigations have shown that the cumulative doses to the rectum and bladder do not always correspond to the clinical complication rate (ESCHE et al. 1987).

Individual treatment requires also that the current gynecological status is evaluated by a thorough manual examination before each afterloading fraction. This is an important element of the cooperation between the gynecologist and the radiotherapist and enables the therapeutic approach to be varied as necessary.

It is worthwhile to compare the described technique and the previously cited possible combinations of applicators, nuclides, source arrangements, and dose rates with regard to the extent to which they meet requirements for adequate brachytherapy, summarized earlier in this section.

1. Forms of Applicator. The progress in computer-controlled treatment planning for HDR brachytherapy of gynecological tumors has created the possibility of optimizing the dose distribution. There are many different ways to achieve this aim (HERBOLSHEIMER 1993), but a general requirement for such individual planning is a suitable form and shape of the applicator.

Comparing the source distribution of uterine packing techniques with rigid applicators, whatever their type (single tube, double shaped tube, combined tube and vaginal colpostats), packing allows better individual adaptation of the dose distribution because the uterine cavity has no regular shape, especially in those cases in which an exophytic tumor is present. Moreover, when treatment planning is combined with MRI, the information regarding myometrial infiltration and an irregular outer shape of the uterus can be translated to a different weighting of the capsules. Techniques based on rigid applicators cannot react sufficiently to such individual anatomical circumstances. Only the applicator developed by BAUER et al. (1981), which bears a resemblance to a besom, the so-called bulb technique of BJÖRNSSON and SORBE (1982), the flexible intrauterine tube combined with vaginal ovoids used by ALDRICH et al. (1989), and the so-called endouterine umbrella used by PERNOT et al. (1994) represent a certain compromise regarding an individual dose distribution because they can be considered as semiflexible applicators.

There are some authors who perform uterine packing in a manner similar to the procedure described above (NORI et al. 1982; PEREZ et al. 1985; GRIGSBY and PEREZ 1989); sometimes a combination with a tandem for the lower uterine segment and ovoids for the vaginal vault (ROSE et al. 1993) is used.

It should be mentioned that in seldom special cases of stage II endometrial cancer with extensive exophytic tumoral involvement of the cervix, one can use a combination of capsules sparing the lower uterine segment and a ring, which is routinely used in cervical cancer in conjunction with a uterine tube. This special combination, which delivers an adequate dose to both the exophytic tumor and the uterine serosa, is another element of an individual treatment. Of course, external beam therapy is adapted to the altered brachytherapy treatment volume in such cases.

For users of one tube applicator for intracavitary treatment, Vahrson has presented a technique involving hysterography with an indwelling applicator (see Chap. 3. Sect. 3.6.8).

2. *Choice of Nuclide.* Remote uterine packing requires applicators with narrow tubes because a cervical dilatation exceeding Hegar 12 is usually not tolerated (large cavities have to be packed with 15 applicators or more). Thus a sufficiently small source that passes the tubes without disturbance is necessary.

The chosen source must have a high activity guaranteeing a high dose rate at the reference points, with avoidance of clinical complications, patient discomfort, shifting of sources, and consequently insufficient dosimetry due to long treatment times. Finally, the nuclide should have a low gamma energy.

WALSTAM (1977) suggested cesium-137 to be the most suitable nuclide for brachytherapy in general. However, if we consider the requirements for a modified packing technique we find a different situation. Comparing radium-226, cesium-137, cobalt-60, and iridium-192 with regard to size, specific activity, and gamma energy, iridium-192 best meets the three requirements. Its short half-life is a disadvantage that requires a relatively frequent change of the source; on the other hand, examination of sealing and mechanical injury is not necessary.

3. *Arrangement of Sources.* It is not possible to provide a uniform answer to the question as to the most suitable source arrangement of an afterloading machine, i.e., whether to use source pellets or a single source that is moved in steps or is oscillating. We think that a single source moved in steps is adequate in order to produce individual isodoses: a great variation of reproducible isodose curves can be provided simply; moreover no further source is necessary.

4. *Dose Rate.* There is no general agreement over whether a low, medium, or high dose rate is to be preferred for remote-control afterloading brachytherapy of gynecological cancer.

As is well known, the reason for the replacement of manual radium applications by remote afterloading techniques was the lack of radiation protection and not the ineffectiveness of radium therapy. As a consequence of this many radiotherapists saw no reason to abandon the principle of protraction when using afterloading equipment, given that there was no great experience in a therapy that demanded a totally different dose-time relation. Using LDR afterloading therapy the reference dose rate could be kept near 50 cGy/h, which was the dose rate in classical radium treatment. Under HDR conditions, however, radiotherapists had to deal with an increase in dose rate by a factor of more than 100 (the rate sometimes exceeded 180 Gy/h). Thus the temporal differences ranged between about 160 h (Manchester or Paris System) and only a few minutes (HDR procedures).

Both high- and low-dose afterloading techniques have certain advantages (Table 10.6). An important advantage of LDR techniques is the greater therapeutic breadth in comparison to HDR regimens. This is based on the repair capacity of involved normal tis-

Table 10.6. Comparison of high- and low-dose-rate remote control afterloading

Advantages of low-dose-rate techniques
1. Great therapeutic breadth
2. No requirement for specially shielded rooms
3. Easy transfer of radium experiences to afterloading strategies

Advantages of high-dose-rate techniques
1. Short treatment and immobilization times
2. Reproducible geometry of source positions
3. Possibility of optimizing spatial dose distribution
4. High patient frequency, creating the possibility of outpatient treatment with reduced health care costs

sue; sublethal radiation damage can be repaired during the exposure time if the dose rate to the organs at risk is similar to that with classic radium therapy (KUMMERMEHR 1990). The sparing of normal tissue under LDR conditions can compensate for the lack of constant and reproducible source positions which is associated with the long treatment time.

Experimental trials suggested that unfractionated irradiation with dose rates higher than 12 Gy/h would produce up to a 60% increase in radiobiological effects (FOWLER and STERN 1963; JOSLIN et al. 1967; LIVERSAGE 1973; ELLIS and SORENSEN 1974). Such effects have been confirmed by well-known observations in various clinical situations (THAMES et al. 1990), and especially concern late responding tissues, which are more efficiently spared by fractionation than early reacting tissues. The reduced therapeutic breadth of HDR treatment in comparison with LDR brachytherapy therefore requires adequate fractionation on the basis of calculation models relating to the time-dose relationship and taking into account the time factor for repair of normal tissue (ELLIS 1963; FOWLER and STERN 1963; COHEN 1968; KIRK et al. 1971; LIVERSAGE 1971, 1973, 1978; ORTON and ELLIS 1973; ORTON and WEBBER 1977; BARENDSEN 1982; KELLERER 1984; DALE 1985; STITT et al. 1992). Moreover, ORTON (1981) suggested that the total doses in HDR treatment, as calculated using various time-dose relationship models, should be reduced by at least 20% in order to avoid a higher frequency of complications.

The problem of calculating an adequate temporal dose distribution for HDR irradiation is demonstrated by the great variety of parameters that influence the modelling formulas. ORTON (1987), WARMELINK et al. (1989), and DALE (1990) pointed out that special care has to be taken when choosing the parameters used in the calculation of biological effects, and SCALLIET (1993) recommended the use of calculation formulas equating LDR with HDR with caution.

There are many variable influences that hinder the achievement of constant tumor control without increased side-effects:

1. Different times and amounts of repair of radiation damage (LIVERSAGE 1966)
2. Variations in the reoxygenation, proliferation, and redistribution of radiated cells
3. The number of hypoxic cells (TROTT 1974, 1975, 1978)

In addition to the aforementioned specific facts concerning the radiosensitivity of different tissues, consideration must be given to patient-related circumstances such as general health and age, as well as to volume effects (BUSCH et al. 1977).

From among the different calculation models, the linear-quadratic formula basing on the investigations of FOWLER and STERN (1963) seems to be the most suitable. It is widely accepted because it allows differentiation between late and early normal tissue reactions, which are represented by the alpha-beta term. The alpha/beta ratio models the fractionation sensitivity of the tissue at which alpha/beta rates of 10 Gy or more represent acute effects and alpha/beta rates lower than 5 Gy, late effects. The biological effect calculated by this model is expressed by the term BED (biological effect dose). It indeed displays relatively good agreement with the clinical data obtained in daily routine, but only if the special nature of brachytherapy is taken into account.

What is meant by the "special nature of brachytherapy"? It has been shown that high single doses result in an increased rate of late side-effects (DEORE et al. 1991; HALL and BRENNER 1991), which, of course, can be avoided by adequate fractionation. This means that – according to theoretical considerations in radiobiology – an HDR treatment should be split into about 10–30 fractions (DALE 1985; FOWLER 1989a). For example: Replacing a radium treatment with a total dose of 60 Gy given in 5 days by an HDR modality with a dose rate of more than 100 Gy/h to the reference isodose, we would have to apply 30 fractions of 2 Gy within 40 days according to the linear-quadratic formula in order to achieve the same effects in the tumor and in the normal tissue. But 30 fractions are absolutely unrealistic in clinical practice! Our fractionation of modified Heyman packing with 5 times 10 Gy as well as our temporal dose distribution in other gynecological tumors is far removed from this theoretical requirement of radiobiology. Indeed, this obviously holds true for every clinician performing HDR brachytherapy.

According to the linear-quadratic model, five fractions applied under these conditions would result in overdosing late reaction tissues by about 33% (FOWLER 1989b). However, our own complication rates and those reported in the literature (see Sect. 10.11) indicate that side-effects are not increased. It is well known that about four to eight fractions (the number chosen in clinical practice by the majority of clinicians) result in a much lower complication rate than that predicted by the linear quadratic model. This surprising but obvious discrepancy between theory and practice cannot be explained by the easily reproducible applicator position in HDR schemes or by the computer-controlled therapy planning alone. Rather the explanation lies in the already mentioned nature of brachytherapy, which results in a very high integral tumor dose with good sparing of the organs at risk.

Due to the steep dose gradient the doses delivered to the rectum or bladder are normally much lower than those to the tumor (DALE 1990). In calculating fractionation we should therefore refer not to the prescription dose - which is, for example, 10 Gy to the reference isodose in our treatment regimen for endometrial carcinoma - but rather to the doses applied to the reference points of the organs at risk as defined in the ICRU Report 38 (1985). This inhomogeneous dose distribution of brachytherapy, in contrast to external beam therapy, should indicate the use of some kind of dose reduction or sparing factor. Such a factor k has already been introduced in the modelling formula (BAIER 1989; WARMELINK et al. 1989). It should not be confused with the already mentioned reduction factor for the total dose (ORTON 1981), which was created in order to maintain constant biological effects when changing from radium to HDR afterloading or changing the number of fractions within HDR treatment schemes.

An analysis of 30 applications using modified Heyman packing showed that the doses applied to the reference point of the organs at risk were, on average, 30% in comparison with our prescription dose of 10 Gy. Thus the reduction factor k was 0.3. In order to assess its influence on the calculation of late side-effects we integrated k into the linear-quadratic formula and reduced the number of fractions under constant tumor control: In a range from 30 to 3 fractions we calculated an almost equal rate of late side-effects in the organs at risk. Thus our fractionation of 5 times 10 Gy within 40 days cannot lead to an increased rate of side-effects. This conclusion agrees with our complication rate, which will be presented later (see 10.11). In this context it should be mentioned that the dosage and fractionation of modified packing have been derived from former radium applications, and this was also true of our afterloading technique with a double-shaped applicator, employed between 1972 and 1988. In this period the rate of side-effects in 327 patients amounted to 7%; as with our current treatment, these effects were restricted to mild inflammatory signs, without any evidence of rectal fistulas or ulcers.

The correlation between the doses to the target volume and those to the organs at risk and its influence on late damage with different numbers of fractions is shown in Fig. 10.12.

To summarize: If the reduction factor k is taken into account, the linear-quadratic model is reliable in predicting the rate of side-effects, and the alleged discrepancy between calculations and clinical results does not arise. As a consequence of k, high fraction numbers can be avoided if the organs at risk have a certain distance from the target volume. Only in those cases where k is about 0.9–1.0 because of an unfavorable position of the organs at risk are an increased number of fractions needed. Fortunately, in many cases this can be avoided by an appropriately placed vaginal tamponade and by optimizing the dose distribution in computerized treatment planning.

However, it must not be forgotten that each radiobiological formula has a restricted range, i.e., the linear-quadratic model is no longer valid when calculating doses higher than about 10 Gy per fraction (BAIER 1993). In a randomized study, KOB et al. (1988) compared tumor control and side-effects of

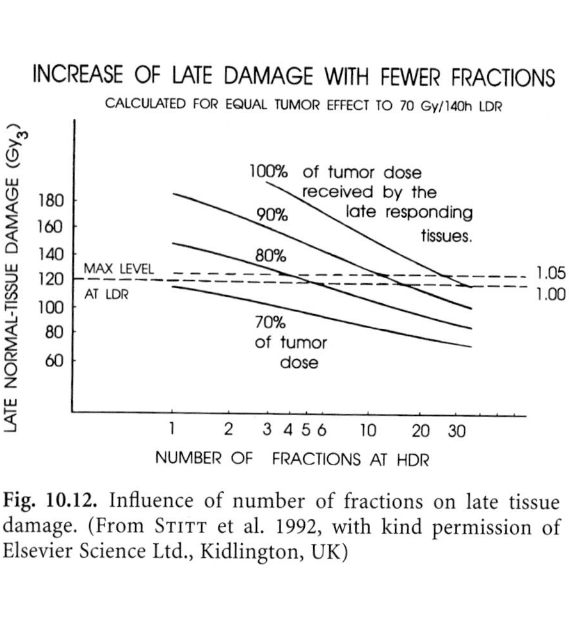

Fig. 10.12. Influence of number of fractions on late tissue damage. (From STITT et al. 1992, with kind permission of Elsevier Science Ltd., Kidlington, UK)

three fractionation schedules: 4 × 10 Gy, 5 × 8 Gy, and 8 × 5 Gy. According to the linear-quadratic formula, the greatest tumor effect should be expected with a fraction dose of 10 Gy. However, the clinical data showed a worse tumor regression after treatment with four fractions of 10 Gy than after the other two fractionation schedules. There were no differences in the rate of side-effects. This suggests that the linear-quadratic formula overestimates the effectiveness of high single doses in achieving tumor control. Similar results were obtained by ROTTE (1985) in cervical cancer stage III: after changing from three to five fractions tumor control increased significantly.

Nevertheless, the question, "Which treatment form should be preferred – HDR LDR afterloading?", cannot be answered. As already pointed out (Table 10.5), both strategies have their specific advantages, and the published clinical studies comparing HDR and LDR treatment show heterogeneous results in regard to local tumor control as well as to side-effects. In general, they confirm the suggestion that there is no significant difference between the two modalities of brachytherapy (GLASER 1980; ROTTE 1980; PEREZ et al. 1983, 1984; HIMMELMANN et al. 1985; JACOBS 1988; KOB et al. 1988; BATES 1989; VAHRSON 1989, 1991, 1992; LADNER 1990; ORTON et al. 1991; ARAI et al. 1992; OKAWA et al. 1992; HERRMANN et al. 1993).

Since 1971 intracavitary afterloading has been performed under HDR conditions in the Universitäts-Frauenklinik Würzburg. We have been able to show that when computer-controlled treatment planning is carried out on the basis of imaging procedures systematically performed for each patient and each fraction, which allows the dose distribution to be modified when necessary, there is no significant difference in the treatment results achieved by HDR as compared with LDR procedures (ROTTE 1980, 1990, 1992). Another way to combine the favorable therapeutic ratio of LDR and the possibility of optimizing the dose distribution is the use of pulsed dose rate (PDR) techniques: A single iridium-192 source of medium-strength activity (37 GBq) simulates an LDR treatment by means of multiple pulses of short duration, the source being moved in steps. Experimental studies employing, for instance, pulses of 10 min in each hour, delivering 1 Gy or less per hour, and keeping the same overall dose and total treatment time, showed this method to be an alternative to classical LDR treatments (BRENNER and HALL 1991; FOWLER 1993; FRITZ et al. 1992; MAZERON et al. 1994).

Like HDR brachytherapy, PDR techniques permit a more precise application of the prescribed dose to the treatment volume. Though it is possible to uncouple the patients from the machine during the intervals between pulses, there is restricted mobility in comparison with HDR techniques, which has to be considered a certain disadvantage.

In comparison with LDR techniques there are at least three advantages of PDR techniques:

1. The provision of a sufficient therapeutic ratio
2. The possibility of optimizing the dose distribution
3. The periodical replacement of only one source

At present the PDR technique, which was derived from trials in external beam therapy (PIERQUIN et al. 1978), is in use at only a few institutes and has not yet been generally introduced in daily routine. In comparison with continuous LDR treatment, first clinical results show no significant differences concerning both acute toxicity and preliminary tumor control (ADLER et al. 1994; MCLEAN 1994; SWIFT et al. 1994).

We prefer the HDR technique without exception when performing intracavitary brachytherapy (in contrast to our LDR interstitial implants to the tumor bed in breast cancer) because the lesser therapeutic breadth can be compensated by the already discussed advantages (more exact geometry, i.e., the reproducible position of applicators, dose optimization by means of computer-controlled planning, the possibility of practicable and adequate fractionation, and the absence of risk of complications related to long treatment times).

An overview of combined irradiation with interstitial brachytherapy for locally advanced gynecological malignancies is presented by MARTINEZ et al. (1985, 1989), who use a transperineal technique. Though the indications for such treatment of the female genital tract were restricted to cervical and vaginal cancer, the use of this technique might also be considered in inoperable advanced endometrial carcinoma. SYED and PUTHAWALA (1987) and DONATH et al. (1992) have reported successful attempts to increase local tumor control in cancer of the gynecological tract by the use of interstitial implants. The interstitial version of brachytherapy as a boost to tumor infiltrations after combined intracavitary and percutaneous radiation or for the treatment of recurrences after irradiation plays an important role because it is usually the sole possibility to apply sufficient tumor dose without exceeding the tolerance dose of the connective normal tissue and of the organs at risk. We have used interstitial brachytherapy for this purpose for several years. But, as already pointed out by HORIOT et al. (1989), this method requires some experience and one has to be aware of complications such as bleeding and inflammation.

10.7.2 Teletherapy

In primary irradiation our intracavitary applications are scheduled within the course of megavoltage treatment to the pelvic lymphatics, which are irradiated using 10-MeV photons from a linear accelerator utilizing bisegmental arc techniques with two isocenters. The lower margin of the portals is at the inferior border of the obturator foramen, the upper margin at the L4/5 space. We apply 25 fractions of 2 Gy to the maximum point, and the target volume must be enclosed within the 80% isodose. If the total treatment time is prolonged, for instance by intervening public holidays, the total dose is changed according to a modified linear-quadratic formula (BAIER 1987).

Planning is supported by computed tomography in several slice positions. The target volumes are defined with regard to the individual anatomy and to the area that is irradiated by afterloading.

In general the adaptation of individual dose distributions of brachytherapy and external beam irradiation gives rise to considerable problems, especially because of the well-known mobility of the uterus, which varies from patient to patient and from application to application. In spite of this we do not consider brachytherapy as a boost which is applied after homogeneous external beam irradiation of the whole pelvis up to, for instance, 30 Gy or even more. We distinguish two separate target volumes (Fig. 10.13): a volume of first rank, in which only brachytherapy is involved, and a volume of second rank, which is covered by external beam therapy. This concept has already been reported by GAUWERKY (1977, 1980). As external beam therapy delivers no relevant doses to the center of the pelvis, we can apply high brachytherapy doses there, which means we can utilize the full scope of the intracavitary treatment. We are convinced that use of brachytherapy which is not limited by dose contributions of external beam irradiation is the reason for the very good results in gynecological radiotherapy in general, since it allows the delivery of high central doses surrounded by steep dose gradients.

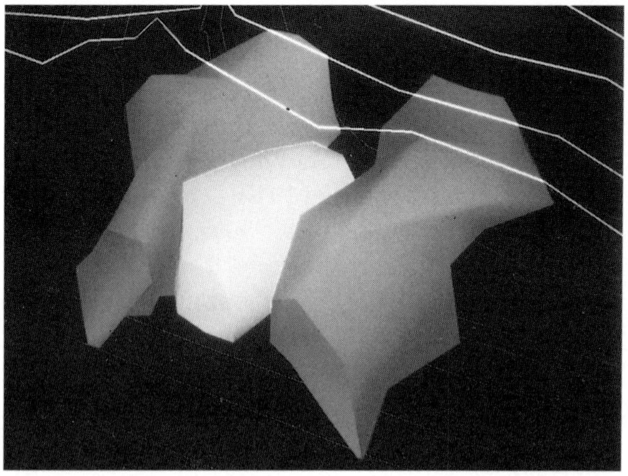

Fig. 10.13. Three-dimensional computer reconstruction of target volumes in primary irradiation of endometrial cancer. The first-rank target volume (defined for brachytherapy) in the center is flanked by the second-rank target volumes (defined for external beam therapy)

We use no shielding of the target volume treated by brachytherapy when we perform external beam irradiation, but rather a biaxial arc technique; this allows us to react better to the assumed mobility of the uterus, because sharp dose profiles at the borderline of the two target volumes are avoided. Additionally we think this relatively smooth dose profile to be a suitable adaptation to parametrial tumor infiltration.

We ensure that the maximum teletherapy dose to the reference volume of brachytherapy is about 10 Gy. In some stage II and stage III tumors, however, the uterus is often fixed in an eccentric position because the involved parametrium is shortened. Though we react to this situation when defining the target volumes of teletherapy in the different CT slices, we tolerate a somewhat higher dose to the involved side. This means that physical doses up to a total of 80 Gy have to be expected in a marginal region of about 1 cm where overlapping of the reference volumes takes place. This region is represented by the outer part of the myometrium and by the paracervical tissue which is immediately adjacent to the cervix. Estimation of the volume effect by a radiobiological model entails difficulties, but this can be neglected from the clinical point of view because in such cases the aforementioned margin is preponderantly infiltrated by tumorous tissue and the volume of overdosaged normal tissue is very restricted. Thus this relative overdosage can even be desirable with regard to tumor control, and it is not surprising that our clinical data show no increase in side-effects. Above all, we have seen no cases of "frozen pelvis," i.e., fibrotic stricture of the ureter.

By comparison with the use of opposite isocentric anteroposterior and posteroanterior portals with central shielding or a box technique, a rotation arc technique results in more sparing of the skin. As a consequence of this the rate of erythema is almost nil. Our technique with four segments of 30° and two isocenters is similar to those long-established techniques which have been employed by others in cervical cancer in order to compensate skin reactions due to the smaller build-up effect of telecobalt (SURMONT et al. 1956; HEINZEL 1961; FRISCHBIER and HASSE 1965).

The described strategies (with respect to both brachytherapy and teletherapy) that we use in primary radiotherapy of endometrial cancer are related to stage I–III disease. In stage IV disease it is our policy to consider the individual situation. It depends on the specific case whether brachytherapy alone or a combination of brachytherapy and external beam therapy is performed, and this also holds true with respect to the doses applied. Sometimes only a symptomatic treatment is chosen, which can be restricted to one to three fractions of brachytherapy or to teletherapy alone. In these cases the only aim is to control discharge or pelvic pain in order to improve the quality of life. All patients in stage IV are candidates for systemic therapy. We consider general policies of management not to be practicable.

The management and special aspects of para-aortic treatment will be discussed in the following section.

10.8 Pre- and Postoperative Irradiation

Preoperative irradiation aims (a) to decrease the opportunity for viable tumor cells seeded in the operative field to develop into local recurrence, (b) to render the malignant cells nonviable and decrease the risk of distant tumor dissemination, and (c) to irradiate the area of infiltrated lymph nodes that are not removed at the time of surgery. On the other hand, postoperative irradiation is an element of the different adjunctive treatment modalities. Its role can be defined clearly: The domain of surgery is the removal of macroscopic (sometimes gross) tumor masses but there is insufficient eradication of surrounding microscopic tumor cells. Especially these cells are the domain of radiotherapy, which on the other hand is usually unsuitable for large tumor volumes. Thus the combination of the modalities results in a locoregional control which cannot be achieved by surgery or radiation alone.

Preoperative radiotherapy, sometimes combined with an additional postoperative irradiation, is or has been a common treatment at several institutions (OHLSEN et al. 1977; UNDERWOOD et al. 1977; SALAZAR et al. 1978a; SPANOS et al. 1978; GAGNON et al. 1979; FLETCHER et al. 1980; RITCHER et al. 1981; BEDWINEK et al. 1984; GRIGSBY et al. 1985; PESCHEL et al. 1989; GLASSBURN et al. 1992; PERNOT et al. 1994).

GLASSBURN et al. (1992) performed intrauterine and intravaginal insertions in stage II tumors about 1 week before hysterectomy. This short interval was chosen in order to use the pathological features which are helpful for further treatment strategies. If surgery were to be performed after some weeks, these features would be more difficult to evaluate although a higher degree of tumor sterilization would be observed (HOMESLY et al. 1977; UNDERWOOD et al. 1977).

DEVITA et al. (1993) proposed adding external beam irradiation with a midline shielded block after preoperative intrauterine brachytherapy, followed by hysterectomy and bilateral salpingo-ophorectomy if the myometrial infiltration exceeds 50%. The doses were 20 Gy to the whole pelvis and 30 Gy to the parametria with central shielding. A boost was indicated for residual tumor.

GRIGSBY et al. (1985) performed preoperative intrauterine brachytherapy in patients with stage II tumors showing only microscopic involvement of the endocervix. If there was gross involvement of the ectocervix, in addition to the intracavitary treatment, external beam irradiation was performed, the doses being 20 Gy to the whole pelvis and 30 Gy to the parametria. Hysterectomy was carried out about 1 month later.

REISINGER et al. (1992) reported on a small series of patients with gross cervical infiltration (stage II tumors) in whom preoperative external radiation with 50 Gy was combined with intracavitary brachytherapy.

RUBIN et al. (1992) employed a combination of preoperative external beam therapy and postoperative intracavitary radiation. In patients with stage II tumors this procedure resulted in a disease-free survival of about 75% at 8 years. However, as more than two-thirds of the patients had only detached fragments of carcinoma in the cervical fraction of the curettage and only one-third real involvement of cervical stroma, the classification as stage II has been considered rather liberal (Bertelsen and Jakobsen 1993).

We do not perform preoperative irradiation as a standard practice, because the evaluation of histopathological prognostic features and their influence on further treatment modalities, which is one of the main advantages of surgery, would become much more difficult (Berman et al. 1980). Moreover, the value of preoperative radiotherapy is controversial (Piver et al. 1979; Eifel et al. 1983; Bedwinek 1984; Käser 1986). Piver et al. (1979) compared surgery alone with preoperative and postoperative treatment schemes. Though the survival rate was equal in all groups, there were no vaginal recurrences in the group that was treated postoperatively, in contrast to the other groups. Among the patients of Klötzer et al. (1992), the combination of preoperative uterine irradiation and facultative postoperative irradiation by HDR afterloading was not superior to surgery and facultative postoperative radiotherapy. de Waal and Lochmüller (1982) saw no improvement in results after preoperative radium therapy of the vagina, and according to David et al. (1983) vaginal irradiation before surgery does not prevent vaginal recurrences. This is logical considering the possibility that during hysterectomy endometrial tumor cells might be detached, leading to their implantation into the vaginal wall, though again, there is no general agreement as to this hypothesis. Especially paraurethral lesions are suggested to be due to lymphatic spread (deVita et al. 1993; Elliot et al. 1994). Thus, in agreement with Grigsby and Perez (1989), we normally treat patients with unresectable tumors by radiotherapy alone instead of preoperative management, as reported above. This also applies generally to most stage III tumors.

Postoperative irradiation includes vaginal brachytherapy and external beam therapy of the pelvis. There is no general agreement as to which patients should undergo adjuvant radiotherapy and which need no further treatment. Especially the indication for combined brachy- and teletherapy is disputed, whereas vaginal applications are widely accepted. The latter subject, and especially sole vaginal irradiation, will be considered in detail in Sect. 10.8.1. There are different opinions concerning the use of teletherapy for the treatment of stage I tumors.

In many institutions it is policy to add external beam pelvic irradiation in stage I only if the tumor infiltration extends beyond the inner third or the inner half of the myometrium, or in grade 3 disease (Onsrud et al. 1976; Joslin et al. 1977; Aalders et al. 1980; Mandell et al. 1985a; Marchetti et al. 1986; von Fournier et al. 1987; Kucera and Weghaupt 1988; Poulsen and Roberts 1988; Kucera et al. 1989; Piver and Hempling 1990; Glassburn et al. 1992; Elliot et al. 1994).

In a prospective and randomized clinical trial (Aalders et al. 1980) the effect of postoperative external pelvic irradiation was evaluated in 540 patients with stage I endometrial carcinoma. One group received only vaginal brachytherapy after primary surgery. The other was treated by a combination of vaginal brachytherapy and external high-voltage irradiation to the pelvis; these patients received 40 Gy to the entire pelvis with a central shielding at 20 Gy. In this study a highly significant improvement in pelvic control was obtained after 6 years in patients receiving additional external irradiation, confirming the findings of a former preliminary survey (Onsrud et al. 1976) that showed a reduction in the number of pelvic recurrences after external irradiation. Aalders et al. (1980) showed that especially in histological grade 3 tumors the difference was clear: The group treated with additional teletherapy showed a recurrence rate of 3%, as compared with 14% in the control group. This is all the more remarkable because 40 Gy is a somewhat low dose, especially in unfavorable histological subtypes. On the other hand pelvic irradiation was followed by a higher incidence of distant metastases, which led to equal survival data in the two groups.

In the study of Elliot et al. (1994), which included 811 stage I and 116 stage II tumors, the frequency of vaginal, pelvic, and distant metastases was considerably lowered in patients with high-risk tumors after postoperative brachytherapy and external beam treatment.

In patients with stage I tumors Joslin et al. (1977) also reported a significant reduction of pelvic failure after postoperative intravaginal and percutaneous treatment in comparison with postoperative vaginal brachytherapy alone. Again, this was particularly true of the deeply invasive cases. In contrast to Aalders et al. (1980), the 5-year survival was improved from 67% for surgery alone to about 90% for combined surgery and radiotherapy.

With regard to the rate of distant metastases in the trial of Aalders et al. (1980), which was increased after postoperative external beam irradiation to the whole pelvis, one could speculate about the influence of irradiation on the immunological defence system.

However, the significance of these data is unclear. Thus such speculation should not lead to a decision not to use pelvic irradiation, with the accompanying risk of poorer local control. This risk is higher than the unproven risk of an increased rate of distant metastases. And it must not be forgotten that the effectiveness of treatment of recurrences is restricted, whatever the treatment form (Barber and Brunschwig 1968; Höckel 1990; Kucera et al. 1983). It should also be considered that others (Joslin et al. 1977; Elliot et al. 1994) have observed a clear benefit from postoperative external beam therapy, which was related not only to the incidence of pelvic recurrences but also to the survival rate. Kucera et al. (1990b), who perform postoperative irradiation that is strictly related to prognostic criteria (and above all to the myometrial infiltration depth), achieved results in cases with a poor prognosis by external beam irradiation which were similar to those in patients who did not undergo teletherapy due to their good prognosis. A similar tendency was reported by Vahrson (1992): after postoperative radiation in patients with myometrial infiltration, improved survival was obtained in comparison with patients who had no infiltration and consequently were not irradiated. Our results confirm these observations and are reported in Sect. 10.11.

All clinical data show that treatment of endometrial cancer with deep myometrial infiltration must go beyond removal of the primary and irradiation of the vaginal tissue; thus a decision not to use external beam therapy of the pelvis can only be justified if surgery is equivalent to a Wertheim operation. It is known, however, that the majority of patients suffering from endometrial cancer are far from being in a good condition and that radical surgery still entails an increased risk in spite of improvements in anesthesia and surgical management. Moreover, it has not been proved that a radical operation significantly increases survival in patients with stage I tumors. The question of quality of life should be considered, too.

According to our treatment policy, postoperative external beam irradiation is indicated in stage I if the myometrial infiltration is 3 mm or more. This strategy is widely accepted, as shown above. Myometrial infiltration is of greater prognostic significance than other parameters (DiSaia et al. 1985) and shows a clear positive correlation with the degree of differentiation (Creasman et al. 1976; Thipgen et al. 1986). The seeming contrast with institutions which measure the depth of infiltration not in millimeters but as a proportion of the myometrial thickness is only of a theoretical nature. Nevertheless, we prefer a specification in millimeters (Rotte 1975) because we think it is better related to the size of the tumor mass: A patient with tumoral invasion of 7 mm and a myometrium of 2.5 cm will undergo adjuvant external beam treatment according to our criteria. By contrast, such a patient would not receive external beam treatment at an institution that has a borderline of one-third or one-half of myometrial thickness; on the other hand a patient with the same infiltration depth and a myometrial thickness of only 2 cm would be treated. Our indications for teletherapy are not related to the differentiation of the tumor, because grading alone has a much smaller influence on prognosis than myometrial infiltration. Kucera and Vavra (1991) reported that even in the case of high-grade carcinomas restricted to the endometrium no lymph node involvement could be found, and this was also true for malignancies with only slight myometrial infiltration (Kucera and Vavra 1991). Moreover, grade 3 tumors with a low infiltration depth are not very frequent. Other investigators also think that histological grade alone is of no significant value (Bruckman et al. 1980; Greer and Hamberger 1983; Mackillop and Pringle 1985; Stokes et al. 1986), though their data refer to higher stages.

In cases with an unfavorable histomorphology (serous-papillary, clear cell, or adenosquamous carcinoma), external beam irradiation should be considered whatever the infiltration. Normally, however, deep infiltration is present in such cases. Advanced age alone should not influence the indication for radiation procedures because acute side-effects or late toxicity of radiotherapy are not increased compared with younger patients (Rotte 1975; Sturm 1977; Rustowski and Kupsc 1982; Huguenin et al. 1992). We think the condition of the patient is more important than her age. Thus, even in stage I, external beam therapy can be indicated in patients of advanced age if their condition is good. It must not be forgotten that these patients have been classified as operable and it would seem rather strange for there to be discussion over the appropriateness of radiotherapy after they have got over surgery well.

At higher tumor stages there is agreement that postoperative irradiation is generally required, especially in those patients with a stage III tumor who have undergone operation (Kucera and Vavra 1991; Glassburn et al. 1992; DeVita et al. 1993; Greven et al. 1993). All our stage II tumors are irradiated after operation, as are those stage III outpatients who are operated on.

All these strategies refer to the usual situation which dose not allow performance of diagnostic lymphadenectomy, as is recommended by FIGO. The general state of health of typical patients with endometrial carcinoma usually does not allow adequate lymphadenectomy in the pelvic or higher lymph nodes but only sampling of a small number of lymph nodes. The latter cannot be considered an adequate investigation. It must be stressed that it is absolutely inadequate only to palpate lymph nodes: small infiltrated lymph nodes cannot be detected and not each enlarged lymph node is infiltrated. According to Pfleiderer (1991) at least 15–20 lymph nodes must be examined.

If pelvic lymphadenectomy has been performed without reliable information on the para-aortic state one should have a special look at the relation between the number of dissected and number of involved lymph nodes before deciding whether adjuvant pelvic irradiation should be performed. Several constellations are possible:

1. More than 30 lymph nodes are dissected and less than five are infiltrated. In this case the staging lymphadenectomy should be considered therapeutic because the situation resembles the state after Wertheim's operation and the effect of adjuvant irradiation would be uncertain; moreover, one could expect increased side-effects.
2. Only 15–20 lymph nodes are dissected and most of them are infiltrated. Irradiation of the pelvis is necessary. If the patient is in a good general state of health we would also treat the para-aortic lymph nodes because the risk of lymph node infiltration in this region is at least 40% in such a constellation (Creasman et al. 1987). This is one of the few instances where adjuvant para-aortic irradiation would be indicated. Normally we perform such additional radiation therapy only if there is histological proof of lymph node metastases or at least suspicion thereof on the basis of imaging procedures. Regardless of such involvement, we agree with the recommendation of Averette et al. (1987) that in all patients who are to undergo extended field radiation therapy, scalene node biopsy should be performed. A positive result will contraindicate curative para-aortic radiation; moreover, one should consider changing the general radiation management and foregoing adjunctive irradiation procedures completely.
3. About 15–20 or more lymph nodes are dissected and no metastases have been found. No adjuvant teletherapy is necessary even if the prognosticators (e.g., myometrial infiltration, grading, ploidy, histological subtype, progesterone receptor) indicate a so-called high-risk case. The aforementioned factors prognosticate the risk of lymph node metastases and their value is diminished if there is no histological proof of infiltration.
4. Less than 15 lymph nodes are dissected and no metastases have been found. These patients should be treated in the same way as those without any lymph node sampling, i.e., radiation therapy should depend on the usual prognosticators. Examinations in cervical cancer (Kreienberg et al. 1990) have shown that the risk of pelvic metastases is considerably underestimated if only about 20 lymph nodes are dissected. It can be suggested that this is also true for endometrial cancer.

Adjuvant external beam therapy of the pelvis is, of course, indicated if there is infiltration of blood or lymph vessels, whatever the nodal state. If teletherapy is indicated we employ a biaxial monosegmental arc technique (Fig. 10.14) using 10-MeV photons. Twelve fractions of 2 Gy are applied to the whole pelvis, followed by 13 fractions of 2 Gy to the pelvic lymphatics using the same technique as in primary irradiation. The dose refers to the maximum point; at least the 80% isodose encloses the target

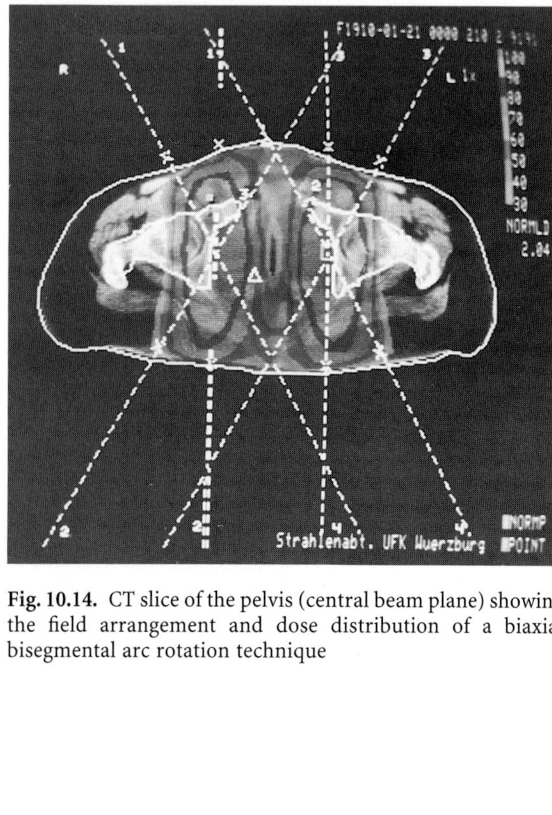

Fig. 10.14. CT slice of the pelvis (central beam plane) showing the field arrangement and dose distribution of a biaxial bisegmental arc rotation technique

volume. The technique is suitable for sparing the organs at risk and the skin. Additionally we define the target volumes individually in several CT slices, which supports the planning procedure. The center of the pelvis is spared in order to avoid overlapping doses resulting from brachytherapy of the vaginal stump. The intracavitary treatment amounts to 3 times 8 Gy applied in 30 days to the applicator surface (for details see Sect. 10.8.1). One can suppose that this technique might deliver too low a dose to the upper center of the pelvis, but analysis of recurrences (see Sect. 10.11) shows no reason to irradiate the whole pelvis homogeneously. Only in cases at risk, e.g., if lymphangiosis carcinomatosa is verified, do we perform a homogeneous irradiation of the whole pelvis utilizing a box technique. Twenty-five fractions of 2 Gy are applied and the brachytherapy volume is shielded. There is no standard therapy for patients with peritoneal tumor spread.

Teletherapy of the abdomen plays little role though it is sometimes performed even as adjuvant treatment (GREER and HAMBERGER 1983; LOEFFLER et al. 1988; POTISH 1989). The effect of such irradiation is restricted because tumor cells between the diaphragm and the liver cannot be sterilized sufficiently due to the tolerance doses of the organs at risk in this region. Some authors recommend intraperitoneal application of radiopharmaceuticals (SOPER et al. 1985; HEATH et al. 1988). PIVER et al. (1988) administered progesterone acetate, which seems to be the most suitable treatment.

It is widely accepted that para-aortic lymphatics should be irradiated only if they are involved in metastatic spread (ROSE et al. 1992; DEVITA et al. 1993; GREVEN et al. 1993) and not as an adjuvant treatment. We regard this procedure as justified only in rare cases owing to the poor benefit, the relatively severe discomfort (partial involvement of the small bowel and stomach), the decreased tolerance to irradiation which results from a pelvic plus para-aortic treatment volume, the sometimes poor general state of health in combination with advanced age, a risk of nephritis, and the possible partial exposure of the spinal cord (unfavorable relation between treatment volume and angulated target volume).

The radiation technique, which may be a combination of fixed fields, sometimes in conjunction with wedge filters or arc rotation therapy, has hardly any influence in these circumstances. We apply a maximum dose of 25 × 2 Gy using 10-MeV photons, and at least the 80% isodose encloses the target volume.

The prognosis is in general poor (MORROW et al. 1991).

10.8.1 Postoperative Brachytherapy of the Vaginal Stump Only

The incidence of vaginal metastases after hysterectomy and bilateral salpingo-oophorectomy ranges between 5% and 20% if no postoperative radiation is performed (RUTLEDGE et al. 1958; PRICE et al. 1965; GRAHAM 1971; FRICK et al. 1983; SORBE and SMEDS 1990; DEVITA et al. 1993). The median rate is about 10% (LEIBEL and WHARHAM 1980; MANDELL et al. 1985a). Many authors report a considerable reduction in this rate after vaginal irradiation (GAUWERKY and OBRANOVIC 1967; ROTTE 1969; SHAH and GREEN 1972; ONSRUD et al. 1976; JOSLIN et al. 1977; AALDERS et al. 1980; LEIBEL and WHARHAM 1980; LADNER 1983; BEDWINEK et al. 1984; PIPARD et al. 1985; MANDELL et al. 1985a; PEREZ et al. 1985; NORI et al. 1987; KUCERA and WEGHAUPT 1988; PETTERSSON et al. 1989; SORBE and SMEDS 1990; PFLEIDERER 1991; VAVRA et al. 1991; SCHULZ-WENDTLAND et al. 1993; ELLIOT et al. 1994), but the value of vaginal irradiation is nevertheless sometimes doubted (MALKASIAN et al. 1980; HORDING and HANSEN 1985).

Analyses of rates of vaginal recurrence after surgery alone and postoperative brachytherapy showed no vaginal recurrences in the irradiated groups whereas in control groups recurrence rates of 12% (GRAHAM 1971) and 8% (PIVER 1980) were seen. Similar results in patients with stage I tumors, whatever the grade, have been reported by others (REDDY et al. 1979; BOND 1985; MARCHETTI et al. 1986).

In a retrospective study of recurrences in patients with stage I endometrial carcinoma (VAVRA et al. 1991), the value of vaginal irradiation was obvious. In the group without postoperative irradiation, 90% of the relapses were of vaginal origin, whereas in the irradiated group the ratio of vaginal and extravaginal recurrences was 1:1. After irradiation only 8 of 360 patients showed a vaginal recurrence. The rate of vaginal recurrences after brachytherapy averages about 1% (GAUWERKY and OBRANOVIC 1967; GAUWERKY 1980; JOSLIN et al. 1977; ROTTE 1969; KUCERA and WEGHAUPT 1988; PESCHEL et al. 1989).

The Annual Report documented by PETTERSSON (1991) showed an increased survival rate in women treated postoperatively by vaginal brachytherapy as compared with women undergoing only surgery. This was especially true of cases with an unfavorable grade. Though this was a retrospective analysis, it can be regarded as persuasive owing to the great number of cases considered. Further aspects of the treatment results will be considered later in Sect. 10.11.

We agree with GRAHAM (1971), GOODMAN and HELLMAN (1974), and KUCERA et al. (1986) and perform vaginal stump irradiation in all patients who have undergone surgery for endometrial carcinoma, whatever the stage and the risk factors. This liberal indication is based on the fact that with such a policy we observe both a considerable reduction in vaginal recurrences and no early or late side-effects. There is nearly unanimous agreement on this point among the cited authors, and it is thus justified to treat about 90% of the patients unnecessarily. There is still a lack of adequate prognosticators that allow definition of certain groups at low risk so that the number of irradiated patients can be reduced. Moreover, it is known that vaginal recurrences occur even in women with low-risk tumors after surgery alone (PRICE et al. 1965; JOSLIN et al. 1967; SHAH and GREEN 1972; AALDERS et al. 1980; KLEINE et al. 1982). In spite of the favorable results of vaginal brachytherapy, several authors have renounced postoperative irradiation because they suppose that removal of a larger vaginal cuff at hysterectomy would have the same effect (BERMAN et al. 1980). However, this argument has not taken into consideration those recurrences which are located paraurethrally. In contrast to lesions in the upper vagina, which are assumed to be metastases to the vagina resulting from surgery, the paraurethral lesions are probably due to metastatic spread through submucosal venous and lymphatic plexuses (DEVITA et al. 1993; ELLIOT et al. 1994). Thus we also irradiate the lower vagina up to the hymenal ring. A similar procedure has been reported by others (GRAHAM 1971; SHAH and GREEN 1972; JOSLIN et al. 1977; BOND 1985; MANDELL et al. 1985a; DEVITA et al. 1993; ELLIOT et al. 1994), whereas PIPARD et al. (1985) and PERNOT et al. (1994) do not recommend irradiation of the entire length of the vagina because they suggest that this poses a potential risk to healthy tissues. A special policy is preferred by KINDERMANN (1981), who inserted a vaginal wick irrigated with alcohol at hysterectomy in order to prevent the implantation of tumor cells to the upper part of the vagina. In regard to the risk of suburethral metastases, he recommends additional brachytherapy that is restricted to the lower two-thirds of the vagina.

It must not be forgotten that the treatment outcomes of vaginal relapses are poor (LEIBEL and WHARHAM 1980; PHILLIPS et al. 1982; CURRAN et al. 1988; KUTEN et al. 1989; SORBE and SMEDS 1990), whatever the treatment form (surgery or intracavitary or interstitial brachytherapy).

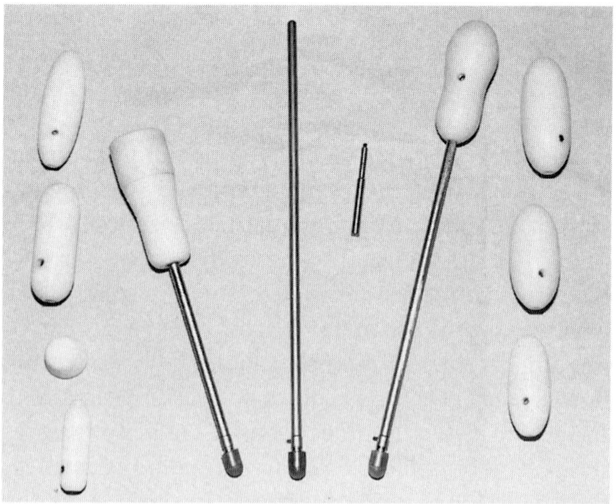

Fig. 10.15. Individually manufactured vaginal applicators for use in remote-controlled afterloading

Our plastic vaginal applicators are manufactured in our workshop. Their size and form are designed according to the individual situation (Fig. 10.15). We apply three fractions of 8 Gy to the surface of the applicator. The fractions are delivered 10 days apart if external beam therapy is performed simultaneously and 7 days apart if it is not. Treatment planning is without exception based on digitized orthogonal radiographs, as in primary radiation of endometrial cancer. As we place the reference isodose to the surface of the applicator, and not to any defined depth in the paravaginal tissue, the applied doses are normalized both to the site of recurrences and to the site of eventual side-effects. We tolerate 7 Gy per fraction to the organs at risk in patients being treated by a combination of external beam radiation and brachytherapy, or a total dose of 60 Gy within 6 weeks, as already recommended in former times (NEEFF 1941; FRISCHKORN 1983).

10.9 Hormones

As already pointed out, hormone response depends on the receptor status, and especially on the progesterone receptor (EHRLICH et al. 1981; QUINN et al. 1985). The content of progesterone receptors is correlated with the histological grade, and well-differentiated tumors respond more frequently to a hormonal therapy than do poorly differentiated lesions, as is well known. EHRLICH et al. (1981) reported that nearly 90% of progesterone-responsive tumors were receptor-positive and that more than 90% of nonresponders were receptor-negative. Commonly medroxyprogesterone acetate is applied. One has to distinguish between treatment of recurrences or metastases and adjuvant therapy.

10.9.1 Progesterone Therapy in Recurrent or Metastatic Cases

In general, response rates of about 15%–30% are reported with progesterone therapy for recurrences or metastases (PIVER et al. 1980b, KLEINE et al. 1990; MOORE et al. 1991; GLASSBURN et al. 1992). About 70% of recurrent or metastatic endometrial carcinomas are receptor-negative (KLEINE et al. 1990), which is surely one of the reasons for the relatively poor results.

Several studies have shown responses to be associated with prolonged survival. Median survival for women responding to hormonal therapy is about 1.5 years in comparison with only ca. 6 months for nonresponders (REIFENSTEIN 1971; KNEALE 1986; GLASSBURN et al. 1992). The response to hormones is increased in patients with a long disease-free interval (2–3 years), and it seems to be more common in vaginal or lung metastases than in pelvic recurrences. If hormonal therapy is not limited by venous thrombosis it should be continued indefinitely until progression is found (DEVITA 1993), especially since premature termination of therapy can provoke a rebound phenomenon (ROTTE 1975).

Several investigators have stressed the value of progesterone therapy after the irradiation of vaginal recurrences (VON FOURNIER et al. 1981; KUCERA and WEGHAUPT 1988).

A second-line systemic therapy is the administration of tamoxifen, which results in a median response rate of lower than 20% (HALD et al. 1983). As already mentioned (see Sect. 10.5), attempts have been made to enhance the effects of hormonal treatment by additional tamoxifen administration (GURPIDE 1981; CARLSON et al. 1984), which can increase the progesterone receptor level (JÄNNE et al. 1979, POLLOW et al. 1986). The response rates have not differed significantly from those achieved with sole progesterone treatment, however (CARLSON et al. 1984). This is also true for combinations with estradiol or aminoglutethimide (SCHULZ and KAISER 1983; RENDINA et al. 1984; QUINN et al. 1985). PIVER et al. (1988) reported use of progesterone therapy in cases with a peritoneal tumor spread. This treatment seems to be superior to postoperative irradiation of the whole pelvis and to intraperitoneal nuclide application.

10.9.2 Adjuvant Progesterone Therapy

The use of progesterone as an adjunctive modality in cases of endometrial cancer is considered controversial. Some authors recommend its use in high-risk cases (GUSBERG 1980; DEPALO et al. 1983; KNEALE 1986); others, however, have failed to observe any benefit (LEWIS et al. 1974; MALKASIAN and DECKER 1978; MACDONALD et al. 1988; VERGOTE et al. 1989; KAUFMANN et al. 1990). In their randomized study, moreover, VERGOTE et al. (1989) saw an increased rate of cardiovascular diseases in patients treated with progesterone. An adjuvant hormone therapy is not common in our clinic. In patients with recurrent or disseminated disease, the use of progesterone depends on the risk of venous thrombosis. In addition, other side-effects such as increasing obesity and a negative influence on diabetes mellitus should be taken into account; of course, these side-effects are relatively mild and cannot be compared to those of polychemotherapy.

According to RENDINA (1984) the most effective dose seems to be 1000 mg a week. Lower doses are considered to be ineffective. KUCERA (1993) recommended a median dose of 600 mg daily. Usually we begin with an intramuscular injection of 1000 mg twice a week for 4 weeks, after which the dose is reduced to one application a week. If we employ oral administration, 500 mg is administered daily.

10.10 Role of Chemotherapy, Sensitizers, and Hyperthermia

Patients in whom hormone therapy fails may be considered for chemotherapy with palliative intent. Trials examining the effect of single-agent chemotherapy in endometrial carcinoma show that only a few drugs, such as doxorubicin, hexamethylmelamine, and cisplatin, have a certain activity. The response rates are in the range of 15%–30% (SESKI et al. 1981, 1982; DEPPE et al. 1984). Reasonable response rates have only been achieved when the agents have been applied at high doses as a first-line treatment. In general, the duration of single-agent responses has been only a few months.

Combination chemotherapy appears to display a degree of enhanced activity. In patients with advanced or recurrent disease, studies employing doxorubicin and cisplatin or doxorubicin, cisplatin, and cyclophosphamide produced higher response rates (about 40%–60%) compared with doxorubicin alone (PASMANTIER et al. 1985; HANCOCK et al. 1986; CHAUVERGNE et al. 1986). In a randomized study a combination of melphalan and 5-fluorouracil or 5-fluorouracil, doxorubicin, and cyclophosphamide yielded response rates of more than 80% in advanced tumor stages (COHEN et al. 1984). These results, however, must be confirmed in larger trials. Moreover, in most trials there has been no survival benefit and no longer duration of response compared with the results of single-agent therapy. The increased toxicity of combination chemotherapy also has to be considered, especially in typical patients suffering from endometrial cancer. Thus single-agent carboplatin may be a reasonable alternative (KAVANAGH and KUDELKA 1993). According to VADON (1992), regional chemotherapy with doxorubicin, mitomycin-C, and 5-fluorouracil may be another alternative regimen in patients with recurrences, producing tumor regression with reduced side-effects, though he conceded that it is only temporarily effective. Moreover, the results refer to a small number of patients and mostly to cervical cancer. Similar points can be made regarding intraperitoneal applications of mitomycin C in the treatment of peritoneal carcinomatosis (MONK et al. 1988). The combination of ifosfamide and mesna showed some activity in refractory endometrial adenocarcinoma failing platinum-based therapy (SUTTON et al. 1994). Treatment with palliative intention using interferons (KUDELKA et al. 1993) and gonadotropin-releasing hormones (GALLAGHER et al. 1991) has also shown some effect, though a benefit in terms of survival has not been reported. Studies of combined hormonal therapy and systemic chemotherapy similarly failed to show improved survival rates (PIVER et al. 1986).

Undifferentiated, hormone receptor-negative and clear cell or papillary serous tumors are suggested to be more sensitive to chemotherapy (GREVEN et al. 1993), but even in these groups the results are poor in general. Chemotherapy as an adjuvant modality appears to be of no value. In a randomized trial there was no benefit of additional chemotherapy with doxorubicin after surgery and postoperative radiation (MORROW et al. 1990).

Reports on chemotherapeutic agents as radiation sensitizers in patients with pelvic tumors are sparse. Sensitization is sometimes confused with synergism between cytotoxic drugs and irradiation. The important feature of a radiation sensitizer is its low or missing effect if it is applied as a single agent. A natural sensitizer is, of course, oxygen. The well-known term "oxygen enhancement ratio," which is based on the studies of GRAY et al. (1953), refers to the fact that anoxygenic tissue has to be irradiated with a threefold dose to obtain the same effect as in oxygenic tissue. Among the different drugs which have been considered to be sensitizers of radiation therapy, 5-fluorouracil, hydroxyurea, misonidazole, and metronidazole and their breakdown products should be mentioned. According to experimental data, 5-fluorouracil is suggested to synchronize tumor cells in the most sensitive phase of the cell cycle. Misonidazole and metronidazole enhance selectively the radiosensitiveness of hypoxic cells (HALL and ROIZIN-TOWLE 1975; DISCHE et al. 1978; MAGDON 1980). The clinical results in this area are generally disappointing (DISCHE 1985). Reports on uterine malignancies are sparse and are mostly related to small groups of patients with cervical cancer (PIVER et al. 1974; HRESHCHYSHYN et al. 1979; STEHMAN et al. 1988).

In experimental studies, synergism of hyperthermia and irradiation (SURWIT et al. 1983; JORRITSMA et al. 1985; RAFLA et al. 1989) and enhancement of the cell-killing effect of cytotoxic drugs by hypertermia (MELLA 1985) have been demonstrated. Hyperthermia is not dependent on the presence of oxygen, and it can thus overcome radioresistance of hypoxic tissues. Moreover, tumor cells in the late S phase are supposed to be sensitive to hyperthermia, in contrast to radiotherapy (HETZEL 1989). However, because of the technological limitations to the delivery of adequate heat to large parts of the body, such as the pelvis, few results are available in respect of hyperthermia in the treatment of gynecological tumors. Reports on the combination of pelvic irradiation and hyperthermia are mostly related to nongynecological tumors, and there is a lack of clinical trials documenting its efficacy in uterine cancer. The rare reports are restricted to advanced or recurrent cervical cancer (SURWIT et al. 1983; HORNBACK et al. 1986; STEINDORFER et al. 1987; VORA et al. 1988; SHARMA et al. 1989; GOFFINET et al. 1990; BLOSS et al. 1992), and have revealed no significant improvement in disease-free intervals or survival rates in comparison with radiotherapy alone. The improved tumor response rates reported by SHARMA et al. (1989) in their prospective randomized study are based on a group of only 50 patients including the control group. Reports on the use of combined hyperthermia and irradiation for endometrial cancer refer to single patients with vaginal recurrences (BELCH et al. 1990; STÜCKLSCHWEIGER et al. 1991).

10.11 Five-Year Results and Complications

10.11.1 Primary Irradiation

In the Röntgen- und Strahlenabteilung der Universitäts-Frauenklinik Würzburg from May 1988 up to December 1994, 68 patients were treated according to the described protocol of modified Heyman packing. Thus, as five fractions are required by the protocol, the total number of applications during this period was 340. Those patient who received a treatment that aviated from the protocol with respect to fractionation, total dose, overall time, or teletherapy, for whatever reason, are not taken into account in this analysis. The median observation time was 38 months. The mean age of the patients was 78 years.

As shown in Table 10.7, to date there have been two local recurrences. The relapse of a stage III tumor occurred within 12 months after treatment and was associated with rapidly progressing metastases to the lung and pleural effusion. The patient died a few weeks later. Three other women developed diffuse metastatic seeding into the lung and/or the liver within 8–24 months. Nine patients died intercurrently. In comparison with our historical patient group, which was treated between 1972 and 1988 by radium packing or HDR afterloading with a rigid applicator, the results of our current regimen show a considerable improvement, even taking into account the different periods of follow-up (Table 10.8). Of course, long-term results are necessary to confirm this clear-cut trend. But, as dosage and fractionation in the 327 patients treated up to 1988 were nearly identical to those in our current patient group, we have no reason to expect worse results in a regimen which is much more individual and which shows a higher geometrical precision than the old techniques.

A comparison of data reported in the literature is difficult because of patient selection factors, differences in technique and dosage, and inexact staging. In women who have undergone both brachytherapy and external beam irradiation, survival after 5 years ranges between 60% and 80% in stage I tumors and between 35% and 60% in stage II tumors; it averages about 60% in all stages (LANDGREN et al. 1976;

Table 10.7. Results of primary radiation therapy of endometrial carcinoma with high-dose-rate afterloading simulating Heyman packing, 1988–1994

FIGO	No.	3-year actuarial survival	Local recurrences	Distant metastases	Side-effects[a]
I	24	23/24 (95.8%)	1 (4.2%)	–	–
II	31	24/31 (77.4%)	–	1 (3.2%)	–
III	13	9/13 (69.2%)	1 (7.7%)	3 (23.1%)	–
Total	68	56/68 (82.4%)	2 (2.9%)	4 (5.9%)	–

[a] Fistulas, ulcers, stenoses.

Table 10.8. Results of primary radiotherapy for carcinoma of the corpus uteri (n = 395) at UFK Würzburg (observation period 1972–1994)

Stage	Radium-226 (LDR), 1972–1982: 5-year crude survival	Double-rod-shaped applicator (HDR), 1972–1987: 5-year crude survival	Heyman capsules (HDR), 1988–1994: 3-year actuarial survival
I	76.9% (= 30/39)	72.7% (= 72/99)	95.8% (= 23/24)
II	73.9% (= 34/46)	72.4% (= 76/105)	77.4% (= 24/31)
III	28.5% (= 6/21)	35.3% (= 6/17)	69.2% (= 9/13)

GRIGSBY et al. 1985; ROTTE 1985; VARIA et al. 1986; KUCERA and WEGHAUPT 1988; VAHRSON 1991; DUBOIS et al. 1992; ROSE et al. 1993; PERNOT et al. 1994).

All data, as well as those in respect of our historical patient group (Table 10.8), have been worse than the results of surgery and postoperative irradiation in early stage cancer. This difference does not represent proof of the superiority of hysterectomy but is rather due to several influences: patients who are irradiated primarily are considerably older, normally in a worse general state, and suffer from more advanced disease. These factors ultimately lead to the decision to treat them by radiotherapy. In primary irradiation, rates of deaths due to intercurrent disease of between 45% and 60% are reported (LANDGREN et al. 1976; VARIA et al. 1986). All these circumstances stress the need to evaluate corrected survival data (VAHRSON 1991; ROSE et al. 1993; PERNOT et al. 1994).

This has been done in a case-controlled study of more than 700 patients by ROSE et al. (1993): 64 stage I and II patients treated by primary radiation therapy were matched with surgically treated controls for clinical stage, histological grade, and time of diagnosis, and no statistical difference was observed in respect of survival. Our preliminary findings indicate the results achieved with the modified Heyman packing protocol to be equivalent to those of surgery, even without any correction. These are only two examples, but they show that it is not justified to underestimate the efficacy of primary radiotherapy though surgery followed by tailored irradiation has become the widely accepted therapy for early stage endometrial cancer.

Nevertheless, since the FIGO Committee agreed upon the system for surgical staging in 1988, the comparison of surgery plus radiotherapy and radiotherapy alone has become more difficult. This is also true for comparisons between current and former surgical procedures. Moreover, results in respect of preoperative irradiation are no longer comparable. Further aspects of surgical staging will be discussed after presentation of the results of postoperative radiotherapy.

The reported rates of pelvic recurrences and distant metastases after primary irradiation vary considerably. According to GLASSBURN et al. (1992), DE VITA et al. (1993), and PERNOT et al. (1994), who summarized the literature data, the frequency of relapses ranges between 8% and 25% in stage I and II disease. The rate of distant metastases is about 30%–35%.

In our series acute side-effects are restricted to mild cystitis or diarrhea. They are seen in about 70% of our patients, the diarrhea primarily being related to external beam irradiation. Severe early complications have not occurred to date, nor have there been severe late side-effects (of course, only those patients who have a follow-up of more than 24 months can be considered) – in particular, there have been no cases of fistulas or ulcers. As shown in Table 10.9, we found no difference between the current and the historical regimen with regard to either early or late reactions (in contrast to the differences in respect of survival and recurrence rate).

These observations agree with numerous reports in literature where late toxicity after irradiation of gynecological malignancies has rarely been observed. Intestinal ulcerations, fistulas to the rectum or bladder, vaginal necrosis or stenosis, ureteral stricture, and contracted bladder are reported in about 1%–3% of patients (BÖTTCHER et al. 1983; KUCERA et al. 1990a; HUGUENIN et al. 1992; WILLGEROTH 1992; ROSE et al. 1993; PERNOT et al. 1994).

We suggest the modest rate of sequelae in our patient group to be due to the individual dose distribution of brachytherapy, the smaller target volume of the rotation arc technique in comparison with standing opposite fields or a box technique, and the adaptation of the dose distribution of the first- and second-rank target volumes. Using MRI for treatment planning, we can adapt the irradiated (and not only the treated) volume to the uterine size, which helps to avoid overdosage of the small bowel, and especially of those segments which are possibly immobile and adherent to the uterine surface. The significance of this must not be underestimated because typical patients suffer from diabetes and hypertension, which can increase the risk of damage in intestinal vessels.

Thus a general requirement for the avoidance of severe side-effects is the use of computerized treat-

Table 10.9. Side-effect in the bladder and rectum in patients treated with primary radiotherapy for carcinoma of the corpus uteri (n = 395) at UFK Würzburg (observation period 1972–1994)

Radium-226 (LDR)		Iridium-192 (HDR)	
Bladder:	1.8%	Bladder.	1.7%
Rectum:	5.6%	Rectum:	5.2%
Total of lesions: 7.5%		Total of lesions: 7.0%	

Note: No vesicovaginal or rectovaginal fistulas were observed.

ment planning on the basis of suitable imaging procedures which provides the possibility to visualize a three-dimensional dose distribution. However, these dose-related aspects have to be regarded only as a part of an interplay of factors influencing side-effects (HEILMANN and BÜNEMANN 1987), such as the general state of the patient and concomitant diseases. This may explain the lack of correspondence that sometimes exists between cumulated doses to the organs at risk and the clinical complication rate (ESCHE et al. 1987). Irrespective of these consideration, it is known that severe early reactions are not significantly associated with late complications or vice versa (THAMES 1983).

General recommendations regarding the treatment of the heterogeneous side-effects are not meaningful. Individual administration of local or systemic drugs (e.g., corticosteroids), adequate alimentation, and other symptom-alleviating measures should be taken.

In achieving the therapeutic aim, side-effects cannot be avoided totally. However, experience and specialization in gynecological radiotherapy can help to reduce them.

10.11.2 Postoperative Irradiation

In the Röntgen- und Strahlenabteilung der Universitäts-Frauenklinik Würzburg, 894 women with endometrial cancer (including five with a mixed müllerian tumor and ten with different forms of sarcoma) were treated by radiation therapy from January 1983 to December 1992. Among these, 637 patients suffering from endometrial carcinomas with complete clinical and histopathological data were irradiated after abdominal hysterectomy and bilateral oophorectomy in accordance with the surgical and radiotherapeutic treatment protocol mentioned above. Only these 637 patients were analysed; lost cases and patients for whom the cause of death is unknown have been registered as dead of endometrial cancer.

Table 10.10. Stage distribution of endometrial cancer treated with postoperative irradiation at UFK Wüzburg, 1983–1992

Stage	No.	%
I	459	72
II	108	17
III	64	10
IV	6	1
Total	637	100

Table 10.11. Degrees of differentiation of endometrial carcinoma treated with postoperative irradiation at UFK Würzburg, 1983–1992

Grade	No.	%
1	248	39
2	274	43
3	102	16
Unknown	13	2
	637	100

The mean age of the patients was 68 years. More than 75% showed an adenocarcinoma of the endometrioid type, about 10% showed papillary forms, 10% had serous, or adenosquamous types, and the remaining 5% displayed various other lesion types, especially clear cell carcinoma. The stage distribution and the degree of differentiation are shown in Tables 10.10 and 10.11. The relatively high rate of stage III tumors is due to the fact that our group includes patients transferred from other clinics for postoperative radiation therapy. According to the interdisciplinary approach of our clinic, many of these women would have been candidates for primary irradiation.

A total of 141 patients with stage I tumors, myometrial infiltration less than 3 mm, and a highly differentiated endometrioid adenocarcinoma were treated by vaginal irradiation alone. The rest underwent additional external beam therapy. The median observation time until December 1993 was 74 months (minimum 13 months, maximum 131 months). The crude survival is presented in Fig. 10.16. The 3-year survival rate by all stages and all histological subtypes of carcinoma is 83%, and the 5-year survival rate is 79%. About 20% of the deaths were intercurrent.

Our results are comparable to the survival data shown in Table 10.12 and to those of other series of postoperative irradiation reported in the literature (MANDELL et al. 1985a; LYBEERT et al. 1989; VAHRSON 1991; PERNOT et al. 1994). It should be mentioned that PERNOT et al. (1994) obtained favorable results by preoperative irradiation in stages I–III; follow-up related to a treatment period between 1973 and 1988, and overall survival after 10 years was 71%.

In stage I endometrial carcinoma NORI et al. (1987) reported a corrected 5-year survival rate of 91% ($n = 300$) after surgery and radiotherapy versus only 73% ($n = 376$) after surgery alone.

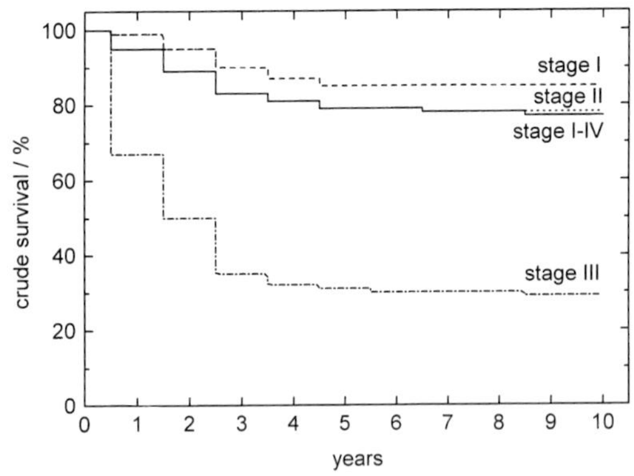

Fig. 10.16. Crude survival according to stage and duration of observation for patients with endometrial carcinoma treated with postoperative irradiation at UFK Würzburg

Table 10.12. Survival at 5 years after surgery and radiation for endometrial carcinoma. (Modified from GLASSBURN et al. 1992)

Investigators	Stage	No.	%
GRAHAM (1971)	I	123	74
BRADY et al. (1974)	I	99	88
FRICK et al. (1983)	I	239	78
GRIGSBY et al. (1991)	I	858	89
ONSRUD et al. (1982)	II	40	85
GRIGSBY et al. (1985)	II	90	78
ANDERSEN (1990)	II	54	71
MACKILLOP and PRINGLE (1985)	III	62	38

Table 10.13. Vaginal recurrences after adjuvant brachytherapy. (Modified from ELLIOT et al. 1994)

Authors	No.	Vaginal recurrences
Low-risk stage I tumors		
GRAHAM (1971)	51	0
JOSLIN et al. (1977)	88	1
BOND (1985)	481	0
MARCHETTI et al. (1989)	117	0
SORBE and SMEDS (1989)	335	0
PIVER and HEMPLING (1990)	92	0
ELLIOT et al. (1994)	163	1
Total	1327	2
High-risk stage I and II tumors		
GRAHAM (1971)	25	0
JOSLIN et al. (1977)	168	2
MARCHETTI et al. (1986)	41	1
SORBE and SMEDS (1990)	69	1
ELLIOT et al. (1994)	127	1
Total	440	5

Our low-risk group treated by vaginal brachytherapy alone showed an 85% survival rate after 5 years. The same rate was achieved in the other stage I tumors, and the results in stage II tumors were not essentially worse. This stresses the efficacy of external beam therapy in cases carrying a worse prognosis. Similar conclusions were drawn by KUCERA et al. (1989). In their group of 544 patients with stage I tumors they compared the results of sole brachytherapy in low-risk cases (G1 tumors, myometrial infiltration less than one-third) and combined brachytherapy and external beam therapy in high-risk cases (G2/3, deep infiltration) and found no significant difference (survival at 5 years-91% vs 88%). JOSLIN et al. (1977) achieved improved results in deeply invasive stage I tumors by combined brachytherapy and external beam therapy in comparison with surgery alone (survival at 5 years-90% vs 67%).

Normally the results in patients with stage III tumors are poor, i.e., the overall survival is less than 50% (Table 10.12). Significantly better results have, however, been reported by GREVEN et al. (1993), who reported a 5-year disease-free survival rate of 64% in a series of 105 patients. Similar favorable results have been presented by GREER and HAMBERGER (1983), GENEST et al. (1987), GRIGSBY et al. (1987), and POTISH (1989), in small groups of patients. Possibly these results are a consequence of aggressive (in some cases, whole abdominal) radiotherapy.

A site of predilection for recurrences is the vaginal stump (INGERSOLL 1971; ROTMAN et al. 1988), and above all the vault and the upper third of the vagina (SALAZAR et al. 1977; AALDERS et al. 1980). On average, vaginal recurrences are reported in about 10% of patients after surgery alone (LEIBEL and WHARHAM 1980; MANDELL et al. 1985a). The efficacy of adjuvant brachytherapy of the whole vagina in low- and high-risk cases is undoubted, and has been demonstrated in several published studies of large numbers of patients (Table 10.13). In low-risk patients vaginal recurrences can be almost entirely eliminated and in high-risk cases radiotherapy will significantly reduce their incidence (GAUWERKY and OBRANOVIC 1967; GAUWERKY 1980; ROTTE 1969; GRAHAM 1971; JOSLIN et al. 1977; REDDY et al. 1979; PIVER 1980; BOND 1985; MARCHETTI et al. 1986; KUCERA and WEGHAUPT 1988; PESCHEL et al. 1989; VAVRA et al. 1991). These reports are in agreement with our own results, which show a vaginal recurrence rate of about 1%, whatever the stage.

Table 10.14 shows the patterns of recurrences after postoperative radiation therapy in stage I and II

Table 10.14. Pattern of recurrences after surgery and irradiation

Stage I	Own patient group (n = 459)	Summary of other authors' groups[a] (n = 1635)
Vagina	2 (0.4%)	–
Pelvis	11 (2.4%)	46 (2.8%)
Vagina + pelvis	2 (0.4%)	–
Distant metastases	41 (8.9%)	116 (7.1%)
Vagina/pelvis + distant metastases	–	30 (1.8%)

Stage II	(n = 108)	(n = 214)
Vagina	1 (0.9%)	2 (0.9%)
Pelvis	4 (3.7%)	5 (2.3%)
Vagina + pelvis	1 (0.9%)	4 (1.8%)
Distant metastases	11 (10.2%)	20 (9.4%)
Vagina/pelvis + distant metastases	5 (4.6%)	7 (3.2%)

[a] Cited from GLASSBURN et al. (1992).

tumors. In stage III disease, 45% (29/64) of our patients developed distant metastases (including para-aortic lymph node metastases), which were associated with pelvic failure in 12 cases. Not only this high rate of distant metastases, which influenced the survival rate considerably, but also the pelvic recurrences (14/64) remain a problem. Even in studies presenting a favorable survival rate (see above), pelvic failure is reported in 15%–30%.

About 80% of our relapses by all stages occurred within 36 months, and this rate is confirmed by others (BROWN et al. 1968; ROTTE 1969; SALAZAR et al. 1977; REDDY et al. 1979; LEIBEL and WHARHAM 1980; PEREZ and CAMEL 1982; CURRAN et al. 1988; PIVER and HEMPLING 1990; VAVRA et al. 1991). Among patients with stage I or stage II tumors, pelvic failure was not significantly more frequent in low-risk cases than in those showing deep infiltration. We think this to be a consequence of external beam therapy; the effectiveness of the latter in preventing vaginal and pelvic recurrences (which is comparable to its effect on survival) has been stressed by the well-known prospective study of AALDERS et al. (1980) in stage I carcinoma.

The already mentioned prognostic influence of histological subtypes was obvious in our patients: In about 50% of distant, regional, or local recurrences papillary or adenosquamous types were found, whereas they occurred only in 20% of the whole group. Moreover, about 30% of the recurrent endometrioid carcinomas were poorly differentiated, whereas grade 3 tumors were present in only 16% of all patients. Especially the recurrences of papillary carcinomas were associated with distant metastases, whatever the stage. Similar observations have been reported by others (MANDELL et al. 1985b).

Severe side-effects after postoperative irradiation are somewhat more frequent than after vaginal brachytherapy alone, but their incidence is reported to be less than 3%; among these severe effects, vaginal necrosis, fistulas, and ulcers are of interest (NORI et al. 1987; KUCERA and WEGHAUPT 1988; ELLIOT et al. 1994). Early side-effects such as mild colpitis, cystitis, and enteritis are all transient.

In our patients vaginal complications did not occur at all, irrespective of whether sole brachytherapy or combined brachytherapy and external beam therapy was used. Pelvic side-effects were all mild and transient and did not differ from those reported after primary irradiation. Special aspects of the treatment and the avoidance of complications have already been mentioned above in the section dealing with primary irradiation. Of course, the complication rate is influenced by surgery. It is known that the incidence of late bowel reactions is increased after pelvic lymph node dissection followed by external beam therapy (DALY et al. 1989; LEWANDOWSKI et al. 1990; POTISH and DUSENBERY 1990; PFLEIDERER 1991). The low grade of pelvic side-effects in our patients can be explained by the fact that most of them did not undergo such surgical treatment because of their general state.

As already mentioned, the agreement by the FIGO Committee on the system for surgical staging had the disadvantage that many results are no longer comparable. On the other hand, surgical staging has the advantage of providing better individual information on the tumor volume and spread, and it can thus improve adjuvant treatment modalities. Moreover, it has been suggested that para-aortic lymphadenectomy may represent not only a diagnostic but also a therapeutic advance (PFLEIDERER 1991), though this remains to be proven in further studies. Nevertheless, the value of surgical staging is a matter of debate for reasons other than the already mentioned problems in comparing results. While the information on the nodal state that is provided by pelvic and para-aortic lymphadenectomy is indeed one of the most important advantages of surgical staging (assuming a sufficient number of lymph nodes are examined), this extended surgery has some problematic aspects:

1. It cannot be performed in many cases because of the patient's general state. This drawback has been evident in our patient group. Laparoscopic staging may be a safe and feasible solution to this problem in patients who are not or are incompletely surgically staged, as recommended by CHILDERS et al. (1994). Sole palpation of lymph nodes is no alternative, as already mentioned.
2. There is no general agreement as to the morbidity of lymphadenectomy. HOMESLY et al. (1992) and LARSON et al. (1992) found no increase in morbidity in patients who underwent hysterectomy and pelvic and para-aortic lymphadenectomy in comparison with those who had only hysterectomy, but CLARKE-PEARSON et al. (1991) did observe such a difference. It should be mentioned that some investigations reporting tolerance of surgery refer only to lymph node sampling and not to radical lymphadenectomy (MOORE et al. 1989). There is a need for further investigations.
3. In patients who are treated by radiotherapy after lymphadenectomy, increased morbidity has to be expected (DALY et al. 1989; LEWANDOWSKI et al. 1990; POTISH and DUSENBERY 1990; PFLEIDERER 1991).
4. The risk of an increased morbidity would be justified only if the rate of, for instance, para-aortic lymph node metastases were relatively high, but this is not true in endometrial cancer.
5. The relative value of the different surgical procedures for the removal of lymph nodes is not yet established (WILLGEROTH 1994), and the benefits for patients are not yet obvious (VAHRSON 1991). Simple lymph node sampling, at least, yields no improvement in survival (JONES 1975; CREASMAN et al. 1976). Moreover, the prognosis of patients with para-aortic lymph node metastases is poor in general (MORROW et al. 1991), whatever the management.

For all these reasons it is difficult to estimate the value of surgical staging. At present it is not absolutely certain whether the majority of the patients will profit from such staging.

10.12 Management of Recurrences

10.12.1 Literature Data and the Würzburg Experience

To avoid confusion in terminology, the term "recurrence" must be defined. It is only justified to speak of a recurrence if there is a disease-free interval of at least 6 months after the completion of the primary treatment; in the absence of such an interval one is dealing with a progressive primary (ROTTE 1969; KUCERA 1990). About two-thirds of recurrences occur within 24 months after therapy, and nearly 90% within 36 months (BROWN et al. 1968; ROTTE 1969; SALAZAR et al. 1977; REDDY et al. 1979; LEIBEL and WHARHAM 1980; GLASSBURN 1981; PEREZ and CAMEL 1982; CURRAN et al. 1988; PIVER and HEMPLING 1990; VAVRA et al. 1991).

The sites of predilection for recurrences are (depending of the primary management) the uterus, the vaginal cuff, and the ovaries (ROTTE 1969, 1975; KUCERA et al. 1990a). The site and the incidence depend on the already mentioned prognosticators such as stage, grading, histological type, myometrial infiltration, receptor status, infiltration of vessels, and lymph node involvement (see Sects. 10.4 and 10.5), and, of course, on the therapeutic management of the primary. About 25% of all treatment failures are located in the vagina after hysterectomy alone (INGERSOLL 1971; ROTMAN et al. 1988). Two-thirds of them are isolated recurrences (JOSLIN and SMITH 1971; PHILLIPS et al. 1982; GREVEN and OLDS 1987). Para-aortic involvement is observed in about 30% of high-risk cases (CREASMAN et al. 1976), whereas the rate of pelvic recurrences in stage I tumors after surgery and radiation has been reported to be only 7% (PEREZ et al. 1983). These results are slightly different from those summarized in Table 10.14. The influence of the different prognostic features on the survival rate has been stressed by SUTTON et al. (1989). Endometrioid carcinomas tend to recur locally, whereas early generalization is common to secretory carcinomas, and especially those of the papillary subtype (MANDELL et al. 1985b; CHRISTOPHERSON 1986; BURKE et al. 1990; WILSON et al. 1990; VAVRA et al. 1991).

According to the literature, the 3-year survival rate of patients with recurrences is about 40%–50% (BROWN et al. 1968; REDDY et al. 1979; VAVRA et al. 1991), whereby previous irradiation appears to be of no influence (VAVRA et al. 1991). The 5-year progression-free survival of patients with an isolated vaginal recurrence treated by radiation is about 30% (AALDERS et al. 1984b; GREVEN and OLDS (1987). Patients with distant metastases have a 5-year survival rate of less than 10% (GLASSBURN et al. 1992). In our historical patient group, 10% of the recurrences were associated with distant metastases (ROTTE 1969).

The management of recurrences has to consider the individual circumstances. General directions, which should be considered only as guidelines, are summarized in Table 10.15. It is not wise to use standard strategies, because the treatment is influenced by many variables, and above all by the site of the recurrence. A limited central recurrence (including local relapses after primary irradiation) can be removed by surgery, taking into account the doses of previous radiation therapy. Normally, however, irradiation or re-irradiation is performed. We treat isolated vaginal recurrences by sole brachytherapy with individually adapted applicators (Figs. 10.15, 10.17). In women who have been previously irradiated a special shielded applicator (Fig. 10.17a) or a flattened applicator (Fig. 10.17b) is used in order to spare those areas which are not macroscopically infiltrated. The applicator containing a one-sided iron shield allows a reduction in dose to the shielded segment of 35%; in the plain part of the one-sided flattened applicator the dose increase ranges up to 250% according to the square-distance law. The treatment planning procedure, which is the same as in adjuvant vaginal brachytherapy, allows us to apply about 50 Gy to the macroscopic lesion and to spare the other previously irradiated vaginal parts considerably. A selective dose reduction of 30%–50% is possible. In the case of relapses after surgery alone, we apply five fractions of 11 Gy once a week to

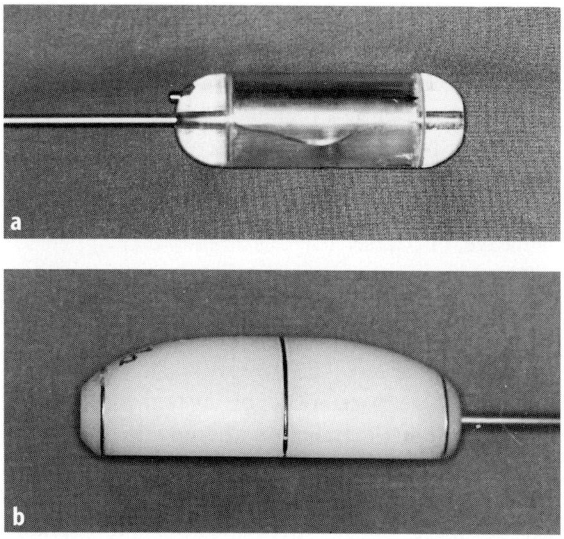

Fig. 10.17 a,b. Special vaginal applicators for use in remote-controlled afterloading. **a** One-sided iron-shielded applicator; **b** one-sided flattened applicator

the surface of the applicator. These doses are absolutely necessary because the prognosis is relatively poor and is not dependent on the grade of risk which is related to the primary (RUBIN et al. 1963; PRICE et al. 1965; LONG et al. 1972; LEIBEL and WHARHAM 1980). The prognosis is worse in recurrences in the lower vagina (RUTLEDGE et al. 1958; BROWN et al. 1968; GOODMAN and HELLMAN 1974; JOHNSSON 1979; REDDY et al. 1979; MANDELL et al. 1985b; ROTMAN et al. 1988) and the more recent the treatment (RUBIN et al. 1963; INGERSOLL 1971; PEREZ and CAMEL 1982; SORBE and SMEDS 1990).

If the recurrence has been removed and there is only microscopic tumor infiltration of the vagina, we reduce the single dose to 8 Gy, irrespective of previous irradiation.

If there is a pelvic recurrence after surgery alone which is outside of the reference volume of brachytherapy, we perform percutaneous treatment of the whole pelvis. Fractionation and dosage are the same as in adjuvant therapy, with an additional boost of about 20 Gy to the residual tumor. This strategy is only adopted if the recurrence cannot be operated on. In patients who have been previously irradiated by teletherapy, the target volume is restricted to the macroscopic tumor. If its site is paravaginal or central above the vaginal cuff, interstitial treatment may be indicated. A similar strategy was reported by PUTHAWALA et al. (1982).

HÖCKEL et al. (1989, 1990, 1993) reported a novel approach in the treatment of local recurrences to the pelvic side wall after previous irradiation in selected

Table 10.15. General directions for the treatment of recurrences of endometrial carcinomas

Site	Previous irradiation	Treatment
1. Vagina	–	Surgery or brachytherapy (macroscopic residual tumor after excision or brachytherapy alone: 5 × 11 Gy, otherwise 5 × 8 Gy)
2. Vagina	+	Brachytherapy, dosage depending on local situation (e.g., 3–5 × 8–11 Gy)
3. Pelvis	–	Surgery and external pelvic irradiation (25 × 2 Gy) or external pelvic irradiation (25 × 2 Gy) and percutaneous or interstitial[a] boost to the tumor (20 Gy minimal dose)
4. Pelvis	+	External irradiation to the tumor (25 × 2 Gy) or interstitial[a] brachytherapy (6 × 6 Gy HDR or 50 Gy LDR)
5. Vagina + pelvis	–/+	Combination of modalities 1–4, adapted to the individual situation

[a] Central or paravaginal site.

patients. After subtotal tumor resection, interstitial afterloading therapy is performed, with hollow plastic tubes being inserted at the tumor site during surgery and covered by a regional muscle flap in order to create a protective distance between the applicators and radiosensitive pelvic structures. In spite of the reported tumor remissions the strategy remains palliative, of course.

The intraperitoneal application of yttrium-90 in patients suffering from peritoneal tumor spread has been abandoned. In these cases a systemic treatment should be preferred.

If there are para-aortic or distant metastases, only symptomatic radiation therapy in combination with hormone therapy is performed. Usually medroxyprogesterone acetate is applied if possible, i.e., if there is no predisposition to venous thrombosis. Otherwise tamoxifen is chosen as a second-line therapy. In nearly all cases combined or single-agent chemotherapy as described above (see Sect. 10.10) is not possible due to the patient's state of health. Naturally, the management also depends on the site. The efficacy of progesterone acetate, above all in visceral metastases, has already been pointed out. The response rate was about 30% in the study of CAFFIER et al. (1982). Bone metastases can be treated by a combination of radiation therapy and bisphosphonates. One should distinguish between radiation for pain, with a few fractions of high single doses (e.g., 4 × 5 Gy total dose within 1 week), and for consolidation, with a normal fractionation (e.g., 20–25 × 2 Gy total dose within 4–5 weeks) in order to avoid fractures or paraplegia in cases of vertebral destruction. It is known that radiation therapy is less effective than for metastases of breast cancer.

The survival rates reported after radiation in the diverse groups of patients ranges up to about 30%, as already indicated; thus the treatment is palliative, except in patients with isolated vaginal recurrences.

It should be stressed again that each recommended approach in the treatment of recurrences is only a guideline and depends on individual circumstances. Above all, the quality of life and the life expectancy have to be considered.

Unfortunately the incidence of recurrences is increased by inadequate or uncommon diagnoses or forms of pretreatment. Incomplete histological findings, lack of abdominal exploration, failure to perform curettage followed by vaginal hysterectomy for lesions expected to be benign, and supracervical amputation without oophorectomy are well-known pitfalls. Follow-up examinations have to take into account such factors because these women should be managed as high-risk cases.

10.12.2 The Freiburg Experience

H.-A. LADNER, A. PFLEIDERER, J. BAHNSEN, and S. LADNER

10.12.2.1 Definitions

The following rules were used to classify follow-up tumor events: An isolated vaginal recurrence (VR) is a tumor up to 20 mm in size, limited to the vaginal mucosa, and not occurring within 6 months after primary therapy. The definition of isolated vaginal recurrence was adopted from PEREZ and CAMEL (1982), modified according to newer publications (CURRAN et al. 1988; SEARS et al. 1994; ELLIOTT et al. 1994). Vaginal recurrence of maximally 20 mm was distinguished from combined vaginal and pelvic recurrence (VPR) with a vaginal tumor and a histologically proven metastasis in the central pelvis or at the pelvic wall more than 6 months after therapy. Vaginal recurrence also has to be differentiated from primary vaginal involvement (PVI), after FIGO from 1988 (stage IIIB or IV). Recurrence within 6 months or primary failure of therapy was grouped under tumor progression (TP). Pelvic recurrence (PR) is defined as tumor growth limited to the pelvis and not involving the vagina 6 months or later after treatment of the primary. Distant metastasis (DM) was assumed in cases of histologically or cytologically proven tumor growth (e.g., lung, bone, brain) 6 months or later after treatment.

10.12.2.2 Patients

From 1969 to 1990 2519 patients with endometrial cancer were treated in the Universitäts-Frauenklinik (UFK) Freiburg, Germany. In 924 women primary surgery was performed in Freiburg. In 1206 patients surgery was carried out in other institutions in the southern part of Baden but radiotherapy was performed in the Department of Radiotherapy of the UFK Freiburg. Seventy-eight percent of the patients underwent surgery and postoperative radiotherapy, while 15.6% (389 women) were irradiated primarily without major surgery.

10.12.2.3
Surgery

The standard procedure was hysterectomy including the vaginal vault and both adnexa. Bilateral pelvic lymphadenectomy was performed in selected cases. The frequency of lymphadenectomy increased after 1979 (Pfleiderer 1992; Käser 1987). In gynecological departments outside the UFK Freiburg, surgery of lymph nodes was less radical and less frequent for fear of complications. Para-aortic nodes were very seldom resected. The percentage of patients receiving radiotherapy without major surgery declined rapidly after 1979.

10.12.2.4
Radiotherapy

Brachytherapy and teletherapy were performed as follows: From 1969 to 1983 radium-226 sources were used for brachytherapy of the vagina and the uterus. Between 80 and 100 mg radium within a plastic tube was positioned in the vagina for 18–20 h. Dose maximum to the rectum was measured individually and application was stopped after a rectal dose of 20 Gy; the application time was reduced to 1000 mgelh in 12–15 h in the case of additional teletherapy. From 1984 onward, HDR iridium-192 afterloading was given four times with a dose of 4 × 10 Gy measured at a distance 20 mm from the applicator axis. In the case of teletherapy, the afterloading dose was reduced to 21 Gy. The position of the applicator was documented by x-ray in two planes from 1973 onward. Teletherapy was performed with a cobalt-60 machine. Total dose at the pelvic wall was 30 Gy in 1969, 40 Gy from 1970 to 1983, and 50 Gy after 1984. From 1984 teletherapy was intensified to 56 Gy in the presence of several risk factors (Ladner 1983). In some cases additional para-aortic teletherapy with a maximum of 44 Gy was given in FIGO stages II–IV (Ladner 1992). In radiotherapy without major surgery a Heyman pack with radium ovoids was inserted. Since 1984 an afterloading method with iridium-192 has been used, with an afterloading dose of 60 Gy at the uterine surface. Additional teletherapy has been given using central shielding.

10.12.2.5
Follow-up

Control data were collected until 31 December 1995. Follow-up sources were the registration office, physicians, and clinical records. In 2450 of 2519 women the course of the disease was evaluated.

A further 50 women had a medical record 5–10 years after therapy. In 30 cases follow-up did not exceed 2–3 years. Survival data were calculated with the life table method according to Kaplan and Meier, using the statistical package of SPSS/PC.

10.12.2.6
Results

Follow-up of the 2519 women showed a 5-year crude survival of 72.7%. The period from 1969 to 1978 was distinguished from 1979 to 1990 because the therapeutic strategy changed from primary irradiation to the preference for primary surgery. Analysis of the 5-year survival revealed a figure of 72.8% in 1056 cases of the first period and 72.6% in 1464 cases of the second period. Mean follow-up was 10.6 years versus 10.9 years. It may be concluded that the extensive use of surgery did not improve the overall survival rate (see also Vahrson 1991; Hourvitz et al. 1995).

From 1969 to 1990 52 isolated vaginal recurrences and 65 combined vaginal and pelvic recurrences were treated at the UFK Freiburg (Table 10.16). A further 68 women had primary involvement of the vagina, FIGO IIIB and IV (2.5%). In total, 184 women had primary involvement or recurrent vaginal tumor (7.3%). Pelvic recurrence without vaginal involvement was seen in 43 cases (1.7%). Distant metastasis occurred in 103 women (4.1%).

FIGO STAGE

The main prognostic factor is FIGO stage (Creasman et al. 1987; Morrow and Townsend 1987; Morrow et al. 1991). In the Freiburg series, 4.2% of patients with stage II disease had isolated vaginal recurrences, which was more than in FIGO I (1.7%). Combined vaginal and pelvic recurrence was also more frequent in FIGO II patients, 3.1% versus 2.4% (Tables 10.16, 10.17).

We found that some histologic features are associated with a high rate of vaginal recurrences (Table 10.18). Prognostically unfavorable histologic subtypes were observed in 4.5% of vaginal recurrences (14.8% in all cases with recurrences). Grade 3 was overrepresented in vaginal recurrences (2.9% versus

Table 10.16. Frequency of isolated vaginal recurrences (VR) and of combined vaginal and pelvic recurrences (VPR) in patients with endometrial cancer, UFK Freiburg, 1969–1990

Stage, location of recurrences	UFK Freiburg: Primary operation	UFK Freiburg: Primary irradiation	Primary operation in other hospitals	Total
Stage I: VR	0.7% (5/676)	0.8% (2/238)	2.5% (24/943)	1.7% (31/1857)
VPR	1.0% (7/676)	2.5% (6/238)	3.4 (32/943)	2.4% (45/1857)
VR + VPR: St. I	1.7% (12/676)	3.3% (8/238)	5.9% (56/943)	4.1% (76/1857)
Stage II: VR	3.8% (4/105)	4.9% (4/81)	3.9% (4/103)	4.2% (12/289)
VPR	2.9% (3/105)	0 (0/81)	5.8% (6/103)	3.1% (9/289)
VR + VPR: St. II	6.7% (7/105)	4.9% (4/81)	9.7% (10/103)	7.3% (21/289)
Stage III: VR	2.9% (3/104)	0 (0/47)	3.0% (4/133)	2.5% (7/284)
VPR	1.9% (2/104)	2.1% (1/147)	3.0% (4/133)	2.5% (7/284)
VR + VPR: St. III	4.8% (5/104)	2.1% (1/47)	6.0% (8/133)	4.9% (14/284)
Stage IV: VR	5.1% (2/39)	0 (0/23)	0 (0/27)	2.2% (2/89)
VPR	2.5% (1/39)	0 (0/23)	11% (3/27)	4.5% (4/89)
VR + VPR: St. IV	7.6% (3/39)	0% (0/23)	11% (3/27)	6.7% (6/89)
Total	2.9% (27/924)[a]	3.3% (13/389)[a]	6.4% (77/1206)	4.6% (117/2519)

[a] Total for primary operation and primary irradiation at UFK Freiburg: 40/1313 = 3.0%.

Table 10.17. Frequency of recurrences in endometrial cancer, FIGO stages I–IV, at the UFK Freiburg, 1969–1990

Localization of recurrences	No.	Stage I	Stage II	Stage III	Stage IV
Isolated vaginal recurrence	52	31 (1.7%)	12 (4.2%)	7 (2.5%)	2 (2.2%)
Vaginal and pelvic recurrence	65	45 (2.4%)	9 (3.1%)	7 (2.5%)	4 (4.5%)
Pelvic recurrence	43	33 (1.8%)	6 (2.1%)	3 (1.0%)	1 (1.1%)
Distant metastasis	103	52 (2.8%)	14 (4.8%)	28 (9.9%)	9 (10.1%)
All recurrences	263	161 (8.7%)	41 (14.2%)	45 (15.8%)	16 (17.9%)
Tumor progression (TP)	306	144 (7.8%)	46 (15.9%)	74 (26.0%)	58 (65.2%)
All recurrences (with TP)	570	306 (16.5%)	87 (30.1%)	119 (41.9%)	74 (83.1%)

Table 10.18. Frequency of recurrences following primary therapy in patients with adverse histologic subtypes, grade 3, or deep (>2/3) invasion of the myometrium, UFK Freiburg, 1969–1990

Localization of recurrences or metastases	Adverse histologic subtypes		Grade 3		>2/3 infiltration of myometrium		Adverse subtypes/ grade 3/ >2/3 myometrial inf.		All patients	
	No.	%	No.	%	No.	%	No.	%	No.	%
Vaginal recurrences	7	4.5	14	2.9	10	2.2	31	2.8	52	2.1
Vaginal and pelvic recurrences	7	4.5	26	5.3	19	4.2	52	4.7	65	2.6
Pelvic recurrences	3	1.9	12	2.4	15	3.3	29	2.6	43	1.7
Distant metastases	6	3.9	22	4.5	34	7.5	62	5.6	103	4.1
Primary vaginal involvement	13	8.4	35	7.1	26	5.7	73	6.6	68	2.7
Tumor progression (TP)	30	19.3	126	25.7	81	17.8	237	21.5	306	12.1
All recurrences	23	14.8	73	14.9	78	17.1	175	15.9	264	10.5
All recurrences and TP	53	34.2	199	40.5	159	34.9	412	37.8	570	22.6
All patients in UFK Freiburg	155	100	491	100	455	100	1101	100	2519	100

2.1% of all patients). Deep invasion of myometrium of more than two-thirds had no influence on the frequency of vaginal recurrence (2.2% versus 2.1%). A similar overrepresentation was seen in cases of combined vaginal and pelvic recurrences (VPR). The frequency of grade 3 was 5.3% in VPR (19.5% in all cases), and that of deep myometrial invasion, 4.2% in VPR (18.1% in all cases). Of all recurrences, 117 were vaginal or vaginal and pelvic, 43 were pelvic, and 103 were distant metastases. In all subgroups there were more cases with unfavorable prognostic factors.

PROGNOSTIC FACTORS

In the Freiburg series, early FIGO stages were very strongly represented among the recurrences: 61% of all recurrences, 69% of vaginal and pelvic recurrences, 77% of pelvic recurrences, and more than 50% of distant metastases were FIGO I. Of all patients with FIGO stages I and II, 11.4% developed recurrences. Because the percentage showing recurrence is remarkably high, the influence of risk factors in early stages will be analyzed (Table 10.19).

Histologic Grade 3. The 5-year survival rate in patients with endometrial cancer of grade 3 after hysterectomy and vaginal brachytherapy was 74.6%, while after combined irradiation (brachy- and teletherapy) it was 73.8%; the 10-year survival was 49.8% and 63%, respectively.

Adverse Histologic Subtypes. Adenosquamous, clear cell, and serous-papillary carcinomas were considered adverse subtypes, and accounted for 6.1% of all cases. These subtypes had an increased proportion of isolated vaginal recurrences (4.5% vs 2.1%), of combined vaginal and pelvic recurrences (4.5% vs 2.6%), and of pelvic recurrences (1.9% vs 1.7%). The rate of distant metastasis was little affected by histologic type (3.9% vs 4.1%). The 5-year survival among patients with adverse histologic subtypes was reduced by 12.2%, and the 10-year survival rate by 6.7%.

Myometrial Infiltration of the Carcinoma. Infiltration of the outer third of the uterine wall was more frequent in cases of primary vaginal involvement (FIGO IIIB and IV: 7.0%), and of subsequent pelvic recurrence (2.2%). Deep myometrial infiltration was present in 4.2% of patients with combined vaginal and pelvic recurrence, and 3.3% of patients with pelvic recurrence alone. The Freiburg experience shows a rate of 10.5% for all recurrences. The 5-year survival rate was reduced by 6.7% in cases with deep myometrial infiltration compared to all cases of stage I (10 years: 10.6%).

Age. In general, outcome was inferior in very old women: the 5-year survival rate was 81.6% (10-year rate: 68.9%) in 61- to 70-year-old women, and 67.8% (10-year rate: 41%) in 71- to 80-year-old women.

Table 10.19. Five and 10-year survival rates and influence of therapeutic modalities and prognostic factors in cases of FIGO stage I endometrial cancer at UFK Freiburg, 1969–1990

Therapeutic modalities, prognostic factors	No.	5-year survival (%)	Difference from the median survival (%)	10-year survival (%)	Difference from the median survival (%)
Surgery + BT + HV	973	84.8	+4.8	72.0	+5.9
Surgery + BT	551	82.5	+2.5	79.8	+13.7
Age:					
50–60 years	500	91.1	+11.1	84.6	+18.5
61–70 years	719	81.6	+1.6	68.9	+2.8
71–80 years	455	67.8	–12.2	41.0	–25.1
>80 years	72	40.3	–39.7	20.4	–45.7
FIGO stage I	*1869*	*80.0*	*0*	*66.1*	*0*
Stage I, surgery alone	83	58.8	–21.2	48.2	–17.9
FIGO stage II	286	65.1	–14.9	48.9	–17.2
Histologic grade 3	288	65.9	–14.1	53.9	–12.2
>2/3 invasion of the myometrium	261	73.3	–6.7	55.5	–10.6
Adverse histologic subtypes	155	67.8	–12.2	59.4	–6.7
Primary radiotherapy:					
High-voltage irradiation	47	71.4	–8.6	66.4	+0.3
Brachytherapy alone	202	55.8	–24.2	31.2	–34.9

BT, brachytherapy; HV, high-voltage irradiation.

Advanced age (over 70 years) led to increased recurrence rate and reduced survival.

THERAPY AND PROGNOSIS OF RECURRENCE

The prognosis of recurrence depends on the location. Isolated vaginal recurrence has a favorable prognosis, with a 5-year survival of 56.5% (10 years: 39.8%), while only 28.4% of patients with combined vaginal and pelvic recurrences survived 5 years (10 years: 16.8%). Similar results were obtained in cases with primary vaginal involvement (Table 10.20).

In cases with distant metastasis following primary therapy we saw a 5-year survival rate of 44.3% (10 years: 20.2%). The high survival rate may be due to the delay before distant metastasis following primary therapy. Thus 5-year survival after distant metastasis was only 21% (10 years: 15%). The good results in isolated vaginal recurrence demand appropriate radiotherapy and/or surgery. Even in cases of distant metastasis the remaining life span may be several years, and sufficient palliation is necessary.

Table 10.20. Five-year survival rates after radiotherapy of isolated vaginal recurrences and mean duration of follow-up, as reported in the literature from 1984 to 1995

Study, observation period, and stages	No.	Follow-up (years)	Survival (%)
Aalders et al. 1984 (1960–1976), all stages	42	3–19	24
Mandell et al. 1985[a] (1969–1980), stage I	12	4	40
Nori 1987[a] (1969–1979), stage I	18	4	50
Greven and Olds 1987 (1970–1982), stages I and II	18	3–10	33
Curran et al. 1988[a] (1970–1985), all stages	55	5	31
Kuten et al. 1989[a] (1959–1986), all stages	17	4.8	40
Vavra et al. 1993 (1973–1987), stages I–III	40	3 (!)	54 (3 yr)
Morgan et al. 1993 (1964–1987), stages I and II	34	2 (!)	60[b]
Elliot et al. 1994[a] (1964–1985), stages I and II	27	10	23 (5 yr) 10 (10 yr)
Sears et al. 1994[a] (1973–1991), all stages	45	7	44
UFK Freiburg, present series[a] (1969–1990), all stages	52	10.6	56 40 (10 yr)
Weighted mean (a only)	226	<5	41.1

[a] Weighted mean used.
[b] Disease-free survival.

There is no reason for fatalism in recurrent endometrial cancer!

10.12.2.7 Discussion

It should first be noted that extensive use of surgery between 1979 and 1990 did not improve the overall survival rate (Vahrson 1991; Hourvitz et al. 1995). The adopted definition of isolated vaginal recurrence (Perez and Camel 1982: a tumor smaller than or equal to 20 mm with no infiltration beyond the mucosa) has been used in recent publications (Curran et al. 1988; Sears et al. 1994; Ellott et al. 1994); results are consequently now more comparable, and the effect of improved therapy can be measured. The recurrence rate in Freiburg was 10.4% in all stages (cf. 11.2%: Aalders et al. 1984a,b; 14%: Poulsen and Roberts 1988; 15%: Disaia and William 1986). Excluding primary vaginal involvement (stages IIIB and IV) in Freiburg 20% of recurrences were restricted to the vagina, 25% were combined vaginal and pelvic recurrences, 16% were pelvic recurrences without vaginal involvement, and 39% were distant metastases. Similar results were obtained by Kuten et al. (1989): In a multicenter study from 1959 to 1986 51 recurrences were analyzed; 33% were vaginal recurrences, 24% combined vaginal and pelvic recurrences, 7% pelvic recurrences without vaginal involvement, and 29% distant metastases. The distribution of recurrences varied with institution and mode of therapy.

The frequency of isolated vaginal recurrence in the Freiburg area was 1.5% in all stages. Other authors have found rates of 3.2% (Curran et al. 1988) to 6.7% (Greven and Olds 1987) in endometrial carcinoma of all FIGO stages. Selecting early cases, reported rates were 2.4% in FIGO I (Mandell et al. 1985), 2.2% in FIGO II (Lanciano et al. 1994), and 6.5% in FIGO I and II after hysterectomy (Elliott et al. 1994). The relation of vaginal and pelvic recurrences varies. Thus Poulsen and Roberts (1988) observed 36 vaginal and 57 pelvic recurrences in all stages. Sorbe and Smeds (1990) found a recurrence rate of 13% in stage I endometrial cancer treated by surgery, as compared with 29% following radiotherapy. In Freiburg we found a rate of 13% following radiotherapy.

FIGO Stage II. Similar results to the Freiburg observations were obtained by Prem et al. (1979), Philipps et al. (1982), Nori et al. (1987), Poulsen and ROBERTS (1989), VAVRA et al. (1993), SEARS et al. (1994), and LEMINEN et al. (1995): FIGO II tumors resulted in more recurrences, especially vaginal recurrences and distant metastases (24%: LEMINEN et al. 1995).

FIGO Stage I. Because about 70% of all endometrial cancers are FIGO I, this subgroup has been of special interest for gynecologists (LOTOCKI et al. 1983; DISAIA et al. 1985; ROTMAN et al. 1988; MARZIALE et al. 1989; SORBE and SMEDS 1989; LURAIN et al. 1993; ANGEL et al. 1993).

Histological Grade 3. BEDWINEK et al. (1984) reported a recurrence rate of 20.4% (distant metastasis mainly) and a 5-year survival rate of 71%. AALDERS et al. (1980) and HENDRIKSON et al. (1982) found a recurrence rate of 22%. The introduction of brachytherapy and megavoltage teletherapy improved survival in several institutions (PIVER et al. 1979; LOTOCKI et al. 1983; SUTTON et al. 1989; GREVEN et al. 1993; MORROW et al. 1991; LURAIN et al. 1993). The same effect can be demonstrated with the results of Freiburg. Data from the Annual Report, vol. 21, also show a benefit from radiotherapy after hysterectomy in stage I, grade 3 tumors (75.5% versus 68.1%). Consequently many institutions have accepted the indication for postoperative radiotherapy in FIGO I, grade 3 cases (Table 10.19).

Adverse Histologic Subtypes. WILSON et al. (1990) reported similar results to those obtained in Freiburg. The survival rate in adverse subtypes was 33% lower than in typical adenocarcinoma of the corpus. For clear cell carcinoma the reduction of survival was 20%–64% (KURMAN and SCULLY 1976; WEBB and LAGIOS 1987; PETTERSSON 1991). Patients with serous papillary tumors had a survival rate of 50%–60% compared to a rate of 70%–90% in patients with endometrioid carcinomas (CHRISTOPHERSON et al. 1983; GALLION et al. 1989; ROSENBERG et al. 1993).

Myometrial Infiltration by the Carcinoma. An increased frequency of recurrence in cases with deep myometrial infiltration was found by PRICE et al. (1965), LOTOCKI et al. (1983), and DISAIA et al. (1985). In 46% of cases with infiltration of the outer third, a subsequent distant metastasis occurred (DISAIA et al. 1985). In stage I cancer the 5-year survival rate dropped by 20%–25% in cases with deep infiltration.

Inferior results in isolated vaginal recurrence were reported by AALDERS et al. (1984: 24%), MANDELL et al. (1985: 40%), GREVEN and OLDS (1987: 33%), and KUTEN et al. (1989: 33%). The application of brachytherapy, teletherapy, and surgical vaginal resection was individualized (LEIBEL and WHARAM 1980; LADNER 1983; ROTMAN et al. 1988; PFLEIDERER 1992; VAVRA et al. 1993; SEARS et al. 1994; ELLIOTT et al. 1994).

Summary. The experiences of the UFK Freiburg show that surgery and postoperative irradiation of the whole vagina or primary irradiation with brachy- and teletherapy can reduce the risk of vaginal, pelvic, and distant recurrences in cases of high-risk endometrial cancer. Individualized treatment of patients with different localizations of recurrence yields a considerable improvement in long-term survival rates.

10.13 Follow-up Examinations

M. HERBOLSHEIMER and K. ROTTE

The task of follow-up examinations is the recognition of recurrences, metastases, second primaries, and side-effects of treatment. Additionally they play a role in overcoming psychosocial problems and, of course, in general medical care. The importance of the last point is often underestimated though it is well-known that old patients with sufficiently treated low-risk tumors sometimes have a higher life expectancy than the comparable group within the general population.

General agreement is lacking as to the appropriate frequency of follow-up examinations. Irrespective of the individual degree of risk of the primary, we recommend that these examinations be performed in asymptomatic patients every 3 months in the first 2 years after therapy, since about 70% of relapses occur within this period. Up to the fifth year an interval of 6 months seems sufficient, and after this period only yearly controls are indicated. Except for the first 2 years after therapy we consider these recommendations only as a guideline which should be modified in accordance with the individual circumstances.

A careful gynecological and a general physical examination are obligatory elements of follow-up examinations, together with documentation of the findings and the interval since the last examination. Cystoscopy must be performed within 4 weeks after therapy. Periodical imaging procedures can be restricted to mammography at least every 2 years and to chest radiography at each follow-up examination. Recently the value of periodical chest radiography for the early detection of distant metastases has been questioned. We do not use this examination in most tumor entities, but in the case of endometrial cancer we recommend the aforementioned high frequency of chest radiography even in asymptomatic patients, because lung metastases have therapeutic consequences in the form of progesterone therapy (CAFFIER et al. 1982), which yields satisfactory response rates. Sonography, urography, skeletal scinitigraphy, CT, and MRI are only indicated if there are clinical signs of relapse.

If primary irradiation has been performed, several authors recommend control curettage within 6 months after treatment (GAUWERKY 1957; KUCERA et al. 1984).

As already pointed out (see Sect. 10.5), tumor markers are relatively unspecific. Carcinoembryogenic antigen (CEA) can be helpful in assessing the clinical course (KREIENBERG 1989), but in future we shall not use tumor markers in general in asymptomatic patients as an essential component of each follow-up examination.

Recurrences should be proven by histological or at least cytological procedures, for instance by a control abrasion about 6 months after primary irradiation. But it should be mentioned that according to KUCERA et al. (1984) only about 60% of the recurrences could be detected by second-look curettage.

The already listed prognosticators of the primary, such as grading, stage, and myometrial infiltration (see Sect. 10.4) obviously influence the rate of recurrences (DISAIA et al. 1985). About 10% of patients who have not undergone postoperative vaginal irradiation are suggested to suffer from a vaginal recurrence (LEIBEL and WHARHAM 1980; MANDELL et al. 1985a).

As reported above, we observed no severe side-effects after primary or postoperative irradiation; in particular, fistulas did not occur, and acute reactions were restricted to mild diarrhea or cystitis.

It is known that there is no correlation between the degree of acute side-effects and the range of late reactions. Thus it is worthwhile to perform endoscopy if there are clinical signs of inflammation of the rectum or bladder, especially if they occur later than 1 year after radiation.

The specific treatment possibilities for side-effects and complications have already been discussed (see Sect. 10.11).

About 10% of patients with endometrial carcinoma develop a metachronous second primary, above all neoplasms of the colon and the breast (SCHÜNEMANN and JOURDAIN 1989). Thus the value of the already mentioned mammography is obvious.

Postirradiation malignancies (e.g., sarcomas, leukemia, mixed müllerian tumors) are sometimes reported (WILLIAMSON and CHRISTOPHERSON 1972), but the number of patients is very small and no definite conclusions can be drawn (DE VITA et al. 1993).

There are no clear guidelines regarding the administration of estrogen in younger patients with a treated endometrial carcinoma who are suffering from postmenopausal syndromes, though CREASMAN et al. (1986) saw no increase in the rate of relapses after estrogen substitution in their retrospective study.

There is some confusion in the literature concerning the role of tamoxifen. As mentioned above (see Sects. 10.5 and 10.9), several authors recommend that tamoxifen be administered as a component of hormonal therapy in order to enhance the hormonal effects (GURPIDE 1981; CARLSON et al. 1984). On the other hand, VAN LEEUWEN et al. (1994) report an increased risk of endometrial cancer after tamoxifen treatment of breast cancer. It can be supposed that a similar risk exists in regard to endometrial recurrence, but the reported risk related only to long-term treatment (>2 years) with tamoxifen, whereas tamoxifen administration as a stimulus for the progesterone receptor level is of short duration. Moreover, it must not be forgotten that the advantages of giving the drug after breast cancer exceed the risk of an endometrial recurrence, and that normally tamoxifen is not given for longer than 2 years as an adjunct in the treatment of breast cancer. Nevertheless, in patients receiving tamoxifen, ultrasound examinations of the endometrium should be performed routinely to minimize the cancer risk, given the well-known residual estrogenic potency of tamoxifen.

Psychological aspects are always important in cancer patients. After oncological treatment of the genital tract various sexual problems have to be considered; this also applies to endometrial cancer even though it mostly occurs in old women. The self-confidence of every women is related to her intact body and her intact sexual function: this is not a question of age. Symptoms such as dyspareunia, loss of libido, neurotic fixation, and reactive depression are usually consequences of a psychosomatic interplay: Treatment sequelae such as an operatively shortened vagina or adhesive vaginal walls after high-dose irradiation in combination with the psychological effects of diagnosis and therapy of cancer can disturb sexuality in general and especially copulation, which also has a negative influence on the partner, of course. Many patients are confronted with the prejudice that disease and sexuality are incompatible, which leads to isolation of the patient and intensification of the fear of cancer (REICHENBERGER 1992). This vicious circle has to be detected early, and it is the task of follow-up examinations not to treat somatic symptoms alone but also to discuss such problems with the patient and her partner. As physicians are sometimes overtaxed by psychological problems, the advisory center of a hospital should be involved if necessary.

10.14 Clinical Trials and Outlook

The Gynecologic Oncology Group designed trials of systemic agents for recurrent or advanced endometrial carcinoma, evaluating the effects of weekly application of vincristine, comparing doxorubicin with a combination of doxorubicin and cisplatin, and evaluating the use of tumor necrosis factor.

DE VITA et al. (1993) have reported on randomized studies evaluating surgery versus surgery plus adjunctive whole-pelvis irradiation for patients with intermediate-risk stage I endometrial carcinoma. In patients with stage III or IV endometrial carcinoma and with all stages of papillary serous and clear cell carcinomas of the endometrium, the efficacy of total abdominal radiation therapy has been demonstrated. Such trials have been based on the promising results of pilot studies with whole-abdominal irradiation in such high-risk patients.

Except for the study of AALDERS et al. (1980), there are still few reliable data on the efficacy of adjuvant irradiation in endometrial cancer. The well-known discrepancy between a decreased rate of pelvic recurrences and an increased rate of distant metastases, which of course influenced the survival rate in this trial, requires large prospective and randomized studies. The Gynecologic Oncology Group is performing such a randomized trial, testing the efficacy of adjuvant radiotherapy in patients with an unfavorable prognosis after surgical staging. Such a study is of great importance, but it cannot solve the problem that typical patients cannot be staged as desired (lymph node dissection!); especially in these (not seldom) cases further studies are necessary because there is still no general agreement on how to manage the postoperative treatment.

The study of ELLIOT et al. (1994) showed a significant reduction of vaginal, pelvic, and distant metastases after postoperative radiation of the whole pelvis in comparison with surgery alone. This is especially important in regard to the results of the historic trial of AALDERS et al. (1980), where some confusion was caused by a higher incidence of distant metastases after pelvic irradiation. By contrast, a clear benefit with respect to survival following postoperative radiation could not be established in the study of KADAR et al. (1992b).

Studies of high-risk tumors are thus highly desirable: Surgery or irradiation in patients with cancers which are restricted to the uterus yield 5-year survival rates of more than 80%, but in cases showing extrauterine tumor spread the results are generally poor. A statistically significant benefit can only be expected in such high-risk cases; moreover, these cases are a great challenge for therapy. It is now obvious that improved results can only be achieved by aggressive treatment, and controlled studies are necessary to prove the efficacy of such treatment in relation to the complication rate. Several other studies in advanced tumor stages have already been mentioned in this chapter (see Sect. 10.10).

In a retrospective case-controlled study, ROSE et al. (1993) saw no significant difference in survival between patients treated with primary irradiation (using a modified packing technique) and those who received surgery plus postoperative irradiation; this held true even in early tumor stages. Our results to date confirm these observations. In order to show that primary irradiation is a true alternative to surgery, however, more studies of large patient groups are desirable.

Clinical trials of intraoperative irradiation (electron beam therapy, permanent and temporary interstitial techniques utilizing afterloading systems) coupled with external beam therapy have shown impressive local control in the management of primaries and recurrences (NORI et al. 1989; NORI and WILLIAMS 1992; LUKAS et al. 1993). Though gynecological tumors play only a minor role in these studies, intraoperative techniques may be a promising modality for cancers of the uterine cervix or corpus, especially in advanced stages or recurrences (HÖCKEL 1990; HÖCKEL et al. 1989, 1993).

We should also remember the possibility of an interstitial boost to incomplete tumor regression after combined radiation or to recurrences in a pretreated area, as already discussed (see Sect. 10.7.2). This is surely a promising modality which should be used more often.

Three-dimensional displays of dose distribution based on the reconstruction of multiple axial CT slices (Fig. 10.13) are becoming increasingly popular. We agree with HILARIS et al. (1992) that detailed images showing the entire volume of the tumor as well as the volume of the surrounding tissue are helpful in optimizing the dose distribution. Nevertheless, they can only support individualization by improved visualization of the treatment site. The dose optimization itself depends above all on a suitable imaging procedure (MRI, for instance), flexible source arrangements, and reproducible source positions, as already discussed in detail.

The technical progress in producing new radioactive sources has led, for instance, to the clinical use of small iridium-192 sources, which enables an individual dose distribution to be performed. The search for an ideal nuclide with a suitable half-life and low beta or gamma energy is continuing and has yielded new sources (e.g., palladium-103, samarium-145, americium-241, and ytterbium-169). A short summary has been presented by BATTISTA and MASON (1992).

MARUYAMA et al. (1994) report on the use of the neutron emitter californium-252 in endometrial carcinomas. Because of its low oxygen enhancement ratio and its high biological effectiveness, this nuclide seems very suitable for (mostly hypoxic) recurrent or advanced tumors. The outcomes were satisfactory; however, the number of patients (n = 31) was low, and further studies are required. As to the use of new nuclides in general, the question of practicability in daily routine has to be confronted.

The problem of how to combine brachy- and teletherapy in regard to the spatial overlapping and to radiobiological end points remains to be solved; moreover, greater consideration needs to be given to dose-volume histograms.

Although there is a clear tendency in favor of HDR brachytherapy, LDR techniques will retain their place in the treatment of gynecological tumors because the advantages of HDR treatment forms are not predominantly related to tumor control. In addition, further development of pulsed dose rate therapy certainly appears worthwhile. Agreement is lacking with regard to optimal dose rates. If we compare the various opinions in the literature, which are discussed in detail in Sect. 10.7.1 and are summarized in a short paper by BATTERMANN (1992), only one conclusion can be drawn: The question as to future dose rates remains open.

It is a well-known fact that early diagnosis, which helps to avoid advanced stages and to detect high-risk cases, is of more importance than the treatment approach. In order to achieve early diagnosis it is necessary to educate the general population as to the clinical signs of a malignant tumor of the genital tract: women have to be encouraged to take vaginal bleeding seriously, for instance.

Table 10.21. Summary of management in endometrial cancer

Prophylaxis
Education of population
Gynecological check-up for cancer detection free of charge

Diagnosis
Fractionated abrasion for tumor classification, grading, receptor status, ploidy
Cytology (facultative)
Clinical staging by physical examination and imaging procedures
Laboratory examinations including tumor markers

Therapy
1. Surgery
   - Hysterectomy plus bilateral oophorectomy
   - Lymph node dissection if possible
   - Histopathological staging
   - Vaginal brachytherapy based on orthogonal radiographs and computerized planning
   - Simultaneous pelvic irradiation based on three-dimensional planning (facultative)
   - Simultaneous irradiation of para-aortic metastases (facultative)
   - Hormone therapy, cytostasis (facultative)
2. Primary radiation therapy
   - Insertion of flexible uterine afterloading applicators and of measurement tubes
   - Orthogonal radiographs and MRI if possible
   - Computerized brachytherapy planning and optimization of dose distribution
   - Three-demensional planning of external beam therapy
   - Definition of separated first- and second-rank target volumes
   - Adaptation of the different target volumes
   - Simultaneous performance of brachy- and pelvic teletherapy
   - Simultaneous irradiation of para-aortic metastases (facultative)
   - Hormone therapy, cytostasis (facultative)

Follow-up examinations
1. Asymptomatic patients
   - Periodical physical examinations
   - Cystoscopy within 4 weeks after therapy
   - Periodical chest radiography and mammography
   - Determination of tumor markers (facultative)
   - Treatment of psychosomatic sequelae
   - Complete documentation
2. Symptomatic patients
   - Treatment of complications/side-effects
   - Restaging of cases suspicious of a relapse
   - Curative, palliative, or symptomatic treatment of recurrences/distant metastases
   - Complete documentation
   - Individual managment of the further follow-up

Another requirement is careful and accurate histopathological staging including lymph node dissection in probable high-risk cases. Of course, biochemical examination of the tumor tissue in order to determine the hormone receptor status must not be neglected.

Finally it should be stressed again that it is the interaction of four elements which leads to a decrease in cancer mortality: prophylaxis, detection, therapy, and follow-up examinations. Recommendations concerning their use in the management of endometrial neoplasms are summarized in Table 10.21.

Technical advances in diagnosis and treatment, improved knowledge of tumor biology, specialization in oncology, and interdisciplinary cooperation have already improved prognosis in general, and it is realistic to expect further improvements. Unfortunately, however, it is a fact that the various possibilities of cancer management are sometimes not known or not exhausted.

References

Aalders JG, Abeler V, Kolstad P, Onsrud M (1980) Postoperative external irradiation and prognostic parameters in stage I endometrial carcinoma: clinical and histopathologic study of 540 patients. Obstet Gynecol 56:419–426

Aalders JG, Abeler V, Kolstad P (1984a) Clinical (stage III) as compared to subclinical intrapelvic extrauterine tumour spread in endometrial carcinoma: a clinical and histopathological study of 175 patients. Gynecol Oncol 17:64–74

Aalders JG, Abeler V, Kolstad P (1984b) Recurrent adenocarcinoma of the endometrium: a clinical and histopathological study of 379 patients. Gynecol Oncol 17: 85–103

Adler GF, Karolis C, Kramer W, Sun EC, Yuile PG (1994) Initial PDR brachytherapy experience at Sydney, Australia. Nucletron Activity Report 5:11–14

Aldrich JE, Filbee JF, Tompkins MG (1989) Flexible applicators for the treatment of gynaecological malignancies: early clinical results. In: Mould RF (ed) Brachytherapy 2. Nucletron International, Leersum, pp 272–276

Ambros RA, Kurman RJ (1992) Identification of patients with stage I uterine endometrioid adenocarcinoma at high risk of recurrence by DNA ploidy, myometrial invasion, and vascular invasion. Gynecol Oncol 45:235–239

Andersen ES (1990) Stage II endometrial carcinoma: prognostic factors and the results of treatment. Gynecol Oncol 38:220–223

Anderson B, Marchant DJ, Munzenrider JE, Moore JP, Mitchell GW (1976) Routine noninvasive hysterography in the evaluation and treatment of endometrial carcinoma. Gynecol Oncol 4:354–367

Angel C, Du Beshter B, Dawson AE, Keller J (1993) Recurrent stage I endometrial adenocarcinoma in the nonirradiated patients: preliminary results of surgical "staging". Gynecol Oncol 48:221–226

Antunes CMF, Stolley PD, Rosenheim NB, et al. (1979) Endometrial cancer and estrogen use. N Engl J Med 300:9–13

Arai T, Nakano T, Morita S, Sakashita K, Nakamura YK, Fukuhisa K (1992) High dose rate remote afterloading intracavitary radiation therapy for cancer of the uterine cervix. Cancer 69:175–180

Averette HE, Donato DM, Lovecchio JL, Sevin B (1987) Surgical staging of gynecological malignancies. Cancer 60:2010–2020

Ayhan A, Yarali H, Ayhan A (1991) Endometrial carcinoma: a pathologic evaluation of 142 cases with and without associated endometrial hyperplasia. J Surg Oncol 46:182–184

Baier K (1987) Ein biologisches Planungssytem für die routinemäßige klinische Strahlentherapie. Röntgen-Berichte 16:180–191

Baier K (1989) HDR Afterloading und biologische Therapieplanung. In: Leetz HK (ed) Medizinische Physik. Deutsche Gesellschaft für medizinische Physik, pp 75–79

Baier K (1993) Philosophy and practice of HDR and LDR gynaecological brachytherapy. In: Mould RF, Müller R-P (eds) Brachytherapy in Germany. Nucletron International, Veenendaal, pp 12–28

Baltzer J, Lohe KJ (1986) Präneoplasien und Karzinome des Endometriums. In: Wulf K-H, Schmidt-Matthiesen H (eds) Spezielle gynäkologische Onkologie I. Urban & Schwarzenberg, München, pp 232–263 (Klinik der Frauenheilkunde und Geburtshilfe, vol XI)

Baltzer J, Maaßen V (1991) Malignome des Corpus uteri. In: Bender HG (ed) Gynäkologische Onkologie. Thieme, New York, pp 208–240

Baram A, Figer A, Inbar M, Levy E, Peyser MR, Stein Y (1985) Endometrial carcinoma stage I – comparison of two different treatment regimes – evaluation of risk factors and its influence on prognosis: suggested step by step treatment protocol. Gynecol Oncol 22:294–301

Barber HR, Brunschwig H (1968) Treatment and results of recurrent cancer of corpus uteri in patients receiving anterior and total pelvic exenteration 1947–1963. Cancer 22: 949–955

Barendsen GW (1982) Dose fractionation, dose rate and iso-effect relationships for normal tissue responses. Int J Radiat Oncol Biol Phys 8:1981–1997

Bates TD (1989) Historical review and critical evaluation of different techniques of intracavitary brachytherapy for carcinoma of the cervix from the clinical standpoint. In: Rotte K, Kiffer J (eds) Changes in brachytherapy. Wachholz, Nürnberg, pp 29–34

Battermann JJ (1992) Dose rates of the future. In: Mould RF (ed) International brachytherapy. Nucletron International, Veenendaal, pp 128–131

Battista JJ, Mason DLD (1992) New radionuclides for brachytherapy. In: Mould RF (ed) International brachytherapy. Nucletron International, Veenendaal, pp 125–127

Bauer M, von Fournier D, Fehrentz F, Kuttig H, zum Winkel K, Neidner F (1981) Afterloading-Methode zur Simulation der intrauterinen Packmethode beim Korpuskarzinom. Strahlentherapie 157:793–800

Bauknecht T, Kohler M, Janz I, Pfleiderer A (1989) The occurrence of epidermal growth factor receptors and the characterization of EGF-like factors in human ovarian, endometrial, cervical, and breast cancer. J Cancer Res Clin Oncol 115:193–199

Bedwinek JM, Galaktos AE, Camel HM, Kao MS, Stokes S, Perez CA (1984) Stage I, grade III adenocarcinoma of the endometrium treated with surgery and irradiation. Cancer 54:40–47
Belch RZ, Ryan TP, Taylor JH, Coughlin CT (1990) Interstitial microwave hyperthermia combined with brachytherapy in the treatment of malignancies involving the gynecologic organs. Endocurie Hypertherm Oncol 6:159–165
Belloni C, Vigano R, del Maschio A, Sironi S, Taccagni G, Vignali M (1990) Magnetic resonance imaging in endometrial carcinoma staging. Gynecol Oncol 37:172–177
Benraad TJ, Friberg LG, Koenders AJM, Kullander S (1980) Do estrogen and progesterone receptors (E2R and PR) in metastasizing endometrial cancers predict the response to gestagen therapy? Acta Obstet Gynecol Scand 59:155–159
Berchuck A, Soisson A, Olt G, Soper J, Clarke-Pearson D, Bast R, McCarthy K (1989) Epidermal growth factor receptor expression in normal and malignant endometrium. Am J Obstet Gynecol 161:1247–1252
Berchuck A, Rodriguez G, Kinney RB, Soper JT, Dodge RK, Clarke-Pearson DL, Bast RC Jr (1991) Overexpression of HER-2/*neu* in endometrial cancer is associated with advanced stage disease. Am J Obstet Gynecol 164:15–21
Berman ML, Ballon SC, Lagasse LD, Watring WG (1980) Prognosis and treatment of endometrial cancer. Am J Obstet Gynecol 136:679–688
Bertelsen K, Jakobsen A (1993) Radiotherapy for gynecologic cancer. Curr Opin Oncol 5:885–890
Björnsson M, Sorbe B (1982) Intracavitary irradiation of endometrial carcinomas of the uterus in stage I using a "bulb technique": physical basis. Br J Radiol 55:56–59
Bloss JD, Berman ML, Syed N, Puthawala A, Manetta A, Rafie S, DiSaia PJ (1992) Treatment of advanced carcinoma of the uterine cervix with interstitial radiotherapy and hyperthermia. Endocurie Hypertherm Oncol 8:145–150
Bond WH (1985) Early uterine body carcinoma: has postoperative vaginal irradiation any value? Clin Radiol 36:619–623
Boner JA, Kacl GM, Trinkler M, Meyenberger C, Schär G, Krestin GP (1994) Hochauflösende Magnetresonanztomographie des kleinen Beckens mittels Endorektalspule. Fortschr Röntgenstr 160:546–554
Boronow RC (1969) Carcinoma of the corpus. In: Cancer of the uterus and ovary. Year Book Medical Publishers, Chicago, pp 35–61
Boronow RC (1976) Endometrial cancer: not a benign disease. Obstet Gynecol 47:630–634
Boronow RC, Morrow CP, Creasman WT, et al. (1984) Surgical staging in endometrial cancer: clinical-pathologic findings of a prospective study. Obstet Gynecol 63:825–832
Bosari S, Viale G, Radaelli U, Bossi P, Bonoldi E, Coggi G (1993) p53 accumulation in ovarian carcinomas and its prognostic implications. Hum Pathol 24:1175–1179
Böttcher HD, Schütz J, Mathei B (1983) Nebenwirkungen bei der Therapie des Kollumkarzinoms. Strahlenther Onkol 159:334–343
Brady LW, Lewis GJ, Antoniades J, et al. (1974) Evolution of radiotherapeutic techniques. Gynecol Oncol 2:314–323
Brandner P, Gnirs J, Neis KJ, Hettenbach A, Schmidt W (1991) Der Stellenwert der Vaginosonographie in der noninvasiven Beurteilung des Endometriums am postmenopausalen Uterus. Geburtshilfe Frauenheilkd 51: 734–740
Brenner DJ, Hall EJ (1991) Conditions for the equivalence of continuous to pulsed low dose rate brachytherapy. Int J Radiat Oncol Biol Phys 20:181–190
Brinton LA, Berman ML, Mortel R, et al. (1992) Reproductive, menstrual, and medical risk factors for endometrial cancer. Results from a case-control study. Am J Obstet Gynecol 167:1317–1325
Britton LC, Wilson TO, Gaffey TA, Lieber MM, Wieand HS, Podratz KC (1989) Flow cytometric DNA analysis of stage I endometrial carcinoma. Gynecol Oncol 34:317–322
Brown JM, Dockerty MB, Symmonds RE, Banner EA (1968) Vaginal recurrence of endometrial carcinoma. Am J Obstet Gynecol 100:544–549
Bruckman JE, Bloomer WD, Marck A, Ehrmann RL, Knapp RC (1980) Stage III adenocarcinoma of the endometrium: two prognostic groups. Gynecol Oncol 9:12–17
Burke TW, Heller PB, Woodward JE, Davidson SA, Hoskins WJ, Park RC (1990) Treatment failure in endometrial carcinoma. Obstet Gynecol 75:96–101
Busch M, Makoski B, Schulz U, Sauerwein K (1977) Das Essener Nachlade-Verfahren für die intrakavitäre Strahlentherapie. Strahlentherapie 153:581–588
Butler EB (1976) The early diagnosis of cancer of the endometrium. Clin Obstet Gynecol 3:389–405
Cacciatore B, Lehtovirta P, Wahlström T, Ylöstalo R (1989) Preoperative sonographic evaluation of endometrial cancer. Am J Obstet Gynecol 160:133–137
Caffier H, Horner G, Baum J (1982) Treatment of advanced or recurrent endometrial adenocarcinoma with progestins, including medroxyprogesterone acetate. In: Cavalli F, McGuire WL, Pannuti F, Pelegrini S, Robustelli G (eds) Proceedings of the international symposium on medroxy progesterone acetate. Excerpta Medica, Amsterdam, pp 389–396
Carlson JJ, Allegra JC, Day TJ, Wittliff Jl (1984) Tamoxifen and endometrial carcinoma: alterations in estrogen and progesterone receptors in untreated patients and combination hormonal therapy in advanced neoplasia. Am J Obstet Gynecol 149:149–153
Chauvergne J, Granger C, Mage P, Pigneux J, David M (1986) Palliative chemotherapy of endometrial cancer. Value of combinations with doxorubicin and cisplatin. Rev Fr Gynecol Obstet 81:547–551
Childers JM, Spirtos NM, Brainard P, Surwit EA (1994) Laparoscopic staging of the patient with incompletely staged early adenocarcinoma of the endometrium. Obstet Gynecol 83:597–600
Christopherson WM (1986) The significance of the pathologic findings in endometrial cancer. Clin Obstet Gynecol 13: 673–693
Christopherson WM, Alberhasky RC, Conelly PJ (1982) Carcinoma of the endometrium. II. Papillary adenocarcinoma: a clinical pathological study of 46 cases. Am J Clin Pathol 77:534–540
Christopherson WM, Connelly PJ, Alberhasky RC (1983) Carcinoma of the endometrium: an analysis of prognosticators with favorable subtypes and stage I disease. Cancer 51:1705–1709
Clarke-Pearson D, Cliby J, Soper A, et al. (1991) Morbidity and mortality of selective lymphadenectomy in early stage endometrial cancer. Gynecol Oncol 40:168–178
Cohen CJ, Bruckner HW, Deppe G, Blessing JA, Homesley H, Lee JH (1984) Multidrug treatment of advanced and recurrent endometrial carcinoma: a Gynaecologic Oncology Group study. Obstet Gynecol 63:719–756
Cohen L (1968) Theoretical "iso-survival" formulae for fractionated radiation therapy. Br J Radiol 41:522–528
Cook GB (1966) A comparison of single and multiple primary cancers. Cancer 19:959–966

Cramer DW, Cutter SJ, Christine B (1974) Trends in the incidence of gynecological cancer in the United States. Gynecol Oncol 2:130–143
Creasman WT (1992) Prognostic significance of hormone receptors in endometrial cancer. Cancer 71:1467–1470
Creasman WT, Weed FC (1981) Carcinoma of endometrium (FIGO stages I and II): clinical features and management. In: Coppleson M (ed) Gynecologic oncology. Churchill Livingstone, Edinburgh
Creasman WT, Boronow RC, Morrow CP, DiSaia PJ, Blessing J (1976) Adenocarcinoma of the endometrium: its metastatic lymph node potential. Gynecol Oncol 4:239–243
Creasman WT, McCarty KS, Barton TK (1980) Clinical correlates of estrogen- and progesterone-binding proteins in human endometrial adenocarcinoma. Obstet Gynecol 55: 363–370
Creasman WT, Soper JT, McCarty KS Jr, McCarty KS Sr, Hinshaw W, Clarke-Pearson DL (1985) Influence of cytoplasmic steroid receptor content on prognosis of early stage endometrial carcinoma. Am J Obstet Gynecol 151: 922–932
Creasman WT, Henderson D, Hinshaw W, Clarke-Pearson DL (1986) Estrogen replacement therapy in patients treated for endometrial cancer. Obstet Gynecol 67:326–330
Creasman WT, Morrow CP, Bundy BN, Homesley HD, Graham JE, Heller PB (1987) Surgical-pathologic spread patterns of endometrial cancer. A Gynecologic Oncology Group study. Cancer 60:2035–2041
Crombach G, Würz H, Antczak W, Reusch K, Herrmann F, Bolte A (1986) Wertigkeit des tumorassoziierten Antigens CA 15-3 beim Mammakarzinom. In: Greten H, Klapdor R (eds) Klinische Relevanz neuer monoklonaler Antikörper. Thieme, Stuttgart, pp 184–194
Curran WJ, Whittington R, Peters AJ, Fanning J (1988) Vaginal recurrences of endometrial carcinoma: the prognostic value of staging by a primary vaginal carcinoma system. Int J Radiat Oncol Biol Phys 15:803–808
Dale RG (1985) The application of the linear-quadratic dose-effect equation to fractionated and protracted radiotherapy. Br J Radiol 58:515–528
Dale RG (1990) The use of small fraction numbers in high dose-rate gynaecological afterloading: some radiobiological considerations. Br J Radiol 63:290–294
Daly NJ, Izar F, Bachaud JM, Delannes M (1989) The incidence of severe chronic ileitis after abdominal and/or pelvic external irradiation with high energy photon beams. Radiother Oncol 14:287–295
David C, Figge P, Otto M, Tamini HK, Greer BE (1983) Treatment variables in the management of endometrial cancer. Am J Obstet Gynecol 146:495–500
Davies JL, Rosenshein NB, Antunes CMF, Stolley PD (1981) A review of the risk factors for endometrial carcinoma. Obstet Gynecol Surv 36:107–116
Delclos L, Fletcher GH, Moore EB, Sampiere VA (1980) Minicolpostats, dome cylinders, other additions and improvements of the Fletcher-Suit afterloadable system: indication and limitations of their use. Int J Radiat Oncol Biol Phys 6:1195–1206
Demopoulos RI (1977) Carcinoma of the endometrium. In: Blaustein A (ed) Pathology of the female genital tract. Springer, Berlin Heidelberg New York
Deore SM, Shrivastava SK, Viswanathan PS, Din-Shaw KA (1991) The severity of late rectal and recto-sigmoid complications related to fraction size in irradiation treatment of carcinoma cervix stage IIIB. Strahlenther Onkol 167: 638–642
DePalo G, Spatti GB, Bandieramonte G, Luciani L (1983) Pilot study with adjuvant hormone therapy in FIGO stage I endometrial carcinoma with myometrial invasion. Tumori 69:65–67
Deppe G (1990) Chemotherapy for endometrial cancer. In: Deppe G (ed) Chemotherapy of gynecologic cancer, 2nd edn. Wiley-Liss, New York, pp 155–174
Deppe G, Malviya VK, Zbella E (1984) Nonhormonal chemotherapy in endometrial cancer – a review. Wien Klin Wochenschr 96:757–756
de Vita VT Jr, Hellman S, Rosenberg SA (1993) Cancer. Principles and practice of oncology, 4th edn. Lippincott, Philadelphia, pp 1195–1225
de Waal J, Lochmüller H (1982) Präoperative Kontaktbestrahlung beim Endometriumkarzinom. Geburtshilfe Frauenheilkd 42:394–396
DiSaia PJ, William CT (1986) Management of endometrial adenocarcinoma stage I with surgical staging followed by tailored adjuvant radiation therapy. Clin Obstet Gynecol 13 (4)
DiSaia PJ, Creasman WT, Boronow RC, Blessing JA (1985) Risk factors and recurrent patterns in stage I endometrial cancer. Am J Obstet Gynecol 151:1009–1015
Dische S (1985) Chemical sensitizers for hypoxic cells: a decade of experience in clinical radiotherapy. Radiother Oncol 3:97–115
Dische S, Saunders MI, Flockhart IR (1978) The optimum regime for the administration of misonidazole and the establishment of multi-center clinical trials. Br J Cancer 37 (Suppl 3):318–321
Donath D, Clark B, Kaufmann C, Evans MDC, Stanimir G (1992) HDR interstitial brachytherapy of lower gynaecological tract cancer. In: Mould RF (ed) International brachytherapy. Nucletron International, Veenendaal, pp 219–225
Dubois JB, Gely S, Pourquier H (1992) La radiotherapie exclusive des cancers de l'endometre. Bull Cancer Radiother 79:506 (cited by Pernot M et al. 1994)
Duk MJ, Aalders JG, Fleuren GJ, de Bruijn HWA (1986) CA 125, a useful marker in endometrial cancer. Am J Obstet Gynecol 155:1097–1102
Dyroff R, Michalzik K (1957) Wichtige Gesichtspunkte bei der Nachuntersuchung bestrahlter Genitalkarzinome der Frau. Strahlenther 103:376–382
Ehrlich CE, Young PC, Cleary RE (1981) Cytoplasmic progesterone and estradiol receptors in normal, hyperplastic, and carcinomatous endometria: therapeutic implications. Am J Obstet Gynecol 141:539–546
Ehrlich CE, Young PCM, Stehman FB, Sutton GP, Alford WM (1988) Steroid receptors and clinical outcome in patients with adenocarcinoma of the endometrium. Am J Obstet Gynecol 158:796–807
Eifel P, Ross J, Hendrickson M, Cox RS, Kempson R, Martinez A (1983) Adenocarcinoma of the endometrium. Analysis of 256 cases with disease limited to the uterine corpus: treatment comparisons. Cancer 52:1026–1031
Elliot P, Green D, Coates A, et al. (1994) The efficacy of postoperative vaginal irradiation in preventing vaginal recurrence in endometrial cancer. Int J Gynecol Cancer 4:84–93
Ellis F (1963) Dose-time relationships in clinical radiotherapy. In: Raven RW (ed) Cancer Progress 1963. Butterworth, London, pp 163–176
Ellis F, Sorensen A (1974) A method of estimating biological effect of combined intracavitary low dose rate radiation with external radiation in carcinoma of the cervix uteri. Radiology 110:681–686

Englmeier K-H, Hecker R, Hötzinger H, Thiel H (1985) Automatische Kontursuche und Segmentierung von sonographischen Transversalschnittbildern des Uterus hinsichtlich einer optimierten Isodosengestaltung bei Korpuskarzinomen. Strahlentherapie 161:275–280

Esche BA, Crook JM, Horiot JC (1987) Dosimetric methods in the optimization of radiotherapy for carcinoma of the cervix. Int J Radiat Oncol Biol Phys 13:1183–1192

Fischer G, Matthaei D, Carduck HP, Machinek R, Fietkau R, Dühmke E (1994) Use of surface markers for MR radiotherapy planning. Strahlenther Onkol 170:169–173

Fleming WP, Peters WA, Kumar NB, Morley GW (1984) Autopsy findings in patients with uterine sarcoma. Gynecol Oncol 19:168–172

Fletcher GH, Stovall M, Sampiere V (1962) Carcinoma of the uterine cervix, endometrium and ovary, vol 69. Year Book Medical Publishers, Chicago

Fletcher GH, Rutledge FN, Delclos L (1980) Adenocarcinoma of the uterus. In: Fletcher GH (ed) Textbook of radiotherapy, 3rd edn. Lea & Febiger, Philadelphia, pp 789–808

Fowler JF (1989a) The radiobiology of brachytherapy. In: Martinez AA, Orton CG, Mould RF (eds) Brachytherapy HDR and LDR. Nucletron International, Leersum, pp 121–137

Fowler JF (1989b) The linear quadratic formula and progress in fractionated radiotherapy: a review. Br J Radiol 62:99–112

Fowler JF (1993) Why shorter-half times of repair lead to greater damage in pulsed brachytherapy. Int J Radiat Oncol Biol Phys 26:353–356

Fowler JF, Stern BE (1963) Dose-time relationships in radiotherapy and the validity of cell survival curve models. Br J Radiol 36:163–173

Frick HC, Munnell EW, Richart RM, Berger AP, Lawry MF (1983) Carcinoma of the endometrium. Am J Obstet Gynecol 115:663–676

Frischbier HJ, Hasse J (1965) Die biaxiale Telekobalt-Pendelbestrahlung des Kollumkarzinoms. Dosisverteilung, Herddosisberechnung und klinische Erfahrungen. Strahlenther 126:481–494

Frischkorn R (1983) Die Strahlentherapie des Endometriumkarzinoms. Gynäkologe 16:104–113

Fritz P, Weber KJ, Frank C, Spyropoulos B, Flentje M (1992) In-vitro investigations concerning pulsed brachytherapy. In: Mould RF, Müller RP (eds) Brachytherapy in Germany. Nucletron International, Veenendaal, pp 271–277

Gagnon JD, Moss WT, Gabourel LS, Stevens KR (1979) External irradiation in the management of stage II endometrial carcinoma. Cancer 44:1247–1251

Gallagher CJ, Oliver RT, Oram DH, et al. (1991) A new treatment for endometrial cancer with gonadotropin releasing hormone analogue. Br J Obstet Gynecol 98:1037–1041

Gallion HH, van Nagel JR, Powell DF, et al. (1989) Stage I serous papillary carcinoma of the endometrium. Cancer 63:2224–2228

Gallup DG, Stock RJ (1984) Adenocarcinoma of the endometrium in women 40 years of age or younger. Obstet Gynecol 64:417–420

Gauwerky F (1957) Standardisierung und individuelle Anpassung bei der Strahlenbehandlung der Gebärmutter- und Scheidenkarzinome. Strahlentherapie 103:16–47

Gauwerky F (1977) Kurzzeit-Afterloading-Curietherapie gynäkologischer Karzinome. Technik und Problematik. Strahlenther 153:793–801

Gauwerky F (1980) Weibliche Genitalorgane. In: Scherer E (ed) Strahlentherapie - Radiologische Onkologie, 2nd edn. Springer, Berlin Heidelberg New York, pp 661–722

Gauwerky F, Obranovic J (1967) Probleme der radiologischen Behandlung des Uteruskarzinoms. Sonderband Teil B Strahlentherapie 66:15–30

Genest P, Drouin P, Girard A, Gerig L (1987) Stage III carcinoma of the endometrium: a review of 41 cases. Gynecol Oncol 26:77–86

Glaser FH (1980) Decatron remote afterloading therapy with high activity sources. In: Bates TD, Berry R (eds) High dose rate afterloading in the treatment of cancer of the uterus, Special Report no 17. British Institute of Radiology, London, pp 51–58

Glaser FH, Rauh G, Grimm D, Salewski D, Muth C-P, Heider K-M, Kraft M (1977) Das Decatron-remote Afterloading mit hoher Dosisleistung in der Kontakt-Curie-Therapie. Radiobiol Radiother (Berl) 18:707–716

Glaser FH, Grimm D, Heider KM (1984) Zum Einfluß der zeitlichen Dosisverteilung bei protrahierter und fraktionierter Brachytherapie gynäkologischer Tumoren. Mathematisch formulierte Modellvorstellungen und klinische Erfahrungen beim fraktionierten Kurzzeit-Afterloading mit hohen Dosisraten. Radiobiol Radiother (Berl) 25:231–240

Glassburn JR (1981) Carcinoma of the endometrium. Cancer 48:575–581

Glassburn JR, Brady LW, Grigsby PW (1992) Endometrium. In: Perez CA, Brady LW (eds) Principles and practice of radiation oncology, 2nd edn. Lippincott, Philadelphia, pp 1203–1221

Glatsein E, Lichter AS, Fraas AF, Kelly BA, Van de Geijn J (1985) The imaging revolution and radiation oncology: use of CT, ultrasound, and NMR for localization, treatment planning and treatment delivery. Int J Radiat Oncol Biol Phys 11:299–314

Goffinet DR, Prionas SD, Kapp DS, et al. (1990) Interstitial Ir-192 flexible catheter radiofrequency hyperthermia treatments of head and neck and recurrent pelvic carcinomas. Int J Radiat Oncol Biol Phys 18:199–210

Goodman R, Hellman S (1974) The role of postoperative irradiation in carcinoma of the endometrium. Gynecol Oncol 2:354–361

Graham J (1971) The value of pre-operative or post-operative treatment by radium for carcinoma of the uterine body. Surg Gynecol Obstet 132:855–860

Gray LH, Conger AO, Ebert M, Hornsey S, Scott OC (1953) The concentration of oxygen dissolved in tissue at the time of irradiation as a factor in radiotherapy. Br J Radiol 26:638–643

Greer BE, Hamberger AD (1983) Treatment of intraperitoneal metastatic of the endometrium by the whole-abdomen moving-strip technique and pelvic boost irradiation. Gynecol Oncol 16:365–373

Greven KM, Olds W (1987) Isolated vaginal recurrences of endometrial adenocarcinoma and their management. Cancer 60:419–421

Greven KM, Lanciano RM, Corn B, Case D, Randall ME (1993) Pathologic stage III endometrial carcinoma: prognostic factors and patterns of recurrence. Cancer 71:3697–3702

Grigsby PW, Perez CA (1989) Intracavitary and external beam irradiation for endometrial carcinoma In: Mould RF (ed) Brachytherapy 2. Nucletron International, Leersum, pp 252–267

Grigsby PW, Perez CA, Camel HM, Kao MS, Galaktos AE (1985) Stage II carcinoma of the endometrium: results of therapy and prognostic factors. Int J Radiat Oncol Biol Phys 11:1915–1923

Grigsby PW, Perez CA, Kuske RR, Kao MS, Galaktos AE (1987) Results of therapy, analysis of failures, and prognostic fac-

tors for clinical and pathologic stage III adenocarcinoma of the endometrium. Gynecol Oncol 27:44–57
Grigsby PW, Perez CA, Kuten A, et al. (1991) Clinical stage I endometrial cancer: results of adjuvant irradiation and patterns of failure. Int J Radiat Oncol Biol Phys 21:379–385
Grimm D, Grimm I, Schindler J, Hänsgen G, Glaser FH, Salewski D, Rauh G (1992) DNA-Verteilung bei gynäkologischen Tumoren nach High-dose-rate-Afterloadingtherapie. In: Grimm D, Eichhorn M, Hänsgen G (eds) Fortschritte in der intrakavitären und interstitiellen Afterloadingtherapie. Sauerwein, Haan, pp 19–24
Gurpide E (1981) Hormonereceptors in endometrial cancer. Cancer 48:638–641
Gusberg SB (1947) Precursors of corpus carcinoma estrogens and adenomatous hyperplasia. Am J Obstet Gynecol 54:905–927
Gusberg SB (1976) The individual at high risk for endometrial carcinoma. Am J Obstet Gynecol 1:535–542
Gusberg SB (1980) Current concepts in cancer: the changing nature of endometrial cancer. N Engl J Med 302:729–731
Gusberg SB (1988) Diagnosis and principles of treatment of cancer of the endometrium. In: Gusberg SB, Shingleton HM, Deppe G (eds) Female genital cancer. Churchill Livingstone, New York, pp 337–360
Hald I, Salimtschik M, Mouridsen HT (1983) Tamoxifen treatment of advanced endometrial carcinoma. A phase II study. Eur J Gynaecol Oncol 4:83–87
Hall EJ, Brenner DJ (1991) The dose-rate effect revisited: radiobiological considerations of importance in radiotherapy. Int J Radiat Oncol Biol Phys 21:1403–1414
Hall EJ, Roizin-Towle L (1975) Hypoxic sensitizers: radiobiological studies at the cellular level. Radiology 117:453–457
Hancock KC, Freedman RS, Edwards CL, Rutledge FN (1986) Use of cisplatin, doxorubicin, and cyclophosphamide to treat advanced and recurrent adenocarcinoma of the endometrium. Cancer Treat Rep 70:789–791
Hanson MB, Van Nagell JR, Powell DE, et al. (1985) The prognostic significance of lymph-vascular space invasion in stage I endometrial cancer. Cancer 55:1753–1757
Harouny VR, Sutton GP, Clark SA, Geisler HE, Stehman FB, Ehrlich CE (1988) The importance of peritoneal cytology in endometrial carcinoma. Obstet Gynecol 72:394–398
Heath R, Rosenman J, Varia M, Walton L (1988) Peritoneal fluid cytology in endometrial cancer: its significance and the role of chromic phospate (32-P) therapy. Int J Radiat Oncol Biol Phys 15:815–822
Heilmann HP, Bünemann H (1987) Weibliche Genitalorgane. In: Scherer E (ed) Strahlentherapie. Springer, Berlin Heidelberg New York, pp 783–862
Heinzel F (1961) Über die Notwendigkeit der Rotationsbestrahlung in der Telekobalttherapie. Strahlenther 116:180–187
Hendricks DH, Callendine GW, Morton JL (1955) A bead packing technique for the application of uniform irradiation to the endometrial cavity. Am J Obstet Gynecol 69:1039–1050
Hendrikson M, Ross J, Eifel P, Martinez A, Kempson R (1982) Uterine papillary serous carcinoma: a highly malignant form of endometrial adenocarcinoma. Am J Surg Pathol 6:93–108
Henschke UK, Hilaris BS, Mahan GD (1963) Afterloading in interstitial and intracavitary radiation therapy. Am J Roentgenol 90:386–395
Henschke UK, Hilaris BS, Mahan GD (1966) Intracavitary radiation therapy of uterine cervix by remote afterloading with cycling sources. Am J Roentgenol 96:45–51
Herbolsheimer M (1989) Intrauterine packing by remote HDR afterloading in endometrial carcinoma. In: Rotte K, Kiffer J (eds) Changes in brachytherapy. Wachholz, Nürnberg, pp 130–138
Herbolsheimer M (1993) Is individual treatment planning in gynaecological brachytherapy necessary? In: Mould RF, Müller R-P (eds) Brachytherapy in Germany. Nucletron International, Veenendaal, pp 145–155
Herbolsheimer M, Romen W, Richter E, Schmitt R (1987) Bericht über ein Fünffachmalignom. Onkologie 10:284–289
Herbolsheimer M, Baier K, Gall P, Löffler E, Rotte K (1988) Fernegesteuerte intrauterine Nachlade-Packmethode beim Endometriumkarzinom. Röntgen-Berichte 17:226–234
Herbolsheimer M, Baier K, Götz-Gersitz U, Güllenstern M-L, Rotte K, Sauer O (1991) Endometrial carcinoma remote HDR afterloading using modified Heyman packing. Activity Selectron Brachytherapy Journal 1:17–20
Herbolsheimer M, Sauer O, Rotte K (1992) Primary irradiation of endometrial cancer: technical aspects, individual treatment planning, and first results in a modified Heyman packing with high dose rate afterloading. Endocurie Hypertherm Oncol 8:11–18
Herrmann T, Christen N, Alheit H-D (1993) Gynäkologische Brachytherapie – von Low-dose-rate zu High-tech. Strahlenther Onkol 169:141–151
Hetzel FW (1989) Biologic rationale for hyperthermia. Radiol Clin North Am 27:499–508
Heuck A, Sittek H, Seelos K, Kreft B, Hermanns M, Reiser M (1994) MRT des weiblichen Beckens: Turbo-Spin-Echo-(TSE)-Sequenzen im Vergleich mit konventionellen Spin-Echo-Sequenzen bei 0,5 Tesla. Fortschr Röntgenstr 160: 538–545
Heyman J (1935) The so-called Stockholm method and the results of treatment of uterine cancer at Radiumhemmet. Acta Radiol 16:129–148
Heyman J, Reuterwall O, Benner S (1941) The Radiumhemmet experience with radiotherapy in cancer of the corpus of the uterus: classification, method of treatment and results. Acta Radiol 22:11–98
Hilaris BS, Tenner M, High M, Shih L, Silvern D (1992) Three-dimensional brachytherapy treatment planning. In: Mould RF (ed) International brachytherapy. Nucletron International, Veenendaal, pp 117–118
Himmelmann A, Holmberg E, Oden A, Skogsberg K (1985) Intracavitary irradiation of carcinoma of the cervix stage IB and IIA. Acta Radiol Oncol 24:139–144
Höckel M (1990) Experimentelles intraoperatives Konzept zur Behandlung von Beckenwandrezidiven. In: Baier K, Herbolsheimer M, Sauer O (eds) Interdisziplinäre Behandlungsformen beim Mammakarzinom und bei gynäkologischen Malignomen. Bonitas-Bauer, Würzburg, pp 150–159
Höckel M, Kutzner J, Bauer H, Friedberg V (1989) Eine neue experimentelle Methode zur Behandlung von Beckenwandrezidiven gynäkologischer Malignome. Geburtshilfe Frauenheilkd 49:981–986
Höckel M, Knapstein PG, Hohenfellner R, Rösler HP, Kutzner J (1993) Die kombinierte operative und radiotherapeutische Behandlung (CORT) von Beckenwandrezidiven: Erfahrungsbericht nach 3 Jahren. Geburtshilfe Frauenheilkd 53:169–176
Homesley HD, Boronow RC, Lewis JJ (1977) Stage II endometrial adenocarcinoma. Memorial Hospital for Cancer 1949–1965. Obstet Gynecol 49:604–608
Homesley HD, Kadar N, Barret RJ, Lentz SS (1992) Selective pelvic and periaortic lymphadenectomy does not increase

morbidity in surgical staging of endometrial carcinoma. Am J Obstet Gynecol 167:1225–1230
Hording U, Hansen U (1985) Stage I endometrial carcinoma. A review of 140 patients primarily treated by surgery only. Gynecol Oncol 22:51–58
Horiot JC, Pourquier H, Schraub S, Pigneux J, Brosens M, Loiseau D (1989) Current status of the management of cancer of the cervix in daily practice and in clinical research. In: Mould RF (ed) Brachytherapy 2. Nucletron International, Leersum, pp 199–214
Hornback NB, Shupe RE, Shidnia H, Marshall CU, Lauer T (1986) Advanced stage III-B cancer of the cervix treated with hyperthermia and radiation. Gynecol Oncol 23:160–167
Hourvitz A, Menczer J, Chetrit A, Modan B (1995) Surgical vs. clinical staging of endometrial carcinoma. The impact on treatment modification, morbidity, and survival. Eur J Gynecol Oncol 16:357–362
Hreshchyshyn MM, Aaron BS, Boronow RC, Franklin E, Shingleton HM, Blessing JA (1979) Hydroxyurea or placebo combined with radiation to treat stages IIIB and IV cervical cancer confined to the pelvis. Int J Radiat Oncol Biol Phys 5:317–322
Hricak H, Stern JL, Fisher MR, Shapeero LG, Winkler ML, Lacey CG (1986) Endometrial carcinoma staging by MR imaging. Radiology 162:297–305
Hricak H, Rubinstein LV, Gherman GM, Karstaedt N (1991) MR imaging evaluation of endometrial carcinoma: results of an NCI cooperative study. Radiology 179:829–832
Huguenin PU, Glanzmann C, Hammer F, Lütolf UM (1992) Endometrial carcinoma in patients aged 75 years or older: outcome and complications after postoperative radiotherapy or radiotherapy alone. Strahlenther Onkol 168: 567–572
Ingersoll FM (1971) Vaginal recurrence of carcinoma of the corpus: management and prevention. Am J Surg 121:473–477
ICRU. International Commission on Radiation Units and Measurements (1985) Dose and volume specification for reporting intracavitary therapy in gynaecology, vol 38. ICRU, Bethesda, pp 11–12
Iversen OE, Segadal E (1985) The value of endometrial cytology. A comparative study of the Gravlee Jet-Washer, Isaacs Cell Sampler and Endoscan versus curettage in 600 patients. Obstet Gynecol Surv 40:14–20
Iversen OE, Utaaker E, Skaarland E (1988) DNA ploidy and steroid receptors as predictors of disease course in patients with endometrial carcinoma. Acta Obstet Gynecol Scand 67:531–537
Jacobs H (1988) Experiences with interstitial HDR afterloading therapy in genital and breast cancer. In: Vahrson H, Rauthe G (eds) High Dose Rate afterloading in the treatment of cancer of the uterus, breast and rectum. Urban & Schwarzenberg, München, pp 258–262
Jänne O, Kauppila A, Kontula K, Syrjälä P, Vihko R (1979) Female sex streoid receptors in normal, hyperplastic, and carcinomatous endometrium. The relationship to serum steroid hormones and gonadotropins and changes during medroxyprogesterone acetate administration. Int J Cancer 24:545–554
Jones HW (1975) Treatment of adenocarcinoma of the endometrium. Obstet Gynecol Surv 30:147–169
Johnsson JE (1979) Recurrences and metastases in carcinoma of the uterine body correlated to the size and location of the primary tumors. Acta Obstet Gynecol Scand 58:405–408
Jorritsma JBM, Kampinga HH, Scaf AHJ, Konings AWT (1985) Strand break repair, DNA polymerase activity, and heat radiosensitization in thermotolerant cells. Int J Hyperthermia 1:131–147
Joslin CAF (1991) A place for high dose rate brachytherapy in gynecological oncology: fact or fiction? Activity Selectron Brachyther J Suppl 2:3–4
Joslin CAF, Smith CW (1971) Postoperative radiotherapy in the management of uterine corpus carcinoma. Clin Radiol 22:118–124
Joslin CAF, O'Connell D, Howard NW (1967) The treatment of uterine carcinoma using Cathetron III: clinical considerations and preliminary reports on treatment results. Br J Radiol 40:899–904
Joslin CAF, Vaishampayan GV, Mallik A (1977) The treatment of early cancer of the corpus uteri. Br J Radiol 50:38–45
Joslin CAF (1989) Henschke memorial lecture. Endocurie Hypertherm Oncol 5:69–81
Kadar N, Homesley HD, Malfetano JH (1992a) Positive peritoneal cytology is an adverse factor in endometrial carcinoma only if there is other evidence of extrauterine disease. Gynecol Oncol 46:145–149
Kadar N, Malfetano JH, Homesley HD (1992b) Determinants of survival in surgically staged patients with endometrial carcinoma histologically confined to the uterus: implications for therapy. Obstet Gynecol 80:655–659
Käser O (1986) Kommentar zu: "Die primär operative Therapie des Korpuskarzinoms". Gynäkologe 19:94–95
Käser O (1987) Endometriumkarzinom Stadium I und II-Chirurgische Behandlung. Arch Gynecol 242:19–25
Kauppila A (1984) Progestin therapy of endometrial, breast, and ovarian carcinoma: a review of clinical observations. Acta Obstet Gynecol Scand 63:441–450
Kaufmann M, Abel U, Brunnert K, et al. (1990) Adjuvant treatment with tamoxifen (TAM) or medroyprogesteroneacetate (MPA) or observation only in pathological stage I endometrial carcinoma. In: Salmon S (ed) Adjuvant therapy of cancer, VI. Saunders, Philadelphia, pp 522–526
Kauppila A, Sipila P, Koivula A (1987) Intracavitary irradiation of endometrial cancer of large uteri using a two-phase afterloading technique. Br J Radiol 60:1093–1097
Kavanagh JJ, Kudelka AP (1993) Systemic therapy for gynecologic cancer. Curr Opin Oncol 5:891–899
Kellerer AM (1984) Verallgemeinerung des NSD-Konzeptes auf Multifraktionierung, sowie intrakavitäre und interstitielle Therapie. In: Schmidt T (ed) Medizinische Physik. Deutsche Gesellschaft für Medizinische Physik, pp 384–392
Kempson RL, Bari W (1970) Uterine sarcomas. Classification, diagnosis, and prognosis. Hum Pathol 1:331–349
Kindermann G (1981) Zur Therapie des Endometriumkarzinoms. Geburtshilfe Frauenheilkd 41:650
Kirk J, Gray WM, Watson ER (1971) Cumulative radiation effect. I. Fractionated treatment regimes. Clin Radiol 22:145–155
Kjörstadt KE, Örjaseter H (1977) Studies on carcinoembryonic antigen levels in patients with adenocarcinoma of the uterus. Cancer 40:2935–2956
Kleine W (1984) Rezeptorverhalten beim Endometriumkarzinom. In: Nagel GA, Robustelli Della Cuna G, Lanius P (eds) Medroxyprogesteronacetat (MAP) in der Therapie hormonsensibler Tumoren. Kehrer, Freiburg, pp 55–64
Kleine W, Fuchs A, De Gregorio G, Geyer H (1982) Östrogen- und Progesteronrezeptoren beim Korpuskarzinom und ihre klinische Bedeutung. Geburtshilfe Frauenheilkd 42:884–887

Kleine W, Maier T, Geyer H, Pfleiderer A (1990) Estrogen and progesterone receptors in endometrial cancer and their prognostic relevance. Gynecol Oncol 38:59–65

Klötzer K-H, Kob D, Günther R, Sommer H, Retzke U (1992) Ist die präoperative Afterloading-Kontaktstrahlentherapie (AL-KT) bei Patienten mit Endometriumkarzinom zur Verbesserung der Therapieergebnisse geeignet? In: Grimm D, Eichhorn M, Hänsgen G (eds) Fortschritte in der intrakavitären und interstitiellen Afterloadingtherapie. Sauerwein, Haan, pp 50–55

Kneale BL (1986) Adjunctive and therapeutic progestin in endometrial cancer. Clin Obstet Gynaecol 13:789–809

Knörr K, Knörr-Gärtner H, Beller FK, Lauritzen C (1989) Geburtshilfe und Gynäkologie, 3rd edn. Springer, Berlin Heidelberg New York, p 703

Kob D, Kloetzer KH, Kriester A, Sommer H (1988) Prospektive randomisierte Studie zur Fraktionierung der Afterloading-Therapie von Zervix- und Endometriumkarzinomen. Strahlenther Onkol 164:708–713

Kohorn EJ (1976) Gestagens and endometrial cancer. Gynecol Oncol 4:398–411

Kolles H, Stegmaier C, von Seebach HB, Ziegler H (1989) Deskriptive Epidemiologie und Prognose maligner gynäkologischer Tumoren. Geburtshilfe Frauenheilkd 49:573–578

Kreienberg R (1989) Allgemeine und spezifische Laborparameter im Rahmen der Tumornachsorge bei gynäkologischen Malignomen und bei Mammakarzinomen. Gynäkologe 22:55–62

Kreienberg R, Ebert J, Beck T (1990) Die Therapie des Zervixkarzinoms in der Universitäts-Frauenklinik Mainz. In: Teufel G, Pfleiderer A, Ladner H-A (eds) Therapie des Zervixkarzinoms. Springer, Berlin Heidelberg New York, pp 134–146

Kucera H (1990) Therapieformen und -techniken bei der Bestrahlung des Korpuskarzinoms. In: Baier K, Herbolsheimer M, Sauer O (eds) Interdisziplinäre Behandlungsformen beim Mammakarzinom und bei gynäkologischen Malignomen. Bonitas-Bauer, Würzburg, pp 125–129

Kucera H (1993) Das Karzinom des Corpus uteri. In: Roth SL, Böttcher HD (eds) Gynäkologische Strahlentherapie (Bücherei des Frauenarztes, vol XLIV). Enke, Stuttgart, pp 48–54

Kucera H, Vavra N (1991) Ein Risiko-Score für das operierte Endometriumkarzinom und seine Bedeutung für die adjuvante Strahlentherapie. Geburtshilfe Frauenheilkd 51:798–805

Kucera H, Weghaupt K (1988) Die postoperative Bestrahlung des Carcinoma corporis uteri mit der Iridium-Afterloading Technik. Strahlenther Onkol 164:501–507

Kucera H, Gerstner G, Pateisky N, Weghaupt K (1983) Zur Strahlentherapie des Korpuskarzinomrezidivs. Geburtshilfe Frauenheilkd 43:107–111

Kucera H, Vytiska-Binstorfer E, Weghaupt K (1984) Erfahrungen mit der Second-Look-Curretage nach primär bestrahltem Korpuskarzinom. Konsequenzen in der Tumornachsorge. Geburtshilfe Frauenheilkd 44:286–290

Kucera H, Ünel N, Weghaupt K (1986) Nebenwirkungen der postoperativen High-dose-rate-Iridium- und Low-dose-rate- Radium-Bestrahlung beim Korpuskarzinom. Strahlenther Onkol 162:111–114

Kucera H, Vavra N, Weghaupt K (1989) Zum Wert der postoperativen Bestrahlung beim Endometriumkarzinom im pathohistologischen Stadium I. Geburtshilfe Frauenheilkd 49:618–624

Kucera H, Vavra N, Weghaupt K (1990a) Zum Wert der alleinigen Bestrahlung des allgemein inoperablen Endometriumkarzinoms mittels High-Dose-Rate-Iridium-192. Geburtshilfe Frauenheilkd 50:610–613

Kucera H, Vavra N, Weghaupt K (1990b) Benefit of external radiation in pathologic stage I endometrial carcinoma: a prospective clinical trial of 605 patients who received postoperative vaginal irradiation and additionally pelvic irradiation in the presence of unfavourable prognostic factors. Gynecol Oncol 38:99–104

Kudelka AP, Freedman RS, Edwards CL, Lippman SM, Tornos CS, Krakoff IH, Kavanagh JJ (1993) Metastatic adenocarcinoma of the endometrium treated with 13-cis-retinoic acid plus interferon-alpha. Anticancer Drugs 4:335–337

Kühn W, Kaufmann M, Feichter GE, Rummel HH, Abel U, Heep J, v. Minckwitz G (1989) Prognostische Bedeutung zellkinetischer Parameter beim Endometriumkarzinom. Geburtshilfe Frauenheilkd 49:787–792

Kumar NB, Hart WR (1982) Metastases to the uterine corpus from extragenital cancers – a clinicopathologic study of 63 cases. Cancer 50:2163–2169

Kumar PP, Good RR (1985) A new intracavitary cervix applicator. Review of existing intracavitary techniques. Endocurie Hypertherm Oncol 1:247–255

Kummermehr J (1990) Strahlenbiologische Grundlagen der Brachytherapie. In: Baier K, Herbolsheimer M, Sauer O (eds) Interdisziplinäre Behandlungsformen beim Mammakarzinom und bei gynäkologischen Malignomen. Bonitas-Bauer, Würzburg, pp 29–54

Kurman RJ, Scully RE (1976) Clear cell carcinoma of the endometrium. An analysis of 21 cases. Cancer 37:872

Kuten A, Grigsby PW, Perez CA, Fineberg B, Carcia DM, Simpson JR (1989) Results of radiotherapy in recurrent endometrial carcinoma: a retrospective analysis of 51 patients. Int J Radiat Oncol Biol Phys 17:29–34

Ladner H-A (1983) Zur Prognose und Strahlentherapie des Korpuskarzinoms. Radiologe 23:12–19

Ladner H-A (1988) Some aspects of afterloading therapy in endometrium cancer. In: Vahrson H, Rauthe G (eds) High Dose Rate afterloading in the treatment of cancer of the uterus, breast and rectum. Urban & Schwarzenberg, München, pp 40–42

Ladner H-A (1990) Therapieformen und -techniken bei der Bestrahlung des Kollumkarzinoms. In: Baier K, Herbolsheimer M, Sauer O (eds) Interdisziplinäre Behandlungsformen beim Mammakarzinom und bei gynäkologischen Malignomen. Bonitas-Bauer, Würzburg, pp 129–135

Ladner H-A (1992) Zur Strahlentherapie des Endometriumkarzinoms. In: Ladner HA, Pfleiderer A, Profous CZ (eds) Gynäkologische Radiologie. Springer, Berlin Heidelberg New York, pp 35–44, 112–119

Lanciano RM, Corn BW, Schultz DJ, Kramer CA, Rosenblum N, Hogan WM (1993) The justification for a surgical staging in endometrial carcinoma. Radiother Oncol 28:189–196

Landgren RC, Fletcher GH, Delclos L, Wharton JT (1976) Irradiation of endometrial cancer in patients with medical contraindication to surgery or with unresectable lesions. Am J Roentgenol 126:148–154

Larson DM, Johnson K, Olson KA (1992) Pelvic and para-aortic lymphadenectomy for surgical staging of endometrial cancer: morbidity and mortality. Obstet Gynecol 79:998–1001

Lee KR, Belinson JL (1991) Recurrence in non-invasive endometrial carcinoma. Relationship to uterine papillary serous carcinoma. Am J Surg Pathol 15:965–973

Lee KR, Scully R (1989) Complex endometrial hyperplasia and carcinoma in adolescent and young women 15–20 years of age. A report of 10 cases. Int J Gynecol Pathol 8:201–213
van Leeuwen FE, Benraadt J, Coebergh JW, et al. (1994) Risk of endometrial cancer after tamoxifen treatment of breast cancer. Lancet 343:448–452
Leibel SA, Wharham MD (1980) Vaginal and para-aortic lymphnodes in carcinoma of the endometrium. Int J Radiat Oncol Biol Phys 6:893–914
Leminen A, Forss M, Lehtorvita P (1995) Endometrial adenocarcinoma with clinical evidence of cervical involvement: accuracy of diagnostic procedures, clinical course, and prognostic factors. Acta Obstet Gynecol Scand 74:61–66
Leung Y, DePetrillo AD (1993) Etiology, epidemiology, risk and prognostic factors, screening and imaging of gynecologic cancers. Curr Opin Oncol 5:869–876
Lewandowski G, Torrisi J, Potkul RK, Holloway RW, Popescu G, Whitfield G, Delgado G (1990) Hysterectomy with extended surgical staging and radiotherapy in stage I endometrial cancer: a comparison of complication rates. Gynecol Oncol 36:401–404
Lewis BV, Stallworthy JA, Cowdell R (1970) Adenocarcinoma of the body of the uterus. J Obstet Gynaecol Br Commonw 77:343–348
Lewis GJ, Slack NH, Mortel R, Bross ID (1974) Adjuvant progestogen therapy in the primary definitive treatment of endometrial cancer. Gynecol Oncol 2:368–376
Lindahl B, Gullberg B (1991) Flow cytometrical DNA- and clinical parameters in the prediction of prognosis in stage I–II endometrial carcinoma. Anticancer Res 11:783–788
Lindahl B, Willen R (1991) Endometrial hyperplasia: clinicopathological considerations of a prospective randomized study after abrasion only or high-dose gestagen treatment. Anticancer Res 11:403–406
Lindahl B, Alm P, Ferno M, Killander D, Langstrom F, Norgren A, Trope C (1989) Prognostic value of steroid receptor concentration and flow cytometrical DNA measurements in stage I–II endometrial carcinoma. Acta Oncol 28:595–599
Liversage WE (1966) The application of cell survival theory to high dose-rate intracavitary therapy. Br J Radiol 39:338–349
Liversage WE (1971) A critical look at the ret. Br J Radiol 44:91–100
Liversage WE (1973) Radiotherapy of carcinoma of the cervix: relevance of dose-rate. Proc R Soc Med 66:940–941
Liversage WE (1978) A comparison of the predictions of the CRE, TDF and Liversage formulae with clinical experience. (Special Report No. 17). Br J Radiol 182–189
Liversage WE, Martin-Smith P, Ramsey NW (1967) The treatment of uterine carcinoma using the Cathetron. II. Physical measurements. Br J Radiol 40:888–894
Lochmüller H (1978) Kumulative Überlebensrate verschieden therapierter Kollektive. In: Lochmüller H (ed) Das Endometriumkarzinom als chronische Erkrankung. Wachholz, Nürnberg, pp 98–100
Loeffler JS, Rosen EM, Niloff JM, Howes AE, Knapp RC (1988) Whole abdominal irradiation for tumors of the uterine corpus. Cancer 61:1332–1335
Long RTL, Sala JM, Spratt JA (1972) Endometrial carcinoma recurring after hysterectomy. A study of 64 cases with observation on effective treatment modalities and implications for alteration of primary therapy. Cancer 29:318–321
Lotocki RJ, Copeland LJ, DePetrillo AD, Murhead W (1983) Stage I endometrial carcinoma: treatment results on 835 patients. Am J Obstet Gynecol 146:141–146
Lukas P, Schröck R, Rupp N, et al. (1986) MR-Tomographie bei gynäkologischen Erkrankungen im kleinen Becken. Fortschr Röntgenstr 144:159–165
Lukas P, Ries G, Stepan R, et al. (1993) Intraoperative brachytherapy. In: Mould RF, Müller R-P (eds) Brachytherapy in Germany. Nucletron International, Veenendaal, PP 209–214
Lundberg LM, Mattson O, Ragnhult I (1989) Remote afterloading of the uterine cavity using a MicroSelectron-LDR unit. In: Mould RF (ed) Brachytherapy 2. Nucletron International, Leersum, pp 521–529
Lurain JR (1992) The significance of positive peritoneal cytology in endometrial cancer. Gynecol Oncol 46:143–144
Lurain JR, Rice BL, Rademaker AW, Poggensee LE, Schink JC, Miller DS (1993) Prognostic factors associated with recurrence in clinical stage I adenocarcinoma of the endometrium. Obstet Gynecol 78:63–69
Lybeert M, Vanputten W, Ribot J, Crommelin M (1989) Endometrial carcinoma: HDR brachytherapy in combination with external irradiation: a multivariate analysis of relapses. Radiother Oncol 16:245–252
MacDonald RR, Thorogoog J, Mason MK (1988) A randomized trial of progestagens in the primary treatment of endometrial carcinoma. Br J Obstet Gynaecol 95:166–174
Mackillop WJ, Pringle JF (1985) Stage III endometrial carcinoma: a review of 90 cases. Cancer 56:2519–2523
MacMahon B, Austin JH (1969) Association of carcinomas of the breast and corpus uteri. Cancer 23:275–280
Mäentausta O, Boman K, Isomaa V, Stendahl U, Bäckström T, Vihko R (1992) Immunhistochemical study of the human 17β-hydroxysteroid dehydrogenase and steroid receptors in endometrial adenocarcinoma. Cancer 70:1551–1555
Magdon E (1980) Zum gegenwärtigen Stand des Einsatzes von Radiosensitizern in der Strahlentherapie aus strahlenbiologischer Sicht. Radiobiol Radiother (Berl) 21:778–787
Malkasian GD, Decker DG (1978) Adjuvant progesterone therapy for stage I endometrial carcinoma. Int J Gynaecol Obstet 16:48–49
Malkasian GD, Annegers JF, Fountain KS (1980) Carcinoma of the endometrium stage I. Am J Obstet Gynecol 136:872–888
Mandell LR, Nori D, Anderson L, Hilaris BS (1985a) Postoperative vaginal radiation in endometrial cancer using a remote afterloading technique. Int J Radiat Oncol Biol Phys 11:473–478
Mandell LR, Nori D, Hilaris BS (1985b) Recurrent stage I endometrial carcinoma: results of treatment and prognostic factors. Int J Radiat Oncol Biol Phys 11:1103–1109
Marchetti DL, Piver MS, Tsukada Y, Reese P (1986) Prevention of vaginal recurrence of stage I endometrial adenocarcinoma with postoperative vaginal radiation. Obstet Gynecol 67:399–402
Marth C, Koza A, Müller-Holzner E, Hetzel H, Fuith LC, Dapunt O (1990) Prognostisch relevante Faktoren beim malignen Müllerschen Mischtumor. Geburtshilfe Frauenheilkd 50:605–609
Martinez A (1989) Interstitial and external beam therapy for the treatment of locally advanced cancers of the female genital tract. In: Rotte K, Kiffer J (eds) Changes in brachytherapy. Wachholz, Nürnberg, pp 154–163
Martinez A, Edmundson GK, Cox RS, Gunderson LL, Howes AE (1985) Combination of external beam irradiation and multiple-site perineal applicator (Mupit) for treatment of locally advanced or recurent prostatic, anorectal, and gynecologic malignancies. Int J Radiat Oncol Biol Phys 11:391–398

Maruyama Y, Yoneda J, Wierzbicki J (1994) Californium-252 neutron brachytherapy for endometrial adenocarcinoma. Endocurie Hypertherm Oncol 10:1–13

Marziale P, Atlante G, Pozzi M, Diotallevi F, Iacovelli A (1989) 426 cases of stage I endometrial carcinoma: a clinicopathological analysis. Gynecol Oncol 32:278–281

Mazeron JJ, Boisserie G, Gokarn N, Baillet F (1994) Pulsed LDR brachytherapy, current clinical status, Paris, France. Nucletron Activity Report 5:24–28

McCarty KS, Barton TK, Fetter BF, Creasman WT (1979) Correlation of estrogen and progesterone receptors with histologic differentiation in endometrial adenocarcinoma. Am J Pathol 96:171–184

McDonald TW, Malkasian GD, Gaffey TA (1977) Endometrial cancer associated with feminizing ovarian tumor and polycystic ovarian disease. Obstet Gynecol 49:654–658

McLean M (1994) Initial PDR brachytherapy experience at Toronto, Canada. Nucletron Activity Report 5:6–10

Mecke H, Lüttges J, Lehmann-Willenbroock E, Kunstmann P, Freys I (1994) Treatment of precursors of endometrial cancer. Gynecol Obstet Invest 37:130–134

Mella A (1985) Combined hyperthermia and cis-diaminedichlor platinum in BD IX rats with transplanted BT-4 A tumors. Int J Hyperthermia 1:171–185

Mestwerdt W, Kranzfelder D (1980) Gegenwärtige Gesichtspunkte zur Epidemiologie und Ätiologie des Korpuskarzinoms. Med Klin 75:333–338

Mestwerdt W, Kranzfelder D (1983) Neue diagnostische Möglichkeiten beim Endometriumkarzinom und seinen Vorstufen. Gynäkologe 16:87–92

Milosevic MF, Dembo AJ, Thomas GM (1992) The clinical significance of malignant peritoneal cytology in stage I endometrial carcinoma. Int J Gynaecol Cancer 2:225–235

Monk BJ, Surwit EA, Alberts DS, Graham V (1988) Intraperitoneal mitomycin C in the treatment of peritoneal carcinomatosis following second-look surgery. Semin Oncol 15:27–31

Moore DH, Fowler WC, Walton LA, Droegemueller W (1989) Morbidity of lymph-node sampling in cancers of the uterine corpus and cervix. Obstet Gynecol 74:180–184

Moore TD, Philips PH, Nerenstone SR, Cheson BD (1991) Systemic treatment of advanced and recurrent endometrial carcinoma: current status and future direction. J Clin Oncol 9:1071–1088

Morrow PC, Townsend DE (1987) Tumors of the endometrium, synopsis of gynecologic oncology, 3rd edn. John Wiley, New York, pp 159–205

Morrow PC, DiSaia SP, Townsend DE (1973) Current management of endometrial carcinoma. Obstet Gynecol 42:399–406

Morrow PC, Bundy BN, Homesley HD, Creasman WT, Hornback NB, Kurman R, Thipgen JT (1990) Doxorubicin as an adjuvant following surgery and radiation therapy in patients with high-risk endometrial carcinoma. Stage I and occult stage II: a Gynecologic Oncology Group study. Gynecol Oncol 36:166–171

Morrow PC, Bundy BN, Kurman RJ, Creasman WT, Heller PB, Hoemsley HD, Graham JE (1991) Relationship between surgical-pathological risk factors and outcome in clinical stage I and II carcinoma of the endometrium: a Gynecologic Oncology Group study. Gynecol Oncol 40:55–65

Mortel R, Zaino R, Satyaswaroop PG (1984) Heterogeneity and progesterone-receptor distribution in endometrial adenocarcinoma. Cancer 53:113–116

Morton M, Barnes AC, Hendricks DH, Callendine GW (1953) Irradiation of cancer of the uterine cervix with radioactive cobalt 60 in guided aluminium needles and in plastic threads. Am J Roentgenol 69:813–825

Mould RF (1993) A century of X-rays and radioactivity in medicine: with emphasis on photographic records of the early years. Institute of Pysics Publishing, Bristol, Philadelphia.

Müller JH (1951) Beiträge zur medizinisch-therapeutischen Verwendung der Künstlichen Radioaktivität. Strahlentherapie 85:87–125

Nazeer T, Malfetano JH, Rosano TG, Ross JS (1992) Correlation of tumor cytosol cathepsin-D with differentiation and invasiveness of endometrial adenocarcinoma. Am J Clin Pathol 97:764–769

Neeff TC (1941) Die Bestimmung der Radium-Toleranzdosen auf Grund der Nebenwirkungen an der Harnblase bei der Strahlenbehandlung des Gebärmutterkrebses. Strahlentherapie 70:11–70

Neumannova M, Kauppila A, Kivinen S, Vihko R (1985) Short-term effects of tamoxifen, medroxyprogesterone acetate, and their combination on receptor kinetics and 17β-hydroxysteroid dehydrogenase in human endometrium. Obstet Gynecol 66:695–700

Niloff JM, Klug TL, Schaetzl E, Zurawski VJ, Knapp RC, Bast RJ (1984) Elevation of serum CA 125 in carcinomas of the fallopian tube, endometrium, and endocervix. Am J Obstet Gynecol 148:1057–1058

Nori D, Williams H (1992) Intraoperative brachytherapy: rationale and future directions. In: Mould RF (ed) International brachytherapy. Nucletron International, Veenendaal, pp 132–137

Nori D, Hilaris BS, Anderson L, Lewis JL (1982) A new endometrial applicator. Int J Radiat Oncol Biol Phys 8:941–945

Nori D, Hilaris BS, Tome M, Lewis JL Jr, Birnbaum S, Fuks Z (1987) Combined surgery and radiation in endometrial carcinoma: An analysis of prognostic factors. Int J Radiat Oncol Biol Phys 13:489–498

Nori D, Bains M, Hilaris BS, et al. (1989) New intraoperative brachytherapy techniques for positive or close surgical margins. J Surg Oncol 42:54–59

O'Connell D, Joslin CA, Howard N, Ramsey NW, Liversage WE (1967) The treatment of uterine carcinoma using the Cathetron. I. Technique. Br J Radiol 40:882–887

Ohlsen JO, Johnsom GH, Stewart JR, Eltringham JR, Stenchever MA (1977) Combined therapy for endometrial carcinoma: preoperative intracavitary radiation followed promptly by hysterectomy. Cancer 39:659–664

Okawa T, Sakata S, Kita-Okawa M, et al. (1992) Comparison of HDR versus LDR regimens for intracavitary brachytherapy of cervical cancer: Japanese experience. In: Mould RF (ed) International brachytherapy. Nucletron International, Veenendaal, pp 13–17

Onsrud M, Kolstad P, Normann T (1976) Postoperative external pelvic irradiation in carcinoma of the corpus stage I: a controlled clinical trial. Gynecol Oncol 4:222–231

Onsrud M, Aalders J, Abeler V, Tailor P (1982) Endometrial carcinoma with cervical involvement (stage II): prognostic factors and value of combined radiological-surgical treatment. Gynecol Oncol 13:76–86

Orton CG (1981) Radiobiological dose rate considerations with remote afterloading. In: Shearer DR (ed) Recent advances in brachytherapy physics. American Institute of Physics, New York, pp 190–200

Orton CG (1987) What minimum number of fraction is required with high dose-rate remote afterloading? Br J Radiol 60:300–301

Orton CG, Ellis F (1973) A simplification in the use of the NSD concept in practical radiotherapy. Br J Radiol 46:529–537
Orton CG, Webber BM (1977) Time-dose factor (TDF) analysis of dose rate effects in permanent implant dosimetry. Int J Radiat Oncol Biol Phys 2:55–60
Orton CG, Seyedsadr M, Somnay A (1991) Comparison of high and low dose rate remote afterloading for cervix cancer and the importance of fractionation. Int J Radiat Oncol Biol Phys 21:1425–1434
Pasmantier MW, Coleman M, Silver RT, Mamaril AP, Quiguyan CC, Galindo AJ (1985) Treatment of advanced endometrial carcinoma with doxorubicin and cisplatin: effects on both untreated and previously treated patients. Cancer Treat Rep 69:539–542
Park RC, Grigsby PW, Muss HB, Norris HJ (1992) Corpus: epithelial tumors. In: Hoskins WJ, Perez CA, Young RC (eds) Principles and practice of gynecologic oncology. Lippincott, Philadelphia, pp 664–665
Paterson R, Parker HM (1934) A dosage system for gamma-ray therapy. Br J Radiol 7:592
Perez CA, Camel HM (1982) Long-term follow-up in radiation therapy of carcinoma of the vagina. Cancer 49:1308–1315
Perez CA, Beaux S, Madox-Jones H, Bedwinek JM, Camel HM, Purdi JA, Walz BJ (1983) Radiation therapy alone in the treatment of carcinoma of the uterine cervix. I. Analysis of tumor recurrence. Cancer 51:1393–1402
Perez CA, Beaux S, Bedwinek JM, Madox-Jones H, Camel HM, Purdi JA, Walz BJ (1984) Radiation therapy alone in the treatment of carcinoma of the uterine cervix. II. Analysis of complications. Cancer 54:235–246
Perez CA, DiSaia PJ, Knapp RC (1985) Gynecologic tumors. In: DeVita VT, Hellmann S, Rosenberg SA (eds) Cancer: principles and practice of oncology. Lippincott, Philadelphia, pp 1013–1081
Pernot M, Hoffstetter S, Peiffert D, et al. (1994) Pre-operative, post-operative and exclusive irradiation of endometrial adenocarcinoma. Strahlenther Onkol 170:313–321
Persson I, Adami HO, Bergkvist L (1989) Risk of endometrial cancer after treatment with estrogens alone or in conjunction with progestagen: results of a prospective study. BMJ 298:147–151
Peschel RE, Healey GA, Smith RJ, et al. (1989) High dose rate remote afterloading for endometrial cancer. Endocurie Hypertherm Oncol 5:209–214
Pettersson B, Jansson H, Nilsson A, Schmidt M, Stenson S (1989) Prophylactic vaginal irradiation with low dose afterloading technique in women with endometrial cancer. In: Mould RF (ed) Brachytherapy 2. Nucletron International, Leersum, pp 240–244
Pettersson F (1991) Annual report on the results of treatment in gynecological cancer. Statements of results obtained in patients 1982 to 1986, vol 21. Elsevier, Amsterdam, pp 132–237
Pfändner K, Atzinger A, Breit A (1993) MR treatment planning in brachytherapy. In: Mould RF, Müller R-P (eds) Brachytherapy in Germany. Nucletron International, Veenendaal, pp 215–221
Pfleiderer A (1991) Die Therapie des Endometriumkarzinoms. Geburtshilfe Frauenheilkd 51:787–797
Pfleiderer A (1992) Die Operationen beim Endometriumkarzinom. In: Ladner HA, Pfleiderer A, Profous CZ (eds) Gynäkologische Radiologie. Springer, Berlin Heidelberg New York, pp 13–25
Pfleiderer A, Kleine W, Maier T, Schwörer D, Geyer H, Kaufmehl K (1989) Prognostic factors and endometrial carcinoma. Eur J Gynaecol Oncol 10:186–191
Phillips GL, Prem KA, Adcock LL, Twiggs LB (1982) Vaginal recurrence of adenocarcinoma of the endometrium. Gynecol Oncol 13:323–328
Pierquin B, Muller BK, Baillet F (1978) Low dose irradiation of advanced head and neck tumors: present status. Int J Radiat Oncol Biol Phys 4:565–572
Pierquin B, Wilson JF, Chassagne D (1987) Modern brachytherapy. Masson, New York
Pipard G, Milsztajn M, Jacquet P, Sentenac I (1985) Low dose-rate postoperative irradiation for adenocarcinoma of the endometrium, treating all or part of the vagina. In: Mould RF (ed) Brachytherapy 1984. Nucletron International, Leersum, pp 29–31
Piver MS (1980) Stage I endometrial carcinoma: the role of adjunctive radiation therapy. Int J Radiat Oncol Biol Phys 6:367–368
Piver MS, Hempling RE (1990) A prospective trial of postoperative vaginal radium/cesium for grade 1–2 less than 50% myometrial invasion and pelvic radiation therapy for grade 3 or deep myometrial invasion of surgical stage I endometrial adenocarcinoma. Cancer 66:1133–1138
Piver MS, Barlow JJ, Vongtama V, Webester J (1974) Hydroxyurea and radiation therapy in advanced cervical cancer. Am J Obstet Gynecol 120:969–972
Piver MS, Yazigi R, Blumenson L, Tsukada Y (1979) A prospective trial comparing hysterectomy, hysterectomy plus vaginal radium and uterine radium plus hysterectomy in stage I endometrial carcinoma. Obstet Gynecol 54:85–89
Piver MS, Barlow JJ, Lurain JR, Blumenson LE (1980) Medroxyprogesterone acetate versus hydroxyprogesterone caproate in women with metastatic endometrial adenocarcinoma. Cancer 45:268–272
Piver MS, Lele SB, Patsner B, Emrich LJ (1986) Melphalan, 5-fluouracil, and medroxyprogesterone acetate in metastatic endometrial carcinoma. Obstet Gynecol 63:557–560
Piver MS, Lele SB, Gamarra M (1988) Malignant peritoneal cytology in stage I endometrial adenocarcinoma: the effect of progesterone therapy (a preliminary report). Eur J Gynaecol Oncol 9:187
Plentl AA, Friedman EA (1971) Lymphatic system of the female genitalia: the morphologic basis of oncologic diagnosis and therapy. Saunders, Philadelphia, pp 116–152
Podratz KC, Wilson TO, Gaffey TA, Cha SS, Katzmann JA (1993) Desoxyribonucleic acid analysis facilitates the pretreatment identification of high-risk endometrial cancer patients. Am J Obstet Gynecol 168:1206–1215
Pollow K, Schmidt-Gollwitzer M, Pollow B (1986) Normal-Endometrium und Endometriumkarzinom: Steroidhormon-Rezeptoren und Steroidmetabolismus. In: Nagel GA, Schulz KD, Kreienberg R, Pollow K (eds) Neue Erkenntnisse über den Wirkmechanismus von Medroxyprogesteronazetat. Zuckschwerdt, München, pp 32–48
Poulsen MG, Roberts ST (1988) The salvage of recurrent endometrial carcinoma in the vagina and pelvis. Int J Radiat Oncol Biol Phys 15:809–813
Potish RA (1989) Abdominal radiotherapy for cancer of the uterine cervix and endometrium. Int J Radiat Oncol Biol Phys 16:1453–1458
Potish RA, Dusenbery KE (1990) Enteric morbidity of postoperative pelvic beam and brachytherapy for uterine cancer. Int J Radiat Oncol Biol Phys 18:1005–1010
Prem KA, Adcock LI, Okagaki T, Jones TK (1979) The evaluation of a treatment program for adenocarcinoma of the endometrium. Am J Obstet Gynecol 133:803–813

Price J, Hahn GA, Romingor DJ (1965) Vaginal involvement in endometrial carcinoma. Am J Obstet Gynecol 91:1060–1065

Puthawala AA, Syed AMN, Fleming PA, DiSaia PJ (1982) Re-irradiation with interstitial implant for recurrent pelvic malignancies. Cancer 50:2810–2814

Quinn MA, Couchi M, Fortune D (1985) Endometrial carcinoma: steroid receptors and response to medroxyprogesterone acetate. Gynecol Oncol 21:314–319

Rabe T (1990) Gynäkologische Erkrankungen. In: Rabe T (ed) Gynäkologie und Geburtshilfe. Medizin VCH, Weinheim, pp 220–272

Rafla S, Parikh K, Tchelebi M, Youssef E, Selim H, Bishay S (1989) Recurrent tumors of the head and neck, pelvis and chest wall: treatment with hyperthermia and brachytherapy. Radiology 172:845–850

Ratanatharathorn V, Powers WE (1990) Overview of uterine body malignancy. In: Martinez AA, Orton CG, Mould RF (eds) Brachytherapy HDR and LDR. Nucletron Corporation, Maryland, pp 59–67

Rauthe G, Vahrson H, Giers G (1988) Five-year results and complications in endometrium cancer – HDR afterloading vs. conventional radium therapy. In: Vahrson H, Rauthe G (eds) High Dose Rate Afterloading in the Treatment of Cancer of the Uterus, Breast and Rectum. Urban & Schwarzenberg, München, pp 240–245

Reddy S, Lee M-S, Hendrickson FR (1979) Pattern of recurrences in endometrial carcinoma and their management. Radiology 133:737–740

Regaud C (1922) Services de Curietherapie. Radiophysiologie et radiotherapie recuil de travaux biologiques, techniques et therapeutiques. In: Regaud C, Lacassagne A, Ferroux R (eds) Archives de l'Institut du Radium de l'Universite de Paris et de la Fondation Curie, vol 2. Les Presses Universitaires de France, (cited by Mould RF 1993)

Reichenberger I (1992) Sexuelle Probleme nach gynäkologisch-onkologischer Therapie. Gynäkologe 25:76–81

Reifenstein EC (1971) Hydrogesterone caproate therapy in advanced endometrial cancer. Cancer 27:485–502

Reisinger SA, Staros EB, Feld R, Mohiuddin M, Lewis GC (1992) Preoperative radiation therapy in clinical stage II endometrial carcinoma. Gynecol Oncol 45:174–178

Rendina GM (1984) Die hochdosierte Medroxprogesteronacetat-Therapie des Endometriumkarzinoms. In: Nagel GA, Robustelli Della Cuna G, Lanius P (eds) Medroxyprogesteronacetat (MAP) in der Therapie hormonsensibler Tumoren. Kehrer, Freiburg, pp 173–190

Rendina GM, Donadio C, Fabri M, Mazzoni P, Nazzicone P (1984) Tamoxifen and medroxyprogesterone therapy for advanced endometrial carcinoma. Eur J Obstet Gynecol Reprod Biol 17:258–291

Riippa P, Kivinen S, Kauppila A (1985) Comparison of Heyman packing and Cathetron afterloading methods in the treatment of endometrial cancer. Br J Radiol 58:437–441

Ritcher N, Lucas WE, Yon JL, Sanford GD (1981) Preoperative whole pelvic external irradiation – stage I endometrial cancer. Cancer 48:58–62

Rose PG, Cha SD, Tak WK, Fitzgerals T, Reale F, Hunter RE (1992) Radiation therapy for surgically proven para-aortic node metastasis in endometrial carcinoma. Int J Radiat Oncol Biol Phys 24:229–233

Rose PG, Baker S, Kern M, et al. (1993) Primary radiation therapy for endometrial carcinoma: a case controlled study. Int J Radiat Oncol Biol Phys 27:585–590

Rosenberg P, Risberg B, Askmalm L, Simonsen E (1989a) The prognosis in early endometrial carcinoma. The importance of uterine serous papillary carcinoma (UPSC), age, FIGO grade and nuclear grade. Acta Obstet Gynecol Scand 68: 157–163

Rosenberg P, Wingren S, Simonsen E, Stal O, Risberg B, Nordenskjöld B (1989b) Flow cytometric measurements of DNA index and S-phase on paraffin embedded early stage endometrial cancer: an important prognostic indicator. Gynecol Oncol 35:50–54

Rosenberg P, Blom R, Högberg T, Simonsen E (1993) Death rate and recurrence pattern among 841 clinical stage I endometrial cancer patients with special reference to uterine papillary serous carcinoma. Gynecol Oncol 51:311–315

Roth G, Vahrson H, Rauthe G (1985) Die Hysterographie bei liegendem Afterloading-applikator. Strahlentherapie 161:336–342

Rotman M, Aziz H, Kuruvilla A (1988) Vaginal recurrences in endometrial cancer. Int J Radiat Oncol Biol Phys 15:1043–1044

Rotte K (1969) Das Rezidiv beim Karzinom des Collum- und Corpus uteri. Strahlentherapie 137:637–645

Rotte K (1975) Das Endometriumkarzinom. Med Klin 70:169–173

Rotte K (1980) A randomized clinical trial comparing a high dose rate with a conventional dose rate technique. In: Bates TD, Berry R (eds) High Dose Rate Afterloading in the Treatment of Cancer of the Uterus. British Institute of Radiology, London, Special Report No 17, pp 75–79

Rotte K (1985) Klinische Ergebnisse der Afterloading-Kurzzeittherapie im Vergleich zur Radiumtherapie. Strahlentherapie 161:323–328

Rotte K (1988) Long-time results of HDR afterloading in comparison with radium therapy in endometrial cancer in Würzburg. In: Vahrson H, Rauthe G (eds) High Dose Rate Afterloading in the Treatment of Cancer of the Uterus, Breast and Rectum. Urban & Schwarzenberg, München, pp 218–221

Rotte K (1990) Technique and results of HDR afterloading in cancer of the endometrium. In: Martinez AA, Orton CG, Mould RF (eds) Brachytherapy HDR and LDR. Nucletron Corporation, Columbia, pp 68–79

Rotte K (1992) HDR for endometrial cancer. In: Mould RF (ed) International brachytherapy. Nucletron International, Veenendaal, pp 20–24

Rotte K, Linka F, Felder KD (1973) Intrakavitäre Bestrahlung des Uteruskarzinoms durch ein Afterloading-Gerät mit punktförmiger Iridium-192-Quelle. Strahlentherapie 145: 523–528

Rubin P, Gerle RD, Quick RS, Greenlaw RH (1963) Significance of vaginal recurrence in endometrial carcinoma. Am J Roentgenol 89:91–100

Rubin SC, Hoskins WJ, Saigo PE, Nori D, Mychalczak B, Chapman D, Lewis JL (1992) Management of endometrial adenocarcinoma with cervical involvement. Gynecol Oncol 45:294–298

Rustowski J, Kupsc W (1982) Factors influencing the results of radiotherapy in cases of inoperable endometrial cancer. Gynecol Oncol 14:185–193

Rutledge FN, Delclos L (1980) Adenocarcinoma of the uterus. In: Fletcher GH (ed) Textbook of radiotherapy, 3rd edn. Lea & Febiger, Philadelphia, pp 798–808

Rutledge FN, Tan SK, Fletcher GH (1958) Vaginal metastases from adenocarcinoma of the corpus uteri. Am J Obstet Gynaecol 75:167–174

Salazar OM, Feldstein ML, DePapp EW, et al. (1977) Endometrial carcinoma: analysis of failures with special emphasis on the use of initial preoperative external pelvic radiation. Int J Radiat Oncol Biol Phys 2:1101–1107

Salazar OM, Feldstein ML, DePapp EW, Bonfiglio TA, Keller BE, Rubin P, Rudolph JM (1978a) Management of clinical stage I endometrial carcinoma. Cancer 41:1016–1026

Salazar OM, Bonfiglio TA, Patten SF (1978b) Uterine sarcomas: natural history, treatment and prognosis. Cancer 42:1152–1160

Sauer OA, Götz-Gersitz U, Güllenstern M-L, Baier K, Herbolsheimer M (1994) Precision of the dose calculated for bladder and rectum in HDR gynecological brachytherapy. Endocurie Hypertherm Oncol 10:79–82

Scalliet P (1993) Radiobiology of brachytherapy. In: Mould RF, Müller R-P (eds) Brachytherapy in Germany. Nucletron International, Veenendaal, pp 1–11

Schindler AE (1977) Endometriumkarzinome und extraglanduläre Östrogenbiosynthese. Geburtshilfe Frauenheilkd 34:186–194

Schulz KD, Kaiser R (1983) Gegenwärtiger Stand der medikamentösen Behandlung des Endometriumkarzinoms. Gynäkologe 16:114–118

Schulz-Wendtland R, Bauer M, Teufel G, Freudenberg H (1993) The role of brachytherapy in the management of endometrial carcinoma: University of Freiburg 1982–1986. In: Mould RF, Müller R-P (eds) Brachytherapy in Germany. Nucletron International, Veenendaal, pp 111–125

Schünemann H, Jourdain M (1989) Mehrfachtumoren beim Endometriumkarzinom. Geburtshilfe Frauenheilkd 49: 743–746

Sears JD, Greven KM, Hoen HM, Randall ME (1994) Prognostic factors and treatment outcome for patients with locally recurrent endometrial cancer. Cancer 74:1303–1308

Seski JC, Edwards CL, Copeland LJ, Gershenson DM (1981) Hexamethylmelamine chemotherapy for disseminated endometrial cancer. Obstet Gynecol 58:361–363

Seski JC, Edwards CL, Herson J, Rutledge FN (1982) Cisplatin chemotherapy for disseminated endometrial cancer. Obstet Gynecol 59:225–228

Shah CA, Green TH (1972) Evaluation of current management of endometrial carcinoma. Obstet Gynaecol 39:500–509

Sharma S, Patel FD, Sandhu APS, Gupta BD, Yadav NS (1989) A prospective randomized study of local hyperthermia as a supplement and radiosensitizer in the treatment of carcinoma of the cervix with radiotherapy. Endocurie Hypertherm Oncol 5:151–159

Silverberg SG, Makowski EL, Roche WD (1977) Endometrial carcinoma in women under 40 years of age. Cancer 39:592–398

Simon N, Silverstone SM (1976) Afterloading with miniaturized 137-Cs sources in the treatment of cancer of the uterus. Int J Radiat Oncol Biol Phys 1:1017–1021

Sironi S, Colombo E, Villa G, Taccagni G, Belloni C, Garancini P, del Maschio A (1992) Myometrial invasion by endometrial carcinoma: assessment with plain and gadolinium-enhanced MR-imaging. Radiology 185:207–212

Smith DC, Prentice R, Thompson DJ, Herrmann WL (1975) Association of exogenous estrogen and endometrial carcinoma. N Engl J Med 293:1164–1167

Snelling P (1977) The use of radium substitutes and of after and remote loading techniques in intracavitary therapy. Strahlentherapie 153:594–597

Soper JT, Creasman WT, Clarke-Pearson DL, Sullivan DC, Vergadoro F, Johnston WW (1985) Intraperitoneal chromic phosphate 32-P suspension therapy of malignant peritoneal cytology in endometrial carcinoma. Am J Obstet Gynecol 153:101

Sorbe BG, Smeds AC (1990) Postoperative vaginal irradiation with high dose rate afterloading technique in endometrial carcinoma stage I. Int J Radiat Oncol Biol Phys 18:305–314

Spanos WJ, Fletcher GH, Wharton JT, Gallager HS (1978) Patterns of pelvic recurrence in endometrial carcinoma. Gynecol Oncol 6:495–502

Steck T, Gille J, Beier H, Albert P (1991) Endometriumkarzinom: Zuverlässigkeit des immunzytochemischen Östrogenrezeptor Nachweises gegenüber der biochemischen Analyse. Gynäkol Prax 15:87–92

Stehman FB, Bundy BN, Keys H, Currie JL, Mortel R, Creasman WT (1988) A randomized trial of hydroxyurea versus misonidazole adjunct to radiation therapy in carcinoma of the cervix. Am J Obstet Gynecol 159:87–94

Steindorfer P, German R, Schneider G, Rehak P, Giebler A, Wolf G, Uranüs S (1987) Our experiences with an annular phased array hyperthermia system in the treatment of advanced recurrences of the pelvis. Strahlenther Onkol 163:439–442

Stitt JA, Fowler JF, Thomadsen BR, Buchler DA, Paliwal BP, Kinsella TJ (1992) High dose rate intracavitary brachytherapy for carcinoma of the cervix: the Madison System. I. Clinical and radiobiological considerations. Int J Radiat Oncol Biol Phys 24:335–348

Stokes S, Bedwinek J, Perez CA, Camel HM, Kao MS (1986) Hysterectomy and adjuvant irradiation for pathologic stage III adenocarcinoma of the endometrium. Int J Radiat Oncol Biol Phys 12:335–338

Stücklschweiger G, Arian Schad K, Handl-Zeller L, Leitner H, Poier E, Hackl A (1991) Interstitielle Ir-192-Afterloading therapie mit sequentieller Warmwasserhyperthermie. Strahlenther Onkol 167:98–104

Sturm W (1977) Die Strahlenbehandlung des Uteruskarzinoms im Greisenalter. Inaugural-Dissertation. Fachbereich Medizin der Julius-Maximilians-Universität, Würzburg, pp 1–56

Suit HD, Moore EB, Fletcher GH, Worsnop MA (1963) Modification of Fletcher ovoid system for afterloading using standard-sized radium tubes (milligram and microgram). Radiology 81:126–131

Surmont J, Guy E, Fajbisowicz S, Dutreix A (1956) Possibilites de coordination correcte de la curie et de la roentgentherapie dans le traitement du cancer du col. J Radiol Electrol 37:252–259

Surwit EA, Manning MR, Aristizabal SA, Oleson JR, Cetas TC (1983) Interstitial thermoradiotherapy in recurrent gynecologic malignancies. Gynecol Oncol 15:95–102

Sutton GP, Geisler HE, Stehman FB, Young PC, Kimes TM, Ehrlich CE (1989) Features associated with survival and disease-free survival in early endometrial cancer. Am J Obstet Gynecol 160:1385–1393

Sutton GP, Blessing JA, Homesley HD, McGuire WP, Adcock 1 (1994) Phase II study of ifosfamide and mesna in refractory adenocarcinoma of the endometrium. A Gynecologic Oncology Group study. Cancer 73:1453–1455

Swift PS, Fu KK, Phillips TL, Roberts LW, Weaver KA (1994) Pulsed LDR interstitial and intracavitary therapy, clinical experience at USCF, San Francisco, USA. Nucletron Activity Report 5:29–31

Syed AMN, Puthawala AA (1987) Interstitial-intracavitary Syed-Neblett applicator in the treatment of carcinoma of the cervix. In: Nori D, Hilaris BS (eds) Radiation therapy of gynecologic cancer. Liss, New York, pp 297–307

Takahashi Y, Matsumoto H, Wakuda K, Ishiguro T, Yoshida Y (1991) Analysis of cell cycle kinetics using flow cytometry from paraffin-embedded tissues in endometrial adenocarcinoma. Asia Oceania J Obstet Gynaecol 17:73-81

Teshima T, Inoue T, Ikeda H, Murayama S, Yamasaki H, Sasaki S (1993) The Inoue applicator for endometrial brachytherapy. Activity Selectron Brachytherapy Journal 1:17-18

Thames HD (1983) Early and late gastrointestinal complications following radiotherapy for carcinoma of the cervix. Int J Radiat Oncol Biol Phys 9:1583-1584

Thames HD, Bentzen SM, Turesson I, Overgaard M, van den Bogaert W (1990) Time-dose factors in radiotherapy: a review of the human data. Radiother Oncol 19:219-236

Thigpen JT, Morrow CP, Blessing JA (1986) Adjuvant chemotherapy in high risk endometrial carcinoma. The Gynecologic Oncology Group experience. In: Bolla M et al. (eds) Endometrial cancers. Karger, Basel, pp 223-232

Tod MC, Meredith WJ (1938) A dosage system for use in the treatment of cancer of the uterine cervix. Br J Radiol 11:809-824

Trott K-R (1974) Strahlenbiologische Grundlagen der Strahlenbiologie unter besonderer Berücksichtigung der Therapie mit Korpuskularstrahlung. Strahlentherapie 148: 451-462

Trott K-R (1975) Strahlenbiologische Überlegungen bei der Wahl der Dosisleistung in der intrakavitären Strahlentherapie. Strahlentherapie 150:261-265

Trott K-R (1978) Der Einfluß der Dosisleistung auf die therapeutische Wirkung von 60-Co-Gammabestrahlung beim Adenokarzinom der Maus. Strahlentherapie 154: 656-658

Underwood PJ, Lutz MH, Kreutner A, Miller M, Johnson RJ (1977) Carcinoma of the endometrium: radiation followed immediately by operation. Am J Obstet Gynecol 128:86-98

Vadon G (1992) Regionale Chemotherapie im Kleinen-Becken-Bereich. In: Grimm D, Eichhorn M, Hänsgen G (eds) Fortschritte in der intrakavitären und interstitiellen Afterloadingtherapie. Sauerwein, Haan, pp 75-78

Vahrson H (1970) Umwelt und konstitutionelle Faktoren beim weiblichen Genitalkarzinom. Z Geburtsh Gynäk 172:94-106

Vahrson H (1989) Clinical experience with fractionated high dose rate afterloading brachytherapy in carcinoma of the cervix. In: Rotte K, Kiffer J (eds) Changes in brachytherapy. Wachholz, Nürnberg, pp 108-117

Vahrson H (1991) Die Strahlentherapie des Korpuskarzinoms. In: Künzel W, Kirschbaum M (eds) Giessener gynäkologische Fortbildung. Springer, Berlin Heidelberg New York, pp 163-179

Vahrson H (1992) Die primäre HDR-Al-Bestrahlung des Endometriumkarzinoms - Probleme, Technik, Ergebnisse. In: Grimm D, Eichhorn M, Hänsgen G (eds) Fortschritte in der intrakavitären und interstitiellen Afterloadingtherapie. Sauerwein, Haan, pp 63-74

van Nagell JR, Donaldson ES, Wood EG (1977) The prognostic significance of carcino-embryonic antigen in the plasma and tumors of patients with endometrial adenocarcinoma. Am J Obstet Gynecol 128:308-313

Varia M, Rosenman J, Halle J, Walton L, Currie J, Fowler W (1986) Primary radiation therapy for medically inoperable patients with endometrial carcinoma stage I-II. Int J Radiat Oncol Biol Phys 13:11-15

Vavra N, Kucera H, Weghaupt K (1991) Rezidive des Endometriumkarzinoms im Stadium I: Einfluß von Prognosefaktoren auf das Therapieergebnis. Geburtshilfe Frauenheilkd 51:267-271

Vavra N, Denison U, Kucera H, Barrada M, Kurz C, Salzer H, Sevelda P (1993) Prognostic factors related to recurrent endometrial carcinoma following initial surgery. Acta Obstet Gynecol Scand 72:205-209

Vecchia C, Franceschi S, Parazzini F, Colombo E, Colombo F, Liberati A, Mangioni C (1983) Ten-years survival in 290 patients with endometrial cancer: prognostic factors and therapeutic approach. Br J Obstet Gynaecol 90:654-661

Vergote I, Kjorstad K, Abeler V, Kolstad P (1989) A randomized trial of adjuvant progestagen in early endometrial cancer. Cancer 64:1011-1016

Vergote I, Kjorstad K, Abeler V, Vossli S (1991) Postoperative vaginal irradiation by high dose-rate cobalt afterloading in stage I endometrial cancer: experience from the Norwegian Radium Hospital. In: Kleine W, Meerpohl H-G, Pfleiderer A, Profous CZ (eds) Therapie des Endometriumkarzinoms AGO-Reihe. Springer, Berlin Heidelberg New York, pp 103-107

von Essen CF, Seay DG, Moeller MS, Hilbert JW (1974) Fractionated intracavitary radiation therapy with the brachytron: general techniques and preliminary results in the treatment of cervix cancer. Am J Roentgenol 120:101-110

von Fournier D, Kubli F, Bauer M, Weber E (1981) Hochdosierte Gestagen-Langzeittherapie beim Korpuskarzinom, Einfluß auf die Überlebenszeit. Geburtshilfe Frauenheilkd 41:266-269

von Fournier D, Junkermann H, Anton HW (1987) Indikationen zur Radiotherapie beim Kollum- und Korpuskarzinom nach Operation. Gynäkologe 20:222-227

Vora NL, Luk KH, Forell B, et al. (1988) Interstitial local current field hyperthermia for advanced cancers of the cervix. Endocurie Hypertherm Oncol 4:97-106

Walstam R (1962) Remotely-controlled radiotherapy apparatus. Phys Med Biol 7:225-228

Walstam R (1977) Strahlenphysikalische Voraussetzungen der ferngesteuerten Afterloadingbestrahlung. Strahlentherapie 153:802-806

Warmelink C, Ezzell G, Orton CG (1989) Use of time-dose fractionation model to design high dose-rate fractionation schemes. In: Mould RF (ed) Brachytherapy 2. Nucletron International, Leersum, pp 41-48

Waterhouse I, Muir C, Correa P, Powell I (1977) Cancer incidence in five continents, vol III/15. IARC Scientific Publications, Lyon (cited by Baltzer J and Lohe KJ 1986)

Webb GA, Lagios MD (1987) Clear cell carcinoma of the endometrium. Am J Obstet Gynecol 156:1486-1491

Willgeroth F (1992) Komplikationen der Strahlentherapie in der gynäkologischen Onkologie. Gynäkologe 25:82-88

Willgeroth F (1994) Adjuvante Brachy- und perkutane Strahlentherapie beim primär operierten Endometriumkarzinom. Gynäkologe 27:76-83

Williams KE, Waters ED, Woolas RP, Hammond IG, McCartney AJ (1994) Mixed serous-endometrioid carcinoma of the uterus: pathologic and cytopathologic analysis of a high-risk endometrial carcinoma. Int J Gynecol Cancer 4:7-18

Williamson EO, Christopherson WM (1972) Malignant mixed mullerian tumors of the uterus. Cancer 29:585-592

Wilson TO, Podratz KC, Gaffey TA, Malkasian GD Jr, O'Brien PC, Naessens JM (1990) Evaluation of unfavourable histologic subtypes in endometrial adenocarcinoma. Am J Obstet Gynecol 162:418–426 (discussion 423–426)

Wolff JP, Pejovic MH, Michel G, Gerbaulet A, Prade M, George M (1986) New treatment procedure for stage I endometrial carcinoma. Gynecol Oncol 23:51–58

Wolfson JP, Sightler SE, Markoe AM, Schwade JG, Averette HE, Ganjei O, Hilsenbeck SG (1992) The prognostic significance of surgical staging for carcinoma of the endometrium. Gynecol Oncol 45:142–146

11 Malignancies of the Ovaries

H.W. Vahrson, U. Nitz, and H.G. Bender

CONTENTS

H.W. Vahrson, MD, Professor, Leiter der Abteilung für Gynäkologische Onkologie und Strahlentherapie, Frauenklinik, Klinikum der Justus-Liebig-Universität, Klinikstraße 32, D-35385 Gießen, Germany

U. Nitz, MD, PD, Universitäts-Frauenklinik, Moorenstraße 5, D-40225 Düsseldorf, Germany

H.G. Bender, MD, Professor, Direktor, Universitäts-Frauenklinik, Moorenstraße 5, D-40225 Düsseldorf, Germany

11.1 Epidemiology and Risk Factors

H.W. Vahrson

11.1.1 Incidence, Race, and Religion

The ovaries are the sixth leading site of cancer in females after the breast, lung, colon, rectum, and endometrium. Extreme differences (by a factor of 7!) exist in the incidence of ovarian cancer between (a) developing countries and rural areas of Japan, where the incidence is 2–4 per 100000 population, and (b) Scandinavia, where it is 13.9–15.3 per 100000. The United Kingdom, Switzerland, France, and Germany show an intermediate incidence of 7.8–13.2 per 100000. The annual age-adjusted incidence in the United States is 12–13 per 100000. Race and religion seem to have an impact on the age-adjusted ovarian cancer incidence in the United States: white women have a higher incidence than black women. The difference between whites and blacks diverges progressively with increasing age due to epithelial cancers. In younger women below age 45 the incidence is higher in blacks than in whites due to nonepithelial tumors (Harlap 1993). Generally, however, racial differences in ovarian cancer incidence concern epithelial cancers only, with nonepithelial tumors (germ cell or stromal tumors) tending to be equal in incidence among the races (Pfleiderer 1986).

Jewish women in New York have the highest incidence among all groups. In Israel a great difference between natives and immigrants has been reported: immigrants from Europe and America had the highest age-adjusted incidence of about 35 per 100000, while the rates for immigrants from Asia, immigrants from Africa, Israelis, and the non-Jewish population were about 12, 10, 18 and 8 per 100000, respectively (Schenker and Mazzor 1978). The incidence among Japanese women in Japan is 3.3 per 100000 (Okayama), but in San Francisco it is 6, as compared to 13.2 in whites. In the United States there is a remarkable adaptation of the incidence among second-generation Japanese women to that among white women (Dunn 1975). Mormons and Adventists in the United States have very low incidence rates (Lyon et al. 1980; Enstrom 1979).

11.1.2 Mortality Rates

Approximately 20000 women are diagnosed with ovarian cancer in the United States each year and about 12000 die because of it (Whittemore 1994). In France in 1991, 3175 deaths from ovarian cancer were registered (Rezvani and Lê 1994). The authors found a 72% increase in mortality during the study period 1968–1991, which could be entirely explained by an increase in mortality among women over age 60.

La Vecchia et al. (1992) analyzed the trends in ovarian cancer mortality for 25 European countries from 1955 to 1989. They found an increase in age-adjusted mortality rates in most European countries, the exceptions being Denmark, Sweden, and Switzerland, where certified mortality was already elevated in the late 1950s. The peak rate in these countries was reached in the 1960s (about or above 10/100000). During the last decade the trend has been downward in Nordic countries, Germany, Austria, Switzerland, and Czechoslovakia but still upward in southern Europe, Great Britain, and Ireland. Trends have been more favorable in women aged 35–64 years and, to a greater extent, in women aged 20–44 years. The younger age group has shown a decline in mortality in most European countries, approaching 50% in Great Britain and Scandinavia. The data may represent the European trend in general, but for Germany they are not supported by recent data. In Germany in 1992, 6352 deaths from cancer of the ovaries (and adnexa) occurred in a female population of 41.4 millions. If one considers the falling incidence of cervical cancer and its better prognosis (>50% 5-year survival) and the rising incidence of endometrial cancer, which has a still better prognosis (>60% 5-year survival), then ovarian cancer, with the worst prognosis (<40% 5-year survival) still deserves its bad reputation as the "number one ladykiller" among the genital cancers in Western industrialized countries. Recent data (Statistisches Bundesamt 1994) reveal that the age-adjusted death rate for cancer of the ovaries and the adnexa is 15.2 per 100000 female population in Germany (Table 11.1).

In China between 1973 and 1975 the age-adjusted mortality of ovarian cancer was very low. While cervical cancer ranked second in mortality (18.39%), after stomach (18.72%) and before esophageal cancer (18.15%), ovarian and endometrial cancers were not among the nine leading forms of cancer; rather they were subsumed among "others" (11.66%). Differences between the provinces were, however, important (ATLAS of CANCER MORTALITY 1979).

Table 11.1. Age-adjusted deaths from malignant diseases per 100000 female population in Germany, 1992. (From Statistisches Bundesamt 1994)

All malignancies	250.1
Breast	43.4
Colon/rectum	41.1
Stomach	19.0
Lymphatic/hemopoietic system	17.8
Lung/bronchus	17.7
Ovaries and adnexa	15.2
Uterus	13.9
Urinary tract	11.7

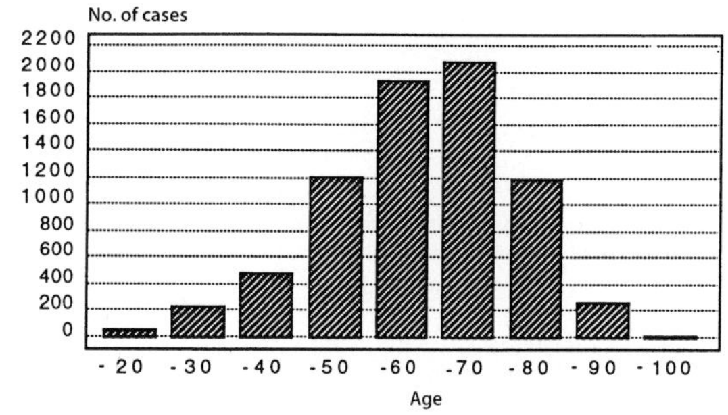

Fig. 11.1. Distribution by age of obviously malignant epithelial ovarian carcinomas in 7509 patients, 1987–1989. (From Annual Report, vol. 22; PETTERSSON 1994)

11.1.3 Age

Age is an important risk factor for ovarian cancer. According to cancer registries in former West Germany (Baden-Württemberg, Hamburg, Saarland), former East Germany, Israel, and Connecticut, age-adjusted incidence rates increase nearly continuously up to age 70 and then seem to decline slightly (Fig. 11.1) (BENDER and ROBRA 1983). The mortality rates are slightly lower but parallel the incidence rates.

The higher life expectancy for the female population is accompanied by an increase in ovarian cancers. At the ZFG Giessen, three different periods could be compared with respect to the age distribution of ovarian cancers at the time of diagnosis (Table 11.2). After a nearly constant age distribution from 1918 to 1968, (v. DELFT 1941; VAHRSON 1970), the recent data from 1979–1993 show a clear shift to the age groups 60–69 (maximum) and 70–79 (LESCHINGER 1995).

11.1.4 Risk Factors

From an overview of 20 studies, HANKINSON et al. (1992) reported the relative risk for ever users of oral contraceptives to be 0.64 (95% confidence interval 0.57–0.73). The risk decreased with increasing duration of contraceptive use to 50% after 5 years' use. This reduced risk persisted for at least 10 years after cessation of use. After 10 or more years the relative risk was still 0.60 (95% confidence interval 0.42–0.86). In the Oxford Family Planning Association contraceptive cohort study (VESSEY and PAINTER 1995) the relative ovarian cancer risk for ever oral contraceptive users vs nonusers was 0.4 (95% confi-

Table 11.2. Age distribution (%) of ovarian cancers at the time of diagnosis in different periods at the ZFG Giessen

Author (year) and period	No.	Age (years)						
		<30	31–39	40–49	50–59	60–69	70–79	80<
v. DELFT (1941) 1918–1935	116	4.3	9.5	27.6	38.8	7.3	2.6	0
VAHRSON (1970) 1957–1968	250	5.2	10.0	29.2	39.2	13.2	2.8	0.4
LESCHINGER (1996) 1979–1983	721	0.02	4.5	15.0	28.0	31.8	17.2	1.4

dence interval 0.2–0.8). Furthermore, the age-adjusted rate of the disease was 29 in nulliparous versus 13 in parous women per 100000 woman-years.

Many risk factors (nulliparity, white race, Protestant religion, immigration to high-risk countries, high socioeconomic status) and protective factors (multiparity, lactation, use of oral contraceptives, Catholic and Methodist religions, black race, low socioeconomic status) seem to have one common feature: the number of ovulatory cycles during a woman's lifetime (PFLEIDERER 1984, 1986; HARLAP 1993; BARBER 1993). The "incessant ovulation" hypothesis postulates that the risk of epithelial ovarian cancer is a function of the epithelial tearing and regeneration during each ovulation. Furthermore, surface epithelium can grow vertically downwards to form crypts and inclusion cysts, which indicates a high absorptive activity, and can also form superficial papillary excrescences. Metaplastic transformation of the various types of müllerian epithelium can occur (DIETL and MARZUSCH 1993). This surface activity and cell turnover – the dividing cells being vulnerable to mutations caused by carcinogens – support this theory (WOODRUFF 1979; PRESTON-MARTIN et al. 1991).

An opposing hypothesis suggests that the risk of mutation is "turned off" at some stage by events in a woman's reproductive life (GWINN et al. 1990), and postulates a role for gonadotropins. Several agents such as premature ovarian failure caused by damage to oocytes through infection (mumps), cytotoxic drugs, radiation, and environmental toxins may result in a breakdown of the normal ovarian-hypothalamic feedback, leading to an excess of gonadotropins.

In a case-control study in 56 Japanese women over the age of 50 who had primary ovarian cancer, a significant association was found between daily meat consumption and the occurrence of ovarian cancer. The attributable risk was 19.2% in elderly Japanese women (MORI and HIYAKE 1988). Recently in a case-control study from Cracow, Poland, concerning the consumption of alcohol, cigarettes, fat, dairy products, and vegetables, the only factor found to have an impact on ovarian cancer risk was the frequent consumption of legumes (peas, beans, broadbeans), which had a significant protective effect (PAWLEGA et al. 1994). Other suggested risk factors are postmenopausal estrogen therapy, talc (and/or asbestos as a contaminant), coffee, alcohol, smoking, and lactose intolerance, but their role is controversial and minor at most (HARLAP 1993).

11.1.5
Irradiation

SPEERT (1952) found one ovarian cancer in 958 women who had previously undergone termination of menstrual flow by x-ray irradiation. In another series of 590 consecutive patients (343 with ovarian cancers and 247 with ovarian cystadenomas), 17 had a record of previous pelvic irradiation for benign conditions. WEST (1966) examined the milliroentgens delivered to the ovaries by diagnostic and therapeutic abdominal x-ray irradiation as one variable and found no influence on the development of ovarian cancers. These studies refute any influence of low-dose irradiation on the ovaries, but the role of high-dose therapeutic pelvic irradiation is still to be established.

11.1.6
Second Primaries

Cancer of the ovaries is sometimes associated with endometrial and/or breast cancer. Women with breast cancer have twice the risk of developing a second primary ovarian cancer (BARBER 1993). The second primaries can occur before, simultaneously with, or after ovarian cancer. In a previous report on a series of 35 advanced ovarian cancers, there were prior cancers of the breast in four cases (11.4%) (VAHRSON 1973).

Among 346 patients with 738 multiple primary tumors at the ZFG Giessen (1957–1992), 214 were diagnosed at the same time (synchronous). Of these 214 tumors, 56 were ovarian cancers with 35 (62.5%) second primaries in the endometrium, six in the breast (10.7%), six in the cervix (10.7%), two in the tuba uterina (3.6%), two in the pancreas (3.6%), and one in the vagina (1.8%). In addition, 134 patients had primary genital cancers which were followed by a second or multiple primaries (metachronous). In 16 cases the ovary was the first site of tumor; of the metachronous tumors, four were in the breast (25%), two in the colon/rectum (12.5%), two in the skin (12.5%), and one (6.25%) in each of the endometrium, cervix, ovary, vulva, vagina, urinary bladder, lung, and head and neck (SCHNEIDER 1995).

11.1.7 Ratio of Genital Cancers

In cases from the first decades of this century reviewed by HINSELMANN (1930), a ratio of 15:1 was found between cervical and endometrial cancers (n = 21493 and 1458, respectively).

The cervical:endometrial:ovarian cancer ratio can be calculated from clinical data from two centers. At the UFK Göttingen from 1933 to 1943, 901 cervical, 211 endometrial, and 140 ovarian (including fallopian tube) cancers were reported (MARTIUS 1943), yielding a ratio of 4.3:1:0.7. The ratio at the ZFG Giessen from 1957/58 to 1987/88 (Table 11.3) shows a clear change in the cervical to endometrial cancer ratio but a fairly constant endometrial to ovarian cancer ratio, the overall ratio being 1:0.7–1:0.8. We must assume that some risk factors must be identical for endometrial and ovarian cancer.

11.1.8 Cancer Families

In contrast to sporadic ovarian cancer (without a family history), familial ovarian cancer is defined as being present when two or more first- or second-degree relatives have the disease, without regard to the age of onset or associated cancer. Its etiology is multifactorial and/or due to chance. LYNCH et al. (1990) concluded that, "The empirical risk to a first-degree relative of an ovarian cancer affected individual in the familial setting is threefold that which exists for patients who lack a familial background of ovarian cancer." They also pointed out that, "Hereditary ovarian cancer is characterized by a pattern within a particular family which shows autosomal dominant segregation of ovarian cancer but which may also show other forms of integrally related cancers such as breast cancer in the breast/ovarian syndrome." These families show an early age of cancer onset and an excess of ovarian and multiple primary cancers. Heterogeneity is significant in hereditary ovarian cancer. Ovarian cancers have shown an association with several familial precancer disorders, including Turner's syndrome (XO/XY mosaicism, dysgerminoma, or gonadoblastoma) and PEUTZ-Jegher's syndrome (nevi, intestinal polyposis). In families with site-specific ovarian cancer or breast–ovarian cancer syndrome, the lifetime risk for ovarian cancer is close to 50% (HARLAP 1993). In these families, the hereditary factor is linked to the breast–ovarian cancer susceptibility gene BRCA 1 on chromosome 17q21 in 78% of cases of site-specific ovarian cancer and in 100% of cases of breast plus ovarian cancer (STEICHEN-GERSDORF et al. 1994).

Table 11.3. Trends in numbers of patients per year with invasive cancers of the cervix, endometrium, and ovaries over 3 decades at the ZFG Giessen (numbers averaged out over 2 years)

Years	Site of cancer			Ratio (endometrium = 1)
	Cervix	Endometrium	Ovaries	
1957/58	91	31	24	2.9:1:0.8
1967/68	103	49	38	1.8:1:0.8
1977/78	120	68	47	1.8:1:0.7
1987/88	49	71	56	0.7:1:0.8

Linkage also exists between another hereditary syndrome involving ovarian, endometrium, breast, and nonadenomatous colon cancer, called the Lynch family cancer syndrome II, and the Kidd blood group, mapped on chromosome 18, q11–q12 (Hoskins and Ostrer 1993).

In the so-called Gilda Radner Familial Ovarian Cancer Registry, 1000 ovarian cancer families were registered. Of these, 724 families had two, 178 families had three, and 98 families had four to ten cases of ovarian cancer. These was a total of 2425 ovarian cancers, 400 breast cancers, 78 breast and ovarian cancers, and 154 colon cancers (54% in females and 46% in males). There was a significantly higher percentage of serous cancers (40% vs 25%) and a significantly lower percentage of mucinous cancers (3% vs 12%) as compared with nonfamilial ovarian cancers from the SEER Program (Piver et al 1996).

11.1.9 Hysterectomy and Oophorectomy

A third hypothesis regarding the etiology of ovarian cancer postulates the direct penetration of carcinogens from the vagina and uterus through the tubes to the peritoneal and ovarian surface. Talc has been investigated best in this context (Cramer et al. 1982). This hypothesis is consistent with the results of Irwin et al. (1991), Whittemore et al. (1992), and Hankinson et al. (1993) that tubal sterilization and hysterectomy have a protective effect against ovarian cancer.

In a recent study of 721 consecutive patients with epithelial cancers from 1979 to 1993 at the ZFG Giessen, 112 (15.5%) had had a previous hysterectomy for benign diseases (95.9%) or cervical/endometrial neoplasias (4.1%). Among them were 29 with unilateral oophorectomy. For comparison, a group of 474 patients from corresponding age groups treated in the same period (1979–1993) for nongynecological and nonmalignant diseases at the Medizinische Universitäts-Klinik Giessen was evaluated. This group had had 132 (27.8%) previous hysterectomies. The difference – 15.5 vs 27.8% – was highly significant ($P < 0.00001$). The risk of developing an ovarian cancer for hysterectomized women is 0.7 (95% confidence interval 0.6–0.8) (Leschinger 1996).

"Prophylactic oophorectomy" is a topic of great controversy. Disregarding the possible complaints in pre- and perimenopausal age groups, bilateral oophorectomy could prevent a considerable percentage of ovarian cancers. Gibbs (1971) presented a series of 236 patients with ovarian cancers, 28 of whom had previously undergone hysterectomy. He added 13 patients with previous breast and colon cancer, who in his opinion could have been oophorectomized to prevent metastases, and a further eight patients who had had pelvic irradiation to induce menopause instead of oophorectomy, giving a total of 49 of the 236 patients (20.7%). From this group of cases he concluded, "that over 20% could have been prevented by radical surgical pelvic procedures in patients over the age of 35."

According to Pfleiderer (1984), prophylactic bilateral oophorectomy is to be favored beyond age 45–48 and to be urgently recommended beyond age 50 if laparotomy is performed for other reasons.

Accessory or supernumerary ovaries (see Sect. 11.2.5) can be rare causes of peritoneal carcinomatosis arising after bilateral oophorectomy for histologically proven nonmalignant ovaries (Wharton 1959; Lynch et al. 1986). In a series of 28 women at risk in cancer-prone families who underwent prophylactic oophorectomy with histologically normal ovaries, three women presented with intra-abdominal carcinomatosis within a follow-up period ranging from 1 to 20 years (Tobacman et al. 1982). This leads to the hypothesis that these cancers arise from the common coelomic epithelium covering the ovaries and the pelvic wall.

11.2 Histopathological Classification and Grading

H.W. Vahrson

The ovaries represent only small flattened ovoids about 2 × 4 cm in diameter but they produce a great variety of histologically different benign, semi-malignant, and malignant tumors, some of which show endocrine activity. A description of the different histological tumor types would be beyond the scope of this chapter. (For comprehensive information see Clement, Russel, Young and Scully, and Talerman in Kurman (ed) Blaustein's pathology of the female genital tract, 4th edn. Springer, New York, 1994.) Therefore this discussion will be confined to the international classification according to FIGO/

WHO and to special points of importance for diagnosis and therapy.

11.2.1 Primary or Secondary Cancers

Primary ovarian cancers are those in which tumor growth begins in the ovaries. Secondary ovarian cancers are those cancers where secondary metastatic spread to the ovaries from other tumor sites is obvious. These sites include the endometrium, fallopian tube, peritoneum, breast, gastrointestinal (Krukenberg tumor) and colorectal tracts, pancreas, liver, and urinary tract.

In older German literature the definitions were quite different. Primary ovarian cancers were those in which tumor was malignant from the beginning. Secondary cancers were cystomas where, in mainly benign structures, a small volume of malignant growth was found, which was thought to represent secondary malignant degeneration in statu nascendi in a primary benign cystoma (Kepp 1952; Hofmann 1963; Frischkorn 1976).

In spite of all attempts, differentiation between primary and secondary ovarian cancer may be impossible, especially in cases of inoperable widespread anaplastic cancers. In their Annual Report vol. 21, FIGO recommended that such cases be classified as carcinoma abdominis (Pettersson 1991).

11.2.2 Second and Multiple Primaries

Second primaries are malignant tumors of different histological type occurring in other sites. They can be synchronous or metachronous (see Sect. 11.1.6). The differentiation between second primary or metastatic disease is often difficult when ovarian, endometrial, breast, or adeno-matous colorectal cancers are involved.

When metachronous tumors of this group are diagnosed at different institutions it is important that both of the histological slides are referred to the same institution for comparison. In this way some misdiagnoses of ovarian cancer (with or without peritoneal carcinomatosis) occurring after breast cancer can be corrected to what they really are: secondary ovarian cancers, i.e., metastatic recurrences of breast cancer.

11.2.3 WHO Classification and Nomenclature of Ovarian Tumors

The classification of common epithelial, sex cord-stromal, and germ cell tumors by WHO is combined in Table 11.4 (Serov et al. 1973; Scully 1975; Barber 1993).

For modifications of the histological classification of sex cord-stromal tumors as presented by Young and Scully (1992, 1994), see Sect. 11.16.1. The lipid (lipoid) cell tumors are now called steroid cell tumors and allotted to the sex cord-stromal tumors (see Sect. 11.1.8).

The common epithelial tumors account for 85% of all primary malignant tumors. Of the other groups, only the granulosa cell tumor, with about 10%, is of major therapeutic interest.

11.2.4 FIGO Histological Classification of Primary Epithelial Ovarian Tumors

For reporting results of therapy in common epithelial ovarian cancer to the Annual Report (Editorial office: Radiumhemmet, S-10401 Stockholm, Sweden) the committee recommends the use of the classification shown in Table 11.5.

The distribution of primary epithelial ovarian borderline tumors and cancers by histological subtype and stage in 7563 patients is shown in Table 11.6. Among the different histological subtypes, prognosis is best for mucinous cancers, and

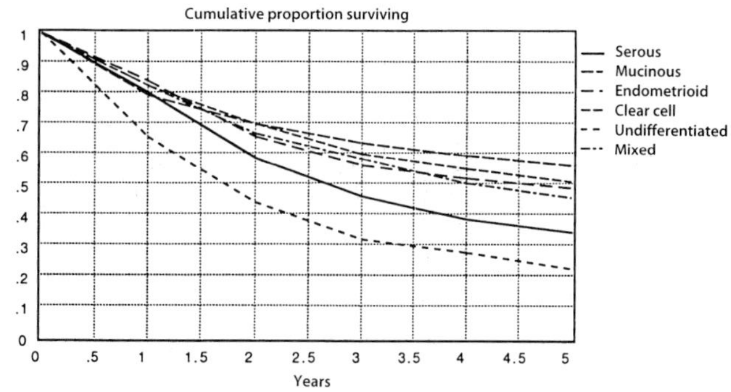

Fig. 11.2. Obviously malignant ovarian carcinoma of all stages: cumulative proportion of patients surviving by histopathological class. At 5 years survival was best for mucinous tumors, followed in descending order by clear cell, endometrioid, mixed, serous, and undifferentiated subtypes. (From Annual Report, vol. 22; Pettersson 1994)

Table 11.4. WHO classification of and nomenclature for ovarian tumors

I. Common epithelial tumors
A. Serous tumors
1. Benign
a) Cystadenoma and papillary cystadenoma
b) Surface papilloma
c) Adenofibroma and cystadenofibroma
2. Borderline malignancy (carcinomas of low malignant potential)
a) Cystadenoma and papillary cystadenoma
b) Surface papilloma
c) Adenofibroma and cystadenofibroma
3. Malignant
a) Adenocarcinoma, papillary adenocarcinoma, and papillary cystadenocarcinoma
b) Surface papillary carcinoma
c) Malignant adenofibroma and cystadenofibroma
B. Mucinous tumors
1. Benign
a) Cystadenoma
b) Adenofibroma and cystadenofibroma
2. Borderline malignancy (carcinomas of low malignant potential)
a) Cystadenoma
b) Adenofibroma and cystadenocarcinoma
3. Malignant
a) Adenocarcinoma and cystadenocarcinoma
b) Malignant adenofibroma and cystadenofibroma
C. Endomertrioid tumors
1. Benign
a) Adenoma and cystadenoma
b) Adenofibroma and cystadenofibroma
2. Borderline malignancy (carcinomas of low malignant potential)
a) Adenoma and cystadenoma
b) Adenofibroma and cystadenofibroma
3. Malignant
a) Carcinoma
i) Adenocarcinoma
ii) Adenoacanthoma
iii) Malignant adenofibroma and cystadenofibroma
b) Endometrioid stromal sarcomas
c) Mesodermal (müllerian) mixed tumors, homologous and heterologous
D. Clear cell (mesonephroid) tumors
1. Benign: adenofibroma
2. Borderline malignancy (carcinomas of low malignant potential)
3. Malignant: carcinoma and adenocarcinoma
E. Brenner tumors
1. Benign
2. Borderline malignancy (proliferating)
3. Malignant
F. Mixed epithelial tumors
1. Benign
2. Borderline malignancy
3. Malignant
G. Undifferentiated carcinoma
H. Unclassified epithelial tumors
II. Sex cord-stromal tumors
A. Granulosa-stromal cell tumors
1. Granulosa-cell tumors
2. Tumors in the thecoma-fibroma group
a) Thecoma
b) Fibroma
c) Unclassified
B. Androblastomas; Sertoli-Leydig cell tumors
1. Well differentiated
a) Tubular androblastoma; Sertoli cell tumors (tubular adenoma of Pick)
b) Tubular androblastoma with lipid storage; Sertoli cell tumor with lipid storage (*folliculome lipidique* of Lecene)
c) Sertoli-Leydig cell tumor (tubular adenoma with Leydig cells)
d) Leydig cell tumor; hilus cell tumor
2. Intermediate differentiation
3. Poorly differentiated (sarcomatoid)
4. With heterologous elements
C. Gynandroblastoma
D. Unclassified
III. Lipid (lipoid) cell tumors
IV. Germ cell tumors
A. Dysgerminoma
B. Endodermal sinus tumor
C. Embryonal carcinoma
D. Polyembryoma
E. Choriocarcinoma
F. Teratomas
1. Immature
2. Mature
a) Solid
b) Cystic
i) Dermoid cyst (mature cystic teratoma)
ii) Dermoid cyst with malignant transformation
3. Monodermal and highly specialized
a) Struma ovarii
b) Carcinoid
c) Struma ovarii and carcinoid
d) Others
G. Mixed forms
V. Gonadoblastoma
A. Pure
B. Mixed with dysgerminoma or other forms of germ cell tumor
VI. Soft tissue tumors not specific to ovary
VII. Unclassified tumors
VIII. Secondary (metastatic) tumors

worst for serous and undifferentiated cancers (Fig. 11.2).

Tumors of *borderline malignancy* (low malignant potential) are tumors with malignant cells in the epithelium, which do not infiltrate the underlying stroma. Most of them are classified as stage I, grade 1. They can spread, but even in advanced stages they have a much better prognosis than obviously malig-

Table 11.5. Histological classification of the common primary epithelial tumors of the ovary

1. *Serous cystomas*
   a) Serous benign cystadenomas
   b) Serous cystadenomas with proliferating activity of the epithelial cells and nuclear abnormalities, but with no infiltrative destructive growth (borderline cases; low potential malignancy)
   c) Serous cystadenocarcinomas

2. *Mucinous cystomas*
   a) Mucinous benign cystadenomas
   b) Mucinous cystadenomas with proliferating activity of the epithelial cells and nuclear abnormalities, but with no infiltrative destructive growth (borderline cases; low potential malignancy)

3. *Endometrioid tumors*
   (similar to adenocarcinoma in the endometrium)
   a) Endometrioid benign cysts
   b) Endometrioid tumors with proliferating activity of the epithelial cells and nuclear abnormalities, but with no infiltrative destructive growth (borderline cases; low potential malignancy)
   c) Endometrioid adenocarcinomas

4. *Clear cell tumors (mesonephroid tumors)*
   a) Benign mesonephroid tumors
   b) Mesonephroid tumors with proliferating activity of the epithelial cells and nuclear abnormalities, but with no infiltrative destructive growth (borderline cases; low potential malignancy)
   c) Mesonephroid cystadenocarcinomas

5. *Undifferentiated carcinoma*
   A malignant tumor of epithelial structures that is too poorly differentiated to be placed in any of the groups 1–4 or 6

6. *Mixed epithelial tumors*
   Tumors composed of a mixture of two or more of the malignant groups 1c, 2c, 3c, or 4c described above, where none of them is predominant. Thus, a case should be listed as mixed epithelial tumor only if it is not possible to decide which is the predominant structure. The pathologist should always try to find out which is the leading structure and classify the case according to that element

7. *No histology or unclassifiable*
   Cases where explorative surgery has shown that obvious ovarian epithelial malignant tumor is present, but where no biopsy has been taken, or where the specimen is unclassifiable because of, for instance, necrosis

nant ovarian cancers (Fig. 11.3). The ongoing discussion on this intermediate category between benign and malignant tumors should be brought to an end by the use of flow cytometry or other methods. It should then become possible to separate euploid benign tumors from aneuploid malignant cancers. Vergote et al. (1992a) studied DNA ploidy in a series of 321 patients and found diploidy in 293 tumors and aneuploidy in 28. Of the 26 patients who died of disease, nine had diploid and 17 aneuploid tumors. A multivariate analysis revealed DNA ploidy to be the most important prognostic factor. Transformation of borderline malignant to obvious malignant tumors is rare. In a literature review of 1500 serous borderline tumors, Kurman and Trimble (1993) calculated the transformation rate to carcinoma to be less than 1%.

11.2.5 Ovarian Cancers Originating from Extraovarian Sites

There are some histologically typical serous, mucinous, endometrioid, or other ovarian carcinomas which occur in patients without or with minor ovarian involvement or after previous bilateral oophorectomy because of benign lesions. This phenomenon may have two main causes, as outlined below.

11.2.5.1 Eutopic Ovaries with Additional or Remaining Ovarian Tissue

The following subtypes are recognized:

1. Accessory ovary
2. Supernumerary ovary

Both of these additional ovarian tissues are less than 1 cm in size and can be attached to the normal ovary (1) or situated with or without a connection to the ovary in the pelvis or retroperitoneally (2). These

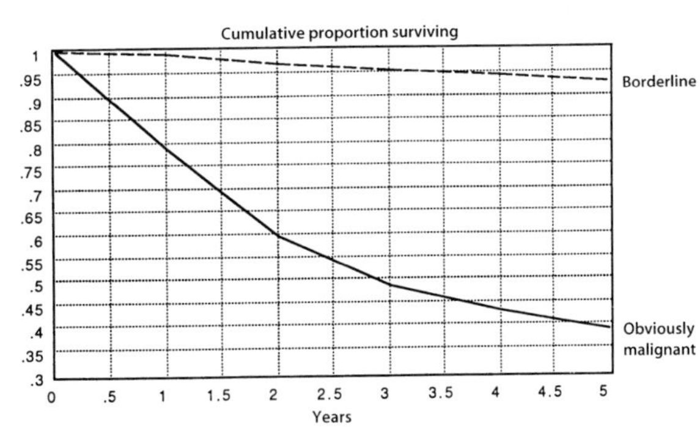

Fig. 11.3. Carcinoma of the ovary, all stages: cumulative proportion of patients surviving with borderline tumors as compared with those with obviously malignant cases. (From Annual Report, vol. 22; Pettersson 1994)

Table 11.6. Carcinoma of the ovary: stage by histopathological subtype

	Stage				Total
	I	II	III	IV	
Serous borderline	197	36	53	2	288
Row %	68.40%	12.50%	18.40%	0.69%	100.00%
Serous cystadenocarcinoma	646	398	2149	787	3980
Row %	16.23%	10.00%	53.99%	19.77%	100.00%
Mucinous borderline	142	4	16	1	163
Row %	87.12%	2.45%	9.82%	0.61%	100.00%
Mucinous cystadenocarcinoma	382	66	246	83	777
Row %	49.16%	8.49%	31.66%	10.68%	100.00%
Endometrioid borderline	11	0	5	0	16
Row %	68.75%	0.00%	31.25%	0.00%	100.00%
Endometrioid adenocarcinoma	407	193	397	159	1156
Row %	35.21%	16.70%	34.34%	13.75%	100.00%
Clear cell borderline	5	1	0	0	6
Row %	83.33%	16.67%	0.00%	0.00%	100.00%
Clear cell adenocarcinoma	184	49	88	41	362
Row %	50.83%	13.54%	24.31%	11.33%	100.00%
Undifferentiated	43	54	313	131	541
Row %	7.95%	9.98%	57.86%	24.21%	100.00%
Mixed epithelial	36	27	67	12	142
Row %	25.35%	19.01%	47.18%	8.45%	100.00%
Unclassifiable	36	8	43	45	132
Row %	27.27%	6.06%	32.58%	34.09%	100.00%
Column total	2089	836	3377	1261	7563

tissues may go unrecognized during transabdominal or transvaginal oophorectomy.

3. Ovarian remnant syndrome (ovarian implant syndrome). This syndrome is due to remaining ovarian tissue after oophorectomy which is complicated by extensive periovarian adhesions after previous inflammatory pelvic disease. The remaining ovarian tissues may cause absence of menopausal symptoms, a cystic pelvic mass, – and malignant degeneration (CLEMENT 1994a).

11.2.5.2
Lesions of the Secondary Müllerian System

1. Extraovarian serous papillary carcinomas can involve the pelvic peritoneum, the omentum, and, less commonly, the abdominal peritoneum. They resemble borderline lesions with psammoma bodies or psammo-carcinomas, when infiltrative. They have a good prognosis.
2. Another invasive type arising from the pelvic peritoneum with lesser differentiation is the so-called serous surface papillary carcinoma or serous papillary carcinoma of the peritoneum, which can involve the ovarian surface by implantation. Some of these cases may occur in patients after bilateral oophorectomy.
3. Mucinous cystadenocarcinomas of the ovarian type are rare and typically found in the retroperitoneum.
4. Endometrioid carcinoma is the most common tumor arising in patients with endometriosis (70% of cases). The second most common is clear cell carcinoma (17% of cases); other types such as serous cystadenocarcinoma, mucinous adenocarcinoma, squamous cell carcinoma, and the very malignant mesodermal mixed tumor are rare (CLEMENT 1994a; GARAM-VOELGYI et al. 1994).

In some advanced cancers, histology shows the typical serous adenocarcinoma of peritoneal tumor spread but no or minimal involvement of the peritoneal surface of the ovaries. Such cases are described as "multifocal extraovarian serous carcinoma."

11.2.6 Histological Grading

The histological grade of differentiation is the most important prognostic factor besides stage of tumor growth and residuals of epithelial cancer of the ovaries (CAREY et al. 1993).

In contrast to the former classification, which used four grades (BRODERS 1926; DECKER et al. 1975), the recent classification has been reduced to the following three grades (DAY et al. 1975; BARBER 1993):

Grade 1: well differentiated
Grade 2: moderately differentiated
Grade 3: poorly differentiated, undifferentiated

It must be taken into account that the criteria for histological grading may differ from pathologist to pathologist, as no obligatory and generally accepted rules exist. Nevertheless the three grades indicate a quite different prognosis, as shown in cases of serous cancer (Fig. 11.4). BARBER (1993) uses three categories for grading:

1. *Histological grading*, which is based on:
   a) Uniformity or lack of uniformity of the cells
   b) Whether the nucleus is regular
   c) The number and size of the nucleoli
   d) The number of mitoses per high-power field.
2. *Nuclear grade*
   Grade 1: marked and enlarged, irregular in outline with chromatin clumping and prominent nucleoli
   Grade 2: intermediate degree of differentiation
   Grade 3: similar in size and appearance to each other and to normal ovarian tissue when present.
   (It must be noted that with histological grading the better differentiated tumors are grade I and the least differentiated grade III, whereas when grading the nuclei, grade 1 is the most anaplastic and grade 3 the least anaplastic.)
3. *Stromal reactions* (according to the number of lymphocytes, plasma cells, and polymorphonuclear leukocytes present). Lymphocyte, plasma cell, and polymorphonuclear infiltration in the stroma and around small veins is graded:

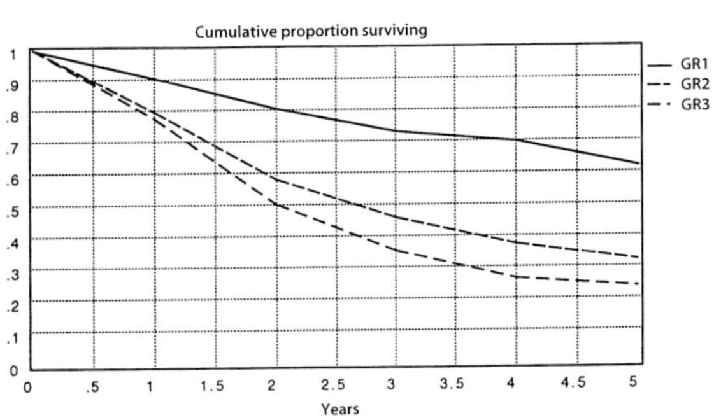

Fig. 11.4. Serous cystadenocarcinoma of the ovary (class 1c): cumulative proportion of patients surviving by degree of differentiation. (From Annual Report, vol. 22; PETTERSSON 1994)

   0: none
   1: minimal
   2: moderate
   3: marked

It would be quite understandable for a non-histopathologist that the weighting of these categories must lead to different results in grading. Nevertheless, the following important conclusions were drawn by DECKER et al. (1975):

1. All epithelial ovarian carcinomas are equally lethal when compared by stage and grade.
2. The low-grade tumors become increasingly lethal as the stage increases.
3. High-grade, low-stage tumors should be treated differently than low-grade, low-stage lesions.
4. Grading, when therapy is uniform within a stage, is of prognostic value to both the patient and the physician.

The following conclusions were drawn by BARBER (1993):

1. Low grade is associated with low stage.
2. More mucinous and endometrioid lesions than serous or solid lesions are low grade and low stage.
3. If serous and mucinous lesions are compared stage for stage and grade for grade, they are of equal lethal potential.

There were insufficient data to develop such comparisons for the endometrioid or solid lesions.

11.3 FIGO and TNM Stages in Primary Epithelial Cancer of the Ovaries

H.W. VAHRSON

The FIGO definition of the stages is most frequently used, but the TNM nomenclature of the UICC and the AICC nomenclature correspond to it.

In contrast to the clinical staging of carcinoma of the cervix and vagina, the Committee on Gynecological Oncology of FIGO recommends that the clinical staging of primary carcinoma of the ovary should be based on findings of laparoscopy or laparotomy as well as on the usual clinical examination and roentgen studies. Thus, laparotomy and resection of ovarian masses, as well as hysterectomy, form the basis for staging. Biopsies of all suspicious sites, such as the omentum, mesentery, liver, diaphragm, and pelvic and para-aortic nodes, are required. The final histological findings after surgery (and cytological findings when available) are to be considered in the staging. In order to evaluate the impact on prognosis of the different criteria for allotting a case to stage Ic or IIc, it is of value to know whether the source of malignant cells detected was peritoneal washings or ascites, and whether the rupture of the capsule was spontaneous or caused by the surgeon. Clinical studies, if carcinoma of the ovary is diagnosed, include routine radiography of the chest. Computed tomography (CT) may be helpful in both the initial staging and the follow-up of tumors.

In cases of strong adhesions or fixation of an ovarian tumor to other pelvic structures (bladder, intestine, pelvic wall, omentum) it is sometimes very difficult to decide whether the case should be allotted to stage I or stage IIb when there is unclear extension of malignant growth to these structures. Since recommendations of FIGO are absent from the volumes of the Annual Report, a more or less subjective allocation to either stage I or stage II has been practised depending on the accuracy of the operation report. For these cases KOTTMEIER (1968) suggested allocation to stage I when the fixation can be separated by hand, and to stage IIb when it can only be separated by sharp preparation. It is of importance for the radiotherapist that this uncertainty in the allocation of cases can influence the reported results in stages I and II, because strong adhesions have a worse prognosis. In a recent study on prognostic factors in stage I ovarian cancer, DEMBO et al. (1990) found grading to be the most powerful predictor of relapse, followed by dense adherence, which resulted in outcomes equivalent to stage II, and large-volume ascites. Beyond these three factors no other factors analyzed were predictive. These findings underline the unfavorable prognosis of adherence. Since this study all early ovarian cancers with dense adherence should be allotted to stage II (preferably IIb) when the dense adhesions can only be dissected by knife. HOSKINS et al. (1995) practised this upstaging in their study.

Table 11.7. Definitions of the stages in primary carcinoma of the ovary (correspondence of TNM categories and FIGO stages)

TNM category	FIGO stage	
T1	Stage I	Growth limited to the ovaries.
T1a	Stage Ia	Growth limited to one ovary; no ascites. No tumor on the external surface, capsule intact.
T1b	Stage Ib	Growth limited to both ovaries; no ascites. No tumor on the external surfaces, capsules intact.
T1c	Stage Ic[a]	Tumor either stage Ia or Ib, but with tumor on surface of one or both ovaries or with capsule ruptured or with ascites present containing malignant cells or with positive peritoneal washings.
T2	Stage II	Growth involving one or both ovaries with pelvic extension.
T2a	Stage IIa	Extension and/or metastases to the uterus and/or tubes.
T2b	Stage IIb	Extension to other pelvic tissues.
T2c	Stage IIc[a]	Tumor either stage IIa or IIb but with tumor on surface of one or both ovaries or with capsule ruptured or with ascites present containing malignant cells or with positive peritoneal washings.
T3	Stage III	Tumor involving one or both ovaries with peritoneal implants outside the pelvis and/or positive retroperitoneal or inguinal nodes. Superficial liver metastasis equals stage III. Tumor is limited to the true pelvis but with histologically proven malignant extension to small bowel or omentum.
T3a	Stage IIIa	Tumor grossly limited to the true pelvis with negative nodes but with histologically confirmed microscopic seeding of abdominal peritoneal surfaces.
T3b	Stage IIIb	Tumor involving one or both ovaries with histologically confirmed implants of abdominal peritoneal surfaces, none exceeding 2 cm in diameter. Nodes are negative.
T3c/N1	Stage IIIc	Abdominal implants greater than 2 cm in diameter and/or positive retroperitoneal or inguinal nodes.
M1	Stage IV	Growth involving one or both ovaries with distant metastases. If pleural effusion is present there must be positive cytology to allot a case to stage IV. Parenchymal liver metastasis equals stage IV.

[a] In order to evaluate the impact on prognosis of the different criteria for allotting a case to stage Ic or IIc, it is of value to know whether the source of malignant cells detected was peritoneal washings or ascites, and whether rupture of the capsule was spontaneous or caused by the surgeon.

NX	Regional lymph nodes cannot be assessed
N0	No regional lymph node metastasis
N1	Regional lymph node metastasis

Distant metastasis (M)

TNM	FIGO	Definition
MX		Presence of distant metastasis cannot be assessed
M0		No distant metastasis
M1	IV	Distant metastasis (excludes peritoneal metastasis)

Stage grouping	T	N	M
IA	T1a	N0	M0
IB	T1b	N0	M0
Ic	T1c	N0	M0
IIA	T2a	N0	M0
IIB	T2b	N0	M0
IIC	T2c	N0	M0
IIIA	T3a	N0	M0
IIIB	T3b	N0	M0
IIIC	T3c	N0	M0
	Any T	N1	M0
IV	Any T	Any N	M1

Problems of inadequate staging may exist in many radiation centers where primary postoperative treatment is carried out following surgery at other institutions, but only some authors are aware of this problem (Dembo 1985; Lindner et al. 1990).

The FIGO classification from the Annual Report volume 21 (Pettersson 1991) and the corresponding TNM categories are shown in Table 11.7.

11.4 Growth Pattern

G. Crombach and M.W. Beckmann

11.4.1 Routes of Tumor Spread

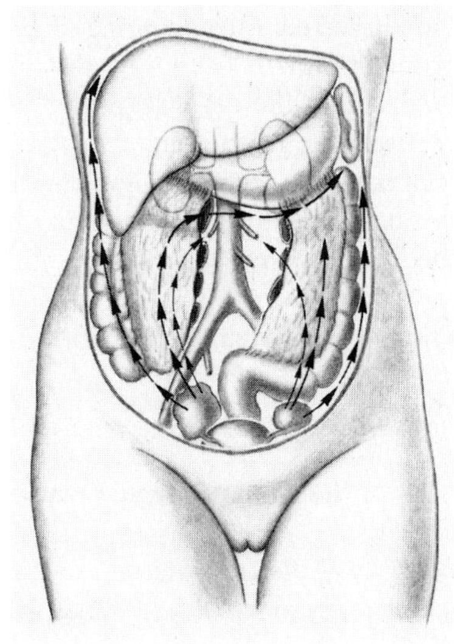

Fig. 11.5. Intra- and retroperitoneal spread of ovarian cancer. (From Sevin 1988)

The spread of ovarian cancer is more dependent on the biological characteristics of the tumor (grade, ploidy, invasiveness) than on its size. Small undifferentiated cancers usually give rise to more extensive spread than do large circumscribed tumors.

Even during the early development of ovarian cancer, malignant cells may become detached by exfoliation from superficial papillary tumor formations, or by penetration of the intact capsule of a cyst containing the primary tumor. The detached tumor cells collect in the pouch of Douglas, involving the parietal as well as the visceral peritoneum of the pelvis. Intraperitoneal spread is favored by intestinal peristalsis and the negative hydrostatic pressure below the diaphragm which is enhanced by inspiration. Exfoliated tumor cells follow the intra-abdominal fluid stream passing the paracolic gutters and implant on the parietal (diaphragm) and visceral peritoneum (liver surface, small and large bowel, mesentery, greater omentum) of the abdomen (Fig. 11.5). The tendency of tumor spread to occur into the right lobe of the liver and to the undersurface of the right hemidiaphragm is due to the upwards directed peristalsis of the ascending colon and to the position of the small and large intestine mesentery (Averette et al. 1983; Buchsbaum et al. 1989; Hoskins 1989; Pickel et al. 1989; Sevin 1989). Cancer cells may obstruct the penetrating lymphatic channels of the diaphragm. This obstruction is probably the main reason not only for the production of ascites but also for the long-term limitation of tumor spread to the peritoneal cavity (Pickel 1993). Intra-abdominal spread leads to miliary involvement of the peritoneum, or to larger tumor masses displacing, fixing, compressing, and/or obstructing the intestines, especially the large bowel. Rarely, a tumor may infiltrate the sigmoid colon, rectum, and vagina.

Implantation may not be the only way in which ovarian cancer affects the peritoneum. Tumors can arise multifocally, leading to miliary occurrence as peritoneal carcinomatosis. These types of cancer originate from embryonal coelomic epithelium which persists in certain peritoneal areas and is transformed into the müllerian duct epithelium with malignant determination (Pickel et al. 1989). Primary ovarian cancers may also induce such a mechanism (August et al. 1985).

In recent years lymphatic spread has been established as another essential mode of tumor dissemination. The lymphatic capillaries of the ovarian parenchyma converge upon the hilus to form the subovarian lymphatic plexus. The lymphatic spread starts from this plexus and principally follows two different routes (Barber 1989):

1. Six to eight lymphatic vessels accompany the ovarian blood vessels up to the para-aortic nodes between the bifurcation of the aorta and the renal arteries.
2. The plexus also drains via the broad ligament towards the hypogastric and the external iliac lymph nodes.

Another route which is clinically less important follows the round ligament to the inguinal nodes. The different groups of pelvic and para-aortic nodes are closely interconnected, thus enabling ante- and retrograde dissemination.

Tumor cells from the diaphragmatic lymph vessels may penetrate into the pleural cavity, causing pleural carcinomatosis. The lymphatic fluid from the para-aortic nodes, diaphragm, and pleura is drained via the mediastinal, supraclavicular, and scalene nodes into the cisterna chyli of the thoracic duct, a portal leading to the systemic circulation.

11.4.2 Involvement of the Contralateral Ovary

The involvement of the contralateral ovary may develop synchronously or metachronously. In general, the rate of bilaterality for stage I ovarian cancer is half that for stage III (e.g., 67% vs 33% in serous carcinomas). The more frequent bilaterality associated with higher stage of disease reflects metastatic spread by implantation rather than independent primary tumor formation in the two ovaries (OZOLS et al. 1992; WILLIAMS et al. 1992). Whereas epithelial ovarian cancer is often bilateral (Table 11.8), most malignant germ cell and stromal tumors are unilateral (>95%); dysgerminoma (10%–20% bilaterality) and the rare gonadoblastoma being the only exceptions (WILLIAMS et al. 1992; MICHAEL and ROTH 1993).

11.4.3 Intraperitoneal Tumor Spread

Ovarian cancer is a disease of the peritoneal surface. In an autopsy study peritoneal tumor deposits were found in 83% of cases. The small and large intestines were affected in 44% and 50% of patients (ROSE et al. 1989). Even in early ovarian cancer (apparently stage I) subclinical metastases were found at the diaphragm (11%) and in the omentum (3%). In 31% of cases free-floating tumor cells could be detected after peritoneal washing (PIVER 1983). Patients undergoing surgery for stage III/IV cancer had a 70% rate of carcinomatosis peritonei. While isolated omental metastases were found more often in stage III (46% vs 9%), superficial liver metastases predominated in stage IV (16% vs 55%). Obviously, stage IV cancer reflects the biological characteristics of the tumor rather than progression of stage III disease (PICKEL et al. 1989).

Intestinal metastases have been found in 26%–39% of all surgically treated ovarian cancer patients. Clinically three types of intestinal metastases may be distinguished (WU et al. 1989). The first type is characterized by multiple, small and superficial nodules (<2 cm) resulting from the implantation of cancer cells in the peritoneal cavity (81% of small bowel metastases). The second type is rare (less than 10% of all intestinal metastases) and shows extremely extensive infiltration of the intestine and mesentery resulting in a stiff, rigid intestinal tract and a shortened mesentery. The third type is characterized by the local involvement of an extended area (tumor diameter >2 cm) of the intestinal wall, especially the large bowel. The rectosigmoid (95%) and the transverse colon (21%) are the most frequently affected sites.

Table 11.8. Frequency of bilateral involvement of the ovaries in epithelial ovarian cancer. (OZOLS et al. 1992; WHEELER 1993)

Histological type	LMP tumor	Carcinoma
Serous	25%–35%	35%–70%
Mucinous	5%–10%	5%–15%
Endometrioid	5%–10%	20%–35%
Clear cell	?	10%–20%
Brenner tumor	?	5%–10%
Undifferentiated	ND	40%–50%

LMP, low malignant potential; ND, not defined as LMP tumor.

11.4.4 Lymphatic Dissemination

The lymphatic spread is usually confined to the pelvic and para-aortic nodes. BERGMAN (1966) and ROSE et al. (1989) found positive pelvic and para-aortic nodes in 48%–80% and 58%–78% of autopsy cases, respectively. The overall incidence of lymph node involvement in surgically treated patients is dependent on the site and extent of lymphadenectomy, increasing to up to 60% after radical procedures (WU et al. 1989a,b; BURGHARDT et al. 1991). The pelvic nodes appear to be involved slightly more often (47%–58%) than the aortic ones (38%–51%). Among the pelvic nodes, most metastases are seen in the external and common iliac nodes. In most patients just one or two node groups are involved, these groups usually containing no more than one to three positive nodes (PICKEL et al. 1989; BURGHARDT et al. 1991). The frequency of

Table 11.9. Incidence of lymph node metastases after radical pelvic and para-aortic lymphadenectomy (LA) related to intraperitoneal tumor stage of ovarian carcinoma. (Wu et al. 1989b: LA up to a. mesenterica inferior; Burghardt et al. 1991; LA up to v. renalis)

Tumor stage (FIGO)	Wu et al. (1989b)	Burghardt et al. (1991)
I	1/7 (14%)	9/37 (24%)
II	3/8 (37%)	7/14 (50%)
III	38/59 (64%)	84/114 (74%)
IV	3/3 (100%)	11/15 (78%)
Total	45/77 (58%)	111/180 (62%)

node involvement increases with intraperitoneal tumor extent (Table 11.9).

Systematic retroperitoneal lymphadenectomy showed that the pelvic and para-aortic nodes were both positive in 28%–44% and simultaneously negative in 35%–44% of patients. Involvement of either the pelvic or the aortic nodes alone was found in 12%–19% and 9%–10%, respectively (Wu et al. 1989a,b; Burghardt et al. 1991). According to Burghardt et al. (1991) the involvement of the aortic nodes alone was found only in stages II and III. These data demonstrate that ovarian cancer may spread directly to either the pelvic or the para-aortic nodes, or to both.

A study in a limited number of patients ($n = 37$) showed that the scalene lymph nodes are involved only in advanced ovarian cancer. Positive nodes were found in 12% and 57% of stage III and IV patients, but not in women having stage I/II disease (Petru et al. 1991).

Hematogenous spread is uncommon in ovarian carcinoma. Metastases in distant organs are more likely to be attributable to local lymphatic and/or capillary invasion by the tumor. According to the results of an autopsy study, liver (48%), lung (34%), and pleura (28%) are the most frequently involved organs (Rose et al. 1989).

11.5 Molecular Prognostic Factors in Ovarian Cancer

M.W. Beckmann and D. Niederacher

Specific pathological findings and distinct genetic hereditary or somatic alterations seem to be major factors somehow linked with the risk of developing ovarian neoplasms and, at a later stage, spread of the disease. Over recent years the model of multistep carcinogenesis of cancer, combining specific pathological findings and distinct genetic alterations, has become a central paradigm of cancer biology (Busch 1990; Hartwell and Kastan 1994; Ford and Easton 1995). As long ago as 1855 Virchow alluded indirectly to molecular genetics when he noted from cell theory not only "*Omnis cellula e cellula*" – that all cells come from cells –, but also "*Omnis cellulae e cellula ejusdem generis*" – that all cells come from the cells of the same type. In the case of cancer, a single cell could be the genesis of the whole malignant process. Cancer cells differ from normal cells in many important characteristics, including loss of differentiation, uncontrolled growth, immortalization, loss of contact inhibition, increased invasive capacity, ability to evade the host immune surveillance processes and the apoptotic signal restraints, and induction of neo-angiogenesis (Berchuck et al. 1993; Baker 1994). As the individual cell acquires these necessary cellular functions or loses these inhibitory signals, it will eventually be the origin of a monoclonal malignant focus. Although clonality does not equate with malignancy, it is interesting to note on the basis of loss of heterozygosity studies that some ovarian cancers show clonality (Sato et al. 1991; Gallion et al. 1996). Advanced tumors still show heterogeneity at the molecular level, one of the most notable features of cancer (Sato et al. 1991; Fox 1993; Muto et al. 1995). Molecular heterogeneity within different parts of a tumor reflects concomitant or successive development of various foci and indicates that malignant transformation is a dynamic process with sequential multistep evolution (Beckmann et al. 1993; Fox 1993; Muto et al. 1995; Scully 1995).

Detailed pathological knowledge of the development of adenomas and carcinomas in the context of colorectal carcinogenesis has led to various investigations into the genetic alterations occurring during this process. While longitudinal observation of these changes is not practicable, cross-sectional analyses, involving the careful pathological examination of large numbers of adenomas and carcinomas for their changes, have pointed to the most common sequence of genetic events and their timing. Fearon and Vogelstein (1990) detected (1) APC mutation or loss in normal mucosa and hyperproliferative epithelium, (2) KRAS mutation in adenoma, (3) DCC loss in adenoma increasing in size and with dysplasia, and finally (4) TP53 loss in invasive and metastatic cancer. These genetic alterations encompass two different classes of genes: those activating cell proliferation (oncogenes), and those inhibiting cellular functions (tumor suppressor genes). For the first time the interdependence between pathology and genetics of a specific cancer type could be demonstrated, but to date the transfer of these key results to other common carcinomas has not been straightforward. In contrast to the case with colorectal cancer, pathological findings in ovarian cancer are very variable, indicating the importance of considering molecular abnormalities in the context of tumor pathology (Fox 1993; Baker 1994; Scully 1995).

Biochemical, cytogenetic, and molecular genetic analysis of ovarian cancer samples suggest that the development of human ovarian cancer is based (1) on the alteration of physiological regulatory cellular pathways (transmembrane or intracellular) (CA-125, ER/PgR) and (2) on the accumulation of various genetic alterations (Masood et al. 1989; Berns et al. 1992; Kenemans et al. 1994; Schutter et al. 1994; Ford and Easton 1995; Dietl 1996). Some of the factors analyzed in the context of multistep carcinogenesis of ovarian cancer have been discussed both as prognostic and as predictive factors.

Glycoproteins and glycolipids are components of normal cell membranes and may be expressed or released during cell proliferation. In the case of malignant growth patterns they increase in concentration in the circulation. Various markers have been studied, including the carcinoembryonic antigen (CEA), lipid-associated sialic acid (LASA), alphafetoprotein (AFP), human chorionic gonadotropin (hCG), placental alkaline phosphatase (PLAP), cancer antigens (CA) 125, 19-9, 72, 15-3, and CYFRA 21-1, and cancer-associated serum antigen (CASA) (Olt et al. 1990; Schutter et al. 1994; Kenemans et al. 1994; Jacobs 1994; Dietl 1996).

In 1981/83, Bast et al. introduced CA-125 in the evaluation of therapeutic effect and course in serous and other histological types of ovarian cancer. The use of CA-125 is supported by the following considerations:

1. Elevated serum levels (>65 U/ml) before treatment enable the control of the effectiveness of any treatment modality.
2. Four weeks after primary surgery the serum level of CA-125 is an indicator for residual disease. Immediately after surgery the serum level may be disturbed by the extent of the surgical trauma (Avall-Lundquist et al. 1992; Mogensen et al. 1993).
3. The half-life of CA-125 in human serum is 4.8 days. Thus changes in serum levels correlate with the tumor mass, indicating the effectiveness of treatment (Canney et al. 1984; Crombach and Würz 1985).
4. As long as the serum level of CA-125 is elevated, no clinically complete remission has been achieved (even though other clinical parameters may suggest clinical remission).

To quantify CA-125 serum levels as an indicator of the final outcome of treatment, Münstedt and Vahrson (1993) introduced the CA-125 ratio:

$$\text{CA-125 ratio} = \frac{\text{CA-125 after therapy}}{\text{CA-125 before therapy}}.$$

Ratios lower than 1 indicate tumor regression, ratios above 1 indicate tumor progression, and ratios equal to 1 indicate stability of disease (no change). In a retrospective analysis of 37 patients with stage III ovarian cancer who received sandwich radio-chemotherapy, CA-125 levels were documented at 4-week intervals before each treatment step. Evaluation of the CA-125 ratios showed that 22/37 patients (60%) were sensitive to both radiotherapy and chemotherapy, 6/37 (16%) were sensitive to radiotherapy, 6/37 (16%) were sensitive to chemotherapy, and 3/37 (8%) were resistant to both treatment modalities (Vahrson et al. 1993; Münstedt and Vahrson 1995). For practical use Table 11.10 may assist in the calculation of the expected number of therapy steps (i.e., cycles of chemotherapy or radiotherapy) required to approach normal CA-125 levels starting from levels at 500, 1000, 2000, and 3000 U/ml with CA-125 ratios 0.1, 0.5, and 0.7. Looking at the extremes it can be easily recognized that a CA-125 ratio of 0.1 leads to a normal level within two steps (cycles), independent of the level at the start of therapy, whereas a high level, such as 3000 U/ml, before treatment and a CA-125 ratio of 0.7 would require 13 steps for a normal level to be reached. In fact, 13 steps would be rather unrealistic, as resistance will be acquired after only a few steps (cycles).

Our clinical experience during the past decade has shown that a CA-125 ratio >0.7 indicates insufficient sensitivity, and that first-line treatment must be replaced by a non-cross-resistant second-line treatment. Ratios ≤0.5 indicate a good to moderate sensitivity, and the treatment should be continued. It must be noted that a ratio of ≤0.5 represents the

Table 11.10. Number of treatment steps required for a normal CA-125 level (<35 U/ml) to be approached, according to the level at start of treatment and the CA-125 ratio. (Vahrson and Münstedt 1995)

CA-125 ratio	0.1				0.5				0.7			
Level at start (U/ml)	500	1000	2000	3000	500	1000	2000	3000	500	1000	2000	3000
1st treatment step	50	100	200	300	250	500	1000	1500	350	700	1400	2100
2nd treatment step	5	10	20	30	125	250	500	750	245	490	980	1470
3rd treatment step					63	125	250	375	172	343	686	1029
4th treatment step					32	63	125	188	120	240	480	720
5th treatment step						32	63	94	84	168	336	504
6th treatment step							32	47	59	118	235	353
7th treatment step								24	41	82	165	247
8th treatment step									29	57	115	173
9th treatment step										40	80	121
10th treatment step										28	56	85
11th treatment step											39	59
12th treatment step											7	42
13th treatment step												29

minimal requirement for a possible successful outcome of treatment. The prognostic significance of stratification to ratio <1 or >1 can be shown in a first series of 14 patients with advanced ovarian cancer (Fig. 11.6) who received taxol monotherapy as second-line treatment (Vahrson HW, Münstedt K, Kirsch K, unpublished work, 1996). A ratio of about 0.1 indicates excellent sensitivity. The first-line treatment should be continued for some cycles after reaching normal levels, resulting in a considerable number of clinically and histopathologically complete remissions. Thus Table 11.10 may be of value in recognizing a successful treatment regimen that should be continued or an unfavorable treatment regimen requiring second-line treatment before complete resistance becomes obvious.

Steroid hormone receptors are expressed in the majority of ovarian cancers (Masood et al. 1989; Kommoss et al. 1991; Berns et al. 1992), but the prognostic or therapeutic value of their determination has not been established.

Ovarian cancers show a high prevalence of aneuploidy. The prognostic value of the measurement of DNA ploidy has been analyzed in retrospective and prospective studies. Tumor DNA aneuploidy is to some extent correlated with a higher S-phase fraction (SPF), high FIGO stage, high tumor bulk, presence of residual tumor, low PgR content, and high histological grade. Data on the prognostic value of DNA ploidy or SPF in multivariate analysis are nevertheless contradictory (Van Dam et al. 1992; Dietl 1996).

Molecular abnormalities of ovarian cancer may be classified into two types: gain-of-function genetic events that activate proto-oncogenes by DNA mutations, rearrangements, or amplifications, and loss-of-function defects reflecting putative tumor suppressor genes that have been inactivated by DNA mutation and unmasked by deletion or allelic loss (Beckmann et al. 1993; Ford and Easton 1995; Dietl 1996). Tumor suppressor genes were first identified as the target of inactivating mutations in inherited cancer, while mutations of the dominantly acting oncogenes have been associated with somatic alterations in the developing tumor. In ovarian tumors the chromosomal sites of oncogenes are mainly marked by regions of DNA amplification. Usually the whole chromosome or a chromosomal arm is involved and amplified as a contiguous unit. In the case of smaller regions, megabases of DNA are amplified. In ovarian cancer oncogene amplification is

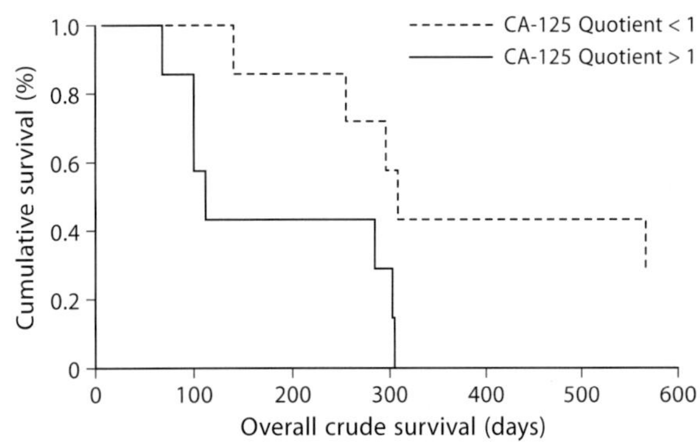

Fig. 11.6. Response to single-agent taxol as second-line chemotherapy after cisplatin, epirubicin, and cyclophosphamide pretreatment in 14 patients with recurrences of advanced ovarian cancer, stratified according to whether the CA-125 ratio was more than or less than 1 (Kaplan-Meier functional survival). (From Vahrson HW, Münstedt K, and Kirsch K, unpublished work, 1996)

the common mechanism. Amplification of various oncogenes, i.e., c-*mos*, c-*fms*, c-*myb*, c-*erb*B-2, *int*-2, and c-*myc*, and chromosomal regions, i.e., 1p31, 1q21–24, 5p13–14, and 11p12–14 (Zheng et al. 1991; Slamon et al. 1989; Sasano et al. 1990; Berchuck et al. 1990; Barletta et al. 1992; Berns et al. 1992; Bast et al. 1993; Hruza et al. 1993; Fischer et al. 1994; Beckmann et al. 1996) has been described, but only a few oncogenes or overexpression of oncoproteins have been evaluated with regard to their prognostic value: the epidermal growth factor receptor (EGFR), c-*erb*B-2, and c-*myc* (Bauknecht et al. 1988; Slamon et al. 1989; Berchuck et al. 1990, 1991; Berns et al. 1992; Hruza et al. 1993; Fischer et al. 1994; Rubin et al. 1993; Beckmann et al. 1996). In 1971 Knudson proposed the two-hit theory about inactivation of a tumor suppressor gene. Loss of normal tumor suppressor protein function can occur through sequential gene mutation events (somatic alteration) or through a single mutational event of a remaining normal copy, when a germline mutation is present. In the case of inherited cancer this second event uncovers the constitutional recessive mutation. The second event is usually chromosome loss, mitotic recombination, or partial chromosome deletion (LOH) (Beckmann et al. 1993; Baker 1994). The consistently mutated gene in ovarian cancer is the tumor suppressor gene p53 (Marks et al. 1991; Berchuck et al. 1994), detected via either direct sequencing or altered protein analysis. An incidence of LOH – the second hit of gene inactivation – of less than 10% may be interpreted as unimportant for ovarian tumor development, resulting merely from genetic instability associated with tumor development and progression. This has to be balanced, however, against the heterogeneity in nuclear pleomorphism seen in different tumors and the variable degree of differentiation (Van Dam et al. 1992; Berchuck et al. 1993; Bast et al. 1993). Allelic loss of chromosome regions 1, 3, 6, 11, and 17, at which potential tumor suppressor genes (Rb, HIC, E-cadherin) are located (Sato et al. 1991; Jacobs et al. 1993; Berchuck et al. 1993; Baker 1994), has been described, but in no instance was analyzed for prognostic value. In summary, multivariant analyses have not proven various molecular genetic alterations to be of greater prognostic value in sporadic ovarian cancer than established prognostic factors, e.g., residual disease. Consequently different oncogenes and tumor suppressor genes, as well as their specific analytical methods, are still under intensive investigation.

11.6 General Management of Primary Epithelial Cancers and Borderline Malignancies

H.W. Vahrson

11.6.1 Malignant Invasive Tumors

After thorough clinical examination and appropriate imaging procedures, surgical intervention is the first treatment step for intraoperative staging, complete removal or debulking of tumor, and histopathological classification. In primary ovarian cancers the most important prognostic factors – stage, histological grade and type, and tumor residuals – are decisive for the choice of postoperative treatment.

Only stage I, grade I cases (low risk) need no further treatment. Today, chemotherapy is the predominant treatment in intermediate and high-risk cases, but radiotherapy still has a place in postoperative treatment. Different volumes of percutaneous irradiation (pelvic, whole abdominal, para-aortic fields) and intraperitoneal radionuclides may be selected. Irradiation is in competition with chemotherapy (preferably platinum-containing combinations and/or taxotere/taxol) postoperatively and in the treatment of progression or recurrence. Both irradiation and chemotherapy can be applied as a single treatment modality or in combination. In advanced stages after successful chemotherapy, surgical second-look interventions are required. Depending on the intraoperative findings and histopathological evaluation of tumor residuals, irradiation can be applied as consolidation or salvage therapy as an alternative to second- or third-line chemotherapy.

Combined treatment modalities integrating radiotherapy into the first cycles of chemotherapy in patients with intermediate and high-risk tumors have proved effective in Giessen.

Until now hormonal therapy has been of minor importance in primary treatment but can be useful in the palliative treatment of progressive or recurrent cancer. Control of tumor markers in serum, especially CA-125 in cases of serous ovarian cancer, is a sensitive method for the evaluation of treatment and the early diagnosis of cancer recurrence.

11.6.2
Tumors of Low Malignant Potential

The histological diagnosis of tumors of low malignant potential is still controversial. Most cases have a very good prognosis and need no postoperative treatment. Therefore besides stage, grade, and histological typing, flow cytometric examination of the nuclear DNA content is required to identify the aneuploid cases which need further treatment. These cases may undergo irradiation (preferably intraperitoneal radionuclide instillation) and/or chemotherapy.

11.7
Surgery for Ovarian Cancer

U. Nitz and H.G. Bender

11.7.1
The Role of Surgery in Different Stages of Ovarian Cancer

In ovarian cancer, surgery is usually accepted as the first-line treatment. The purpose of the initial surgical procedure is to define the extent of disease, to establish the histology of the tumor, and to reduce tumor bulk if present.

The extent of surgery depends on the stage of disease. Stage I ovarian cancer is generally cured by bilateral salpingo-oophorectomy; additional surgery is only done to exclude tumor spread (with regard to staging laparotomy, see Sect. 11.7.3). In advanced ovarian cancer additional surgery must be performed for therapeutic reasons (debulking). Griffiths (1975) was the first to demonstrate the impact of optimal surgery on survival. In stage IV ovarian cancer, surgery is generally palliative.

In recurrent or persistent disease the role of secondary surgical interventions (second-look laparotomy, secondary cytoreduction) has to be defined individually. Outside of clinical trials, second-look laparotomy is recommended only if therapeutic benefits will result. In recurrent or persistent disease, considerable benefit from secondary cytoreduction is demonstrable only in cases with optimal debulking. Results in patients with macroscopic tumor after repeat laparotomy are disappointing.

11.7.2
Preoperative Management

Advanced ovarian cancer demands a multidisciplinary surgical approach. For optimal preoperative planning, information on bowel and urinary tract involvement is required. Table 11.11 gives an overview of routine preoperative tests.

In contrast to clinical examination, ultrasonography displays a high sensitivity in the detection of small pelvic masses. Nevertheless, findings are nonspecific. Only unilocular simple cysts up to 5 cm are generally benign (Goldstein et al. 1989). Other sonographic criteria, such as irregular borders, the presence or absence of solid formations, septations, etc., do not allow precise evaluation of lesion status though usual patterns for many ovarian neoplasms do exist. For example, serous cystadenocarcinoma typically shows solid and cystic structures with multiple septa and papillary projections. By contrast the association of a pelvic mass with extraovarian sonographic findings such as ascites and/or peritoneal tumor is highly predictive for ovarian carcinoma (Conte et al. 1990). CT scans and magnetic resonance imaging generally do not provide additional information.

Intravenous pyelography and cystoscopy are useful to detect retroperitoneal disease with displacement of the ureters and/or bladder involvement (Buchsbaum et al. 1989).

Procto(sigmoido)scopy and barium enema provide additional information on lower gastrointestinal tract involvement or even primary colorectal carcinoma. These tests are recommended by most authors (Curtin 1993). Upper gastrointestinal series are usually demanded in symptomatic cases only. As preoperative examinations cannot exclude bowel involvement with certainty, preoperative bowel preparation (laxatives, antibiotics) is necessary.

Table 11.11. Routine preoperative studies in cases of suspected ovarian cancer

Clinical examination, baseline preoperative studies + CA-125
Vaginal ultrasonography
Abdominal ultrasonography (CT scan?)
Intravenous pyelography
Cysto/procto(sigmoido)scopy
(Barium enema)
Chest x-ray

Liver ultrasonography and chest x-ray are obligatory to exclude stage IV disease.

11.7.3
Surgery for Early Ovarian Cancer: Operative Staging

In early ovarian cancer, staging laparotomy should follow the steps cited in Table 11.12. Surgical exploration begins with a median vertical laparotomy from the symphysis up to the umbilicus. If preoperative diagnosis is confirmed, the incision is extended as far as necessary to allow proper exploration of the upper abdomen and the subdiaphragmatic spaces. Transverse abdominal sections normally do not meet these needs. Unfortunately, detection of early ovarian cancer will often be an unexpected finding when transverse laparotomy or laparoscopy is carried out for other reasons. The data from McGowan et al. (1985) show that only 75% of patients referred with supposedly early disease had an incision that allowed full exploration of the abdominal cavity. At proper restaging about one-third of these patients had to be upstaged.

If ascites is present the volume is estimated and a sample is taken for cytological examination. In the absence of ascites, peritoneal smears or biopsies from the pouch of Douglas, the paracolic gutters, and the subdiaphragmatic regions are taken before any further manipulation of the abdominal organs. The next step is the inspection of the pelvic cavity itself. Tumor volume, integrity of the ovarian capsule, and adhesions to or invasion of the surrounding structures should be recorded because they are of prognostic significance. The abdomen is then thoroughly explored in order to detect any tumor metastasis outside the pelvis (stage III ovarian cancer). For this purpose the presence or absence of tumor on the peritoneal surfaces, the diaphragm, the liver, the spleen, the gallbladder, and the large and small bowel must be carefully documented. The same should be done for the omentum majus and minus and the retroperitoneal structures. If suspicious lesions are present, they should be excised and sent for frozen section. When there is no apparent tumor spread to the abdominal cavity, the diagnosis is confirmed by frozen section of the adnexal mass from adnectomy samples.

Table 11.12. Staging laparotomy in early ovarian cancer

Median vertical laparotomy
Cytology from ascites or peritoneal washings from the pouch of Douglas, the paracolic gutters, and the subdiaphragmatic spaces
Biopsies from the bladder, pouch of Douglas, and subdiaphragmatic and paracolic peritoneum
Bilateral salpingo-oophorectomy + hysterectomy
Omentectomy
Pelvic (para-aortic) lymphadenectomy

Frozen section in ovarian cancer may give misleading results; in particular, the differentiation of low-grade tumors and tumors of low malignant potential is difficult. As the staging procedure remains the same in both cases, the course of the operation is not altered. The same is not true when a fertility-conserving operation is intended and when frozen section cannot correctly identify the histological type (adenocarcinoma, germ cell, or stromal cell tumor). In this setting further surgery must be postponed until final histological evaluation is available (see Sect. 11.7.4.2).

In other cases frozen section may not be able to identify the origin of the tumor. Tumors most often associated with metastasis to the ovary are stomach, colon, breast, and endometrial cancers. With the exception of breast cancers all these tumors may clinically resemble advanced ovarian cancer.

If the diagnosis of ovarian cancer is confirmed by frozen section, bilateral salpingo-oophorectomy and hysterectomy follow. In cases with no macroscopically suspicious lesions in the upper abdominal cavity, random samples from the bladder, the pouch of Douglas, the mesentery, the bowel, and the paracolic and subdiaphragmatic peritoneum are removed and infracolic omentectomy is performed routinely to exclude stage III disease.

For the same reason pelvic and para-aortic lymphadenectomy is recommended by most authors. The radicality of this procedure is the subject of much controversy and will be discussed separately.

11.7.4
Controversies in Surgery for Early Ovarian Cancer

11.7.4.1
Lymphadenectomy in Early Ovarian Cancer

In 1985, FIGO recommended evaluation of retroperitoneal lymph nodes in the staging of ovarian cancer. According to current FIGO criteria, any cancer with retroperitoneal lymph node involvement is classified as stage III disease.

The frequency of pelvic and para-aortic lymph node involvement in early disease stages, as described in the literature, varies over a broad range, probably due to varying radicality of surgical management. In small series, lymph node involvement has been reported to be associated with reduced overall survival (KNAPP and FRIEDMANN 1974; LANZA et al. 1988).

Data from different studies (KNAPP and FRIEDMANN 1974; DI RE et al. 1990; CHEN and LEE 1983; AVERETTE et al. 1983; PICKEL et al. 1989; BUCHSBAUM et al. 1989) are summarized in Table 11.13. Omission of lymphadenectomy would have caused a considerable (4%–23%) incidence of misstaging in these patients. On the other hand, radical pelvic and para-aortic lymphadenectomy is associated with considerable morbidity. PETRU et al. (1994) reported on 40 patients who underwent total abdominal hysterectomy, bilateral salpingo-oophorectomy, omentectomy, and systematic radical lymphadenectomy. Resection of the inferior mesenteric artery occurred in 17.5%, bleeding from the renal vein in 2.5%, febrile morbidity in 12.5%, deep venous thrombosis in 2.5%, lymphoceles in 33%, and lymphedema in 5%. No significant difference in recurrence rates in the two surgical groups (with and without lymphadenectomy) was reported (PETRU et al. 1994). Most authors therefore do not question the value of lymphadenectomy itself; rather the major point of discussion is the radicality of the procedure.

With the intent of individualizing the extent of lymphadenectomy, different aspects of lymphatic spread in early ovarian cancer have been studied. Some investigators (PIVER et al. 1978) have described lymph node involvement in early ovarian cancer predominantly in undifferentiated, stage Ic serous cystadenocarcinoma. By contrast others have demonstrated that the morphological patterns correlating with lymph node involvement are by no means uniform (PETRU et al. 1994). Both PETRU et al. and WU et al. (1986) described cases of contralateral lymph node involvement in stage Ia ovarian cancer. If only lymph nodes suspicious at intraoperative palpation are resected (sampling), nodal status is misdiagnosed in 33%–60% (PETRU et al. 1994).

Table 11.13. Frequency of lymph node involvement in early-stage ovarian cancer

Author	Stage I	Stage II
Knapp	5/26 (19%)	–
Di Re	16/134 (12%)	–
Chen	2/11 (18%)	2/10 (20%)
Averette	1/11 (9%)	5/17 (29%)
Pickel	7/28 (23%)	4/13 (31%)
Buchsbaum	4/95 (4%)	8/41 (19.5%)
Total	35/305 (11.5%)	19/81 (23.4%)

In conclusion, therefore, neither extirpation of clinically suspicious lymph nodes nor ipsilateral lymphadenectomy nor lymphadenectomy in specific histologically defined subgroups guarantees exact staging. Bilateral pelvic lymphadenectomy and para-aortic lymphadenectomy of variable radicality are recommended. In fact the impact of even radical lymphadenectomy on survival remains to be defined. The morbidity of "radical" lymphadenectomy may outweigh the potential benefit for the individual patient.

11.7.4.2 Fertility-Conserving Surgery for Early Ovarian Cancer

Conservative surgery (generally unilateral salpingo-oophorectomy) may be demanded by young women, who strongly wish to preserve fertility. As MUNELL (1969) showed in a review of literature, most authors report small nonrandomized series and/or their personal clinical judgement. His own series of 46 conservatively treated patients and 144 patients treated with bilateral salpingo-oophorectomy and hysterectomy without lymphadenectomy and omentectomy summarizes the results from the literature. Except for mucinous tumors, which are rarely bilateral, 5-year survival was slightly but not significantly reduced in the group treated with conservative surgery. In the control group, which included tumors of different histological types (serous and mucinous carcinoma, granulosa cell tumors), the risk of involvement of the contralateral ovary was 12%–13%.

A more recent series of patients who had been staged according to FIGO criteria, including stage Ia–c tumors, was described by COLOMBO et al. (1994). There were three recurrences (all stage la) in the conservatively operated group ($n = 56$) and five recurrences in the radically operated group ($n = 43$) after a median follow-up of 75 months. Wedge excision of the noninvolved ovary, which has been proposed because of the high incidence of bilaterality of some ovarian cancers (see Sect. 11.2), was not advised by COLOMBO et al. (1994): fertility of the remaining ovary may be compromised by this procedure (WEINSTEIN and POLISHUK 1975).

In conclusion, the few heterogeneous data from the literature cannot exclude an adverse impact of fertility-conserving surgery on survival. Such surgery therefore remains an experimental modality used only in a very small group of patients and, if performed, it should in no case prevent a proper staging procedure. Secondary contralateral salpingo-oophorectomy and hysterectomy after childbirth are recommended by the majority of authors.

11.7.5 Surgery for Advanced Ovarian Cancer

Surgery for advanced ovarian cancer grossly follows the same steps as already outlined for staging laparotomy. In contrast to the surgical staging carried out in early ovarian cancer, there is no need for cytological examination of ascites or peritoneal washings or sampling from the peritoneum if macroscopic disease is present in the abdominal cavity. Every suspicious lesion should be resected as completely as possible with the general aim of leaving behind no tumor with a diameter greater than 1 or 2 cm. As Table 11.14 shows, there is a strong correlation between long-term survival and the diameter of the largest residual tumor (NEIJT et al. 1984; VOGL et al. 1983; POHL et al. 1984; DELGADO et al. 1984; CONTE et al. 1986; PIVER et al. 1988; REDMAN et al. 1986). A similar correlation was demonstrated for the overall residual tumor volume (REDMAN et al. 1986). The data are clearly in favor of aggressive surgical techniques even if the gastrointestinal or urinary tract is involved and if continence of these organs cannot always be preserved. A primary exenterative procedure, on the other hand, is generally not recommended because of the bad prognosis of such aggressively infiltrating tumors.

The extent of lymphadenectomy in advanced ovarian cancer depends on the degree of debulking obtained. When optimal cytoreduction is achieved within the abdominal cavity, radical lymphadenectomy is indicated; however, if large tumor residuals remain in the abdomen, this procedure may cause superfluous morbidity.

Table 11.14. Survival (months) in patients with different postoperative tumor loads;[a] numbers of patients are shown in parentheses

Authors	Residual <1 cm	Residual >1 cm	Chemotherapy regimen
NEIJT et al. (1984)	40 (88)	21 (219)	CHAP vs CP
	Residual <2 cm	Residual >2 cm	
VOGL et al. (1983)	>40 (32)	16 (68)	CHAP
POHL et al. (1984)	45 (37)	16 (57)	Various
DELGADO et al. (1984)	45 (21)	16 (51)	Various
CONTE et al. (1986)	>40 (37)	16 (38)	PAC vs CP
PIVER et al. (1988)	48 (35)	21 (5)	PAC
	Residual <3 cm	Residual >3 cm	
REDMAN et al. (1986)	38 (34)	26 (51)	PAC

C, cyclophosphamide; A, adriamycin; P, cisplatin; H, hexamethylmelamine.
[a] The diameter of the largest residual tumor is shown.

11.7.6 Second-Look Laparotomy

The concept of second-look laparotomy (SLO) was introduced by Wangensteen and Arhelger (ARHELGER et al. 1957) primarily to assess disease status as part of ongoing surgical management in colorectal carcinoma. In ovarian cancer, by contrast, the term "second-look laparotomy" refers to a systematic surgical reexploration in clinically complete responders after primary surgery and chemotherapy. Normal preoperative clinical examination and normal sonographic and radiologic tests cannot reliably predict negative SLO, as demonstrated by remission rates from chemotherapy trials (see Sect. 11.10.3.1). The aim of SLO is therefore to identify those patients with complete clinical remissions who have not achieved complete pathological remission and need further treatment.

In the 1970s two events led to the widespread near-routine use of SLO: (1) long-term use of alkylating agents was shown to be leukemogenic and (2) platinum-based chemotherapy regimens had higher complete clinical remission rates. However, as the influence of SLO on survival has never been demonstrated by a prospective randomized trial, the role of SLO in the routine treatment of ovarian cancer has been challenged during recent years. Below an attempt is made to provide an overview of the ongoing discussion. For didactic reasons data from negative SLO and data for secondary cytoreduction at the time of SLO are discussed separately.

11.7.6.1
Technique of Second-Look Laparotomy

Second-look laparotomy follows the same technique as previously described. All macroscopic tumor is excised if there is a realistic chance of minimizing tumor burden. In patients with no apparent macroscopic tumor, inspection and palpation should be followed by multiple biopsies from high-yield sites. These sites include the right hemidiaphragm, the peritoneum anterior to the superior pole of the right kidney, the right colic gutter and pelvis, the bladder, the vaginal apex, the left pelvis and colic gutter, the mesentery of the distal small bowel and sigmoid colon, and serosa from the distal ileum and sigmoid colon. The retroperitoneum should be carefully palpated and any palpable draining lymph node excised.

11.7.6.2
Negative Second-Look Laparotomy

In an overview of data from 2309 patients reported from 1981 to 1990, RUBIN (1993) shows that in 46% of the cases SLO was negative, with a range from 85% for stage I disease to 34% for stage IV disease. The most reliable predictors of the negative outcome of SLO are initial early tumor stage, low histological grade, and small residual tumor at the time of initial laparotomy (PODRATZ and KINNEY 1993). Normal CA-125 levels are a poor predictor of the absence of disease, whereas elevated levels may reliably predict persistent disease at the time of SLO (RUBIN and LEWIS 1988).

One of the major points in the ongoing discussion is whether negative SLO reliably predicts cure so that treatment can be discontinued. Among the numerous publications dealing with this question, three relatively large single-institution reviews have focused specifically on the issue. The surgical procedures in these reviews were comparable but pretreatment and time to SLO differed. The results are summarized in Table 11.15 (GERHENSON et al. 1985b; PODRATZ et al. 1988; RUBIN et al. 1991). The recurrence rates from Memorial Sloan-Kettering center are the highest rates reported in the literature. Nevertheless, even median recurrence rates of about 35% after negative SLO remain high. The great majority of authors (SMITH et al. 1976; DAUPLAT et al. 1986; CHAMBERS et al. 1988; CREASMAN et al. 1989; OMURA et al. 1989) report having discontinued treatment after negative SLO.

High initial tumor stage and postoperative tumor residuals >2 cm may help to identify patient subsets with a high risk of recurrence after negative SLO. If further treatment is considered, the different biological significance of negative SLO after platinum-based chemotherapy and single alkylating agent therapy must be considered. Possible treatment options are intraperitoneal platinum (see Sect. 11.13), platinum non-cross-resistant drugs such as taxol, whole abdomen irradiation, or intraperitoneal phosphorus-32 instillation.

11.7.6.3
Positive Second-Look Findings; Secondary Cytoreduction at the Time of SLO

About 80% of patients with tumor identified at SLO will have grossly persistent tumor masses. In cases where cytoreduction yielding <2 cm tumor residuals has been achieved at the time of initial surgery, this reflects resistance to platinum chemotherapy. Until the 1990s no effective non-cross-resistant drugs were available, so that cytoreduction was the therapy of choice.

The influence of secondary cytoreduction on survival is demonstrated by the data from different trials (DAUPLAT et al. 1986; HOSKINS et al. 1989; CHAMBERS et al. 1988; PODRATZ et al. 1988), which

Table 11.15. Recurrence rates after negative SLO in stage III/IV ovarian cancer

Institution (*n*)	% negative SLO	% platinuum-based CHT	Number of CHT cycles	Median follow-up (mos.)	Recurrence rate	Time to recurrence (mos.)
M.D. Anderson (85)	35	27	12	>60	24	18.5
Mayo Clinic (50)	37	88	12	41	30	14
Memorial Sloan-Kettering (63)	–	>86	6	55	54	24

CHT, chemotherapy.

Table 11.16. Secondary cytoreduction at SLO and survival

Author	No. of patients	Survival: microscopic disease	Survival: optimally debulked	Survival: suboptimally debulked	Adjuvant treatment
DAUPLAT et al. (1986)	51	–	Significantly better survival ($P < 0.05$)		2nd-line chemotherapy, +/– radiotherapy
HOSKINS et al. (1989)	67	63 months	21 months	16 months	2nd-line chemotherapy, intraperitoneal therapy, irradiation
CHAMBERS et al. (1988)	101	–	No survival difference		2nd-line chemotherapy, 3x irradiation
PODRATZ et al. (1988)	250	55% at 4 yrs	21% (<5 mm) ($P < 0.01$)	14% (>5 mm)	Irradiation, intraperitoneal ^{32}P, chemotherapy

are shown in Table 11.16. Significant improvement of survival rates is generally limited to patients in whom optimal cytoreduction is possible. In cases with suboptimal debulking the impact on survival is minor, and the morbidity of the procedure may outweigh the potential benefit for the patient. When performed by experienced surgeons, SLO is associated with relatively little serious morbidity (CHEN and BOCHNER 1985). In a review, RUBIN et al. (1988) reported no deaths in 682 operations. The most commonly reported complications were infections of the surgical wound (6.3%), of the urinary tract (5.6%), and of the lungs (2.8%). Gastrointestinal injury occurred in 1.6% of the patients, with a 0.4% incidence of postoperative intestinal obstruction.

In conclusion, no prospective randomized trial has evaluated the impact of SLO on survival. In early-stage ovarian cancer SLO will only exceptionally be proposed, because of high cure rates. In stage III/IV ovarian cancer more than half of the patients will have residual disease. Tumor volume is one of the most important prognosticators. If SLO is positive, cytoreduction precedes further individual therapy. An influence on overall survival is usually reported in cases with optimal cytoreduction. In cases with negative SLO the value of the operation will depend on the therapeutic consequences that can be drawn; these will be determined by individual tumor biology, individual pretreatment, and individual history. With the advent of new therapeutic options such as taxol and high-dose chemotherapy, the value of SLO needs to be redefined.

11.7.7 Conclusions

Operative strategies in ovarian cancer can be summarized as follows:

- In early stages, proper staging laparotomies including median laparotomy, bilateral salpingo-oophorectomy, omentectomy, lymphadenectomy, and peritoneal biopsies from high-yield sites are obligatory to prevent misstaging and undertreatment. Fertility-conserving surgery can only be used exceptionally in these stages.
- In advanced ovarian cancer, optimal debulking is associated with prolonged survival.
- The role of routine SLO is unclear: Negative SLO is correlated with prolonged survival and may identify patients in whom treatment can be discontinued. Positive SLO may help to optimize further treatment, especially in view of the availability of new drugs like the taxanes. Subgroups of patients in whom optimal debulking is achieved at the time of SLO will benefit from surgery.

11.8 Postoperative Irradiation in Primary Epithelial Ovarian Cancer

H.W. VAHRSON

The rationale for any kind of locoregional treatment is based on the special growth and spread pattern of the tumor. After rupture of or penetration through the capsule, primary epithelial ovarian cancer spreads rapidly to the pelvic and abdominal surfaces, the omentum, the diaphragm, and intraperitoneal and retroperitoneal lymph nodes by certain favored pathways (see Sect. 11.4). However, for a long time, and even in advanced stages, tumor growth is confined to intraperitoneal organs and retroperitoneal nodes, prior to spread to extraperitoneal organs. A study in 137 patients who died in Munich with malignant ovarian tumors revealed that 56% had solely intraperitoneal metastases at autopsy (REMBERGER 1984). Hematogenous metastases without intraperitoneal spread occurred in only 2%. In a study of 100 patients who died with ovarian cancers in Rochester, N.Y., metastases were found in extraperitoneal organs in less than 50% of cases (DVORETSKY et al. 1988). In both studies lymph nodes were involved in 70% of cases. From these studies and practical experiences we draw two conclusions:

1. Ovarian cancer is not a pelvic disease but a disease of the abdominal cavity.
2. Tumor growth is confined to the abdominal cavity and retroperitoneum in the majority of cases even in advanced stages and at autopsy.

The target volumes for irradiation of ovarian cancers are the following: (a) pelvis, (b) peritoneal surface, (c) whole abdomen, (d) para-aortic lymph nodes, and (e) combinations thereof. Generally the indications for irradiation, as for any other therapy, are: postoperative therapy, consolidation therapy, salvage therapy, and therapy for recurrences. Postoperative therapy comprises treatment for no residual (R_0), microscopic residual (R_{micro}), or macroscopic residual (R_{macro} <2 cm/>2 cm) tumor after primary (initial) surgery. Consolidation therapy is defined as treatment after a second-look procedure (laparoscopy/laparotomy) with negative histopathological findings. Salvage therapy is defined as treatment after second-look procedures with R_{micro} or R_{macro}.

11.8.1 Pelvic Irradiation

Pelvic irradiation was in use as the sole postoperative treatment for decades during the x-ray era. Under high-voltage conditions, 50–60 Gy can be applied to 15 × 15 cm–16 × 16 cm opposing fields including the foramina obturatoria and lumbar vertebra 5. In thicker patients a box technique or, better, a biaxial pendulum technique should be used. Today pelvic irradiation is no longer indicated as a sole postoperative treatment, but in combination with intraperitoneal radionuclides, whole abdominal irradiation, and/or chemotherapy it can still be useful. In combination with intraperitoneal instillation of radionuclides (radiophosphorus) the percutaneously applied dose must be reduced to 30 Gy; doses from 40 to 45 Gy in combination with 10–20 mCi radiophosphorus resemble "a toxic combination" (KLAASEN et al. 1985). When, in abdominopelvic irradiation, a whole abdominal dose of 22.5–30 Gy is applied, pelvic irradiation of 20–25 Gy can be added to yield a total dose of 45–50 Gy (midline).

11.8.2 Irradiation of Para-aortic Lymph Nodes

The pelvic lymph nodes, including the common iliac lymph nodes, are irradiated whenever sole pelvic irradiation or a pelvic boost within abdominopelvic radiotherapy (APRT) is applied with the upper border at L4/L5. However, routine irradiation of the para-aortic lymph nodes is not performed.

Several recent reports on primary surgery or second-look surgery (SLS) with lymphadenectomy have stressed the negative role of lymph node metastases. LAHOUSEN (1994) reported the incidence of lymph node metastases at pelvic and/or para-aortic lymphadenectomy during primary surgery in 267 patients treated at Graz: 19% in stage I, 27% in stage II, 74% in each of stage III and IV, and 58% in stages I–IV. The controversies regarding lymphadenectomy have already been described (see Sect. 11.7.4.1).

DI RE (1990) found lymph node metastases in 58% of cases when lymphadenectomy was performed at primary surgery in 101 stage III and IV patients, as compared with 46% when lymphadenectomy was performed at SLS after platinum-based chemotherapy in 89 stage II–IV ovarian cancer patients. TULUSAN et al. (1990) found lymph node metastases in 57% of cases when lymphadenectomy was performed at primary surgery in 72 patients, as compared with 58% at SLS after chemotherapy. In addition in 30% of cases the latter authors found only microscopic or minimal residual disease at SLS, with the pelvic or para-aortic lymph node metastases being larger than the intraperitoneal residual tumor. On the basis of a literature review (including reports by the above-mentioned authors and the patients from Graz), LAHOUSEN (1994) reported the frequency of lymph node metastases to be 59% in stage III cancer patients at SLS. In patients with no residual tumor after primary surgery he found that 6%–40% of the recurrences were located exclusively in the retroperitoneum.

The following conclusions may be drawn: (a) the frequency of retroperitoneal lymph node metastases increases with stage and (b) these metastases seem to be resistant to platinum-containing chemotherapy.

The role of radiotherapy in the treatment of para-aortic lymph node metastases has not yet been established, either after or instead of lymphadenectomy. Kuipers (1976) published a retrospective analysis of ovarian cancer patients who received radio-chemotherapy with or without lumboaortic irradiation. In stage I and II serous ovarian cancer patients he found a significantly better 4- to 5-year survival when pelvic and lumboaortic irradiation (50 Gy) was performed, as compared with pelvic irradiation only (Fig. 11.7). In stage III and IV patients he found that whether or not a lumboaortic boost (20–25 Gy) was added to APRT (pelvic dose 50 Gy, abdominal dose 20–25) made no difference. These results suggest a benefit of para-aortic lymph node irradiation in early-stage ovarian cancer without lymphadenectomy.

Further recommendations on the use of irradiation of the para-aortic lymph nodes, and reports of experiences with the technique, are scarce in the literature. Martinez et al. (1985) added a boost with a pelvic, para-aortic, and medial diaphragm field to whole abdominal irradiation (to a total dose of 42 Gy in the para-aortic nodal region) as sole postoperative treatment. Subsequently, Schray et al. (1988) reported the toxicity of this Martinez technique in 77 patients with genital cancers (25 ovarian cancers). Eleven patients (14%) developed bowel obstruction, among whom six (8%) were free of progression. Very interesting is the fact that four patients (5%) developed chylous ascites with negative cytology and no known liver or retroperitoneal abnormalities. The chylous ascites was attributed to the para-aortic nodal boost, which included most of the small bowel mesentery, provided that mesenteric lymphatic channel obstruction was the causal mechanism. Furthermore, the authors supposed that any increase in myelosuppression may have been related to the para-aortic nodal boost, which included a substantial bone marrow volume.

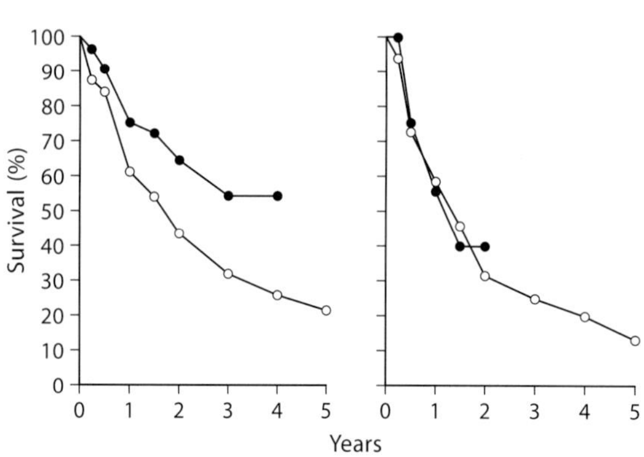

Fig. 11.7. Survival curves of patients irradiated for serous ovarian carcinoma. *Left* mainly stage I and II patients: ○–○ pelvic irradiation only (100 patients); ●–● pelvic irradiation with lumbo-aortic boost (32 patients). *Right* mainly stage III and IV patients: ○–○ whole abdominal irradiation only; ●–● whole abdominal irradiation with lumbo-aortic boost (71 patients). (From Kuipers 1976)

Huget and Debois (1990) supported lumboaortic irradiation with 25 Gy in addition to 45 Gy pelvic irradiation for stage III ovarian cancer, provided surgery was aggressive.

11.8.3 The Intraperitoneal Use of Radiocolloids

As long ago as 1945 Müller of Zürich employed a semicolloidal suspension of radioactive zinc (^{63}Zn) for intraperitoneal instillation and in 1949 he became the first to use radioactive gold (^{198}Au) colloid systematically in abdominal and pleural malignancies (Müller 1956, 1968). Hahn et al. (1947) of Nashville first reported that radioactive colloidal gold remained in the peritoneal cavity, this report being based on two experimental intraperitoneal applications in a man and a woman, each presenting with hypernephroma. Jones et al. (1944) developed a chemically inert colloidal form of ^{32}P. According to Hilaris and Clark (1971) in 1955 Henschke of New York was the first to use colloidal radioactive chromic phosphate (^{32}P) postoperatively in ovarian cancer; but there is an earlier report by Root et al. (1954) on intracavitary administration. The radioactive colloids were originally introduced to treat interstitial tumor spread and malignant effusions in the peritoneal and pleural cavity, but Müller (1968), Keettel et al. (1966), Hofmann (1960, 1963), Ariel et al. (1966), Frischkorn et al. (1973), and Rotte and Feltmann (1969) also used radioactive colloids (predominantly ^{198}Au colloids) in advanced stages of ovarian cancer without effusions.

The "prophylactic use of radioactive gold" was introduced into therapy when Keettel and Elkins (1956) undertook peritoneal washings and cytological examinations in patients with stage I and II ovarian cancer with obviously intact tumor capsules and found tumor cells in 50%. Radiogold has not been available in Germany since Amersham-Buchler stopped delivery in September 1989. The reasons were its gamma component and its late toxicity in producing severe adhesions and intestinal obstructions in some cases. Particularly in the United States, the use of radioactive chromic phosphate was emphasized because of its pure β-emission, longer half-life, and higher β-energy (Table 11.17). Besides

Table 11.17. Physical data in respect of colloidal isotopes

Isotope	$t_{1/2}$ (days)	E $\beta_{max.}$ / $\bar{E}$ β	E_γ	Max. penetrative depth[a]*	Relative depth dose at 1.5 mm[b]
^{198}Au	2.7	0.96 MeV 0.32 MeV	0.41 MeV (95%) 0.68 MeV (1%)	3.8 mm	β 18.4%
^{90}Y	2.7	2.27 MeV 0.90 MeV		10.3 mm	β 33.5%
^{32}P	14.3	1.71 MeV 0.70 MeV		7.5 mm	β 22.2%

[a] In tissue $\rho = 1.05\,g/cm^3$.
[b] 100 mCi in 1000 ml, fluid layer of 1.3 mm thickness (according to JONES 1961).

Table 11.18. Particle size of colloidal nuclides (as indicated by the producers)

Nuclide	Particle size
^{198}Au colloid	5–20 nm[a]
^{90}Y silicate	ca. 100 nm[a]
^{32}P-chromic phosphate	600–4000 nm[6] 0.6–1.3 µm (74.4%) 1.4–2.0 µm (16.6%) 2.1–4.0 µm (7.0%)

[a] AMERSHAM-BUCHLER.
[b] MALLINCKRODT.

the physical data, the size of the radioactive particles (Table 11.18) is important because with small particles a more even distribution on the surfaces and better transport in lymphatic vessels can be assumed. Chromic phosphate particles are about 100 times larger than radiogold particles, as they comprise clumps or aggregates of hundreds or thousands of chromic phosphate molecules (VAN NORSTRAND and SILBERSTEIN 1985). Therefore in terms of particle size, chromic phosphate is far from being an ideal radionuclide for intraperitoneal therapy.

11.8.3.1
Dose Distribution and Calculation

There are only a small number of reports in which calculations are made of the doses delivered to the peritoneal surfaces, retroperitoneal lymph nodes, and organs at risk. At autopsy of a patient with intraperitoneal tumor masses and ascites due to an adenocarcinoma, who died 7 days after instillation of 150 mCi radiogold colloid, MÜLLER (1956) calculated the following doses by neutron activation analysis: peritoneum 4000 cGy, omentum 6000 cGy, and retroperitoneal mediastinal and mesenteric lymph nodes an average of 7000 cGy with probable maxima up to 10 000–30 000 cGy for the β-component (Table 11.19). For the γ-component he added 750 cGy. These nearly ideal therapeutic doses were contradicted by REED et al. (1961), who used a scintillation counter at autopsy to measure the activity in the organs of two patients (one female and one male) who died on the 5th and 12th days, respectively, after instillation of 140 mCi radiogold colloid. Their estimates showed the highest doses in the liver (male: 404 cGy) or in the spleen (female: 593 cGy), while the dose in the para-aortic lymph nodes was found to be

Table 11.19. Measured or calculated doses (in cGy) delivered by intraperitoneal radionuclide instillation

Authors (year)	Nuclide	Dose	Peritoneum	Diaphragm	Omentum	Retroperitoneal Ln.	Mesenteric Ln.	Thoracic Ln.
MÜLLER (1956)	^{198}Au	150 mCi	4000[a]		6000[a]		10 000–30 000[a]	
CURRIE et al. (1981)	^{32}P	5 mCi: GM	70	57–60	960	25–28	300	
		TLD	71–12 453[b]	149–33 156	285–5456	16–94	124–7475	8738

GM, GEIGER-MÜLLER counter; TLD, thermoluminescent dosimetry; Ln., Lymph nodes.
[a] Measured/calculated at one autopsy, 8 days following instillation in stage IV cancer: figure refers to retroperitoneal, mesenteric, and thoracic lymph nodes.
[b] Measured/calculated in 16 healthy dogs (15–25 kg) 14.3 days following instillation.

only 20.6–53.0 and 3.2–13.0 cGy, respectively. After instillation of radiogold colloid the maximum uptake of activity was measured after 1–2 h by VEBERSIK and DVORAK (1967). These authors described a blockade in lymph node function after 2 h which had resolved by the 4th day or later, depending on the patient's age.

These contrasting results may derive from whether or not lymphatic vessels and nodes are already blocked by tumor cells, as we know from lymphography that completely infiltrated lymph nodes have lost their storing capacity and are bypassed by the lymphatic fluid. Using a gamma camera, BOYE et al. (1984) studied the whole body distribution after intraperitoneal instillation of 7–10 mCi ^{32}P-chromic hydroxide in patients operated on for early-stage ovarian cancer and found a fairly uniform distribution. They estimated the dose averaged over the whole peritoneal surface to be about 30 Gy and concluded that a higher dose should be given.

JACKSON and BLOSSER (1981) applied 15–20 mCi ^{32}P-chromic phosphate to 178 patients for malignant ascites, 22 of the patients having two instillations. LEICHNER et al. (1981) measured the distribution and effectiveness of intraperitoneally applied ^{32}P-chromic phosphate by means of autoradiography in New Zealand white rabbits and in vitro in cell lines. They found an uneven distribution of radioactivity in the anterior abdominal wall, with most of the activity concentrated near the midline and in the pelvic region, but a more uniform distribution in the diaphragm. Regarding the dose required to kill the tumor cells in vitro, LEICHNER et al. concluded that 75–150 mCi ^{32}P is necessary in ovarian cancer patients.

CURRIE et al. (1981) measured the dose distribution of ^{32}P-chromic phosphate in dogs and in ovarian cancer patients by different methods. In dogs the intraperitoneal activity was freely movable in the abdominal cavity after instillation and after 1 day appeared to be fixed. From day 3 to day 5 the thoracic nodes showed more activity. Geiger-Müller measurements showed subtherapeutic doses, but autoradiographs and thermoluminescent dosimetry of peritoneal surfaces, organ specimens, and lymph nodes showed that peritoneal surfaces received therapeutic doses of radiation, the infradiaphragmatic areas a higher dose, and the contiguous thoracic lymph nodes the highest dose, while the retroperitoneal lymph nodes failed to receive a therapeutic dose (Table 11.19).

From these experimental data we must draw the conclusion that 15 mCi of ^{32}P-chromic phosphate should be the lowest amount of activity applied. At the ZFG Giessen the dose ranges from 15 to 16.5 mCi depending on the day of application: 15 mCi at the reference date, 15.75 mCi 1 day earlier, and 16.5 mCi 2 days earlier.

11.8.3.2 Time and Mode of Application

Suitable times for insertion of the catheter into the peritoneal cavity and instillation of the radioactivity range from immediately after the primary surgical procedure up to within 6 weeks. Insertion of the catheter immediately after surgery and instillation of the activity within hours up to 1 day was done by HILARIS and CLARK (1971), JACKSON and BLOSSER (1981), BOYE et al. (1984), POTTER et al. (1989), VERGOTE et al. (1992b) in a randomized trial, and SPANOS et al. (1992). BUCHSBAUM and KEETTEL (1975) recommended the 6th–10th postoperative day for the instillation of radiogold, and SOPER et al. (1985) the 7th–14th day for radiophosphorus. PIVER et al. (1982) recommended instillation of activity within 4 weeks, PEZNER et al. (1978) within 3–6 weeks, and VERGOTE et al. (1993b) within 6 weeks. The supporters of immediate instillation cite substantial advantages: insertion of the catheter under direct vision, absence of adhesions, and placement of two catheters to the diaphragm and pelvic wall for better distribution. SPANOS et al. (1992) reported significantly fewer complications when ^{32}P-chromic phosphate was given on the same day as surgery than when administration was delayed for more than 12 h following surgery. Nevertheless, the supporters of delaying instillation until some weeks after surgery also have convincing arguments: possible postoperative complications (including rupture of the abdomen) will have subsided, there will be no leakage from the scar, patients can easily rotate to permit an even distribution, and only one catheter needs to be placed. At the ZFG Giessen we prefer the insertion of the catheter about 4 weeks after surgery. Adhesions and possible violations of the intestine at the place of puncture can easily be prevented by ultrasound examination of the intestinal mobility. In this way intraperitoneal placement of the catheter can be managed as safely as during surgery.

11.8.3.3 Imaging of Radionuclide Distribution

If the catheter for instillation of the radiocolloid is not inserted intraoperatively and the radionuclide is to be instilled immediately after finishing the operation, an imaging procedure must precede the instillation. The bremsstrahlung of radiophosphorus can be scanned with a gamma camera, but with activities below 0.5 mCi no reliable scans can be taken. When intracavitary doses above 5 to the usual 15 mCi are instilled, the bremsstrahlung is sufficient to give good scans (Covington and Hilaris 1973; Barber 1993). However, almost the complete activity must be instilled before a loculation can be detected.

A gamma camera scan after instillation of 1–2 mCi ^{99m}Tc-sulfur colloid has been employed by Alderman et al. (1977), Sullivan et al. (1983), Spanos et al. (1992), Tulchinsky and Eggli (1994), and Pattillo et al. (1995).

Peritoneography with a usual water-soluble contrast medium gives more detailed information on the correct position of the catheter and the intraperitoneal distribution (Keettel et al. 1966; Doench et al. 1973; Piver et al. 1982, 1988; Rosenshein 1983; Bakri et al. 1985; Walton et al. 1991, using fluoroscopy). At the ZFG Giessen we use peritoneography with 250 ml of contrast medium (Fig. 11.8). In a previous report on 157 peritoneographies from Giessen and 184 peritoneographies from Göttingen we demonstrated a low complication rate: only two intestinal punctures (one into the colon and one into the small intestine) (Joswig et al. 1976). For the metallic ^{198}Au suspension and ^{32}P-chromic phosphate, but not for ^{90}Y-silicate, the usual water-soluble contrast media could be used immediately before instillation. The ionic and anionic contrast media contain ethylene diamine tetra-acetic acid (EDTA) as a stabilizer, a substance which dissolves the ^{90}Y-silicate complex completely. Rapid resorption from the peritoneal cavity then leads to renal clearance or bone deposition (bone seeker!). Until now peritoneography preceding ^{90}Y-silicate instillation has had to be performed at least 24 h before the instillation of the nuclide, but a recently introduced nonionic contrast medium, iomeprol (Imeron, Byk Gulden, Konstanz), contains no EDTA and can be used immediately before ^{90}Y instillation.

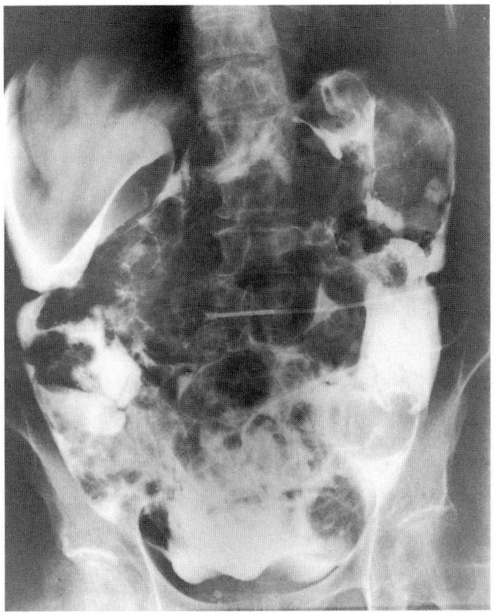

Fig. 11.8. Peritoneogram after abdominal puncture and instillation of 250 ml of radiopaque fluid. Good distribution is seen

11.8.3.4 Instillation Volume and Movement of the Patient

Generally the total instilled volume must be large enough to achieve an even surface distribution but not so large as to cause pains, leakage, and/or immobilization of the patient during the following hours. The reported total volume (radiopaque contrast medium and ^{32}P colloid infusion) has variously been cited as 500 ml (Klaassen et al. 1985), 350–750 ml (Potter et al. 1989), 750 ml (Piver et al. 1988), 1250 ml (Walton et al. 1991), 1500 ml (Sullivan et al. 1983), 2000 ml Taylor et al. (1974), and 2200 ml (Boye et al. 1984). At the ZFG Giessen we use 250 ml of radiopaque contrast medium followed by 1000 ml of 0.9% sodium chloride or Ringer solution, to which the radiocolloid is continuously added, resulting in a total volume of 1250 ml.

Vigorous premixture of the ^{32}P colloid with the saline solution has been emphasized since Currie et al. (1981) described the very weak dispersion of the nuclide when the saline solution is only poured over it.

After instillation, removal of catheter, and closure of the puncture canal, the patient has to move continuously for at least 15 min around her long axis (head down), and during the following 5 h (in a horizontal position) she has to change her position in a 15-min rhythm: back, left side, front, right side, and so on. For the rest of the day the patient has to move occasionally. This regimen prevents uneven distribution and fixation on the peritoneal surfaces.

Sufficient volume, vigorous mixture with the radioactivity, and appropriate movement of the patient for many hours are thus of great importance in order to avoid complications related to the technique of instillation.

Tbale 11.21. Intraperitoneal instillations of colloidal radionuclides in ovarian malignancies from 1957 to 1994 at the ZFG Giessen

Period	Nuclide	Single dose	No.
1957–1989	^{198}Au	100–150 mCi	1600
1987–1994	^{90}Y	50–100 mCi	37
1988–1994	^{32}P	15–16.5 mCi	303
			1940

11.8.4 Radiogold in Postoperative Therapy

Encouraging results following radioactive gold administration in optimally and suboptimally operated patients in disease stages I–III were reported in the 1970s from the Norwegian Radium Hospital, Oslo (Aure et al. 1971; Kolstad et al. 1977). The last update of a clinical study of patients randomized to receive either 100 mCi radiogold + 3000 cGy pelvic megavoltage irradiation or 5000 cGy pelvic megavoltage irradiation was presented by Kolstad et al. (1977). The results are shown in Table 11.20. In stage I the combination radiogold + pelvic irradiation resulted in a 14.9% mortality due to cancer, as against 23.9% with sole pelvic irradiation, a significant difference. Unfortunately this advantage was outweighed by a 4.6% rate of deaths due to complications and a 6.9% rate of intercurrent deaths in the radiogold group, as compared with 0% and 1.1%, respectively, in the sole pelvic irradiation group, resulting in 5-year survival rates of 73.6% and 75.0%, respectively. In stage II the 5-year survival rate was

Table 11.20. Actuarial 5-year survival rates and complications in a prospective randomized trial of ^{198}Au + pelvic irradiation (PEL) versus pelvic irradiation alone. (Modified from Kolstad et al. 1977)

	100 mCi ^{198}Au + 3000 cGy PEL		5000 cGy PEL	
Stage I				
5-year survival	87 pat.	73.6%	88 pat.	75.0%
Cancer deaths	$n = 13$	14.9%	$n = 21$	23.9%
Died of complications	$n = 4$	4.6%	$n = 0$	0%
Intercurrent deaths	$n = 6$	6.9%	$n = 1$	1.1%
Stage II				
5-year survival	74 pat.	54.1%	86 pat.	40.0%
Cancer deaths	$n = 26$	35.1%	$n = 38$	44.2%
Died of complications	$n = 4$	5.4%	$n = 1$	1.2%
Intercurrent deaths	$n = 1$	1.4%	$n = 3$	3.5%

54.1% in the radiogold group versus 40.0% in the sole pelvic irradiation group. But again mortality due to complications was 5.4% in the radiogold group as against only 1.2% in the sole pelvic irradiation group. One of the consequences of this study was the use of radiophosphorus instead of radiogold in the 1980s.

The era of radiogold has now passed. Nevertheless, the author, who himself used radiogold for 25 years in several hundred patients until production was discontinued by Amersham in September 1989, may be permitted a brief reminiscence. From 1957 to 1989 about 1600 instillations were done at the ZFG Giessen for ovarian malignancies (Table 11.21). Up to 1969 the dosage was 2 × 150 mCi (!) at an interval of 8 weeks; this was applied to all stages if possible. Starting from 1970 the dose was reduced successively to 1 × 150 and then to 1 × 130 mCi. The results of this historical treatment are shown in Tables 11.22 and 11.23.

The late complications of treatment with radiogold consisted in extensive serous peritoneal surface fibrosis, described as frosting-like (Hofmann 1960), porcelain-like, or greasy peritoneum, leading to conglomerate tumors (Johannssen 1965; Keettel et al. 1966; Heilmann et al. 1983), pseudocysts (Vahrson and Steckenmesser 1970), and bowel obstruction (Decker et al. 1973; Kolstad et al. 1977). A very thorough investigation was carried out by Gieselberg (1974) at the ZFG Giessen in order to ascertain whether metastatic growth or complications of radiogold treatment were the cause of obstructions. At that time a majority of the obstructions were operated on by the gynecologists at the ZFG, who intensively looked for hidden metastases in a conglomerate tumor and for the typical alterations caused by radiogold. Retrospective evaluation revealed 51 obstructions at surgery among 397 patients with previous intraperitoneal radiogold treatment (Table 11.24); at first sight this rate, 12.8%, appeared unacceptably high, but only 1.5% of the obstructions could be completely attrib-

Table 11.22. Crude 3- and 5-year survival rates in 423 patients with malignant ovarian tumors (including granulosa cell and secondary ovarian cancers) by FIGO stage and in 329 patients with primary epithelial ovarian cancers (not separately staged) treated between 1957 and 1969 at the ZFG Giessen

FIGO stages	No.	%	3-year survival		FIGO stages	No.	%	5-year survival	
			No.	%				No.	%
I	133	31	94	71	I	105	32	69	66
II	120	28	62	52	II	98	30	42	43
III	132	31	10	8	III	90	28	2	2
IV	38	9	1	3	IV	32	10	0	–
All malignancies	423	100	167	39	All malignancies	325	100	113	35
Primary epithelial cancer	329		137	42	Primary epithelial cancer	239		91	38

Table 11.23. Crude 3- and 5-year survival rates in 331 primary epithelial ovarian cancers according to type of histology, treated between 1959 and 1969 at the ZFG Giessen

Histological type	No.	%	3-year survival		Histological type	No.	%	5-year survival	
			No.	%				No.	%
Serous	172	52	66	38	Serous	131	55	40	31
Mucinous	55	17	41	75	Mucinous	41	17	30	73
Endometrioid	45	14	24	53	Endometrioid	32	13	16	50
Undifferentiated	59	18	9	15	Undifferentiated	35	15	4	11
All types	331	100	140	42	All types	239	100	90	38

Table 11.24. Cause of 51 intestinal obstructions at surgery among 397 patients who received radiogold instillation between 1957 and 1970 at the ZFG Giessen. (Modified from Gieselberg 1974)

Cause of obstruction	No.	%
Cancer growth without adhesions: no ^{198}Au involvement	32	8.1
Cancer growth and intensive adhesions: ^{198}Au involvement possible	12	3.0
Intensive adhesions and serosal fibrosis without cancer growth: ^{198}Au damage	6	1.5
Funicular adhesion without cancer growth: perforation following radium	1	0.25
Total obstructions	51	12.8
Obstructions with cancer growth	44	11.0
Obstructions without cancer growth: pure therapy damage	7	1.8

uted to radiogold, with a further 3% being partially attributable to it.

Some surgeons, not knowing the typical alterations of the peritoneal surface, look only at the conglomerate tumor and not at the hidden obstructing metastasis in it and diagnose "radiation damage." This must be kept in mind when comparing the complications of different therapeutic modalities.

11.8.5 Radiophosphorus in Postoperative Therapy

Colloidal radioactive chromic phosphate is now the most commonly used radionuclide for postoperative abdominal instillation for early ovarian cancers of stages I and II. Positive results were initially published by Hilaris and Clark (1971), Pezner et al. (1978), Piver et al. (1982), Kjorstad (1986), and Potter et al. (1989) for early-stage disease and by Jackson and Blosser (1981) for the treatment of ascitic fluid; these results gave rise to two prospective randomized studies, in each of which one treatment arm was ^{32}P colloid.

In the first study the Ovarian Cancer Study Group together with the Gynecologic Oncology Group randomized 141 patients with poorly differentiated stage I or stage II cancers after comprehensive staging at surgery to receive either intraperitoneal ^{32}P-chromic phosphate (15 mCi) or melphalan (0.2 mg/kg body weight daily for 5 days, repeated every 4–6 weeks for 10–12 cycles). The results were published by YOUNG et al. (1990) and the complications were reported separately by WALTON et al. (1991). The 5-year overall survival rate (78% in the ^{32}P arm vs 81% in the melphalan arm) and the 5-year disease-free survival (89% in each arm) showed no significant differences after a median follow-up of more than 6 years (minimum 3 years). Two deaths occurred in in the melphalan group, one from preleukemia and one from acute myelogenous leukemia. In the ^{32}P arm one patient sustained an injury to the ileum at laparoscopic catheter placement; laparotomy was required to repair the injury. A further four patients (6%) required surgical intervention, one for bowel perforation and diffuse peritonitis and three with stage II disease for bowel obstruction without cancer growth. The authors concluded "that the group receiving the single dose of intraperitoneal ^{32}P, with its limited toxicity (and no known risk of leukemia), is the preferred standard group for subsequent study." This study is unique because of the comprehensive intraoperative staging. Nevertheless, some points deserve criticism:

1. Twenty-four patients (17%; 14 in the ^{32}P arm and ten in the melphalan arm) had borderline malignancies later diagnosed by a reference pathology institution.
2. Time to instillation of ^{32}P ranged from 5 days after definitive surgery to 106 days after surgery.
3. The dose of ^{32}P changed from 7–16 mCi initially to a uniform 15 mCi after 1979. In the initial group, doses were: 7 mCi (1), 7.5 mCi (7), and 10 mCi, 12 mCi, 12.8 mCi, 13.6 mCi, 14.4 mCi, and 16 mCi (1 each); thus 13 of the 69 patients (18.8%) receiving ^{32}P had an underdosage down to 50%.
4. The study was joined by 21 institutions, only six of which contributed five or more patients. It was not reported how many institutions applied the ^{32}P instillations, or how much experience they had with the technique. It is possible that points 2–4 negatively influenced the outcome of the ^{32}P arm and the complication rate.

The second study was conducted by the group of the Norwegian Radium Hospital, Oslo (VERGOTE et al. 1992b). The study comprised 340 evaluable patients under age 70 with invasive epithelial cancer or borderline tumor stages I–III with no residual tumor after bilateral salpingo-oophorectomy and hysterectomy (BSOH) and infracolic omentectomy who had been operated on within 6 weeks before entry into the study. The patients were randomized to receive either (n = 169) 7–10 mCi ^{32}P-chromic hydroxide (CIS Bio-International, Gif-sur-Yvette, France) or (n = 171) six cycles of cisplatin (50 mg/m^2 intravenously in repeated courses every 3 weeks). Twenty-eight patients randomized to the ^{32}P arm who had intraperitoneal adhesions were treated with abdominopelvic irradiation (22 Gy to the whole abdomen in 20 fractions/5 days a week and 22 Gy in 11 fractions/4 days a week to the pelvis). The median follow-up was 62 months (minimum 24 months).

No significant differences were found between the two arms in the estimated crude 5-year survival (^{32}P group 83% vs cisplatin group 81%) or the estimated disease-free 5-year survival (^{32}P group 81% vs cisplatin group 75%). After exclusion of the borderline cases, the 5-year disease-free survival rate in stage I was 82% after ^{32}P, 94% after abdominopelvic irradiation, and 79% after cisplatin. In stage II the 5-year disease-free survival rate was 55% in the ^{32}P group compared with 68% in the cisplatin group. In neither stage were the differences significant.

Severe toxicity consisted in an 11% rate of bowel obstruction in the ^{32}P group [9% after ^{32}P and 21% (!) after abdominopelvic irradiation], as compared with only 2% in the cisplatin group. The percentage of patients with bowel obstruction requiring surgery was 1% in the cisplatin group, 4.5% after ^{32}P, and 10.7% after abdominopelvic irradiation. In the cisplatin group treatment had to be discontinued in 12 patients because of neurotoxicity (4), skin rash (3), or nausea and vomiting (5), all of these complications being reversible. From these results the authors suggested that "cis-platin, with its limited toxicity, should be the standard treatment for future controlled trials," and regarding the unusual high rate of bowel obstructions, they commented, "whole abdominal irradiation therefore is not recommended as adjuvant treatment in patients with intraperitoneal adhesions."

In conclusion, there have been two important prospective studies on numerous patients with optimally operated stage I and II (III) ovarian cancers, each randomized to a ^{32}P arm or a chemotherapy arm. In each of the studies the survival results were similar in both arms, as were the complications in the ^{32}P arms. But, depending only on the toxicity of different cytotoxic drugs (melphalan causing leukemia), the authors come to different conclusions as to whether ^{32}P-chromic phosphate should be used as a standard treatment in future trials.

Between 1988 and 1992 we instilled ^{32}P-chromic phosphate (Mallinckrodt Media Inc., St. Louis) in

107 patients using activities in the range of 15–16 mCi in single doses. As this treatment is only one part of the sandwich radiotherapy regimen at the ZFG Giessen (see Sect. 11.13.5), the results are presented later (see Sect. 11.13.5.3).

11.8.6 Radiophosphorus in Consolidation Therapy

The rationale for consolidation of a histopathologically negative finding at second-look laparotomy (SLL) after primary surgery and chemotherapy is the fact that an increasing proportion of patients will relapse during the following years.

In a review of survival data from 18 institutions, VARIA et al. (1988) reported a combined relapse rate of 90/548 (16%) with a median follow-up of 3 years or less in most of the studies. VERGOTE et al. (1993b) found relapses in 19 of 68 cases (28%) after a median follow-up of 65 months (range: 36–111). In the literature, SPENCER et al. (1989) found a range of recurrences after negative SLL from 5.9% to 50%.

The survival results of four studies are discrepant (Table 11.25). SPENCER et al. (1989) and ROGERS et al. (1990) found better results in patients treated with ^{32}P-chromic phosphate after histopathologically negative SLL in comparison with untreated controls. These studies were retrospective and among the controls were patients with adhesions not suited for intraperitoneal application of the nuclide. PETERS et al. (1992) obtained disappointing results in 34 patients without controls. Eighteen of the 34 patients (53%) relapsed during the follow-up period. The disease-free survival rate was 40%. VERGOTE et al. (1993b) reported the results of a prospective randomized trial in 25 patients receiving ^{32}P-chromic hydroxide and 25 controls receiving no further therapy. They found four relapses in the treatment group and one in the control group. Therefore PETERS et al. (1992) and VERGOTE et al. (1993b) found radiophosphorus not to be an effective consolidation therapy after negative SLL.

The rate of intestinal complications without relapse in these four studies was in the range of 6% (ROGERS et al. 1990) to 15% (PETERS et al. 1992). The latter authors had to reduce the ^{32}P activity from 15 to 12 mCi after five bowel injuries occurred in the terminal ileum, with the higher dose being used in 23 patients (rate = 22%!). After reduction to 12 mCi they observed no bowel injuries in the following 11 patients.

VERGOTE et al. (1993b) applied only mini-activities ranging from 7 to 10 mCi of ^{32}P depending upon the body weight, believing that reducing the activity would enable results to be maintained while reducing complications. However, the fact that bowel obstruction occurred in 7% in spite of the mini-activities, as well as the observation of nearly the same rate following 15 mCi of ^{32}P in the two above-mentioned studies, suggests that other mechanisms may be the cause of the complications (technique of instillation, mixture of the radiocolloid in the instilled volume, movement of the patient,

Table 11.25. Results of ^{32}P colloid instillation as consolidation therapy after negative SLL

Authors (year)	Stages Grades	No. with ^{32}P No without ^{32}P	Dosage of ^{32}P	Disease-free survival	Overall survival	^{32}P-related Complications	Median and minimum follow-up
SPENCER et al. (1989)	I–III	14	15 mCi	100% $P = 0.076$	100%	2 unrelated deaths (1 from AML, 1 from natural cause) 1 bowel obstruction	7 years 2 years
		17	0	76%	76%		
ROGERS et al. (1990)	I–III 1–3	50	15 mCi	86% $P = 0.05$	90%	4 bowel obstructions (1 with recurrence)	58 months 18 months
		18	0	67%	78%		
PETERS et al. (1992)	Ic–III 1–3	34	23 × 15 mCi 11 × 12 mCi	40%	64%	5 terminal ileum complications (3 obstructions, 2 ileovaginal fistulae)	31 months 19 months
		–		–	–		
VERGOTE et al. (1993b)	Ia G2,3–IV 1–3	25	7–10 mCi	ca. 83%[a]		7% bowel obstructions without recurrence	65 months 36 months
	8 LMP	25	0	96%			

LMP, low malignant potential/borderline tumor.
[a] Taken from figure.

etc., as mentioned in Sect. 11.8.3). The foregoing chemotherapy (number of cycles, dose intensity, use of multiple drugs, use of platinum compounds), additional radiotherapy, and the SLL itself may play a major role in predisposing towards radionuclide-induced complications. This is partly supported by PETERS et al. (1992), who observed a bowel complication rate of only about 5% in patients receiving adjuvant radiophosphorus therapy with 15 mCi.

In conclusion, the role of ^{32}P-chromic phosphate suspension in consolidation therapy is still undefined. Taking into account the dependence of relapses on stage, grade (and to a lesser extent the histology) of the primary cancer, residual disease after initial surgery, and accuracy of examination at SLL, the treatment has to be individualized. It must be borne in mind that ^{32}P-chromic phosphate instillation takes a few days of hospitalization only, causes less bone marrow toxicity than abdominopelvic irradiation or chemotherapy, is well tolerated by the elderly, and can be safely applied with tolerable toxicity by experienced therapists.

11.8.7 Radiophosphorus in Salvage Therapy

When, after initial surgery and chemotherapy, microscopic (R_{micro}) or macroscopic residual tumors (R_{macro}) are found, the prognosis is very unfavorable, whatever second-line treatment is applied.

Reports concerning ^{32}P colloid salvage therapy are scarce and there have been no prospective randomized trials. SOPER et al. (1987) and POTTER et al. (1989) subdivided residual tumors into R_{micro}, R_{macro} completely resected, and R_{macro} < 5 mm not resected at SLL. R_{micro} and R_{macro} completely resected had not dissimilar disease-free survival (DFS) rates of 36% and 46%/47%, respectively (Table 11.26). ROGERS et al. (1990) reported the results obtained in 30 patients with R_{micro} and R_{macro} < 2 cm combined. The 5-year actuarial disease-free survival rate was 38% for those receiving ^{32}P-chromic phosphate and 0% for those who did not. In contrast SOPER et al. (1987) and POTTER et al. (1989) found no DFS in the small number of nine patients (together) with R_{macro} < 5 mm.

It may be concluded that ^{32}P colloid salvage therapy should be restricted to R_{micro} residuals. R_{macro} residuals are unsuited for such therapy except when their size is within the range of the penetration depth of the ^{32}P electrons, i.e., 1–1.5 mm. For R_{macro} residuals other options such as abdominopelvic irradiation or second-line systemic or intraperitoneal chemotherapy should be preferred.

11.8.8 Special Indications for Radiocolloids

11.8.8.1 Radioyttrium as a Substitute for Radiophosphorus

Of the colloidal preparations ^{90}Y-phosphate, ^{90}Y-fluoride, ^{90}Y-hydroxide, and ^{90}Y-silicate (WALTER et al. 1961), only the suspension of colloidal yttrium-silicate [$^{90}Y_2(SiO_3)_3$] gained some importance in the

Table 11.26. Results of ^{32}P colloid instillation as salvage therapy after positive SLL

Authors (year)	Stages Grades	No. of patients	Findings at SLL	Dose of ^{32}P	Disease-free survival		Overall survival	^{32}P-related complications	Median and minimum follow-up
SOPER et al. (1987)	Ib–IV 1–3	10	R_{micro}	15 mCi	36%	27%	57%	3 bowel obstructions (13%) without recurrence; 1 unrelated death	36 months 5 months (4-year survival rates)
		8	R_{macro} resected	15 mCi	36%				
		5	R_{macro} <5 mm	15 mCi +chemotherapy/ radiation	0%				
POTTER et al. (1989)	I–III 1–3	13	R_{micro}	10–15 mCi	46%			7% surgical interventions	37 months
		15	R_{macro} resected		47%	$P < 0.01$			
		4	R_{macro} >5 mm		0%				
ROGERS et al. (1990)	I–III 1–3	30	R_{micro} and R_{macro} >2 cm	15 mCi	38%	$P < 0.01$		3.5% bowel obstructions (incl. recurrence)	58 months 18 months (5-year survival rates)
		17	R_{micro} and R_{macro} >2 cm	0	0%				

treatment of malignant pleural and peritoneal effusions.

Ariel et al. (1966) reported that such treatment was beneficial in 77% of 30 patients with urogenital cancers and peritoneal effusions. Lang and Riccabona (1974) reported a prolongation of puncture intervals from 10 days before to 68 days after instillation of ^{90}Y-silicate, corresponding with a remission rate of 68.5%.

As regards physical properties, ^{90}Y-silicate has a tenfold smaller particle size and a higher β-energy than ^{32}P-chromic phosphate, but little is known about the fixation of the particles to the surfaces. Walter et al. (1961) found a ca. 50% reduction in the concentration of ^{90}Y in the peritoneal fluid after 2 days, which may indicate a 50% fixation to the peritoneum or the draining lymph nodes. In view of these properties, the abdominal use of ^{90}Y-silicate should be confined to patients:

1. Who have no major adhesions and/or loculation
2. who are receiving palliative treatment only
3. Who have received no previous or planned percutaneous radiation
4. In whom previous systemic or intraperitoneal chemotherapy has been ineffective
5. In whom puncture intervals are too short for the use of ^{32}P colloid.

11.8.8.2 Pseudomyxoma Peritonei

Pseudomyxoma peritonei of ovarian (or appendiceal) origin presenting with mucinous residuals after surgery is still an incurable disease. Patients die within a few years while suffering from cachexia and ileus, having been subjected to repeated surgical interventions to remove as much of the mucin as possible. In 1963 Hofmann mentioned some patients with pseudomyxoma peritonei who, after intraoperative removal of the mucinous masses, received a high single dose of radiogold colloid (200 mCi!) and survived for several years without recurrence. After the production of radiogold was stopped in 1989, we continued the intraperitoneal treatment using 100–150 mCi of ^{90}Y-silicate in several cases and obtained similar results.

In view of the above, it is clear that prevention of pseudomyxoma peritonei is necessary after rupture of a mucinous benign (or malignant) ovarian cystoma. Since the 1960s we have treated 52 patients after spontaneous or intraoperative rupture or puncture of a benign mucinous cystoma – until 1988 with a single dose of 130–150 mCi of ^{198}Au colloid, and since 1988 with 15 mCi of ^{32}P-chromic phosphate. Until now only one patient has developed an intraperitoneal pseudomyxoma, but we have found two cases of what can be called an "ectopic pseudomyxoma." The first patient presented with a mucinous benign cystic tumor 3 × 4 cm in diameter in the extraperitoneal tissues between the pouch of Douglas and the vaginal stump. The mucin was removed by transvaginal puncture but the cyst recurred. After a second puncture, an artificial canal was dilated to insert a radium tube (60 mgel for 10 h). The cystic tumor shrank to a diameter of less than 2 cm, the canal persisted due to radium-induced fibrosis, and the patient reported the passing of "plugs" through the vagina at about monthly intervals. The second patient presented with a pelvic cystic tumor of 10 cm in diameter with the caudal part 2–3 cm above the vaginal stump. The mucin was drained by repeated transvaginal punctures. In neither patient was there evidence of intraperitoneal pseudomyxoma.

These two cases bear witness to the effectiveness of intraperitoneal radionuclide instillation in preventing intraperitoneal pseudomyxoma, but ectopic pseudomyxoma may develop outside of the peritoneal cavity, presumably due to the inoculation of mucinous cells at surgery. It should also be mentioned that during the same period we received 30 patients for treatment of a manifest pseudomyxoma peritonei at varying times after surgery performed in other institutions where no prophylaxis had been done.

If ^{32}P-chromic phosphate proves to be as effective as radiogold, its use for the prevention of pseudomyxoma peritonei can be supported.

11.8.8.3 Malignant Pleural Effusions

The efficacy of intrapleural infusions of radionuclides in patients with malignant pleural effusions was studied, as already mentioned, by Walter et al. (1961), Ariel et al. (1966), and Lang and Riccabona (1974) using ^{90}Y colloids. The results were very similar to those reported after intraperitoneal infusion for malignant ascites. Scheer (1964) reported results from Heidelberg and London after radiogold colloid instillation in malignant pleural effusions from breast and bronchial cancers. He found a good effect (no puncture required within 6 weeks following instillation) in 44%–58% and a moderate effect (puncture required within 6 weeks but less frequently) in 0%–19% after a single or a second application of 80–120 mCi of ^{198}Au colloid.

The substitute for radiogold is now ^{90}Y-silicate. ^{32}P-chromic phosphate is not suitable for fast effusion producing pleural carcinosis because of its longer half-life of 14.3 days. Indications for intrapleural ^{90}Y-silicate instillation are malignant pleural effusions with positive cytology originating from bronchial, breast, ovarian and other genital cancers, or pleural mesothelioma. A conditio sine qua non is the exclusion of adhesions or loculation by an x-ray film in the ipsilateral position. The single dose of ^{90}Y-silicate is 50 mCi (1850 GBq). The treatment can be repeated 4–6 weeks later using the same dose.

Experience at the ZFG Giessen indicates that ^{90}Y-silicate is as effective as radiogold. Continued pleural effusion will be stopped after the second dose at the latest. Intensive adhesions between pleura visceralis and parietalis (= pleurodesis) will occur. Austgen and Trendelenburg (1987) used single doses of 50–75 mCi ^{90}Y-silicate and found complete remission in 58% after one instillation and in 100% after up to five instillations. The median survival was 286 days. With regard to long-term palliation, the pleurodesis following ^{90}Y-silicate is more effective than pleurodesis by insufflation of talc or instillation of tetracyclines. The latter drugs produce partial adhesions and loculation and have no impact on the tumor cells or survival. A comparable antineoplastic effect and pleurodesis can only be achieved by repeated intrapleural instillations of the cytostatics doxorubicin (Kefford et al. 1980), bleomycin (Ruckdeschel et al. 1991), or mitoxantrone (Musch et al. 1992) or of the cytokine tumor necrosis factor (TNF; Schönig et al. 1991).

11.8.9 Intraperitoneal Instillation of Radioisotope–Monoclonal Antibody Conjugates

Intracavitary radioimmunotherapy, first employed by Epenetos and co-workers (Courtenay-Luck et al. 1984; Epenetos et al. 1986, 1987), has attracted increasing interest since it was shown to be efficacious in phase I and II trials, and it is now progressing to phase III trials.

The effector system (isotope, chelator, and antibody) combines the efficacy of an isotope (^{131}I, ^{90}Y, ^{186}Re) with that of a monoclonal antibody [IgG or the fragments Fab and F(ab′)$_2$], which are linked by iodinated tyrosine in the case of ^{131}I immunoglobulin or by chelates [such as diethylene triamine penta-acetic acid (DTPA)] in the case of metallic radioisotopes. The aim of this combination is to direct the radioactivity more specifically to the tumor cells, with reduction of the dose to normal tissues, unlike in the classical intraperitoneal application of ^{32}P/^{90}Y colloids.

Hnatowich et al. (1988) used 1 mCi of ^{90}Y-labeled OC-125 F(ab′)$_2$ coupled with DTPA prior to SLS in five ovarian cancer patients. They found an average urinary excretion of 7% of the administered radioactivity and levels in tumor specimens of between 3% and 25%, while the normal tissues showed a mean accumulation of 8% in serum, 10% in liver, 7% in bone marrow, and 19% in bone, with large patient to patient variations. The calculated dose delivered by 1 mCi ^{90}Y to normal tissue was ≅8 cGy and to tumor ≅ 50 cGy. The dose to bone marrow was considered the limiting factor.

Rosenblum et al. (1991) studied the pharmacology and tissue distribution of the ^{90}Y-labeled monoclonal antibody B72.3 with DTPA against high-molecular-weight tumor-associated glycoprotein (TAG-72) in nine patients with ovarian carcinoma or papillary serous carcinoma of the peritoneum. The activities ranged from 0.5 to 1.2 (mean 0.8) mCi. Analysis of total ^{90}Y in plasma showed that about 60% of the ^{90}Y label was absorbed into the circulation after intraperitoneal administration. Urinary excretion of the total ^{90}Y label accounted for 11% of the injected activity within 3 days, of which the majority (6.7%) consisted of low-molecular-weight ^{90}Y-labeled metabolite. The lowest concentration of ^{90}Y-labeled B72.3 (<0.002% of the injected dose per gram) was found in bone marrow, fat, and rectus abdominis muscle. Higher concentrations (0.003%–0.007%) were found in the peritoneum, liver, bone, and normal lymph nodes. The highest concentrations were found in normal omentum (0.017%) and in samples from histologically confirmed tumor tissue. The uptake of ^{90}Y into various tumor tissues was highly variable in the same patient as well as between patients. There was no significant correlation between TAG-72 expression and uptake of ^{90}Y isotope.

Epenetos et al. (1987) used the ^{131}I-labeled antibodies HMFG1, HMFG2, AUA1, and H17E2 in 24 patients with persistent ovarian cancer after chemotherapy ± external beam irradiation (!). Eight patients with R > 2 cm did not respond and died of progression within 9 months of treatment. Of the 16 patients with R < 2 cm, initially nine responded, of whom four had a DFS of 6 months to 3 years. Besides mild acute toxicity a subphrenic abscess occurred, requiring surgical intervention. The low rate of complications is noteworthy because some of the patients had previously received external irradiation. Doses > 140 mCi were more effective than lower doses. The authors concluded that the intraperitoneal administration of 140 mCi or more of ^{131}I-labeled MAbs represented a new and effective treatment for patients with small-volume stage III ovarian cancer.

Kavanagh et al. (1992) used subtherapeutic doses of ^{90}Y-labeled B72.3-MAb with DTPA intraperitoneally (10–15 mCi). Thrombocytopenia initially limited the dose to 15 mCi ^{90}Y, but concurrent intravenous administration of EDTA resulted in myeloprotection. Analysis of bone content showed a tenfold lower concentration of ^{90}Y with EDTA than without EDTA (0.0017% vs 0.14% of injected dose per gram tissue) and no thrombo-cytopenia occurred up to 30 mCi ^{90}Y, warranting further dose escalation. The authors suggested ^{90}Y-B72.3-DPTA as an attractive alternative to intraperitoneal ^{32}P.

Hird et al. (1993) used intraperitoneal ^{90}Y-anti-HMFG1 antibody treatment in 21 stage Ic-IV ovarian cancer patients in complete remission after surgery and chemotherapy for consolidation. The authors found a significant reduction in the rate of recurrence in comparison with a historical control group.

Muto et al. (1992) conducted a phase I therapeutic trial using escalating doses of ^{131}I-labeled MAb OC-125 for salvage therapy in 28 evaluable patients. They found hematological and gastrointestinal toxicity. Hematological toxicity (neutropenia and thrombocytopenia) occurred in 5/14 (36%) patients receiving 18–87 mCi and in 12/14 (71%) receiving 100–144 mCi ^{131}I. At doses ≥100 mCi patients developed nausea, vomiting, or chronic ileus. This toxicity occurred mainly in patients with protracted urinary excretion. The authors concluded that ^{131}I-labeled OC-125 can be safely administered intraperitoneally.

Mahé and Chatal (1995), in a review of the literature, considered 136 patients with ovarian tumors who received ^{131}I radioimmunotherapy in single or repeated injections. In patients with R_{macro} a complete remission (cR) rate of 2% and a partial remission (pR) rate of 7% were obtained, whereas in patients with R_{micro} a cR of 65% was achieved.

Crippa et al. (1995) used ^{131}I-labeled MOv18 intraperitoneally in 16 evaluable patients with minimal residual disease (R < 5 mm or R_{micro}) after SLS for salvage. The mean dose was 100 mCi ^{131}I. Upon clinical follow-up or third-look evaluation performed 90 days after radioimmunotherapy (RIT) the authors found cR in 5/16 (31%), no change in 6/16 (38%) and disease progression in 5/16 (31%) of the patients; but follow-up showed only one long-term cR at 34 months, the remaining four cases having relapsed. Only mild toxicity occurred. The production of human-anti-mouse antibodies (HAMA) was found in 15/16 (94%) of the patients.

HAMA responses seem to be a major problem when murine-derived MAbs are used, as they can block effective targeting and rule out the possibility of two or more RIT applications. After two or three Mab doses, 90% of patients develop a HAMA response. The incidence of this immune response can be reduced by using recombinant = chimeric human or humanized antibodies. On the other hand the intravenous administration of HAMA at the time of intraperitoneal RIT may allow a more rapid clearance of any antibody absorbed into the systemic circulation and provide a means of enhancing the therapeutic ratio (Harrington and Epenetos 1994). Radioactive rhenium in a ^{186}Re-labeled Mab was used intraperitoneally in single doses of 25–150 mCi by Jacobs et al. (1993) in a phase I study in 17 patients with residual or recurrent disease. Objective response occurred in 4/17 (24%) of the patients presenting with R < 1 cm. Myelosuppression was the limiting toxicity.

Epenetos (1994) initiated a phase III trial in ovarian cancer patients in clinically and laparoscopically confirmed complete remission after initial surgery and platinum-based chemotherapy, the patients receiving either 18 mCi/m^2 ^{90}Y-HMFG1 intraperitoneally or no further treatment.

The choice of the isotope appropriate for tumor deposits of different sizes has to take into account the maximum penetration depth of the highly energetic β-particles in tissue (Larson 1991) and the relative depth dose. The maximum penetration depth of ^{90}Y is 10.3 mm and the depth dose at 1.5 mm is 33.5% (see Table 11.17), which makes this isotope more suitable for macroscopic tumors <1 cm in diameter. The maximum penetration depth of the β-particles of ^{131}I is 2.4 mm, which makes this isotope suitable for microscopic or very small visible tumors up to 1–2 mm large.

Experimental in vitro and in vivo data indicate that other radionuclides may be useful for RIT, examples being the α-emitters lead-212 (^{212}Pb), bismuth-212 (^{212}Bi), astatine-211 (^{211}At), and the Auger electron emitter bromine-80m (^{80m}Br) (Rotmensch et al. 1989a,b, 1990, 1991).

In conclusion: Intraperitoneal RIT is an exciting means of delivering radiotherapy more selectively to intraperitoneal tumors than is possible with classical colloidal radionuclide instillation. The results to date have been promising, but many problems remain to be resolved and further clinical studies are needed. According to Harrington and Epenetos (1994), before radical RIT can be achieved "it will be necessary to improve specific tumor cell targeting and to increase both the initial dose rates and the total dose delivered to the tumor deposits. Until that time, it is likely that RIT will be incorporated into multimodality protocols to deliver a moderate (10–20 Gy) tumour boost, or in an adjuvant setting in patients with minimal residual disease."

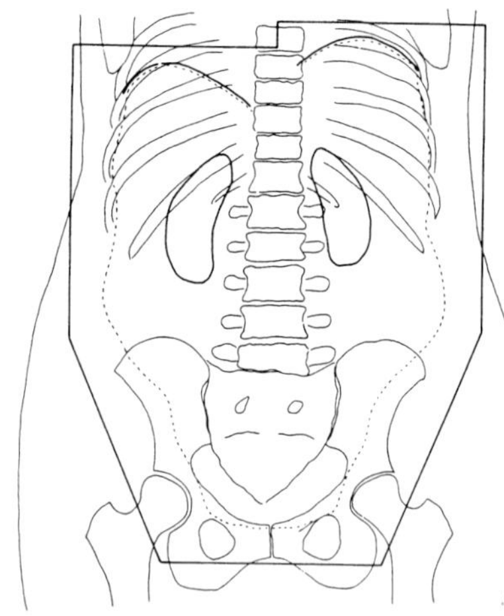

Fig. 11.9. Abdominopelvic radiotherapy using the open-field technique, posteroanterior projection. [From Dembo (1985), Cancer 55:2285–2290. Copyright American Cancer Society. Reprinted by permission of Wiley-Liss, Inc., a subsidiary of John Wiley & Sons, Inc.]

11.9 Whole Abdominal Irradiation

H.W. Vahrson

11.9.1 Moving Strip or Open-Field Technique?

Whole abdominal irradiation (WAI) can be delivered by the moving strip technique, the open-field technique, or by modified techniques using three or more fields (see Chap. 4). The moving strip technique was introduced at the M.D. Anderson Hospital, Houston in 1957. This technique was described as not changing the patient's weight during the treatment and in combination with additional pelvic irradiation as being superior to the other methods of irradiation Delclos and Smith 1975). The technique was adopted by many centers (Perez et al. 1975; Bush et al. 1977; Haas et al. 1980; Nevin et al. 1983). Two prospective randomized studies compared the moving strip and the open-field techniques: Fazekas and Maier (1974) compared delivery of 30 Gy in 10 days using the moving strip technique and delivery of 40 Gy in 56 days to the entire abdomen using the open-field technique and found no significant difference in length of survival or local tumor control in spite of the biologically larger dose of the moving strip irradiation (1400 rets vs 1060 rets).

Dembo and co-workers (Dembo et al. 1983; Dembo 1984) compared two techniques of abdominopelvic irradiation: the moving strip (22.5 Gy in 10 fractions) and the open field (22.5 Gy in 22 fractions). A pelvic boost dose (22.5 Gy in 10 fractions) was given in each case before the WAI. Survival, relapse-free rates, and failure patterns were identical for both techniques but there was less late toxicity with the open-field technique: bowel obstructions requiring surgery occurred in 6% of patients treated with the moving strip technique, versus 1.2% treated with the open-field technique. Because of these results and the simplicity of application and the shorter treatment duration (6–7 weeks vs 11–13 weeks), the open-field technique was adopted as the standard technique at the Princess Margaret Hospital (PMH), Toronto. Later, Files et al. (1992) from PMH Toronto published an analysis of complications following abdominopelvic radiotherapy (APRT). After use of the moving strip technique these authors found the following complication rates: 7% bowel obstructions, 23% chronic diarrhea, 37% pneumonitis, 2% jaundice, and 2% gastrointestinal deaths; after use of the OF technique these rates were 4.3%, 13%, 12%, 0%, and 0.6% respectively.

One important point should be mentioned here. With regard to tumor cell movement along the intra-abdominal pathways (see Sect. 11.4) it can be assumed that each day thousands of mobile tumor cells are outside the irradiated strip volume, provided that free flow of the peritoneal fluid is possible and mobile malignant cells are present. Bearing this in mind, at ZFG Giessen we instilled colloidal radiogold

Table 11.27. Principles of abdominopelvic radiotherapy as sole postoperative treatment. (Dembo 1985, 1992)

1. The technique should be used only in patients with no macroscopic disease in the upper abdomen and small macroscopic (less than 2–3 cm) or no macroscopic residual disease in the pelvis.
2. The entire peritoneal cavity must be encompassed. Radiological verification is required.
3. No liver shielding is used. This limits the upper abdominal dose to 2500–2800 cGy in 100- to 120-cGy daily fractions.
4. Partial kidney shielding is used to keep the renal dose at 1800–2000 cGy.
5. The true pelvis is given a boost dose in 180- to 220-cGy fractions to a total dose of 4500 cGy.
6. Parallel opposing portals should be used, with beam energy sufficient to ensure a dosage variation no greater than 5%.
7. The field should extend outside the iliac crests.
8. The field should extend outside the peritoneum (indicated by a dotted line in Fig. 11.9), with a generous margin.
9. A 1–2 cm margin should be allowed above the diaphragm in expiration.

(130 mCi) as pretreatment to eradicate the mobile tumor cells 4 weeks before application of moving strip irradiation. We stopped this pretreatment when we adopted the open-field technique according to the PMH as our standard technique of WAI (Fig. 11.9).

The decisive factor for the efficacy of APRT is the exact definition of the borders of the abdominal volume. Dembo (1985, 1992) defined these borders on the basis of the principles shown in Table 11.27. Violations of this protocol lead to intraperitoneal recurrences and poor survival rates. Dembo (1992) reported survival rates in relation to a violation score (concerning the borders of the pelvic and abdominal fields and the probability of underdosage), based on the NCI of Canada randomized study (Klaassen et al. 1988): APRT patients with a score of 0 had a 76% 5-year survival rate, those with a score of 1–5 (minor violations) had a rate of 67%, and those with a score ≥6 (major violations) had a rate of only 33%.

11.9.2 Whole Abdominal Irradiation as Sole Postoperative Therapy

Many publications from PMH Toronto (Bush et al. 1977; Dembo et al. 1979; Dembo and Bush 1982; Dembo 1984, 1985, 1992; Lederman et al. 1991; Whelan et al. 1992; Files et al. 1992; Carey et al.

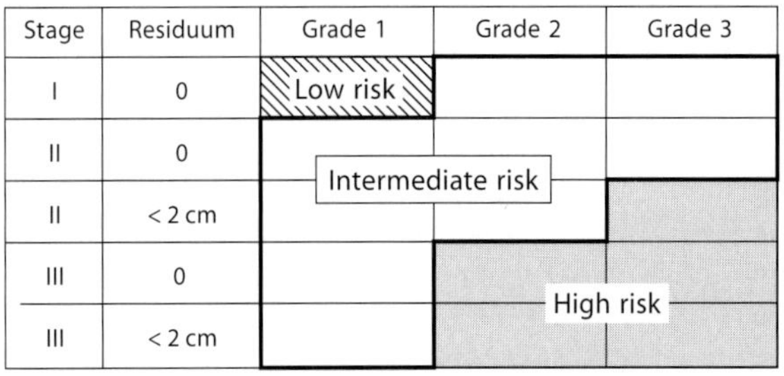

Fig. 11.10. Prognostic subgroupings according to stage, residuum, and grade in patients with stages I through III and small or no tumor residuum. [From Dembo (1992) Int J Radiat Oncol Biol Phys 22:835–845, with permission of Elsevier Science Inc.]

1993) show that postoperative WAI using the open-field technique with pelvic boost (APRT) has become established as the sole adjuvant postoperative therapy in a well-defined group of patients. The definition of this group of "intermediate risk" patients was originally based on stage, histological type and grade of differentiation, and tumor residual at first surgery (Dembo and Bush 1982). However, when the prognostic value of the combined histology-grade variable (Carey et al. 1993) and of the grade alone was tested in two historical groups, it was found that there was no major advantage to using one classification rather than the other for clinical applications. For this reason, and because of its simplicity, the classification based on only stage, grade and tumor residual classification has been favored for stratification of patients into risk categories (Fig. 11.10). Low-risk patients need no further therapy after surgery, while intermediate-risk patients can be treated with sole APRT and in high-risk patients chemotherapy should be added to radiotherapy. The 5-and 10-year survival rates of patients treated between 1971 and 1981 at PMH were published by Dembo (1985), and are shown in Fig. 11.11. In the intermediate group the overall survival rates after 5 years were 75% and after 10 years 68%, while in the high-risk group they were 32% and 19% respectively. In this period APRT was used as sole postoperative therapy. These results are among the best ever published.

Goldberg and Peschel (1988) used the PMH classification and applied APRT as sole postoperative therapy to 74 patients with invasive ovarian cancer stage I–III after BSOH and debulking procedures (residual <2 cm). For the "favorable" group ($n = 60$) the actuarial 10-year survival rate was 77% (±10%), as compared with only 7% in the "unfavorable"

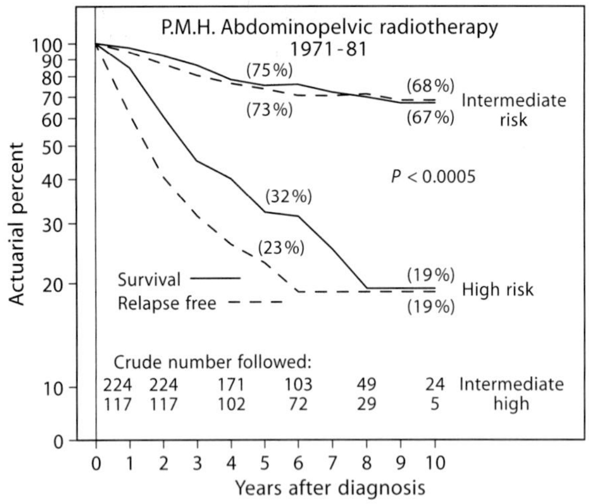

Fig. 11.11. Survival rates (including all causes of death) and relapse-free rates in 341 intermediate- and high-risk patients. Percentages of 5- and 10-year rates in parentheses. [From DEMBO (1985) Cancer 55:2285–2290. Copyright American Cancer Society. Reprinted by permission of Wiley-Liss, Inc., a subsidiary of John Wiley & Sons, Inc.]

group (n = 10). Interruption of radiotherapy was necessary in 18%. Severe late side-effects (bowel obstruction) occurred in 7% of the patients.

A German prospective study in 79 patients with classification into risk groups according to the PMH recommendations was conducted by LINDNER et al. (1990). APRT was applied with the moving strip technique in 43 patients and with the open-field technique in 36 patients. The median follow-up time was 57 months (3–136 months), and the mean follow-up was 55.8 + 24.8 months. The authors reported a DFS of 75% and a crude 5-year survival rate of 78% (life table method according to Kaplan-Meier). The corresponding survival rates for the high-risk group were 16% and 22% respectively (Table 11.28). The survival rates are very similar to those from PMH. The acute side-effects were moderate and comprised hematotoxity, nausea and vomiting, and diarrhea of WHO grades I–III. In ten patients radiotherapy had to be interrupted because of hematotoxity. Other acute side-effects were cystitis (8), vaginitis (2), and pains (4). Late side-effects occurred in two patients: one with ureteral obstruction and one with a lethal small intestine obstruction following a 52.5 Gy pelvic dose.

HAMMOND et al. (1992) treated 59 patients with WAI after primary cytoreductive surgery in stages I–III (residual <2 cm), including 26 patients with stage I ovarian carcinoma. The median survival was 53 months. Serious morbidity developed in 8%; one

Table 11.28. Five-year survival rates (KAPLAN-MEIER) after sole postoperative abdominopelvic radiotherapy in 79 patients. (Modified from LINDNER et al. 1990)

	Crude survival (%)	Disease-free survival (%)
All cases (n = 79)	66 ± 6	63 ± 6
Intermediate risk	78 ± 7	75 ± 7
High risk	22 ± 11	16 ± 10
Stage I	85 ± 7	86 ± 7
Stage II	64 ± 10	52 ± 10
Stage III	34 ± 13	39 ± 13
G1	93 ± 6	83 ± 11
G2	61 ± 9	60 ± 9
G3	58 ± 13	56 ± 11
R_0	70 ± 7	67 ± 7
R_1, R_2	40 ± 15	40 ± 15

R_1 = <2 cm, R_2 = >2 cm residual.

Table 11.29. Five-year DFS rates following postoperative sole abdomino-pelvic irradiation in 345 patients with ovarian cancer at the Maria Sklodowska-Curie Memorial Institute, Cracow. (Modified from REINFUSS et al. 1993)

	No. of patients	5-year DFS survival	
		No.	%
Histology:			
Serous carcinoma	162	65	40.1
Mucinous carcinoma	79	43	54.4
Undifferentiated carcinoma	48	9	18.8
Endometrioid carcinoma	43	24	55.8
Clear-cell carcinoma	13	3	23.1
Differentiation:			
G1	125	85	68.0[a]
G2	140	41	29.3
G3	80	18	22.5
Clinical stage:			
Ia	80	68	85.0[a]
Ib	25	17	68.0
Ic	39	22	56.4
IIa	20	11	55.0
IIb	28	11	39.3
IIc	7	3	42.9
III	146	12	8.2
Residuals at first surgery:			
R_0	115	84	73.0
R_{micro}	30	21	70.0
R ≤ 3 cm	90	36	40.0
R ≥ 3 cm	110	3	2.7
Total	345	144	41.7

[a] Statistically significant differences (log-rank test).

patient died from liver failure attributed to radiotherapy and four patients had bowel obstruction.

REINFUSS et al. (1992) treated 345 patients with ovarian cancer of stages I–III with postoperative sole APRT (Table 11.29). The 5-year DFS rate was 41.7%. While the results in stages Ia–IIc were very good and comparable to those of DEMBO (1985), the DFS rate in stage III was only 8.2% and in patients with gross tumor residuals (>3 cm) at first surgery only 2.7%. The results in stage III patients and those with gross residual disease demand the use of chemotherapy. Severe late side-effects occurred in 2.3%, including bowel obstruction in 1.7%.

11.10 Chemotherapy of Epithelial Ovarian Cancer

U. NITZ and H.G. BENDER

11.10.1 Introduction

Chemotherapy after surgery has evolved to become one of the standard primary treatment procedures for two principal reasons: (a) approximately two-thirds of women have stage III and IV disease, which is not surgically curable and (b) even in the one-third of patients apparently presenting with localized disease, relapse rates may be as high as 40%.

During recent decades drug treatment has changed from long-term therapy with a single alkylating agent to more aggressive, shorter, platinum-based polychemotherapy protocols. Because of reduced tumor load and theoretically high growth fractions after debulking procedures, the optimal time for commencement of chemotherapy seems to be early after the operation.

Table 11.30. Single-agent activity in advanced ovarian cancer

Drug	Patients	Response rates (%)
Alkylating agents	1371	33
Ifosfamide	37	22
Cisplatin	190	32
Doxorubicin	102	33
5-Fluorouracil	126	29
Methotrexate	34	18
Mitomycin C	49	16
Hexamethylmelamine	215	24
Prednimustine	36	28
Taxol	41	36

Table 11.31. Prognostic factors in early ovarian cancer

Good prognosis	Poor prognosis
Intact capsule	Ruptured capsule
No tumor excrescences	Tumor excrescences
Stage Ia,b disease	Stage Ic–II disease
Grade 1 disease	Grade 2–3 disease
	Clear-cell histology
	Tumor residuum

Table 11.30 provides an overview of the active agents and the clinical response rates after single-agent therapy for advanced disease (THIGPEN 1985; THIGPEN et al. 1990; SUTTON et al. 1990). Even if these data show that ovarian cancer is very chemosensitive, the majority of stage III and IV patients are not cured with the existing therapies. Early development of drug resistance is a major cause of therapy failure. As new modalities to overcome drug resistance have become available in recent years, we are hoping for an improvement in survival data within the next decade.

11.10.2 Chemotherapy of Early-Stage Ovarian Cancer

11.10.2.1 General Considerations

Published 5-year survival rates range from 50% to 95% for stage I patients and from 30% to 80% for patients with stage II disease (YOUNG 1993). Chemotherapy in early-stage ovarian cancer is generally adjuvant in character since in most cases tumor can be resected completely.

The number of cures achieved by operation alone varies considerably, so that in subgroups with a good prognosis, the proportion of patients at risk of recurrence (who might benefit from adjuvant therapy) will be very low. On the other hand with routine chemotherapy 2%–5% of patients will develop irreversible platinum toxicity (neurotoxicity/nephrotoxicity) and there will be rare cases of secondary leukemia. Therefore in clinical practice it is difficult to advise routine adjuvant chemotherapy in early disease. Benefit will be maximal in patients at high risk of recurrence. There is a good body of evidence allowing the identification of high-risk subgroups with conventional prognostic parameters. Table 11.31 gives an overview of the known prognostic factors (BJORKHOLM et al. 1982; DEMBO and BUSH 1982; MARTINEZ et al. 1985; YOUNG et al. 1990).

11.10.2.2
Early-Stage Patients Not Requiring Adjuvant Treatment

Patients with stage IaIb G1 tumors and patients with stage I tumors of low malignant potential with none of the above-mentioned high-risk factors do not receive adjuvant treatment. Data for these patients derive mainly from two prospective randomized trials. The first compares adjuvant radiotherapy versus no treatment (see Sect. 11.9) and the second, adjuvant melphalan versus no treatment (YOUNG et al. 1990). Results from the latter trial are summarized in Table 11.32. No difference was detected between the two treatment arms.

Results from these protocols are of further interest because central pathology review led to the conclusion that 51 patients had borderline lesions. Within this group no patient died directly from ovarian cancer. These results were confirmed by another trial with stage I borderline tumors randomized to no therapy, adjuvant radiation, or intermittent oral melphalan; of the 55 randomized patients only one had a recurrence (CREASMAN et al. 1982).

11.10.2.3
Early-Stage Patients Requiring Adjuvant Therapy

A number of retrospective and prospective trials in early-stage ovarian cancer have compared radiation therapy, intraperitoneal radioisotope instillation, and single alkylating agent chemotherapy (see Sect. 11.9).

Since the 1970s there has been increasing interest in platinum-based (poly)chemotherapy for early disease. The Italian Interregional Cooperative Group for Gynecologic Oncology (BOLIS et al. 1989, 1991) randomized stage Ia,b and grade 2–3 tumors to receive either cisplatin (50 mg/m^2 CDDP q4w × 6) or no treatment. At 5 years 85% overall survival was observed in both arms. Within the same trial stage Ic cancers were randomized to receive the same cisplatin regimen or instillation of ^{32}P. Adjuvant platinum was significantly better than radionuclide instillation (disease-free survival 82% vs 70%).

A very similar trial at the Norwegian Radium Hospital (VERGOTE et al. 1992b) included 347 patients with stage I–III tumors without postoperative tumor residuals. Estimated 5-year disease-free survival for stage I patients in this nonrandomized study was equal in the two treatment groups. Late bowel complications were significantly higher in the radionuclide arm, so that the authors preferred cisplatin as standard adjuvant therapy.

Since data from the literature cannot provide conclusive information on this point, two further prospective randomized trials in stage I/G3, Ic, and II tumors comparing intraperitoneal ^{32}P with cyclophosphamide/cisplatin (1000 mg/m^2/100 mg/m^2 three times at monthly intervals) have been activated by the GOG (protocol # 91) and the EORTC. Results will be available within the next few years and will allow better definition of the "standard" adjuvant regimen for this subgroup of patients.

Table 11.32. GOG protocol 7601

Patient characteristics	Treatment	Recurrence-free survival (%) at 5 years
Ia,b; G1–2	Melphalan	91
Ia,b; G1–2	Control	98

11.10.3
Chemotherapy of Advanced Ovarian Cancer

11.10.3.1
History

Until the 1960s most chemotherapic regimens used in patients with ovarian cancer consisted in the long-term administration of an alkylating agent such as melphalan, busulfan, or cyclophosphamide. Later anthracycline-containing polychemotherapy regimens were preferred because they yielded better remission rates and better long-term survival (OMURA et al. 1983, 1986, 1989). In 1970 another compound, cisplatin, which to date is considered to be the most active agent against ovarian cancer, was introduced by Wiltshaw's group (WILTSHAW et al. 1979). The GOG protocols 22 and 47 (see Table 11.33) demonstrate the historical development (OMURA et al. 1986, 1989).

With regard to its side-effects, cisplatin has some major disadvantages in the therapy of potentially curable disease. There is a rate of irreversible peripheral neurotoxicity (peripheral polyneuropathy, ototoxicity) of about 2%–5% and a comparable rate of irreversible renal damage. Application demands extensive prehydration and is highly emetogenic. An alternative platinum compound, carboplatin, has the advantage of low nephro-and neurotoxicity, is moderately emetogenic, rarely causes alopecia, and is easily applicable in daily routine. The substance has been widely tested in ovarian cancer and has been found in different combinations to be as effective as cisplatin at a dose of 400 mg/m² versus 100 mg/m² (see Table 11.34). At this dose level carboplatin causes mainly hematotoxic side-effects. Like the cisplatin compound, the substance is excreted mainly by the kidney, so that dosage should be adjusted to renal function as characterized by glomerular filtration rate (CALVERT et al. 1989). Table 11.34 shows the outcome of the most important trials testing carboplatin against cisplatin (ALBERTS et al. 1989, 1992; PATER 1990; TEN BOKKEL HUINNK et al. 1988; EDMONDSON et al. 1989). Today the two substances are widely accepted as equivalent alternatives in the treatment of epithelial ovarian cancer.

11.10.3.2 *Evaluation of Outcome of Chemotherapy*

Pathological complete remission (pCR) at the time of second-look surgery is the most reliable short-term parameter in evaluating the outcome of chemotherapy or new chemotherapy trials. More than 60% of patients with pCR will be cured, whereas the survival differences of patients with partial remissions at this time are only in the range of several months.

Table 11.33. GOG protocols no. 22 and 47, and results

Parameter	GOG 22		GOG 47	
	L-PAM	AC	AC	PAC
No.	64	72	120	107
CR (%)	20	32	26	51
pCR (%)			3	12
Overall response rate (%)	37	49	48	76
Median survival (months)	12	14	16	19

L-PAM, melphalan; A, adriamycin; C, cyclophosphamide; P, platinum.

Tumor-related predictors of pCR after surgery and chemotherapy may be expressed as a prognostic index including FIGO stage, grade, and Karnofsky status, as proposed by NEIJT et al. (1995). Therapy-related predictors are the use of platinum-based chemotherapy (The Ovarian Cancer Meta-analysis Project 1991) and especially the amount of residual disease after primary surgery. The outstanding importance of residual disease after primary surgery is documented by the cumulated data from different trials with various chemotherapeutic regimens (OMURA et al. 1983, 1986; EHRLICH et al. 1979; GRECO et al. 1981; GALL et al. 1986). If the maximum postoperative tumor residual exceeds 2 cm in diameter, chemotherapy is only rarely curative (Table 11.35).

A rapid decline in pretherapeutically elevated CA-125 levels (after two courses of chemotherapy) (LAWTON et al. 1994; VAHRSON and MUNSTEDT 1994) represents another very sensitive marker of the efficacy of chemotherapy in the individual case.

11.10.3.3 *Today's "Standard" Therapy*

As Table 11.33 shows, even if remission rates after different chemotherapeutic regimens vary widely, the corresponding differences in median survival are small. Therefore the advantage of a prolongation of survival measurable only in months must outweigh the higher toxicity of more aggressive polychemotherapy. The results of an Italian study group (Gruppo Interregionale Cooperativo Onco-

Table 11.34. Carboplatin versus cisplatin in first-line combination chemotherapy of epithelial ovarian cancer

Agent	Dose (mg/m²)	Combination partner (mg/m²)	No.	CR (%)	Median survival (months)
Cisplatin	100 q4w	C 600	342	27 (cCR)	168
Carboplatin	300 q4w			34 (cCR)	20
Cisplatin	75 q4w	C 600	447	18 (pCR)	23
Carboplatin	300 q4w			13 (pCR)	24
Cisplatin	100 q4w	C (1400, p.o.)/ H (2100, p.o.)/A (35)	339	23 (cCR)	108 wks
Carboplatin	350 q4w			24 (cCR)	107 wks
Cisplatin	60 q4w	C 1000	103		27
Carboplatin	150 q4w				20

C, cyclophosphamide; H, hexamethylmelamine; A, adriamycin; cCR, clinical complete remission; pCR, pathological complete remission.

logico Ginecologia 1987) (Table 11.36) suggest that the three alternative standard therapies (P, PC, PAC) differ markedly with respect to response rates but not significantly with respect to pCR rates. For example, the median survival advantage of combination chemotherapy was only about 4 months compared with cisplatin monotherapy. On the other hand there were two deaths due to infections in the polychemotherapy arm. There were no significant differences between the three treatment arms with regard to pCR the most sensitive parameter for potential cure.

A meta-analysis done by The Advanced Ovarian Cancer Trialist's Group (1991) showed a marginally significant advantage for the PAC protocol. Nevertheless, the authors could not decide from the existing data whether this was due to a higher platinum dose intensity in the PAC protocols or to adriamycin. Furthermore, the survival difference was only in the range of several months, so that at present there is not a definitive standard regimen.

There is an ongoing international multicenter trial (ICON) with a planned number of about 2000 patients testing carboplatin (400 mg/m^2) versus PAC (350/60/600 mg/m^2), which will provide further information on this point.

Table 11.35. Residual disease and response to chemotherapy

Regimen	Minimal residual disease	Bulky residual disease
	pCR (%)	*pCR (%)*
PAC (*n* = 137)	33%	12%
PAC (*n* = 17)	30%	13%
HCAP (*n* = 21)	86%	10%
	Median survival	*Median survival*
PAC	42 months	19 months
L-PAM	33 months	13 months

P, platinum; C, cyclophosphamide; A, adriamycin; H, hexamethylmelamine; L-PAM, melphalan.

11.10.3.4 New Strategies

Survival data after chemotherapy in advanced ovarian cancer remain to be improved. At the moment there are two main strategies which seem to be of some interest in the clinical setting: (a) the concept of dose intensification, principally of the platinum derivatives, and (b) the use of non-cross-resistant drugs.

The concept of dose intensification was extensively discussed in the 1980s, when LEVIN and HRYNIUK (1987a,b) showed that there is a positive correlation between survival rate and dose intensity (dose/m^2 per week) for the existing platinum-based polychemotherapies. LEVIN and HRYNIUK concluded that this is due to the existence of a steep dose-response curve for platinum derivatives but not for cyclophosphamide or adriamycin. Though this meta-analysis has been criticised for its statistical methods, a number of clinical trials comparing different platinum dose intensities have been initiated.

There are two randomized studies supporting the hypothesis of a steep dose-response curve for cisplatin. In the Hong Kong Ovarian Carcinoma Study Group (1989) study, patients (n = 60) were treated with 50 or 100 mg/m^2 cisplatin in combination with cyclophosphamide 750 mg/m^2. Recurrence-free survival was significantly higher in the "high-dose" subgroup. The low-dose treatment arm of a very similar trial conducted by KAYE et al. (1992) had to be closed for ethical reasons.

Table 11.36. Randomized comparison of P, PC, and PAC in advanced ovarian cancer (toxicity data and survival data)

	P (50)[a]	PC (50/650)[a]	PAC (50/50/650)[a]
Thrombopenia °3	2.5%	2.5%	7%
Leukopenia °3	2%	3%	8%
Deaths during therapy	0	0	2 (general infections, low performance status
Neurotoxicity °2	4%	6%	4%
Intractable vomiting	20%	15%	23%
Overall response	49%	56%	66%
pCR	20%	21%	26%
Median survival (months)	19.4	21.4	23.8

P, Platinum (cisplatin); C, cyclophosphamide; A, adriamycin.
[a] Figures in parentheses show dose in mg/m^2.

Table 11.37. High-dose carboplatin: results from phase I–II trials

Author	OZOLS et al. (1986)	TEN BOKKEL HUININK et al. (1989)	GEORGE et al. (1988)	REED et al. (1990)	PERREN et al. (1988)
Carboplatin	800 mg/m² q5w	800 mg/m² q5w	800 mg/m² q5w	800 mg/m² + GM-CSF q5w	0.52–1.0 g/m² q4–5w
Stage	Advanced, platinum refractory	Platinum refractory <1 year	III/IV	Advanced, platinum refractory	IV
Clinical CR		18%	61%		29%/19%
OR	35%	39%	84%	35%	50%/62%

CR, complete response; OR, overall response.

On the other hand a prospective randomized GOG trial comparing 4 times cisplatin 100 mg/m² and cyclophosphamide 1000 mg/m² given at 3-week intervals versus cisplatin 50 mg/m² and cyclophosphamide 500 mg/m² given 8 times at 3-week intervals ($n = 450$) showed no significant difference in disease-free or overall survival (McGuire et al. 1995). The received/projected dose intensity in this trial was 0.46/0.52 in the low-dose arm and 0.90/1.03 for the high-dose arm. Similarly, an Italian trial of 50 mg/m² cisplatin q1w × 9 versus 75 mg/m² q3w × 6 did not show any significant difference between the two treatment arms (Colombo et al. 1993).

Since these trials were conducted, two new clinically relevant alternatives to dose intensification have become available. Hematotoxicity, which is generally dose limiting with carboplatin and alkylating agents, can be reduced by the use of hematopoietic growth factors or stem cell support. Table 11.37 shows preliminary data from phase I–II trials of "high-dose" carboplatin with or without growth factor support (Ozols et al. 1986; ten Bokkel Hiunink et al. 1989; George et al. 1988; Reed et al. 1990; Perren et al. 1988). The dose intensities reported in these trials are twice the conventionally used ones. Response rates as high as 35% in platinum-refractory cancer (defined as progressive disease during or relapse within 6–12 months after conventionally dosed platinum-based polychemotherapy) support the hypothesis of steep dose-response curves for higher dose intensities. Data from phase I trials show that with growth factor support, weekly doses of 200 mg/m² of carboplatin can be administered safely if dose intensification is achieved by shortening therapy intervals (Nitz et al. 1994; Lind et al. 1993).

As most of the agents active against ovarian cancer (e.g., carboplatin, alkylators such as cyclophosphamide, melphalan, thiotepa, etc.) show threatening extramedullary toxicity only at high doses, they are ideal partners in a high-dose setting with stem cell support. Thiotepa, for example, can be escalated by a factor of 20–40 without important extramedullary toxicity. Carboplatin is limited by relevant nephro- and neurotoxicity at doses >2000 mg/m² (Shea et al. 1989). Up to now data refer to small phase I–II high-dose chemotherapy trials with autologous stem cell support in recurrent and advanced ovarian cancer with a poor prognosis.

Table 11.38. World survey of high-dose chemotherapy with autologous hematopoietic progenitor cell support for poor-prognosis ovarian cancer. (Shpall et al. 1995)

Country	No.	Response rate (%)	Median duration (mo)	Median survival (mo)
United States	146	71	6	12
Netherlands	21	60	10	NR
Italy	13	82	NR	NR
France	55	NE	NE	40
Japan	42	NE	NE	48
Total	277			

NR, not recorded; NE, not evaluated.

Table 11.38 gives data from a world survey published by Shpall et al. (1995). Overall response rates are as high as 89% (Stiff et al. 1995) in relapsed and refractory disease and 75% (Shpall et al. 1990) in patients with >3 cm postoperative residuals of stage III/IV disease; response duration is short in these cases. In patients with minimal tumor burden (microscopic disease after initial surgery), 4-year survival rates of 70% have been described (Shinozuka et al. 1991). As the data from the world survey show, the results are promising but highly preliminary (Thigpen 1995). Currently the Southwest Oncology Group is investigating a phase 2 protocol comparing thiotepa/cyclophosphamide/cisplatin and mitoxantrone/cyclophosphamide/carboplatin in patients with residual disease after platinum-containing induction therapy. A phase III trial has not yet been initiated.

As already mentioned, a second possible means of "improving" standard therapy of ovarian cancer consists in the administration of drugs that are non-cross-resistant to platinum and its analogs. The most promising drug in this context is taxol, a diterpene from the Western yew *Taxus brevifolia*. This substance enhances microtubule polymerization and stabilizes preformed microtubules. In more than 1000 patients with platinum-refractory ovarian cancer who were treated with taxol, an overall response rate of 22% was observed (EINZIG 1993).

In the early phase 1 trials of taxol, allergy and cardiotoxicity seemed to be the limiting adverse effects. Anaphylaxis is effectively prevented by premedication with corticoids, antihistamines, and H_2-blockers. In the case of allergy, prolongation of infusion time usually reduces it to a tolerable extent (MEERPOHL 1993). Cardiac monitoring has shown that even with longer infusion schedules, bradycardia appears in about 3% of patients; as it is asymptomatic in the great majority of patients, cardiac monitoring is no longer advised routinely. Data dealing with 3- and 24-h infusion schedules show that grade III–IV (WHO) peripheral neuropathy and hematotoxicity are the most important side-effects after administration of taxol. Peripheral neuropathy may be irreversible and seems to be dose dependent. At conventional doses of taxol (135–175 mg/m^2), neuropathy is observed in 36%–51% of patients, with a 0.5%–1% incidence of grade III–IV (WHO) toxicity (MEERPOHL 1993). Hematotoxicity is mainly confined to neutrophils. Neutropenia correlates with dose and duration of infusion schedule. With the above-mentioned doses, grade IV neutropenia is observed in 42%–51% of patients, with febrile neutropenia in 6%–7%. If the drug is administered within 3 h, grade IV neutropenia is observed in only 19% of patients. As there is no concomitant thrombocytopenia, severe hematological side-effects can be effectively prevented by prophylactic administration of hematopoietic growth factors like G-CSF.

Especially in the treatment of ovarian cancer, pharmacological interventions with cisplatin require optimal scheduling when given in combination with taxol. If cisplatin is given before taxol infusion, there may be a loss of activity of the combination and more severe neutropenia may result. A similar but less marked effect is described for the simultaneous administration of taxol and adriamycin.

In refractory ovarian cancer, a European and Canadian group studied two different doses (135 mg/m^2 and 175 mg/m^2) of taxol and two different infusion schedules (3 h and 24 h). The data are in favor of the higher dosage, but are not conclusive at this point.

In conclusion, it is impossible at present to decide on the optimal dose and scheduling and the dose-response relationship of this new agent in ovarian cancer. Nevertheless, data are already available from a phase III trial comparing taxol/cisplatin and cyclophosphamide/cisplatin (MCGUIRE et al. 1993) in

Table 11.39. Taxol/cisplatin (135/75 mg/m^2) versus cyclophosphamide/cisplatin (750/75 mg/m^2) in suboptimally debulked ovarian cancer (phase III trial; MCGUIRE et al. 1993)

Parameter	Taxol/cisplatin (n = 196)	Cyclophosphamide/ cisplatin (n = 214)
Clinical CR	54%	33%
Pathological CR	25%	20%
Allergy (grade 3/4)	3/2	0/0
Gastroint. toxicity (grade 3/4)	23/6	16/7
Renal toxicity (grade 3/4)	1/0	2/1
Neurotoxicity (grade 3/4)	9/0	6/3

CR, complete response.

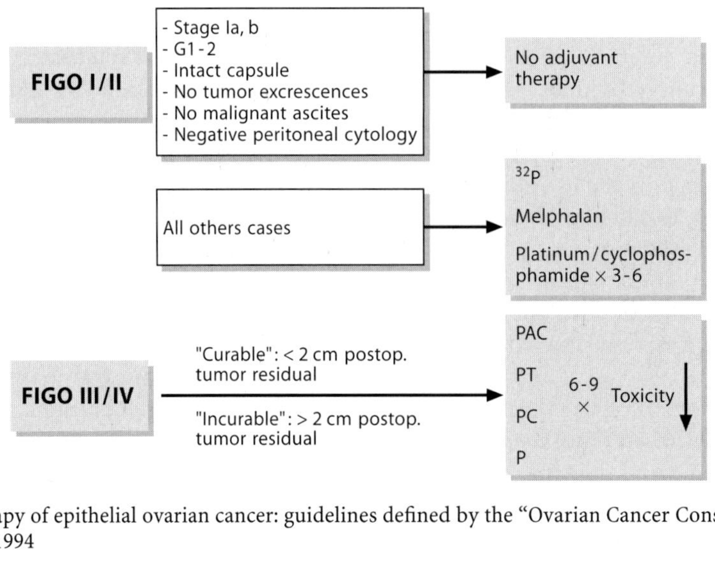

Fig. 11.12. Chemotherapy of epithelial ovarian cancer: guidelines defined by the "Ovarian Cancer Consensus Meeting", Washington D.C., February 1994

patients with a postoperative tumor residual of more than 1 cm (Table 11.39). A significant advantage for the taxol/cisplatin regimen is evident, so that this combination is assumed to be the new standard regimen (ASCO 1994).

11.10.4 Conclusions

Data from the text can be summarized by the guidelines defined during the "Ovarian Cancer Consensus Meeting" in February 1994 in Washington D.C. (Fig. 11.12):

1. FIGO Ia, Ib, G1 tumors require no adjuvant chemotherapy.
2. Stage I, G3 tumors and clear cell carcinoma require adjuvant chemotherapy.
3. Every ovarian cancer > stage IB requires postoperative chemotherapy.
4. Platinum + cyclophosphamide is the "standard" regimen; early data suggest that the combination of cisplatin and taxol is superior to the combination of cisplatin and cyclophosphamide.
5. Carboplatin is preferable to cisplatin.
6. In FIGO stage III and IV tumors, chemotherapy should be continued for 6–9 cycles.

Special points of interest for further research in chemotherapy of ovarian cancer are optimal scheduling of taxol therapy and evaluation of high-dose chemotherapy with autologous stem cell support.

11.11 The Role of Intraperitoneal Chemotherapy

U. Nitz and H.G. Bender

11.11.1 Rationale for Intraperitoneal Chemotherapy: Preclinical and Early Clinical Data

Ovarian cancer, even when advanced, is often confined to the abdominal cavity and rarely represents systemic disease. Therefore very early in the 1950s the idea that administration of drugs to the region of the body containing the cancer might be more effective than systemic chemotherapy was common. In the late 1970s Dederick et al. (1978) studied a pharmacokinetic model for regional chemotherapy that strongly suggested a considerable pharmacological advantage for direct application of the cytostatics to the body cavity. This advantage is maximal if the drug meets the following criteria:

1. It is active in ovarian cancer, with a steep dose-response curve.
2. It is active without requiring activation by different metabolic steps.
3. There is low clearance from the intra-abdominal compartment and high clearance from the systemic circulation (high first-pass effect).
4. It is well tolerated by the peritoneal lining even at high concentrations.

The most widely used drugs in ovarian cancer are alkylating agents, platinum analogs, paclitaxel, mitoxantrone, and anthracyclines. Most of the alkylating agents have to be activated in the liver and/or act through their metabolites, so that these agents are not appropriate for intraperitoneal chemotherapy. Anthracyclines, on the other hand, cause a significant amount of local irritation, so that they are of minor importance in intracavitary chemotherapy. For these reasons platinum analogs, paclitaxel, and mitoxantrone are the best investigated drugs.

Table 11.40 gives the most important preclinical and clinical data for the above-mentioned cytostatics (Markman 1986; Pfeiffer et al. 1990; Levin and Hryniuk 1987a,b; Markman et al. 1990, 1991a, 1991d; Schuler and Ehinger 1990; Alberts et al. 1985). The carboplatin analog causes more profound systemic side-effects, such as myelosuppression, than does cisplatin. Furthermore, a preclinical model suggested that carboplatin has a lower degree of tissue penetration than cisplatin (Los et al. 1989). Therefore cisplatin is generally preferred in intraperitoneal chemotherapy. Combination with i.v. carboplatin is feasible without excessive toxicity. In cases with resistance to systemic platinum therapy, response rates seem to be low (Markman et al. 1991c). Mitoxantrone is well tolerated locally and the systemic drug concentration is low at conventional doses (25 mg/m^2) (Hilfrich et al. 1989; Schuler and Ehninger 1990); in several trials it has been effective even in platinum-resistant disease (Markman et al. 1990, 1991a).

Up to now paclitaxel has been evaluated mainly in phase 1 trials. The pharmacological advantage of i.p. administration is considerable; even in a heavily pretreated population with bulky peritoneal disease there was evidence of antitumor activity (McGuire 1995). There are practically no data concerning dose-response effects. The ongoing GOG (Gynecologic

Table 11.40. Characteristics of cytostatics used in intraperitoneal chemotherapy

Agent	Peak peritoneal cavity/plasma concentration ratio	Local side-effects at conventional doses	Systemic side-effects	Dose-response curve	Remission rates (small-volume disease)
Cisplatin	20	(+) (100 mg/m^2)	(+)	Steep	25%–30% pCR
Carboplatin	18	(+) (400 mg/m^2)	++ Myelo-suppression	Steep	25% pCR
Mitoxantrone	620	++ (25–30 mg/m^2)	(+)	Steep	25% pCR
Paclitaxel	1000	++ (<125 mg/m^2)	(+)	?	20%–30% pCR

pCR, pathological complete remission.

Oncology Group) phase II trials recommend doses of 60 mg/m^2 (weekly) (McGuire 1995). Until more data are available, paclitaxel is recommended especially in platinum-resistant disease.

The cytotoxics are generally applied by single use or permanent indwelling catheters directly into the peritoneal cavity (see Sect. 11.13.2). In contrast to systemic drug delivery, the systemic drug uptake from the peritoneal cavity occurs by the mechanism of free surface diffusion. Experimental models with different cytotoxic drugs have confirmed that the ability of drugs to penetrate into tissue ranges from several cell layers to 1–2 mm (Ozols et al. 1979; Los et al. 1989). In heavily preoperated patients or patients who have already had i.p. chemotherapy, drug distribution may be restricted by adhesion formation, causing suboptimal activity of therapy. On a theoretical basis, therefore, i.p. chemotherapy will be most effective in patients with few adhesions and small-volume residual disease.

11.11.2 Technique of Intraperitoneal Chemotherapy

Intraperitoneal chemotherapy requires repeated paracentesis or insertion of a semipermanent catheter either sub- or transcutaneously. Paracentesis is performed under local anesthesia in an area where no intestinal adhesions to the abdominal wall are suspected (clinical and/or ultrasound verification). If there is no ascites, entrance to the cavity is usually felt as a loss of resistance when the syringe fluid passes freely into the abdominal cavity. Generally aspiration is recommended to exclude inadvertent entry into a bowel loop. If greater volumes of fluid pass easily, good distribution is probable, but most authors recommend confirmation by injection of a water-soluble radio-opaque dye or radioactive material suitable for external imaging. In the absence of outflow obstruction, peritoneal lavage with warm isotonic saline should be performed to prevent protein binding of the cytostatics. To allow optimal distribution of the therapeutic agents, volumes of 1–1.5 l are needed.

The most commonly reported complication is inflow obstruction of semipermanent catheters, which occurs in 2.1%–8.8% of the cases. Injury of the bowel or vascular structures is infrequent (0.0%–3.5%) (Vaccarello and Hoskins 1995). In a series of 227 patients, Davidson et al. (1991) reported an 8.8% incidence of infections due to semipermanent catheters, with a peritonitis rate of 0.9%. Catheter placement at the time of surgery does not seem to cause higher infection rates (Braly et al. 1986; Davidson et al. 1991). Subcutaneously implanted systems are superior to transcutaneous catheters with regard to infections.

Overall, i.p. therapy may be employed in selected patients with reasonable morbidity. Subcutaneous implantation of a semipermanent device allows repeated access to the peritoneal cavity and minimizes the risk of infection.

11.11.3 Impact on Survival of Salvage and Initial Postoperative Therapy

There are no prospective randomized trials evaluating the impact of salvage i.p. regimens in refractory or recurrent ovarian cancer. Results from a phase I–II study (Howell et al. 1987) showed long-term survival (median survival >4 years) especially for patients with small-volume disease (<2 cm largest residual tumor diameter). In patients with larger residual tumor masses a median survival of less than 1 year was documented. These data have been confirmed for patients with small-volume residual disease (n = 58) treated with three different regimens (cisplatin + etoposide/cisplatin + cytarabine/mitoxantrone) at the Memorial Sloan-Kettering

Hospital (REICHMANN et al. 1989; MARKMAN et al. 1991b). In patients responding to i.p. therapy, median survival was 40 months, compared to 19 months for nonresponders.

For primary postoperative i.p. therapy, on the other hand, a phase III trial has recently been published (ALBERTS et al. 1995). This trial compares i.p. cisplatin + cyclophosphamide versus i.v. cisplatin + cyclophosphamide in patients with optimally debulked stage III ovarian cancer. The pathologically documented complete remission rates for the i.p. regimen were 40% versus 31% in the i.v. arm (P = 0.10) and survival was significantly longer in the i.p. arm (49 vs 41 months of median survival, 560 eligible patients).

11.11.4 Conclusion

Due to theoretical considerations, i.p. chemotherapy will be effective only in patients with small-volume residual disease. Thus this approach will be confined to patients with small-volume residual disease after operation (phase III data available) or patients with minimal or no evidence of disease after postoperative systemic chemotherapy (phase I–II data available). Agents used in intracavitary chemotherapy should be well tolerated locally, should have steep dose-response curves, and should be slowly eliminated from the peritoneal cavity and quickly eliminated from the systemic circulation. Agents that have been evaluated and meet these demands are platinum analogs, mitoxantrone, and probably paclitaxel. In disease resistant to systemic platinum therapy, platinum analogs should not be used.

11.12 Hormonal Therapy

G. EMONS and K.-D. SCHULZ

11.12.1 Introduction

Platinum-based chemotherapy and radical surgical concepts have significantly increased short- and medium-term survival in patients with advanced epithelial ovarian cancer. Substantially improved cure rates, however, have not been achieved during the past decade despite the early promise of high response rates to cisplatin chemotherapy, and the overall effects on survival have been modest (OZOLS et al. 1992). In particular, after failure of platinum compounds, available second- or third-line chemotherapic agents, including paclitaxel, achieve only modest response rates of around 20% at best (OZOLS et al. 1992; TRIMBLE et al. 1993; TEN BOKKEL HUININK et al. 1993; HOSKINS and SWENERTON 1994). Chemotherapy regimens conventionally used in ovarian cancer patients have relevant acute toxicity. In addition, long-term sequelae, such as secondary myelodysplasia and leukemia, have to be considered (KALDOR et al. 1990; CHERUKU et al. 1993; COLON-OTERO et al. 1993).

In the treatment of breast and endometrial cancers, endocrine manipulations have been a mainstay for decades due to their minimal toxicity combined with satisfactory efficacy (SANTEN et al. 1990; SCHULZ et al. 1987, 1991; EMONS and SCHULZ 1994). Correspondingly, many authors have studied the use of endocrine manipulations of epithelial ovarian cancer, which appears plausible, as these tumors express receptors for steroid, protein, and peptide hormones (Table 11.41). In addition, receptors for a variety of growth factors, other cytokines, and related oncogene products have been demonstrated in ovarian cancers, which might allow for novel therapeutic approaches (BERCHUK et al. 1992; GODWIN et al. 1992; BAST et al. 1993; MALIK and BALKWILL 1991).

11.12.2 Attempts at Endocrine Manipulation of Ovarian Cancer Through Steroid Receptors

Since the beginning of the 1970s, extensive studies have been performed on the expression of steroid receptors in ovarian cancers. In two recent reviews

Table 11.41. Theoretical endocrine manipulations for epithelial ovarian cancer

Hormone receptor in epithelial ovarian cancers	Possible endocrine manipulation
Estrogen receptor (ER)	Estrogens, antiestrogens, aromatase inhibitors
Progesterone receptor (PR)	Progestagens
Androgen receptor (AR)	Androgens, antiandrogens
Gonadotropin receptors (LH-R, FSH-R)	Estrogen/progestagens, LH-RH analogs
Luteinizing hormone-releasing hormone receptor (LH-RH-R)	LH-RH analogs

(Slotman 1990; Rao and Slotman 1991), 65 original papers regarding this topic were discussed, summarizing the data of more than 2000 patients. Approximately 60% of epithelial ovarian cancers expressed estrogen receptors (ER), 50% progesterone receptors (PR), and 69% androgen receptors (AR). In 36% of ovarian cancers both ER and PR were expressed, while only 25% of these tumors had neither ER nor PR (Slotman 1990; Rao and Slotman 1991).

Many authors have tried to correlate steroid receptor status in ovarian cancers with parameters like FIGO stage, histological type, and grading. However, only uncertain or contradictory relationships have been identified. At best, it could be demonstrated that in diploid tumors PR and/or high concentrations of AR are expressed with a higher frequency (Rao and Slotman 1991). In addition, the value of steroid receptors as prognostic factors has been assessed. Regarding ER, results are contradictory (Rao and Slotman 1991; Kieback et al. 1993). High PR and/or AR concentrations are significantly correlated with longer survival times, but only the PR concentration can be considered an independent prognosticator (Slotman et al. 1990).

In view of the high frequency of steroid receptor-positive ovarian cancers, many clinical trials have been performed with steroids or their respective antagonists aiming at these receptors. In these studies, basically the approaches proven to be effective in the endocrine treatment of breast and endometrial cancer have been applied.

11.12.2.1 Antiestrogens, Aromatase Inhibitors

Tamoxifen has been studied in a series of phase II clinical trials in patients with advanced relapsed ovarian cancer (Myers et al. 1981; Schwartz et al. 1982; Landoni et al. 1985; Shirey et al. 1985; Slevin et al. 1986; Weiner et al. 1987; Hatch et al. 1991; van der Burg et al. 1993; Ahlgren et al. 1993). Overall, a 9.1% rate of objective remissions (30 out of 328 patients) was achieved. While some of these studies observed no objective remissions at all (0 out 99 patients, Landoni et al. 1985; Shirey et al. 1985; Slevin et al. 1986), in a recent trial performed by the Gynecologic Oncology Group (Hatch et al. 1991) a response rate of 17% (18 of 105 patients) in women who relapsed after cisplatin treatment was seen. Also Ahlgren et al. (1993), evaluating the efficacy of high-dose tamoxifen (80 mg/day for 30 days, then 40 mg/day) in 29 patients with chemoresistant ovarian cancer, obtained five responses (17%), two of them exceeding 5 years in duration. In some of the aforementioned trials, high frequencies of disease stabilization during tamoxifen treatment were seen: 35% (Landoni et al. 1985), 80% (Shirey et al. 1985) and 28% (Hatch et al. 1991). So far no controlled trials have been performed on the use of tamoxifen as a single agent in ovarian cancer. The combination of tamoxifen with chemotherapy (cisplatin plus adriamycin) has been evaluated in a prospective randomized trial in 100 patients: the addition of tamoxifen to the chemotherapy had no beneficial effect (Schwartz et al. 1989).

In a phase II clinical trial on the efficacy of the aromatase inhibitor aminoglutethimide, no objective remissions were seen among 15 patients with advanced refractory ovarian cancer (Ahlgren et al. 1993).

11.12.2.2 Progestagens

Since the beginning of the 1960s, various progestagens have been tested in different dosages in patients with advanced ovarian cancer. The published data show an overall response rate of 13% (66 of 507 patients). In addition, approximately 10% patients experienced a stabilization of disease (Slotman 1990; Rao and Slotman 1991; van der Burg et al. 1993; Ahlgren et al. 1993; Malfetano et al. 1993).

A trial in patients suffering from well-differentiated endometrioid ovarian cancers (Rendina et al. 1982) resulted in a response rate of 55% (18 of 33 patients). In other trials with large numbers of cases, however, only modest response rates were seen, e.g., 2% (1 of 41 patients: EORTC-Gynecological Cancer Cooperative Group, Hamerlynck et al. 1985) or 9% (Northern California Oncology Group, Sikic et al. 1986). Controlled trials evaluating single-agent progestagens in ovarian cancer have not been performed so far. Controlled trials assessing the effect of the addition of a progestagen to polychemotherapy failed to demonstrate an improvement in response rates (Slotman 1990) or survival time (Jeppson et al. 1987) in comparison to patients receiving only chemotherapy.

No matter whether or not progestagens have specific antitumor effects in ovarian cancer, high doses of these compounds (e.g., 500 mg medroxyprogesterone acetate orally per day) can have positive general effects on the patients' well-being. In women suffering from tumor cachexia, high-dose progestins can increase appetite and weight and often improve the patients' mood (SCHULZ 1991). These positive effects of high-dose progestagen treatment, however, are limited by the adverse effects of these steroids (diabetogenic activity, hypertension) (SCHMIDT-RHODE 1991). In particular, thromboembolic events can be a major pitfall of high-dose progestagens in patients with advanced ovarian cancer, as these women already have an increased risk of this complication due to their primary disease (SCHMIDT-RHODE 1991).

11.12.2.3 Combinations of Progestagens with Estrogens or Antiestrogens

Estrogens can induce PR in ovarian cancer cells (HAMILTON et al. 1984). On this theoretical basis, cyclic estrogen-progestin therapy might be superior to single-agent progestagens in ovarian cancer. FREEDMAN et al. (1986) studied the sequential administration of ethinylestradiol (50–100 µg/day) and medroxyprogesterone acetate (100–200 mg/day) in 65 patients with advanced chemotherapy-resistant ovarian cancer. Nine women (14%) experienced objective remissions and 13 (20%), disease stabilization. Nine patients, however, suffered from relevant nausea and vomiting during this therapy, and three had vascular complications, including one case of hemiplegia (FREEDMAN et al. 1986). In a subsequent trial, using a reduced estrogen (50 µg ethinylestradiol/day on days 1–7) and an increased progestin dose (400 mg medroxyprogesterone acetate/day on days 8–25), FROMM et al. (1991) observed four partial remissions (17%) among 25 patients with refractory epithelial ovarian cancer with positive estrogen receptors. In addition, two "incomplete remissions" and 11 cases of stable disease were seen. No relevant adverse effects occurred in this trial with reduced estrogen doses.

The combination of progestagens with tamoxifen, which might also induce PR, yielded discouraging results. No objective remissions were obtained by JAKOBSEN et al. (1987), BELINSON et al. (1987), comparing single-agent megestrol acetate (MGA) with a combination of MGA plus tamoxifen, did not observe any remission in either group of patients. Twenty-one percent of women treated with single-agent MGA and 53% of patients receiving MGA plus tamoxifen had stable disease, but overall progression-free intervals did not differ between the two groups.

11.12.2.4 Hormone Replacement Therapy

Bilateral oophorectomy is, with very few exceptions, an obligatory component of primary therapy for ovarian cancer. Many patients, in particular premenopausal women, suffer significantly from the estrogen deficiency caused by this procedure. Due to the high frequency of ER- and/or PR-positive ovarian cancers, many physicians have considered hormone replacement therapy (HRT) to be hazardous for these patients. The biological function of ER and PR in epithelial ovarian cancers, however, seems to be different from that in breast and endometrial cancer (EMONS and SCHULZ 1994), a phenomenon which might also explain the poor response rates of ovarian cancer to (anti)steroidal treatments. Therefore, on a theoretical basis, some authors have recommended HRT in patients with ovarian cancer (e.g., LAURITZEN 1990; BRECKWOLDT 1993; EMONS et al. 1993c). Recently, a retrospective epidemiological study on 373 patients aged 50 years or younger who had undergone bilateral oophorectomy for epithelial ovarian cancer demonstrated that HRT (mainly conjugated estrogens ± norgestrel) was unlikely to have a detrimental effect on the prognosis of these patients. On the contrary, even a trend (not statistically significant) towards longer relapse-free intervals and survival was seen in patients receiving HRT (EELES et al. 1991). The authors concluded that randomized controlled trials should clarify whether or not there is a beneficial effect of HRT. In the meantime, ovarian cancer patients should receive HRT if necessary, as its benefits (HARLAP 1992) are certainly greater than a putative negative effect (EELES et al. 1991).

11.12.2.5 Androgens, Antiandrogens

In view of the high frequency of AR-positive ovarian cancers and the known efficacy of androgens in breast cancer, KAVANAGH et al. (1987) studied the use of the androgen fluoxymestrone in 16 patients with advanced refractory ovarian cancer. No objective response was seen.

As ovarian cancers produce large amounts of androgens, RAO and SLOTMAN (1991) speculated that these steroids might stimulate tumor proliferation through the AR which are expressed by many of these carcinomata. Based on this hypothesis, these authors examined the in vitro effects of the 3-hydroxysteroid-dehydrogenase inhibitor epostan and of several antiandrogens. These compounds inhibited the proliferation of AR-positive ovarian cancer cell lines as well as of 60% of primary cultures derived from ovarian carcinomata (Slotman and Rao 1989a,b). These findings stimulated a phase II trial by the Gynecological Cancer Cooperative Group of the EORTC on the efficacy of the antiandrogen flutamide in patients with refractory advanced ovarian cancer (Rao and Slotman 1991). So far, however, only two responses (6%) among 33 patients have been reported from this trial (van der Burg et al. 1993).

11.12.3 Attempts at Endocrine Manipulation of Ovarian Cancer Through Gonadotropin Receptors

A large body of epidemiological and experimental data exists to suggest that epithelial ovarian cancer could be dependent on gonadotropin secretion (Emons et al. 1990a,b, 1992a,b; Foekens and Klijn 1992; Emons and Schally 1994). If this were the case, suppression of endogenous gonadotropins should have beneficial effects in ovarian cancer patients. This suppression of secretion of luteinizing hormone and follicle-stimulating hormone is most elegantly achieved by the selective medical hypophysectomy obtained after chronic administration of superactive analogs of luteinizing hormone-releasing hormone (LH-RH) (Schally et al. 1990; Emons and Schally 1994). Parmar et al. (1985) reported on a patient with advanced ovarian cancer who had relapsed after surgery, chemotherapy, and radiotherapy and who was then treated with the LH-RH agonist triptorelin. Concomitantly with the suppression of gonadotropins there was a marked shrinkage of the tumor mass which lasted for 12 months. This encouraging report stimulated a series of phase II trials on the use of LH-RH agonists in patients with advanced refractory ovarian cancer (Parmar et al. 1988a,b; Kullander et al. 1987; Jäger et al. 1989; Kavanagh et al. 1989; Vavra et al. 1990; Lind et al. 1992; van der Burg 1993). In these trials, 21 objective remissions (12%) and 32 cases of stable disease (19%) were observed among 171 evaluable patients. Duration of response varied between 26 and 98+ weeks (Emons and Schulz 1994).

In a multicenter controlled phase III trial, investigators from Finland, Sweden, Israel, and Germany have tried to corroborate these findings (Emons et al. 1990a). The study was performed in patients in whom advanced ovarian cancer of FIGO stages III or IV have been diagnosed for the first time. After conventional surgical treatment and staging, the patients were randomized into two groups receiving either monthly injections of a long-acting preparation of the LH-RH agonist triptorelin or placebo (double blinded) for up to 4 years or until death. For ethical reasons, all patients received a first-line platinum-based polychemotherapy and, if necessary, second- or third-line chemotherapies. A total of 130 patients has been accrued. Though suppression of gonadotropin levels was consistently seen in patients treated with triptorelin, no beneficial effect on survival could be achieved by the LH-RH administration (Decapeptyl-Ovarian Cancer Group, in preparation). It is true that the results of this trial do not absolutely preclude a marginal effect of single-agent LH-RH agonists in ovarian cancer, but they suggest that these agents are of limited clinical efficacy, even in the absence of simultaneous chemotherapy, as many of the patients in our trial had long periods when they received only the LH-RH agonist and no chemotherapy. It should be mentioned, however, that the other endocrine therapies showing some activity in phase II trials in patients with ovarian cancer (tamoxifen, progestagens, estrogen–progestagen combinations) have not been subjected to prospective controlled trials. Also the chemotherapic agents presently used in second- and third-line treatment have not been evaluated in randomized phase III trials assessing whether or not they really have a beneficial effect on survival.

A few anecdotal case reports suggest that the suppression of endogenous gonadotropins by LH-RH agonists could be of clinical use in patients with malignant granulosa cell tumors (Kauppila et al. 1990) or with androgen-producing ovarian tumors (Lamberts et al. 1982; Kennedy et al. 1987; Emons et al. 1992c). This issue, however, requires further systematic studies (Emons and Schally 1994).

11.12.4 Attempts at Endocrine Manipulation of Ovarian Cancer Through LH-RH Receptors

Apart from its function as a key hormone in the hypothalamic-pituitary-gonadal axis, LH-RH is probably also involved in the regulation of extrapituitary tissues. In human placenta, an autocrine system based on LH-RH has been convincingly demonstrated (MERZ et al. 1991). Such LH-RH based autocrine systems have also been detected in breast, prostate, and endometrial cancer (HARRIS et al. 1991; LIMONTA et al. 1993; EMONS et al. 1993a).

Approximately 80% of epithelial ovarian cancers express specific binding sites for LH-RH (EMONS et al. 1989; PAHWA et al. 1989). Several groups have reported that the in vitro proliferation of human ovarian cancer cell lines could be inhibited by analogs of LH-RH (OHTANI et al. 1990; THOMPSON et al. 1991; EMONS et al. 1993b). Ovarian cancer cell lines and biopsies from primary ovarian cancers express specific high-affinity binding sites for LH-RH and the mRNA for the human LH-RH receptor (EMONS et al. 1993b; IRMER et al. 1994).

In addition, the production of LH-RH and the expression of its mRNA could be demonstrated in human ovarian cancer cell lines (OHNO et al. 1993; IRMER et al. 1994). These findings strongly support the concept of an autocrine regulatory system based on LH-RH in epithelial ovarian cancer. So far, however, no easy clinical exploitation of this autocrine system appears realizable, as much higher concentrations of LH-RH analogs are necessary for direct inhibition of ovarian cancer cells than are achieved with the presently available depot preparations. It needs to be emphasized that the LH-RH analogs used at present in clinical medicine have been designed to exert maximal activity at the pituitary level. The development of LH-RH analogs with maximal activities at extrapituitary sites or of LH-RH analogs with cytotoxic activity (SCHALLY et al. 1990; EMONS and SCHALLY 1994) might allow for an effective clinical exploitation of direct LH-RH effects on ovarian cancer in the future.

11.12.5 Growth Factors and Other Cytokines

Growth factors such as epidermal growth factor, insulin-like growth factor-1, macrophage colony-stimulating factor (M-CSF), and platelet-derived growth factor, the receptors for these growth factors, and related oncogene products, e.g., the HER-2/neu protein or the fms protein, play an important role in the regulation of proliferation of ovarian cancer (BERCHUK et al. 1992; GODWIN et al. 1992; BAST et al. 1993; KACINSKI 1993; HENRIKSEN et al. 1993; HOFMANN et al. 1994). Also interleukin-6 (IL-6) is suggested to be an autocrine growth factor for epithelial ovarian cancer (WATSON et al. 1993). The role of tumor necrosis factor-α (TNF-α) in ovarian cancer is controversial. Some authors have shown that i.p. injections of this compound effectively reduce malignant ascites in the palliative situation, though not prolonging survival (KAUFMANN et al. 1990; MARKMAN and BEREK 1993; KARCK et al. 1993). Other authors, in contrast, point out that TNF promotes proliferation of ovarian cancer and its invasive capacity and therefore suggest the therapeutic use of TNF antagonists (MALIK and BALKWILL 1991; WU et al. 1993; NAYLOR et al. 1993). So far, the picture is still obscure and much work remains to be done before the complex network of cytokines and growth factors will be sufficiently understood, especially regarding ovarian cancer. Possible therapeutic applications might evolve from the use of antibodies to growth factor receptors and related oncogene products, their use for targeting toxins or radioisotopes, or the application of antisense oligonucleotides for growth factors or cytokines (SCHRÖDER and BENDER 1992; RODRIGUEZ et al. 1993; WATSON et al. 1993; BECKMANN et al. 1993). It is true that many of the tumor-promoting effects of hematopoietic growth factors (M-CSF) or cytokines (TNF, IL-6) observed in experimental systems might not be of relevance in the clinical situation (SCHRÖDER and BENDER 1992). Before the exact mechanism of action of this complex network is sufficiently understood, however, uncritical applications of these compounds should be avoided (SCHRÖDER and BENDER 1992).

11.12.6 Conclusions

In spite of the intensive efforts of many investigators, no endocrine therapy for ovarian cancer has thus far been developed which has an efficacy comparable to that of hormonal manipulations of breast and endometrial cancer (Table 11.42). Addition of endocrine treatments (tamoxifen, progestins, LH-RH analogs) to chemotherapy does not increase the efficacy of the cytotoxic drugs. The response rates obtained with endocrine salvage therapies in patients with advanced refractory ovarian cancer are in the range of 10% on average and 17% at best (HATCH et al. 1991; AHLGREN et al. 1993) and have not been corroborated by controlled trials. It needs to be emphasized, however, that even the most active chemotherapeutic agent for the salvage situation, paclitaxel, has response rates of approximately 20%, and response durations of a few months in ovarian cancer patients refractory to platinum compounds (TEN BOKKEL HUININK et al. 1993; TRIMBLE et al.

Table 11.42. Status of hormonal treatments of advanced refractory ovarian cancer

Therapy	Efficacy
Antiestrogens	0%–17% objective responses (mean = 9%), often stable disease, no relevant toxicity
Progestagens	0%–55% objective responses (mean = 13%), about 10% stable disease; possible adverse effects at high doses
Estrogen/progestin combinations	Approximately 15% objective remissions, often stable disease; possible adverse effects
LH-RH agonists	0%–22% objective remissions (mean = 12%), about 20% stable disease, no relevant toxicity
Antiandrogens	About 6% objective remissions in a pilot study
Androgens	None
Aromatase inhibitors	None

Table 11.43. Recommended hormonal therapies in advanced refractory ovarian cancer

Agent	Dose
Tamoxifen	40 mg orally/day or 80 mg orally/day for 30 days, then 40 mg/day
Medroxyprogesterone acetate (MPA)	200–500 mg orally/day
LH-RH analogs, e.g. leuprorelin, triptorelin, goserelin	One depot injection or depot implantation/4 weeks

1993). Other second- or third-line chemotherapeutic agents such as hexamethylmelamine, ifosfamide, or etoposide also achieve response rates of 20% at best and short progression-free intervals (Ozols et al. 1992; Hoskins and Swenerton 1994).

None of these chemotherapeutic agents have been evaluated in controlled trials in the salvage situation. Thus, though the efficacy of endocrine therapy in relapsed refractory ovarian cancer is definitely poor, the results of the available chemotherapeutic alternatives, including paclitaxel, are not strikingly superior. In addition, the toxicity of the chemotherapeutic regimens, which is very often striking in these moribund patients, has to be considered. Finally, the costs of these salvage chemotherapies, which are probably in vain in up to 80% and more of the truly platinum-refractory cases, must be taken into account. Therefore, endocrine therapies (Table 11.43) which are devoid of relevant toxicity (except for high-dose progestins and high-dose estrogen/progestin combinations), which are available at reasonable expense, and which can be applied without interfering with in-patient procedures still remain a viable therapeutic option for patients who have failed cytotoxic chemotherapy or cannot tolerate its effects (Ozols et al. 1992). Unless the unspecific effects of high-dose progestins (improvement of appetite and mood) are desired, these compounds should be avoided due to their potential risks. LH-RH analogs, though virtually having no adverse effects, are not cheap, require injections, and are of doubtful efficacy at the present dosages. In our opinion, tamoxifen, which has been shown to have a reasonable activity in two recent trials (Hatch et al. 1991; Ahlgren et al. 1993), is probably the best buy regarding response rates, lack of toxicity, and reasonable costs. Future research on the direct effects of LH-RH analogs, antiandrogens, and the growth factor/cytokine system might open up new perspectives for efficacious hormonal treatments of ovarian cancer.

11.13 Combined Treatment Modalities

H.W. Vahrson

Combined treatment modalities comprising primary surgery (PS), chemotherapy (CT), staging or cytoreductive second-look operation (SLO), and radiotherapy (RT) have been used in many centers. The employed methods differ with respect to the sequence of chemotherapy and radiotherapy. To better describe these methods, the following subdivision may be used:

1. Sequential: PS – CT – SLO – RT
2. Sandwich: PS – CT – RT – CT ± SLO or
PS – RT – CT – RT – CT ± SLO
3. Simultaneous: PS – CT + RT ± SLO

These combined treatment modalities were introduced in an attempt to achieve results in advanced stages superior to those which could be achieved by RT or CT alone. However, it must be stressed that all of the combined treatment modalities considerably elevate the risk of acute and late side-effects which may cause interruption or discontinuation of treatment or necessitate surgical intervention.

11.13.1 Sequential Chemo-radiotherapy for Consolidation

When, after initial cytoreductive surgery and several cycles of chemotherapy in advanced ovarian cancer patients, second-look surgery (SLS) reveals a histopathological complete remission, the likelihood of recurrence is still about 50% (Rubin et al. 1988). As the abdominal cavity is the predominant site of recurrence, it has seemed reasonable to continue treatment with consolidative whole abdominal irradiation (WAI). The moving strip and/or open field technique with or without pelvic boost (APRT), as well as special modifications of these techniques, have been used for consolidation. An analysis of available reports on WAI following initial surgery, platinum-containing chemotherapy, and SLS is presented in Table 11.44. The 2- to 5-year disease-free survival (DFS) is 73%. Considering the range of 2–5 years, this result is not so different from the expected 50% 5-year DFS with no further treatment after SLS. The acute and late side-effects of WAI are discussed elsewhere (see Sect. 11.9).

Recently, Sorbe et al. (1996) reported on the results of a prospective multicenter trial of the Swedish-Norwegian Ovarian Cancer Study Group in stage III ovarian cancer patients with complete surgical remission who were randomized to receive either APRT or chemotherapy as consolidation treatment. Pretreatment consisted in four cycles of cisplatin/doxorubicin (50 mg/m^2 each). Of the 172 patients found to be in surgically complete remission at SLS, 98 had pathological complete remission (pCR) and 74 R_{micro}. The pCR group was randomized to (a) APRT (20 Gy WAI without shielding +20 Gy pelvic boost), (b) chemotherapy (six cycles of adriamycin and cyclophosphamide), or (c) no further treatment. The R_{micro} group was randomized to (a) APRT or (b) chemotherapy (as above). Median follow-up was 53 months (range 24–98 months). In the pCR group the 3-year overall survival (OS) rate was 83% after APRT, 76% after chemotherapy, and 73% after no further treatment. In the R_{micro} group the 3-year OS rate was 46% after APRT and 56% after chemotherapy. Progression-free survival was significantly better in the APRT group than in the control group but not significantly different from that in the chemotherapy group. The rate of recurrences was lowest in the APRT group. Both treatments were well tolerated by the patients. The authors concluded that after pCR consolidation radio- or chemotherapy

Table 11.44. Two- to 5-year DFS in stage III and IV ovarian cancer patients treated with primary surgery, platinum-containing chemotherapy, and cytoreductive SLS, who received WAI for consolidation or salvage. Subsets according to residual disease after completion of SLS

	No residual	R_{micro}	R ≤ 1 cm	R ≤ 2 cm	R > 2 cm	Comment
Hainsworth et al. (1983)	–	3/11	0/5	0/1	–	
Greiner et al. (1985)	20/24	1/4	0/8	0/3	0/2	
Hacker et al. (1985)	–	4/16	2/6[a]	0/8[b]	–	[a]≤5 mm, [b]6–15 mm
Hoskins et al. (1985)	–	0/1	0/6	–	0/1	
Rizel et al. (1985)	7/10	4/12	–	–	0/6	
Rosen et al. (1986)	4/4	2/3	1/2	0/4	0/1	
Cain et al. (1988)	–	5/9	0/1[a]	–	–	[a]2 mm
Green et al. (1988)	9/10		[a]	[a]	[a]	[a]No precise differentiation
Kersh et al. (1988)	1/4	3/3	7/10	1/4		
Kuten et al. (1988)	5/5	12/18	–	1/14	–	
Schray et al. (1988)	–	8/22	6/31[a]	–	–	[a]Incl. ≤2 cm (minority)
Bolis et al. (1990)	–	6/18[a]	0/8	–	–	[a]≤5 mm
Kucera et al. (1990)	–	2/10	0/4	0/2	–	2 DFS, no precise details
Eifel et al. (1991)	–	3/25	–	0/12	–	Twice-daily split-course
Rothenberg et al. (1992)	5/12	–	2/9[a]	–	–	[a]≤5 mm
Reddy et al. (1993)	–	9/22	–	1/22[a]	–	[a]Included R_{macro} 6 cm
Ben-Baruch et al. (1994)	6/10	0/4	–	0/4	–	
Fein et al. (1994)	–	8/11	–	6/17[a]	–	[a]Incl. resected
Chapet et al. (1995)	–	9/26[a]	–	0/6	–	[a]Incl. Ro
Total	57/79 (72%)	79/215 (37%)	18/90 (20%)	9/97 (9%)	0/10	

Note: R_{micro} includes all of the tumors which where resected from R_{macro} to no macroscopic residual at SLS.

seemed to improve progression-free survival (PFS) compared with no further treatment but long-term OS was not significantly different. In the R_{micro} group APRT and chemotherapy seemed to be similarly effective with regard to OS and PFS.

Intraperitoneal instillation of radioactive ^{32}P-chromic phosphate is an alternative to WAI for consolidation, as described above (see Sect. 11.8.6) and is preferred at the ZFG Giessen because of its advantages in application and tolerance.

11.13.2 Sequential Chemo-radiotherapy for Salvage

When no macroscopic residual is found at SLS but when peritoneal washings and/or biopsies from the peritoneal surfaces reveal microsopic residual disease (R_{micro}) it has been supposed that WAI with or without pelvic boost can destroy the cancer cells. The same has been assumed for macroscopic tumor residuals which can be completely removed at SLS. As these completely resected residuals seem to have a similar prognosis, they have been attributed to R_{micro} in most reports and in Table 11.44. In 215 patients the 2- to 5-year DFS was 37%, which is very disappointing. For $R \leq 1$ cm we calculated a 2- to 5-year DFS of 20% in 90 patients, and for $R \leq 2$ cm, a rate of 9% in 97 patients. For $R > 2$ cm no survival was reported.

Mychalczak and Fuks (1993) analyzed reports on stage III ovarian cancer patients from the literature between 1983 and 1990; this analysis included some of the same studies as are detailed in Table 11.44, but with different subsets of tumor size. They found that the 2- to 5-year DFS in 157 patients with "microscopic or no residual tumors" combined was 44%, while it was 27% in 130 patients with "residual tumors <1 cm" and 4% in 51 patients with "larger residual tumors >1 cm." [In the group of tumors >1 cm an incorrect number of 18 instead of 8 in the citation of Hacker et al. (1985) has emerged. After correction the 2- to 5-year DFS of this group was 5%.] The results are very similar to those in Table 11.44. From these results was must conclude that WAI as salvage treatment is only effective in R_{micro}/R completely resected and in some $R \leq 1$ cm tumors at SLS. Thomas (1993), who reviewed 28 clinical trials reporting the results of WAI for consolidation or salvage, also came to the conclusion that WAI should only be used in R_0 and R_{micro} residuals. For macroscopic residuals $R > 1$ cm/$R \leq 2$ cm, the DFS results are so disappointingly low that other treatment modalities (second-line chemotherapy or intraperitoneal application) should be considered.

The possible reasons why patients with microscopic or minimal residual disease have done so poorly are diverse:

1. The overall treatment time was rather long in some reports, due to the technique of WAI or to interruptions because of acute side-effects such as vomiting, diarrhea, or myelosuppression. Prolonged treatment time may be associated with accelerated proliferation of clonogenic tumor cells (stem cells), as mentioned by Dembo (1992). He pointed to the results of Withers et al. (1988) with different fractionation schemes in head and neck cancers. They found the proliferation rates of the stem cells to be constant for the first 4 weeks of a course of fractionated radiotherapy, but after this time the rate of proliferation seemed to accelerate, requiring a higher dose per fraction.
2. In some of the reports the patients received less than 25–30 Gy to the upper abdomen, and a pelvic boost to a total dose of 45–50 Gy was given to only some of the patients. Furthermore, nearly every report includes patients in whom WAI had to be discontinued because of acute side-effects or patient refusal.
3. Tumor cells have an inherently low radiosensitivity. In culture, the radiosensitivity of ovarian cancer cells has been found to be similar to that of mesothelial and fibroblast cells (Rotmensch et al. 1989a,b).
4. The use of a prolonged treatment regimen with more than six cycles of platinum-containing chemotherapy (Fuks et al. 1988) or a dose-intensive treatment regimen (Rothenberg et al. 1992) before WAI may have induced pleiotropic drug-resistant tumor clones which are cross-resistant to radiation. Louie et al. (1985) found that pleiotropic resistance could be induced by stepwise incubation with drugs in a formerly drug-sensitive cell line, and other pleiotropic drug-resistant cell lines could be established from drug-refractory ovarian cancer patients; all of these cell lines were cross-resistant to irradiation. From these experimental data the authors considered the sequential use of radiotherapy following chemotherapy to be less effective than a combined modality approach integrating radiation and chemotherapy prior to the development of drug resistance and cross-resistance to irradiation.

11.13.3 Side-effects of Sequential Chemo-radiotherapy

As already mentioned, the rate of acute and late side-effects of WAI/APRT is higher when WAI/APRT is applied for consolidation or salvage than when it is used as sole postoperative treatment. WHELAN et al. (1992) from PMH Toronto reported the side-effects in their own series of 105 patients who received APRT following chemotherapy with or without previous SLS. *Acute side-effects* mainly consisted in cramps or diarrhea (77%), nausea or vomiting (77%), leukopenia <2000 (32%) or <1000 (2%), and thrombocytopenia <100 000 (42%) or <50 000 (16%); these effects led to treatment delay in 16% and incomplete treatment in 15%. These results differ favorably from those of other authors. FUKS et al. (1988) reported treatment interruptions lasting more than 2 weeks in 5/29 (17%) patients because of diarrhea and vomiting and in 12/29 (41%) because of myelosuppression. A further three (9%) patients could not complete the planned course of radiotherapy. GREINER et al. (1985) reported different rates of interruption or discontinuation depending on the technique of WAI. In the period when the moving strip technique (median treatment time 104 days!) was used, interruptions were required in 15/28 (54%) patients and discontinuation in 7/28 (25%) patients. The corresponding rates with the open-field technique were 4/19 (21%) and 3/19 (16%) respectively.

Late side-effects mainly consist in bowel obstruction, but chronic diarrhea, chronic repeat bleeding, radiation-induced basal lung fibrosis, cystitis, and transient alkaline phosphatase elevation may occur. WHELAN et al. (1992) found bowel obstruction in 12/105 (11%) patients without progressive disease at 5 years of follow-up, of whom nine (9%) needed surgery. A further four obstructions in patients with progressive disease were not considered to represent radiation-induced damage. In their review of the literature, WHELAN et al. calculated a total of 44 (10%) obstructions in 425 patients without progression or recurrence and 15 (33%) obstructions in 45 patients in whom it was not ascertained whether progression or recurrence was present or not at the time of obstruction.

The obstruction rates requiring surgery range from 0% to 30% in the literature (HACKER et al. 1985). These obstruction rates differ unfavorably from the figure of 25/598 (4.2%) reported by FILES et al. (1992) after sole postoperative APRT, of which only 16 (2.7%) required surgery.

The possible reasons for the higher complication rate following WAI for consolidation or salvage include:

1. One or more instance of cytoreductive SLS, causing adhesions
2. More than six cycles of chemotherapy, causing cross-resistance
3. Action of adriamycin and platinum as radiosensitizers in normal tissues
4. Doses >25 Gy to the abdominal and/or >45 Gy to the pelvic field

11.13.4 Hyperfractionated Whole Abdominal Irradiation

Attempts have been undertaken to increase the tolerated dose and decrease the toxicity of salvage WAI in ovarian cancer by means of hyperfractionation. KONG et al. (1988) from M.D. Anderson Hospital, Houston described the method. These authors gave two fractions of 1 Gy each daily with an interval of at least 4 h between the fractions, to a total of 15 Gy over $1\frac{1}{2}$ weeks. After 3 weeks' rest an identical course of 15 Gy was given to a final dose of 30 Gy WAI using the open-field technique. Thus WAI was separated into two segments. The usual posterior shielding of the kidneys to less than 20 Gy and anterior-posterior shielding of the right lobe of the liver to less than 28 Gy was carried out.

EIFEL et al. (1991) published an update in 37 patients who received this twice-daily split-course WAI following SLS with positive findings (R_{micro} 25, R_{macro} 12) after six cycles of cisplatin–cyclophosphamide. Eleven patients also had a boost of 9–20 Gy to sites of gross residual disease after completion of WAI. Only one patient did not complete therapy and two had 1-week prolongation because of hematological toxicity. However, at 3 years all of the 12 patients with gross residual disease prior to WAI had relapsed and died of the disease. Only 5 of the 25 patients (20%) with R_{micro} at SLS were free of disease. Fourteen patients (38%) had bowel obstructions with progressive disease. According to EIFEL et al., it must be concluded that twice-daily split-course WAI is well tolerated and enables a dose intensification (30 Gy/3 weeks). The outcome was not better than in other studies with conventional radiation shedules.

In a recent study, FEIN et al. (1994) from the University of Florida College of Medicine reported on 28 stage III ovarian cancer patients presenting with persistent disease at SLS after they had received between six and 28 (mean 12) courses of cisplatin-based chemotherapy. Patients with gross residual R > 2 cm were excluded. The authors applied split-course WAI using the open-field technique, delivering 0.8 Gy twice daily with a 6 h interval between fractions on 5 days per week. Total dose ranged from 26 to 35.2 Gy; 21 patients received 30.4 Gy. The kidneys were shielded but the liver was not. A pelvic boost with twice-daily fractionation using 0.8–1.2 Gy per fraction to a total boost dose of 3.6–20 Gy (mean 14.54 Gy) was applied to 20 patients after WAI. Two patients (7%) had treatment breaks because of thrombocytopenia. In the 11 patients with R_{micro} at SLS the 2-year and 5-year OS were 73% and 27% and the 3-year and 5-year DFS were 52% and 31% (?) respectively. Two deaths occurred (7%). Four patients (14%) developed small bowel obstruction requiring surgery, of whom two (7%) had no evidence of disease. According to the authors no patient was successfully salvaged in this series.

Conclusion: Twice-daily split-course open-field WAI and twice-daily open-field WAI are well tolerated and have only moderate late toxicity but there is no advantage in survival in comparison to conventional WAI.

11.13.5 Sandwich Radio-chemotherapy at the ZFG Giessen

11.13.5.1 Introduction

Sandwich radio-chemotherapy has been a historical development at the ZFG Giessen. As postoperative treatment traditionally started with one of the two radiation modalities it was an obvious option to administer interim chemotherapy followed by the second radiation modality, and then continuation of chemotherapy. There is a strong argument for sandwich radio-chemotherapy, i.e., integration of radiotherapy into the first cycles of chemotherapy: Presuming that radiotherapy is effective in minimal residual disease (R_{micro}–R <2 cm) it seems unreasonable to wait for the completion of six or more cycles of chemotherapy until WAI is commenced. During chemotherapy, resistance to chemotherapy may already have developed, accompanied by cross-resistance to radiotherapy. This problem of acquired cross-resistance to irradiation does not exist during the first cycles of chemotherapy.

Another point is the poor tolerance of WAI when it is applied for consolidation or salvage, leading to a high percentage of interruptions for more than 2 weeks or to discontinuation. This unfavorable aspect of irradiation can be avoided or even converted to a treatment strategy when a series of WAI is interrupted half way through (e.g., after 15 Gy WAI given within 3 weeks) for 1 week, followed by a cycle of chemotherapy; 3–4 weeks later the second half of the WAI (again 15 Gy, with liver and kidney shielding) is then completed.

The treatment policy, difficulties, and outcome of sandwich radio-chemotherapy will be presented in detail below.

11.13.5.2 Patients and Methods

Patients. From 1970 to 1992, 1086 patients with primary epithelial ovarian cancer were treated at the ZFG Giessen. Of these, 904 patients, treated between 1970 and 1988, had at least 5-years' follow-up. Borderline cases and recurrent disease were excluded but second or multiple primaries were included. The age of the patients ranged from 13 to 89 years (mean 57.9 years).

Primary Surgery and Staging. Primary surgery was performed at the ZFG Giessen in 33% of cases, at associated academic hospitals in 14%, and at other institutions, mainly small departments of gynecology and obstetrics, in 53%, i.e., only one-third of the patients were operated on at the ZFG and two-thirds were transferred to our institution for postoperative primary treatment after initial surgery elsewhere.

Surgery ideally consisted in BSOH and omentectomy and/or tumor debulking in operable cases or staging laparotomy in inoperable cases. The final staging was done at the ZFG according to the rules of the Annual Report, i.e., allocation to the lower stage, but treatment was performed for a higher risk. This downstaging to stage I is obvious when we compare the stage distribution at the ZFG Giessen, where a reoperation was rarely performed, with the UFK Freiburg, where nearly every patient was reoperated on and reevaluated by stage and histology (Table 11.45). This extremely thorough re-evaluation resulted in a reduction of stage I to 6.3% at the UFK Freiburg compared with 34.8% at the ZFG Giessen. Conversely, stage III was found in 50% and stage IV in 28.5% at the UFK Freiburg; the corresponding rates at the ZFG Giessen were 33.9% and 11.6% respectively. The general stage distributions found at German centers reporting their results to the Annual Report can be taken from Table 11.55 (see Sect. 11.15).

Historical Sandwich Radio-chemotherapy. Instead of a description of the many historical and obsolete therapeutic regimens, which changed rapidly due to the introduction of new cytostatic agents in the period in question, only one historical therapy plan for stage III ovarian cancer (optimally cytoreduced) will be presented (Fig. 11.13).

Current Sandwich Radio-chemotherapy. Stage Ia G1 receives no further therapy when accurately staged by the surgeon.

Table 11.45. Relative stage distribution of ovarian cancers at primary surgery at the UFK Freiburg, 1977–84 (Teufel 1986), and the ZFG Giessen, 1979–85 (Vahrson et al. 1991)

	UFK Freiburg		ZFG Giessen	
	No.	%	No.	%
Stage I	17	6.3	117	34.8
Stage II	41	15.2	66	19.6
Stage III	135	50.0	114	33.9
Stage IV	77	28.5	39	11.6
Stage I–IV	270	100.0	336	100.0

Stages Ib, Ic and IIa (intermediate risk cancers) receive ^{32}P combined with a cyclophosphamide push (60 mg/kg) on the 8th day after instillation. Four weeks after the cyclophosphamide push in higher risk cases a series of 30 Gy pelvic irradiation (5 × 1.8 Gy/week) with 18-MV photons from a linear accelerator is administered, completed by two applications of a 10 Gy surface dose to the vaginal stump by HDR-afterloading brachytherapy. With this brachy-/teletherapy combination the total dose to the vaginal wall is 50 Gy and at the site of risk after removal of the uterus, i.e., the space between the pouch of Douglas and the vaginal stump, a dose of about 40 Gy is delivered. The pelvic dose applied by external beam therapy should not exceed 30 Gy when combined with 15–16.5 mCi ^{32}P, which is supposed to add another 30–40 Gy to the pelvic surfaces.

Stage IIb or c (optimally resected) patients without adhesions first receive ^{32}P, to prevent further spilling of tumor cells, followed by a cyclophosphamide push (60 mg/kg) on the 8th day. Four weeks after the push dose, a series of 30 Gy pelvic irradiation (as above) is applied. This is followed by five to six cycles of chemotherapy (PEC: 50 mg/m^2 cisplatin, 60 mg/m^2 epirubicin, 500 mg/m^2 cyclophosphamide each on day 1) at 4-week intervals. Dose intensification by 3-weekly cycles cannot be recommended when the two radiation modalities are integrated.

Operation: Complete BSOH + omental resection

Irradiation:
100-150 mCi ^{198}Au
intraperitoneally

Chemotherapy:
Induction push with 2 of the following cytostatics:

Cyclophosphamide	Adriamycin	Cisplatin
60 mg/kg	100-150 mg/m^2	100 mg/m^2

40 Gy
pelvis

Further therapy with 5-10 AC cycles:

1st day: 40 mg/m^2 adriamycin i.v.
300 mg/m^2 cyclophosphamide i.v.
2nd day: 300 mg/m^2 cyclophosphamide i.v.
3rd day: 300 mg/m^2 cyclophosphamide i.v.
4th day: 300 mg/m^2 cyclophosphamide i.v.

Fig. 11.13. Historical treatment regimen (1980) in stage IIIb ovarian cancers. The sandwich radio-chemotherapy was applied in order from top to bottom. *Left* irradiation; *right* chemotherapy

Stage IIIa–c (optimally and suboptimally resected) and *stage IV* (liver metastasis) patients are the domain of sandwich radio-chemotherapy with WAI (Fig. 11.14), starting with one or two cycles of PEC, followed by the first series of 15 Gy open-field irradiation. Then one PEC cycle is interposed. Treatment is continued with the second series of 15 Gy open-field irradiation, followed by three or more PEC cycles.

In some stage III and IV cases, when there is a rapid fall in the CA-125 level (CA-125 ratio <0.3) and appropriate changes in clinical status during the first PEC cycles, indicating a very high sensitivity to chemotherapy, WAI will be omitted and chemotherapy continued to clinically complete remission. After SLS resulting in R_0 or R_{micro}, in suitable cases ^{32}P is applied for consolidation or salvage treatment. In cases unsuited for ^{32}P instillation (due to adhesions), WAI is given. The sandwich modification of combined radio-chemotherapy as used at the ZFG Giessen has not yet gained acceptance at other centers. This is rather surprising since as long ago as 1985 Louie et al., on the basis of experimental data, suggested the early integration of radio- and chemotherapy prior to the development of resistance and cross-resistance.

Hoskins et al. (1995) reported on a retrospective, nonrandomized study in "high-risk" stage I–III ovarian cancer patients who could be optimally cytoreduced to R_0 at first surgery. In regimen A 75 mg/m^2 cisplatin and 600 mg/m^2 cyclophosphamide were given intravenously every 4 weeks for six cycles, with APRT "sandwiched" between cycles 3 and 4. APRT was initiated 3 weeks after the third cycle with 22.5 Gy mid-plane pelvic irradiation in ten fractions within 2 weeks, followed by 22.5 Gy open-field irradiation in 22 fractions over 4.5 weeks from a 4-MV linear accelerator, using full posterior kidney shields to limit the renal dose to 15 Gy. Regimen B provided only monotherapy with 75 mg/m^2 cisplatin intravenously every 3 weeks for six cycles. The median follow-up time for 131 evaluable patients was 3.7 years (range 0.5–8.4 years). Five-year overall survival and failure-free survival for regimens A and B were 82% vs 48% and 68% vs 48% respectively. In the 63 patients receiving APRT in regimen A, chronic APRT-associated toxity occurred in 17 (27%), with small bowel obstruction requiring surgery in two (3%) and malabsorption syndrome in two (3%). The remaining 13 (21%) had intermittent bloating, cramps, or diarrhea. Two of the 63 patients (3%) did not complete APRT. The results of this study demonstrate the su-

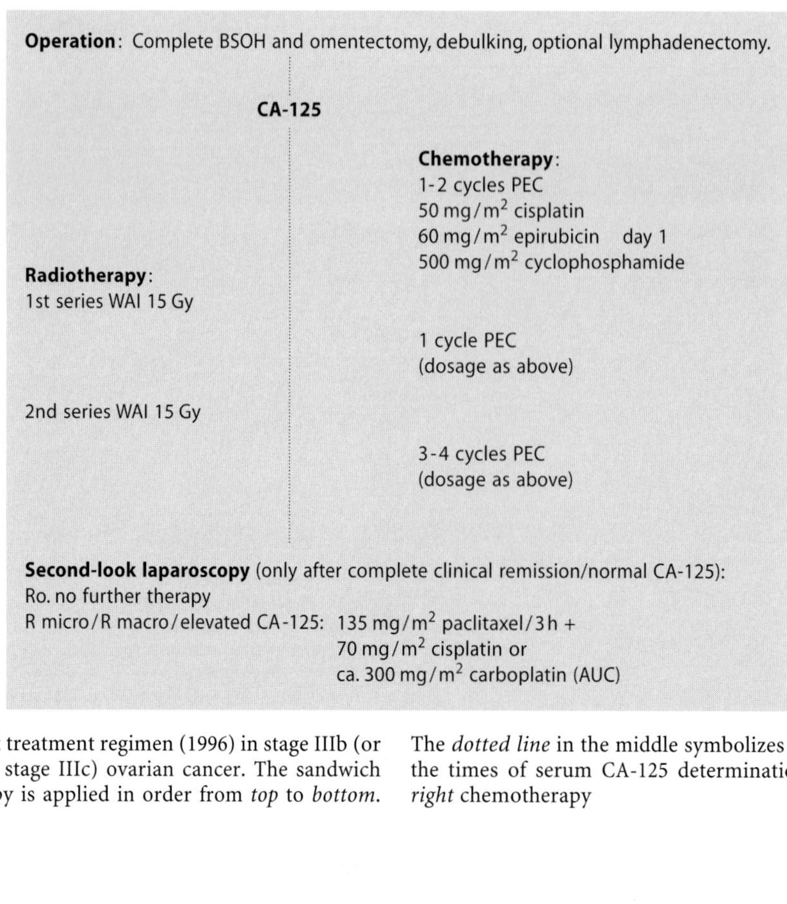

Fig. 11.14. Current treatment regimen (1996) in stage IIIb (or optimally resected stage IIIc) ovarian cancer. The sandwich radio-chemotherapy is applied in order from *top* to *bottom*. The *dotted line* in the middle symbolizes the central role and the times of serum CA-125 determination. *Left* irradiation; *right* chemotherapy

periority of regimen A with cisplatin/cyclophosphamide chemotherapy and APRT interposed between cycles 3 and 4. The serious late toxicity rate of 6%, including a 3% rate of bowel obstruction needing surgery, is very low in comparison to the 10% incidence of bowel obstruction reported in the literature when APRT is added after completion of chemotherapy and SLS (WHELAN et al. 1992).

11.13.5.3 Results of Sandwich Radio-chemotherapy

The results and complications in 1415 patients with primary epithelial ovarian cancer treated in four consecutive periods from 1957 to 1992 are presented.

1. In the first period, 1957–1969, a total of 329 patients could be evaluated for survival and complications. No sandwich therapy was used. The absolute 5-year OS was 38% for all stages, but only 2% for stage III and 0% for stage IV.
2. From 1970 to 1979 a total of 478 patients were treated. Instillations of radiogold were sandwiched with consecutive push doses of two of three cytostatics – cyclophosphamide (60 mg/kg), adriamycin (100–150 mg), and cisplatin (100 mg) – and with pelvic irradiation (40 Gy). Cycles of AC combinations followed (see Fig. 11.13). The results by stage and by type of histology are shown in Tables 11.46 and 11.47.
3. From 1980 to 1988 a total of 426 patients were treated. Radiogold was reduced to one instillation of 130 mCi for early stages or consolidation, sandwiched with two induction push doses of cyclophosphamide and adriamycin or cisplatin (dosage as above). Adriamycin (100 mg) was subsequently replaced by an equitoxic epirubicin dose (150 mg) (VAHRSON and KIRSCHBAUM 1985). The 3-year and 5-year survival rates increased slightly in all stages and histological types (Tables 11.48, 11.49). Stage III OS increased successively from 2% to 13% to 18% during the three periods, and stage IV OS rose from 0% to 3% to 6%. There was a

Table 11.46. Crude 3- and 5-year survival rates by FIGO stage in 478 patients with primary epithelial ovarian cancers treated between 1970 and 1979 at the ZFG Giessen

FIGO stage	No.	%	3-year survival		5-year survival	
			No.	%	No.	%
I	150	31	105	70	88	59
II	85	18	52	61	40	47
III	163	34	33	20	22	13
IV	61	13	5	8	2	3
S	19	4	1	5	1	5
Total	478	100	196	41	153	32

S, special group without surgery.

Table 11.47. Crude 3- and 5-year survival rates by type of histology in 478 patients with primary epithelial ovarian cancers treated between 1970 and 1979 at the ZFG Giessen

Histological type	No.	%	3-year survival		5-year survival	
			No.	%	No.	%
Serous	274	57	113	41	84	31
Mucinous	75	16	48	64	40	53
Endometrioid	21	4	9	43	8	38
Clear cell	3	1	1	–	1	–
Undifferentiated	100	21	23	23	18	18
Mixed epithelial	5	1	2	–	2	–
All types	478	100	196	41	153	32

Table 11.48. Crude 3- and 5-year survival rates by FIGO stage in 426 patients with primary epithelial ovarian cancers treated between 1980 and 1988 at the ZFG Giessen

FIGO stage	No.	%	3-year survival		5-year survival	
			No.	%	No.	%
I	137	32	113	82	94	69
II	81	19	48	59	35	43
III	161	38	50	31	29	18
IV	47	11	5	11	3	6
Total	426	100	216	51	161	38

Table 11.49. Crude 3- and 5-year survival rates by type of histology in 426 patients with primary epithelial ovarian cancers treated between 1980 and 1988 at the ZFG Giessen

Histological type	No.	%	3-year survival		5-year survival	
			No.	%	No.	%
Serous	272	64	137	50	95	35
Mucinous	53	12	33	62	30	57
Endometrioid	36	8	19	53	15	42
Clear cell	21	5	14	67	10	48
Undifferentiated	37	9	10	27	8	22
Mixed epithelial	7	2	3	–	3	–
All types	426	100	216	51	161	38

marked increase in 3-year OS from 42% to 41% to 51%, reflecting the prolonged survival time of incurable cancer patients achieved with more effective chemotherapywithin the context of sandwich radio-chemotherapy. The 5-year OS was identical in the first and third periods, at 38%, but this rate was slightly better than in the second period (32%).

4. From 1989 to 1992 a total of 182 patients were treated. As the deadline for the last evaluation was 31 December 1992, only 88 patients could be evaluated for 3-year OS and 36 for 4-year OS. The 3-year OS rate of 88 patients is 43% and the 4-year survival rate of 36 patients, 42% (Table 11.50). Thus the expected 5-year OS will not be better than in the previous period.

Complications Following Radiogold Instillation. The complications following high activities of ^{198}Au colloid (2 × 150 mCi) in the first period, 1957–1969, have already been described (see Sect. 11.8.4). At the ZFG Giessen bowel obstruction occurred in 12.8% of cases during this period, but only 1.5% could be completely and 3% partially (= total of 4.5%) attributed to radiogold. For this reason it was very interesting to investigate the complications in the following period, when radiogold was reduced from 2 × 150 mCi to 1 × 130–150 mCi.

From 1970 to 1988 a total of 562 patients were treated with radiogold instillations. Among these, 37 intestinal obstructions (6.6%) occurred, as shown in Table 11.51. We found five obstructions (0.9%) in the group with no obvious cancer progression, all of which needed surgical intervention, and 32 (5.7%) in the group with cancer progression, 24 (4.3%) of which needed surgical intervention. In 79 patients treated with exclusive postoperative radiogold instillation, no bowel obstructions occurred in the group without progression, and two (2.5%) in the group with progression not requiring surgery. From the top of the table (exclusive radiogold in low- or intermediate-risk patients without tumor residuals) to the bottom (radiogold + chemotherapy + WAI – preferably with the moving strip technique – in high-risk patients with tumor residuals outside the pelvis) there is a successive increase in stage, deterioration of prognosis, and bowel obstruction. Thus the higher rate of bowel obstruction in combined treatment modalities reflects tumor growth rather than treatment complications.

Table 11.50. Crude 1- to 4-year survival rates in 182 patients with primary epithelial ovarian cancers treated between 1989 and 1992 at the ZFG Giessen

No. of pts. treated	Survival	No.	%
182	1 year	150	82
136	2 years	82	60
88	3 years	38	43
36	4 years	15	42

Complications Following Radiophosphorus Instillation. From 1988 to 1992 a total of 107 patients were treated with 1 × 15–16.5 mCi ^{32}P-chromic phosphate. Three patients (2.8%) experienced complications: one patient had a puncture of the colon, in one case

Table 11.51. Evaluation of bowel obstructions and therapy required in 562 patients with primary epithelial ovarian cancer treated with radiogold + chemotherapy and other irradiation between 1970 and 1989 at the ZFG Giessen

Treatment	No.	Obstruction, no progression			Obstruction with progression		
		Total	Therapy	No.	Total	Therapy	No.
Radiogold exclusively	79	0			2 (2.5%)	Conservative Surgical	2 0
Radiogold + Chemo	229	3 (1.3%)	Conservative Surgical	0 3	8 (3.5%)	Conservative Surgical	0 8
Radiogold + PEL	18	0			1 (5.6%)	Conservative Surgical	0 1
Radiogold + Chemo + PEL	210	2 (1.0%)	Conservative Surgical	1 1	15 (7.1%)	Conservative Surgical	3 12
Radiogold + Chemo + WAI[a]	26	0			6 (23.1%)	Conservative Surgical	3 3
All modalities	562	5 (0.9%)	Conservative Surgical	1 4	32 (5.7%)	Conservative Surgical	8 24

Chemo, chemotherapy; PEL, pelvic irradiation; WAI, whole abdominal irradiation.
[a] WAI was preferably applied using the moving strip technique.

Table 11.52. Evaluation of bowel obstructions and therapy required in 107 patients with primary epithelial ovarian cancer treated with ^{32}P-chromic phosphate between 1988 and 1992 at the ZFG Giessen

Treatment	No.	Obstruction, no progression			Obstruction with progression		
		Total	Therapy	No.	Total	Therapy	No.
^{32}P colloid exclusively	25	0			0		
^{32}P colloid + Chemo	34	0			0		
^{32}P colloid + PEL	3	0			1	Conservative	1
					(33.3%)	Surgical	0
^{32}P colloid +	41	1	Conservative	0	2	Conservative	0
Chemo + PEL		(2.4%)	Surgical	1	(4.9%)	Surgical	2
^{32}P colloid +	4	0			1	Conservative	0
Chemo + OF					(25.0%)	Surgical	1
All modalities	107	1	Conservative	0	4	Conservative	1
		(0.9%)	Surgical	1	(3.8%)	Surgical	3

Chemo, chemotherapy; PEL, pelvic irradiation; OF, open-field irradiation.

the catheter was cut off with a residual segment in the peritoneal cavity, and one patient suffered abdominal cramps after completion of the instillation procedure. The patient in whom a part of the catheter was cut off had to be operated on later because of psychological stress and the segment was removed. One patient (0.9%) suffered bowel obstruction without tumor progression and underwent surgery; four patients (3.8%) suffered bowel obstruction with tumor progression, of whom one underwent conservative and three surgical treatment (Table 11.52). It must be noted that 25 patients who received ^{32}P instillations as the only adjuvant treatment and a further 34 patients who received ^{32}P and chemotherapy had no obstruction. In contrast, in the remaining 48 patients who received additional therapy (irradiation + chemotherapy), there was one case of surgically treated obstruction without progression (2.1%) and four obstructions with tumor progression (8.3%); in three of the latter cases, surgery was performed.

Complications Following Percutaneous Irradiation (PEL, WAI). From 1970 to 1992 a total of 560 patients received either PEL or WAI or combinations of the two modalities. In seven patients (1.2%) irradiation had to be discontinued because of ileus in three, reduced status in three, and acute lumbago in one. Acute and late complications occurred in five patients (0.9%): two with transient epitheliolysis, one with a rectovaginal fistula, and two with ulcerations, (one of the rectum, one of the abdominal wall). All of them had pelvic irradiation sandwiched with chemotherapy and intraperitoneal radionuclide instillation.

All Complications. From 1970 to 1992, of a total of 1005 patients who received percutaneous irradiation, radionuclide instillation, chemotherapy, or combinations thereof (sandwich radio-chemotherapy), 105 (10.4%) had treatment complications (including discontinuation) without obvious tumor progression. When discontinuation of treatment was excluded, the overall complication rate was below 10%.

11.13.6 Simultaneous Radio-chemotherapy

Few attempts have been made to treat ovarian carcinoma with simultaneous radio- and chemotherapy. In 1972 at the ZFG Giessen we began to apply a push dose of 60 mg/kg *cyclophosphamide* as a bolus intravenously during a series of high-voltage irradiation using pelvic opposing fields or extended fields including the groins and lower para-aortic lymph nodes (5 × 2 Gy/week). The planned midline dose was 40–50 Gy (pelvic field) or 46 Gy (extended field). After a dose of usually 12 Gy (range 9–39 Gy) the cyclophosphamide push dose was applied. Two days later irradiation was continued. In a study on 21 stage II and III ovarian cancer patients submitted to this treatment between 1972 and 1976 (Wolf et al. 1976) we found considerable acute toxicity. Seven (33%) patients suffered from septic neutropenia, of whom one (5%) died of extreme leukopenia and thrombocytopenia in spite of repeated transfusions. A second patient presenting with reversible cardiac failure, lung edema, and pleural and pericardial effusions recovered very slowly. Only in two patients did the disease progress; the remaining 18 patients showed a response up to complete clinical remission.

In another five patients 100–150 mg/m² *doxorubicin* (adriamycin) was given intravenously as a bolus during a series of irradiation. Three presented with stage III ovarian cancer, one with a second abdominal recurrence of a breast cancer (pretreated with 2 × 150 mCi radiogold intraperitoneally and triple drug push chemotherapy), and one after initial surgery of a leiomyosarcoma in the parametrium. Two of the five patients had the usual transient leukopenia and thrombocytopenia, while three had life-threatening toxicities to which the leiomyosarcoma patient succumbed. She received 20 Gy by opposing pelvic fields and 2 days later 150 mg/m² adriamycin. During the following 14 days she developed thrombocytopenia <12 000, peripheral cyanosis, anuria, necrosis of a 20-cm terminal ileum segment, and multiple, in some cases perforating ulcers of other intestinal parts. The necrosis and all of the ulcers were located within the irradiated volume. After this experience we stopped giving the highly toxic simultaneous radio-chemotherapy with doxorubicin. However, when applying consecutive sandwich radio-chemotherapy we never had a case of intestinal necrosis when using adriamycin or any other drug in a single push dose or in combination.

Szepesi et al. (1979) treated stage III and IV ovarian cancer patients with simultaneous radio-chemotherapy and subsequent early SLS in a prospective study. The authors applied a 40 Gy surface dose to the pelvis and then 60 Gy to the abdomen by positive grid telecobalt fields (5–6 × 3 Gy surface dose/week). Simultaneously two cycles of *adriamycin* 20 mg/m² i.v. on days 1–3 and *bleomycin* 15 mg/m² i.v. on days 1–5 were applied. In the 8th–9th week SLS was performed. Starting with the 11th week, biaxial telecobalt pendulum irradiation was given, delivering 35 Gy axis dose (45 Gy central dose) to a total dose (grid fields + pendulum fields) of 60 Gy. Simultaneously with this second part of irradiation, four cycles of adriamycin 20 mg/m² i.v. on days 1–3 and *5-fluorouracil* 500 mg/m² once per week per os or per infusion were applied. According to the later publication from 1982, bleomycin must have been replaced by *cyclophosphamide* instead of 5-fluorouracil. Chemotherapy was continued with a consolidation regimen with 5-fluorouracil 500 mg/m² per infusion on days 1–3 and *chlorambucil* 5 mg/m² on days 2–6 every 4 weeks up to the 12th cycle and then every 8 weeks for cycles 13–18. The consolidation regimen additionally contained megestrol acetate 60 mg daily and permanently.

This rather complicated but very logical simultaneous radio-chemotherapy regimen was re-evaluated by Szepesi et al. in 1982. Among 55 treated patients (45 stage III and 10 stage IV) the authors found a response rate of 94%, comprising 33/52 (63%) clinical complete responses (cCR) and 16/52 (31%) clinical partial responses (cPR). In stage III cCR occurred in 32/43 (74%) cases and cPR in 11/43 (26%); the corresponding rates for stage IV were 11% and 56% respectively. The three nonresponders had stage IV disease. The response rate for R > 2 cm at initial surgery was 37/40 (92%), including cCR in 21/40 (52%).

The high response rates were corrected by the survival rates. In stage III the survival rates after 1, 2, 3, and 4 years were 82%, 42%, 30%, and 20%, respectively (median 18 months). In stage IV the survival rate was 20% after 1 year. The toxicity of this simultaneous treatment regimen consisted in small bowel obstruction/sigmoid stenosis in six patients (11%) without recurrence, requiring surgery. Furthermore three patients (5%) died of internal or urological complications. The high complication rate led the authors to discontinue the simultaneous treatment regimen in 1981.

In conclusion, there is no place for simultaneous radio-chemotherapy in ovarian cancer with one exception: single push cyclophosphamide with 60 mg/kg as an i.v. bolus can be applied on the 8th day after instillation of radiophosphorus (15–16.5 mCi) without any major acute or late toxicity.

11.14 Management of Progression and Recurrences: Second-Line Treatments

U. Nitz, H.G. Bender, and H.W. Vahrson

11.14.1 General Considerations

Factors associated with a high risk of recurrence have been discussed extensively in the preceding sections.

Just like the diagnosis of primary ovarian cancer, the diagnosis of progressive or recurrent ovarian cancer may be difficult to establish by clinical, radiological, or ultrasound examination only. A persistently high level of CA-125 or the reappearance of pathological serum concentrations of this protein reliably predicts recurrence. On the other hand, the absence of pathological CA-125 levels even in primarily tumor marker-positive disease does not exclude recurrent disease (RUBIN et al. 1989).

Therapeutic options are the same as described for primary disease, with the difference that second-line therapy is only exceptionally curative. Recurrence-free survival correlates best with overall survival, thus indicating that the biological behavior of the tumor will determine the outcome to a much greater extent than the therapy. Patients with primarily progressive disease or recurrences within 6 months after primary therapy generally do not survive the 2-year limit. In this context prognosis is exceptionally bad for patients with platinum-resistant disease (progression during or <6 months after the end of primary platinum chemotherapy).

11.14.2 Secondary Cytoreduction

Although there is little doubt as to the value of primary cytoreductive surgery for advanced ovarian cancer, the value of secondary cytoreduction is not as clearly established. In patients with progressive disease after primary therapy, results are especially poor. MICHEL et al. (1989) operated on 77 patients with recurrence prior to the planned second-look operation (SLO), the great majority of whom had received platinum-based chemotherapy for 6–12 months. They found that in these cases, whatever surgery was performed, the results were the same. As MICHEL et al. reported a high rate (57%) of optimally debulked patients in their series, the results probably did not reflect a lack of surgical skill but the inherent biological aggressiveness of the tumor.

Other authors, however, have found that secondary cytoreduction is beneficial, especially when optimal debulking (microscopic residuals) is achieved. In such cases survival rates of 55% at 4 years (PODRATZ et al. 1988) or 51% at 5 years (HOSKINS et al. 1989) have been reported.

There are very few data for patients presenting with late, isolated recurrences of ovarian carcinoma. MUNKARAH et al. (1996) report on very high rates of optimal debulking (72%) and promising early survival rates in this situation.

To summarize, data from the literature suggest that secondary cytoreduction should be restricted to carefully selected patients. The maximum benefit will be achieved in patients who are in good general medical condition, have no evidence of ascites, have not yet received platinum-containing polychemotherapy, have a partial response to alkylating chemotherapy, and have a reasonably long interval (>9–12 months) from diagnosis. If the patient has previously received platinum, outcome is better in cases where disease-free survival exceeds 24 months (HOSKINS et al. 1989). The goal of secondary debulking is to remove all gross tumor or to reduce the metastatic tumor burden to <5 mm maximum dimension.

11.14.3 Second-Line Chemotherapy

During the past decade, platinum-based polychemotherapy has become a standard primary treatment of advanced epithelial ovarian cancer (NIH 1994). Reinduction with platinum-containing regimens is more effective, the longer the disease-free interval. MARKMAN et al. (1990) describe response rates to platinum reinduction of 28%–58% at intervals of 5–12 and >24 months after primary chemotherapy.

Disease progression on platinum therapy or recurrence within 6–12 months after platinum therapy is defined as platinum-resistant ovarian cancer. Paclitaxel is the best investigated drug in this situation. MCGUIRE (1995) reported a response rate of 22% and a median survival of 9 months in patients with refractory ovarian carcinoma (three prior chemotherapy regimens). Similar response rates have been described within smaller trials of oral etoposide (ROSE et al. 1996) and topotecan (CARMICHAEL et al. 1996), a promising experimental agent in the treatment of epithelial ovarian malignancies. Dose intensification of platinum [i.v. administration (±G-CSF) or i.p. administration (REICHMANN et al. 1989) may represent another alternative with comparable effectiveness (see Sect. 11.2.3).

In platinum-sensitive recurrences, platinum-based polychemotherapy seems to be superior to single-agent paclitaxel. COLOMBO et al. (1996) have reported response rates of 49% and 54% with single-agent paclitaxel (group A) and cyclophosphamide, adriamycin, and cisplatin (group B), respectively. Progression-free survival was 7.3 months in group A and 18.9 months in group B. The value of additional paclitaxel in a platinum-based regimen in this situation remains to be defined.

In the very near future the question of what to do when platinum/paclitaxel has been given for primary chemotherapy will arise. One of the few drugs investigated in this situation is topotecan. Response rates of 13% and 14.5% have been reported for second- and third-line therapy with this agent in patients mostly resistant to paclitaxel or cisplatin (GORDON et al. 1996). As in other series, response duration for third-line therapy was in the range of weeks (mean: 11 weeks).

In summary, in cases of platinum-resistant ovarian carcinoma response rates vary between 20% and 35%, but response duration is short. In platinum-sensitive recurrences, platinum-based second-line therapy (i.v. or i.p.) with or without paclitaxel results in about 20% of patients surviving the 2–3 year limit. Third-line therapies are generally of limited benefit.

11.14.4 The Role of Radiotherapy

Radiotherapy is of very limited efficacy in progressive ovarian cancer and can only have a palliative intent. Second- or third-line chemotherapy is the treatment of choice, and if resistance to platinum and/or paclitaxel-based chemotherapy has occurred, this pleiotropic drug resistance is commonly linked with cross-resistance to irradiation, as already pointed out (see Sect. 11.13.2).

In recurrences, i.e., after a disease-free interval of at least 6 months since last treatment, chemotherapy is again the therapy of choice for a widespread recurrence, but in isolated small local or metastatic recurrences radiotherapy may be superior.

DAVIDSON et al. (1993) reported their experiences with limited-field pelvic or para-aortic irradiation with 40–70 Gy (median 46 Gy) to the pelvis, para-aortic retroperitoneum, or vaginal cuff in 35 patients with progressions or recurrences. All of the patients completed therapy, five (14%) with treatment breaks. Median actuarial and disease-free survival were 40 and 14 months; late bowel complications occurred in three patients (9%).

CORN et al. (1994) irradiated 33 patients with recurrent ovarian cancer to 47 sites with a *hypofractionated treatment regimen* based on the biological effective dose (BED). The sites included the pelvis (33), abdomen (5), chest (4), brain (3), and others (2). The median fraction size was 2.5 Gy (range 1–5 Gy). Median total dose was 35 Gy (range 7.5–75 Gy). The most frequently used palliative regimen was 14 × 2.5 Gy = 35 Gy. Complete symptomatic response was achieved in 51% and an overall symptomatic effect in 70%. The overall response rates by symptom were as follows: control of vaginal bleeding in nine of ten (90%) patients, control of rectal bleeding/obstruction in 11 of 13 (85%), pain relief in 15 of 18 (83%), pulmonary symptom relief in three of four (75%), and control of other symptoms in 50%. However, median survival for the entire series was only 4 months. Thus palliation of symptoms until death was achieved in 90%.

In rare cases high intentionally palliative doses may produce long-term survival or even cure. KLOETZER et al. (1978) described a patient who was disease-free at 76 months after 60 Gy telecobalt irradiation delivered to metastases of both ossa ilia. In our experience, especially if local recurrence is confined to the pouch of Douglas as the sole manifestation and adhesions prevent spillage of cancer cells to the abdominal cavity, the delivery of a 50–60 Gy tumor dose by pendulum or limited pelvic opposing fields can result in tumor control and long-term survival.

In conclusion, radiotherapy – either in progressive or in recurrent ovarian cancer – should preferably be applied to a small volume not previously irradiated, where 40–60 (70) Gy can be tolerated.

11.15 Five-Year Results in Primary Epithelial Ovarian Cancer

H.W. VAHRSON

The volumes of the FIGO Annual Report (last editor Folke Pettersson, Stockholm) are the best source of results of treatment in gynecological cancer.

Table 11.53. Carcinoma of the ovary: mode of treatment by stage of disease. (Annual Report vol. 22)

Stage	Surg.	Surg. + rad.	Chemo.	Surg. + chemo. + rad.	Surg. + chemo.	Total
I	829	344	13	238	654	2078
II	98	96	9	236	402	841
III	380	70	111	889	1973	3423
IV	169	12	62	158	635	1036
Total	1476	522	195	1521	3664	7378

Surg., surgery; rad., radiotherapy; chemo., chemotherapy.

The mode of treatment by stage of 7378 ovarian cancers treated between 1987 and 1989 is shown in Table 11.53. Surgery alone was the treatment in 1476 patients (27.8%). Surgery + chemotherapy was the most common treatment, being employed in 3664 patients (49.7%). Radiotherapy after surgery was applied to 522 patients (7.1%) and combination surgery, chemotherapy, and radiotherapy was applied to 1521 patients (20.6%); thus radiotherapy was applied to 2043:7378 (27.7%) of the patients (Annual Report vol. 22: Pettersson 1994).

Table 11.54. Carcinoma of the ovary (obviously malignant cases; all histopathological classes): 5-year actuarial survival by stage (Annual Report vol. 22)

Stage	No.	5-year survival (%)
Ia	845	83.5
Ib	188	79.3
Ic	606	73.1
IIa	140	64.6
IIb	272	54.2
IIc	336	61.3
IIIa	171	51.7
IIIb	366	29.2
IIIc	1903	17.7
IV	1291	14.3
	6118	

From the same volume 22 the actuarial 5-year survival rates by stage of 6118 patients can be shown (Table 11.54). The range is from 83.5% in stage Ia to 14.3% in stage IV.

Volume 21, issued in 1991 (Pettersson 1991), was the last one presenting detailed crude 5-year overall survival (OS) rates by stage from each of the collaborating centers. Table 11.55 presents the survival rates of 14 German institutions taken from this report. The crude 5-year OS is 637:1879 (34%).

Three survival curves – (a) by histological type of cancer, (b) by borderline vs obvious malignant cancer and (c) by grade of differentiation in serous cancer – from Annual Report vol. 21 have already been presented earlier (see Sect. 11.2).

All of the contributors to the Annual Report can only hope very intensely that this tremendously

Table 11.55. Crude 5-year survival rates according to stage of 1879 ovarian cancer patients treated between 1982 and 1986 at 14 German hospitals (including 12 Universitäts Frauenkliniken: UFK). (Taken from Annual Report vol. 21, 1991) ($n < 10$ are not given in %)

Institution (authors)	Stage							
	Ia	Ib	Ic	I	II	III	IV	I–IV
UFK Freiburg (Pfleiderer et al.)	20/21 (95%)	1/1	5/7	26/29 (90%)	19/27 (70%)	25/124 (20%)	5/46 (11%)	75/226 (33%)
FK Fulda (Göltner and Kraus)	3/4	1/2	2/3	6/9	1/5	4/22 (18%)	1/9	12/45 (27%)
UFK Giessen (Vahrson et al.)	27/39 (69%)	3/4	32/49 (65%)	62/92 (67%)	23/51 (45%)	18/91 (20%)	2/26 (8%)	105/260 (40%)
UFK Greifswald (Göretzlehner and Gürtler)	5/8	1/1	0	6/9	1/3	5/15 (33%)	3/14 (21%)	15/41 (37%)
UFK Göttingen (Kuhn et al.)	8/12 (67%)	2/3	2/7	12/22 (55%)	20/38 (53%)	29/133 (22%)	6/53 (11%)	67/247 (27%)
FK Hannover (Kühnle and Zech)	8/10 (80%)	1/1	2/3	11/14 (79%)	6/10 (60%)	6/33 (18%)	0/10	23/67 (34%)
UFK Heidelberg (v. Fournier and Bastert)	10/10 (100%)	0/1	5/5	15/16 (94%)	7/9	3/18 (17%)	0/16	25/59 (42%)
UFK Jena (Nöschel and Stech)	4/5	0	7/11 (64%)	11/16 (69%)	5/10 (50%)	11/42 (26%)	2/14 (14%)	29/82 (35%)
UFK Kiel (Weisner)	30/34 (88%)	13/16 (81%)	10/17 (59%)	53/67 (79%)	14/20 (70%)	13/49 (27%)	1/41 (2%)	82/178 (46%)
UFK Leipzig (Bilek and Richter)	11/17 (65%)	1/2	3/3	15/22 (68%)	7/11 (64%)	8/79 (10%)	2/15 (13%)	32/127 (25%)
I. UFK München (Kürzl)	14/22 (64%)	5/9	16/27 (59%)	35/58 (60%)	19/47 (40%)	13/85 (15%)	1/37 (3%)	69/227 (25%)
UFK München Großhadern (Heyn)	9/13 (69%)	1/1	13/20 (60%)	23/34 (68%)	3/14 (21%)	27/95 (14%)	3/22 (14%)	56/165 (34%)
UFK Rostock (Schwarz et al.)	11/13 (85%)	1/1	6/9	18/23 (78%)	0/2	6/29 (21%)	0/8	24/62 (39%)
UFK Würzburg (Wulf and Rotte)	9/12 (75%)	4/6	1/3	14/21 (67%)	3/8	6/36 (17%)	1/28 (4%)	24/93 (26%)
Total	169/220 (77%)	34/48 (71%)	104/164 (63%)	307/432 (71%)	128/255 (50%)	174/851 (20%)	27/339 (8%)	636/1877 (34%)

important work will be continued after Folke Pettersson has retired as the editor.

11.16 General Management and the Role of Irradiation in Malignant Sex Cord-Stromal Tumors of the Ovaries

I.B. Vergote and D. Timmerman

Sex cord-stromal tumors are ovarian neoplasms that contain granulosa cells, theca cells, Sertoli cells, Leydig cells, and fibroblasts of gonadal stromal origin, singly or in various combinations and in varying degrees of differentiation. The classification used here is similar to that formulated by the International Society of Gynecological Pathologists under the auspices of the World Health Organization (Young and Scully 1992) (Table 11.56). Steroid cell tumors are traditionally included under the general heading of sex cord-stromal tumors but are now recognized as a separate entity, and will be discussed in Sect. 11.18.

Sex cord-stromal tumors account for approximately 8% of all ovarian tumors and fibromas account for approximately half of these cases (Young and Scully 1984b). The development of our understanding of the natural history and management of sex cord-stromal tumors has been limited by their scarcity. Hence, a good deal of the literature consists of retrospective surveys of nonuniform treatment spanning many decades. In the last decade, a considerable improvement in pathological classification of these tumors has been achieved, and this will probably make it possible to adapt the management of these rare tumors more precisely to their behavior. With regard to the histopathology of the sex cord-stromal tumors see Sect. 11.2. Here, we will review their clinical features and management.

Table 11.56. Classification of sex cord-stromal tumors (as formulated by the International Society of Gynecological Pathologists under the auspices of the World Health Organization). (Young and Scully 1992)

1. Granulosa-stromal cell tumors
   A. Granulosa cell tumor
      (i) Adult type
      (ii) Juvenile type
   B. Thecoma-fibroma group
      (i) Thecoma
         a) Typical
         b) Luteinized
      (ii) Fibroma-fibrosarcoma
         a) Fibroma[a]
         b) Cellular fibroma
         c) Fibrosarcoma
      (iii) Stromal tumor with minor sex cord elements[a]
      (iv) Sclerosing stromal tumor[a]
      (v) Unclassified
2. Sertoli-stromal cell tumors
   A. Sertoli cell tumor
   B. Leydig cell tumor[b]
   C. Sertoli-Leydig cell tumor
      (i) Well differentiated
      (ii) Of intermediate differentiation
      (iii) Poorly differentiated
      (iv) With heterologous elements
      (v) Retiform variant
      (vi) Mixed
3. Gynandroblastoma
4. Sex cord-stromal tumor with annular tubules
5. Unclassified

[a] Benign tumors.
[b] More logically regarded as a steroid cell tumor and discussed in Sect. 11.18.

11.16.1 Granulosa-Stromal Cell Tumors

Granulosa-stroma cell tumors are subdivided into granulosa cell tumors and tumors in the thecoma-fibroma group (Table 11.56). Adult-type granulosa cell tumors differ both clinically and pathologically from the much rarer juvenile type. The names of these two tumors reflect only a strong tendency for them to occur at certain ages. Adult granulosa cell tumors, however, do occur very rarely in children, and juvenile granulosa cell tumors have been encountered very rarely in women over 30 years of age (Young et al. 1984a).

11.16.1.1 Granulosa Cell Tumors

ADULT GRANULOSA CELL TUMORS

Epidemiology and Clinical Features. Adult granulosa cell tumors account for 1%–2% of all ovarian tumors (Young and Scully 1992; Fox and Buckley 1992). Reviewing the literature on 818 cases, the average age of occurrence is 53 years (Table 11.57) (Goldston et al. 1972; Fox et al. 1975; Anikwue et al. 1978; Pankratz et al. 1978; Stenwig et al. 1979; Evans et al. 1980; Bjorkholm and Silversward 1981; Schweppe and Beller 1982; Bartl et al. 1984; Scharl et al. 1988; Baumann et al. 1992;

Table 11.57. Age, frequency of stage I disease, and bilaterality in granulosa cell tumors

Author	Cases	Mean age	Bilateral (all stages)	Stage I/ total[a]	Bilateral stage I/ stage I
Norris and Taylor (1968)	97	NR	2	NR	NR
Goldston et al. (1972)	41	53	7	28/41	0/28
Fox et al. (1975)	92	53	7	NR	NR
Schwartz and Smith (1976)	37	NR	NR	26/37	1/26
Anikwue et al. (1978)	32	50	NR	NR	NR
Stage and Grafton (1977)	29	NR	0	25/29	0/29
Stenwig et al. (1979)	118	54	6	92/118	NR
Pankratz et al. (1978)	61	50	5	31/61	NR
Evans et al. (1980)	118	51	3	93/118	0/93
Antolic et al. (1980)	28	NR	2	NR	NR
Bjorkholm and Silversward (1981)	198	53	5	181/198	NR
Schweppe et al. (1982)	36	48	NR	29/36	7/29
Ohel et al. (1983)	172	NR	NR	77/143	NR
Bartl et al. (1984)	27	54	NR	16/26	3/16
Scharl et al. (1988)	26	51	2	20/26	2/26
Baumann et al. (1992)	15	57	13	6/15	4/6
Malmstrom et al. (1994)	54	57	NR	47/54	3/47
Total	1181	53[b]	52/823 (6%)	671/902 (74%)	20/300 (7%)

NR, not recorded.
[a] Only the patients with known stage are included.
[b] Weighted mean in 818 patients with age recorded.

Malmstrom et al. 1994). However, in many older series a small number of juvenile granulosa cell tumors have been included.

Granulosa cell tumors are more often diagnosed in early-stage disease than epithelial ovarian carcinomas. In a compilation of the literature on 902 granulosa cell tumors, 74% were diagnosed in FIGO stage I disease (Table 11.57), although it must be remembered that accurate and complete surgical staging as we conceive it today is not available in most older series. Indeed, 394 out of 475 patients (83%) in series which included patients before 1940 had stage I disease, versus 119 of 210 (57%) in series including patients treated after 1960 only.

Many older series only quoted a frequency of involvement of both ovaries for all stages. This frequency is low (6%, Table 11.57). More recent studies have shown that for stage I disease, bilaterality is similar compared with the total group (7%, Table 11.57). The tumors vary in size from microscopic lesions to masses measuring 40 cm in diameter, with an average of about 12 cm (Fox et al. 1975). Only about 15%–25% of the tumors are larger than 15 cm (Stenwig et al. 1979; Stage and Grafton 1977; Ohel et al. 1983).

About two-thirds of the patients present with abnormal vaginal bleeding related to estrogen production in the tumor (Fox et al. 1975; Schwartz and Smith 1976; Stage and Grafton 1977; Anikwue et al. 1978; Pankratz et al. 1978; Stenwig et al. 1979; Schweppe and Beller 1982; Malmstrom et al. 1994). In premenopausal patients the tumor may be associated with a variety of menstrual disorders including menorrhagia, metrorrhagia, oligomenorrhea, and even amenorrhea. After the menopause, postmenopausal bleeding is the typical presenting symptom. In the absence of abnormal vaginal bleeding, patients usually present with abdominal distention or abdominal pain. Androgenic granulosa cell tumors have been reported but occur in only 1%–2% of the patients (Schweppe and Beller 1982; Nakashima et al. 1984; Zaydon et al. 1989). Hormone production by granulosa cell tumors has been documented by changes in serum hormone levels during treatment (Marsh et al. 1962; Witt et al. 1992), by direct measurements on the tumors (Kurman et al. 1979), and by the demonstration of stimulation by gonadotropins of the steroidogenesis by the tumor cells in vitro (Hahlin et al. 1991). However, although circulating estradiol has been used as a tumor marker of granulosa cell tumors for many decades, its use has been hampered by the fact that about one-third of the primary tumors and many recurrences do not produce the hormone. Recently, it has been shown that serum inhibin levels are more accurate as a marker for primary as well as recurrent granulosa cell tumors (Lappohn et al. 1989).

Another frequent result of the estrogen production in the tumor is the occurrence of endometrial hyperplasia and even frank carcinoma. In the original Gusberg series (Gusberg and Kardon 1971) on thecomas, granulosa cell tumors, and granulosa-thecoma cell tumors, 21% of the patients had an endometrial carcinoma. However, in more recent series on granulosa cell tumors the incidence of endometrial carcinoma is as low as 9%, while atypical hyperplasia is found in 8% and cystic hyperplasia in 55% of the patients (Table 11.58). It has been suggested that patients with granulosa cell tumors have an increased incidence of breast cancer (Evans et al. 1980; Scharl et al. 1988; Ohel et al. 1983), but this remains unsure.

Recurrences most often occur intraperitoneally and tend to displace rather than to invade (Norris and Taylor 1968; Fox et al. 1975; Pankratz et al. 1978; Anikwue et al. 1978; Stenwig et al. 1979; Evans et al. 1980). Death is often caused by tumor hemorrhage or malignant ascites. Hepatic, lung, spleen, and cerebral metastases have been reported, but are rare (Norris and Taylor 1968; Fox et al. 1975; Anikwue et al. 1978; Evans et al. 1980; Margolin et al. 1985; Ebel et al. 1993). Lymph node metastases occur less often than in epithelial ovarian carcinoma (Norris and Taylor 1968; Fox et al. 1975; Anikwue et al. 1978; Stenwig et al. 1979; Evans et al. 1980). At autopsy, Diddle (1952) found positive lymph nodes in only 8% of 110 cases in which granulosa cell tumors caused death. Another interesting feature of granulosa cell tumors is their propensity to display an indolent nature and late recurrence. The mean time to recurrence ranges from 2 to 9 years (Norris and Taylor 1968; Fox et al. 1975; Schwartz and Smith 1976; Anikwue et al. 1978; Stenwig et al. 1979; Evans et al. 1980; Bjorkholm and Silversward 1981; Scharl et al. 1988; Malmstrom et al. 1994). These differences may be due to different durations of follow-up. Certainly there are many reports of recurrences 10–25 years after primary diagnosis.

Prognosis. Due to the late recurrences observed in granulosa cell tumors, a true estimate of the malignancy of these tumors can only be achieved by prolonged surveillance, probably lifelong but for at least 20 years. In a number of studies the 20-year corrected survival of adult-type granulosa cell tumors has been about 50%–60% (Fox et al. 1975; Pankratz et al. 1978; Stenwig et al. 1979; Schweppe and Beller 1982; Ohel et al. 1983), though a considerably higher survival rate was observed in one older study (Norris and Taylor 1968). It should be clear, therefore, that all granulosa cell tumors should be regarded as being at least potentially malignant. Conversely, extraovarian spread is the only absolute indication of a poor prognosis (Goldston et al. 1972; Fox et al. 1975; Pankratz et al. 1978; Stenwig et al. 1979; Evans et al. 1980; Bjorkholm and Silversward 1981; Ohel et al. 1983; Malmstrom et al. 1994). The 10-year cor-

Table 11.58. Endometrial hyperplasia and adenocarcinoma in patients with granulosa cell tumors

Author	Cystic hyperplasia	Atypical hyperplasia	Adenocarcinoma
Norris and Taylor (1968)	15/38	2/38	4/38
Goldston et al. (1972)	24/30	1/30	2/30
Fox et al. (1975)	24/59	5/59	6/59
Schwartz and Smith (1976)	6/18	4/18	0/18
Anikwue et al. (1978)	NR	NR	1/26
Pankratz et al. (1978)	NR	NR	3/24
Stenwig et al. (1979)	41/64	1/64	2/64
Antolic et al. (1980)	14/28	3/28	4/28
Bjorkholm and Silversward (1981)	66/101	5/101	11/101
Schweppe and Beller (1982)	NR	NR	2/27
Ohel et al. (1983)	37/63	0/63	7/63
Bartl et al. (1984)	1/12	0/12	1/12
Scharl et al. (1988)	9/19	0/19	2/19
Baumann et al. (1992)	2/5	0/5	1/5
Malmstrom et al. (1994)	30/54	16/54	5/54
Total	269/491 (55%)	37/491 (8%)	51/568 (9%)

NR, not recorded.

rected survival in stage I disease ranges from 75% to 92%, with a weighted mean on 393 patients with stage I disease of 89% (PANKRATZ et al. 1978; STENWIG et al. 1979; EVANS et al. 1980; BJORKHOLM and SILVERSWARD 1981). There seems to be agreement in most large studies that a high number of mitoses is of strict relevance for the prognosis (FOX et al. 1975; STENWIG et al. 1979; OHEL et al. 1983; MALMSTROM et al. 1994). Other prognostic factors such as nuclear atypia (STENWIG et al. 1979; BJORKHOLM and SILVERSWARD 1981), size (FOX et al. 1975; BJORKHOLM and SILVERSWARD 1981), rupture (BJORKHOLM and SILVERSWARD 1981), and bilaterality (FOX et al. 1975) have been proposed but are still debatable. The type of histological pattern seen in the tumor is not prognostically relevant.

The incidence of aneuploidy seems to be lower than in epithelial ovarian cancer, and unlike in the case of epithelial tumors, DNA ploidy does not seem to be of prognostic value (HITCHCOCK et al. 1989; CHADHA et al. 1990; SUH et al. 1990; VERGOTE et al. 1993a). Only in one study was it suggested that S-phase and ploidy were predictors of survival (KLEMI et al. 1990). Trisomies 12, 4, and 14 have been reported in ovarian granulosa cell tumors, but the prognostic significance of this finding remains unknown (LEUNG et al. 1990; FLETCHER et al. 1991; GORSKI et al. 1992).

Management. Surgery is the cornerstone of therapy of granulosa cell tumors of the ovary. Adequate treatment must be defined as total hysterectomy, bilateral adnexectomy, omentectomy, and complete cancer staging, as is recommended in epithelial ovarian carcinoma. Routine para-aortic and pelvic lymphadenectomy do not seem to be indicated because the incidence of lymph node metastases appears to be low (see above). In the occasional younger woman who wishes to preserve her fertility a unilateral salpingo-oophorectomy may be considered if complete staging shows no evidence of spread. Dilatation and curettage, and preferentially also hysteroscopy to rule out endometrial pathology, should be performed. When deciding to treat the patient conservatively one should bear in mind that the frequency of bilaterality is 7% in stage I disease (Table 11.57) and that two studies suggested that unilateral adnexectomy might result in a higher death rate (PANKRATZ et al. 1978; EVANS et al. 1980). When childbearing is no longer desired, total hysterectomy and contralateral adnexectomy appear to be mandatory.

The role of adjuvant radiotherapy in stage I disease cannot be established because no randomized studies exist with a no-treatment arm. Some authors have suggested that adjuvant radiotherapy improves survival rates (SCHWARTZ and SMITH 1976; PANKRATZ et al. 1978; KIETLINSKA et al. 1993). KIETLINSKA et al. (1993) observed four failures in ten radically operated patients versus 15 (17%) relapses in 88 radically operated patients treated with postoperative radiotherapy. However, in most series no advantage has been shown (GOLDSTON et al. 1972; FOX et al. 1975; STENWIG et al. 1979; EVANS et al. 1980; BJORKHOLM and SILVERSWARD 1981; OHEL et al. 1983; SCHARL et al. 1988). Furthermore, it appears that most patients with stage I disease based on optimal surgical staging have a very low risk of recurrence since the corrected 10-year survival rates in older studies with probably incomplete staging, as we conceive it today, were as high as 89% (see above).

Little information is available concerning the use of radiotherapy in advanced or recurrent granulosa cell tumors. Many reports include patients treated with irradiation, but the lack of proper staging, standardized treatment regimens, response evaluation, and long-term follow-up make the results uninterpretable.[1] Also the literature concerning the use of

[1] *Editor's note.* In the series of 543 patients with ovarian malignancies treated at the ZFG Giessen between 1957 and 1969, 465 were primary malignancies with accurate histological evaluation. Of these, 37 (8%) were granulosa cell tumors. Their stage distribution was as folows: stage I, 21 (53.8%); stage II, seven (18.0%); stage III, seven (18.0%); and stage IV four (10.2%). The overall crude 5-year survival rate was only 37%, obviously due to undertreatment. In comparison, the crude 5-year survival rate for primary epithelial serous cancers was 30.5%, that for mucinous cancers 73.2%, and that for endometrioid cancers 50.5%. Thus granulosa cell tumors had the second worst survival rate, quite near to that of serous cancers. Therefore the clinical course of the majority of the granulosa cell tumors was far away from that of merely a potentially malignant tumor. Furthermore, late recurrence after 5–10 years seems to be a special feature of this tumor. An investigation of the reason for these bad results in granulosa cell tumors revealed that at the ZFG Giessen, as in other operative departments, in most cases no postoperative treatment was given, which was followed by progression or recurrence. The malignant potential of the granulosa cell tumors seemed to be underestimated. For these reasons at the ZFG Giessen postoperative irradiation is widely used, nowadays preferably with intraperitoneal ^{32}P chromic phosphate instillation, depending on the risk factors stage, grade, and residuals as are used in primary epithelial ovarian cancers. Chemotherapy is added in stages II, III, and IV. The results of an evaluation of this treatment policy in the years 1970–1992, which has been started at the ZFG Giessen, are awaited.

chemotherapy in advanced or recurrent disease is sparse. Anecdotal response has been reported with alkylating agents (SMITH and RUTLEDGE 1970; MALKASIAN et al. 1974; LUSCH et al. 1978; SCHWARTZ and SMITH 1976; EVANS et al. 1980), doxorubicin (DISAIA et al. 1978), and actinomycin D/fluorouracil/cyclophosphamide (SCHWARTZ and SMITH 1976). In recent years, combination chemotherapy including cisplatin has proven to be more effective. Seven out of nine patients treated with cisplatin/doxorubicin/cyclophosphamide showed a response (CAMLIBEL and CAPUTO 1983; KAYE and DAVIES 1986; SCHULMAN et al. 1974; GERSHENSON et al. 1987). JACOBS et al. (1982a) observed two responses in two patients treated with cisplatin/doxorubucin. Most experience has been gained with the cisplatin/vinblastine/bleomycin (PVB) regimen. Of a total of 31 patients reported, 25 (81%) showed a response (16 complete responses and nine partial responses) (COLOMBO et al. 1986; ZAMBETTI et al. 1990; PECORELLI et al. 1988). This is impressive, especially in the series of COLOMBO et al. (1986), because all of the six complete responses were pathologically confirmed, and all but one remained free of disease. However, it should be noted that all complete responses were obtained in patients with residual disease less than 2 cm, that the follow-up was relatively short, and that the PVB regimen is associated with severe toxicity, particularly bone marrow, pulmonary, and peripheral neurotoxicity. Because of its lower toxicity, we recommend the use of the bleomycin/etoposide/cisplatin regimen (BEP) instead of PVB for the treatment of recurrent or advanced granulosa cell tumors (see also Sect. 11.17). Because bleomycin is known to induce lung fibrosis and even toxic deaths, and because of the good prognosis of stage I disease, we use the etoposide/cisplatin (EP) regimen as adjuvant treatment in patients with unfavorable prognostic characteristics (see below).

Recently, the use of gonadotropin-releasing hormone agonists (KAUPPILA et al. 1992) or progesterone (MALIK and SLEVIN 1991) has been advocated in recurrent or advanced disease. In recurrent disease, salvage surgery should always be considered because of the indolent nature of the disease and because the metastases are often not deeply infiltrating.

In conclusion, surgery is the cornerstone of therapy. Adjuvant treatment has no proven value in stage I disease and is unnecessary in most patients. In stage I patients with more than three mitoses per ten high power fields and with severe nuclear atypia, adjuvant radiotherapy to the whole abdomen or adjuvant EP chemotherapy may be considered. In patients with more advanced disease, especially with residual tumor following surgery, we prefer the use of BEP chemotherapy.

JUVENILE GRANULOSA CELL TUMORS

Clinical Features. The juvenile granulosa cell tumor was described by SCULLY (1977) as a granulosa cell tumor that occurs before the age of normal puberty and that has the distinctive microscopic features of a juvenile granulosa cell tumor. In the series from Massachusetts General Hospital (YOUNG et al. 1984a) with 125 of these neoplasms, 44% occurred in the first decade, 34% in the second decade, 19% in the third decade, and only 3% beyond the age of 30 years. In addition to the different age distribution, juvenile granulosa cell tumors show more immature follicles, less Call-Exner bodies, darker nuclei which are rarely grooved, more frequent luteinization, and a higher mitotic index than the adult type.

In prepubertal girls, the presence of a juvenile granulosa cell tumor typically results in isosexual pseudoprecocity (YOUNG et al. 1984a; LACK et al. 1981; ZALOUDEK and NORRIS 1982; VASSAL et al. 1988; BISCOTTI and HART 1989). In older patients, it results in menometrorrhagia or amenorrhea. With very rare exceptions a granulosa cell tumor causing precocity is palpable, at least on rectal examination (YOUNG and SCULLY 1984b). Some ovarian germ cell tumors producing human chorionic gonadotrophin (HCG) and estrogen-secreting Sertoli cell tumors may also cause sexual precocity. The presence of HCG rules out a juvenile granulosa cell tumor. Juvenile granulosa cell tumors are, like the adult type, associated with increased serum inhibin levels (NISHIDA et al. 1991). There is a suggestion of a specific, though weak, association with Ollier's disease (endochondromatosis) or Maffucci's syndrome (Ollier's disease with multiple hemangiomas) (VELASCO-OSES et al. 1988).

At operation spread beyond one ovary is unusual. According to YOUNG et al. (1984b), only 3% of the tumors were bilateral at the time of diagnosis and involvement of the contralateral ovary became apparent in an additional 2% within 1 year postoperatively. The tumors are usually relatively large, averaging approximately 12.5 cm in diameter. The appearance is often solid and cystic in which the solid component is typically yellow-tan or gray.

Prognosis and Treatment. Approximately 5% of juvenile granulosa cell tumors behave in a malignant fashion (LACK et al. 1981; ZALOUDEK and NORRIS

1982; Young et al. 1984a); such cases are usually, but not invariably, those showing the greatest degree of atypia and mitotic activity. The indolent course followed by the adult type is not, however, mirrored by the juvenile form, for these tend to behave aggressively at relapse, with wide dissimination in the whole abdominal cavity within 2 years.

Unilateral salpingo-oophorectomy is adequate therapy for most stage Ia cases. Because of the rarity of this tumor, very few patients have received radiotherapy or chemotherapy. Obviously more experience is necessary to evaluate these forms of therapy.

11.16.1.2 Thecoma-Fibroma Group

Thecomas. There is a continuous morphological spectrum between a fibroma, composed almost entirely of fibroblastic collagen-producing cells, and a thecoma, formed largely of plump lipid-containing cells, and this makes the drawing of boundaries between these two neoplasms often a largely arbitrary exercise. Thecomas can be divided into typical and luteinized forms (Table 11.56). Together the thecomas are about one-third as frequent as granulosa cell tumors (Bjorkholm and Silversward 1980). Typical thecomas occur most often in postmenopausal patients (mean age 59 years), and are characteristically accompanied by estrogenic manifestations (endometrial carcinoma in about 20% of the patients) (Bjorkholm and Silversward 1980). Fibromas or thecomas containing luteinized cells have been called luteinized thecomas. These tumors occur in a younger age group (30% younger than 30 years) than the typical thecomas. Half of the luteinized thecomas are estrogenic, 40% nonfunctioning, and 10% androgenic (Zhang et al. 1982). Typical and luteinized thecomas are usually unilateral and benign. Unilateral oophorectomy with sampling of the endometrium is generally the preferred treatment in patients desiring to preserve their fertility. Hysterectomy with bilateral salpingo-oophorectomy is recommended in the other patients. The number of malignant thecomas reported in the literature is very small. In the absence of established criteria for malignancy, the same criteria as are helpful in distinguishing between cellular fibromas and fibrosarcomas, namely the degree of mitotic activity and nuclear atypicality, have been used (Young and Scully 1984b).

Fibroma/Cellular Fibroma/Fibrosarcoma. These tumors probably arise from ovarian stromal cells rather than from nonspecific fibrous stroma within the ovary and therefore merit inclusion within the sex cord-stromal group of neoplasms (Fox 1985). Fibromas are benign and most of them occur in patients over 40 years of age, with an average of 48 years (Dockerty and Masson 1944). Young women with the basal cell nevus syndrome often have ovarian fibromas, which are usually calcified, multinodular, and bilateral (Young and Scully 1984b). Fibromas may be associated with ascites and pleural effusions (Meigs' syndrome; Meigs 1954) in about 1% of the cases. Meigs' syndrome is associated with elevated serum CA-125 levels (Timmerman et al. 1995).

Some fibromatous tumors are more cellular and mitotically active than the usual fibroma. In a study of 17 of these tumors it was found that those tumors with an average of less than three mitotic figures per ten high power fields in the most cellular areas generally behaved in a clinically benign manner (cellular fibromas), whereas those with a higher mitotic activity typically had a malignant course (fibrosarcomas) (Prat and Scully 1981). Some cellular fibromas may be malign, especially when they are adherent to the pelvic wall or ruptured. However, nonadherent intact cellular fibromas also may rarely behave in a malignant fashion (Young 1991). Little is known about the preferred treatment of malignant cellular fibromas and fibrosarcomas.

Stromal Tumor with Minor Sex Cord Elements. Occasionally thecomas and fibromas have a minor (<5%) component of sex cord cells. The features and clinical behavior of these tumors are more similar to those of fibroma or thecoma than to those of a granulosa cell tumor or Sertoli-Leydig cell tumor (Young 1991).

Sclerosing Stromal Tumor. The sclerosing stromal tumors are rare neoplasms of ovarian stromal origin which occur at a younger age (most commonly in the third decade) than the typical thecomas and fibromas (Chalvardjian and Scully 1973; Fox 1985; Young 1991). In contrast to the typically functioning thecomas, the sclerosing stromal tumor has been associated with estrogenic secretion only occasionally and evidence of androgen secretion has rarely been present. All sclerosing stromal tumors encountered to date have been unilateral and benign.

11.16.2 Sertoli-Stromal Cell Tumors

Sertoli-Leydig cell tumors account for less than 0.2% of all ovarian neoplasms (Young and Scully 1984b). Approximately 40%–50% of the patients present with hirsutism or virilization (Young and Scully 1984b; Young and Scully 1985). Sertoli-Leydig cell tumors are sex cord-stromal tumors that exhibit a testicular direction of differentiation, and were originally designated as arrhenoblastomas or androblastomas. The term Sertoli-Leydig cell tumor is more appropriate for several reasons (Young and Scully 1985): (a) "arrhenoblastoma" or "androblastoma" connotes masculinization, but more than half of the tumors are nonfunctioning or even estrogenic; (b) numerous other ovarian tumors may be androgenic; (c) the designation Sertoli-Leydig cell is parallel to that used for the sex cord-stromal tumors that exhibit an ovarian direction of differentiation, the granulosa-stromal cell tumors. According to the classification proposed by the International Society of Gynecological Pathologists, these tumors are divided into three subgroups: Sertoli cell tumors, Leydig cell tumors, and Sertoli-Leydig cell tumors (Table 11.56).

11.16.2.1 Pure Sertoli Cell Tumors

Pure Sertoli cell tumors are rare, with fewer than 30 well-documented examples in the literature (Young and Scully 1984a; Young 1993b). In contrast to the more frequently observed Sertoli-Leydig cell tumors, pure Sertoli tumors produce estrogens in two-thirds of cases. Enigmatically, Sertoli cell tumors have accounted for three of the small number of ovarian neoplasms associated with renin production resulting in hypertension (Ehrlich et al. 1963; Korzets et al. 1986; Aiba et al. 1990). All tumors have been unilateral and only one has behaved in a clinically malignant manner (Young and Scully 1984a).

11.16.2.2 Leydig Cell Tumors

The Leydig cell tumors are more logically regarded as steroid cell tumors and will be discussed in Sect. 11.18.

11.16.2.3 Sertoli-Leydig Cell Tumors

Sertoli-Leydig cell tumors are divided into five categories: well differentiated, intermediately differentiated, poorly differentiated, tumors with a retiform pattern, and tumors with heterologous elements. In the largest study on 207 cases, 11% were well differentiated, 54% were of intermediate differentiation, 13% were poorly differentiated, and 22% contained heterologous elements. In most of the latter tumors the heterologous elements consist of intestinal-type epithelium, and in some cases of cartilage or skeletal muscle. A prominent retiform pattern was present in 15% (Young and Scully 1985). About 97% of the tumors are in stage I and only 1.5% are bilateral (Roth et al. 1981; Zaloudek and Norris 1984; Young and Scully 1985). They are encountered at all ages but their peak incidence is during the early reproductive years, with an average of 25 years (Young and Scully 1985).

The most important prognostic factor is the degree of differentiation. In the study of The Massachusetts General Hospital (Young and Scully 1985), none of the well-differentiated tumors recurred, while relapse was observed in 11% of the tumors with intermediate differentiation and in 59% of the poorly differentiated tumors. Relapse was noted in 19% of the tumors with heterologous elements, mainly in the group with cartilage or skeletal muscle as the heterologous part. Other unfavorable prognostic factors are rupture, a mitotic index higher than 15 per ten high power fields, a tumor size larger than 15 cm, and advanced stage of disease (Roth et al. 1981; Zaloudek and Norris 1984; Young and Scully 1985).

The standard treatment of Sertoli-Leydig cell tumors in older patients is total abdominal hysterectomy, bilateral salpingo-oophorectomy, and omentectomy. In younger patients wishing to preserve their fertility, the low frequency of bilaterality justifies the performance of a unilateral oophorectomy if the tumor is in stage Ia. Para-aortic and pelvic lymphadenectomy might be justified in undifferentiated stage I tumors. Subsequent adjuvant therapy has been advocated for any undifferentiated or poorly differentiated tumor higher than stage Ia, and stage Ia undifferentiated tumors (Young and Scully 1985). In older series the use of adjuvant radiotherapy has been proposed in patients with residual tumor <2 cm and chemotherapy in patients with residual tumor >2 cm (Schwartz and

SMITH 1976). Newer studies suggest that these tumors are very sensitive for combination chemotherapy, especially when cisplatin is included (SCHWARTZ and SMITH 1976; YOUNG and SCULLY 1983, 1984b, 1985; ROTH et al. 1981; ZALOUDEK and NORRIS 1984;). Although the optimal form of adjuvant therapy is not established at the present time, we prefer the use of the bleomycin, etoposide, and cisplatin (BEP) regimen in patients with residual tumor or stage I disease with an unfavorable prognosis because of its lower long-term toxicity compared with radiotherapy.

11.16.3 Gynandroblastoma

The term "gynandroblastoma" has been used in a somewhat indiscriminate fashion but should be restricted to neoplasms in which both granulosa-thecal and Sertoli-Leydig cell elements are present, the diagnosis being a purely morphological one and lacking any endocrinological connotations (FOX 1985). Because of the relative frequency with which extensive sampling of a Sertoli-Leydig cell tumor demonstrates very small foci of granulosa cells and vice versa, the diagnosis of gynandroblastoma should be reserved for those tumors that contain at least 10% of the second tumor type (YOUNG and SCULLY 1984b). If this strict definition is used, gynandroblastoma is extremely rare and not enough examples have been accumulated for the biological behavior of these neoplasms to be defined.

11.16.4 Sex Cord-Stromal Tumors with Annular Tubules

The sex cord-stromal tumor with annular tubules is a clinically and pathologically distinctive lesion first described in 1970 (SCULLY 1970a). One-third of the cases of sex cord-stromal tumor with annular tubules are associated with Peutz-Jeghers syndrome (gastrointestinal polyposis, oral and cutaneous melanin pigmentation). Almost all patients with the Peutz-Jeghers syndrome whose ovaries have been examined microscopically have had sex cord-stromal tumors with annular tubules. The lesions are multifocal and bilateral in most such patients, smaller than 3 cm, and behave in a benign fashion. In contrast, in patients without Peutz-Jeghers syndrome, the tumors are almost always unilateral, usually form a palpable mass, and are clinically malignant in at least one-fifth of the patients (YOUNG and SCULLY 1984b; FOX 1985). These tumors are estrogenic in 40% of the cases.

Unilateral salpingo-oophorectomy is the therapy of choice in young patients without Peutz-Jeghers syndrome. The possible role of chemotherapy or radiotherapy in clinically malignant cases needs further evaluation.

11.16.5 Unclassified Sex Cord-Stromal Tumors

Approximately 10% of the patients with sex cord-stromal tumors have patterns and cell types intermediate between those of Sertoli-Leydig cell tumors and granulosa cell tumors. Such tumors are placed in the unclassified category (YOUNG and SCULLY 1984b). Sex cord-stromal tumors from pregnant patients are particularly likely to be placed in this category (YOUNG et al. 1984b).

11.17 General Management and the Role of Irradiation in *Germ Cell Tumors* of the Ovaries

I.B. VERGOTE and D. TIMMERMAN

Germ cell neoplasms are the second most common group of ovarian tumors after the epithelial tumors. In Europe and North America, germ cell neoplasms account for approximately 20% of all ovarian tumors. The great majority of ovarian germ cell tumors are benign and consist of mature cystic teratomas. The latter account for more than 90% of ovarian germ cell tumors (TALERMAN 1992). In the subgroup of malignant ovarian tumors, germ cell neoplasms are also the second most frequent group, and account for about 2%–3% of all ovarian cancers.

In this chapter we will use the World Health Classification of ovarian germ cell tumors (Table 11.59), and only the management of malignant germ cell tumors will be discussed.

Modern therapy has changed an almost universally fatal disease to one that is highly curable. The marked improvement during recent decades in the prognosis of yolk sac tumors, immature teratomas, and mixed germ cell tumors is rivalled only in gyne-

Table 11.59. Classification of ovarian germ cell tumors as formulated by the World Health Organization. (Talerman 1992)

1. Dysgerminoma
2. Yolk sac tumor (endodermal sinus tumor)
3. Embryonal carcinoma
4. Polyembryoma
5. Choriocarcinoma (nongestational)
6. Teratoma
   A. Immature
   B. Mature
      (i) Solid[a]
      (ii) Cystic
         a) Mature cystic teratoma (dermoid cyst)[a]
         b) Mature cystic teratoma with malignant transformation
   C. Monodermal
      (i) Struma ovarii
      (ii) Carcinoid
      (iii) Strumal carcinoid
      (iv) Others (e.g., mucinous, neuroectodermal, sebaceous)
7. Mixed germ cell tumors (tumors composed of types 1 through 6 in any possible combination)
8. Gonadoblastoma

[a] Benign tumors.

cological oncology by the almost complete curability of gestational trophoblastic disease. If managed correctly, a young woman with a malignant germ cell tumor now has a better than 85% chance of being cured and a good chance of remaining fertile (Rustin 1987). Germ cell tumors are the most frequently encountered ovarian tumors in childhood and adolescence. Gynecologists and pediatricians should be aware that an ovarian mass with solid areas on ultrasonography may be a malignant germ cell tumor.

11.17.1 Clinical Features of Germ Cell Tumors

11.17.1.1 Dysgerminoma

In older series, dysgerminoma was the most common malignant ovarian germ cell tumor (Scully 1979). Nowadays more dysgerminomas are found to be combined with other neoplastic germ cell tumors and are included in the category of mixed germ cell tumors (Gershenson et al. 1984; Talerman 1992). Dysgerminoma differs from the epithelial ovarian tumors in many respects (Thomas et al. 1987): It mainly occurs in a much younger age group, with 85% of the patients being less than 29 years old and the mean age being 22 years (Asadourian and Taylor 1969); its principal mode of dissemination is nodal rather than transperitoneal (Asadourian and Taylor 1969; De Palo et al. 1984); and its extreme radiosensitivity and chemosensitivity much more closely resembles that of the equivalent male tumor, seminoma, than that of epithelial ovarian cancer. Furthermore, dysgerminomas, unlike epithelial ovarian carcinomas, are confined to one ovary (stage Ia) in about 75% of the cases at the time of diagnosis. Macroscopically, dysgerminoma is usually unilateral, although it may be bilateral microscopically in 10%–15% of cases (Gordon et al. 1981; Bjorkholm et al. 1990). In this respect it differs from the other malignant germ cell tumors, which are virtually never bilateral. The median tumor diameter is 15 cm (Asadourian and Taylor 1969), with approximately half of the tumors being more than 10 cm in one study (De Palo et al. 1984). Its external surface is generally smooth and lobulated. On cut surface it is solid pink or tan, and has focal hemorrhage or necrosis. Abdominal enlargement is the most frequent presenting symptom (Gordon et al. 1981; Bjorkholm et al. 1990).

Although dysgerminoma is the most common germ cell tumor encountered in subjects with gonadal maldevelopment and chromosomal abnormalities, only 5%–10% of dysgerminomas occur in such patients (Vergote et al. 1983). Most of these patients have a female phenotype. Between 8% and 10% of dysgerminomas contain syncytiotrophoblastic giant cells, which have been conclusively shown to produce beta-human chorionic gonadotropin (β-HCG) (Zaloudek et al. 1981). These tumors may be accompanied by hyperestrinism resulting in menstrual disturbances in postpubertal women and isosexual pseudoprecocity in prepubertal female patients. Pure dysgerminomas are also often associated with increased serum placental alkaline phosphatase (Vergote et al. 1987) and lactic dehydrogenase levels (Pressley et al. 1992). Dysgerminoma is the second most common ovarian neoplasm after small cell carcinomas associated with hypercalcemia (Fleischhacker and Young 1994). Dysgerminomas are almost always diploid (Kommoss et al. 1990).

11.17.1.2 Yolk Sac Tumor (Endodermal Sinus Tumor)

Yolk sac tumor is the second most common malignant ovarian germ cell neoplasm occurring in pure form, and is also a frequent component of mixed germ cell tumors (TALERMAN 1992). The development of treatment principles has been hindered by the confusion regarding terminology and the multiplicity of histological patterns. Ten histological patterns have now been described (microcystic, endodermal sinus, papillary, glandular-alveolar, solid, myxomatous, macrocystic, polyvesicular vitelline, hepatoid, and primitive intestinal) (TALERMAN 1992). Only recently has the presence of perivascular formations (Schiller-Duval bodies), a hallmark of yolk sac tumors, no longer been considered a prerequisite for the diagnosis.

Yolk sac tumors are most frequently encountered in the second and third decades, followed by the first and fourth (TEILUM 1965; KURMAN and NORRIS 1976b; SCULLY 1979; LANGLEY et al. 1981). Yolk sac tumors are unilateral and to date no well-documented cases of bilateral primary tumors have been reported. Patients with yolk sac tumors usually present with abdominal enlargement and pain, or both (KURMAN and NORRIS 1976b). Grossly these neoplasms are usually encapsulated, smooth, and lobulated. The cut surface has a variegated aspect.

Although an elevated serum alpha-fetoprotein (AFP) level in a young woman with an ovarian tumor is very suggestive of a yolk sac tumor, patients with embryonal carcinomas, immature teratomas, Sertoli-Leydig cell tumors, clear cell carcinomas, and mucinous carcinomas occasionally present with elevated serum AFP levels (TALERMAN 1992; YOUNG 1993a). Yolk sac tumors are generally aneuploid (KOMMOSS et al. 1990).

A yolk sac tumor is rapidly growing and highly malignant, invading the surrounding structures and metastasizing early via the lymphatic route and by hematogenous spread to lungs, liver, and other organs.

11.17.1.3 Embryonal Carcinoma

Although recognized in the 1973 World Health Organization classification (SEROV et al. 1973), only in recent years has embryonal carcinoma been characterized as a separate clinicopathological entity (KURMAN and NORRIS 1976a). Previously the terms "embryonal carcinoma" and "endodermal sinus tumor" were used interchangeably. Although embryonal carcinoma is a rare component of mixed germ cell tumors, it is extremely rare in the pure state. Embryonal carcinomas occur in the same age group and have the same presenting signs as yolk sac tumors. However, elevated serum β-HCG levels resulting in pseudoprecocity or menstrual disorders are frequently observed. Elevated AFP levels have been reported. It has been suggested that patients with embryonal carcinoma have a somewhat better prognosis than patients with yolk sac tumors (KURMAN and NORRIS 1976a).

11.17.1.4 Polyembryoma

Polyembryoma is an extremely uncommon primitive germ cell tumor, which is composed entirely or in large part of embryoid bodies that histologically mimic embryos of about 1–2 weeks' gestation (PEYRON 1939; TAKEDA et al. 1982; KING et al. 1991). Usually the tumor is combined with other malignant germ cell elements and classified as a mixed germ cell tumor. Polyembryomas are malignant and should be treated in the same way as the other nondysgerminomatous germ cell tumors.

11.17.1.5 Choriocarcinoma (Nongestational)

Choriocarcinoma of the ovary, like its testicular counterpart, rarely occurs in a pure histological form (JACOBS et al. 1982b; AXE et al. 1985; VANCE and GEISINGER 1985). The presence of choriocarcinoma in a premenarchal girl or its occurrence with other germ cell elements eliminates the possibility of gestational origin. Choriocarcinoma typically occurs under the age of 20 years and because of elevated HCG levels there may be isosexual pseudoprecocity, menstrual disorders, or pseudopregnancy. Choriocarcinomas are unilateral, rapidly growing, and had a bad prognosis prior to the advent of modern combination chemotherapy.

11.17.1.6 Teratoma

Teratomas are germ cell tumors composed of derivatives of the three primitive germ layers, ectoderm, mesoderm, and endoderm. In the ovary the overwhelming majority (99%) of teratomas are mature and cystic (TALERMAN 1992). They are classified as mature cystic teratomas or dermoid cysts and by virtue of complete maturity of the constituent tissues are benign, and will not be discussed in this chapter.

Immature Teratoma. To investigate the relation of immature teratomas to dermoid cysts, a study of 350 cases of immature teratoma was recently conducted and disclosed that 26% of the former contained one or more grossly visible dermoid cyst, that 10% were associated with a contralateral dermoid cyst, and that 2.6% occurred in patients with a history of resection of an ipsilateral dermoid cyst (Yanai-Inbar and Scully 1987). The authors concluded that a patient with a history of resection of a dermoid cyst is at slightly increased risk for the subsequent development of an immature teratoma. In a combined experience involving 108 patients with stage I immature teratomas, none of the tumors were bilateral (Vergote et al. 1990). The median age at the time of diagnosis is about 19 years (Norris et al. 1976; Nogales et al. 1976; Nielsen et al. 1986; Vergote et al. 1990). Abdominal pain and discomfort are common symptoms caused by rupture or torsion of the tumor.

A strong correlation exists between the degree of immaturity of the tumor and its behavior. This has led to the formulation of a grading system proposed by Thurlbeck and Scully (1960), which was later adapted and extended by Norris et al. (1976).

Immature teratoma is often a part of a mixed germ cell tumor. Elevated serum HCG or AFP levels should alert the pathologist to sample an immature teratoma liberally to identify less favorable germ cell components such as yolk sac tumors, embryonal carcinoma, or choriocarcinoma. It should be noted, however, that AFP levels may be increased in pure immature teratomas. Survival was poor in the prechemotherapy era (Norris et al. 1976), but has improved substantially during the last 2 decades (see Sect. 11.17.2).

Mature Cystic Teratoma with Malignant Transformation. Malignant transformation of a mature cystic teratoma (dermoid cyst) occurs in 1%–2% of the cases (Scully 1979; Peterson 1957). Unlike the vast majority of patients with malignant germ cell tumors who are younger than 30 years, most of the patients with this tumor are postmenopausal. The most common tumor is a squamous cell carcinoma. The tumor responds poorly to chemotherapy or radiotherapy and has a very poor prognosis (Talerman 1992).

Monodermal Teratomas. The tumors that make up this group are composed entirely or predominantly of a single tissue and are considered to represent one-sided development of a teratoma. Some of these tumors may be malignant and are usually treated according to their differentiation and not like the other malignant germ cell tumors. Struma ovarii is the best known and widely recognized member of this group of neoplasms (Scully 1979). Occasionally these tumors are malignant (Young 1993a). Ovarian carcinoid tumors are the second most common type of monodermal teratoma, and are classified as insular carcinoid, trabecular carcinoid, or mucinous carcinoid. Insular carcinoid tumors behave as neoplasms of low-grade malignancy, and the treatment of choice is excision (Robboy et al. 1975; Scully 1979). Trabecular carcinoid tumors have not been associated with metastases and have an excellent prognosis (Talerman 1984). Mucinous carcinoid tumors are more malignant than the other types of ovarian carcinoid tumors. Response to chemotherapy has been poor in this group of tumors (Alenghat et al. 1986). Ovarian strumal carcinoid tumor is composed of thyroid tissue intimately admixed with carcinoid tumor, and is the second most common type of ovarian carcinoid after the insular type (Robboy and Scully 1980; Snyder and Tavassoli 1986). Excision of the tumor has resulted in complete cure.

Recently four other types of monodermal teratomas have been recognized: monodermal teratoma with neuroectodermal differentiation, ependymoma, monodermal teratoma composed of vascular tissue, and sebaceous tumors. Malignant monodermal teratomas with neuroectodermal differentiation pursue an aggressive course and have a poor prognosis (Aguirre and Scully 1982). The prognosis of patients with pure ovarian ependymomas is much more favorable, even when the tumors have metastasized (Kleinman et al. 1984). Monodermal teratomas with immature vascular tissue behave in a less aggressive manner than high-grade immature teratomas and hemangioendothelial sarcomas of the ovary (Talerman 1992). Also sebaceous carcinomas generally have a favorable prognosis (Chumas and Scully 1991).

11.17.1.7 Mixed Germ Cell Tumors

Mixed germ cell tumors comprise all germ cell tumors composed of more than one germ cell element. The therapy depends on the germ cell elements found in the tumor.

11.17.1.8
Gonadoblastoma

Gonadoblastomas are composed of germ cells and admixed with sex cord-stromal derivatives. Gonadoblastomas are almost exclusively seen in patients with gonadal dysgenesis. Most patients are young phenotypic females (80%) and some (20%) are phenotypic male pseudohermaphrodites (SCULLY 1970b). The most common karyotypes observed are 46,XY and most of the remainder have been mosaics with 45,XO/46,XY. Gonadoblastoma is frequently admixed with dysgerminoma and sometimes with other types of malignant germ cell tumors. In the former cases the prognosis is very good, while in the latter group the surgical removal of the tumor has to be followed by the combination chemotherapy used to treat nondysgerminomatous malignant germ cell tumors. The therapy of pure gonadoblastomas in patients with dysgenetic gonads is bilateral adnexectomy because of the high malignant potential and because the gonads are nonfunctional.

11.17.2
Treatment of Malignant Germ Cell Tumors

11.17.2.1
Diagnosis

Once the diagnosis of malignant germ cell tumor of the ovary is suspected, preoperative evaluation should include serological tumor markers (HCG, AFP, and LDH isoenzymes), ultrasonography of the pelvis, chest x-ray, and computed tomography of the abdomen. Optional studies would include barium enema and intravenous pyelography. It is important to perform karyotyping on all premenarchal girls with a suspected ovarian tumor, because germ cell tumors have a propensity to occur in dysgenetic gonads.

11.17.2.2
Operative Management

In patients suspected of having a malignant germ cell tumor it is best to perform a laparotomy through a vertical midline incision. Ascites or saline washings of the pelvis and paracolic gutters should be sent for cytological analysis. As in epithelial ovarian carcinomas, a complete evaluation of the whole abdomen and an omentectomy should be performed. If the ovarian pathology is unilateral, a unilateral salpingo-oophorectomy may be performed because most patients are young, and malignant germ cell tumors are almost always unilateral, except for dysgerminomas (see Sect. 11.17.1). As will be discussed in Sect. 11.17.2.3, dysgerminomas are extremely sensitive to chemotherapy at the time of relapse. Therefore we do not biopsy the contralateral ovary if it appears normal, even when the frozen section reveals the presence of a dysgerminoma. Any suspicious or palpable retroperitoneal lymph nodes should be biopsied, but there is no indication for a formal pelvic and para-aortic lymphadenectomy because of the chemo- and radiosensitivity of dysgerminomas, and because of the chemosensitivity and rapid hematogenous spread in the nondysgerminomatous malignant germ cell tumors (GERSHENSON 1985; WILLIAMS 1991; PFLEIDERER 1993). In dysgerminoma, cytoreductive surgery does not seem to be important, while in nondysgerminomatous malignant germ cell tumors there might be a correlation between tumor response to chemotherapy and volume of residual disease (WILLIAMS et al. 1989b). However, because germ cell tumors are generally more sensitive to chemotherapy than epithelial tumors, the added benefit of very aggressive cytoreductive surgery has been questioned. In patients with nondysgerminomatous malignant germ cell tumors we favor a reasonable attempt at surgical debulking, and we try to preserve the reproductive organs when they are not clearly involved (WILLIAMS et al. 1991).

11.17.2.3
Postoperative Management of Dysgerminoma

Dysgerminoma differs from its nondysgerminomatous counterpart in several respects. First, it is probably more likely to be localized to the ovary at the time of diagnosis. Second, bilateral involvement is more frequent. Third, spread to retroperitoneal lymph nodes is probably more frequent and hematogenous spread less frequent. Fourth, the tumor is substantially more sensitive to radiotherapy. And fifth, dysgerminoma is probably more curable at the time of relapse.

Until the mid-1980s the recommendation for therapy after surgical removal of the tumor, which usually included bilateral salpingo-oophorectomy and hysterectomy, was postoperative irradiation (KREPART et al. 1978; GERSHENSON 1985; THOMAS et al. 1987). Once patients with nondysgerminomatous tumors were excluded, the treatment results for surgery and radiation therapy in pure dysgerminomas were excellent, with a survival rate of approximately 83% (GORDON et al. 1981). Three large series, however, have examined the results of conservative surgery without postoperative irradiation in 145 patients (ASADOURIAN and TAYLOR 1969; GORDON et al. 1981; MALKASIAN and SYMMONDS 1964). In spite of the fact that meticulous staging was not performed and that effective chemotherapy was not available at that time, the 10-year survival was as high as 91%. Salvage therapy consisting of reoperation alone, radiation alone, or both was successful in 65% of the patients.

Recently the extreme sensitivity of pure dysgerminoma to platinum-based combination chemotherapy has been reported, with a cure rate of 96% in patients with advanced or recurrent disease (NEWLANDS et al. 1982; SMALES and PECKHAM 1987; GERSHENSON et al. 1990a; WILLIAMS et al. 1991; ZINSER et al. 1990; KUMAR et al. 1993; SEGELOV et al. 1994). In the study of the Gynecologic Oncology Group (WILLIAMS et al. 1991), 19 patients out of 20 with advanced or recurrent dysgerminoma were cured with platinum-based chemotherapy. In another study from M.D. Anderson, 14 dysgerminoma patients received similar chemotherapy and all were disease-free (GERSHENSON et al. 1990b). In an Australian study, 13 out of 14 patients were cured with platinum-based chemotherapy (SEGELOV et al. 1994).

The most frequently used regimen is bleomycin, etoposide, and cisplatin (BEP) (WILLIAMS et al. 1991). However, fatal bleomycin pulmonary toxicity has been observed in patients (about 0.5%–1%) treated for malignant ovarian germ cell tumors (TAYLOR et al. 1985; SINGH et al. 1987; SEGELOV et al. 1994), and the use of etoposide has been associated with an increased risk of leukemia (PEDERSEN-BJERGAARD et al. 1991; NICHOLS et al. 1993; BOSHOFF et al. 1995). This risk is estimated to be very low (0.02%) when giving a total dose of less than $2000\,mg/m^2$, and as high as 8% when giving more than $2000\,mg/m^2$. Most patients treated with BEP receive less than this dose ($300–500\,mg/m^2$ etoposide per course).

It appears that almost all patients with malignant germ cell tumors treated with platinum-based combination chemotherapy can anticipate normal menstrual function and a reasonable probability of having normal offspring (GERSHENSON 1988; RUSTIN et al. 1988; VERGOTE et al. 1990; WU et al. 1991).

Based on the good prognosis of stage I dysgerminoma, the high curability of relapses, and the long-term side-effects of chemo- or radiotherapy, we advocate no adjuvant treatment in stage 1 disease. Patients with recurrent or advanced disease are treated with etoposide and cisplatin (EP). Tumors resistant to chemotherapy might be cured by surgery and radiotherapy. Second-look surgery is not performed, but the patients are followed closely both clinically and with CT scanning.

11.17.2.4 Postoperative Management of Nondysgerminomatous Tumors

Only 10%–15% of stage I patients with nondysgerminomatous malignant germ cell tumors treated with surgery alone will survive. Equally dismal survival has resulted from postoperative radiotherapy or single alkylating agent treatment (GERSHENSON 1985). Many patients with nondysgerminomatous malignant germ cell tumors that have not metastasized have been treated with vincristine, actinomycin D, and cyclophosphamide (VAC), and about 70% have survived long term (SLAYTON et al. 1985; GERSHENSON et al. 1985a). The largest experience with VAC as adjuvant treatment in patients with nondysgerminomatous malignant germ cell tumors without residual tumor was obtained in a Gynecologic Oncology Group trial. In this study 76 out of 100 patients remained tumor-free (WILLIAMS et al. 1989a). In patients with advanced disease treated with VAC, sustained remissions were observed in 45% of cases (SLAYTON et al. 1985; GERSHENSON et al. 1985). Subsequently, because of the experience in testicular germ cell tumors, cisplatin-based regimens have been used in these patients. Patients with advanced or recurrent nondysgerminomatous malignant germ cell tumors treated with cisplatin, vinblastine, and bleomycin (PVB) appeared to have a better prognosis. The largest study was performed by the Gynecologic Oncology Group (WILLIAMS et al. 1989b) and showed that 47 of 89 patients (53%) were disease-free with a median follow-up of 52 months, and the 4-year survival was 70%.

In cases of testicular cancer, it was shown that etoposide was actually superior to vinblastine (WILLIAMS et al. 1987). The same appears to be true for nondysgerminomatous malignant germ cell tumors (GERSHENSON et al. 1990b; WILLIAMS et al. 1994). In the Gynecologic Oncology Group study (WILLIAMS et al. 1994), 93 patients with nondysgerminomatous malignant germ cell tumors without residual tumor following surgery were treated with three courses of bleomycin, etoposide, and cisplatin (BEP). Ninety-one patients (98%) were disease-free with a follow-up ranging from 4 to 90 months. One patient developed leukemia.

Frequently discussed are the need for the inclusion of bleomycin in the regimen and the optimum duration of chemotherapy. One randomized study from the Eastern Cooperative Oncology Group suggested that the omission of bleomycin in patients with favorable-prognosis disseminated germ cell tumors was deleterious to outcome (LOEHRER et al. 1991). However, in another randomized trial initiated by the Memorial Sloan-Kettering Cancer Center, the addition of bleomycin did not confer any survival advantage in good-prognosis germ cell tumors (BOSL et al. 1988). Another randomized study of the Southeastern Cancer Study Group showed that three courses of BEP was as effective as four courses in favorable-prognosis disseminated germ cell tumors.

Based on the above-mentioned findings we use three courses of BEP as adjuvant therapy for nondysgerminomatous malignant germ cell tumors. Patients with residual tumors receive more courses, dependent on the serum tumor marker levels and the observed response on clinical and CAT scan examination. The only exception to these guidelines is the immature teratomas. It is well established that grade I stage I immature teratomas do not need any adjuvant therapy and that these tumors are more chemosensitive than the other nondysgerminomatous malignant germ cell tumors. Stage I grade 2 and 3 immature teratomas are treated with single-agent doxorubicin because all our patients treated in this way have survived without any major side-effects (VERGOTE et al. 1990). Patients with residual tumor of pure immature teratoma are treated with etoposide and cisplatin (EP). In a review of the literature we presented the results of 85 patients with immature teratoma treated after operation with chemotherapy who underwent a second-look laparotomy (VERGOTE et al. 1990). Only three patients had residual tumor. These three patients had residual grade 3 lesions after primary surgery. Based on these findings we only perform second-look surgery in patients with residual immature teratoma after primary surgery. Another interesting feature is the maturation of residual immature teratoma by chemotherapy. None of 38 patients with mature teratomatous tissue at second-look surgery developed recurrent disease (VERGOTE et al. 1990). Therefore we discontinue therapy when only mature tissue is found at second-look surgery. Based on the large Gynecologic Oncology Group experience with 127 second-look laparotomies in patients with malignant germ cell tumors, it was concluded that second-look surgery is not necessary in patients without residual tumor after primary surgery. Furthermore, only patients with residual tumor that contains immature teratoma benefitted from this procedure.

Nongestational choriocarcinoma (pure or as part of a mixed germ cell tumor) is preferentially treated with BEP. Patients with progression on this regimen may benefit from regimens used for gestational trophoblastic disease such as high-dose methotrexate (JACOBS et al. 1982b).

11.18 General Management and the Role of Irradiation in Steroid Cell Tumors of the Ovary

I.B. VERGOTE and D. TIMMERMAN

Steroid cell tumors, formerly known as lipid or lipid cell tumors, are now subclassified into three major types: (a) stromal luteoma, (b) Leydig cell tumor (hilus cell tumor and Leydig cell tumor, nonhilar type), and (c) steroid cell tumor not otherwise specified.

Stromal luteomas account for approximately 25% of steroid cell tumors, are located within the ovarian stroma, and lack crystals of Reinke. They occur most often in postmenopausal patients. About two-thirds of the patients present with abnormal uterine bleeding due to estrogen production by the tumor. No convincing example of malignant stromal luteoma has been observed (HAYES and SCULLY 1987a).

Leydig cell tumors account for 15% of steroid cell tumors and are also usually encountered in postmenopausal patients. They are characteristically small, circumscribed noduli centered in the ovarian hilus. Androgen manifestations are present in 80% of the cases. Malignant behavior is very rare (STEWART and WOODWARD 1962; ECHT and HADD 1968; PARASKEVAS and SCULLY 1989).

The third type is the steroid cell tumor, not otherwise specified. This tumor occurs at a somewhat younger age than the former tumors (median age, 43 years). These tumors are typically androgenic and may induce heterosexual pseudoprecocity in children. The tumor may also be estrogenic, or produce cortisol. About 30% of these tumors are malignant. A high number of mitoses, a high grade of nuclear atypia, necrosis, and large size correlate with malignant behavior. The tumor is rare and little is known of its chemosensitivity or radiosensitivity (Hayes and Scully 1987b).

11.19 Follow-up Examinations

H.W. Vahrson

The follow-up examinations in patients treated for ovarian cancer do not fundamentally differ from the follow-up for other genital cancers (see Chap. 3). They are a common task of the cancer center, hospital, gynecologist, radiologist, and family doctor, into which the family members and social services must be integrated. Comprehensive follow-up has the following intentions (Vahrson 1983):

1. Diagnosis and therapy of therapy-related side-effects
2. Early diagnosis of recurrence
3. Performance and surveillance of treatment in outpatients
4. Psychological care of the patients and their families
5. Aid in social rehabilitation
6. Long-term control and documentation of the results of treatment

Gynecological examination has to investigate thoroughly the side-effects of surgery, percutaneous irradiation/intraperitoneal nuclide instillation, and chemotherapy. The scale of examinations beyond the gynecological examination (specula, bimanual, rectal) depends on the previous extent of the disease, prognosis, completeness of surgery and postoperative treatment, current status and complaints of the patient, and skill of the examiner. In patients with a good prognosis, very few additional examinations have to be carried out: weight control, measurement of abdominal circumference, blood sedimentation rate (BSR), blood count, and serum CA-125 level. The interval between examinations should be individualized according to the situation.

In the presence of an advanced stage, incomplete surgery, reduced status, and findings suspicious for recurrence, the entire spectrum of clinical diagnostic methods may be helpful to discover the recurrence:

1. Gynecological examination, weight control, control of abdominal circumference
2. Blood chemistry: BSR, blood count, Aph, LDH, GOT, GPT, γ-GT, urea, creatinine, and above all serum CA-125 level (see Sect. 11.5)
3. Transabdominal and transvaginal ultrasonography
4. X-ray films of the chest and bony skeleton, intravenous urography, and abdominal/thoracic CT
5. Phonocardiography (after cardiotoxic chemotherapy)
6. Scintigraphy and immunoscintigraphy for bone and/or soft tissue metastases
7. Magnetic resonance imaging of the abdomen, retroperitoneum, and mediastinum
8. Cerebral CT (in the presence of headache/cerebral symptoms)

The first-choice examinations are at the top of this list; those at the bottom should be used only in special cases.

In the event of incurable progression of the disease, a qualified follow-up must be performed until death occurs. All aid for relief must be given. The following list details such aid according to the presenting problem:

1. Ascites: puncture, instillation of cytostatics/radionuclides for palliation
2. Ileus: anus praeter, intestinal fistula
3. Ureteral obstruction: double-J catheter, renal fistula
4. Pleural effusion: puncture, instillation of cytostatics/radionuclide
5. Bone metastasis: antiosteolytic and bone stabilizing drugs/irradiation
6. Anemia: transfusion of erythrocytes, albumin
7. Tumor cachexia: parenteral nutrition, special diet
8. Tumor pains: morphine schedule or continuous peridural anesthesia by pump, irradiation of bone metastasis
9. Mental depression: estrogens, antidepressive drugs

The family members and or local nursing institution must be informed and instructed to apply drugs and nutrition as long as possible on an outpatient basis. Hospitalization is not the better alternative.

11.20 Clinical Trials and Outlook

U. Nitz, H.G. Bender, and H.W. Vahrson

11.20.1 Prevention and Screening

As ovarian cancer is predominantly diagnosed at advanced incurable stages of disease, one major point of interest will be prevention and improvement of screening. With regard to prevention, the use of oral contraceptives should be studied more systematically. In this context the widespread use of genetic counseling and genetic testing, as has already been achieved for BRCA-1, and further genetic research will allow the identification of subgroups at very high risk of ovarian cancer. Prevention studies should focus on these subgroups. For the entire population, screening must be improved with special emphasis on reducing the proportion of patients who have abnormal screening results as diagnosed by ultrasonography and CA-125 but do not have ovarian cancer. New imaging techniques (color Doppler flow examination, ultrasound contrast media) and new serum markers (OVX-1, M-CSF) should be investigated.

11.20.2 Surgery

In early ovarian cancer with a good prognosis (Ia, G1), the role of fertility-sparing operative techniques should be studied within prospective randomized trials. As primary and second-line chemotherapeutic regimens are changing, there is no possibility of definite evaluation of the role of second-look operation (SLO) in advanced disease at present. The predominant consideration of "SLO-controlled" chemotherapy trials should therefore be the randomized comparison of second-look laparotomy and second-look laparoscopy.

11.20.3 Chemotherapy

For the other early disease stages a prospective randomized EORTC trial is underway to evaluate the role of platinum-based standard chemotherapy (platinum/cyclophosphamide). Patient accrual is ongoing. Trials evaluating the combination of taxol and platin in this situation have not yet been announced.

In advanced disease, research for the moment is concentrating on the role of taxol in the treatment of ovarian carcinoma. Adapted to the risk of recurrence, GOG randomizes patients with advanced disease to two different trials. In optimally debulked ovarian cancer taxol is to be tested versus cisplatin versus cisplatin + taxol (GOG #132). In suboptimally debulked ovarian carcinoma (≤1 cm residual disease) cisplatin/cyclophosphamide is to be tested versus cisplatin/taxol versus sequential carboplatin (AUC 9) × 2 followed by cisplatin i.p./taxol (GOG #114). Another European phase III trial will further elucidate the equipotency of carboplatin/taxol and cisplatin/taxol (German Ovarian Cancer Study Group). The optimal dose level of taxol is being investigated by the GOG (GOG #34) in platinum-resistant clinically measurable ovarian cancer. Results of these trials will be published by the end of the decade.

Scientifically far more interesting will be the development of high-dose chemotherapy regimens with stem cell support. Different phase II trials with the aim of establishing the regimen with optimal response rates/minimal morbidity in advanced ovarian cancer have been announced. The South West Oncology Group (SWOG) will test the combination of high-dose cyclophosphamide/carboplatin and mitoxantrone versus high-dose cyclophosphamide/cisplatin and thiotepa. A German study group will use a sequential design of taxol/cyclophosphamide ×2 → taxol/carboplatin ×2 + peripheral blood stem cells (PBSC) followed by carboplatin/etoposide and melphalan (+ PBSC) in patients with macroscopic residual tumor. The response rates and toxicity of these regimens will be known in the coming years. The question of whether the probably high response rates will translate into higher cure rates will not be answered before the end of the next decade, when phase III trials have been undertaken in patients with potentially curable disease.

11.20.4 Radiotherapy

The role of conventional radiotherapy (APRT, intraperitoneal radiophosphorus) must be newly defined with every advance in chemotherapy or new radiotherapeutic development. Intraperitoneal monoclonal antibody-guided radionuclide therapy may come to substitute for radionuclide-colloid treatment. The combination of WAI (20–25 Gy) and ^{131}I- or ^{90}Y-labeled MAb (30–50 mCi as a boost) may eventually be more effective than APRT.

In 1988 the GOG protocol 95 (SWOG 9047, NCCTG 876102) was started (coordinators: R.C. Young, L. Walton, B. Ned, et al.) as a "randomized trial for the treatment of women with selected stage Ic and II (a,b,c) and selected stage Ia and Ib ovarian cancer (phase III)." The patients were randomized to receive either 15 mCi radiophosphorus in one arm or 3 × cisplatin (100 mg/m^2) + cyclophosphamide (1 g/m^2) every 21 days in the other arm. Up until 9 February 1995 a total of 223 patients had entered the trial, of whom 184 were eligible. One-half of the eligible patients have been followed for at least 23 months. Twenty-two patients have experienced a recurrence of their disease. Until now no comparative results have been published for the two treatment arms.

Given the substantial progress in chemotherapy achieved by the introduction of taxol, and in radiotherapy by the introduction of MAb-targeted radionuclides, future trials should consider these new developments. A trial should be initiated for ovarian cancer patients at intermediate risk, randomized into three arms after optimal initial surgery (R_0, R_{micro}, R_{macro} < 2 cm) to receive:

1. APRT
2. ^{90}Y-labeled MAb (100–150 mCi, residual-adjusted)
3. Taxol + platinum combination (3–6 cycles, residual-adjusted)

For high-risk ovarian cancer patients combined treatment modalities must be favored, including a taxol + platinum combination sandwiched with APRT or ^{90}Y-labeled MAb.

References

Advanced Ovarian Cancer Trialists Group (1991) Chemotherapy in advanced ovarian cancer: an overview of randomized clinicals trials. BMJ 303:884–893

Aguirre P, Scully RE (1982) Malignant neuroectodermal tumor of the ovary, a distinctive form of monodermal teratoma. Report of 5 cases. Am J Surg Pathol 6:283–292

Ahlgren JD, Ellison NM, Gottlieb RJ, et al. (1993) Hormonal palliation of chemoresistant ovarian cancer: three consecutive phase II trials of the Mid-Atlantic Oncology Program. J Clin Oncol 11:1957–1968

Aiba B, Hiryama A, Sakurada M (1990) Spironolactone body-like structure in renin-producing Sertoli cell tumor of the ovary. Surg Pathol 3:143–149

Alberts DS, Young L, Mason N, Salmon S (1985) In vitro evaluation of anticancer drugs against ovarian cancer at concentrations achievable by intraperitoneal administration. Semin Oncol XII, no. 3, Suppl 4:38–42

Alberts DS, Green SJ, Hannigan EV, et al. (1989) Improved efficacy of carboplatin plus cyclophosphamide versus-cisplatin plus cyclophosphamide: preliminary report of the Southwest Oncology Group of a phase III randomized trial in stages III and IV suboptimal ovarian cancer. Proc Am Soc Clin Oncol 8:151

Alberts DS, Green SJ, Hannigan EV, et al. (1992) Improved therapeutic index of carboplatin plus cyclophosphamide versus cisplatin plus cyclophosphamide: final report of the Southwest Oncology Group of a phase III randomized trial in stages II and IV ovarian cancer. J Clin Oncol 10:706–717

Alberts DS, Liu PY, Hannigan EV, et al. (1995) Phase III study of intraperitoneal (IP) cisplatin (CDDP)/intravenous (IV) cyclophosphamide (CPA) vs IV CDDP/IV CPA in patients with optimal disease stage III ovarian cancer. Proc Am Soc Clin Oncol 14:273

Alderman SJ, Dillon TF, Krummermann MS, et al. (1977) Postoperative use of radioactive phosphorus in stage I ovarian carcinoma. Obstet Gynecol 49:659–662

Alenghat E, Okagaki T, Talerman A (1986) Primary mucinous carcinoid tumor of the ovary. Cancer 58:777–783

Anikwue C, Dawood MJ, Kramer E (1978) Granulosa and theca cell tumors. Obstet Gynecol 51:214–220

Antolic ZN, Kovacic J, Rainier S (1980) Theca and granulosa cell tumors and endometrial adenocarcinoma. Gynecol Oncol 10:273–278

Arhelger SW, Jenson CB, Wangensteen OH (1957) Experiences with the "second-look" procedure in management of cancer of the colon and rectum: with special reference to site of residual cancer. Lancet 77:412–417

Ariel IM, Oropeza R, Pack GT (1966) Intracavitary administration of radioactive isotopes in the control of effusions due to cancer. Cancer 19:1096–1102

Asadourian LA, Taylor HB (1969) Dysgerminoma. An analysis of 105 cases. Obstet Gynecol 33:370–379

Asco (1994) Ovarian cancer: screening, treatment and follow-up. Consensus Statement. National Institute of Health

Atlas of cancer mortality in the People's Republic of China (1979) China Map Press, Shanghai, pp 98–99

August CZ, Murad TM, Newton M (1985) Multiple focal extra-ovarian serous carcinoma. Int J Gynecol Pathol 4:11–23

Aure JC, Hoeg K, Kolstad P (1971) Radioactive colloidal gold in the treatment of ovarian carcinoma. Acta Radiol 10:399–407

Austgen M, Trendelenburg F (1987) Die Behandlung der Pleurakarzinose mit ^{90}Y Yttriumsilikat. Prax Klin Pneumol 41:750–751

Avall-Lundquist E, Sjovall K, Hansson L, Eneroth P (1992) Peri- and postoperative changes in serum levels of four markers and three acute phase reactants in benign and malignant gynecological diseases. Arch Gynecol Obstet 251:68–78

Averette HE, Lovecchio JL, Townsend PA, Sevin BU, Gurtanner RE (1983) Cancer campaign: carcinoma of the ovary. Gustav Fischer, Stuttgart

Axe SR, Klein VR, Woodruff JD (1985) Choriocarcinoma of the ovary. Obstet Gynecol 66:111–117

Baker V (1994) Molecular biology and genetics of epithelial ovarian cancer. Obstet Gynecol Clin North Am 21:25–39

Bakri NY, Given FT, Peeples WJ, Frazier AB (1985) Complications from intraperitoneal radioactive phosphorus in ovarian malignancies. Gynecol Oncol 21:294–299

Barber HRK (1989) Spread and treatment of advanced ovarian cancer. Baillière's Clin Obstet Gynaecol 3:23–29

Barber HRK (1993) Ovarian carcinoma. Etiology, diagnosis and treatment, 3rd edn. Springer, Berlin Heidelberg New York

Barletta C, Lazzaro D, Porta RP (1992) C-*myb* activation and the pathogenesis of ovarian cancer. Eur J Gynaecol Oncol 13:53–60

Bartl W, Spernol R, Breitenecker G (1984) Zur Bedeutung klinischer und morphologischer Parameter für die Prognose von Granulosazelltumoren des Ovars. Geburtshilfe Frauenheilkd 44:295–299

Bast RC, Feeny M, Lazarus H, et al. (1981) Reactivity of a monoclonal antibody with human ovarian carcinoma. J Clin Invest 68:1331–1337

Bast RC, Klug TL, Jorn ES, et al. (1983) A radioimmunoassay using monoclonal antibody to monitor the course of epithelial ovarian cancer. N Engl J Med 309:883–887

Bast RC, Boyer CM, Jacobs I, et al. (1993) Cell growth regulation in epithelial ovarian Cancer. Cancer 71:1597–1601

Bauknecht T, Runge M, Schwall M, Pfleiderer M (1988) Occurence of epidermal growth factor receptors in human adnexal tumors and their prognostic value in advanced ovarian carcinomas. Gynecol Obstet 29:147–157

Baumann D, Donat H, Bohme M, Lenz E (1992) Klinische Erfahrungen mit der Behandlung von Granulosazelltumoren. Zentralbl Gynäkol 114:361–364

Beckmann MW, Niederacher D, Schnürch HG, Bender HG (1993) Die erbB-Gen Familie: Bedeutung für die Tumorentwicklung, Prognose und für neue Therapiemodalitäten. Geburtshilfe Frauenheilkd 53:742–753

Beckmann MW, An HX, Niederacher D, et al. (1996) Oncogene amplification in archival ovarian carcinoma detected by fluorescent differential polymerase chain reaction – a routine analytical approach. Int J Gynecol Cancer 6:291–297

Belinson JL, McClure M, Badger G (1987) Randomized trial of megestrol acetate vs. megestol acetate/tamoxifen for the management of progressive or recurrent epithelial ovarian carcinoma. Gynecol Oncol 28:151–155

Ben-Baruch G, Menczer J, Feldman B, et al. (1994) Intraperitoneal cisplatin chemotherapy versus abdomino-pelvic irradiation in ovarian carcinoma patients after second look laparotomy. Eur J Gynaecol Oncol 15:272–276

Bender HG, Robra BP (1983) Incidence and mortality of ovarian cancer in Germany 1968–1979. In: Bender HG, Beck L (eds) Carcinoma of the ovary. Cancer campaign, vol 7. Fischer, Stuttgart

Berchuck A, Kamel A, Whitaker R, et al. (1990) Overexpression of Her-2/neu is associated with poor survival in advanced epithelial ovarian cancer. Cancer Res 50:4087–4091

Berchuck A, Rodriguez GC, Kamel A, et al. (1991) Epidermal growth factor receptor expression in normal ovarian epithelium and ovarian cancer. Am J Obstet Gynecol 164:669–674

Berchuck A, Kohler MF, Bast RC Jr (1992) Oncogenes in ovarian cancer. Hematol Oncol Clin North Am 6:813–827

Berchuck A, Kohler FM, Boente MP, et al. (1993) Growth regulation and transformation of ovarian epithelium. Cancer 71:545–551

Berchuck A, Kohler FM, Marks JR, Wiseman R, Boyd J, Bast RC (1994) The p 53 tumor suppressor gene is frequently altered in gynecological cancers. Am J Obstet Gynecol 170:246–250

Bergman F (1966) Carcinoma of the ovary: a clinical-pathological study of 86 autopsied cases with special reference to mode of spread. Acta Obstet Gynecol Scand 45:211–231

Berns EMJJ, Klijn JGM, Henzen-Logmans SJ, Rodenburg CJ, van der Burg MEL, Foekens JA (1992) Receptors for hormones and growth factors and (onco)-gene amplification in human ovarian cancer. Int J Cancer 52:218–224

Biscotti CV, Hart WR (1989) Juvenile granulosa cell tumors of the ovary. Arch Pathol Lab Med 113:40–46

Bjorkholm E, Silversward C (1980) Theca cell tumors. Clinical features and prognosis. Acta Radiol Oncol Radiat Phys Biol 11:261–274

Bjorkholm E, Silversward C (1981) Prognostic factors in granulosa-cell tumors. Gynecol Oncol 11:261–274

Bjorkholm E, Petterson F, Einhorn N, et al. (1982) Long term follow-up and prognostic factors in ovarian carcinoma: the Radiumhemmet series 1953–1973. Acta Radiol Oncol 21:413–419

Bjorkholm E, Lundell M, Gyftodimos A, Silversward C (1990) Dysgerminoma. The Radiumhemmet series 1927–1984. Cancer 65:38–44

Bolis G, Marsoni S, Chiari N, et al. (1989) Cooperative randomized clinical trial for stage I ovarian carcinoma. In: Conte PF, Ragni N, Rosso R, et al. (eds) Multimodal treatment of ovarian cancer. Raven Press, New York, p 87

Bolis G, Zanaboni F, Vanoli P, et al. (1990) The impact of whole-abdomen radiotherapy on survival in advanced ovarian cancer patients with minimal residual disease after chemotherapy. Gynecol Oncol 39:150–154

Bolis G, Torri V, Babilonti L, et al. (1991) Multicenter controlled trial in patients with stage I ovarian cancer. Gruppo Interregionale Cooperative Oncologia Ginecologica, Milan, Italy. Int Soc Gynecol Cancer Meeting, Cairns, Australia

Boshoff C, Begent RHJ, Oliver RT, Rustin GJ, Newlands ES (1995) Secondary tumours following etoposide containing chemotherapy for germ cell cancer. Ann Oncol 6:35–40

Bosl GJ, Geller NL, Bajorin D, et al. (1988) A randomized trial of etoposide + cisplatin versus vinblastine + bleomycin + cisplatin + cyclophosphamide + dactinomycin in patients with good-prognosis germ cell tumors. J Clin Oncol 6: 1231–1238

Boye E, Lindegaard MW, Paus E, et al. (1984) Whole body distribution of radioactivity after intraperitoneal administration of 32-P-colloids. Br J Radiol 57:395–402

Braly P, Doroshow JH, Hoff S (1986) Technical aspects of intraperitoneal chemotherapy in abdominal carcinomatosis. Gynecol Oncol 25:319–333

Breckwoldt M (1993) Hormonsubstitution bei hormonsensitiven Neoplasien. Gynäkologe 26:137–140

Broders AC (1926) Carcinoma: grading and practical application. Arch Pathol 2:376–380

Bruckner HW, Motwani BT (1989) Treatment of advanced refractory ovarian carcinoma with a gonadotropin-releasing hormone analogue. Am J Obstet Gynecol 161:1216–1218

Buchsbaum HJ, Keettel WC (1975) Radioisotopes in treatment of stage Ia ovarian cancer. Natl Cancer Inst Monogr 42:127–128

Buchsbaum HJ, Brady MF, Delgado G, et al. (1989) Surgical staging of carcinoma of the ovaries. Surg Gynecol Obstet 169:226–232

Burghardt E, Girardi F, Lahousen M, Tamussino K, Stettner H (1991) Patterns of pelvic and paraaortic lymph node involvement in ovarian cancer. Gynecol Oncol 40:103–106

Busch H (1990) The final common pathway of cancer: presidential address. Cancer Res 50:4830–4838
Bush RS, Allt WEC, Beale FA, et al. (1977) Treatment of epithelial carcinoma of the ovary: operation, irradiation, and chemotherapy. Am J Obstet Gynecol 127:692–704
Cain JM, Russel AH, Greer BE, et al. (1988) Whole abdomen radiation for minimal residual epithelial ovarian carcinoma after surgical resection and maximal first-line chemotherapy. Gynecol Oncol 29:168–175
Calvert AH, Newell DR, Gumbrell LA, et al. (1989) Carboplatin dosage: prospective evaluation of a simple formula based on renal function. J Clin Oncol 7:1748–1756
Camlibel TF, Caputo TA (1983) Chemotherapy of granulosa cell tumors. Am J Obstet Gynecol 145:763–765
Canney PA, Moore M, Wilkinson PM, James RD (1984) Ovarian cancer antigen CA 125: a prospective clinical assessment of its role as a tumor marker. Br J Cancer 50:765–769
Carey MS, Dembo AJ, Simm JE, et al. (1993) Testing the validity of prognostic classification in patients with surgically optimal ovarian carcinoma: a 15-year review. Int J Gynecol Cancer 3:24–35
Carmichael J, Gordon AM, Malfetano J, et al. (1996) Topotecan, a new active drug, vs paclitaxel in advanced epithelial ovarian cancer after failure of platinum and paclitaxel: International Topotecan Study Group Trial. Proc Am Soc Clin Oncol 15:283
Chadha S, Cornelisse CJ, Schaberg A (1990) Flow cytometric DNA analysis of ovarian granulosa cell tumors. Gynecol Oncol 36:240–245
Chalvardjian A, Scully RE (1973) Sclerosing stromal tumors of the ovary. Cancer 31:664–670
Chambers SK, Chambers JT, Kohorn E, Schwartz PE (1988) Evaluation of the role of second-look surgery in ovarian cancer. Gynecol Oncol 31:404–408
Chapet S, Berger C, Fignon A, et al. (1995) Abdominopelvic irradiation after second-look laparotomy for stage III ovarian carcinoma. Eur J Obstet Gynecol 62:43–48
Chen S, Lee L (1983) Incidence of paraaortic lymph node metastases in epithelial carcinoma of the ovary. Gynecol Oncol 16:95–100
Chen SS, Bochner R (1985) Assessment of morbidity and mortality in primary cytoreductive surgery for advanced ovarian carcinoma. Gynecol Oncol 20:190–195
Cheruku R, Hussain M, Tyrkus M, Edelstein M (1993) Myelodysplastic syndrome after cisplatin therapy. Cancer 72:213–218
Chumas JC, Scully RE (1991) Sebaceous tumors arising in ovarian dermoid cysts. Int J Gynecol Pathol 10:356–363
Clement PB (1994a) Nonneoplastic lesions of the ovary. In: Kurman RJ (ed) Blausteins' pathology of the female genital tract, 4th edn. Springer, Berlin Heidelberg New York, pp 597–645
Clement PB (1994b) Diseases of the peritoneum. In: Kurman RJ (ed) Blausteins' pathology of the female genital tract, 4th edn. Springer Berlin Heidelberg New York, pp 647–703
Colombo N, Sessa C, Landoni F, Sartori E, Pecorelli S, Mangioni C (1986) Cisplatin, vinblastine, and bleomycin combination chemotherapy in metastatic granulosa cell tumor of the ovary. Obstet Gynecol 67:265–268
Colombo N, Pittelli MR, Parma G, Marzola M, Torri W, Mangioni C (1993) Cisplatin dose-intensity in advanced ovarian cancer: a randomized study of conventional dose versus dose intense cisplatin. Proc Am Soc Clin Oncol 12:806
Colombo N, Chiari S, Maggioni A, Bocciolone L, Torri V, Mangioni C (1994) Controversial issues in the management of early epithelial ovarian cancer: conservative surgery and role of adjuvant therapy. Gynecol Oncol 55:S47–S51
Colombo N, Marzola M, Parma G, Cantu MG, Tarantino G, Fornara G, Gueli-Aletti D (1996) Paclitaxel versus CAP in recurrent platinum sensitive ovarian cancer. Proc ASCO 15:279
Colon-Otero G, Malkasian GD, Edmonson JH (1993) Seondary myelodysplasia and acute leukemia following carboplatin-containing combination chemotherapy for ovarian cancer. J Natl Cancer Inst 85:1858–1860
Conte PF, Bruzzone M, Chiaro S, et al. (1986) A randomized trial comparing cisplatin plus cyclophosphamide versus cisplatin, doxorubicin and cyclophosphamide in advanced ovarian cancer. J Clin Oncol 4:965–972
Conte M, Guariglia L, Panici PL, et al. (1990) Ovarian carcinoma: an ultrasound study. Eur J Gynaecol Oncol 11:33–36
Corn BW, Lanciano RM, Boente M, et al. (1994) Recurrent ovarian cancer. Effective radiotherapeutic palliation after chemotherapy failure. Cancer 74:2979–2983
Courtenay-Luck N, Epenetos AA, Halnan KE, et al. (1984) Antibody guided irradiation of malignant lesions: three cases illustrating a new method of treatment. A report from the Hammersmith Oncology Group and the Imperial Cancer Research Fund. Lancet 1:1441–1443
Covington E, Hilaris B (1973) ^{32}P scans for intracavitary studies. Am J Röntgenol 118:895–899
Cramer DW, Welch WR, Scully RE, Woijciechowsky CA (1982) Ovarian cancer and talc: a case control study. Cancer 50:372–376
Cramer DW, Welch WR, Cassels S, Scully RE (1983) Mumps, menarche, menopause and ovarian cancer. Am J Obstet Gynecol 147:1–6
Creasman WT, Park R, Norris H, et al. (1982) Stage I borderline ovarian tumors, Obstet Gynecol 59:93
Creasman WT, Gall S, Bundy B, Beecham J, Mortel R, Homesley H (1989) Second-look laparotomy in the patient with minimal residual stage III ovarian cancer (a Gynecologic Oncology Group Study). Gynecol Oncol 35:378–382
Crippa F, Bolis G, Seregni E, et al. (1995) Single-dose intraperitoneal radioimmuno-therapy with the murine monolclonal antibody I-131 Mov 18: clinical results in patients with minimal residual disease of ovarian cancer. Eur J Cancer 31:686–690
Crombach G, Würz H (1985) Vergleichende Bestimmung von CA 125, TPA and CEA bei Patienten mit malignen epithelialen Ovarialtumoren. In: Greten H, Klapdor R (eds) Neue tumorassoziierte Antigene. Thieme, Stuttgart, p 167
Currie JL, Bagne F, Harris C, et al. (1981) Radioactive chromic phosphate suspension: studies on distribution dose absorption, and effective therapeutic radiation in phantoms, dogs, and patients. Gynecol Oncol 12:193–218
Curtin JP (1993) Diagnosis and staging of epithelial ovarian cancer. In: Markman L, Hoskins WJ (eds) Cancer of the ovary. Raven Press, New York, p 153
Dauplat J, Ferriere JP, Gorbinet M, et al. (1986) Second-look laparotomy in managing epithelial ovarian carcinoma. Cancer 57:1627–1631
Davidson S, Rubin S, Markman M, et al. (1991) Intraperitoneal chemotherapy: analysis of complications with an implanted subcutaneous port and catheter system. Gynecol Oncol 41:101–106
Davidson SA, Rubin SC, Mychalczak B, et al. (1993) Limited field radiotherapy as salvage treatment of localized persistent or recurrent epithelial ovarian cancer. Gynecol Oncol 51:349–354
Day TG, Gallager HS, Rutledge FN (1975) Epithelial carcinoma of the ovary: prognostic importance of histologic grade.

Symposium on ovarian carcinoma. Natl Cancer Inst Monogr 42:15–18
Decker DG, Webb MJ, Holbrook MA (1973) Radiogold treatment of epithelial cancer of ovary: late results. Am J Obstet Gynecol 115:751–757
Decker DG, Malkasian GD, Taylor WF (1975) Prognostic importance of histologic grading in ovarian carcinomas: symposium on ovarian carcinoma. Natl Cancer Inst Monogr 42:9–11
Dederick RL, Myers CE, Bungay PM, De Vita V (1978) Pharmacokinetic rationale for peritoneal drug administration in the treatment of ovarian cancer. Cancer Treat Rep 62:1–9
Delclos L, Smith JP (1975) Ovarian cancer, with special regard to types of radiotherapy. Natl Cancer Inst Monogr 42:129–135
Delgado G, Oram D, Petrilli ES (1984) Stage III ovarian cancer: the role of maximal surgical reduction. Gynecol Oncol 18:293
Dembo AJ (1984) Radiotherapeutic management of ovarian cancer. Semin Oncol 11:238–250
Dembo AJ (1985) Abdominopelvic radiotherapy in ovarian cancer. A 10-year experience. Cancer 55:2285–2290
Dembo AJ (1992) Epithelial ovarian cancer: the role of radiotherapy. Int J Radiat Oncol Biol Phys 22:835–845
Dembo AJ, Bush RS (1982) Choice of postoperative therapy based on prognostic factors. Int J Radiat Oncol Biol Phys 8:893–897
Dembo AJ, Bush RS, Beale FA, et al. (1979) Ovarian carcinoma: improved survival following abdomino-pelvic irradiation in patients with a completed pelvic operation. Am J Obstet Gynecol 134:793–800
Dembo AJ, Bush RS, Beale FA, et al. (1983) A randomized clinical trial of moving strip vs open field whole abdominal irradiation in patients with invasive epithelial cancer of the ovary (abstract). Int J Radiat Oncol Biol Phys 9:97
Dembo AJ, Davy M, Stenwig AE, et al. (1990) Prognostic factors in patients with stage I epithelial ovarian cancer. Obstet Gynecol 75:263–273
De Palo G, Pilotti S, Kenda R, et al. (1984) Natural history of dysgerminoma. Am J Obstet Gynecol 143:799–807
DeSombre ER, Mease RC, Hughes A, et al. (1988) Bromine-80m labeled estrogens: Auger electron emitting estrogen receptor-directed ligands with potential for therapy of estrogen receptor- positive cancers. Cancer Res 48:899–906
Diddle AW (1952) Granulosa- and theca-cell ovarian tumors: prognosis. Cancer 5:215–228
Dietl J (1996) Typical aspects of ovarian carcinoma. Geburtshilfe Frauenheilkd 56:331–344
Dietl J, Marzusch K (1993) Ovarian surface epithelium and human ovarian cancer. Gynecol Obstet Invest 35:129–135
Di Re F, Fontanelli R, Raspagliesi F, Di Re EM (1990) The value of lymphadenectomy in the management of ovarian cancer. In: Sharp F, Mason WP, Leake RE (eds) Ovarian cancer. Chapman and Hall, London, pp 437–442
DiSaia PJ, Saltz A, Kagan AR, Rich W (1978) A temporary response of recurrent granulosa cell tumor to adriamycin. Obstet Gynecol 52:355–358
Dockerty MB, Masson JC (1944) Ovarian fibromas: a clinical and pathological study of 283 cases. Am J Obstet Gynecol 47:741–750
Doench KF, Frischkorn R, Müller-Heine F, Rosenow F (1973) Die Peritoneographie mit Urovison vor der Radiogoldinstillation. Arch Gynäkol 214:101–102
Dunn JE (1975) Cancer epidemiology in populations of the United States – with emphasis on Hawaii and California – and Japan. Cancer Res 35:3240–3245
Dvoretsky PM, Richards KA, Angel C, et al. (1988) Distribution of disease at autopsy in 100 women with ovarian cancer. Hum Pathol 19:57–63
Ebel H, Villagran R, Conzen M, Schnabel R, Oppel F (1993) Solitare intrakranielle Spatmetatase eines Granulosazelltumors des Ovars. Fallbericht und Literaturubersicht. Neurochir 36:131–134
Echt CR, Hadd HE (1968) Androgen excretion patterns in a patient with a metastatic hilus cell tumor of the ovary. Am J Obstet Gynecol 100:1055–1061
Edmondson JH, McCormack GM, Wieand HS, et al. (1989) Cyclophosphamide-cisplatin versus cyclophosphamide – carboplatin in stage III–IV ovarian carcinoma: a comparison of equally myelosuppressive regimens. J Natl Cancer Inst 81:1500–1504
Eeles RA, Tan S, Wiltshaw E, et al. (1991) Hormone replacement therapy and survival after surgery for ovarian cancer. BMJ 302:259–262
Ehrlich C, Einhorn L, Williams S, et al. (1979) Chemotherapy for stage III–IV epithelial ovarian cancer with cis-dichlordiamineplatinum, adriamycin and cyclophosphamide: a preliminary report. Cancer Treat Rep 63:281–288
Ehrlich EN, Dominguez OV, Samuels LT, Lynch D, Oberhelma Warner NE (1963) Aldosteronism and precocious puberty due to an ovarian androblastoma (Sertoli cell tumor). J Clin Endocrinol Metab 23:358–367
Eifel PJ, Gershenson DM, Delclos L, et al. (1991) Twice-daily split-course abdominopelvic radiation therapy after chemotherapy and positive second-look laparotomy for epithelial ovarian carcinoma. Int J Radiat Oncol Biol Phys 21:1013–1018
Einzig A (1993) Review of phase II trials of paclitaxel in refractory ovarian cancer. Taxol a novel advance in chemotherapy. Taxol-Symposium Munich
Emons G, Schally AV (1994) The use of luteinizing hormone releasing hormone agonists and antagonists in gynaecological cancers. Hum Reprod 9
Emons G, Schulz K-D (1994) New developments in the hormonal treatment of endometrial and ovarian cancer. In: Jonat W, Kaufmann M (eds) Hormone dependent tumors, basic research and clinical studies. Karger, Basel
Emons G, Pahwa GS, Brack C, Sturm R, Oberheuser F, Knuppen R (1989) Gonadotropin releasing hormone binding sites in human epithlial ovarian carcinomata. Eur J Cancer 25:215–221
Emons G, Pahwa GS, Sturm G, Knuppen R, Oberheuser F (1990a) The use of GnRH analogues in ovarian cancer. In: Vickery BH, Lunenfeld B (eds) GnRH analogues in cancer and human reproduction, vol 3. Kluwer, Dordrecht, p 159
Emons G, Pahwa GS, Ortmann O, Knuppen R, Oberheuser F, Schulz K-D (1990b) LH-RH receptors and LH-RH agonist treatment in ovarian cancer: an overview. J Steroid Biochem Mol Biol 37:1003–1006
Emons G, Ortmann O, Phawa GS, Hackenberg R, Oberheuser F, Schulz K-D (1992a) Intracellular actions of gonadotropic and peptide hormones and the therapeutic value of GnRH-agonists in ovarian cancer. Acta Obstet Gynecol Scand 71 (Suppl 155): 31–38
Emons G, Ortmann O, Pahwa GS, Oberheuser F, Schulz K-D (1992b) LHRH agonists in the treatment of ovarian cancer. Recent Results Cancer Res 124:55–68
Emons G, Ortmann O, Pahwa GS, et al. (1992c) in-vivo and in-vitro effects of GnRH anlongues on an ovarian Leydig cell tumor. Geburtshilfe Frauenheilkd 52:487–793
Emons G, Schröder B, Ortmann O, Westphalen S, Schulz K-D, Schally AV (1993a) High affinity binding and direct anti-

proliferative effects of luteinizing hormone-releasing hormone analogs in human endometrial cancer cell lines. J Clin Endocrinol Metab 77:1458–1464
Emons G, Ortmann O, Becker M, et al. (1993d) High affinity binding and direct antiproliferative effects of LHRH analogues in human ovarian cancer cell lines Cancer Res 53:5439–5446
Emons G, Ortmann O, Schulz K-D (1993c) Rolle der endokrinen Therapie beim Ovarialkarzinom. Gynäkologe 26:123–130
Enstrom JE (1979) Cancer mortality among low-risk populations. UCLA Cancer Center Bull 6:3–7
Epenetos AA, Hooker G, Krausz T, et al. (1986) Antibody-guided irradiation of malignant ascites in ovarian cancer: a new therapeutic method possessing specificity against cancer cells. Obstet Gynecol 68 (Suppl):71S–74S
Epenetos AA, Munro AJ, Stewart S, et al. (1987) Antibody-guided irradiation of advanced ovarian cancer with intraperitoneally administered radio-labeled monoclonal antibodies. J Clin Oncol 12:1890–1899
Evans AT, Gaffey TA, Malkasian GD, Annegers JF (1980) Clinicopathologic review of 118 granulosa and 82 theca cell tumors. Obstet Gynecol 55:231–238
Fazekas JT, Maier JG (1974) Irradiation of ovarian carcinomas. A prospective comparison of the open-field and moving-strip techniques. Am J Roentgenol 120:118–123
Fearon ER, Vogelstein B (1990) A genetic model for colorectal tumorigenesis. Cell 61:759–767
Fein DA, Morgan LS, Marcus RB, et al. (1994) Stage III ovarian carcinoma: an analysis of treatment results and complications following hyperfractionated abdominopelvic irradiation for salvage. Int J Radiat Oncol Biol Phys 29:169–176
Files AW, Dembo AJ, Bush RS, et al. (1992) Analysis of complications in patients treated with abdomino-pelvic radiation therapy for ovarian carcinoma. Int J Radiat Oncol Biol Phys 22:847–851
Fischer U, Sattler HP, Bonkhoff H, Hermann M, Wullich B, Meese EU (1994) Amplification on chromosome 1p31, 1q21–24, 5p13–14, and 11p12–14 in ovarian carcinoma detected by reverse chromosome painting. Oncology Reports 1:1069–1073
Fleischhacker DS, Young RH (1994) Dysgerminoma of the ovary associated with hypercalcemia. Gynecol Oncol 52:87–90
Fletcher JA, Gibas Z, Donovan K, et al. (1991) Ovarian granulosa-stromal cell tumors are characterized by trisomy 12. Am J Pathol 138:515–520
Foekens JA, Klijn JGM (1992) Direct antitumor effects of LH-RH analogs. Recent Results Cancer Res 124:7–17
Ford D, Easton DF (1995) The genetics of breast and ovarian cancer. Br J Cancer 72:805–812
Fox H (1985) Sex cord-stromal tumours of the ovary. J Pathol 145:127–148
Fox H (1993) Pathology of early malignant change in the ovary. Int J Gynecol Pathol 12:153–155
Fox H, Buckley CH (1992) Pathology of malignant gonadal stromal tumors of the ovary. In: Coppleson M (ed) Gynecologic Oncology, 2nd edn. Churchill Livingstone, Edinburgh, pp 947–959
Fox H, Agrawal K, Langley FA (1975) A clinicopathologic study of 92 cases of granulosa cell tumor of the ovary with special reference to the factors influencing prognosis. Cancer 35:231–241
Freedman RS, Saul PB, Edwards CL, et al. (1986) Ethinyl estradiol and medroxyprogesterone acetate in patients with epithelial ovarian carcinoma: a phase II study. Cancer Treat Rep 70:369–388
Frischkorn R (1976) Gynäkologische Strahlentherapie. In: Schwalm H, Döderlein G, Wulf KH (eds) Klinik der Frauenheilkunde und Geburtshilfe Vol II, Suppl. Urban & Schwarzenberg, München, p 664/17
Frischkorn R, Siefken E, Doench K, et al. (1973) Versuch einer statistischen Aussage über die Bedeutung der intraperitonealen Radiogoldapplikation. Arch Gynäkol 214:100
Fromm GL, Freedman RS, Fritsche HA, Atkinson EN, Scott W (1991) Sequentially administered ethinyl estradiol and medroxyprogesterone acetate in the treatment of refractory epithelial ovarian carcinoma in patients with positive estrogen receptors. Cancer 68:1885–1889
Fuks Z, Rizel S, Biran S (1988) Chemotherapeutic and surgical induction of pathological complete remission and whole abdominal irradiation for consolidation does not enhance the cure of stage III ovarian carcinoma. J Clin Oncol 6:509–516
Gall S, Bundy B, Beecham J, et al. (1986) Therapy of stage III (optimal) epithelial carcinoma of the ovary with melphalan or melphalan plus corynebacterium parvum (a Gynecologic Oncology Group study). Gynecol Oncol 25:26–36
Gallion HH, de Guarino A, DePriest PD, van Nagell JR, Vaccarello L, Berek JS, Pieretti M (1996) Evidence for a unifocal origin in familial ovarian cancer. Am J Obstet Gynecol 174:1102–1108
Garamvoelgyi E, Guilla L, Gebhard S, et al. (1994) Primary malignant mixed Müllerian tumor (metaplastic carcinoma) of the female peritoneum. Cancer 74:854–863
George M, Kerbrat P, Heron JF, et al. (1988) Phase I-II study of high dose carboplatin as first line chemotherapy of extensive ovarian cancer. Proc Am Soc Clin Oncol 7:539
Gershenson DM (1985) Malignant germ-cell tumors of the ovary. Clin Obstet Gynecol 28:824–837
Gershenson DM (1988) Menstrual and reproductive function after treatment with combination chemotherapy for malignant ovarian germ cell tumors. J Clin Oncol 6:270–275
Gershenson DM, Del Junco G, Copeland LJ, Rutledge FN (1984) Mixed germ cell tumors of the ovary. Obstet Gynecol 64:200–206
Gershenson DM, Copeland LJ, Kavanagh JJ, et al. (1985a) Treatment of malignant nondysgerminomatous germ cell tumors of the ovary with vincristine, dactinomycin, and cyclophosphamide. Cancer 56:2756–2761
Gershenson DM, Copeland LJ, Wharton JT, Atkinson EN, Sneige N, Edwards CL (1985b) Prognosis of surgically determined complete responders in advanced ovarian cancer. Cancer 55:1129–1135
Gershenson DM, Copeland LJ, Kavanagh JJ, Stringer A, Saul PB, Wharton JT (1987) Treatment of metastatic stromal tumors of the ovary with cisplatin, doxorubicin, and cyclophosphamide. Obstet Gynecol 70:765–769
Gershenson DM, Morris M, Cangir A, et al. (1990a) Treatment of malignant germ cell tumors of the ovary with bleomycin, etoposide, and cisplatin. J Clin Oncol 8:715–720
Gershenson DM, Morris M, Cangir A, et al. (1990b) Treatment of malignant germ cell tumors of the ovary with bleomycin, etoposide, and cisplatin. J Clin Oncol 8:715–720
Gibbs EK (1971) Suggested prophylaxis for ovarian cancer. Am J Obstet Gynecol 111:756–765
Gieselberg HG (1974) Die Behandlung des Ovarialkarzinoms an der Universitäts-Frauenklinik Giessen in den Jahren 1957–1970. Inaugural-Dissertation, Giessen 1974
Godwin AK, Perez RP, Johnson SW, Hamaguchi K, Hamilton TC (1992) Growth regulation of ovarian cancer. Hematol Oncol Clin North Am 6:829–841

Goldberg N, Peschel RE (1988) Postoperative abdominopelvic radiation therapy for ovarian cancer. Int J Radiat Oncol Biol Phys 14:425–429
Goldstein SR, Subramanyam B, Snyder JRT, et al. (1989) The postmenopausal cystic adnexal mass: the potential role of ultrasound in conservative management. Obstet Gynecol 73:8–10
Goldston WR, Johnston WW, Fetter BF, Parker RT, Wilbanks GD (1972) Clinicopathologic studies in feminizing tumors of the ovary. I. Some aspects of the pathology and therapy of granulosa cell tumors. Am J Obstet Gynecol 112:422–429
Gordon A, Bookman M, Malmstrom H, et al. (1996) Efficacy of topotecan in advanced epithelial ovarian cancer after failure of platinum and paclitaxel: International Topotecan Study Group Trial. Proc Am Soc Clin Oncol 15:282
Gordon A, Lipton D, Woodruff JD (1981) Dysgerminoma: a review of 158 cases from the Emil Novak Ovarian Tumor Registry. Obstet Gynecol 58:497–504
Health NL (1994) Ovarian cancer: screening, treatment and follow-up. Consensus-Statement
Gorski GK, McMorrow LE, Blumstein L, Faasse D, Donaldson MH (1992) Trisomy 14 in two cases of granulosa cell tumor of the ovary. Cancer Genet Cytogenet 60:202–205
Greco F, Julian C, Richardson R, et al. (1981) Advanced ovarian cancer: brief intensive combination chemotherapy and second look operation. Gynecol Oncol 58:199–205
Green JA, Warenius HM, Errington RD, et al. (1988) Sequential cisplatin/cyclophosphamide chemotherapy and abdominopelvic radiotherapy in the management of advanced ovarian cancer. Br J Cancer 58:635–639
Greiner R, Goldhirsch A, Dreher E, et al. (1985) Die Ganzabdomenbestrahlung nach Kombinationschemotherapie und Second-look-Laparotomie bei der Behandlung des fortgeschrittenen Ovarialkarzinoms. Onkologie 8:364–372
Griffiths CT (1975) Surgical resection of tumor bulk in the primary treatment of ovarian cancer. Natl Cancer Inst Monogr 42:101
Gruppo Interregionale Cooperativo Oncologico Ginecologia (1987) Randomized comparison of cisplatin with cyclophosphamide/cisplatin with cyclophosphamide/doxorubicin/cisplatin in advanced ovarian cancer. Lancet II:353–359
Gusberg SB, Kardon P (1971) Proliferative endometrial response to theca-granulosa cell tumors. Am J Obstet Gynecol 111:633–643
Gwinn ML, Lee NC, Rhodes PH, Layde PM, Rubin GL (1990) Pregnancy, breast feeding and oral contraceptives and the risk of epithelial ovarian cancer. J Clin Epidemiol 43:559–568
Haas JS, Mansfield CM, Hartman GV, et al. (1980) Results of radiation therapy in the treatment of epithelial carcinoma of the ovary. Cancer 46:1950–1956
Hacker NF, Berek JS, Burnison CM, et al. (1985) Whole abdomen radiation as salvage therapy for epithelial ovarian cancer. Obstet Gynecol 65:60–66
Hahlin M, Crona N, Knutsson F, Janson PO (1991) Human granulosa cell tumor: stimulation of steroidogenesis by gonadotropins in vitro. Gynecol Oncol 40:201–206
Hahn PF, Goodell JPB, Sheppard CW, et al. (1947) Direct infiltration of radio-active isotopes as a means of delivering ionizing irradiation to discrete tissues. J Lab Clin Med 32:1442–1453
Hainsworth JD, Malcolm A, Johnson DH, et al. (1983) Advanced minimal residual ovarian carcinoma: abdominopelvic irradiation following combination chemotherapy. Obstet Gynecol 61:619–623
Hamerlynck JVTH, Maskens AP, Mangioni C, van der Burg MEL, Wills AMJ, Vermorken JB, Rotmenz N (1985) Phase II trial of medroxyprogesterone acetate in advanced ovarian cancer: an EORTC gynecological cancer cooperative group study. Gynecol Oncol 22:313–316
Hamilton TC, Behrens BC, Louie KG, Ozols RT (1984) Induction of progesterone receptor with 17β-estradiol in human ovarian cancer. J Clin Endocrinol Metab 59:561–563
Hammond R, Bull C, Houghton CRS (1992) Primary adjunctive whole abdominal radiotherapy in epithelial ovarian cancer: results of 10-years experience. Aust N Z J Obstet Gynecol 32:267–269
Hankinson SE, Colditz GA, Hunter DJ, et al. (1992) A quantitative assessment of oral contraceptive use and risk of ovarian cancer. Obstet Gynecol 89:708–714
Hankinson SE, Hunter DJ, Colditz GA, et al. (1993) Tubal ligation, hysterectomy, and risk of ovarian cancer. JAMA 270:2813–2818
Harlap S (1992) The benefits and risks of hormone replacement therapy: an epidemiologic overview. Am J Obstet Gynecol 166:1986–1992
Harlap S (1993) The epidemiology of ovarian cancer. In: Markman M, Hoskins WJ (eds) Cancer of the ovary. Raven Press, New York, pp 79–93
Harrington KJ, Epenetos AA (1994) Recent developments in radioimmunotherapy. Clin Oncol 6:391–398
Harris N, Dutlow C, Eidne K, Dong KW, Roberts J, Millar R (1991) Gonadotropin-releasing hormone gene expression in MDA-MB-231 and ZR-75-1 breast carcinoma cell lines. Cancer Res 52:2577–2581
Hartwell LH, Kastan MB (1994) Cell cycle control and cancer. Science 266:1821–1828
Hatch KD, Beecham JB, Blessing JA, Creasman WT (1991) Responsiveness of patients with advanced ovarian carcinoma to tamoxifen. Cancer 68:269–271
Hayes MC, Scully RE (1987a) Stromal luteoma of the ovary: a clinicopathologic analysis of 25 cases. Int J Gynecol Pathol 6:313–321
Hayes MC, Scully RE (1987b) Ovarian steroid cell tumor (not otherwise specified): a clinicopathologic analysis of 63 cases. Am J Surg Pathol 11:835–845
Heilmann HP, Petersen F, Seeland M (1983) Postoperative Strahlen-therapie und Radiogoldbehandlung beim Ovarialkarzinom. Strahlen-therapie 159:5–8
Henriksen R, Funa K, Wilander E, Bäckström T, Ridderheim M, Öberg K (1993) Expression and prognostic significance of platelet-derived growth factor and its receptors in epithelial ovarian neoplasms. Cancer Res 53:4550–4554
Hilaris BS, Clark DGC (1971) The value of postoperative intraperitoneal injection of radiocolloids in early cancer of the ovary. Am J Roentgenol 112:749–754
Hilfrich J, Schwarzenau F, Lueck HJ, et al. (1989) Mitoxantron intraperitoneal zur Behandlung des rezidivierenden Aszites beim progredienten Ovarialkarzinom. Aktuelle Onkologie 54:65–69
Hinselmann H (1930) Die Ätiologie, Symptomatologie und Diagnostik des Uteruscarcinoms. In: Stoeckel W (ed) Handbuch der Gynäkologie III, Vol VI I. Bergmann, München, pp 854–953
Hird V, Maraveyas A, Snook D, et al. (1993) Adjuvant therapy of ovarian cancer with radioactive monoclonal antibody. Br J Cancer 68:403–406
Hitchcock CL, Norris HJ, Khalifa MA, Wargotz ES (1989) Flow cytometric analysis of granulosa tumors. Cancer 64:2127–2132

Hnatowich DJ, Chinol M, Siebecker DA, et al. (1988) Patient bio-distribution of intraperitoneally administered Y-90-labeled antibody. J Nucl Med 29:1428–1434

Hofmann D (1960) Die Anwendung von radioaktivem Gold in der gynäko-logischen Strahlentherapie. Grundlagen und klinische Erfahrungen. Strahlentherapie 111:167–181

Hofmann D (1963) Klinik der gynäkologischen Strahlentherapie. Urban & Schwarzenberg, München

Hofmann J, Wegmann B, Hackenberg R, Kunzmann R, Schulz K-D, Havemann K (1994) Production of insulin-like growth factor binding proteins by human ovarian carcinoma cells. J Cancer Res Clin Oncol 120:137–142

Hong Kong Ovarian Carcinoma Study Group: Ngan HYS, Choo YC, et al. (1989) A randomized study of high-dose versus low-dose cis-platinum with cyclophosphamide in the treatment of advanced ovarian cancer. Chemotherapy 35:221–227

Hoskins IA, Ostrer H (1993) Hereditary/familial ovarian cancer. In: Markman M, Hoskins WH (eds) Cancer of the ovary. Raven Press, New York, pp 95–113

Hoskins PJ, Swenerton KD (1994) Oral etoposide is active against platinum-resistant epithelial ovarian cancer. J Clin Oncol 12:60–63

Hoskins PJ, Swenerton KD, Wong F, et al. (1995) Platinum plus cyclophosphamide plus radiotherapy is superior to platinum alone in "high-risk" epithelial ovarian cancer (residual negative and either stage I or II, grade 3, or stage III, any grade). Int J Gynecol Cancer 5:134–142

Hoskins W, Rubin S, et al. (1989) Influence of secondary cytoreduction at the time of second-look laparotomy on the survival of patients with epithelial ovarian carcinoma. Gynecol Oncol 34:365–371

Hoskins WJ (1989) The influence of cytoreductive surgery on progression-free interval and survival in epithelial ovarian cancer. Baillière's Clin Obstet Gynaecol 3:59–71

Hoskins WJ, Lichter AS, Whittington R, et al. (1985) Whole abdominal and pelvic irradiation in patients with minimal disease at second-look surgical reassessment for ovarian carcinoma. Gynecol Oncol 20:271–280

Howell SB, Zimm S, Markman M, et al. (1987) Long-term survival of advanced refractory ovarian carcinoma patients with small volume disease treated with intraperitoneal chemotherapy. J Clin Oncol 5:1607–1612

Hruza C, Dobianer K, Beck A, et al. (1993) *Her*-2 and *int*-2 amplification estimated by quantitative PCR in paraffin-embedded ovarian cancer tissues samples. Eur J Cancer 29A:1593–1597

Huget P, Debois JM (1990) Radiotherapie en ovarium-carcinoom. Ervaring bij 139 patienten. J Belge Radiol 73:113–123

Irmer G, Bürger C, Müller R, Ortmann O, Schulz K-D, Emons G (1994) LH-RH as autocrine regulator of ovarian and endometrial cancer. Exp Clin Endocrinol 102 (Suppl 1):167

Irwin KL, Weiss NS, Lee NC, Peterson HB (1991) Tubal sterilisation, hysterectomy, and the subsequent occurrence of epithelial ovarian cancer. Am J Epidemiol 134:362–369

Jackson GL, Blosser BA (1981) Intracavitary chromic phosphate (^{32}P) colloidal suspension therapy. Cancer 48:2596–2598

Jacobs AJ, Deppe G, Cohen CJ (1982a) Combination chemotherapy of ovarian granulosa cell tumor with cis-platinum and doxorubicin. Gynecol Oncol 14:294–297

Jacobs AJ, Newland JR, Green RK (1982b) Pure choriocarcinoma of the ovary. Obstet Gynecol Surv 37:603–609

Jacobs AJ, Fer M, Su FM, et al. (1993) A phase I trial of rhenium-186-labeled monoclonal antibody administered intraperitoneally in ovarian carcinoma: toxicity and clinical response. Obstet Gynecol 82:586–593

Jacobs I (1994) Genetic, biochemical and multimodal approach to screening for ovarian cancer. Gynecol Oncol 55:S22–S27

Jacobs IJ, Smith SA, Wiseman RW, et al. (1993) A deletion unit on chromosome 17q in epithelial ovarian tumors distal to the familial breast/ovarian cancer locus. Cancer Res 53:1218–1221

Jäger W, Wildt L, Lang N (1989) Some observations on the effects of a GnRH analog in ovarian cancer. Eur J Obstet Gynecol Reprod Biol 32:137–148

Jakobsen A, Bertelsen K, Sell A (1987) Cyclic hormonal treatment in ovarian cancer. A phase II trial. Eur J Cancer Clin Oncol 23:915–916

Jeppson S, Kauppila A, Kullander S, Skryten A (1987) Chemohormonal therapy in advanced ovarian carcinoma. J Steroid Biochem Mol Biol (Suppl) 28:66S

Johannssen H (1965) Spätkomplikationen nach intraperitonealer Radiogold-infusion. Strahlenterapie 127:198–205

Jones JC (1961) Radioactive colloidal yttrium silicate in the treatment of malignant effusions. II. Calculations of tissue dosage. Br J Radiol 34:346–350

Jones HB, Wrobel CJ, Lyons WR (1994) Method of distributing beta-radiation to reticulo-endothelial system and adjacent tissues. J Clin Invest 23:783–788

Joswig EH, Joswig-Priewe H, Frischkorn R, Vahrson H (1976) Erfahrungen mit der Peritoneographie zur Vermeidung primärer Komplikationen bei der intraperitonealen Radiogold-Instillation. Strahlentherapie 151:47–52

Kacinski B (1993) Ovarian carcinoma: tumor- and molecular biology. In: Meerpohl HG, Pfleiderer A, Profous CZ (eds) Das Ovarialkarzinom, vol 1. Springer, Berlin Heidelberg New York, p 7

Kaldor JM, Day NE, Petterson F, et al. (1990) Leukemia following chemotherapy for ovarian cancer. N Engl J Med 322:1–6

Karck U, Meerpohl HG, Kiechle-Schwarz M, Pfleiderer A (1993) Intracavitäre Therapie von Patientinnen mit Aszites oder Pleuraerguß infolge von progredienten gynäkologischen Malignomen. In: Meerpohl HG, Pfleiderer A, Profous CZ (eds) Das Ovarialkarzinom, vol 2. Springer, Berlin Heidelberg New York, p 163

Kaufmann M, Schmid R, Raeth U, et al. (1990) Aszites-Therapie mit Tumornekrosefaktor beim Ovarialkarzinom. Geburtshilfe Frauenheilkd 50:678–682

Kauppila A, Martikainen H, Pentinen J, Reinilä M (1990) GnRH agonist analogue treatment of ovarian granulosa cell malignancies. Gynecol Endocrinol 4 (Suppl 2):97

Kauppila A, Bangah M, Burger H, Martikainen H (1992) GnRH agonist analog therapy in advanced/recurrent granulosa cell tumors: further evidence of a role of inhibin in monitoring response to treatment. Gynecol Endocrinol 6:271–274

Kavanagh JJ, Wharton JT, Roberts WS (1987) Androgen therapy in the treatment of refractory epithelial ovarian cancer. Cancer Treat Rep 71:537–538

Kavanagh JJ, Roberts W, Townsend P, Hewitt S (1989) Leuprolide acetate in the treatment of refractory or persistent epithelial ovarian cancer. J Clin Oncol 7:115–118

Kavanagh JJ, Kudelka AP, Rosenblum MG, et al. (1992) Biomodulation of intraperitoneal monoclonal antibody B72-2-GYK-DTPA ^{90}Y with EDTA in epithelial ovarian cancer. Proc Annu Meet Am Assoc Cancer Res 33: Abstract 2061

Kaye SB, Davies E (1986) Cyclophosphamide, adriamycin, and cis-platinum for the treatment of advanced granulosa cell tumor, using estradiol as a tumor marker. Gynecol Oncol 24:261–264
Kaye SB, Lewis CR, Paul J, et al. (1992) Randomized study of two doses of cisplatin with cyclophosphamide in epithelial ovarian cancer. Lancet 340:329–333
Keettel WC, Elkins HB (1956) Experience with radioactive colloidal gold in treatment of ovarian carcinoma. Am J Obstet 71:553–568
Keettel WC, Fox MR, Longnecker DS, Latourette HB (1966) Prophylactic use of radioactive gold in the treatment of primary ovarian cancer. Am J Obstet Gynecol 94:766-775
Kefford RF, Woods RL, Fox RM (1980) Intracavitary adriamycin, nitrogen mustard and tetracycline in the control of malignant effusions. A randomized study. Med J Australia 2:447–448
Kenemans P, Verstraeten AA, van Kamp GJ, Hilgers J (1994) Tumor markers in gynecology. In: Klapdor R (ed) Current tumor diagnosis: applications, clinical relevance, trends. 7:125–129
Kennedy L, Traub AJ, Atkinson AB, Sheridan B (1987) Short-term administration of gonadotropin-releasing hormone analog to a patient with a testosterone secreting ovarian tumor. J Clin Endocrinol Metab 64:1320–1322
Kepp R, Clemens H (1965) Ergebnisse der postoperativen Radiogoldtherapie bei bösartigen Ovarialtumoren. Strahlentherapie 126:65–69
Kepp RK (1952) Gynäkologische Strahlentherapie – Indikationsstellung, Methodik und ärztliche Betreuung. Thieme, Stuttgart
Kersh CR, Randall ME, Constable WC, et al. (1988) Whole abdominal radiotherapy following cytoreductive surgery and chemotherapy in ovarian carcinoma.
Kieback DG, McCamant SK, Press MF, et al. (1993) Improved predication of survival in advanced adenocarcinoma of the ovary by immunocytochemical analysis and the composition adjusted receptor level of the estrogen receptor. Cancer Res 53:5188–5192
Kietlinska Z, Pietrzak K, Drabik M (1993) The management of granulosa-cell tumors of the ovary based on long-term follow-up. Eur J Gynaecol Oncol 14 (Suppl):118–127
King ME, Hubbell MJ, Talerman A (1991) Mixed germ cell tumor of the ovary with prominent polyembryoma component. Int J Gynecol Pathol 10:88–95
Kjorstad KE (1986) Radiotherapie und Ovarialkarzinom. Gynäkologe 19:170–177
Klaassen D, Starreveld A, Shelly W, et al. (1985) External beam pelvic radiotherapy plus intraperitoneal radioactive chromic phosphate in early stage ovarian cancer: a toxic combination. Int J Radiat Oncol Biol Phys 11:1801–1804
Klaassen D, Shelly W, Starreveld A, et al. (1988) Early stage ovarian cancer: a randomized clinical trial comparing whole abdominal radiotherapy, melphalan, and intraperitoneal chromic phosphate. A National Cancer Institute of Canada Clinical Trials Group report. J Clin Oncol 6:1254–1263
Kleinman GM, Young RH, Scully RE (1984) Ependymoma of the ovary: report of three cases. Hum Pathol 15:632–638
Klemi PK, Joensuu H, Salmi T (1990) Prognostic value of flow cytometric DNA content analysis in granulosa cell tumor of the ovary. Cancer 65:1189–1193
Kloetzer KH, Kob D, Arndt J (1978) Ergebnisse der kombinierten operativ-radiologischen Therapie des Ovarialkarzinoms aus radiologischer Sicht. Zentralbl Gynäkol 100:985–991
Knapp RC, Friedmann EA (1974) Aortic lymph node metastases in early ovarian cancer. Am J Obstet Gynecol 119:1013–1017
Knudson AG (1971) Mutation and cancer: statistical study of retinoblastoma. Proc Natl Acad Sci U S A 68:820–823
Kolstad P, Davy M, Hoeg K (1977) Individualized treatment of ovarian cancer. J Obstet Gynecol 128:617-625
Kommoss F, Bibbo M, Talerman A (1990) Nuclear desoxyribonucleic acid content (ploidy) of endodermal sinus (yolk sac) tumor. Lab Invest 62:223–231
Kommoss F, Pfisterer J, Thome M, Geyer H, Sauerbrei W, Pfleiderer A (1991) Estrogen and progesterone receptors in ovarian neoplasms: discrepant results of immunohistochemical and biochemical results. Int J Gynecol Cancer 1:147–153
Kong JS, Peters LJ, Wharton JT, et al. (1988) Hyperfractioned split-course whole abdominal radiotherapy for ovarian carcinoma: tolerance and toxicity. Int J Radiat Oncol Biol Phys 14:737–743
Korzets A, Nouriel H, Steiner Z, et al. (1986) Resistant hypertension associated with a renin-producing ovarian Sertoli cell tumor. Am J Clin Pathol 85:242–247
Kottmeier HL (1968) Proposals for the standardization of the combined treatment of ovarian cancer. In: Gentil F, Junqueira AC (eds) Ovarian cancer. Springer, Berlin Heidelberg New York
Krepart G, Smith JP, Rutledge F, Delclos L (1978) The treatment for dysgerminoma of the ovary. Cancer 41:986–990
Kucera PR, Berman ML, Treadwell P, et al. (1990) Whole abdominal radiotherapy for patients with minimal residual epithelial ovarian cancer. Gynecol Oncol 36:338–342
Kuipers T (1976) Report on treatment of cancer of the ovary. Br J Radiol 49:526-532
Kullander S, Rausing A, Schally AV (1987) LH-RH agonist treatment in ovarian cancer. In: Klijn JGM (ed) Hormonal manipulation of cancer: peptides, growth factors and new (anti) steroidal agents. Raven Press, New York, p 353
Kumar L, Bhargawa VL, Kumar S (1993) Cisplatin, vinblastine and bleomycin in advanced and relapsed germ cell tumours of the ovary. Asia Oceania J Obstet Gynaecol 19:133–140
Kurman RJ, Norris HJ (1976a) Embryonal carcinoma of the ovary: a clinicopathologic entity distinct of endodermal sinus tumor resembling embryonal carcinoma of the adult testis. Cancer 38:2420–2433
Kurman RJ, Norris HJ (1976b) Endodermal sinus tumor of the ovary. A clinical and pathologic analysis of 71 cases. Cancer 38:2404–2419
Kurman RJ, Trimble CL (1993) The behavior of serous tumors of low malignant-potential: are they ever malignant? Int J Gynecol Pathol 12:120–127
Kurman RJ, Goebelsmann U, Taylor CR (1979) Steroid localization in granulosa-theca tumors of the ovary. Cancer 43:2377–2384
Kuten A, Stein M, Steiner M, et al. (1988) Whole abdominal irradiation following chemotherapy in advanced ovarian carcinoma. Int J Radiat Oncol Biol Phys 14:273–279
Lack EE, Perez-Atayde AR, Murthy ASK (1981) Granulosa theca cell tumors in premenarchal girls. A clinical and pathological study of ten cases. Cancer 48:1846–1854
Lahousen M (1994) Ovarian carcinoma – the way ahead. Onkologie 17:134–140
Lamberts SWJ, Timmers J, Oosterom R, Verleun T, Rommerts FG, deJong FH (1982) Testosterone secretion by cultured arrhenoblastoma cells: suppression by a luteinizing hormone-releasing hormone agonist. J Clin Endocrinol Metab 54:450–454

Landoni F, Epis A, Corga G, Regallo M, Vassena L, Mangioni C (1985) Hormonal treatment in advanced epithelial ovarian cancer. In: Panutti F (ed) Anti-oestrogens in oncology. Past, present and prospects. Excerpta Medica, Amsterdam, pp 262–267

Lang T, Riccabona G (1974) Langzeitergebnisse der intracavitären Isotopentherapie maligner Ergüsse. Nuklearmedizin 13:245–251

Langley FA, Govan ATD, Anderson MC, Gowing NFC, Woodcock AS, Harilal HR (1981) Yolk sac and allied tumors of the ovary. Histopathology 5:389–401

Lanza A, D'Addato F, Valli M, et al. (1988) Pelvic and paraaortic lymph-nodal positivity in the ovarian carcinoma: its prognostic significance. Eur J Gynecol Oncol 9:36–39

Lappohn RE, Burger HG, Bouma J, Bangah M, Krans M, de Bruijn HWA (1989) Inhibin as marker for granulosa-cell tumors. N Engl J Med 321:790–793

Larson SM (1991) Editorial. Choosing the right radionuclide and antibody for intraperitoneal radioimmunotherapy. J Natl Cancer Inst 83:1602–1604

Lauritzen C (1990) Hormonale Kontrazeption und Estrogensubstitution in der Postmenopause im Zusammenhang mit malignen Tumoren. Zentralbl Gynäkol 112:1071–1090

La Vecchia C, Levi F, Lucchini F, et al. (1992) Descriptive epidemiology of ovarian cancer in Europe. Gynecol Oncol 46:208–215

Lawton F, Kelly K, Cassias LJ, Backledge G (1994) Speed of response to platinum-based chemotherapy: implications for the management of epithelial ovarian cancer. Eur J Cancer Clin Oncol 23:1071–1075

Lederman JA, Dembo AJ, Sturgeon JFG, et al. (1991) Outcome of patients with unfavourable optimally reduced cytoreduced ovarian cancer treated with chemotherapy and whole abdominal irradiation. Gynecol Oncol 41:30–35

Leichner PK, Cash SA, Backx C, Durand RE (1981) Effects of injection volume on the tissue dose, dose rate, and therapeutic potential of intraperitoneal ^{32}P. Radiology 141:193–199

Leschinger U (1996) Der Einfluß vorausgegangener Hysterektomien auf die Ent-wicklung, Diagnose, Therapie und Prognose des Ovarialkarzinoms. Inaugural-Dissertation, Giessen

Leung WY, Schwartz PE, Ng HT, Yang-Feng TL (1990) Trisomy 12 in benign fibroma and granulosa cell tumor of the ovary. Gynecol Oncol 38:28–31

Levin L, Hryniuk WM (1987a) The application of dose-intensity to problems in chemotherapy of ovarian and endometrial cancer. Semin Oncol 14 (Suppl 4):12–19

Levin L, Hryniuk WM (1987b) Dose-intensity analysis of chemotherapy regimens in ovarian cancer. J Clin Oncol 5:756–767

Limonta P, Dondi D, Moretti RM, Fermo D, Garattini E, Motta M (1993) Expression of luteinizing hormone-releasing hormone mRNA in the human prostatic cancer cell line LNCaP. J Clin Endocrinol Metab 76:897–800

Lind MJ, Cantwell BMJ, Millward MJ, et al. (1992) A phase II trial of goserelin (Zoladex) in relapsed epithelial ovarian cancer. Br J Cancer 65:621–623

Lind MJ, Gumbrell L, Millward MJ, et al. (1993) A phase I trial of high frequency carboplatin and rhG-CSF in women with epithelial ovarian cancer. Proc Am Soc Clin Oncol 12:365

Lindner H, Willich N, Atzinger A, Schubert-Fritschke G (1990) Die postoperative adjuvante Ganzabdomenbestrahlung beim Ovarialkarzinom. Onkologie 13:260–267

Loehrer PJ, Eldon P, Johnson DH, et al. (1991) A randomized trial of cisplatin plus etoposide with or without bleomycin in favorable prognosis disseminated germ cell tumors: an ECOG study. Proc Am Soc Clin Oncol 10:169 (A 540)

Los G, Mutsaers P, van der Vijgh W, Baldew G, de Graaf P, McVie J (1989) Direct diffusion of cis-diamminedichloroplatinum in intraperitoneal rat tumors after intraperitoneal chemotherapy: a comparison with systemic chemotherapy. Cancer Res 49:3380–3384

Louie KG, Behrens BC, Kinsella TJ, et al. (1985) Radiation survival parameters of antineoplastic drug-sensitive and -resistant human ovarian cancer cell lines and their modification by buthionine sulfoximine. Cancer Res 45:2110–2115

Lusch CJ, Mercurio TM, Runyeon WK (1978) Delayed recurrence and chemotherapy of a granulosa cell tumor. Obstet Gynecol 51:505–508

Lynch HT, Bewtra C, Lynch JF (1986) Familial peritoneal ovarian carcinomatosis: a new clinical entity? Med Hypotheses 21:171–177

Lynch HT, Conway T, Lynch J (1990) Hereditary ovarian cancer. In: Sharp F, Mason WP, Leake RE (eds) Ovarian cancer, biological and therapeutic challenges. Chapman & Hall, London, pp 7–19

Lyon JL, Gardner JW, West DW (1980) Cancer incidence in Mormons and non-Mormons in Utah during 1967–1975. J Natl Cancer Inst 654:1055–1061

Mahé MA, Chatal JF (1995) Radioimmunothérapie des affections malignes. Intéret et perspectives. Presse Med 24:35–38

Malfetano J, Beecham JB, Bundy BN, Hatch KD (1993) A phase II trail of medroyprogesterone acetate in epithelial ovarian cancers. A Gynecologic Oncology Group study. Am J Clin Oncol 16:149–151

Malik S, Balkwill F (1991) Epithelial ovarian cancer: a cytokine propelled disease? Br J Cancer 64:617–620

Malik STA, Slevin ML (1991) Medroxyprogesterone acetate (MPA) in advanced granulosa cell tumours of the ovary – a new therapeutic approach? Br J Cancer 63:410–411

Malkasian GD, Symmonds RE (1964) Treatment of the unilateral encapsulated ovarian dysgerminoma. Am J Obstet Gynecol 90:379–382

Malkasian GD, Webb MJ, Jorgesen GO (1974) Observations of chemotherapy of granulosa cell carcinomas and malignant teratomas. Obstet Gynecol 44:885–888

Malmstrom H, Hogberg T, Risberg B, Simonsen E (1994) Granulosa cell tumors of the ovary: prognostic factors and outcome. Gynecol Oncol 52:50–55

Margolin KA, Pak HY, Esensten ML, Doroshow JH (1985) Hepatic metastases in granulosa cell tumor of the ovary. Cancer 56:691–695

Markman M (1986) Intraperitoneal anti-neoplastic agents for tumors principally confined to the abdominal cavity. Cancer Treat Rev 13:219–242

Markman M, Berek JS (1993) Intraperitoneal administration of the biological agents tumor necrosis factor, gamma interferon, and interleukin 2. In: Meerpohl HG, Pfleiderer A, Profous CZ (eds) Das Ovarialkarzinom, vol 2. Springer, Berlin Heidelberg New York, p 157

Markman M, George M, Hakes T (1990a) Phase 2 trial of intraperitoneal mitoxantrone in the management of refractory ovarian carcinoma. J Clin Oncol 8:146–150

Markman M, Rothman R, et al. (1990b) Second-line cisplatin treatment in patients with ovarian cancer previously treated with cisplatin. Proc Am Soc Clin Oncol ••:599

Markman M, Hakes T, Reichmann B, et al. (1991a) Phase 2 trial of weekly or biweekly intraperitoneal mitoxantrone in epithelial ovarian cancer. J Clin Oncol 9:978–982

Markman M, Hakes T, Reichmann B, Hoskins W, Rubin S, Jones W, Almadrones L, Yordan EL, Eriksson J, Lewis JL (1991b) Intraperitoneal cisplatin and cytarabine in the treatment of refractory or recurrent ovarian carcinoma. J Clin Oncol 9:204–210

Markman M, Reichmann B, Hakes T (1991c) Responses to second-line cisplatin-based intraperitoneal therapy in ovarian cancer: influence of a prior response to intravenous cisplatin. J Clin Oncol 9:1801–1805

Markman M, Rowinsky E, Hakes T (1991d) Phase I study of taxol administered by the intraperitoneal route. Proc Am Soc Clin Oncol 10:185

Marks JR, Davidoff AM, Kerns BJ, et al. (1991) Overexpression and mutation of p53 in epithelial ovarian cancer. Cancer Res 51:2979–2984

Marsh JM, Savard K, Baggett B, Van Wyk JJ, Talbert LM (1962) Estrogen synthesis in a feminizing ovarian granulosa cell tumor. J Clin Endocrinol Metab 22:1196–1200

Martinez A, Schray MF, Hoes AE, Bagshaw MA (1985) Postoperative radiation therapy for epithelial ovarian cancer: the curative role based on a 24-year experience. J Clin Oncol 3:901–922

Martius H (1943) Gynäkologie. In: Auler H, Martius H (eds) Diagnostik der bösartigen Geschwülste. Lehmanns, München, pp 149–183

Masood S, Heitmann J, Nuss RC, Benrubi GI (1989) Clinical correlation of hormone receptor status in epithelial ovarian cancer. Gynecol Oncol 34:57–60

McGowan L, Lesher LP, Norris HJ (1985) Misstaging of ovarian cancer. Obstet Gynecol 65:568

McGuire WP (1995) Ovarian cancer. In: McGuire WP, Rowinski EK (eds) Paclitaxel in cancer treatment. Marcel Dekker, New York, pp 201–221

McGuire WP, Hoskins WJ, Brady MF, et al. (1993) A phase III trial comparing cisplatin/cytoxan and cisplatin/taxol in advanced ovarian cancer. Proc Am Soc Clin Oncol 12: 808

McGuire WP, Hoskins WJ, Brady MF, et al. (1994) A phase III trial of dose intense versus standard dose cisplatin and cytoxan in advanced ovarian cancer. Third Biennial Meeting of the International Gynecologic Cancer Society

McGuire WP, Hoskins WJ, Brady MF, et al. (1995) Assessment of dose-intensive therapy in suboptimally debulked ovarian cancer: a Gynecologic Oncology Group Study. J Clin Oncol 13:1589–1599

McGuire WP, Hoskins WJ, Brady MF, et al. (1995) Taxol and cisplatin (TP) improves outcome in advanced ovarian cancer (AOC) as compared to cytoxan and cisplatin (CP). Proc Am Soc Clin Oncol 14:771

Meerpohl HG (1993) European-Canadian randomized trial of paclitaxel in refractory ovarian cancer. Taxol a novel advance in chemotherapy. Symposium, Munich

Meigs JV (1954) Fibroma of the ovary with ascites and hydrothorax. Am J Obstet Gynecol 67:962–987

Merz WE, Erlewein C, Licht P, Harbarth P (1991) The secretion of human chorionic gonadotropin as well as the α and β-messenger ribonucleic acid levels are stimulated by exogenous gonadoliberin pulses applied to first trimester placenta in a superfusion culture system. J Clin Endocrinol Metab 73:84–92

Michael H, Roth LM (1993) The pathology of ovarian germ cell tumors. In: Rubin SC, Sutton GP (eds) Ovarian cancer. McGraw-Hill, New York, p 131

Michel G, Zarca D, Castaigne D, Prade M (1989) Secondary cytoreductive surgery in ovarian cancer. Eur J Surg Oncol 15:201–204

Mogensen O, Brock, Holm Nyland M (1993) CA 125 measurements in ovarian cancer patients during their first postoperative week. Int J Gynecol Cancer 3:54–56

Mori M, Hiyake H (1988) Dietary and other risk factors of ovarian cancer among elderly women. Jpn J Cancer Res (Gann) 79:997–1004

Müller JH (1956) Zur Dosimetrie des intraperitoneal applizierten kolloidalen Radiogoldes (Au 198) mit spezieller Berücksichtigung der Neutronen-Aktivationsanalyse. Strahlentherapie (Sdbd) 34:177–186

Müller JH (1968) Intraperitoneal colloidal radiogold 198Au therapy in ovarian cancer. In: Gentil F, Junqueira AC (eds) Ovarian cancer. UICC: monograph series, vol 11. Springer, Berlin Heidelberg New York, pp 198–216

Munell E (1969) Is conservative therapy ever justified in stage I (Ia) cancer of the ovary? Am J Obstet Gynecol 103:641–653

Munkarah AR, Gershenson DM, Burke TW, Levenbeck C, Wharton JT, Morris M (1996) Secondary cytoreductive surgery for a clinically apparent solitary intra-abdominal recurrence in patients with epithelial ovarian cancer. Proc Am Soc Clin Oncol 15:295

Münstedt K, Vahrson H (1993) Stellenwert der kombinierten Nachbehandlung des fortgeschrittenen Ovarialkarzinoms (Abstract). Berichte Gynäk Geburtsh 130:196

Münstedt K, Vahrson H (1995) Radio-chemotherapeutic treatment of advanced ovarian cancer. Eur J Gynaecol Oncol 16:174–180

Musch E, Chemaissani A, Eberhardt K, et al. (1992) Intrapleurale Mitoxantron-Therapie zur Behandlung maligner Pleuraergüsse. In: Nagel GA, Fahrtmann EH, Sauer R (eds) Neue Konzepte in der systemischen und lokoregionalen Therapie mit Novantron. Acta Oncol 66:1–17

Muto MG, Finkler NJ, Kassis AI, et al. (1992) Intraperitoneal radioimmunotherapy of refractory ovarian carcinoma utilizing iodine-131-labeled monoclonal antibody OC 125. Gynecol Oncol 45:265–272

Muto MG, Welch WR, Mok SC, et al. (1995) Evidence for a multifocal origin of papillary serous carcinoma of the peritoneum. Cancer Res 55:490–492

Mychalczak BR, Fuks Z (1993) The role of radiotherapy in the management of epithelial ovarian cancer. In: Markman M, Hoskins WJ (eds) Cancer of the ovary. Raven Press, New York, pp 229–241

Myers AM, Moore GE, Major FJ (1981) Advanced ovarian carcinoma: response to antiestrogen therapy. Cancer 48:2368–2370

Nakashima N, Young RH, Scully RE (1984) Androgenic granulosa cell tumors of the ovary. A clinicopathologic analysis of 17 cases and review of the literature. Arch Pathol Lab Med 108:786–791

Naylor MS, Stamp GWH, Foulkes WD, Eccles D, Balkwill FR (1993) Tumor necrosis factor and its receptors in human ovarian cancer, potential role in disease progression. J Clin Invest 91:2194–2206

Neijt JP, van der Burg MEL, Vriesendorp R, et al. (1984) Randomized trial comparing two combination chemotherapy regimens (Hexa-CAF vs CHAP-5) in advanced ovarian carcinoma. Lancet 2:549

Neijt JP, van der Burg MEL, ten Bokkel Huinink WW, et al. (1995) Neuronal nets and prognostic factors in ovarian cancer. Proc Am Soc Clin Oncol 14:739–267

Nevin JE, Pinzon G, Baggerly TJ, et al. (1983) The use of intravenous phenylalanine mustard followed by supervoltage irradiation in the treatment of carcinoma of the ovary. Cancer 51:1273–1283

Newlands ES, Begent RHJ, Rustin GJ, Bagshawe KD (1982) Potential for cure in metastatic ovarian teratomas and dysgerminomas. Br J Obstet Gynaecol 89:555–560

Nichols CR, Breeden ES, Loehrer PJ, et al. (1993) Secondary leukemia associated with a conventional dose of etoposide: review of serial germ cell tumor protocols. J Natl Cancer Inst 85:36–40

Nielsen SN, Gaffey TA, Malkasian GD (1986) Immature ovarian teratoma: a review of 14 cases. Mayo Clin Proc 61:110–117

Nishida M, Jimi S, Haji M, Hayashi I, Kai T, Tasaka H (1991) Juvenile granulosa cell tumor in association with a high serum inhibin level. Gynecol Oncol 40:90–94

Nitz U, Jackisch C, Weise W, Schiller E, Illiger HJ (1994) Doseintensified carboplatinmonotherapy in advanced ovarian cancer. Zentralbl Gynäkol 116:549–554

Nogales FF Jr, Favara BE, Major FJ, Silverberg SG (1976) Immature teratoma of the ovary with a neural component ("solid" teratoma). A clinical pathologic study of 20 cases. Hum Pathol 7:625–632

Norris HJ, Taylor HB (1968) Prognosis of granulosa-theca tumors of the ovary. Cancer 21:255–263

Norris HJ, Zirkin HJ, Benson WL (1976) Immature (malignant) teratoma of the ovary. A clinical and pathologic study of 58 cases. Cancer 37:2359–2372

Ohel G, Kaneti H, Schenker JG (1983) Granulosa cell tumors in Israel: a study of 172 cases. Gynecol Oncol 15:278–286

Ohno T, Imai A, Furui T, Takahashi K, Tamaya T (1993) Presence of gonadotropin-releasing hormone and its messenger ribonucleic acid in human ovarian epithelial carcinoma. Am J Obstet Gynecol 169:605–610

Ohtani K, Sakamoto H, Konbai D (1990) Antagonistic effects of GnRH agonist on gonadotropin stimulated proliferation of human ovarian cancer cell line. Gynecol Endocrinol 4 (Suppl 2):98

Olt G, Berchuck A, Bast RC (1990) The role of tumor markers in gynecologic oncology. Obstet Gynecol Surv 45:570–577

Omura G, Morrow P, Blessing J, et al. (1983) A randomized comparison of melphalan versus melphalan plus hexamethylmelamine versus adriamycin and cyclophosphamide in ovarian carcinoma. Cancer 51:783–789

Omura G, Blessing J, Ehrlich C, et al. (1986) A randomized trial of cyclophosphamide and doxorubicin with or without cisplatin in advanced ovarian carcinoma: a Gynecologic Oncology Group Study. Cancer 57:1725–1730

Omura G, Bundy B, Berek J, Curry S, Delgado G, Mortel R (1989) Randomized trial of cyclophosphamide plus cisplatin with or without doxorubicin in ovarian carcinoma: a Gynecologic Oncology Group study. J Clin Oncol 7:457–465

Ozols RF, Locker G, Doroshow JH, Grotzinger KR, Myers CE, Young RC (1979) Pharmacokinetics of adriamycin and tissue penetration in murine ovarian cancer. Cancer Res 39:3209–3214

Ozols RF, Ostchega Y, Curt G, Young RC (1986) High dose carboplatin in ovarian cancer: potential for replacing high dose cisplatin in the combination therapy of ovarian cancer. Proc Am Soc Clin Oncol 5:461

Ozols RF, Rubin SC, Dembo AJ, Robboy S (1992) Epithelial ovarian cancer. In: Hoskins WJ, Perez CA, Young RC (eds) Gynecologic oncology. Lippincott, Philadelphia, p 731

Pahwa GS, Vollmer G, Knuppen R, Emons G (1989) Photoaffinity labelling of gonadotropin releasing hormone binding sites in human epithelial ovarian carcinomata. Biochem Biophys Res Commun 161:1086–1092

Pankratz E, Boyes DA, White GW, Galliford BW, Fairy RN, Benedet JL (1978) Granulosa cell tumors. A clinical review of 61 cases. Obstet Gynecol 52:718–723

Paraskevas M, Scully RE (1989) Hilus cell tumor of the ovary: a clinicopathologic analysis of 12 Reinke-crystal-positive and 9 crystal-negative cases. Int J Gynecol Pathol 8:299–310

Parmar H, Nicoll J, Stockdale A, Cassoni A, Phillips RH, Lightman SL, Schally AV (1985) Advanced ovarian carcinoma: response to the agonist D-Trp^6-LH-RH. Cancer Treat Rep 69:1341–1342

Parmar H, Rustin F, Lightman SL, Pillips RH, Hanham JW, Schally AV (1988a) Response to D-Trp6-luteinizing hormone-releasing hormone (Decapeptyl) microcapsules in advanced ovarian cancer: BMJ 296:1229

Parmar H, Phillips RH, Rustin F, Lightman SL, Hanham JW, Schally AV (1988b) Therapy of advanced ovarian cancer with D-Trp6-LH-RH (Decapeptyl) microcapsules. Biomed Pharmacother 42:531–538

Pater J (1990) Cyclophosphamide/cisplatin versus cyclophosphamide/carboplatin in macroscopic residual ovarian cancer. Initial results of a National Cancer Institute of Canada Clinical Trials Group trial. Proc Am Soc Clin Oncol 9:155

Pattillo RA, Collier BD, Abdel-Dayem H, et al. (1995) Phosphorus-32-chromic phosphate for ovarian cancer. I. Fractionated low dose intraperitoneal treatments in conjunction with platinum analog chemotherapy. J Nucl Med 36:29–36

Pawlega J, Rachtan J, Dyba T (1994) Ovarian cancer risk with special reference to diet and particularly to legume consumption. Curr Oncol 1:217–220

Pecorelli S, Wagener P, Bonazzi G, et al. (1988) Cisplatin (P), vinblastine (V) and bleomycin (B) combination chemotherapy in recurrent or advanced granulosa cell tumor of the ovary (GCTO): an EORTC Gynecologic Cancer Cooperative Group Study. Proc Am Soc Clin Oncol 7:147

Pedersen-Bjergaard J, Daugaard G, Hansen SW, Philip P, Larsen SO, Rorth M (1991) Increased risk of myelodysplasia and leukaemia after etoposide, cisplatin, and bleomycin for germ cell tumours. Lancet 338:359–363

Perez CA, Walz BJ, Jacobson PL (1975) Radiation therapy in the management of carcinoma of the ovary. Natl Cancer Inst Monogr 42:119–125

Perren TJ, Gore ME, Fryatt I, Wiltshaw E (1988) High dose carboplatin for stage IV ovarian cancer: a preliminary analysis of response, toxicity and survival. Proc Am Soc Clin Oncol 7:568

Peters WA, Smith MR, Cain JM, et al. (1992) Intraperitoneal P-32 is not an effective consolidation therapy after a negative second-look laparotomy for epithelial carcinoma of the ovary. Gynecol Oncol 47:146–149

Peterson WF (1957) Malignant degeneration of benign cystic teratomas of the ovary. A collective review of the literature. Obstet Gynecol Survey 12:793–802

Petru E, Pickel H, Tamussino K, Lahousen M, Heydarfadai M, Posawetz W, Jakse R (1991) Pretherapeutic scalene lymph node biopsy in ovarian cancer. Gynecol Oncol 43:262–264

Pertu E, Lahousen M, Tamussino K, et al. (1994) Lymphadenectomy in stage I ovarian cancer. Am J Obstet Gynecol 170:656–662

Pettersson F (1991) Annual report on the results of treatment in gynecological cancer, vol 21. Radiumhmmet, Stockholm

Pettersson F (1994) Annual report on the results of treatment in gynecological cancer, vol 22. Radiumhemmet, Stockholm

Peyron A (1939) Faits nouveaux relatifs à l'origine et à l'histogénèse des embryomes. Bull Cancer 28:658–672

Pezner RP, Stevens KR, Tong D, Allen CV (1978) Limited epithelial carcinoma of the voary treated with curative intent by the intraperitoneal instillation of radiocolloids. Cancer 42:2563–2571

Pfeiffer P, Bennedaek O, Bertelsen K (1990) Intraperitoneal carboplatin in the treatment of minimal residual ovarian cancer. Gynecol Oncol 36:306–311

Pfleiderer A (1984) Das Ovarialkarzinom. In: Schwalm H, Döderlein G, Wulf KH (eds) Klinik der Frauenheilkunde und Geburtshilfe vol. VIII, Suppl. Urban & Schwarzenberg, München, pp 714/1–174

Pfleiderer A (1986) Epidemiologie maligner Ovarialtumoren in Pfleiderer (ed) Maligne Tumoren der Ovarien. Bücherei des Frauenarztes, vol 23. Enke, Stuttgart, pp 1–12

Pfleiderer A (1993) Therapy of ovarian malignant germ cell tumors and granulosa tumors. Int J Gynecol Pathol 12:162–165

Pickel H (1993) Epithelial ovarian cancer - spread. In: Burghardt E, Webb J, Monaghan JM, Kindermann G (eds) Surgical gynecologic oncology. Thieme, Stuttgart, p 435

Pickel H, Lahoussen M, Stettner H, Girardi F (1989) The spread of ovarian cancer. Ballieres Clin Obstet Gynaecol 3:3–12

Piver MS (1983) Ovarian malignancies: the clinical care of adults and adolescents. In: Piver MS (ed) Current reviews in obstetrics and gynecology, vol 4. Churchill Livingstone, New York, p 74

Piver MS, Barlow JJ, Lele SB (1978) Incidence of subclinical metastasis in stage I and II ovarian carcinoma. Obstet Gynecol 52:100–104

Piver MS, Barlow JJ, Lele SB, et al. (1982) Intraperitoneal chromic phosphate in peritoneoscopically confirmed stage I ovarian adenocarcinoma. Am J Obstet Gynecol 144:836–840

Piver MS, Lele SB, Marchetti DL, et al. (1988) The impact of aggressive debulking surgery and cisplatin chemotherapy on progression-free survival in stage III and IV ovarian carcinomas. J Clin Obstet Cynecol 6:983–989

Piver MS, Goldberg JM, Tsukada Y, et al. (1996) Characteristics of familial ovarian cancer: a report of the first 1000 families in the Gilda Radner Familial Ovarian Cancer Registry. Eur J Gynaecol Oncol 17:169–176

Podratz KC, Kinney WK (1993) Second-look operation in ovarian cancer. Cancer 71:1551–1558

Podratz KC, Schray MF, Wieand HS, et al. (1988) Evaluation of treatment and survival after positive second look laparotomy. Gynecol Oncol 31:9–21

Pohl R, Dallenbach-Hellweg G, Plugge T, et al. (1984) Prognostic parameters in patients with advanced malignant ovarian tumors. Eur J Gynaecol Oncol 3:160

Potter ME, Partridge EE, Shingleton HM, et al. (1989) Intraperitoneal chromic phosphate in ovarian cancer: risks and benefits. Gynecol Oncol 32:314–318

Prat J, Scully RE (1981) Cellular fibromas and fibrosarcomas of the ovary: a comparative clinicopathological analysis of 17 cases. Cancer 47:2663–2670

Pressley RH, Muntz HG, Falkenberry S, Rice LW (1992) Serum lactic dehydrogenase as a tumor marker in dysgerminoma. Gynecol Oncol 44:281–283

Preston-Martin S, Pike MC, Ross RK, Henderson BE (1991) Epidemiologic evidence for the increased cell proliferation model of carcinogenesis. Prog Clin Biol Res 369:21–34

Rao RB, Slotman BJ (1991) Endocrine factors in common epithelial ovarian cancer. Endocr Rev 12:14–26

Reddy S, Lee MS, Yordan E, et al. (1993) Salvage whole abdomen radiation therapy: its role in ovarian cancer. Int J Radiat Oncol Biol Phys 27:879–884

Redman JR, Petroni GR, Saigo PE, Geller NL, Hakes TB (1986) Prognostic factors in advanced ovarian cancer. J Clin Oncol 4:515

Reed E, Janik J, Bookman M, et al. (1990) High dose carboplatin and rhGM-CSF in refractory ovarian cancer. Proc Am Soc Clin Oncol 9:609

Reed GW, Watson ER, Chesters MS (1961) A note on the distribution of radioactive colloidal gold following intraperitoneal injection. Br J Radiol 34:323–326

Reichmann B, Markman M, Hakes T, et al. (1989) Intraperitoneal cisplatin and etoposide in the treatment of refractory/recurrent ovarian carcinoma. J Clin Oncol 7:1327–1332

Reinfuss M, Kojs Z, Skolyszewski J (1993) External beam radiotherapy in the management of ovarian carcinoma. Radiother Oncol 26:26–32

Remberger K (1984) Pathologische Anatomie der Ovarialkarzinome und die Kriterien der Malignität. In: Georgii A (ed) Aspekte der Klinischen Onkologie. Verh Dtsch Krebsges 5:671–682. Fischer, Stuttgart

Rendina GM, Donadio C, Giovannini M (1982) Steroid receptors and progestagenic therapy in ovarian endometroid carcinoma. Eur J Gynaecol Oncol 3:241–246

Rezvani A, Lê MG (1994) Evolution de la mortalité par cancer de l'ovaire en France entre 1968–1991. Bull Cancer (Paris) 81:1091–1095

Rizel S, Biran S, Anteby SO, et al. (1985) Combined modality treatment for stage III ovarian carcinoma. Radiother Oncol 3:237–244

Robboy SJ, Scully RE (1980) Strumal carcinoid of the ovary: an analysis of 50 cases of a distinctive tumor composed of thyroid tissue and carcinoid. Cancer 46:2019–2034

Robboy SJ, Norris HJ, Scully RE (1975) Insular carcinoid primary in the ovary. A clinicopathologic analysis of 48 cases. Cancer 36:404–418

Rodriguez GC, Boente MP, Berchuck A, et al. (1993) The effect of antibodies and immunotoxins reactive with HER-2/neu on growth of ovarian and breast cancer cell lines. Am J Obstet Gynecol 168:228–232

Rogers L, Varia M, Halle J, et al. (1990) 32P following second look laparotomy for epithelial ovarian cancer (abstr)2 Int J Radiat Oncol Biol Phys 19 (Suppl 1):167–168

Root SW, Tyor MP, Andrews GA, Kniseley RM (1954) Distribution of colloidal radioactive chromic phosphate after intracavitary administration. Radiology 63:251–259

Rose PG, Piver MS, Tsukada Y, Lau T (1989) Metastatic patterns in histologic variants of ovarian cancer: an autopsy study. Cancer 64:1508–1513

Rose PG, Blessing JA, Mayer AR, Homesly AB (1996) Prolonged oral etoposide as second-line therapy for platinum resistant and platinum sensitive ovarian carcinoma: a Gynecologic Oncology Group study. Proc Am Soc Clin Oncol 15:282

Rosen EM, Goldberg ID, Rose C, et al. (1986) Sequential multiagent chemotherapy and whole abdominal irradiation for stage III ovarian carcinoma. Radiother Oncol 7:223–232

Rosenblum MG, Kavanagh JJ, Burke TW, et al. (1991) Clinical pharmacology, metabolism and tissue distribution of ^{90}Y-labeled monoclonal antibody B72.3 after intraperitoneal administration. J Natl Cancer Inst 83:1629–1636

Rosenshein NB (1983) Radioisotopes in the treatment of ovarian cancer. Clin Obstet Gynaecol 10:279–295

Roth LM, Anderson MC, Govan ADT, Langley FA, Gowing NFC, Woodcock AS (1981) Sertoli-Leydig cell tumors. A clinicopathological study of 34 cases. Cancer 48:187–197

Rothenberg ML, Ozols RF, Glatstein E, et al. (1992) Dose-intensive induction therapy with cyclophosphamide, cisplatin, and consolidative abdominal radiation in

advanced-stage epithelial ovarian cancer. J Clin Oncol 10:727–734
Rotmensch J, Beckett MA, Toohill P, et al. (1989a) Comparative analysis of the inherent radiosensitivity of ovarian carcinoma. Gynecol Obstet Invest 28:215–218
Rotmensch J, Atcher RW, Hines J, et al. (1989b) The development of α-emitting radionuclide lead 212 for the potential treatment of ovarian carcinoma. Am J Obstet Gynecol 160:789–797
Rotmensch J, Roeske J, Chen G, et al. (1990) Estimates of dose to intraperitoneal micrometastases from alpha and beta emitters in radioimmunotherapy. Gynecol Oncol 38:478–485
Rotmensch J, Schwartz JL, Atcher RW, et al. (1991) Increased nuclear damage by high linear energy transfer radioisotopes applicable for radiodirected therapy against radiologic malignancies. Gynecol Obstet Invest 32:180–184
Rotte K, Feltmann K (1969) Zur Behandlung tumorbedingter Ergüsse mit Radiogold. Med Klin 64:1598–1603
Rubin SC (1993) Second-look laparotomy in ovarian cancer. In: Markman M, Hoskins W (eds) Cancer of the ovary. Raven Press, New York, p 175
Rubin SC, Lewis JJ (1988) Second-look surgery in ovarian carcinoma. Crit Rev Oncol Hematol 8:75–91
Rubin SC, Hoskins WT, Hakes TB, et al. (1988) Recurrence after negative second-look laparotomy for ovarian cancer: analysis of risk factors. Am J Obstet Gynecol 158:1094–1098
Rubin SC, Hoskins WJ, Hakes TB (1989) Serum CA 125 levels and surgical findings in patients undergoing secondary operations for epithelial ovarian cancer. Am J Obstet Gynecol 160:667–671
Rubin SC, Hoskins WJ, Saigo PE, Chapman D, Hakes TB, Markman M, et al. (1991) Prognostic factors for recurrence following negative second-look laparotomy in ovarian cancer patients treated with platinum-based chemotherapy. Gynecol Oncol 42:137–141
Rubin SC, Finstad CL, Wong GY, Almadrones L, Plante M, Lloyd KO (1993) Prognostic significance of Her-2/neu expression in advanced epithelial ovarian cancer: a multivariate analysis. Am J Obstet Gynecol 168:162–169
Ruckdeschel JC, Moores M, Lee JY, et al. (1991) Intrapleural therapy for malignant pleural effusions. A randomized comparison of bleomycin and tetracycline. Chest 100:1528–1535
Russel P (1994) Surface epithelial-stromal tumors of the ovary. In: Kurman RJ (ed) Blausteins' pathology of the female genital tract, 4th edn. Springer, Berlin Heidelberg New York, pp 705–782
Rustin GJ (1987) Managing malignant ovarian germ cell tumors. BMJ 295:869–870
Rustin GJ, Newlands ES, Begent RHJ, Bagshawe KD (1988) Fertility after chemotherapy for ovarian germ cell tumors. J Clin Oncol 6:1520
Santen RJ, Manni A, Harvey HA, Redmond C (1990) Endocrine treatment of breast cancer in women. Endocr Rev 11:221–265
Sasano H, Carleton TG, Wilkinson DS, Silverberg S, Comerford J, Hyde J (1990) Protooncogene amplification and tumor ploidy in human ovarian neoplasms. Hum Pathol 21:382–391
Sato T, Saito H, Morita R, et al. (1991) Allelotype of human ovarian cancer. Cancer Res 51:5118–5122
Schally AV, Srkalovic G, Szende B, et al. (1990) Antitumor effects of analogs of LH-RH and somatostatin: experimental and clinical studies. J Steroid Biochem Mol Biol 37:1061–1067
Scharl A, Vierbuchen M, Kusche M, Bolte A (1988) Zur Klinik und Prognose von Granulosazelltumoren. Geburtshilfe Frauenheilkd 48:567–573
Scheer KE (1964) Die Behandlung maligner Ergüsse mit Radioisotopen. Sdbd Strahlentherapie 55B. Urban & Schwarzenberg, München
Schenker JG, Mazzor M (1978) Cancer of the ovary in Israel (1966–1971). Gynecol Oncol 6:397–410
Schmidt-Rhode P (1991) Kontrolluntersuchungen während und nach einer medikamentösen Tumortherapie -Erkennung und Behandlung von Nebenwirkungen. In: Kaiser R, Schulz K-D, Maass H (eds) Hormonale Behandlung von Genital- und Mammatumoren bei der Frau. Thieme, Stuttgart, p 137
Schneider F Untersuchungen zur Frage der Therapieinduktion von 738 multiplen Malignomen bei 10.461 Patientinnen mit Genitalkarzinomen (1957–1992) am ZFG Giessen. Inaugural-Dissertation, Giessen (in preparation)
Schönig T, Schmid H, Kaufmann M, Bastert G (1991) Intrapleurale Applikationen von rekombinantem humanem Tumornekrosefaktor (rHuTNF) bei malignen Pleuraergüssen. Arch Gynecol Obstet 250:288–289
Schray MF, Martinez A, Howes AE, et al. (1988) Advanced epithelial ovarian cancer: salvage whole abdominal irradiation for patients with recurrent or persistent disease after combination chemotherapy. J Clin Oncol 6:1433–1439
Schray MF, Martinez A, Howes AE (1989) Toxicity of open-field whole abdominal irradiation as primary postoperative treatment in gynecologic malignancy. Int J Radiat Oncol Biol Phys 16:397–403
Schröder W, Bender HG (1992) Pharmakologische Entwicklungen zum therapeutischen Einsatz von Biological-response-Modifiern. Gynäkologe 25:258–267
Schuler U, Ehninger G (1990) Pharmakokinetik bei der intraperitonealen Applikation von Mitoxantron. Aktuelle Onkologie 54:55–59
Schulman P, Cheng P, Cvitkovic E, Golbey R (1974) Spontaneous pneumothorax as a result of intensive cytotoxic chemotherapy. Chest 75:194–196
Schulz K-D (1991) Ovarialkarzinom. In: Kaiser R, Schulz K-D, Maass H (eds) Hormonale Behandlung von Genital- und Mammatumoren bei der Frau. Thieme, Stuttgart, p 94
Schulz K-D, King RJB, Taylor BW (eds) (1987) Endometrial cancer. Zuckschwerdt, München
Schulz K-D, Hofmann J, Hackenberg R, Emons G, Schmidt-Rhode P (1991) Palliative hormonal treatment in endometrial carcinoma. In: Kleine W, Meerpohl HG, Pfleiderer A, Profous CZ (eds) Therapie des Endometriumkarzinoms. Springer, Berlin Heidelberg New York, p 119
Schutter EMJ, Kenemans P, Sohn C, et al. (1994) Diagnostic value of pelvic examination, ultrasound and serum CA 125 in postmenopausal women presenting with a pelvic mass, an international multicenter study. Cancer 74:1398–1406
Schwartz PE, Smith JP (1976) Treatment of ovarian stromal tumors. Am J Obstet Gynecol 125:402–408
Schwartz PE, Keating G, MacLusky N, Naftolin F, Eisenfeld A (1982) Tamoxifen therapy for advanced ovarian cancer. Obstet Gynecol 59:583–588
Schwartz PE, Chambers JT, Kohorn EJ, et al. (1989) Tamoxifen in combination with cytotoxic chemotherapy in advanced epithelial ovarian cancer. Cancer 63:1074–1078
Schweppe KW, Beller FK (1982) Clinical data of granulosa cell tumors. J Cancer Res Clin Oncol 104:161–169
Scully RE (1970a) Sex cord tumors with annular tubules. A distinctive ovarian tumor of the Peutz-Jeghers syndrome. Cancer 25:1107–1121

Scully RE (1970b) Gonadoblastoma. A review of 74 cases. Cancer 25:1340–1356
Scully RE (1975) World Health Organization classification and nomenclature of ovarian cancer: symposium on ovarian carcinoma. Monogr Natl Cancer Inst 42:5–7
Scully RE (1977) Sex cord-stromal tumors. In: Blaustein A (ed) Pathology of the female genital tract. Springer, Berlin Heidelberg New York, pp 505–526
Scully RE (1979) Tumors of the ovaries and maldeveloped gonads. Atlas of tumor pathology, second series, fascicle 16. Armed Forces Institute of Pathology, Washington DC
Scully RE (1995) Early de novo ovarian cancer and cancer developing in benign ovarian lesions. Int J Gynecol Obstet 49:S9–S15
Segelov E, Campbell J, Ng M, et al. (1994) Cisplatin-based chemotherapy for ovarian germ cell malignancies: the Australian experience. J Clin Oncol 12:378–384
Serov SF, Scully RE, Sobin LH (1973) International histological classification of tumours no. 9 histological typing of ovarian tumours. World Health Organization, Geneva
Sevin B-U (1988) Die prätherapeutische Staging-Laparotomie. In: Hepp H, Scheidel P, Monaghan JM (eds) Die Lymphonodektomie in der gynäkologischen Onkologie. Urban & Schwarzenberg, München, p 19
Sevin B-U (1989) Intraoperative staging in ovarian cancer. Baillière's Clin Obstet Gynaecol 3:13–21
Shea TC, Flaherty M, Elias A, et al. (1989) A phase I clinical and pharmacokinetic study of carboplation and autologous bone marrow support. J Clin Oncol 7:651–661
Shirey DR, Kavanagh JJ, Gershenson DM, Freedman RS, Copland LJ, Jones LA (1985) Tamoxifen therapy of epithelial ovarian cancer. Obstet Gynecol 66:575–578
Shinozuka T, Murakami M, Miyamoto T, et al. (1991) High dose chemotherapy with autologous bone marrow transplantation in ovarian cancer. Proc Am Soc Clin Oncol 10:193
Shpall EJ (1990) Preliminary results from the University of Colorado Bone Marrow Transplant Program (unpublished data).
Shpall EJ, Clarke-Pearson D, Soper J, et al. (1990) High dose alkylating agent therapy with autologous marrow support in patients with stage III/IV epithelial ovarian cancer. Gynecol Oncol 38:386–391
Shpall EJ, Cagnoni PJ, Bearman SI, Purdy MH, Jones RB (1995) High-dose chemotherapy with autologous hematopoietic cell support (AHCS) for the treatment of epithelial ovarian cancer. Educational Booklet. Am Soc Clin Oncol, pp 360–364
Sikic BJ, Scudder SA, Ballon SC, et al. (1986) High-dose megestrol acetate therapy of ovarian carcinoma. A phase II study by the Northern California oncology group. Semin Oncol (Suppl 4) 13:26–32
Singh P, Yordan EL, Graham JR, et al. (1987) Combination chemotherapy for immature (malignant) teratomas of the ovary. Asia Oceania J Obstet Gynaecol 13:455–459
Slamon DJ, Godolphin W, Jones LA, et al. (1989) Studies of Her-2/neu protooncogene in human breast and ovarian cancer. Science 244:707–712
Slayton RE, Park RC, Silverberg S, Shingleton H, Creasman W, Blessing J (1985) Vincristine, dactinomycin, and cyclophosphamide in the treatment of malignant germ cell tumors of the ovary. A Gynecologic Oncology Group study (a final report). Cancer 56:243–248
Slevin ML, Harvey VJ, Osborne RJ, Shepherd JH, Williams CJ, Mead DM (1986) A phase II study of tamoxifen therapy in ovarian cancer. Eur J Cancer Clin Oncol 22:309–312
Slotman BJ (1990) Rationale for the use of endocrine therapy in ovarian cancer. Thesis Publishers, Amsterdam, pp 1–175
Slotman BJ, Rao BR (1989a) Response to inhibition of androgen actions of human ovarian cancer cells in vitro. Cancer Lett 45:213–220
Slotman BJ, Rao BR (1989b) Primary human ovarian adenocarcinoma: response to steroids and anti-hormones in vitro. Cancer J 2:373–377
Slotman BJ, Nauta JJP, Rao BR (1990) Survival of ovarian cancer patients: apart from stage and grade, tumor progesterone receptor is a prognostic indicator. Cancer 66:740–744
Smales E, Peckham MJ (1987) Chemotherapy of germ cell ovarian tumours: first line treatment of etoposide, bleomycin and cisplatin or carboplatin. Eur J Cancer 23:469–474
Smith JP, Rutledge F (1970) Chemotherapy in the treatment of cancer of the ovary. Am J Obstet Gynecol 107:691–700
Smith JP, Delgado G, Rutledge F (1976) Second-look operation in ovarian carcinoma. Cancer 38:1438–1442
Snyder RR, Tavassoli FA (1986) Ovarian strumal carcinoid: immunohistochemical, ultrastructural, and clinicopathologic observations. Int J Gynecol Pathol 5:187–201
Soper JT, Creasman WT, Clarke-Pearson DL (1985) Intraperitoneal chromic phosphate P32 suspension therapy of malignant peritoneal cytology in endometrial carcinoma. Am J Obstet Gynecol 153:191–196
Soper JT, Wilkinson RH, Lawrence C, et al. (1987) Intraperitoneal chromic phosphate P32 as salvage therapy for persistent carcinoma of the ovary after surgical restaging. Am J Obstet Gynecol 156:1153–1158
Sorbe B, Tropé C, Nordal R, et al. (1996) Chemotherapy versus radiotherapy a consolidation treatment of ovarian carcinoma stage III at surgical complete remission from induction chemotherapy. Proc Am Soc Clin Oncol ASCO 15 revised: 287 (abstr 780)
Spanos WJ, Day T, Abner A, et al. (1992) Complications in the use of intra-abdominal ^{32}P for ovarian carcinoma. Gynecol Oncol 45:243–247
Speert H (1952) The role of ionizing radiations in the causation of ovarian tumors. Cancer 5:478
Spencer TR, Marks RD, Fenn JO, et al. (1989) Intraperitoneal P-32 after negative second-look laparotomy in ovarian carcinoma. Cancer 63:2434–2437
Stage AH, Grafton WD (1977) Thecomas and granulosa-theca cell tumors of the ovary. An analysis of 51 tumors. Obstet Gynecol 50:21–27
Statistisches Bundesamt (ed) (1994) Statistisches Jahrbuch (1994) für die Bundesrepublik Deutschland.
Steichen-Gersdorf E, Gallion HH, Ford D, et al. (1994) Familial site-specific ovarian cancer is linked to BRCA 1 on 17q 12–21. Am J Hum Genet 55:870–875
Stenwig JT, Hazekamp JT, Beecham JB (1979) Granulosa cell tumors of the ovary. A clinicopathological study of 118 cases with long-term follow-up. Gynecol Oncol 7:136–152
Stewart RS, Woodward DE (1962) Malignant ovarian hilus cell tumor. Arch Pathol 73:91–99
Stiff P, Bayer R, Camarda M, et al. (1995) A phase II trial of high-dose mitoxantrone, carboplatin and cyclophosphamide with autologous bone marrow rescue for recurrent epithelial ovarian carcinoma: analysis of risk factors and clinical outcome. Gynecol Oncol 57:278–285
Suh KS, Silverberg SG, Rhame JG, Wilkinson DS (1990) Granulosa cell tumor of the ovary. Histopathologic and flow cytometric analysis with clinical correlation. Arch Pathol Lab Med 114:496–501

Sullivan DC, Harris CC, Currie IL, et al. (1983) Observation on the peritoneal distribution of chromic phosphate (32-P) suspension for intraperitoneal therapy. Radiology 146: 539–541

Sutton GP, Blessing JA, Photopoulos G, Berman ML, Homesley HD (1990) Gynecologic Oncology Group experience with ifosfamide. Semin Oncol 17(Suppl 4):6–10

Szepesi T, Seitz W, Kogelnik HD, et al. (1979) Simultane Radio-Chemotherapie des fortgeschrittenen Ovarialkarzinoms – Phase I. In: Wannenmacher M, Gauwerky F, Streffer C (eds) Kombinierte Strahlen- und Chemotherapie. Urban & Schwarzenberg, München, pp 180–184

Szepesi T, Kärcher KH, Breitenecker G, et al. (1982) Ansprech- und Überlebensraten von Patientinnen mit fortgeschrittenem Ovarialkarzinom nach Radio-/Chemotherapie in Abhängigkeit von Stadium und Histologie. Strahlentherapie 158:642–652

Takeda A, Ishizuka T, Goto T, et al. (1982) Polyembryoma of the ovary producing alpha-fetoprotein and HCG: immunoperoxidase and electron microscopic study. Cancer 49:1878–1889

Talerman A (1984) Carcinoid tumors of the ovary. J Cancer Res Clin Oncol 107:125–135

Talerman A (1992) Germ cell tumors. Curr Top Pathol 85:165–202

Taylor A Jr, Baily NA, Halpern SE, Asburn WL (1974) Loculation as a contraindication to intracavitary ^{32}P-chromic phosphate therapy. J Nucl Med 16:318–319

Taylor MH, DePetrillo AD, Turner AR (1985) Vinblastine, bleomycin and cisplatin in malignant germ cell tumors of the ovary. Cancer 56:1341–1349

Teilum G (1965) Classification of endodermal sinus tumor (mesoblastoma vitellinum) and so called "embryonal carcinoma" of the ovary. Acta Pathol Microbiol Scand 64:407–429

ten Bokkel Huinink WW, van der Burg MEL, van Oosterom AT, et al. (1988) Carboplatin in combination therapy for ovarian cancer. Cancer Treat Rev 15 (Suppl B):9–15

ten Bokkel Huinink WW, Rodenhuis S, Wanders J, et al. (1989) High dose carboplatin in resistant ovarian cancer. Proc Am Soc Clin Oncol 8:590

ten Bokkel Huinink WW, Eisenhauer E, Swenerton K (1993) Preliminary evaluation of a multicenter, randomized comparative study of TAXOL (paclitaxel) dose and infusion length in platinum-treated ovarian cancer. Canadian-European Taxol cooperative trial group. Cancer Treat Rev 19 (Suppl C):79–86

Teufel G (1986) Primäre operative Therapie maligner Ovarialtumoren. In: Pfleiderer A (ed) Maligne Tumoren der Ovarien. Zeitschr Geburtsh Perinat, Suppl 23. Enke, Stuttgart, pp 159–167

The Ovarian Cancer Meta-analysis Project (1991) Cyclophosphamide plus cisplatin versus cyclophosphamide, doxorubicin, and cisplatin chemotherapy of ovarian carcinoma: a meta-analysis. J Clin Oncol 9:1668–1674

Thigpen JT (1985) Single agent chemotherapy in the management of ovarian carcinoma. In: Alberts DS, Surwit EA (eds) Ovarian carcinoma. Martinus Nijhoff, Boston, p 115

Thigpen JT (1995) High-dose chemotherapy with autologous bone marrow support in ovarian carcinoma: the bottom line, more or less. Gynecol Oncol 57:275–277

Thigpen JT, Blessing J, Ball H, Hummel S, Barret R (1990) Phase II trial of taxol as second-line therapy for ovarian carcinoma: a Gynecologic Oncology Group study. Proc Am Soc Clin Oncol 9:156

Thomas GM (1993) Is there a role for consolidation or salvage radiotherapy after chemotherapy in advanced epithelial ovarian cancer? Gynecol Oncol 51:97–103

Thomas GM, Dembo AJ, Hacker NF, DePetrillo AD (1987) Current therapy for dysgerminoma of the ovary. Obstet Gynecol 70:268–275

Thompson MA, Adelson MP, Kaufman LM (1991) Lupron retards proliferation of ovarian epithelial tumor cells cultured in serum free medium. J Clin Endocrinol Metab 72:1036–1041

Thurlbeck WM, Scully RE (1960) Solid teratoma of the ovary. A clinicopathologic analysis of 9 cases. Cancer 13:805–811

Timmerman D, Moerman PH, Vergote IB (1995) Meigs' syndrome with elevated serum CA 125 levels: two case reports and review of the literature. Gynecol Oncol

Tobacman JK, Tucker MA, Kase R, et al. (1982) Intra-abdominal carcinomatosis after prophylactic oophorectomy in ovarian cancer- prone families. Lancet ii:795–797

Trimble EL, Adams JD, Vena D, et al. (1993) Paclitaxel for platinum-refractory ovarian cancer: results from the first 1000 patients registered to National Cancer Institute Treatment Referral Center 9103. J Clin Oncol 11:2405–2410

Tulchinsky M, Eggli DF (1994) Intraperitoneal distribution imaging prior to chromic phosphate (P-32) therapy in ovarian cancer patients. Clin Nucl Med 19:43–48

Tulusan AH, Adam R, Reinhardt M, et al. (1990) Lymph node metastases in epithelial ovarian cancer. In: Sharp F, Mason WP, Leake RE (eds) Ovarian cancer. Chapman and Hall, London, pp 443–445

v. Delft H (1941) Erfolge der operativen und Strahlentherapie bösartiger Ovarialtumoren. Zentralbl Gynäkol 65:1507–1514

Vaccarello L, Hoskins WJ (1995) Central venous and intraperitoneal access in patients with ovarian cancer. In: Markman M, Hoskins WJ (eds) Cancer of the ovary. Raven Press, New York, pp 205–216

Vahrson H (1970) Umwelt und konstitutionelle Faktoren beim weiblichen Genitalkarzinom. Z Geburtshilfe Gynäkol 172:94–106

Vahrson H (1973) Die Triple-drug-Stoßtherapie bei der Behandlung des fortgeschrittenen Ovarialkarzinoms. Geburtshilfe Frauenheilkd 33:293–296

Vahrson H (1983) Die Nachsorge des Ovarialkarzinoms aus gynäkologischer Sicht. Strahlentherapie 159:267–270

Vahrson H, Kirschbaum M (1985) Erste klinische Erfahrungen mit Epirubicin (Farmorubicin®) bei Ovarialkarzinom im Vergleich zu Adriamycin. In: Nagel CA, Wannenmcher M (eds) Farmorubicin, klinische Erfahrungen. Akt Onkol 15:215–221

Vahrson H, Münstedt K (1995) CA-125 Tumormarkerverläufe zur Beurteilung der Therapieeffizienz bei Radio-Chemotherapie fortgeschrittener Ovarialkarzinome. In: Kreienberg R, Grill HJ, Möbus V, Koldorsky U (eds) Aktuelle Aspekte der Tumorimmunologie in der Gynäkologie. Akt Onkol 86:23–28

Vahrson H, Steckenmesser R (1970) Angiographischer Nachweis einer Pseudozyste nach Radiogoldtherapie eines Ovarialkarzinoms. Strahlentherapie 139:167–172

Vahrson H, Dolzycki E, Münstedt K (1993) Postoperative Strahlentherapie des Ovarialkarzinoms. In: Künzel W, Kirschbaum M (eds) Giessener Gynäkologische Fortbildung 1993. Springer, Berlin Heidelberg New York, pp 287–305

Vance RP, Geisinger KR (1985) Pure nongestational choriocarcinoma of the ovary. Report of a case. Cancer 56:2321–2324

Van Dam PA, Watson JV, Lowe DG, Shepherd JH (1992) Flow cytometric DNA analysis in gynecological oncology. Int J Gynecol Cancer 2:57–65

van der Burg MEL, ten-Bokkel-Huinink WW, Kobiersky A, et al. (1993) Chemotherapy and hormonal treatment in ovarian cancer: experiences of the EORTC gynecological cancer cooperative group. In: Meerpohl HG, Pfleiderer A, Profous CZ (eds) Das Ovarialkarzinom, vol 2. Springer, Berlin Heidelberg New York, p 114

Van Norstrand D, Silberstein EB (1985) Therapeutic uses of ^{32}P. In: Freeman LM, Weissmann HS (eds) Nuclear Medicin Annual 1985. Raven Press, New York, pp 285–344

Varia M, Rosenman J, Venkatraman S, et al. (1988) Intraperitoneal chromic phosphate therapy after second-look laparotomy for ovarian cancer. Cancer 61:919–927

Vassal G, Flamant F, Caillaud JM (1988) Juvenile granulosa cell tumor of the ovary in children. A clinical study of 15 cases. J Clin Oncol 6:990–995

Vavra N, Barrada M, Fritz R, Sevelda P, Baur M, Dittrich C (1990) Goserelin eine neue Form der Hormontherapie beim Ovarialkarzinom. Gynäkol Rundsch 30 (Suppl 1):61–63

Vebersik V, Dvorak O (1967) Zur Verteilung des intraperitoneal applizierten kolloidalen Radiogoldes ^{198}Au in den einzelnen Lymphknoten und deren funktionelle Blockierung. Zentralbl Gynäkol 89:1032–1039

Velasco-Oses A, Alonso-Alvaro A, Blanco-Pozo A (1988) Ollier's disease associated with ovarian juvenile granulosa cell tumor. Cancer 62:222–225

Vergote IB, Dieleman V, Becquart D, Buytaert PH (1983) Dysgerminoma of the ovary in association with XY gonadal dysgenesis. Eur J Obstet Gynecol Reprod Biol 14:385–391

Vergote IB, Onsrud M, Nustad K (1987) Placental alkaline phosphatase as a tumor marker in ovarian cancer. Obstet Gynecol 67:228–232

Vergote IB, Abeler VM, Kjorstad KE, Trope CG (1990) Management of malignant ovarian teratoma. Role of adriamycin. Cancer 66:882–886

Vergote IB, Kaern J, Tropé C (1992a) Adjuvant treatment of stage I ovarian cancer. How can we prevent overtreatment? Proc Am Soc Clin Oncol 11:225

Vergote IB, Vergote-de Vos LN, Abeler VM (1992b) Randomized trial comparing cisplatin with radioactive phosphorus or whole abdomen irradiation as adjuvant treatment of ovarian cancer. Cancer 69:741–749

Vergote IB, Kaern J, Abeler VM, Pettersen EO, De Vos LN, Trope CG (1993a) Analysis of prognostic factors in stage I epithelial ovarian carcinoma: importance of degree of differentiation and desoxyribonucleic acid ploidy in predicting relapse. Am J Obstet Gynecol 169:40–52

Vergote IB, Winderen M, de Vos LN, Tropé CG (1993b) Intraperitoneal radioactive phosphorus therapy in ovarian carcinoma: analysis of 313 patients treated primarily or at second-look laparotomy. Cancer 71:2250–2260

Vessey MP, Painter R (1995) Endometrial and ovarian cancer and oral contraceptives – findings in a large cohort study. Br J Cancer 71:1340–1342

Virchow R (1855) Cellularpathologie. Arch Pathol Anat 8:1–39

Vogl SE, Pagano M, Kaplan BH, et al. (1983) Cisplatin-based chemotherapy for advanced ovarian cancer: high overall response rate with curative potential only in women with small tumor burdens. Cancer 51:2024

Walter J, Jones JC, Fisher M (1961) Radioactive colloidal yttrium silicate in the treatment of malignant effusions. I. Clinical aspects and investigations. Br J Radiol 34:337–346

Walton LA, Yadusky A, Rubinstein L (1991) Intraperitoneal radioactive phosphate in early ovarian carcinoma: an analysis of complications. Int J Radiat Oncol Biol Phys 20:939–944

Watson JM, Berek JS, Martinéz-Maza O (1993) Growth inhibition of ovarian cancer cells induced by antisense IL-6 oligonucleotides. Gynecol Oncol 49:8–15

Weiner SA, Alberts DS, Surwitt EA, Davis J, Grosso D (1987) Tamoxifen therapy in recurrent epithelial ovarian carcinoma. Gynecol Oncol 27:208–213

Weinstein D, Polishuk WZ (1975) The role of wedge excision of the ovary as a cause for mechanical sterility. Surg Obstet Gynecol 134:417–422

West RO (1966) Epidemiologic study of malignancies of the ovaries. Cancer 19:1001–1007

Wharton LR (1959) Two cases of supernumerary ovary and one of accessory ovary, with an analysis of previously reported cases. Am J Obstet Gynecol 78:1101–1119

Wheeler JE (1993) Pathology of malignant ovarian epithelial tumors and miscellaneous and rare ovarian and paraovarian neoplasms. In: Rubin SC, Sutton GP (eds) Ovarian cancer. McGraw-Hill, New York, p 87

Whelan TJ, Dembo AJ, Bush RS, et al. (1992) Complications of whole abdominal and pelvic radiotherapy following chemotherapy for advanced ovarian cancer. Int J Radiat Oncol Biol Phys 22:853–858

Whittemore AS (1994) Characteristics relating to ovarian cancer risk: implications for prevention and detection. Gynecol Oncol 55:15–19

Whittemore AS, Harris R, Itnyre J and the Collaborative Ovarian Cancer group (1992) Characteristics relating to ovarian cancer risk: collaborative analysis of 12 US case control studies. II. Invasive epithelial ovarian cancers in white women. Am J Epidemiol 136:1184–1203

Williams SD (1991) Chemotherapy of ovarian germ cell tumors. Hematol Oncol Clin North Am 5:1261–1269

Williams SD, Birch R, Einhorn LH, et al. (1987) Disseminated germ cell tumors: chemotherapy with cisplatin plus bleomycin plus either vinblastine or etoposide. N Engl J Med 316:1435–1440

Williams SD, Blessing J, Slayton R, et al. (1989a) Ovarian germ cell tumors: adjuvant trials of the Gynecologic Oncology Group. Proc Am Soc Clin Oncol 8:150 (A 584)

Williams SD, Blessing JA, Moore DH, Homesley HD, Adcock L (1989b) Cisplatin, vinblastine and bleomycin in advanced and recurrent ovarian germ cell tumors: a trial of the Gynecologic Oncology Group. Ann Intern Med 111:22–27

Williams SD, Blessing JA, Hatch KD, Homesley HD (1991) Chemotherapy of advanced dysgerminoma: trials of the Gynecologic Oncology Group. J Clin Oncol 9:1950–1955

Williams SD, Gershenson DM, Horowitz CJ, Scully RF (1992) Ovarian germ cell and stromal tumors. In: Hoskins WJ, Perez CA, Young RC (eds) Principles and practice of gynecologic oncology. Lippincott, Philadelphia, p 715

Williams SD, Blessing JA, Liao SY, Ball H, Hanjani P (1994) Adjuvant therapy of ovarian germ cell tumors with cisplatin, etoposide, and bleomycin: a trial of the Gynecologic Oncology Group. J Clin Oncol 12:701–706

Wiltshaw E, Subramarian S, Alexopoulus C, Barker GH (1979) Cancer of the ovary: a summary of experience with cis-dichlorodiammineplatinum (II) at the Royal Marsden Hospital. Cancer Treat Rep 63:1545–1548

Withers HR, Taylor JMG, Maciejewski B (1988) The hazard of accelerated tumor clonogen repopulation during radiotherapy. Acta Oncol 27:131–146

Witt BR, Wolf GC, Wainwright CJ, Thorneycroft IH (1992) Endocrine function of granulosa cell tumors in vivo. Gynecol Obstet Invest 33:59–64

Wolf A, Bork E, Vahrson H (1976) Mögliche Inkompatibilität von Tiefenbestrahlung und hochdosierter Adriamycin- oder Cyclophosphamid-Stoßtherapie bei fortgeschrittenen Genitalmalignomen der Frau. Strahlentherapie 152:422–426

Woodruff JD (1979) The pathogenesis of ovarian neoplasia. Johns Hopkins Med J 144:117–120

Wu PC, Qu J, Lang J, Huang R, Tang M, Lian L (1986) Lymph node metastasis of ovarian cancer: a preliminary survey of 74 cases of lymphadenectomy. Am J Obstet Gynecol 155:1103–1108

Wu PC, Lang JH, Huang RL, Liu J, Tang MY, Lian LJ (1989a) Intestinal metastasis and operation in ovarian cancer: a report on 62 cases. Baillière's Clin Obstet Gynaecol 3:95–108

Wu PC, Lang JH, Huang RL, et al. (1989b) Lymph-node metastasis and retroperitoneal lymphadenectomy in ovarian cancer. Baillière's Clin Obstet Gynaecol 3:143–155

Wu PC, Huang RL, Lang JH, Huang HF, Lian LJ, Tang MY (1991) Treatment of ovarian germ cell tumors with preservation of fertility: a report of 28 cases. Gynecol Oncol 40:2–6

Wu S, Boyer CM, Whitaker RS, et al. (1993) Tumor necrosis factor α as an autocrine and paracrine growth factor for ovarian cancer: monokine induction of tumor cell proliferation and tumor necrosis factor α expression. Cancer Res 53:1939–1944

Yanai-Inbar I, Scully RE (1987) Relation of ovarian dermoid cysts and immature teratomas: an analysis of 350 cases of immature teratoma and 10 cases of dermoid cyst within microscopic foci of immature tissue. Int J Gynecol Pathol 6:203–212

Young RC (1993) Management of early stage ovarian cancer. In: Markman M, Hoskins WJ (eds) Cancer of the ovary. Raven Press, New York, p 359

Young RC, Walton LA, Ellenberg SS, et al. (1990) Adjuvant therapy in stage I and stage II epithelial ovarian cancer. Results of two prospective randomized trials. N Engl J Med 322:1021–1027

Young RH (1991) Ovarian tumors other than those of the surface epithelial-stromal type. Hum Pathol 22:763–775

Young RH (1993a) New and unusual aspects of ovarian germ cell tumors. Am J Surg Pathol 17:1210–1224

Young RH (1993b) Sertoli-Leydig cell tumors of the ovary: review with emphasis on historical aspects and unusual variants. Int J Gynecol Pathol 12:141–147

Young RH, Scully RE (1983) Ovarian Sertoli-Leydig cells tumors with a retiform pattern: a problem in histopathologic diagnosis. Am J Surg Pathol 7:755–771

Young RH, Scully RE (1984a) Ovarian Sertoli cell tumors. A report of 10 cases. Int J Gynecol Pathol 2:349–363

Young RH, Scully RE (1984b) Ovarian sex cord-stromal tumours: recent advances and current status. Clin Obstet Gynaecol 11:93–134

Young RH, Scully RE (1985) Ovarian Sertoli-Leydig cell tumors. A clinicopathological analysis of 207 cases. Am J Surg Pathol 9:543–569

Young RH, Scully RE (1992) Endocrine tumors of the ovary. Curr Top Pathol 85:113–164

Young RH, Scully RE (1994) Sex cord-stromal, steroid cell, and other ovarian tumors with endocrine, paraendocrine, and paraneoplastic manifestations. In: Kurman RJ (ed) Blaustein's pathology of the female genital tract, IVth edn. Springer, New York Berlin Heidelberg, pp 783–847

Young RH, Dickersin GR, Scully RE (1984a) Juvenile granulosa cell tumor of the ovary. A clinicopathological analysis of 125 cases. Am J Surg Pathol 8:575–596

Young RH, Dudley AG, Scully RE (1984b) Granulosa cell, Sertoli-Leydig cell and unclassified sex cord-stromal tumors associated with pregnancy. A clinicopathological analysis of 36 cases. Gynecol Oncol 18:181–205

Zeloudek CJ, Norris HJ (1982) Granulosa tumors of the ovary in children. A clinical and pathological study of 32 cases. Am J Surg Pathol 6:503–512

Zaloudek CJ, Norris HJ (1984) Sertoli-Leydig tumors of the ovary: a clinicopathological study of 64 intermediate and poorly differentiated neoplasms. Am J Surg Pathol 8:405–418

Zaloudek CJ, Tavasolei FA, Norris HJ (1981) Dysgerminoma with syncytiotrophoblastic giant cells. A histopathologically and clinically distinctive subtype of dysgerminoma. Am J Surg Pathol 5:361–367

Zambetti M, Escobedo A, Pilotti S, De Palo G (1990) Cisplatinum/vinblastine/bleomycin combination chemotherapy in advanced or recurrent granulosa cell tumors of the ovary. Gynecol Oncol 36:317–320

Zaydon C, Bogaars HA, Tucci JR (1989) Virilizing granulosa cell tumor responsive to human chorionic gonadotropin and oral contraceptive with 8-year follow-up. Int J Gynecol Obstet 29:87–80

Zhang J, Young RH, Arsenau J, Scully RE (1982) Ovarian stromal tumors containing lutein or Leydig cells (luteinized thecomas and stromal Leydig cell tumors). A clinicopathological analysis of fifty cases. Int J Gynecol Pathol 1:270–285

Zheng J, Robinson WR, Ehlen T, Yu MC, Dubeau L (1991) Distinction of low grade from high grade human ovarian carcinomas on the basis of losses of heterozygosity on chromosomes 3, 6, and 11 and Her-2/neu gene amplification. Cancer Res 51:4045–4054

Zinser JW, Ramirez-Gaytan JL, Lara F, Dominguez-Malagon HR (1990) Ovarian dysgerminoma treated with cisplatin and cyclophosphamide. Report of 15 cases. Proc Am Soc Clin Oncol 9:A631

12 Cancer of the Fallopian Tube

D.M. Ostapovicz and L.W. Brady

CONTENTS

12.1 Embryology

At approximately the fifth week of gestation, genital ridges form on the dorsal wall of the celomic cavity. The paramesonephric duct then arises as a longitudinal fold on the anterolateral surface of the genital ridge. The paramesonephric ducts subsequently become the female genital tract in the absence of müllerian inhibiting substance, by migrating from opposite sides and fusing caudally in a vertical position to form the early uterus and vagina. The remaining horizontal parts of both ducts become the fallopian tubes as they traverse past the mesonephric ducts. The cranial ends of the ducts open into the celomic cavity and eventually form the fimbriated ends of the fallopian tube infundibulum. The ovaries are also derived from the celomic epithelium, mesenchyme, and, in addition, the primordial germ cells. Therefore, the fallopian tubes share a common embryological derivation with the ovary, uterus, and cervix even though they develop under different hormonal influences. In the male embryo, the mesonephric duct differentiates into the genital ducts due to regression of the paramesonephric duct via müllerian inhibiting substance secreted by the fetal testes.

12.2 Anatomy

The fallopian tubes are hollow, muscular viscera positioned horizontally within the superior part of the broad ligament. Each tube extends from its own ovary, communicating with the peritoneal cavity. They project outward, backward, and then downward to open into the superior posterior part of the uterine fundus, where they communicate with the endometrial cavity. Each tube is approximately 11 cm Long and consists of four segments: (a) the interstitial portion, which inserts into the myometrium, (b) the isthmus or horizontal, medial portion, (c) the ampulla, which encloses the ovary, and (d) the infundibulum or fimbrated portion. Histologically, the tubal wall consists of four separate layers: the mucosa, submucosa, muscularis (external longitudinal and inner circular layers), and outer se-

D.M. Ostapovicz, MD, Department of Radiation Oncology, Altoona Hospital, 620 Howard Avenue, Altoona, PA 16602, USA
L.W. Brady, MD, Professor, Department of Radiation Oncology, Allegheny University of the Health Sciences, Broad and Vine Streets, Mail Stop 200, Philadelphia, PA 19102-1192, USA

rosal layer, which is continuous with the visceral peritoneum of the uterus.

The mucosa is intricately folded, the number of folds increasing from the interstitial portion to the ampulla. The epithelium is composed mainly of ciliated cells and secretory cells. Cyclical changes are evident in the tubal epithelium similar to those of the endometrium in response to estrogen and progesterone. The epithelium is the origin of most malignancies, its changes during the menstrual years and postmenopausally possibly playing a role in tumorigenesis.

Arterial blood supply of the fallopian tube is derived from the ovarian artery, which anastomoses with the uterine artery. Venous drainage is via the pampiniform plexus to the ovarian vein along with the uterine plexus. The lymphatics, richly anastomosed with those of the adjacent organs, drain into the ovarian lymphatics and the lumbar lymph nodes (GOMPEL and SILVERBERG 1994). These lymphatics course along the folds of the tubal mucosa where they form a network of intercommunicating lymphatic sinusoids (GOMPEL and SILVERBERG 1994). From this area, they drain into the para-aortic and iliac nodes.

12.3 Epidemiology

The first descriptions of a primary malignancy of the fallopian tube are attributed to Renard and Ricci in 1845 and Orthmann in 1866 and 1888. Since then, less than 1500 cases have been reported. This disease entity is the rarest of the female genital tract malignancies, accounting for only 0.15%–1.8% of all gynecological malignancies (ROSEN et al. 1994; HANTON et al. 1966; MOMATZEE and KEMPSON 1968; ROBERTS and LIFSHITZ 1982; PHELPS and CHAPMAN 1974), with an average of 0.3% (HANTON et al. 1996). The theoretical incidence is 3–3.6/1 000 000 women/year (ROSENBLATT et al. 1989; Texas State Cancer Registry). The reported incidence in whites is 14% higher than in blacks (ROSENBLATT et al. 1989).

The age range of this disease has been reported to be from 18 to 87 years, with most occurrences between the fifth and sixth decades of life. In a review of the literature regarding 393 patients, a mean age of 55 years was reported (BENEDET et al. 1977). This is consistent with the mean age of 56.7 years cited in a recent meta-analysis of 577 patients (NORDIN 1994). The clinical profile of these patients reveals a relatively low parity rate (BROWN et al. 1985; MCMURRAY et al. 1986; DENHAM and MACLENNAN 1984; SEDLIS 1978; PETERS et al. 1988; BOUTSELIS and THOMPSON 1971), with a mean parity of 1–1.7 (NORDIN 1994; BROWN et al. 1985; MCMURRAY et al. 1986). By virtue of the mean age of incidence as mentioned above, most patients are postmenopausal.

12.4 Symptomatology

Unlike ovarian malignancies, tumors of the fallopian tube cause early clinical signs and symptoms. Although several triads of pelvic pain, lower abdominal pain, pelvic mass, leukorrhea, and vaginal bleeding, and vaginal discharge, have been described as pathognomonic, the highest percentage of patients presenting with such a triad of symptoms has been only 11% (HANTON et al. 1966). Another classic sign, "hydrops tubae profluens," which is a sudden emptying of accumulated fluid in the distended fallopian tube causing profuse, watery serosanguinous discharge to be released from the vagina accompanied by a decrease in pelvic mass size on physical examination, was identified in only 9% of 122 patients in a meta-analysis (NORDIN 1994). In many other series it has been specifically reported that neither a triad nor hydrops tubae profluens was present in any of the patients reviewed (SEDLIS 1978; YOONESSI et al. 1988; ROBERTS and LIFSHITZ 1982; BROWN et al. 1985).

Despite these inconsistencies in symptoms, the most common presenting sign is metrorrhagia (SEDLIS 1978; PFEIFFER et al. 1989; PETERS et al. 1988; EDDY et al. 1984b; BROWN et al. 1985; AMENDOLA et al. 1983; BENEDET et al. 1977; MCMURRAY et al. 1986; ASMUSSEN et al. 1988; PODRATZ et al. 1986), followed by pain and vaginal discharge (EDDY et al. 1984b; BENEDET et al. 1977; SEDLIS 1978). The most common physical sign is that of a pelvic mass, occurring in 12%–66% of patients (BENEDET et al. 1977; HANTON et al. 1966; EDDY et al. 1984b; BROWN et al. 1985).

The difference in the reported frequency of these various clinical signs may be related to the appearance of symptoms relative to the course and progression of disease. That is, early bleeding is replaced by pain and accumulated secretions as tumor mass increases, causing distention of the narrow tubal lumen (SEDLIS 1978).

12.5 Preoperative Diagnosis

Because of the rarity of primary malignancies of the fallopian tube and the fact that the range of presenting signs is similar to that seen in patients with salpingitis, ovarian abscess or tumor, pelvic inflammatory disease, and even ectopic pregnancy, it has proved difficult to diagnose most cases before surgical exploration. The delay in correct diagnosis has ranged from 2 to greater than 12 months (EDDY et al. 1984b). Many series report missing the correct diagnosis entirely in their working differential diagnosis (DENHAM and MACLENNAN 1984; MCMURRAY et al. 1986; ROBERTS and LIFSHITZ 1982; RAGHAVAN et al. 1991).

Some authors have reported and advocated the use of PAP smears as a preoperative screening tool in patients with nonspecific symptomatology, with diagnostic results ranging from 0% to 60% (HANTON et al. 1966; ROBERTS and LIFSHITZ 1982; YOONESSI et al. 1988; PETERS et al. 1988; SEDLIS 1978). Few report diagnostic results at the higher end of this range. The use of endometrial sampling has produced equally unpromising results (SEDLIS 1978).

Many different modalities for the detection of fallopian tube cancers are presently under investigation. Some of these have yielded promising results, including various nuclear medicine imaging techniques with radioactive nucleotides, magnetic resonance imaging, ultrasonography, and the use of tumor markers (see text under the corresponding subject headings).

12.6 Natural History of Disease

The primary spread of disease is similar to that of ovarian cancers in that there is local extension of tumor to adjacent structures to involve the peritoneum, omentum, bowel, and ovaries (SCHRAY et al. 1987; EDDY et al. 1984b; ROBERTS and LIFSHITZ 1982; HENDERSON et al. 1987; YOONESSI et al. 1988). However, 70% of patients with fallopian tube tumors at presentation have disease confined to the pelvis, as compared with only 48% of patients with ovarian malignancies (ROBERTS and LIFSHITZ 1982), and up to 50% of patients with fallopian tube tumors are diagnosed as having stage I disease (KONE et al. 1992). This again is probably due to the early presentation of abnormal bleeding and pain with distention of a small tubal lumen which is absent in the anatomy of the ovary.

Many authors believe that local extension is followed in frequency by lymphatic and/or hematogenous spread (ROSEN et al. 1993; SCHRAY et al. 1987). However, in view of inconsistent staging and with the advent of improved surgical resection with exploration and lymph node sampling, it has been suggested that early lymphatic and vascular invasion may play a more prominent role in disease progression than previously thought. That is, periaortic spread may precede intra-abdominal dissemination (TAMINI and FIGGE 1981; MAXSON et al. 1987; JACKSON-YORK and RAMZY 1992). In cases where lymph node involvement has been observed, there has been a wide range of lymph node positivity, i.e., 10%–55%, at the time of diagnosis (AMENDOLA et al. 1983; BENEDET et al. 1977; EDDY et al. 1984b; YOONESSI et al. 1988; TAMINI and FIGGE 1981; SCHRAY et al. 1987). Lymph node positivity has been found in 75% of patients at autopsy (MAXSON et al. 1987). In a review of 67 patients, SEDLIS (1978) reported that tubal musculature was rarely involved when lymphatic metastases were present.

Transcelomic spread is found to have an impact on survival, with a decrease in survival rates as the depth of wall invasion increases (SCHILLER and SILVERBERG 1971). It stands to reason that in cases where the ampulla is obstructed, tumor spread is more likely to occur earlier through direct invasion of the tubal wall and by way of its capillary network and lymphatics. In these instances, periaortic and pelvic lymph nodes would perhaps be involved earlier than contiguous pelvic structures, and involved lymph nodes would be distributed according to the location of the primary tumor within the tube. For example, a portion of the drainage of tumors in the medial portion of the tube is into the lymphatics of the round ligament and from there, into the inguinal region. The majority of the drainage of the remainder of the tube is to the periaortic nodes (TAMINI and FIGGE 1981). When the tubal ampulla is patent or when the serosa is breached by tumor, intra-abdominal seeding and contiguous spread of disease may be a more obvious route of tumor spread. It has been noted that in cases where the tube is obstructed, patients' survival is better (BOUTSELIS and THOMPSON 1971; SCHRAY et al. 1987).

The conclusion which may be inferred here is that spread of disease can occur by way of direct extension through the fallopian tube wall and progress by means of lymphatic or blood vessels and peritoneally along the serosal surface if penetration of serosa has occurred, or by means of luminal travel. Lymph node involvement will depend on the extent of spread via either route.

Far less common in fallopian tube cancer are "distant" metastases to liver and lung, which most often occur by local extension outside of the peritoneal cavity via nodal rather than transdiaphragmatic and hematogenous spread (Schray et al. 1987). Distant metastases are more important as a site of treatment failure in ovarian cancer, where more than 50% of recurrences occur outside of the peritoneal cavity. Given this difference between ovarian and fallopian tube cancer, one could argue for aggressive postsurgical adjuvant treatment in fallopian tube carcinoma (Eddy et al. 1984b).

12.7 Pathology

The most common histopathology of fallopian tube malignancies is serous papillary adenocarcinoma, similar to that found in the ovary. Benign tumors are even less frequent than malignant neoplasms. Rare histological subtypes are found (see Sect. 12.13). Tumors that were previously graded as papillary (pure), papillary-alveolar, or alveolar-medullary (Hu et al. 1950) are now routinely classified as well, moderately, or poorly differentiated (grades I, II, and III respectively) (Markman 1992).

The disease presents bilaterally in approximately 5%–30% of patients at the time of initial diagnosis. This finding is considered as a multicentric primary. Malignancies are distributed equally between the left and right fallopian tubes.

The gross appearance of a fallopian tube with a primary adenocarcinoma without invasion of the serosal lining is usually enlarged and deformed, fusiform, or sausage-like because of the large intraluminal growth of the tumor. It may mimic the appearance of more benign pathological processes such as hydrosalpinx, pyosalpinx, or hematosalpinx (Anbrokh 1970). In more advanced disease with tubal wall invasion, cells may form nodules on the peritoneal surface, mimicking a tubo-ovarian abscess and making the diagnosis of primary organ involvement difficult. Multiple adhesions to surrounding tissue may be found, presumably due to chronic inflammation. The most frequent site is the ampulla, followed by the infundibulum, and the lumen is closed in approximately 50% of cases (Pordatz et al. 1986; Woodruff and Pauerstein 1969).

The lumen is usually filled with necrotic, friable, papillary, or solid tumor affixed to the mucosal surface and accompanied by fluid (Wheeler 1994; Markman 1992).

Microscopically, the papillary configuration of epithelium is usually preserved and diagnosis usually follows the criteria set by Hu et al. (1950). Cells of acute and chronic inflammation are seen. Epithelial hyperplasia is the proliferation of epithelium without the presence of marked cytologic atypia or mitotic activity. These changes may become predominant in the presence of granulomatous inflammation, rendering difficult the distinction from premalignancy (Markman 1992).

Up to 14% of otherwise normal tube specimens show nuclear atypia with nuclear crowding, epithelial stratification, and loss of polarity and should not be classified as carcinoma in situ (Wheeler 1994). Cases thus classified should demonstrate cells with malignant mitotically active nuclei which are still attempting to form papillae (Wheeler 1994). It is thought that adenomatous hyperplasia is a precursor of carcinoma in situ (Gompel and Silverberg 1994).

12.8 Prognostic Factors

In a multivariate analysis, statistically significant prognostic factors were found to be: (a) stage at presentation, (b) age, (c) presence of ascites, (d) amount of residual tumor after primary surgical resection (Peters et al. 1988), and (e) aggressiveness of the treatment program. When computed as single factors, only stage (I vs II) and residual tumor volume were significant (Peters et al. 1988). Although it was earlier thought that a high degree of histological dedifferentiation inferred a worse prognosis (Hu et al. 1950), many authors have found this to be incorrect (Momatzee and Kempson 1968; Hanton et al. 1966; Schray et al. 1987; Denham and MacLennan; Peters et al. 1988). Rosen et al. (1993) discovered a trend for higher grade lesions to correlate with a decrease in survival rates, but this was not statistically substantiated. It was also reiterated that increased age resulted in a decreased survival rate, as did a residual tumor volume >2 cm after primary surgical resection (Rosen et al. 1993).

The presence of vascular or lymphatic invasion in patients with early-stage disease was reported to reduce 5-year survival rates to 29%, as compared with 83% in those without such invasion (Pfeiffer et al.

1989). Comparing mucosal and stromal invasion, significantly lower 5-year survival was found in patients with the former (91%–100% vs 50%–55%): (SCHILLER and SILVERBERG 1971; KLEIN et al. 1994, respectively). Pelvic inflammatory disease and tuberculous salpingitis were once believed to be causative factors in the development of fallopian tube malignancies. If this were the case, one would expect a higher incidence of tubal malignancies given the prevalence of pelvic inflammatory disease. In fact, no study to date has proven this theory.

12.9 Staging

Because carcinoma of the fallopian tube is one of the rarest of all gynecological malignancies and has both close proximity to the ovary and similarities in embryological derivation and histopathology, specific diagnostic criteria were established by HU et al. in 1950. These guidelines to help differentiate fallopian tube malignancies from those of the ovary and other primary sites are listed in Table 12.1.

Table 12.1. Criteria for diagnosis of primary carcinoma of the fallopian tube (HU et al. 1950)

1. Grossly, the main tumor is in the tube
2. Microscopically, the mucosa should be chiefly involved and should show a papillary pattern
3. If the tubal wall is found to be involved to a great extent, the transition between benign and malignant should be demonstrable

The criteria shown in Table 12.1 were later modified (SEDLIS 1978) but the same basic principles were retained. It should be noted, however, that in advanced-stage disease it will still be difficult to determine the site of origin of the primary tumor. Such tumors are more likely to be described as ovarian primaries because of the higher frequency of the latter, thereby causing the incidence of fallopian tube primaries to be underestimated.

Numerous staging classifications have been proposed in the literature, as well as inconsistent and poorly documented staging procedures. In a review of ten patients, EREZ et al. (1967) proposed a staging scheme which closely followed the natural history of spread of ovarian malignancies. Both Momatzee and Dodson subsequently endorsed a similar staging system based on the FIGO staging for ovarian carcinoma (Table 12.2) and demonstrated a direct relationship between the stage of disease and survival (MOMATZEE and KEMPSON 1968; DODSON et al. 1970).

In 1971, a new format based on Duke's classification of rectal cancer was proposed (SCHILLER and SILVERBERG 1971). This was founded on the development of tumor spread and penetration through a hollow viscus with a muscular wall similar to that of the gastrointestinal tract (Table 12.2). The anatomi-

Table 12.2. Comparison of previously used staging systems

	MOMATZEE and KEMPSON (1968)	DODSON et al. (1970)	SCHILLER and SILVERBERG (1971)
Stage 0			Carcinoma in situ (limited to tubal mucosa)
Stage I	Tumor limited to tube mucosa/myometrium	Ia: 1 tube involved; no ascites Ib: 2 tubes involved; no ascites Ic: 1 or 2 tubes involved; ascites present with malignant cells in fluid	Tumor extending into the submucosa and/or muscularis but not penetrating to the serosal surface of the fallopian tube
Stage IIa	Tumor extends through serosa	Extension and/ or metastases to the uterus or ovary	Tumor extending to the serosa of the fallopian tube
Stage IIb	Tumor invading organs in the pelvis or abdomen, including metastasis	Extension to other pelvic tissues	
Stage III	True metastasis to organs outside the pelvis but confined to the abdomen	Growth involving 1 or 2 tubes with widespread intraperitoneal metastasis to the abdomen	Direct extension of the tumor to the ovary and/or endometrium
Stage IV	Metastasis outside the abdomen	1 or 2 tubes involved with widespread intraperitoneal metastasis to the abdomen	Extension of tumor beyond the reproductive organs

cal extent of the tumor when substaged by penetration of mucosa versus submucosa and muscularis was noted to carry significant prognostic implications. Although this system has been less utilized, it allows a distinction between the anatomy of the fallopian tube and the ovary which in all likelihood has important prognostic significance since malignancies in the former organ tend to have earlier symptomatology and are therefore diagnosed at an earlier stage. This may be due to a decreased probability of peritoneal metastasis when the tumor and/or associated inflammation causes obstruction of the ampulla of the tube (Schray et al. 1987; Boutselis and Thompson 1971). The route of spread must then be through the tubal wall, possibly allowing important time to administer more efficacious therapy.

In 1991, an official staging system for carcinoma of the fallopian tube was established by FIGO (Table 12.3). This staging system continues to follow the main directives set for ovarian carcinomas with the addition of guidelines for carcinoma in situ or stage 0 based on the involvement of the interface of the mucosal basement membrane and the tubal stroma (Pettersson 1992). In a recent publication (Klein et al. 1994), a review of patients with stage 0 and invasive stage I disease illustrated prognostic implications and selection of adjuvant therapy in demonstrating an overall improved survival in early-stage disease.

Staging is presently done at the time of surgical exploration. If ascitic fluid is present and cytology is negative, peritoneal washings are performed and subsequent cytology is carried out. The omentum is usually excised and examined for tumor involvement. Areas of bowel, liver, and diaphragm are sampled for metastatic implants and direct tumor invasion is determined by review of these sites as well as the ovaries, uterus, bladder, and rectum.

12.10 Tumor Markers

12.10.1 CA-125

CA-125 is an antigen expressed by epithelial ovarian tumors as well as other cells derived from the müllerian duct and celomic tissues. It has previously been used chiefly for the detection and surveillance of patients with ovarian malignancies. The presence of the antigen in tumors which express it is detected by a murine monoclonal antibody, OC 125.

CA-125 was first described as a tumor marker abnormally elevated in patients with recurrence of fallopian tube carcinoma (Niloff et al. 1984). Within the next several years, numerous authors reported its use as a marker during treatment to monitor re-

Table 12.3. FIGO fallopian tube staging

Stage 0	Carcinoma in situ (limited to tubal mucosa)
Stage I	Growth limited to the fallopian tubes
Stage IA	Growth is limited to one tube, with extension into the submucosa and/or muscularis but without penetration of the serosal surface; no ascites
Stage IB	Growth is limited to both tubes with extension into the submucosa and/or muscularis but without penetration of the serosal surface; no ascites
Stage IC	Tumor of either stage IA or IB, with tumor extension through or onto the tubal serosa, or ascites containing malignant cells or with positive peritoneal washings
Stage II	Growth involving one or both fallopian tubes with pelvic extension
Stage IIA	Extension and/or metastasis to the uterus and/or ovaries
Stage IIB	Extension to other pelvic tissues
Stage IIC	Tumor of either stage IIA or IIB with ascites containing malignant cells or with positive peritoneal washings
Stage III	Tumor involving one or both fallopian tubes with peritoneal implants outside of the pelvis and/or positive retroperitoneal or inguinal nodes. Superficial liver metastasis equals stage III. Tumor appears limited to the true pelvis but there is histologically proven malignant extension to the small bowel or omentum
Stage IIIA	Tumor is grossly limited to the true pelvis with negative nodes but with histologically confirmed microscopic seeding of abdominal peritoneal surfaces
Stage IIIB	Tumor involving one or both tubes with histologically confirmed implants of abdominal peritoneal surfaces, none exceeding 2 cm in diameter. Lymph nodes are negative
Stage IIIC	Abdominal implants greater than 2 cm in diameter and/or positive retroperitoneal or inguinal nodes
Stage IV	Growth involving one or both fallopian tubes with distant metastasis. If pleural effusion is present, there must be positive cytology to be stage IV. Parenchymal liver metastases equal Stage IV

sponse to therapy (Loostsma-Miklosava et al. 1987; Tokunaga et al. 1990; Davies et al. 1991; Kol et al. 1990). One report described two cases of fallopian tube carcinoma 11 and 3 months prior to symptomatology when screening for ovarian cancer revealed elevated CA-125 levels (Davies et al. 1991).

Levels greater than 65 U/ml have been defined as probable for fallopian tube malignancies, with a specificity of 98% and a sensitivity of 75% (Kol et al. 1990). However, serum antigen levels are found to be elevated in both malignant and benign conditions such as endometriosis, pelvic inflammatory disease, and early pregnancy (Davies et al. 1991). Levels below the upper limit were noted in two patients who at second-look laparotomy had disease recurrence (Tokunaga et al. 1990). There has also been a report of a patient who was diagnosed as having stage II disease but expressed a normal CA-125 level (Loostsma-Miklosava et al. 1987). This would suggest that the serum level of CA-125 by itself does not provide enough information for a differential diagnosis or for use as a screening technique for primary carcinoma of the fallopian tube. However, more recent reports suggest that screening with this tumor marker would be more effective if used serially and in combination with ultrasonography, and specifically, transvaginal ultrasonography (see below) (Davies et al. 1991; Podobnik et al. 1993). This would allow for earlier detection and define the normal range for therapeutic effect as compared with the ranges for primary tumors and for recurrences, which may be related to tumor bulk. It might also have a role in monitoring the response to adjuvant treatment postoperatively, serving as a substitute for invasive procedures such as second-look laparotomy which can carry significant morbidity as well as displaying an inability to detect foci of microscopic disease.

It has been suggested that elevated levels of CA-125 in supposed early-stage disease in conjunction with the use of CA-125 immunoscintigraphy may be predictive of metastatic disease (Lehtovirta et al. 1990; Gadducci et al. 1993). Gadducci et al. described a patient who refused a second-look laparotomy after adjuvant chemotherapy for adenocarcinoma of the fallopian tube. The patient continued to have increasing serum levels of CA-125 and immunoscintigraphy revealed a 5-cm area of metastasis in the retroperitoneal area. This also reaffirms the need for adequate surgical staging at the time of initial diagnosis in these patients.

12.10.2 CA 19-9

CA 19-9 is a glycoprotein of normal cells belonging to the Lewis blood group of antigens. It is therefore expressed only by patients with a positive Lewis phenotype. It has been used in monitoring malignancies of the gastrointestinal tract. More recently it was studied for possible expression in gynecological malignancies (Scharl et al. 1991). Although it was found to be expressed in müllerian tissue-derived tumors, its sensitivity is low as it is poorly released into the bloodstream and is expressed more overtly in less-differentiated or anaplastic tumors (Scharl et al. 1991). Scharl et al. concluded that it may have a role in surveillance of patients whose tumors do not express CA-125.

12.11 Radiological Imaging

12.11.1 Hysteroscopy and Hysterosalpingography

Various imaging techniques have been used in diagnosing pathology of the pelvis and genital tract. One of the earliest methods was hysterosalpingography. Although this procedure can diagnose abnormal masses and structures of the fallopian tube, it is very nonspecific and its use may cause intraperitoneal tumor seeding when the ampulla is patient (Hinton et al. 1988); it was therefore never widely used as a diagnostic technique. Unusual hysteroscopic findings were obtained preoperatively in a patient with primary carcinoma of the fallopian tube (Finikiotis et al. 1990). However, this was a nonspecific finding and did not allow a preoperative diagnosis.

12.11.2 Ultrasonography

The introduction of the vaginal ultrasound transducer has allowed more accurate assessment of adnexal pathology than can be achieved with pelvic ultrasonography alone. It is easier to visualize pelvic structures because the transducer is closer to the organs of interest; therefore there is less attenuation and better resolution (Granberg and Jansson 1990; Kol et al. 1990).

Sonograms of fallopian tube carcinoma show solid or cystic adnexal masses with luminal papillary projections (Kol et al. 1990; Ajjimakorn and Bhamarapravati 1991; Podobnik et al. 1993). In one reported case, however, no difference was found between conventional and transvaginal ultrasonography in that the vaginal transducer could not clearly identify the interstitial portion of the fallopian tube. The diagnosis in this case was made by observing the shape and size of the mass accompanied by the passage of free fluid through the uterine cavity ("hydrops tubae profluens").

By combining other screening techniques and modalities, transvaginal sonography (TVS) can be rendered more effective as a screening tool for diagnosis of primary fallopian tube carcinoma. Kol et al. (1990) described a case in which TVS was used to aid in the preoperative diagnosis in conjunction with elevated CA-125 levels. The addition of color flow and Doppler waveform measurements has increased the sensitivity of TVS (Kurjak et al. 1992; Podobnik et al. 1993). In malignant masses, there is typically a decreased amount of muscle in the lining of the tumor vessels, which, combined with increased arterial-venous shunting within the tumor, increases flow and results in abnormal pulsatile and resistance indices compared with those of normal vessels (Podibnik et al. 1993). Use of color flow alone in the imaging of postmenopausal adnexal masses has a reported specificity of only 65% assuming that flow is visible (Kurjak et al. 1992). Kurjak et al. found that the differences in vessel resistance indices between benign and malignant tumors gave a sensitivity of 96% and a specificity of 95% ($P < 0.001$).

The drawbacks to TVS with color flow Doppler concern the experience required of the operator, the quality of instrumentation utilized and the change in imaging characteristics of tumors in accordance with stage (Kurjak et al. 1992). In addition, the costs of screening with ultrasonography in such a rare tumor may preclude its routine use except in cases where a patient's symptomatology or elevated tumor markers arouse suspicion of a fallopian primary malignancy (Granberg and Jansson 1990; Ajjmakorn and Bhamarapravati 1991).

12.11.3 Magnetic Resonance Imaging

Some authors report that magnetic resonance imaging (MRI) is superior to ultrasonography and computed tomography in that it can better differentiate the fallopian tube from other pelvic organs (Thurnher et al. 1990; Kawakami et al. 1993). However, the distinction of benign from malignant processes is difficult, and it has been concluded that ultrasonography is superior to MRI as a screening modality in the evaluation of adnexal tumors (Thurner et al. 1990).

12.11.4 Nuclear Scan Imaging

Radioimaging with a combination of immunolymphoscintigraphy and immunoscintigraphy with iodine-131 labeled F(ab')2 fragments of monoclonal OC 125 antibodies has been shown to improve detection of retroperitoneal lymph node metastases, with a sensitivity of 90% and a specificity of 83% (Lehtovirta et al. 1990). These findings were correlated with abnormally elevated levels of CA-125 which would indicate that those individuals with high circulating levels of this tumor marker are at a higher risk of having metastatic disease.

Based on the biological increase in glucose metabolism in malignant tumors, positron emission tomography (PET) has been used extensively in patients with gliomas of the central nervous system. In a recent report (Karlan et al. 1993), whole-body fluorodeoxyglucose PET scanning was demonstrated to detect sites of metastatic fallopian tube carcinoma in areas of skin nodules and bone discomfort.

Both of the above imaging techniques show promise in allowing earlier detection of disease spread or recurrence and monitoring of adjuvant therapy by serial imaging (Lehtovirta et al. 1990; Karlan et al. 1993).

12.12 Management

Primary treatment of adenocarcinoma of the fallopian tube comprises surgical resection at the time of initial diagnosis. Extensive surgical resection and staging should be performed (total abdominal hysterectomy, omentectomy, and bilateral salpingectomy), as well as sampling of ascitic fluid or peritoneal washings and peritoneal sampling of diaphragm, bladder, and bowel. Recent reports advocate lymph node sampling, as nodal involvement may arise early in the course of disease spread. This may occur even earlier than the extent of pelvic spread may indicate (Tamini and Figge 1981;

Schray et al. 1987). It has been observed by numerous authors that if >2 cm residual tumor is left behind at primary resection, this has grave prognostic implications (Podratz et al. 1986). Some investigators have reported satisfactory results with conservative surgical treatment (unilateral salpingectomy only) in cases where tumor has not invaded beyond the mucosa (Klein et al. 1994). Most patients, however, require some form of adjuvant treatment postoperatively to combat bulk residual disease or to treat assumed microscopic involvement.

It must be remembered in this context that interpreting the literature in search of the most favorable treatment regimens is fraught with difficulties. Most studies reporting results of adjuvant therapy cover the time span of several decades without prospective randomization of patients or employ inconsistent staging schema and poorly reported or performed surgical staging. The authors then suggest on the basis of good responses observed in small numbers of cases that a certain mode of therapy requires further investigation, this mode being outdated by the time investigators can acquire enough patients to make the study statistically significant.

12.12.1 Chemotherapy

One of the first reports of a response of fallopian tube adenocarcinoma to a chemotherapeutic agent was with the alkylating agent Alkeran (Boronow 1973). Hanton et al. (1966) had previously reported that no single agent or combination of agents, including 5-fluorouracil, thiotepa, and nitrogen mustards, had proven useful in obtaining a tumor response.

Later studies utilized treatment regimens developed and noted to have good response rates in the treatment of ovarian cancers, which have been assumed to share similarities with fallopian tube carcinoma in regard to embryological derivation and histopathology. It appears that overall the results have been similar to those observed in ovarian carcinoma.

More recently, combination chemotherapeutic regimens have been used in response to the poor results obtained with single agents. It has been suggested, however, that these initial poor responses were due to the use of the agents for recurrences after primary treatment failure (Rose et al. 1990).

Deppe et al. (1980) was one of the first to report a surgically documented response via second-look laparotomy, using cisplatin-based combination chemotherapy. Another later study retrospectively compared results obtained in patients treated with or without cisplatin, employing combination therapy or single-agent therapy only. They observed a response in 12 out of 14 patients (86%) who received the cisplatin-based regimen (Peters et al. 1988). However, more patients with recurrence and failure received the less aggressive treatment. It should also be noted that 33% of patients who were free of disease at second-look laparotomy subsequently relapsed.

In the only prospective trial, 18 patients receiving cisplatin, doxorubicin, and cyclophosphamide in at least 6–12 cycles showed a response rate of 53%, which is similar to that seen in patients with ovarian carcinoma (Morris et al. 1990). The series, however, was small and had no controls. The authors suggested that current treatment used for ovarian cancer should not simply be used for fallopian tube carcinoma; rather trials should be designed to define the true similarities between the diseases, after which the most appropriate treatment for fallopian tube carcinoma can be established.

Several other authors have cited good response rates utilizing cisplatin-based combination chemotherapy for fallopian tube carcinoma in both localized and disseminated disease (Asmussen et al. 1988; Eddy et al. 1984b; Gurney et al. 1990; McMurray et al. 1986; Peters et al. 1988; Yoonessi et al. 1988; Maxson et al. 1987; Barakat et al. 1990). Some of these authors have mentioned that doxorubicin has not shown any additional benefit when used with cisplatin combined with cyclophosphamide (Barakat et al. 1990; Maxon et al. 1987). These studies did not always provide information regarding surgical staging prior to treatment or data on assessment of tumor response and possible subsequent relapse (Gurney et al. 1990; Barakat et al. 1990; Muntz et al. 1991, Pectasides et al. 1994). Muntz et al. (1991) suggested that prolonged following-up is advisable before recommending adjuvant treatment in stage I.

Since the normal fallopian tube epithelium is known to exhibit cyclic changes in response to the hormonal variations of the menstrual cycle, progesterones have been studied for possible use in treatment of fallopian tube malignancies. This has met with no success (Eddy et al. 1984b; Yoonessi et al. 1988; Boronow 1973; Denham and MacLennan 1984; Podratz et al. 1986), No controlled trials, however, have been performed. It would seem logical that in the evolution of carcinoma, dedifferentiation may result in fewer or aberrant hormone receptors studies should be implemented to address this possibility and thereby further elucidate the biology of fallopian tube malignancies.

12.12.2 Second-Look Laparotomy

Second-look laparotomy is controversial in the treatment of fallopian tube carcinoma, although it has generally been accepted as a tool for the management of ovarian cancer (Eddy et al. 1984a). It is defined as an exploratory laparotomy following a planned treatment program for cancer. Its purpose is to assess tumor status and remove, if possible, residual disease and sample for areas with microscopic involvement. It is supposed to allow for earlier treatment withdrawal to avoid unnecessary toxicity as well as to provide prognostic information pertinent to the use of other treatment modalities. Some also argue that it is of limited benefit when there is no proven second-line treatment, although it is known that reduction of tumor bulk improves the prognosis for survival in patients with ovarian cancer with or without any further treatment. This may also be true for fallopian tube carcinoma.

The likelihood of being free of disease at second-look laparotomy is related to the initial stage and the amount of residual disease after initial surgery (Rubin et al. 1988). The predictive value of the technique in ascertaining whether patients will remain disease free appears to be limited: several authors have reported relapse rates from 19%–40% after a negative second-look operation (Eddy et al. 1984a; Rubin et al. 1988; Barakat et al. 1990).

It has been suggested that higher relapse rates may occur secondary to higher response rates and shorter duration before reexploration in patients achieving a rapid and dramatic response with cisplatin-based chemotherapy. In such patients treatment may be withdrawn prematurely, before the drug can effectively eliminate all microscopic residual disease (Rubin et al. 1988). A controlled trial of various intervals prior to second-look laparotomy and/or specific guidelines would be of value in the study of disease recurrence.

12.12.3 Radiation Therapy

Postoperative radiation therapy has been used as a traditional form of therapy for fallopian tube carcinoma dissemination and recurrence. It has been recommended by some authors and questioned by others (Boutselis and Thompson 1971; Hanton et al. 1966; Momatzee and Kempson 1968; Roberts and Lifshitz 1982). The rarity of this tumor makes it difficult to acquire skill in its management and renders a large study at a single institute difficult. It is also difficult to decipher results of past literature due to variability in respect of staging schema, surgical staging techniques, treatment volume, dosage fractionation, and type of radiation used. All reported studies are retrospective and usually involve small numbers of patients treated over long periods.

Several early small studies observed promising results using techniques similar to those used in treatment of ovarian carcinoma. They suggested that use of whole abdominal external beam radiation or intraperitoneal administration of radioactive colloids (^{32}P, ^{198}Au) results in better survival rates compared with the use of surgery alone (Schray et al. 1987; Podratz et al. 1986; Phelps and Chapman 1974; Henderson et al. 1987). Some investigators have observed that there are too few data to support the use of radioactive colloids and that they have no role in patients with bulky disease (Benedet et al. 1977; Phelps and Chapman 1974; Roberts and Lifshitz 1982).

The best results were achieved with total doses of greater than 50 Gy/5–6 weeks using megavoltage rather than orthovoltage therapy (Amendola et al. 1983; Fogh 1961). McMurray and Brown both stated that recurrence of early-stage disease (I and II) was likely to be upper abdominal if only pelvic irradiation was performed, and that areas at risk such as the abdomen and para-aortics should be included within the initial treatment volume. Other studies noted a 50% relapse rate when treating early-stage disease with surgery alone or surgery + pelvic irradiation as compared with a greater than 50% 5-year survival rate when the abdomen and para-aortic areas were treated (Podratz et al. 1986; Brown et al. 1985; McMurray et al. 1986).

A recent study utilizing the new FIGO staging system for fallopian tube carcinoma compared outcome in carcinoma in situ and in stage I disease with use of either radiation or cisplatin-based chemotherapy (Klein et al. 1994). It was observed that tumor penetration through the basement membrane (invasive carcinoma) decreased the survival rate by 50%. Stage I patients treated by irradiation showed a significantly better prognosis than patients treated by chemotherapy ($P = 0.017$) (Klein et al. 1994). A few studies reported disappointing results using radiation to treat early-stage fallopian tube carcinoma

(ROBERTS and LIFSHITZ 1982; PETERS et al. 1988). However, these studies contained small numbers, utilized treatment to the pelvis only, and had inconsistent or incomplete surgical resection and staging (ROBERTS and LIFSHITZ 1982; PETERS et al. 1988). Many of the series that showed no benefit with radiation used orthovoltage, which is unable to deliver high doses to the deeper pelvic structures (SINGHAL et al. 1991).

A series of 275 patients with carcinoma of the fallopian tube were recently presented in Annual Report volume 22 (PETTERSSON 1994). Overall survival with follow-up for 0–5 years was 46.5%. In this series review, 3.6% were lost to follow-up, 4.7% died of intercurrent disease, and 45% died from their carcinoma. Survival by stage was as follows: stage I, 67.4%; stage II, 44.7%; stage III, 20.5%; and stage IV, 38.4%. Independent variables found to be significant for prognosis were age >50 years and stage. Treatment modalities such as surgery alone and surgery combined with radiation were not found to be significant in patient prognosis.

There is little information regarding combined use of chemotherapy and radiation as postoperative treatment. Most studies have used a single modality and after failure have attempted the other approach (MARKMAN 1992). Since both modalities have shown treatment response when used together or separately (YOONESSI 1988), a randomized, prospective study may be of help in establishing the relative value of the different approaches. Toxicity will, of course, play a role in determining whether an efficacious dose of each treatment can be given.

Although there have been reports of treatment complications with use of radiation (AMENDOLA et al. 1983; KINZEL 1976), most have been small in number and minor in severity. With proper planning and shielding of vital structures during critical portions of treatment, the sequelae should be minimal. It should be noted, however, that patients who have undergone multiple surgical explorations and have extensive disease involving bowel, bladder, and other vital structures will always be at an increased risk for development of complications in any treatment regimen.

Some of the reported results in respect of the 5-year survival rates achieved with radiation therapy and chemotherapy are shown in Table 12.4.

Table 12.4. Five-year survival rates achieved by various authors in patients with fallopian tube carcinoma

Authors	No. of cases	Postoperative treatment						Five-year survival
		Observation	XRT		CTX		XRT + CTX	
			Pelvic	Abdomen[a]	Single	Combination		
Stages I and II								
DENHAM and MACLENNAN (1984)	27	7	20	–	–	–	–	33%–100%
PETERS et al. (1988)	65	21	26	7	6	1	4	29%–61%
GURNEY et al. (1990)	17	6	9	–	–	2	–	50%–80%
SCHRAY et al. (1987)	21	–	10	7	–	–	4	42%–78%
EDDY et al. (1984b)	34	7	20 (NOS)		4 (NOS)		3	35%
AMENDOLA et al. (1983)	20	5	13	–	–	–	2	50%
MEIN et al. (1994)	54	4	26	–	14	–	–	28%–53% (CTX vs XRT)
MCMURRAY et al. (1986)	20	3	6	1	–	6	4	27%–56%
Stages III and IV								
DENHAM and MACLENNAN (1984)	13	3[b]	1	3	–	2	3	0%–18%
PETERS et al. (1988)	29	2	4	1	6	14	2	0%–17%
GURNEY et al. (1990)	13	2	3	–	2	6	–	18%
SCHRAY et al. (1987)	12	6[c]	3	1	–	–	2	33%
EDDY et al. (1984b)	33	2	9 (NOS)		17 (NOS)		5	5%
AMENDOLA et al. (1983)	14	1	5	4	2 (1 NOS)		2	0%–25%
MCMURRAY et al. (1986)	10	–	–	4	2	4	4	0%–14%

NOS, not otherwise specified; XRT, radiation therapy; CTX, chemotherapy.
[a] External beam or intraperitoneal ^{32}p.
[b] Radiation to one metastatic site.
[c] Only six patients treated with curative intent.

12.13 Rare Histological Subtypes of Fallopian Tube Malignancies

The most common malignant primary tumors of the fallopian tube are of adenocarcinomatous histology, 90% of which are papillary serous carcinomas. There are, however, numerous reported cases of rare histological subtypes which, for the sake of completeness, require a brief overview (see Table 12.5 for the WHO classification of fallopian tube malignancies).

12.13.1 Gestational Trophoblastic Disease and Choriocarcinoma

Trophoblastic lesions and choriocarcinomas of the fallopian tube are rare, approximately 76 cases being accepted out of a review of 100 multiple case reports in the literature (OBER and MAIER 1981). They are usually reported in cases of ectopic pregnancies. The incidence of choriocarcinoma of the fallopian tube is theoretically 1 in 5333 tubal pregnancies (HERTIG and MANSELL 1956). Gestational choriocarcinoma may arise from any type of pregnancy: normal term, molar, abortion, and, least frequently, ectopic pregnancy (BAKRI et al. 1992). The rarity of this particular location for this type of malignancy may be due to the early symptoms related to tubal distention and inflammation seen in the typical profile of a patient with an ectopic gestation. The malignancy is then either missed or is not allowed to develop out of the trophoblast. Patients at risk for ectopic pregnancies are those with histories of pelvic inflammatory disease, endometriosis, and other causes of tubal obstruction.

Tubal choriocarcinomas appear to have the same favorable prognosis and responsiveness to chemotherapy as intrauterine gestational choriocarcinomas (BAKRI et al. 1992; KJER et al. 1991; MUTO et al. 1991). It is mentioned, however, that the standard surgical treatment of ectopic pregnancy by conservative methods and not by extensive surgical excision or staging requires careful monitoring of beta-HCG titers after diagnosis and treatment regardless of a diagnosis of concurrent malignancy (BAKRI et al. 1992).

Table 12.5. Malignant tumors of the fallopian tube (WHO classification)

Epithelial tumors
Carcinoma in situ
Serous carcinoma
Mucinous carcinoma
Endometrioid carcinoma
Clear cell carcinoma
Transitional cell carcinoma
Squamous cell carcinoma
Undifferentiated and other
Mixed epithelial-mesenchymal tumors
Adenosarcoma[a]
Mesodermal (müllerian) mixed tumor
Homologous (carcinosarcoma)
Heterologous
Mesenchymal tumors
Leiomyosarcoma
Others

[a] Cases of adenosarcoma have not been reported.

12.13.2 Endometrioid Carcinoma

Endometrioid carcinomas of the fallopian tube are extremely rare, with only a handful of cases having been reported in the literature. They include a large variety of histological subtypes with both benign- and malignant-appearing squamous elements, e.g., adenoacanthoma, adenofibroma, and adenosquamous (DAYA et al. 1992; RORAT and WALLACH 1990; CZERNOBILSKY and CORNOG 1972; SERAJ et al. 1990). The ovary is the most common site of endometrial-appearing adenocarcinomas.

Although endometriosis is a common gynecological entity and a case of endometrioid carcinoma arising from a focus of this tissue has been reported (SERAJ et al. 1990), it does not appear to be a predisposing factor for development of a malignancy in the fallopian tube. Current treatment consists of surgical resection and postoperatine radiation therapy (SERAJ et al. 1990).

12.13.3 Transitional Cell Carcinoma

SILVA et al. (1993) compared cases of transitional cell carcinoma (TCC) primary carcinoma of the fallopian tube with non-TCC-pattern tumors by reference to clinical course and histochemical analyses. They concluded that TCC-pattern tumors are a distinct entity in primary fallopian tube neoplasms; they recurred later after treatment, suggesting a more favorable response to chemotherapy than occurr with the same histopathology in ovarian carcinoma (see also ROBEY et al. 1989).

12.13.4 Teratoma

Teratomas of the fallopian tube are rare, with only about 50 cases reported and only four of these (SWEET et al. 1975; FROST et al. 1989) being of the malignant variety. They more commonly occur in the ovary. They represent histology derived from all three germ layers, possibly by way of some pluripotent properties retained by germ cells that do not reach the ovary during normal migration from the yolk sac. They then develop under different hormonal influences in the fallopian tube. Another theory suggests that there is a process of blastomeric isolation, in which blastula cells that become isolated in the developing gynecological tract later develop into teratomas (LAI and LIM-TAN 1993). The patient profile differs from that seen with most fallopian tube malignancies in that these neoplasms occur during the reproductive years, mostly in the fourth decade (LAI and LIM-TAN 1993; KUTTEH and ALABERT 1991).

12.13.5 Sarcomas

Primary sarcomas of the fallopian tube are exceedingly rare. As of the latest review of the literature, only 34 cases have been reported. Histologically, those pure or mixed neoplasms containing cytologically benign epithelial elements are designated as adenosarcoma. Those containing malignant epithelial components are classified as malignant mixed müllerian tumors (WHEELER 1994) (see Sect. 12.3.6).

Leiomyosarcomas are the predominant type, with even fewer cases being classified as giant cell sarcoma, myxosarcoma, chondrosarcomas, and malignant fibrous histiocytomas (ABRAMS et al. 1958; JACOBY et al. 1993; HALLIGAN 1990; SCHEFFY et al. 1941). Adenosarcomas have not been reported, (WHEELER 1994). Epidemiology of the few cases shows a median age of 47 years with presentation similar to that of adenocarcinoma of the fallopian tube, i.e., pain and vaginal discharge (JACOBY et al. 1993). Overall survival is poor as patients usually present at a late stage and tend to suffer tumor recurrence after surgery despite adjuvant treatment with chemotherapy or radiation, for which there is no standard regimen (JACOBY et al. 1993).

12.13.6 Malignant Mixed Müllerian Tumors

Malignant mixed müllerian tumors (MMMTs) are a rare histological subset of fallopian tube carcinomas with less than 50 reported cases in the literature, accounting for 0.02%–0.04% of all gynecological malignancies (CHIANG et al. 1991; CARLSON et al. 1993). They are defined histologically by malignant epithelial and stromal components present as carcinoma and sarcomatous elements within the same tumor.

Specific histogenesis fails to be completely understood. They are thought to arise from the multipotent mesoderm of the müllerian or paramesonephric duct system (see Sect. 12.1). The cephalad portion of the paramesonephric duct, where the fallopian tube develops, appears to be less active than other areas of the genital tract during developmental stages. Although there are cyclic changes in the epithelium of the tube during the menstrual years, there appears to be no stromal activity and actual loss of tissue save for the number of cilia (VERHEGE et al. 1979). This observation may represent an explanation for the varied incidence of these tumors in different portions of the female genital tract (they are more common in the uterus, ovary, and cervix) (WILLIAMS and WOODRUFF 1963).

The category "MMMT" includes neoplasms in which the malignant mesenchymal elements contain tissue types normally found in this area (smooth muscle, endometrial stromal cells). These are called homologous and are also referred to as carcinosarcomas. Tumors containing tissues not normally found in the tube (striated muscle, cartilage, and bone) are called heterologous. The incidence of these histological subtypes is equal (WEBER et al. 1993). More than 90% of case reports cite adenocarcinoma as the carcinomatous element; the most frequent heterologous components are the rhabdomyoblast and chondroblast, the least common being the osteoblast (LIANG et al. 1990; IMACHI et al. 1992).

The epidemiological profile is similar to that of adenocarcinoma of the fallopian tube. The mean age at diagnosis is 59 years. The most common presenting symptoms are abnormal bleeding and (in order of decreasing incidence) abdominal/pelvic pain, pelvic mass, and increasing abdominal girth.

Watery vaginal discharge, commonly seen in adenocarcinoma, is infrequent. The majority of patients are postmenopausal. Although staging is not consistent in the literature, the majority of cases at the time of diagnosis are beyond the tube (> stage I). Few early-stage lesions are documented.

Prognosis is poor despite various treatments, but the small number of well-documented cases make analysis of postoperative treatment difficult. The most important prognostic factors appear to be stage and spread of disease and no difference has been found between homologous and heterologous subtypes with respect to survival (LIANG et al. 1990; IMACHI et al. 1992).

Mean survival ranges from 18 to 40 months, with some authors noting an increase since the 1970s and 1980s. This may be attributed to an improvement in treatment techniques and drug regimens (MOORE et al. 1992; CARLSON et al. 1993). Surgery is usually followed by adjuvant treatment with radiation and/or chemotherapy. Numerous reports document varied success with either regimen. Most recurrences arise within 2 years of diagnosis and the most common site of failure is within the pelvis (LIANG et al. 1990). This is consistent with the known route of spread and metastatic pattern of adenocarcinoma of the fallopian tube (along intraperitoneal surfaces followed by lymphatic and vascular invasion, with distant metastasis being rare until later in the course of the disease).

Although there is insufficient reporting and lack of documentation of both staging and radiation therapy techniques, it appears that the best results derive from the combined use of radiation and chemotherapy postoperatively (MUNTZ et al. 1989; CARLSON et al. 1993). Also, although radioresistance has been noted for MMMTs of the uterus, ovary, and cervix, increased local control has been documented using 45–50 Gy pelvic irradiation for the treatment of uterine sarcomas (MUNTZ et al. 1989). Because spread of these tumors may involve either stromal or epithelial components, it stands to reason that radiation has a role in adjuvant treatment as in adenocarcinoma of the fallopian tube.

Chemotherapeutic regimens have included the use of cisplatin, vincristine, and doxorubicin, as well as numerous other agents, in small total numbers of patients (MUNTZ et al. 1989; HANJANI et al. 1980; SERAJ et al. 1990; MOORE et al. 1992; CARLSON et al. 1993; IMACHI et al. 1992; WEBER et al. 1993). There appears to be a role for cisplatin-based chemotherapy with or without cyclophosphamide (MOORE et al. 1992; WEBER et al. 1993; IMACHI et al. 1992; MCMURRAY et al. 1986; CARLSON et al. 1993; LIANG et al. 1990; SERAJ et al. 1990; MUNTZ et al. 1989).

It appears that stage I lesions (those in which there is no penetration of the serosa) confer the best survival and may have a decreased ability to spread intraperitoneally when the ampulla is sealed (MUNTZ et al. 1989). However, when the serosa is breached or there is tumor spillage, the disease can no longer be considered local, making surgical resection an inadequate treatment (MUNTZ et al. 1989; CARLSON et al. 1993) even though removal of gross tumor is known to impact on survival.

As noted previously, the fallopian tube is rich in lymphatics, draining the mesosalpinx into the para-aortic lymph nodes. Attention therefore should be directed to the development of better chemotherapeutic regimens and radiation therapy techniques designed not only to control local disease but also to eliminate the possibility of distant failure and metastasis by means of systemic prophylaxis and extension of radiation fields to include the abdominal areas at risk.

12.13.7
Others

There are other scattered cases of extremely rare histological primary malignancies of the fallopian tube, namely lymphoma (HERTIG and MANSELL 1956), glassy cell carcinoma (HERBOLD et al. 1988), clear cell carcinoma (VOET and LIFSHITZ 1992) and squamous cell carcinoma (CHEUNG et al. 1994).

Female adnexal tumors of probable wolffian (mesonephric) duct origin are extratubal. They are usually benign neoplasms that arise within the broad ligament (SCULLY 1979; DAYA et al. 1992). They may be difficult to differentiate from müllerian-derived primary tumors of the fallopian tube and multiple histochemical and ultrastructural analyses may be necessary (DAYA et al. 1992; GOMPEL and SILVERBERG 1994).

12.14
Metastatic Tumors of the Fallopian Tube

Metastatic tumors of the fallopian tube are more common than primary neoplasms. They are most often extensions of primary ovarian, endometrial, or cervical cancers. Metastases from gynecological organs are followed in frequency by metastases from gastrointestinal and breast primaries.

References

Abrams J, Kazal H, Hobbs R (1958) Primary sarcoma of the fallopian tubes. Am J Obstet Gynecol 75:1

Ajjimakorn S, Bhamarapravati Y (1991) Transvaginal ultrasound and the diagnosis of fallopian tube carcinoma. J Clin Ultrasound 19:116–119

Amendola BL, LaRorrere J, Amendola MA, et al. (1983) Adenocarcinoma of the fallopian tube. Surg Gynecol Obstet 157:223

Anbrokh YM (1970) Microscopic characteristics of cancer of the fallopian tube. Neoplasma 17:557

Asmussen M, Karen J, Kjoerstad K, et al. (1988) Primary adenocarcinoma localized to the fallopian tubes; report on 33 cases. Gynecol Oncol 30:183

Bakri Y, Amri A, Mulla J (1992) Gestational choriocarcinoma in a tubal ectopic pregnancy. Acta Obstet Gynecol Scand 71:67–68

Barakat R, Rubin S, Saigo P, et al. (1990) Cisplatin-based combination chemotherapy in carcinoma of the fallopian tube. Gynecol Oncol 42:156–160

Benedet JL, White GW, Fairey RN, et al. (1977) Adenocarcinoma of the fallopian tube. Obstet Gynecol 50:654

Boronow R (1973) Chemotherapy for disseminated tubal caner. Obstet Gyncol 42:62–66

Boutselis JG, Thompson JN (1971) Clinical aspects of primary carcinoma of the fallopian tube: a clinical study of 14 cases. Am J Obstet Gynecol 111:98

Brown MD, Kohorn EI, Kapp DS, Schwartz PE, Merino M (1985) Fallopian tube carcinoma. Int J Radiat Oncol Biol Phys 11:583–590

Carlson J, Ackerman B, Wheeler J (1993) Malignant mixed müllerian tumor of the fallopian tube. Cancer 71:187–192

Cheung A, So KF, Wong LC, et al. (1994) Primary squamous cell carcinoma of fallopian tube. Int J Gynecol Pathol 13:92–95

Chiang A, So KF, Soong YK (1991) Malignant mixed müllerian tumor of the fallopian tube. Case report and review of the literature. Chang Gung Med J 14:259–263

Czernobilsky B, Cornog JL (1972) Squamous predominance in adenocanthema of the adenexa – report of a patient. Obstet Gynecol 37:55–59

Davies AR, Fish A, Woolas R, et al. (1991) Raised serum CA-125 preceding the diagnosis of carcinoma of the fallopian tube; two case reports. Br J Obstet Gynaecol 98:602

Daya D, Young R, Scully R (1992) Endometrial carcinoma of fallopian tube resembling an adnexal tumor of probable wolffian origin: a report of six cases. Int J Gynecol Pathol 11:122–130

Denham JW, MacLennan KA (1984) The management of primary carcinoma of the fallopian tube. Cancer 53:166

Deppe G, Bruckner H, Cohen C (1980) Combination chemotherapy for advanced carcinoma of the fallopian tube. Obstet Gynecol 56:530–532

Dodson MO, Ford JH, Averette HE (1970) Clinical aspects of fallopian tube carcinoma. Obstet Gynecol 36:935

Eddy GL, Copeland LJ, Gershenson DM (1984a) Second-look laparotomy in fallopian tube carcinoma. Gynecol Oncol 19:182

Eddy GL, Copeland LJ, Gershenson DM, et al. (1984b) Fallopian tube carcinoma. Obstet Gynecol 64:546

Erez S, Kaplan AL, Wall JA (1967) Clinical staging of fallopian tube carcinoma. Obstet Gynecol 30:547

Finikiotis G, O'Shea RT, Sanders RR (1990) An unusual hysteroscopic finding in association with primary carcinoma of the fallopian tube. Br J Hosp Med 44:124–125

Fogh IB (1961) Primary carcinoma of the fallopian tube. Cancer 23:1332

Frost RG, Roongpisuthipong A, Cheek BH, Majmudar BN (1989) Immature teratoma of the fallopian tube. A case report. J Reprod Med 34:62–64

Gadducci A, Madrigali A, Ciancia EM, Campani D, Facchino V, Fioretti P (1993) The clinical, serological, pathological and immunocytochemical features of a case of primary carcinoma of the fallopian tube. Eur J Gynaecol Oncol 14:374–379

Gompel C, Silverberg SG (1994) Pathology in gynecology and obstetrics, 4th edn. Lippincott, Philadelphia

Granberg S, Jansson I (1990) Early detection of primary carcinoma of the fallopian tube by endovaginal ultrasound. Acta Obstet Gynaecol Scand 69:667–668

Gurney H, Murphy D, Crouther D (1990) The management of primary fallopian tube carcinoma. Br J Obstet Gynaecol 97:822

Halligan AWF (1990) Malignant fibrous histiocytoma of the fallopian tube. Br J Obstet Gynaecol 97:275–276

Hanjani P, Peterson PO, Bonnell SA (1980) Malignant mixed müllerian tumor of the fallopian tube: report of a case and review of the literature. Gynecol Oncol 9:381–393

Hanton E, Malkasian G, Dahlin D, Pratt J (1966) Primary carcinoma of the fallopian tube. Am J Obstet Gynecol 94:32–839

Henderson SR, Harper RC, Salazar ON, et al. (1987) Primary carcinoma of the fallopian tube. Difficulties of diagnosis and treatment. Gynecol Oncol 5:168

Herbold DR, Axelrod JH, Bobowski SJ, et al. (1988) Glassy cell carcinoma of the fallopian tube. A case report. Int J Gynecol Pathol 7:384–390

Hertig AT, Mansell IT (1956) Tumors of the female sex organs. 1. Atlas of tumor pathology. pp 62–63, Washington, D.C. Armed Forces Institute of Pathology

Hinton A, Bea C, Winfield AC, et al. (1988) Carcinoma of the fallopian tube. Urol Radiol 10:113

Hu CT, Taymon MZ, Hertig AT (1950) Primary carcinoma of the fallopian tube. Am J Obstet Gynecol 59:67

Imachi M, Tsukamoto N, Nakana H, et al. (1992) Malignant mixed müllerian tumor of the fallopian tube; report of two cases and review of literature. Gynecol Oncol 47:114–124

Jackson-York GL, Ramzy L (1992) Synchronous papillary mucinous adenocarcinoma of the endocervix and fallopian tube. Int J Gynecol pathol 11:122

Jacoby AF, Fuller AF, Muntz HG, et al. (1993) Primary leiomyosarcoma of the fallopian tube. Gynecol Oncol 51:404–407

Karlan B, Hoh C, Tse N, et al. (1993) Whole body position emission tomography with (fluorine-18)-2 deoxy-glucose can detect metastatic carcinoma of the fallopian tube. Gynecol Oncol 49:383–388

Kawakami S, Togashi K, Kimura I, et al. (1993) Primary malignant tumor of the fallopian tube; appearance at CT and MR imaging. Radiology 186:503–508

Kinzel GE (1976) Primary carcinoma of the fallopian tube. Am J Obstet Gynecol 125:816

Kjer JJ, Iversen T, Haarstad I (1991) Malignant trophoblastic cell tumor localized to the fallopian tube; a case report. Eur J Obstet Gynecol Reprod Biol 39:163–164

Klein M, Rosen A, Graf A, et al. (1994) Primary fallopian tube carcinoma: a retrospective survey of 51 cases. Arch Gynecol Obstet 255:141–146

Kol S, Gal D, Friedman M, et al. (1990) Preoperative diagnosis of fallopian tube carcinoma by transvaginal sonography and CA-125. Gynecol Oncol 37:129

Kone M, Body G, Calais G, Fynn A, Fetissif F, Lansae J (1992) Adenocarcinoma printif de la trampe. Gynecol Obstet Biol Reprod 21:187–192

Kurjak A, Schulman H, Sosic A, Zalerd I, Shalan H (1992) Transvaginal ultrasound, colon flow and Doppler wave form of the postmenopausal adenexal mass. Obstet Gynecol 80:917–921

Kutteh W, Albert T (1991) Mature cystic teratoma of the fallopian tube associated with an ectopic pregnancy. Obstet Gynecol 78:984–986

Lai SF, Lim-Tan SK (1993) Benign teratoma of the fallopian tube. A case report. Singapore Med J 34:274–275

Lehtovirta P, Kaisemo KJ, Liewendahl K, et al. (1990) Immunolymphoscintigraphy and immunoscintigraphy of ovarian and fallopian tube cancer using F(ab')2 fragments of monoclonal OC125. Cancer Res 50:9375

Liang WW, Lin YN, Lee YN (1990) Malignant mixed müllerian tumor of fallopian tube. Report of a case and review of literature. Chin Med J (Engl) 45:272–275

Loostsma-Miklosava E, Aalders JG, Willemse PHB, et al. (1987) Levels of Ca-125 in patients with carcinoma of the fallopian tube; two case histories. Eur J Obstet Gynecol Reprod Biol 24:231

Markman M (1992) Principles and practice of gynecological oncology. Lippincott, Philadelphia, pp 783–794

Maxson WZ, Stehman FB, Ulbright TM, et al. (1987) Primary carcinoma of the fallopian tube; evidence for activity of cisplatin combination therapy. Gynecol Oncol 26:305

McMurray EH, Jacobs AJ, Perez A, et al. (1986) Carcinoma of the fallopian tube. Management and sites of failure. Cancer 58:2070

Momatzee S, Kempson RL (1968) Primary adenocarcinoma of the fallopian tube. Obstet Gynecol 32:649

Moore D, Taslimi MM, Kasanorich M (1992) Malignant mixed müllerian tumor of the fallopian tube of the heterologous type. J Tenn Med Assoc 513–514

Morris M, Gershinson PM, Burke TW, et al. (1990) Treatment of fallopian tube carcinoma with cisplatin, doxorubicin, and cyclophosphamide. Obstet Gynecol 76:1020

Muntz H, Rutgers J, Fuller A, et al. (1989) Carcinosarcomas and mixed müllerian tumors of the fallopian tube. Gynecol Oncol 34:109–115

Muntz IT, Tarraza H, Golf B, et al. (1991) Combination chemotherapy in advanced adenocarcinoma of the fallopian tube. Gynecol Oncol 40:268–273

Muto M, Lage J, Bernstein M, et al. (1991) Gestational trophoblastic disease of the fallopian tube. J Reprod Med 36:57–60

Niloff JM, Klu TZ, Schaatzel E, et al. (1984) Elevation of CA-125 in carcinomas of the fallopian tube, endometrian and endocervix. Am J Obstet Gynecol 148:1057

Nordin A (1994) Primary carcinoma of the fallopian tube: a 20 year literature review. Obstet Gynecol Surv 49:349–361

Ober WB, Maier RC (1981) Gestational choriocarcinoma of the fallopian tube. Diagn Gynecol Obstet 3:213

Pectasides D, Sintila B, Varthalitis S, et al. (1994) Treatment of primary fallopian tube carcinoma with cisplatin-containing chemotherapy. Am J Clin Oncol 17:68–71

Peters WA, Anderson WA, Hopkins MP, et al. (1988) Prognostic features of carcinoma of the fallopian tube. Obstet Gynecol 71:757

Pettersson F (1992) Staging rules for gestational trophoblastic tumors and fallopian tube cancer. Acta Obstet Gynecol Scand 71:224–225

Pettersson F (1994) Annual report on the results of treatment in gynecological cancer, vol 22. Radiumhemmet, Stockholm

Pfeiffer P, Mogensen H, Amtrup F, et al. (1989) Primary carcinoma of the fallopian tube. A retrospective study of patients reported to the Danish Cancer Registry in a five-year period. Acta Oncol 28:7

Phelps H, Chapman K (1974) Role of radiation therapy in treatment of primary carcinoma of the uterine tube. Obstet Gynecol 43:669–673

Podobnik M, Singer Z, Ciglar S, Bulic M (1993) Preoperative Diagnosis of primary fallopian tube carcinoma by transvaginal ultrasound, cytological finding and CA-125. Ultrasound Med Biol 19:587–591

Podratz KC, Podczaski ES, Gaffey TA, et al. (1986) Primary carcinoma of the fallopian tube. Am J Obstet Gynecol 154:1319

Raghavan S, Chadaya R, Rani R, Aemachigai A, Rajaram P (1991) A review of fallopian tube carcinoma over 20 years (1971–90). Pondicherry 28:188–195

Renard F, Ricci JV (1945) One hundred years of gynecology. Blakiston, Philadelphia

Roberts J, Lifshitz (1982) Primary adenocarcinoma of the fallopian tube. Gynecol Oncol 13:301–308

Robey SS, Silva EG, Gershenson DM, McLemore D, El-Naggar A, Orodonez NG (1989) Transitional cell carcinoma in high-grade, high-stage ovarian carcinoma: an indicator of favorable response to chemotherapy. Cancer 63:839–847

Rorat E, Wallach RC (1990) Endometrial carcinoma of the fallopian tube: pathology and clinical outcome. Int J Gynecol Obstet 32:163–167

Rose PG, Piver MS, Tsukada Y (1990) Fallopian tube cancer. The Roswell Park experience. Cancer 66:2661

Rosen A, Klein M, Lahousen M, Graf AH, Rainer A, Vavra N (1993) Primary carcinoma of the fallopian tube. A retrospective analysis of 115 patients. Br J Cancer 68:605–609

Rosen AC, Swelda P, Klein M, et al. (1994) A comparative analysis of management and prognosis in stage I and II fallopian tube carcinoma and epithelial ovarian cancer. Br J Cancer 69:577–579

Rosenblatt KA, Weiss NS, Schwartz SM (1989) Incidence of malignant fallopian tube tumors. Gynecol Oncol 35:236

Rubin S, Hoskins W, Lewis J, et al. (1988) Recurrence after negative second-look laparotomy for ovarian cancer: analysis of risk factors. Am J Obstet Gynecol 159:1094–1098

Scharl A, Crombach G, Vurbuchen M, et al. (1991) Antigen CA 19-9 presence in mucosa of nondiseased müllerian duct derivatives and marker for differentiation in their carcinomas. Obstet Gynecol 77:580

Scheffy LC, Lang WR, Nugent FB (1941) Clinical and pathologic aspects of primary sarcoma of the uterine tube. Am J Obstet Gynecol 52:904–915

Schiller HM, Silverberg SG (1971) Staging and prognosis in primary carcinoma of the fallopian tube. Cancer 28:389

Schray MF, Podratz KC, Malkasian GD (1987) Fallopian tube cancer: the role of radiation therapy. Radiother Oncol 10:267

Scully RF (1979) Embryology of the ovary. In: Tumors of the ovary and maldeveloped gonads. Armed Forces Institute of Pathology, Washington DC, pp 1–5

Sedlis A (1978) Carcinoma of the fallopian tube. Surg Clin North Am 58:121

Seraj I, King A, Chase D (1990) Malignant mixed müllerian tumor of the oviduct. Gynecol Oncol 37:296–301

Seraj I, Chase D, King A (1991) Endometrial carcinoma of the oviduct. Gynecol Oncol 41:152–155
Silva EG, Robey SS, Smith TL, Gershenson DM (1993) Ovarian carcinomas with transitional cell patterns. Am J Clin Pathol 93:457–465
Singhal S, Sharma S, De S, et al. (1991) Role of radiotherapy in the management of primary carcinoma of the fallopian tube. Indian J Med Sci 45:58
Sweet RL, Selinger HE, McKay DG (1975) Malignant teratoma of the uterine tube. Obstet Gynecol 45:553–556
Tamini HK, Figge DC (1981) Adenocarcinoma of the uterine tube: potential for lymph node metastases. Am J Obstet Gynecol 141:132
Thurner S, Hodler J, Baer S, Marincek B, Von Schultress G (1990) Gadolinium-DOTA enhanced MR Imaging of adnexal tumors. J Comput Assist Tomogr 14:939–949
Tokunaga T, Miyazaki K, Matsuyama S, et al. (1990) Serial measurements of CA-125 in patients with primary carcinoma of the fallopian tube. Gynecol Oncol 36:335
Verherge HG, Bareithu MZ, Jaffe RC, Akbar M (1979) Cyclic changes in ciliation secretion and cell height of the oviductal epithelium in women. Am J Anat 156:505–521
Voet RL, Lifshitz S (1992) Primary clear cell adenocarcinoma of the fallopian tube; light microscopic and ultrastructural findings. Int J Gynecol Pathol 1:292–298
Weber A, Hewett W, Cuny S, et al. (1993) Malignant mixed müllerian tumors of the fallopian tube. Gynecol Oncol 50:239–243
Wheeler JE (1994) In: Kurman RJ (ed) Blaustein's pathology of the female genital tract: diseases of the fallopian tube. Springer, Berlin Heidelberg New York, pp 529–561
Williams T, Woodruff JD (1963) Malignant mixed mesenchymal tumor of the uterine tube. Obstet Gynecol 21:618–621
Woodruff JD, Pauerstein CJ (1969) The fallopian tube. Williams & Wilkins, Baltimore
Yoonessi M, Leberer JP, Crickard K (1988) Primary fallopian tube carcinoma: treatment and spread pattern. J Surg Oncol 38:97

13 Genital Soft Tissue Sarcomas

H.-A. LADNER and U. KARCK

CONTENTS

13.1 Introduction

During recent decades more details regarding the pathology of gynecological sarcomas have become known; this is reflected in the detailed classification of uterine sarcomas in Table 13.1, taken from the interesting review on the pathology of uterine sarcomas by CLEMENT and SCULLY (1981). However, for the gynecologist and radiotherapist working in the hospital it has become more difficult to classify individual cases according to such systems or schemes. Nevertheless, it appears important to discover specific details about the characteristics of different subtypes of uterine sarcomas, especially as this might have therapeutic consequences. Following the classification of Table 13.1, this review will focus on the three most frequently observed subtypes of uterine sarcomas: leiomyosarcomas, endometrial stromal sarcomas, and mixed müllerian or mesodermal sarcomas or tumors, the latter including the adenosarcomas. The WHO (1975) and the Gynecologic Oncology Group (1985) have also suggested classifications concentrating on clinical aspects. In the final section of this contribution we have tried to outline the findings applicable to all uterine sarcomas, again concentrating on clinical aspects.

We hope that we have succeeded in providing a key for the understanding of the complicated field of uterine sarcomas. Mainly reviews and case histories published during the last 10 years have been taken into consideration. For details we recommend the following reviews: PIVER and LURAIN (1981), CLEMENT and SCULLY (1981) (pathology), ANTMANN (1986), MARCHESE and NORI (1987), SILVERBERG (1992) (mixed müllerian tumors), HANNIGAN et al. (1992) and ZALOUDEK and NORRIS (1994). Uterine sarcomas continue to present a challenge to the gynecological oncologist.

13.2 Endometrial Stromal Sarcoma

Endometrial stromal sarcoma (ESS) accounted for 8% of all uterine sarcomas referred to Radiumhemmet (Stockholm, Sweden) during a 46-year period. Endometrial stromal tumors [low grade (LGSS) and high grade (HGSS)] occurred in younger women than leiomyosarcoma, carcinosarcoma, or endometrial carcinoma. Histopathologically, 16 of 28 cases of stromal sarcomas treated from 1936 to 1981 at the Radiumhemmet were classified as high grade and 12 as low grade (LARSON et al. 1990a). A significant relation between mitotic count and relative survival within 10 years of the diagnosis was

H.-A. LADNER, MD, Professor, Im Großacker, 3, D-79249 Merzhausen, Germany
U. KARCK, MD, Universitäts-Frauenklinik, Hugstetter Straße 55, D-79106 Freiburg, Germany

Table 13.1. Classification of uterine sarcomas and related neoplasms

Pure mesenchymal
Homologous
Endometrial stromal
Endolymphatic stromal myosis (ESM)
(low-grade stromal sarcoma, stromatosis)
(High-grade) stromal sarcomas (ESS)
Smooth muscle
Leiomyosarcoma (LMS)
Leiomyoblastoma, malignant
(epitheloid smooth muscle tumor, malignant)
Heterologous
Rhabdomyosarcoma
Chondrosarcoma
Osteosarcoma
Liposarcoma
Of uncertain origin
Malignant müllerian mixed tumors (MMT)
Homologous (carcinosarcoma)
Heterologous
Müllerian adenosarcoma
Lymphoma and leukemia

found ($P < 0.05$) in this study, a more favorable outcome being observed for patients with low counts. More than 50% of patients were premenopausal or perimenopausal, and rare examples of ESS occurred in young woman and girls. There was no association with parity or endometrial risk factors, but a few patients had a history of prior pelvic irradiation.

Endometrial stromal tumors can be divided into three types based on mitotic activity, vascular invasion, and observed differences in prognosis. The endometrial stromal nodule is a lesion confined to the uterus, with less than ten mitoses per ten high power fields (HPF), and no lymphatic or vascular invasion. This is an expansile, noninfiltrating, solitary lesion and should be considered benign. The second type of endometrial stromal tumor is endolymphatic stromal myosis or endometrial stromatosis. This is a low-grade stromal sarcoma differing from true ESS only in the mitotic rate. Vascular and lymphatic invasion is common; therefore this lesion will have infiltrated the myometrium and extended beyond the uterus in 40% of cases at the time of diagnosis. The third type, ESS, is a rapidly lethal neoplasm (Norris and Taylor 1966; Salazar et al. 1978; Piver and Lurain 1981). ESS of grade 2 or 3 infiltrates the myometrium and metastasizes widely. Differential diagnosis of these tumors includes malignant lymphoma or undifferentiated small cell carcinoma of the cervix (Antmann 1986). Belgrad et al. (1975) advocated preoperative radiotherapy for ESS.

The type and extent of the tumor and the type of operation determine the risk of recurrence. The best 5-year survival rates reported in LGSS exceed 50%. The survival is less favorable (40%–50% for LGSS and 0%–50% for HGSS) when there is advanced disease at presentation. Recurrences occur in almost 50% of cases after initial therapy (Norris and Taylor 1966). Krieger and Gusberg (1973) suggested that radical hysterectomy may be the treatment of choice because of the high incidence of parametrial involvement and pelvic recurrence. A beneficial effect of radiation therapy has been reported (Norris and Taylor 1966).

A favorable influence of radiotherapy in ESS has been reported by several authors in cases with extrauterine growth and recurrent disease (Norris and Taylor 1966; Yoonessi and Hart 1977), including when given as adjuvant therapy (Piver and Lurain 1987; Taina et al. 1989; Larson et al. 1990a). In the series of Larson et al. (1990a) radiotherapy was part of the primary treatment. Seventeen out of 20 stage I patients received adjuvant radiotherapy with a 5-year survival of 73% (8/11) for the high-grade tumors. The effect of radiotherapy in low-grade ESS was difficult to evaluate due to the small number of cases and the more protracted course of these tumors. According to others the exact role of postoperative radiotherapy remains unclear (Piver et al. 1984; Taina et al. 1989).

Sutton et al. (1986) found the highest receptor levels in low-grade ESS; therefore progesterone could be supposed to have a beneficial effect in low-grade ESS both as adjuvant treatment and as treatment for recurrent and metastatic disease. Chemotherapy was ineffective in LGSS (Berchuk et al. 1990).

13.3 Leiomyosarcoma (LMS)

13.3.1 Clinical Features and Prognosis

Leiomyosarcomas (LMS) account for 1.3% of uterine malignancies and about one-third of uterine sarcomas (Zaloudek and Norris 1994). The mean age of patients with LMS has been reported to be 52 years (range 40–70 years) (Kahanpäa et al. 1986; Nickie-Psikuta and Gawrychowski 1993).

Compared with patients with ESS or mixed müllerian tumors, a higher percentage of LMS patients will present as stage I. Both age and menopausal status have been shown to influence survival (MARCHESE et al. 1984). It has been reported that premenopausal LMS patients have significantly better survival rates than postmenopausal patients (SILVERBERG 1971; VARDI and TOWELL 1980). In these studies, however, patient age was not correlated with clinical stage. In the series of KAHANPÄÄ et al. (1986), patients younger than 50 years of age had a better prognosis, but most of these patients (82%) had stage I disease. The more favorable prognosis of the premenopausal patients could be explained on the basis of the clinical stage of the disease rather than the patients' age. The use of histological criteria to estimate the prognosis of uterine LMS has been the source of much controversy (SILVERBERG 1971; SAKSELA et al. 1974; VARDI and TOWELL 1980). The histological degree of differentiation has been found to correlate with the mitotic activity as an indicator of prognosis on a statistical basis (SILVERBERG 1971). As with other histological types of sarcoma, extrauterine extention of LMS carries a worse prognosis (SILVERBERG 1971; VONGTAMA et al. 1976; SALAZAR et al. 1978; DINH and WOODRUFF 1982). In the LMS group, a markedly poorer prognosis was observed if the mitotic index was 5.0 or higher (KAHANPÄÄ et al. 1986). The use of mitotic counts is now becoming accepted as the most reproducible and accurate criterion for defining LMS (AARO et al. 1966; SAKSELA et al. 1974). The number of mitoses in the tumor seems to be the most reliable indicator of malignant behavior (SILVERBERG 1971; CHRISTOPHERSON et al. 1972; SALAZAR et al. 1978). TAYLOR and NORRIS (1966) found that none of their 21 patients with tumors having fewer than ten mitoses per ten high power fields died of disease, whereas 31 of the 36 patients with tumors having ten or more mitoses developed metastatic or recurrent disease.

Survival rates of patients with LMS have been reported to be 20%–63% (CHRISTOPHERSON et al. 1972; SAKSELA et al. 1974, 39%; KAHANPÄÄ et al. 1986, 52%; NICKIE-PSIKUTA and GAWRYCHOWSKI 1993). The pattern of tumor spread was to the myometrium, pelvic blood vessels and lymphatics, adjacent pelvic structures, and then distant sites, most commonly the lungs. Survival after recurrence is poor regardless of initial stage or histology. Less than 30% of patients will survive for 1 year and less than 10% for 2 years following local and/or distal tumor recurrence (MARCHESE et al. 1984; MARCHESE and NORI 1987).

SUTTON et al. (1992) found in a phase II groupwide study of the Gynecologic Oncology Group with 52 patients it was found that ifosfamide had modest activity in patients with advanced or recurrent LMS of the uterus. There are four clinicopathological variants: leiomyoblastoma, intravenous leiomyomatosis, metastasizing uterine leiomyoma, and leiomyomatosis peritonealis disseminata (PIVER and LURAIN 1981).

13.3.2 Therapy

Many different methods of treatment have been used, especially in patients with stage III or IV disease. Because the patient groups in all series have been small, it has not been possible to draw conclusions about the relative value of the different treatment methods. However, the effect of postoperative external radiotherapy could be studied in stage I and II leiomyosarcoma patients: 16 of 32 patients studied were alive 5 years after therapy (KAHANPÄÄ et al. 1986). In this study, no additional effect of radiation therapy could be demonstrated. SALAZAR and DUNNE (1980) found that there was a trend towards better 5-year survival results for stage I patients with LMS who were treated with surgery and radiation than for those who were treated with surgery alone (72 patients were analyzed, with 13 surviving longer than 5 years). Due to the small number of patients, however, the difference was not statistically significant.

Postoperative pelvic irradiation delivering 50 Gy to the pelvic axis in 5 weeks followed by intravaginal iridium or other contact therapy to the vaginal surface has been strongly recommended (SALAZAR and DUNNE 1980). The latter should only be applied when the tumor has involved the cervix (stage II), when invasion of more than 50% of the myometrium is found, or when a small surgical cuff has been left at hysterectomy. In a review published in 1987, MARCHESE and NORI demonstrated a 30% improvement in the 5-year survival rate following radiotherapy (77% for the combination of surgery and radiotherapy versus 48% after surgery alone) using the combined results from PEREZ et al. (1979), SALAZAR and DUNNE (1980), and MARCHESE et al. (1984) for their analysis.

In LMS patients the most important factor determining 5-year survival seems to be mitotic activity (LARSON et al. 1990). In cases with low-grade mitotic activity, NICKIE-PSIKUTA and GARWYCHOWSKI (1993) found adjuvant radiotherapy (63.6% survival) to yield better results than surgery alone (54.5% survival). KULLER et al. (1990) emphasized the need to perform biopsy of vulvar LMS during pregnancy.

Other histological types (mainly heterologous): A clinical and pathological staging system for soft tissue sarcomas was described by RUSSELL et al. (1977). The distribution of cases by histological type (rhabdomyosarcoma, liposarcoma, angiosarcoma, etc.) and the 5-year survival rates were analyzed in 1215 cases of 13 types of soft tissue sarcoma, primarily in the extremities.

In the differential diagnosis of uterine sarcomas, retroperitoneal soft tissue sarcoma, with a 5-year survival rate of 36%, is important (CATTON et al. 1994).

13.4 Mixed Müllerian Tumors

The classification scheme of the International Society of Gynecological Pathologists (1989) is reproduced in Table 13.2. The classification of MMT following pathological and anatomical criteria demonstrates the complexity of these tumors, which have to be distinguished from malignant adenosarcomas.

13.4.1 Malignant Mixed Müllerian Tumors

The preferred nomenclature for this lesion in the new classification is carcinosarcoma, but these tumors are commonly known as malignant mixed mesodermal tumors or malignant mixed müllerian tumors. These tumors are uncommon neoplasms, accounting for 1%–3% of all uterine corporal malignant tumors. They are composed of a mixture of a malignant epithelial element (carcinoma) and a malignant mesenchymal element (sarcoma), and the prognosis has been described as uniformly poor. The tumors are subdivided into two types – homologous MMT and heterologous MMT – depending on the presence or absence of heterologous mesenchymal elements such as rhabdomyosarcoma, chondrosarcoma, and osteosarcoma. To date the histogenesis of the mixed tumors, and especially of the heterologous forms, is not entirely clear. Excellent references about the histogenesis can be found in the literature (CHUANG et al. 1970; MORTEL et al. 1974). The oldest theory (COHNHEIM 1875) saw these tumors as evolving from dystopic embryonal germ cells. Other theories followed, suggesting blastomatous degeneration of endometrial stroma (WILLIAM and WOODRUFF 1962) or of epithelial and mesenchymal cells (VELIOS et al. 1962; JOPP 1965) or blastic differentiation of an omnipotent mesenchymal cell lying directly underneath the surface of the endometrium (STERNBERG et al. 1954; KATENKAMP and STILLER 1973; SCHMITT and SCHÄFER 1976).

Table 13.2. Classification of uterine mixed epithelial-nonepithelial tumors according to the International Society of Gynecological Pathologists

Benign
Adenofibroma
Adenomyoma
Variant – atypical polypoid adenomyoma
Malignant
Adenosarcoma
Homologous
Heterologous
Carcinosarcoma (malignant mixed mesodermal tumor; malignant mixed müllerian tumor)
Homologous
Heterologous
Carcinofibroma

13.4.1.1 Prognostic Factors

Premenopausal patients and those younger than 50 years have the best prognosis, particularly for stage I. Patients over 70 have the highest mortality. In the Memorial Hospital series of MMT patients (MARCHESE and NORI 1987), for example, five of five patients who had stage I disease and were premenopausal and younger than 50 survived 5 years. Thirty patients older than 50 had a 49% 5-year actuarial survival and 27 postmenopausal patients had a 46% survival. For stages II–IV, however, the prognosis is uniformly poor. Among stage I patients, those with deep myometrial tumor penetration tend to have a worse prognosis. Stage I patients with tumor infiltration of less than one-third of the myometrium had a 67% 5-year survival, whereas those with deeper infiltration had a 44% 5-year survival in the Memorial Hospital Series.

13.4.1.2 Treatment and Prognosis

Total abdominal hysterectomy with bilateral salpingo-oophorectomy (TAH-BSO) is the accepted method for primary therapy. The most important single factor affecting prognosis is the spread of the tumor at the time of the first treatment. The overall 5-year survival has approximated 30% in most series (SAKSELA et al. 1974; SALAZAR et al. 1978; KAHANPÄÄ et al. 1986).

The important question to be resolved is the role of adjuvant therapy. No prospective randomized trials of adjuvant radiotherapy have been reported. In the literature, SALAZAR and DUNNE (1980) found 990 cases available for 5-year survival analysis. However, only 410 (41%) could be analyzed by stage and only 254 (26%) could be reanalyzed by stage and treatment method. A relatively large series of 72 patients with a single histology (MMS), treated between 1951 und 1981, was analyzed by MARCHESE and NORI (1987). For both stage I and stages II–III (surgically staged), a statistically significant difference in survival was seen in the adjuvant radiotherapy group: 64% versus 41% 5-year survival for stage I, and 49% versus 10% for stages II–III. PEREZ et al. (1979) suggested that patients with stages I and II should be treated with preoperative irradiation (more than 50 Gy) and surgery.

MMT tumors rarely occur in extragenital sites. Twenty-one patients with primary MMT of the peritoneum have been reported in the literature (GARAMVOELGYI et al. 1994). Primary MMT of the female peritoneum is a rare but highly malignant neoplasm occurring in elderly postmenopausal women. The prognosis is gloomy despite the various treatments that have been attempted.

13.4.2 Adenosarcoma

Adenosarcoma most often arises in the endometrium, but also occurs in the cervix or extrauterine pelvic locations such as the fallopian tube, ovary, and paraovarian tissues. Adenosarcoma was first described in 1974 by CLEMENT and SCULLY. Since then, several hundred cases have been reported, with the largest series comprising 100 (CLEMENT and SCULLY 1990), 31 (KAKU et al. 1992) and 25 (ZALOUDEK and NORRIS 1981) cases. Adenosarcoma occurs in patients of all ages. The reported median age is about 57 years, with a range of 14–79 years. Adenosarcoma was not as aggressive as mixed muellerian tumor. Thus adenosarcoma is usually diagnosed in middle-aged or elderly women (IRMSCHER et al. 1995: 81 years), with a mean age between 55 and 60 years, but cases have been seen in younger women and even in children (ZALOUDEK and NORRIS 1981; CLEMENT and SCULLY 1990; SÖLDER et al. 1995). Most tumors arise in the uterine fundus; they are usually solitary, and the average diameter has been reported to be about 5 cm (CLEMENT and SCULLY 1990).

In most series, the majority of cases of adenosarcoma have not invaded the myometrium and have not recurred following surgical excision. In the large series of CLEMENT and SCULLY (1990), recurrences developed in approximately 25% of cases, usually within the vagina, pelvis, or abdomen, and often appeared after an interval of 5 years or more following hysterectomy. In the series of ZALOUDEK and NORRIS (1981), recurrence occurred in 40% of the cases, with a median interval of 5 years. Death from tumor progression occurred in 24%. In the study of KAKU et al. (1992), 30% of cases recurred and 20% of patients died of tumor progression. Recurrence generally occurred in the pelvis or vagina, but distant metastasis occurred in 5% of patients.

In general, the treatment of adenosarcoma has to date been almost exclusively surgical, with some patients receiving radiation or chemotherapy for recurrent disease. Among those cases which have recurred, many of the recurrences have been vaginal, and these have been composed of either pure sarcoma or adenosarcoma; distant metastases have generally been composed of pure sarcoma (CLEMENT and SCULLY 1990).

13.5 Sarcoma and Carcinosarcoma of the Uterine Cervix

Primary sarcoma and carcinosarcoma of the uterine cervix are exceedingly rare neoplasms. Cervival sarcomas account for less than 0.5% (CRAWFORD and TUCKER 1959; CHANG 1957) of all primary cervical malignancies and only about 100 cases have been reported, 12 of them by ABELL and RAMIREZ (1973). Histologically, primary sarcomas of the cervix are classified in the same way as their counterparts in the corpus uteri (ABELL and RAMIREZ 1973; ROTMENSCH et al. 1983; ABDUL-KARIM et al. 1987). The patient's average age has been reported as 54 years, ranging from 15 to 72 years (MIYAZAWA and HERNANDEZ 1986). On physical examination the patients demonstrate polyploid or solid masses replacing the cervix. A simple classification of cervical sarcomas has been proposed by ROTMENSCH et al.

(1983). It divides cervical sarcomas into two mayor groups: leiomyosarcomas and stromal sarcomas. In the view of these authors, mixed müllerian tumors belong to the group of stromal sarcomas. The stromal sarcomas are classified as homologous or heterologous, the homologous subgroup being composed of tissue normally present in the cervix, and the heterologous subgroup with malignant elements basically not found in the cervix. Only 12 cases (ROTMENSCH et al. 1983) of endocervical stromal sarcoma have been reported so far. Most of the described müllerian adenosarcomas have been located in the uterine corpus and have been found in older women (KATZENSTEIN et al. 1977; DAMJANOW et al. 1978). Adenosarcoma of the uterine cervix has been encountered only in five cases (ROTH et al. 1976; FAYEMI et al. 1978; GAL et al. 1988). All patients with cervical adenosarcoma have had a favorable outcome with conservative management only. GAL et al. (1988) described a case in a teenage girl with heterologous elements and with a fatal outcome. The metastases of this tumor are usually homologous and composed of the same tissue as the primary lesion (JAFFE et al. 1985).

Surgery is the main therapy (ABELL and RAMIREZ 1973). More than 50% of patients die during the first 2 years, and only those with well-differentiated lesions survive that period (JAFFE et al. 1985). Only a few patients have been treated by hysterectomy followed by radiation. It is very difficult to decide whether this tumor is relatively radioresistant because the prognosis for patients with this tumor is very poor (JAFFE et al. 1985).

13.6 Carcinosarcoma (Malignant Mixed Mesodermal Tumor) of the Corpus Uteri

The mean age of patients with carcinosarcoma of the corpus uteri has been reported to be 65 years (CHUANG et al. 1970), 67.7 years (KÜHN et al. 1982), 65 years (SHAW et al. 1983), and 63 years (KAHANPÄÄ et al. 1986). The patients are usually 10 years older than woman with leiomyosarcoma of the uterus or patients with endometrial carcinoma. Most women with MMT are postmenopausal. In the series of SALAZAR et al. (1978) and KAHANPÄÄ et al. (1986), MMTs occurred later in life than did leiomyosarcoma or other histological types of uterine sarcoma. This group of patients also had the worst prognosis. The results of these studies were in agreement with most earlier reports.

A pilot study by the Gynecologic Oncology Group found 10 of 28 (35%) stage I mixed müllerian sarcomas to have positive pelvic lymph nodes when sampled at surgery (DI SAIA et al. 1978). Dissection of pelvic lymph nodes revealed metastatic tumor in 17% of cases that appeared to be limited to the uterus. According to the literature, 5-year survival in the mixed müllerian sarcoma group is poor – between 0% and 32%. CHUANG et al. (1970) reported a 30% survival rate among stage I patients, but a 0% survival rate if the disease extended beyond the uterus. SALAZAR et al. (1978) observed a 5-year survival of 62% after radical surgery with pelvic exenteration among stage I patients and 33% among all stages of mixed müllerian tumors. SALAZAR et al. (1978) reported failure of treatment to the pelvis in only 1 of 12 stage I patients. The radiotherapy usually consisted of postoperative external irradiation with bilateral 120° arcs delivering 45 Gy to the pelvic side walls of the pelvis. SPANOS et al. (1984) reported a large series of MMT patients (108 cases) from the M.D. Anderson Hospital, Houston, Texas. Eighty-four patients treated for cure received surgery and radiotherapy. Overall, 5-year disease-free survival was 52% for 50 stage I cases and 28% for 18 stage II–III cases. The 10-year survival figures were significantly worse ($P < 0.05$) in the MMT group (14%) than in the groups with leiomyosarcoma (27%) or endometrial stromal sarcoma (37%) (KAHANPÄA et al. 1986; SALAZAR et al. 1978).

The most important reason for precision in the diagnosis of uterine carcinosarcoma is the extremely unfavorable prognosis of this tumor, with 5-year survival rates in recently reported series ranging between 18% and 39% [KAHANPÄÄ et al. 1986 (37.7%); NIELSEN et al. 1989; DINH et al. 1989; PODCSCASKI et al. 1989; GALLUP et al. 1989 (32%); SCHWEIZER et al. 1990 (38%)]. This largely reflects the fact that most patients present with tumor which has already spread to extrauterine sites. The surgical stage and the depth of myometrial invasion of the tumor have been shown to be important prognostic indicators in almost all large published series, although other pathological factors have been more controversial (SILVERBERG et al. 1990). Only 29% of their patients with mixed müllerian tumor were in stage I (KAHANPÄÄ et al. 1986). MMT may contain estrogen and progesterone receptors (SALAZAR et al. 1978; SUTTON et al. 1986). Increased receptor levels seem to be associated with improved short-term survival, but SUTTON et al. (1986) found that women whose tumors were receptor-positive did not have an improved long-term survival, nor did they respond to hormonal therapy.

In a series of 29 MMT patients, MARTH et al. (1990) demonstrated the prognostic relevance of tumor spread and parity; these findings were supported by CHRISTENSEN et al. (1994) in their study in Essen (24 MMT patients). MAJOR et al. (1993) found that patients with a heterologous component in their sarcomas had a worse prognosis than patients with carcinosarcomas. A similar conclusion was drawn by BARWICK and LIVOLSO (1979). However, MARTH et al. (1990) reported different results. The Essen study underlined the bad prognosis of patients with MMT, citing a 5-year survival rate of less than 30%.

Women with stage II and III MMT are often treated with postoperative pelvic radiation, since in some studies women treated with combined therapy have been shown to have a lower risk of pelvic recurrence (SALAZAR et al. 1978; ECHT et al. 1990).

13.7 Primary Sarcoma of the Fallopian Tube

Primary sarcomas of the fallopian tube are exceedingly rare. Excluding malignant mixed müllerian tumors, only 35 cases have been reported in the literature in more than 100 years (SENGER 1886; BLAIKLEY 1973; JACOBY et al. 1993). The age at diagnosis has varied from 21 to 70 years, with a median of 47 years. Prognosis is poor; however, long-term survivors have been reported. The primary treatment is surgery, but adjuvant radiation or chemotherapy may be of some benefit.

13.8 Malignant Mixed Tumor of the Vagina

Biphasic tumors of the vagina, consisting of both epithelial and mesenchymal elements, are also very rare. OGAGAKI et al. (1976) and SHEVCHUK et al. (1978) each published a case of a biphasic vaginal tumor resembling synovial carcinoma. The tumor reported by SHEVCHUK et al. arose in the upper lateral vagina, probably in mesonephric rests. A similar case was reported by HERTIG and GARE in 1960; that lesion was found on the posterior wall of the vagina just inside the hymenal ring and seemed more benign. The two aforementioned malignant biphasic tumors resembled synovial sarcomas histologically and ultrastructurally.

13.9 Lymphoma

Lymphoma rarely occurs with initial uterine involvement, but when it does, the cervix is the presenting site three times more often than the endometrium. Lymphoma occurs predominantly in women aged 20 years or older. Hodgkin's disease rarely involves the uterus (RAGGIO et al. 1988). An 89% survival rate has been reported in patients with localized (Ann Arbor stage IE) lymphoma of the uterus and vagina (HARRIS and SCULLY 1984). The differential diagnosis includes leiomyoma containing a heavy lymphocytic infiltrate and lymphoma-like lesions (pseudolymphoma). Uterine involvement as an initial manifestation of leukemia is even rarer than lymphoma at this site (HARRIS and SCULLY 1984; ZUTTER and GERSELL 1990).

13.10 Final Remarks and Findings Regarding All Types of Uterine Sarcoma

13.10.1 Staging and Its Significance

Stage is the most important prognostic factor in patients with malignant sarcomas. Staging has generally followed the FIGO (International Federation of Gynecologists and Obstetricians) system for endometrial carcinomas (Annual Report 1992, vol. 20 and 21). When corrected for stage and age, no significant differences in survival can be demonstrated between the three main histological forms. A higher percentage of LMS than of MMS or ESS patients will present as stage I. However, multivariate analysis showed that if similar cases for stage, age and histological grade are compared then mixed mesodermal tumors carry a better prognosis than leiomyosarcomas (OLAH et al. 1992). The results of a retrospective study of 423 cases of uterine sarcomas demonstrated very well the danger of considering each variable in isolation when the relation between variables can lead to spurious significance or lack of significance because of imbalance in numbers between groups of prognostic importance (OLAH et al. 1992). This study underlined the need for an adequate inspection of the intra-abdominal contents at the time of hysterectomy for uterine sarcoma.

It has not been necessary to study all sarcomas of the uterus as one entity, since histological criteria have become well established and the numbers of series of these rare tumors have increased. More recent reports have been confined to one particular subtype (PEREZ et al. 1979; LARSON et al. 1990a,b; SILVERBERG 1992). These studies have been undertaken to reveal clinical differences and prognosis in particular types of uterine sarcoma.

13.10.2 Lymph Node Metastases

The high rate of nodal involvement in patients with stage I sarcoma of the uterus (9 of 20, i.e., 45%, showed pelvic and/or para-aortic lymph node involvement) was associated with deep myometrial invasion, uteri with a cavity larger than 8 cm, patients older than 65 years, and leiomyosarcoma (MAJOR et al. 1987, 1993). Local recurrence in stage I decreased from nine of 22 cases in which operation alone was performed to none of 15 cases in which pelvic radiotherapy was added, but no improvement in the 5-year survival rate was observed (COVENS et al. 1987). Like lymphadenectomy and radiotherapy, the use of chemotherapy for uterine sarcoma has been found to have no impact on survival (COVENS et al. 1987).

13.10.3 Previous Irradiation

The most frequently mentioned risk factor for uterine sarcoma is previous irradiation (7–26 years earlier: BARTSICK et al. 1967; SALAZAR et al. 1978, NICKIE-PSIKUTA and GAWRYCHOWSKI 1993). The relative risk of developing uterine sarcomas following pelvic irradiation has been estimated at 2%. The data obtained from the literature suggest that mixed müllerian tumors are the most frequent mesenchymal tumor to arise after previous irradiation (NORRIS and TAYLOR 1966; MIYAZAWA and HERNANDEZ 1986), though MMT of the female peritoneum also displays this tendency (GARAMVOELGYI et al. 1994).

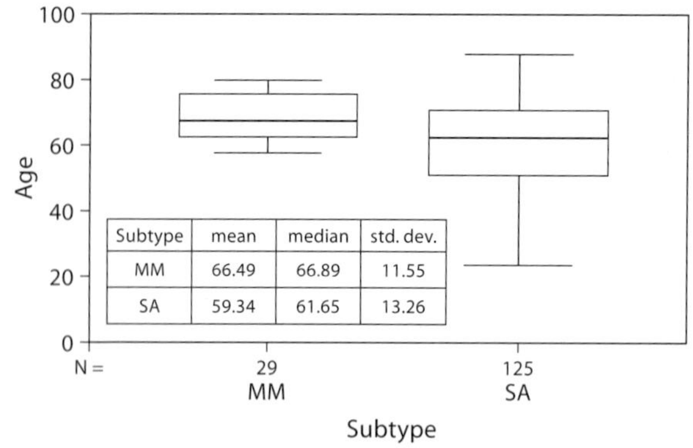

Fig. 13.1. Box plot of the age distribution of 29 patients with MMT and 125 patients with other uterine sarcomas (*SA*). The mean age for MMT patients was 66.5 years, and that for SA patients, 59.3 years. The difference between the two groups is statistically significant (Mann-Whitney *U* test, $P < 0.005$)

13.10.4 Age Distribution

Even though uterine sarcomas can be found in women of all age groups, they tend to occur in peri- and postmenopausal women. MMT generally occurs at a higher age than other uterine sarcomas, as shown by an analysis of a series of 154 women treated at the Freiburg University Women's Hospital (UFK Freiburg) between 1964 and 1992. Figure 1.31 shows a box plot of the age distribution of these patients. Women with an MMT presented at a median age of 66.9 years in comparison to 61.5 years for other sarcoma patients. This difference was statistically significant ($P < 0.005$, Mann Whitney *U* test) and appeared to be mainly due to a wider age distribution in the non-MMT group.

13.10.5 Overall Five-Year Survival

First, we will present the overall survival of patients with uterine sarcomas, including MMT, at the UFK Freiburg. The 50% survival rate was reached after 2.8 years in both groups (MMT and other sarcomas). The 5-year survival was 39.1% and 37% respectively (Fig. 13.2). When looking at both groups together, it is apparent that the survival curve shows a frightening decline during the first 2 years after diagnosis. Thereafter it levels off to run nearly parallel to overall survival curves for controls of the same age group. This observation supports the clinical impression that the therapy of uterine sarcomas appears to constitute an all or

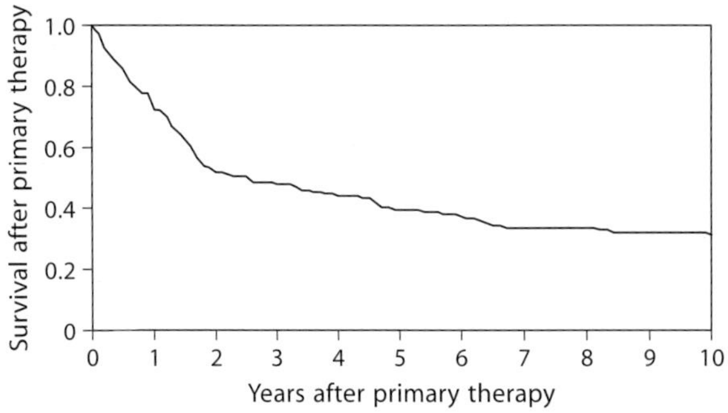

Fig. 13.2. Kaplan-Meier survival estimates of 154 patients with uterine sarcomas treated at the UFK Freiburg between 1964 and 1992. Patients were mainly treated by surgery and postoperative radiotherapy (telecobalt external beam). The survival rates taken from this curve support those reported in smaller series (see text)

nothing situation: either the tumor is removed completely or it will kill its bearer within a very short time. Thus tumor stage, with the question of whether the tumor can be completely removed surgically or not, becomes the most important prognostic factor.

The 5-year survival rates reported in the literature range very widely, from a few percent to 40%. The overall 5-year survival data as presented by the different authors are as follows: 38.3% (WOLF and VAHRSON 1976), 27% (SALAZAR et al. 1978), 40% (TEUFEL et al. 1980), 36% (ATZINGER et al. 1982), 25% (KELLER et al. 1987), 31% (OLAH et al. 1991, 1992), 18% (PEIFFERT et al. 1991), and 34.5% (NICKIE-PSIKUTA and GAWRYCHOWSKI 1993). The single most important factor was reported to be tumor spread at the time of diagnosis (SALAZAR et al. 1978; ATZINGER et al. 1982; TEUFEL et al. 1980; KAHANPÄÄ et al. 1986; MARCHESE and NORI 1987; MAJOR et al. 1993). Therefore survival depends on the proportion of early cases. The number of early cases varied immensely between the studies: half of the patients reported by SALAZAR et al. (1978) were in stage I, and 54% survived 5 years. In the study by TEUFEL et al. (1980), 61% of the patients were in stage I. ATZINGER et al. (1982) had 48% stage I patients and found a 5-year survival rate of 42%.

These overall survival rates provide very little information on the efficacy of different therapies. Even studies with more than 100 patients suffering from certain subtypes of uterine sarcoma provide very little information with regard to the therapies applied, and provide only hints as to the possibility of a positive response to a certain form of therapy. In the larger studies the results obtained for the different subtypes have mainly indicated the differences between these histological entities and not between different therapeutic approaches.

The overall 5-year survival rates in particular subgroups were as follows: 52% in LMS, 30% in ESS, and 20% in MMT and cervical sarcomas (NICKIE-PSIKUTA and GAWRYCHOWSKI 1992). No difference in survival was found between the main histological variants of uterine sarcoma when a univarate analysis was performed (OLAH et al. 1992: LMS 34%, ESS 42%, and MMT 33%, $n = 423$). The multivariate analysis of OLAH et al. (1992) showed that, for patients with a similar stage, age, and grade, mixed müllerian mesodermal tumors had a better prognosis than leiomyosarcomas.

The further course of the disease in stage I and stage II tumors is influenced by the histological grading (AARO et al. 1966). Using survival curves, EBERL et al. (1980) showed that patients in these stages with grade 1 and 2 lesions exhibited a better 5-year survival rate than patients with grade 3 and 4 lesions (77% versus 41%).

HANNIGAN et al. (1983) recommended *reexploration of the abdomen* after therapy for uterine sarcomas (second-look laparotomy), but there is some controversy as to whether the techniques that have evolved for the reexploration of patients with overian carcinoma can be used to evaluate patients with uterine sarcomas. The biological behavior of uterine sarcomas is believed to be dramatically different from that of ovarian tumors. Second-look laparotomy after a period of therapy provided valuable prognostic information for planning of further therapy in 11 patients with uterine sarcomas (HANNIGAN et al. 1983, 1992).

MALMSTROEM et al. (1992) investigated the prognostic importance of *DNA ploidy and S-phase rate* in relation to mitotic count, tumor stage, tumor grade, and histology in 37 patients with uterine sarcomas. The 5-year survival rate was only 11% in aneuploid cases compared with 59% in diploid cases. No significant differences were seen between histological types. There are only a few reports on the value of flow cytometry in uterine sarcoma (NELSON et al. 1987; DE FUSCO et al. 1988; TSUSHIMA et al. 1988; AUGUST et al. 1989).

In an analysis of 15 patients with soft tissue sarcoma, BRIZEL et al. (1995) showed that intrapatient heterogeneity was less than interpatient heterogeneity with respect to *median pO_2 and hypoxic fraction.* This was also true for other histologies and anatomical sites. Recently, NORDSMARK et al. (1994) evaluated the heterogeneity of tumor oxygenation in patients with soft tissue sarcoma. They concluded that intrapatient heterogeneity was less than interpatient heterogeneity with respect to median pO_2 and hypoxic fraction. The aim was to determine the value of tumor oxygen measurement as a predictor of treatment outcome in patients with soft tissue sarcomas.

13.10.6 Radiotherapy

Although often considered radioresistant in the past, more recent studies (GILBERT et al. 1975; KAHANPÄÄ et al. 1986; MARCHESE and NORI 1987) in which significant numbers of patients have received radiotherapy have made a strong argument for *the use of adjuvant radiotherapy* to increase local control and survival.

The patterns of failure have not appeared to vary by histology. More than 80% of tumor recurrences have arisen within the first 2 years. About two-thirds of patients who are initially controlled will fail in the pelvis (SALAZAR et al. 1978; MARCHESE et al. 1984, MARCHESE and NORI 1987).

Reviews of the results reported from the *neutron therapy* centers (WAMBERSIE 1988) and of radiotherapy with pions (THUM et al. 1988) indicated an overall local control rate after neutron therapy of 53% and a 2-year survival rate of 56% for inoperable soft tissue sarcomas. As not only uterine sarcomas were included in the study, it remains to be established whether neutron therapy will provide improved results in patients with uterine sarcomas.

13.10.7 Cytostatic Agents

The limited efficacy of chemotherapeutic agents in the treatment of uterine sarcomas is illustrated by the review by BOKEMEYER et al. (1994). Only a few cytostatic drugs have been used for the treatment of adult soft tissue sarcomas, with adriamycin and ifosfamide being the most active agents, achieving response rates of 20%–35%. In addition, for dacarbazine and cyclophosphamide responses have been reported in 10%–20% of patients. Clinical studies have indicated a dose-response relationship for adriamycin and ifosfamide. However, complete remissions were achieved in only a small proportion of cases, and the overall duration of responses after escalated doses of active agents in soft tissue sarcomas was not longer than for standard therapy. Currently dose-intensified chemotherapy cannot be regarded as standard treatment for soft tissue sarcomas, and its value must be studied in further controlled clinical trials.

References

Aaro LA, Symmonds RE, Dockerty MB (1966) Sarcoma of the uterus. Am J Obstet Gynecol 94:101–109

Abdul-Karim FW, Bazi TM, Sorensen K, Nasr M (1987) Sarcomas of the uterine cervix: clinicopathologic findings in three cases. Gynecol Oncol 26:103–111

Abell MR, Ramirez JA (1973) Sarcomas and carcinosarcomas of the uterine cervix. Cancer 31:1176–1184

Annual report on the results of treatment in gynecological cancer vol. 21 (1992) Pettersson F (ed). Elsevier, Amsterdam

Antmann KH (1986) In: Gynecological oncology. Knapp RC, Berkowitz RS (eds) Uterine sarcomas. Macmillan, New York, pp 297–311

Atzinger A, Ries G, Hötzinger H, Hermans M, Pfänder K (1982) Zur Klinik, Therapie und Prognose des Uterussarkoms. Strahlenther Onkol 158:210–216

August CZ, Bauer KD, Lurain J, Murad T (1989) Neoplasms of endometrial stroma: histopathologic and flowcytometric analysis with clinical correlation. Human Pathol 20:232–237

Bartsich EG, Bowe ET, Moore JG (1968) Leiomyomasarcoma of the uterus. A 50 year review of 42 cases. Obstet Gynecol 32:101–105

Barwick KW, Livolso VA (1979) Malignant mixed müllerian tumor of the uterus, a clinicopathologic assesment of 34 cases. Am J Surg Pathol 3:125–135

Belgrad R, Elbadawi N, Rubin P (1975) Uterine sarcomas. Radiology 114:181–188

Berchuk A, Rubin SC, Hoskins WJ, Saigo PE, Pierce VK, Lewis JL Jr (1990) Treatment of endometrial stromal tumors. Gynecol Oncol 36:60–65

Blaikley JB (1973) Sarcoma of the fallopian tube. J Obstet Gynaecol Br Commonw 80:759–760

Bokemeyer C, Harstrick A, Schmoll HJ (1994) Treatment of adult soft-tissue sarcomas with dose-intensified chemotherapy and haematopoietic growth factors. Onkologie 17:216–225

Brizel DM, Rosner GL, Prosnitz LR, Dewhirst MW (1995) Patterns and variability of tumor oxygenation in human soft tissue sarcomas, cervical carcinomas, and lymph node metastases. Int J Radiat Oncol Biol Phys 32:1121–1125

Catton CN, O'Sullivan B, Kotwall C, Cummings B, Hao Y, Fornasier V (1994) Outcome and prognosis in retroperitoneal soft tissue sarcoma. Int J Radiat Oncol Biol Phys 29:1005–1010

Chen SS (1989) Propensity of retroperitoneal lymph node metastasis in patients with stage I sarcoma of the uterus. Gynecol Oncol 32:215–217

Cheng WF, Lin HH, Chen CK, Chang DY, Huang SC (1995) Leiomyosarcoma of the broad ligament: a case report and literature review. Gynecol Oncol 56:85–89

Christensen B, Annweiler H, Schütte J, Schindler AE (1994) Maligne Müllersche Mischtumoren. Prognose, Verlauf und chemotherapeutische Möglichkeiten bei fortgeschrittenen Tumoren bzw. Rezidiven. Tumordiagn Therapie 15:53–56

Christopherson WM, Williamson EO, Gray LA (1972) Leiomyosarcoma of the uterus. Cancer 29:1512–1527

Chuang JT, van Velden JJ, Graham JB (1970) Carcinosarcoma and mixed mesodermal tumor of the uterine corpus: review of 49 cases. Obstet Gynecol 35:769–780

Clement PB, Scully RE (1974) Müllerian adenosarcoma of the uterus. A clinicopathologic analysis of ten cases of a distinctive type of müllerian mixed tumor. Cancer 34:1138–1149

Clement PB, Scully RE (1990) Müllerian adenosarcoma of the uterus. A clinicopathological analysis of 100 cases with a review of the literature. Hum Pathol 21:363–381

Clement PB, Scully RE (1981) Pathology of uterine sarcomas. In: Coppleson M (ed) Gynecologic oncology. Churchill Livingstone, Edinburgh, pp 591–607

Covens AI, Nisker JA, Chapman WB, Allen HH (1987) Uterine sarcoma: an analysis of 74 cases. Am J Obstet Gynecol 136:370–374

Crawford EJ, Tucker R (1959) Sarcoma of the uterus. Am J Obstet Gynecol 77:286–291

Damajanow J, Casey MJ, Maenza RM, Kennedy AW (1978) Müllerian adenosarcoma of the uterus. Ultrastructure before and after radiation therapy. Am J Clin Pathol 70:96–103

De Fusco P, Gaffey T, Malkasian G, Long H, Cha S, Wieand HS (1988) Endometrial stroma sarcoma: review of the Mayo experience, 1945–1980. Proc Ann Meet Am Soc Clin Oncol 7:A559

Dinh TV, Woodruff JD (1982) Leiomyosarcoma of the uterus. Am J Obstet Gynecol 144:817–823

Dinh TV, Slavin RE, Bhagavan BS, Hannigan EV, Tiamson EM, Yandel BB (1989) Mixed müllerian tumors of the uterus: a clinicopathological study. Obstet Gynecol 74:388–392

Di Saia PJ, Morrow CP, Boronow R, et al. (1978) Endometrial sarcoma: lymphatic spread patterns. Am J Obstet Gynecol 130:104–105

Eberl M, Pfleiderer A, Teufel G, Bachmann F (1980) Sarcomas of the uterus. Morphological criterias and clinical course. Pathol Res Pract 169:165–172

Echt G, Jepson J, Steel J, Langholz B, Luxton G, Hermandez W, Astrahan M, Petrovich Z (1990) Treatment of uterine sarcomas. Cancer 66:35–39

Fayemi A, Ali H, Braun E (1978) Müllerian adenosarcoma of the uterine cervix. Am J Obstet Gynecol 130:734–735

Gal D, Kerner H, Beck H, Peretz A, Eyal A, Paldi E (1988) Müllerian adenosarcoma of the uterine cervix. Gynecol Oncol 31:445–453

Gallup DG, Gable DS, Talledo E, Otken LB (1989) A clinical-pathologic study of mixed muellerian tumors of the uterus over a 16-year period - The Medical College of Georgia experience. Am J Obstet Gynecol 161:533–538

Garamvoelgyi E, Guillou L, Gebhard S, Salmeron M, Seematter RJ, Hadji MH (1994) Primary malignant mixed Müllerian tumor (metaplastic carcinoma) of the female peritoneum. Cancer 74:854–863

Gilbert HA, Kagan AR, Lagasse L, Jacobs MR, Tawa K (1975) The value of radiation therapy in uterine sarcoma. Obstet Gynecol 45:84–88

Hannigan E, Curtin JP, Silverberg SG, Thipgen JI, Spanos WJ (1992) In: Hoskins WJ, Perez CA, Young RC (eds) Gynecologic oncology. Lippincott, Philadelphia, pp 695–714

Hannigan EV, Freedman RS, Elder KS, Rutledge FN (1983) Reexploration after treatment for uterine sarcoma. Gynecol Oncol 16:1–5

Harris NL, Scully RE (1984) Malignant lymphoma and granulocyte sarcoma of the uterus and vagina. A clinicopathological analysis of 27 cases. Cancer 53:2530–2545

Hart WR, Yoonessi M (1977) Endometrial stromatosis of the uterus. Obstet Gynecol 49:393–399

Hertig AT, Gare H (1960) Tumors of the female sex organs. Part 2. Armed Forces Institute of Pathology, Washington, DC, pp 68–83

Irmscher S, Krüger G, Köppe I (1995) Müllersches Adenosarkom des Uterus, eine Kasuistik. Geburtshilfe Frauenheilkd 55:115–117

Jacoby AF, Fuller AF, Thor AD, Muntz HG (1993) Primary leiomyosarcoma of the fallopian tube. Gynecol Oncol 51:404–407

Jaffe R, Altaras M, Bernheim J, Ben Aderet N (1985) Endocervical stroma sarcoma - a case report. Gynecol Oncol 22:105–108

Jopp H (1965) Über Karzino-Sarkome des Endometrium. Zentralbl Gynäkol 87:1268–1277

Kahanpää KV, Wahlström T, Gröhn P, Heinonen E, Neiminen U, Widholm O (1986) Sarcomas of the uterus: a clinicopathologic study of 119 patients. Obstet Gynecol 67:417–424

Kaku T, Silverberg SG, Major FJ, Miller A, Felter B, Brady MF (1992) Adenosarcoma of the uterus. A gynecologic oncology group clinicopathologic study of 31 cases. Int J Gynecol Pathol 11:75–88

Katenkamp D, Stiller D (1973) Heterologe mesodermale (Müllersche) Mischtumoren des Uterus. Zentralbl Allg Pathol 117:478–487

Katzenstein ALA, Askin FB, Feldman PS (1977) Müllerian adenosarcoma of the uterus: an ultrastructural study of four cases. Cancer 40:2233–2242

Keller J, Poulter C, Beecham J, Rubin P (1987) Uterine sarcoma: a ten year experience at the University of Rochester, NY. Proc Am Soc Clin Oncol 17–19 May 1987, Atlanta, Georgia, Nr.454

Krieger PD, Gusberg SB (1973) Endolymphatic stromal myosis; a grade I endometrial sarcoma. Gynecol Oncol 1:299–303

Kühn W, Heberling D, Höffken H, Rummel HH (1982) Morphologie and Klinik der malignen Müller schen Mischtumorea des Corpus uteri. Geburtshilfe Frauenheilkd 42:888–891

Kuller JA, Zucker PK, Peng TCC (1990) Vulvar leiomyosarcoma in pregnancy. Am J Obstet Gynecol 162:164–166

Larson B, Silfverswärd C, Nilsson B, Petterson F (1990a) Endometrial stromal sarcoma of the uterus. A clinical and histopathological study. The Radiumhemmet series 1936–1982. Eur J Obstet Gynecol Reprod Biol 35:239–249

Larson B, Silfverswärd C, Nilsson B, Petterson F (1990b) Mixed Müllerian tumours of the uterus-prognostic factors. A clinical and histopathological study of 147 cases. Radiother Oncol 17:123

Major F, Silverberg S, Morrow P, Blessing JA, Creasman W, Currie J (1987) A preliminary analysis of prognostic factors in uterine sarcoma. A Gynecologic Oncology Group study. Abstracts p 20. 18th Annual Meeting of the Society of Gynecologic Oncology. Miami, Florida, 1–4 February 1987

Major FJ, Blessing JA, Silverberg SG, Morrow CP, Creasman WT, Currie JL, Yordan E, Brady MF (1993) Prognostic factors in early-stage uterine sarcoma. Cancer 71:1702–1709

Malmström H, Schmidt H, Persson PG, Carstensen B, Simonsen E (1992) Flow cytometric analysis of uterine sarcoma: polidy and S-phase rate as prognostic indicators. Gynecol Oncol 44:172–177

Marchese M, Nori D (1987) Role of radiation in the management of uterine sarcoma. In: Nori D, Hilaris BS (eds) Radiation therapy of gynecological cancer. Liss, New York, pp 223–231

Marchese MJ, Liskow AS, Crum CP, et al. (1984) Uterine sarcomas: a clinicopathologic study 1965–1981. Gynecol Oncol 18:299–312

Marth C, Koza A, Müller-Holzner E, Hetzel H, Fuith IC, Dapunt O (1990) Prognostisch relevante Faktoren beim malignen Müllerschen Mischtumor. Geburtshilfe Frauenheilkd 50:605–609

Michalas S, Creatos G, Deligeoroglou E, Markaki S (1994) High-grade endometrial stromal sarcoma in a 16-year-old girl. Gynecol Oncol 54:95–98

Miyazawa K, Hernandez E (1986) Cervical carcinosarcoma: a case report. Gynecol Oncol 23:376–380

Morrow CP, D'Ablang G, Brady LW, Blessing JA, Hreshchyshyn MM (1984) A clinical and pathologic study of 30 cases of malignant mixed müllerian epithelial and mesenchymal ovarian tumors: a Gynecologic Oncology Group study. Gynecol Oncol 18:278–292

Mortel R, Koss LG, Lewis J Jr, D'Urso JR (1974) Mesodermal mixed tumors of the uterine corpus. Obstet Gynecol 43:248–256

Nelson KG, Haskill JS, Sloan S, Siegfried JM, Siegal GP, Walton L, Kaufman DG (1987) Flow cytometric analysis of human uterine sarcomas and cell lines. Cancer Res 47:2814–2820

Nickie-Psikuta M, Gawrychowski K (1993) Different types and different prognosis – study of 310 uterine sarcomas. Eur J Gynaecol Oncol 15 (Suppl):105–113

Nielsen SN, Podratz KC, Scheithauer BW, O'Brien PC (1989) Clinicopathologic analysis of uterine malignant mixed müllerian tumors. Gynecol Oncol 34:372–378

Nordsmark M, Bentzen SM, Overgaard J, et al. (1994) Measurement of human oxygenation status by a polarographic needle electrode: an analysis of inter- and intratumor heterogenity. Acta Oncol 33:383–389

Norris HJ, Taylor HB (1966) Mesenchymal tumors of the uterus. I. A clinical and pathological study of 53 endometrial stromal tumors. III. A clinical and pathologic study of 31 carcinosarcomas. Cancer 19:755–766, 1459–1465

Okagaki T, Ishida T, Hilgers R (1976) A malignant tumor of the vagina resembling synovial sarcoma. Cancer 37:2306–2320

Olah KS, Gee H, Blunt S, Dunn JA, Kelly K, Chan KK (1991) Retrospective analysis of 318 cases of uterine sarcomas. Eur J Cancer 27:1095–1099

Olah KS, Dunn JA, Gee H (1992) Leiomyosarcomas have a poorer prognosis than mixed mesodermal tumours when adjusting for known prognostic factors: the results of a retrospective study of 423 cases of uterine sarcoma. Br J Obstet Gynaecol 99:590–594

Peiffert D, Pernot M, Guillemin F, Luparsi E, Parache RM, Legras B, Bey P (1991) Les tumeurs mixtes mulleriennes de l'endometre. Etude retrospective a visce prognostique, comparant leur evolution a cell des adenocarcinomes de 1 endometre. J Obstet Gynecol 20:933–940

Perez CA, Askin F, Baglan RJ, Kao MS, Kraus FT, Perez BM, Williams CF, Weiss D (1979) Effects of irradiations on mixed muellerian tumors of the uterus. Cancer 43:1274–1284

Piver MS, Lurain JR (1981) Uterine sarcomas: clinical features and management. In: Coppleson M (ed) Gynecologic oncology, vol 2. Churchill Livingstone, Edinburgh, pp 608–618

Piver MS, Rutledge FN, Copeland L, et al. (1984) Uterine endolymphatic stromal myosis – a collaborative study. Obstet Gynecol 64:173–178

Podczaski ES, Woomert CA, Stevens C Jr, et al. (1989) Management of malignant mixed mesodermal tumors of the uterus. Gynecol Oncol 32:240–244

Raggio ML, Bostrom SG, Harden EA (1988) Hodgkin's lymphoma of the uterus presenting as refractory inflammatory disease, a case report. J Reprod Med 33:827–830

Roth LM, Pride GI, Sharma HM (1976) Müllerian adenosarcoma of the uterine cervix with heterologous elements. A light and electron microscopy study. Cancer 37:1725–1730

Rotmensch J, Rosenheim NB, Woodruff JD (1983) Cervical sarcoma: a review. Obstet Gynecol Surv 38:456–460

Russell WO, Cohen J, Enzinger F, et al. (1977) A clinical and pathological staging system for soft tissue sarcomas. Cancer 40:1362–1370

Saksela E, Lampinen V, Procope BJ (1974) Malignant mesenchymal tumors of the uterine corpus. Am J Obstet Gynecol 120:452

Salazar OM, Dunne ME (1980) The role of radiation therapy in the management of uterine sarcomas. Int J Radiat Oncol Biol Phys 6:899–902

Salazar OM, Bonfiglio TA, Patten SF, et al. (1978) Uterine sarcoma. Analysis of failures with special emphasis on the use of adjuvant radiotherapy. Cancer 42:1161–1170

Schmitt K, Schäfer A (1976) Zur Histogenese uteriner Mischtumoren. Österr Z Onkol 3:122–126

Schweizer W, Demopoulos R, Beller U, Dubin N (1990) Prognostic factors for malignant müllerian tumors of the uterus. Int J Gynecol Pathol 9:129–136

Senger E (1886) Über ein primäres Sarkom der Tuben. Zentralbl Gynaekol 10:601–604

Shaw RW, Lynch PF, Wade-Evans T (1983) Muellerian mixed tumour of the uterine corpus: a clinical and histopathological review of 28 patients. Br J Obstet Gynaecol 90:562–569

Shevchuk MM, Fenoglio CM, Lattes R, Frick HC, Richart RM (1978) Malignant mixed tumor of the vagina probably arising in mesonephric rests. Cancer 42:214–223

Silverberg SG (1971) Leiomyosarcoma of the uterus. A clinicopathological study. Obstet Gynecol 38:613–622

Silverberg SG (1992) Mixed müllerian tumors. In: Sasano N (ed) Gynecological tumors. Springer, Berlin Heidelberg New York, pp 35–56

Silverberg SG, Major FJ, Blessing JA, et al. (1990) Carcinosarcoma (malignant mixed mesodermal tumor) of the uterus: a Gynecologic Oncology Group pathologic study of 203 cases. Int J Gynecol Pathol 9:1–19

Sölder E, Huter O, Müller-Holzner E, Brezinka C (1995) Adenofibrom und Adenosarkom des Uterus bei jungen Frauen. Geburtshilfe Frauenheilkd 55:118–120

Spanos WJ, Wharton, JT, Gomez L, et al. (1984) Malignant mixed müllerian tumors of the uterus. Cancer 53:311–316

Spanos WJ Jr, Peters LJ, Oswald MJ (1986) Patterns of recurrence in malignant mixed müllerian tumor of the uterus. Cancer 57:155–159

Sternberg W, Clark WH, Smith RC (1954) Malignant mixed Müllerian tumor (mixed mesodermal tumor of the uterus). A study of twenty-one cases. Cancer 7:704–724

Sutton GP, Stehman FB, Michael H, Young PE, Ehrlich CE (1986) Estrogen and progesterone receptors in uterine sarcomas. Obstet Gynecol 68:709–714

Sutton GP, Blessing JA, Barrett RJ, McGehee R (1992) Phase II trial of ifosfamide and mesna in leiomyosarcoma of the uterus: a Gynecologic Oncology Group study. Am J Obstet Gynecol 166:556–559

Taina E, Maenpää J, Ekkola R, Ikkala J, Söderström O, Vitanen A (1989) Endometrial stromal sarcoma: a report of nine cases. Gynecol Oncol 32:156–162

Taylor H, Norris H (1966) Mesenchymal tumors of the uterus. IV. Diagnosis and prognosis of leiomyosarcomas. Arch Pathol 82:40–49

Teufel G, Frauer A, Eberl M, Pfleiderer A, Neunhoeffer J (1980) Sarcomas of the female genitalia. Pathol Res Pract 169:173–178

Thum P, Greiner R, Blattmann H, Coray A, Zimmermann A (1988) Pionen-Strahlentherapie nichtresektabler Weichteilsarkome am schweizerischen Institut für Nuklearforschung (SIN). Strahlenther Onkol 164:714–723

Tsushima K, Stanhope CR, Gaffey TA, Lieber MM (1988) Uterine leiomyosarcomas and benign muscle tumors: usefulness of nuclear DNA patterns studied by flow cytometry. Mayo Clin Proc 63:248–255

Vardi JR, Tovell HMM (1980) Leiomyosarcoma of the uterus: clinicopathological study. Obstet Gynecol 56:428–436

Velios F, Stander RW, Huber CP (1963) Carcinosarcoma (malignant mixed müllerian tumor) of the uterus. Am J Clin Pathol 39:496–505

Vongtama V, Karlen JR, Piver SM, Tsukada Y, Moore RH (1976) Treatment, results and prognostic factors in stage I and II sarcomas of the corpus uteri. Am J Roentgenol Rad Ther Nucl Med 126:139–147

Wambersie A (1990) Fast neutron therapy at the end of 1988 – a survey of the clinical data. Strahlenther Onkol 166:52–60

William TJ, Woodruff JD (1962) Similarities in malignant mixed mesenchymal tumors of the endometrium. Obstet Gynecol Surv 17:1–18

Wolf A, Vahrson H (1976) Zur Prognose der Genitalsarkome bei der erwachsenen Frau unter besonderer Berücksichtigung der Sarkome des Corpus uteri. Geburtshilfe Frauenheilkd 36:856–861

Yoonessi M, Hart WR (1977) Endometrial stromal sarcomas. Cancer 40:898–906

Zaloudek CJ, Norris HJ (1981) Adenofibroma and adenosarcoma of the uterus: a clinicopathologic study of 35 cases. Cancer 48:354–366

Zaloudek CJ, Norris HJ (1994) Mesenchymal tumors of the uterus. In: Kurman RJ (ed) Blaustein's pathology of the female genital tract, 4th edn. Springer, New York Berlin Heidelberg, pp 487–528

Zutter MM, Gersell DJ (1990) Acute lymphoblastic leukemia, a usual case of primary relapse in the uterine cervix. Cancer 66:1002–1004

14 Gestational Trophoblastic Disease

H.-A. Ladner and S. Ladner

CONTENTS

14.1 Introduction

Gestational trophoblastic disease (GTD) encompasses a heterogeneous group of lesions, including hydatidiform mole, invasive mole, choriocarcinoma, and placental site trophoblastic tumor (Mazur and Kurman 1994). Trophoblastic disease originates from the placental villi. From the standpoint of graft immunity, the disease has the characteristics of a homograft tumor. These tumors produce human chorionic gonatropin (hCG), and the level of hCG is a valuable marker for diagnosis as well as for assessment of therapeutic effect and remission. Radiotherapy has proven to be a valuable adjunct to chemotherapy in the management of selected cases of GTD. Patients who derive the greatest benefit from radiotherapy are those with brain, liver, and vaginal metastases. Radiotherapy is of limited value in the treatment of metastatic disease in other visceral locations. On the other hand, chemotherapy is effective, and even metastatic cases may be cured by chemotherapy alone. The tumors apparently progress from hydatidiform mole to invasive mole to choriocarcinoma, and therefore by controlling the hydatidiform mole stage it is possible to detect early choriocarcinoma or even to prevent its occurrence.

For details we recommend the following reviews: Bagshawe and Begent (1981), Park (1981) (pathology), Berkowitz and Goldstein (1986), Soper et al. (1992), Tomoda et al. (1992), and Mazur and Kurman (1994).

The Japanese Society of Obstetrics and Gynecology published a classification of GTD in 1982 (Tomoda et al. 1992), and the simplified form of the Japanese classification is very similar to the WHO classification (Table 14.1). The frequency of development of a choriocarcinoma following a mole is 2%–3% (Soper et al. 1992).

14.2 Staging and Prognostic Factors

The International Federation of Gynecology and Obstretics (FIGO) uses an anatomic staging system for GTD (Table 14.2).

Four factors are especially important for successful treatment of GTD: (1) level of hCG elevation before therapy, (2) duration of disease before initiation of chemotherapy, (3) absence of CNS and hepatic metastases, and (4) proper administration of chemotherapy (Mazur and Kurman 1994). Adverse prognostic factors include advanced disease at diagnosis, failure of prior chemotherapy, and a pretreatment serum β-hCG titer of more than 40 000 mIU/ml (Weed et al. 1982b; Survit et al. 1984). Metastatic disease limited to the lungs or vagina is not a poor prognostic sign. Although it is difficult to assess precisely the prognostic significance of extrapulmonary metastases, patients with CNS metastases have an approximately 50% remission rate (Weed and Hammond 1980). Patients with hepatic metastases also have a poor prognosis, but multiagent chemotherapy appears to increase the survival rate (Wong et al. 1986). Choriocarcinoma after term gestation generally has a worse prognosis than that after a mole.

H.-A. Ladner, MD, Professor, Im Großacker 3, D-79249 Merzhausen, Germany
S. Ladner, MD, Zentrales Röntgeninstitut, Städtisches Klinikum Karlsruhe, Moltkestraße 14, D-76133 Karlsruhe, Germany

Table 14.1. The WHO classification of GTD (1983)

1. Hydatidiform mole
   a) Complete hydatidiform mole
   b) Partial hydatidiform mole
2. Invasive mole
3. Gestational choriocarcinoma
4. Placental site trophoblastic tumor

Table 14.2. FIGO staging of GTD

Stage	Definition
I	Confined to corpus uteri
II	Metastases to pelvis and vagina
III	Metastases to lung
IV	Distant metastases

Multivariate analysis using these prognostic factors helps to predict the outcome of GTD (Lurain et al. 1991). Several different scoring systems for prognosis have been proposed (Nishikawa et al. 1985), and the WHO scoring system has received the greatest acceptance (Mazur and Kurman 1994).

The role of radiotherapy in the treatment of trophoblastic neoplasms may be characterized as that of a tertiary modality to prevent or control hemorrhage or to provide palliation for patients with drug-resistant tumors beyond the scope of surgery (Jones 1987).

14.3 Metastases

At Nagoya University Hospital, Japan, metastasis was noted at the time of admission in 71% of patients treated from 1957 to 1984. Pulmonary metastases were found in 67% (125), intracranial metastases in 5% (9), intrapelvic metastases in 14% (24), and vaginal metastases in 12% (22).

14.3.1 Lung Metastases

Pulmonary metastases occur in up to 70% of patients with gestational choriocarcinoma. Chemotherapy has been the first-line treatment overall. Regarding surgical intervention for pulmonary metastases, Shirley et al. (1972) operated on four patients and reported remission in three of them. However, they did not recommend surgery because chemotherapy is extremely effective. Xu et al. (1985) reported that from 1962 to 1982 pulmonary metastatic choriocarcinoma was found to be resistant to chemotherapy in 43 of their patients who subsequently underwent surgery with a 5-year survival rate of 50% (16/32). The timing of surgery is very important, and it must be emphasized that satisfactory results will not be achieved if it is performed too early or too late.

14.3.2 Liver Metastases

Liver metastases develop in approximately 10% of patients with metastatic GTD. In most instances liver metastases occur in patients with other high-risk factors and in those who have developed resistant disease in other systemic locations (Bagshawe and Begent 1981). It is generally agreed that multiagent chemotherapy should be the primary modality in the treatment of these patients. The management of hepatic metastases is particularly difficult and problematic. If a patient is resistant to systemic chemotherapy, hepatic arterial infusion of chemotherapeutic agents may induce complete remission in selected cases (Goldstein 1972; Berkowitz and Goldstein 1986).

14.3.3 Brain Metastases

If brain metastases are detected, whole-brain irradiation (30 Gy in 10 fractions or 20 Gy over 7 days) should be promptly instituted (Brace 1968; Jones 1987). A variety of radiation doses and fractionation procedures have been used in the treatment of brain metastases (Cairncross et al. 1980). In a large randomized clinical trial by the Radiation Therapy Oncology Group in which doses to the brain ranging from 20 to 40 Gy were compared, no single treatment schedule could be identified as clearly superior (Borgelt et al. 1980). The risk of spontaneous hemorrhage may be reduced by the concurrent use of combination chemotherapy and brain irradiation. Brain irradiation may be both hemostatic and tumoricidal. Whether radiotherapy can cure intracerebral choriocarcinoma remains unknown. There appeared to be a survival advantage for in a collected series in which the overwhelming majority received adjunctive radiotherapy (37% vs 16%, Jones 1987: literature comparison between nonirradiated and brain-irradiated patients).

14.3.4 Vaginal Metastases

Metastatic vaginal choriocarcinoma is highly responsive to chemotherapy, complete remission rates of greater than 90% being reported in patients who are treated early in the course of their disease. Brace (1968) reported on five patients with vaginal hemorrhage, all of whom had an excellent response to radiotherapy, with cessation of bleeding within a few days after the start of treatment. When the size or location of the vaginal lesions precludes control of the hemorrhage by local measures, bilateral hypogastric artery ligation followed immediately by vaginal irradiation can be effective (15 Gy over a 5-day period through anterior-posterior portals to the vaginal tumor with cessation of bleeding 3 days later). Based on such responses radiotherapy is highly recommended as an adjunct to chemotherapy for local control of metastatic choriocarcinoma complicated by hemorrhage.

14.4 Chemotherapy

In the past, the change from single-agent chemotherapy to combination chemotherapy resulted in a marked increase in curability (Lewis 1980). Multiagent chemotherapy programs that include etoposide (VP-16) have been developed (Schink et al. 1992) and offer an increased rate of sustained remissions for very high-risk patients and for those who have not benefited from other conventional forms of chemotherapy (Weed et al. 1982a).

14.5 Complications of Radiotherapy

The most serious complication of radiotherapy in the treatment of GTD patients is radionecrosis. Pratt et al. (1977) were the first to report on a patient who developed grand mal seizures, collapse, and hemiparesis more than 2 months following 30 Gy whole-brain irradiation and chemotherapy. Weed et al. (1982b) described three surviving patients with neurologic sequelae ("frontal lobe syndrome," grand mal seizure disorder, and atopia, optic atrophy, and seizures). In children, second primary tumors, functional deficits, and mental retardation appear to be common complications but even in these situations the majority of patients are judged to have an acceptable quality of life (Danoff et al. 1982).

References

Bagshawe KD (1987) Chemotherapy and general treatment, current and future developments. In: Takagi S, Friedberg V, Haller U, Knapstein PG, Sevin BV (eds) Gynecologic oncology, surgery and urology. Central Foreign Books, Tokyo, pp 243–249

Bagshawe KD, Begent RHJ (1981) Trophoblastic tumors: clinical features and management. In: Coppleson M (ed) Gynecologic oncology. Fundamental principles and clinical practice. Churchill Livingstone, Edinburgh, pp 757–772

Berkowitz RS, Goldstein DP (1986) Management of molar pregnancy and gestational trophoblastic tumors. In: Knapp RC, Berkowitz RS (eds) Gynecologic oncology. Macmillan, New York, pp 425–443

Borgelt B, Gelber R, Kramer S, et al. (1980) The palliation of brain metastases: Final results of the first two studies by the Radiation Therapy Oncology Group. Int J Radiat Oncol Biol Phys 6:1–9

Brace KC (1968) The role of irradiation in the treatment of metastatic trophoblastic disease. Radiology 91:540–544

Cairncross JG, Kim JH, Posner JB (1980) Radiation therapy for brain metastases. Ann Neurol 7:529–541

Danoff BF, Conchock FS, Marquette C, Mulgrew L, Kramer S (1982) Assessment of the long term effects of primary radiation therpy for brain tumors in children. Cancer 49:1580–1586

Goldstein DP (1972) The chemotherapy of gestational trophoblastic disease. Principles of clinical management. J Am Med Assoc 220:209–213

Jones WB (1987) Gestational trophoblastic disease: the role of radiotherapy. In: Nori D, Hilaris BS (eds) Radiation therapy of gynecological cancer. Alan R.Liss, New York, pp 207–221

Lewis JL Jr (1980) Choriosarcoma: a success story for chemotherapy. Int J Radiat Oncol Biol Phys 6:897–898

Lurain JR, Casanova LA, Miller DS, Rademaker AW (1991) Prognostic factors in gestational trophoblastic tumors: a proposed new scoring system based on multivariate analysis. Am J Obstet Gynecol 164:611–616

Mazur MT, Kurman RJ (1994) Gestational trophoblastic disease and related lesions. In: Kurman RJ (ed) Blaustein's pathology of the female genital tract, 4th edn. Springer, New York Berlin Heidelberg, pp 1049–1093

Nishikawa Y, Kaseki S, Tomoda Y, Ishizuka T, Asai Y, Suzuki T, Ushiuma H (1985) Histopathologic classification of uterine choriocarcinoma. Cancer 55:1044–1051

Park WW (1981) Pathology and classification of trophoblastic tumors. In: Coppleson M (ed) Gynecologic oncology. Fundamental principles and clinical practice. Churchill Livingstone, Edinburgh, pp 745–756

Pratt RA, DiChiro G, Weed JC (1977) Cerebral necrosis following irradiation and chemotherapy for metastatic choriocarcinoma. Surg Neurol 7:117–120

Schink JC, Singh DK, Rademaker AW, Miller DS, et al. (1992) Etoposide, methotrexate, actinomycin-D, cyclophosphamide, and vincristine for the treatment of metastatic, high-risk gestational trophoblastic disease. Obstet Gynecol 80:817–820

Shirley RL, Goldstein DP, Collins JJ (1972) The role of thoracotomy in the management of patients with chest metastases from gestational metastatic disease. J Thorac Cardiovasc Surg 63:545–550

Soper JT, Hammond CB, Lewis JL (1992) Gestational trophoblastic disease. In: Hoskins WJ, Perez CA, Youg RC (eds) Principles and practice of gynecologic oncology. J.B. Lippincott, Philadelphia pp 795–825

Survit EA, Alberts DS, Christian CD, Graham VE (1984) Poor-prognosis gestational trophoblastic disease: an update. Obstet Gynecol 64:21–26

Tomoda Y, Ishizuka T, Goto S, Furushashi Y (1992) Trophoblastic disease. In: Sasano N (ed) Gynecological tumors. Springer, Berlin Heidelberg New York, pp 203–231

Weed JC, Woodward KT, Hammond CB (1982a) Choricarcinoma metastatic to the brain, therapy and prognosis. Semin Oncol 9:208–212

Weed JC, Barnard DE, Currie JL, et al. (1982b) Chemotherapy with the modfified Bagshawe protocol for poor prognosis metastatic trophoblastic disease. Obstet Gynecol 59:377–380

Weed JC, Hammond CB (1980) Cerebral metastatic choriocarcinoma: intensive therapy and prognosis. Obstet Gynecol 55:89–94

Wong LC, Choo YC, Ma HK (1986) Hepatic metastases in gestational trophoblastic disease. Obstet Gynecol 67:107

World Health Organization Scientific Group on Gestational Trophoblastic Disease (1983) Gestational trophoblastic diseease. In: Technical Reports Series 692. WHO, Geneva

Xu LT, Sun CF, Wang YE, Song HZ (1985) Resection of pulmonary metastatic choriocarcinoma in 43 drug-resistant patients. Ann Thorac Surg 39:257–259

15 Management of Reactions and Complications Following Radiation Therapy

G. Rauthe

CONTENTS

15.1 Introduction

Solum dosis fecit venenum. This adage is of significant relevance for radiation-specific toxicity. For both individual doses and the total dosage, the irradiation time frame and the irradiation volume are the most important parameters in clinical practice for comparing the tumoricidal dose with the tolerance dose of normal tissue (Fletcher 1979; Seegenschmiedt and Sauer 1993).

Curves depicting the probability of local tumor control and the risk of causing damage to normal tissue as a function of the total dosage both have sigmoidal shapes (Holthusen 1921; Hübener et al. 1993; Yeoh and Horowitz 1987). The difference between them represents the therapeutic gain (Holthusen 1921; Kinsella and Bloomer 1980). Actions that increase this difference improve the therapeutic gain by increasing the likelihood of local tumor control and/or reducing the risk of severe damage to normal tissue (Kinsella and Bloomer 1980; Yeoh and Horowitz 1987).

The biological effect of ionizing radiation is damage to the intracellular DNA, which is then rendered incapable of replication, resulting in cell death. Hence, those tissues with a rapid cell turnover manifest radiation injury before cells which divide more slowly (Johnson and Carrington 1992). *Early reaction* stems from epithelial necrosis (Johnson and Carrington 1992). During and after radiotherapy, an unstable equilibrium is created between loss and production of epithelial cells. When the balance is disrupted, partial or complete denudation can occur. Patients who have an acute radiation reaction seem more likely to progress to serious chronic radiation damage (Johnson and Carrington 1992).

Chronic radiation injury results from damage to vascular and stromal cells. Vessels undergo endothelial degeneration, fibroid necrosis, transmural inflammation, and fibrosis (Johnson and Carrington 1992; Hasleton et al. 1985). Atrophy is one of the most common delayed effects of therapeutic irradiation. It occurs in all epithelial linings, as well as in all glands and in parenchymatous tissues (Fajardo 1989). Fibrosis is one of the most common delayed manifestations of the stroma. It is much more than a mark of radiation damage, it is damage in itself (Fajardo 1989). The fibrosis may become so extensive that the so-called frozen pelvis may develop (Russel and Welch 1979).

Risk versus benefit considerations in patients undergoing curative radiotherapy pose a complex philosophical and practical problem (Bloomer and Hellman 1975). If a radiation complication is manageable, the dose of irradiation used should maximize tumor control and the higher complication rate should be accepted. Conversely, an intractable and life-threatening complication necessitates the use of a radiation dose that will minimize the risk of having such a complication develop, despite the reduced probability of tumor control (Kinsella and Bloomer 1980).

G. Rauthe, MD, Schloßbergklinik, D-87534 Oberstaufen, Germany

In the palliative situation, the sole purpose of the treatment is the alleviation of an incurable illness (GALLAND and SPENCER 1987). Side-effects which reduce the quality of life of the patient should be prevented whenever possible. The main purpose of managing reactions and complications is not just to keep patients alive, but to allow them to live.

15.2 Classification of Radiation Morbidity

It is impossible to compare the published data on cancer treatment complications owing to the lack of a common language for defining and ranking them (SKENE et al. 1990).

The Radiation Therapy Oncology Group published a meaningful grading system for radiation toxicity (Tables 15.1, 15.2) (PILEPICH et al. 1983; SCHELLHAMMER et al. 1986). The system is based on the effect of the treatment-related morbidity on the patients' performance status and the intervention required (SCHELLHAMMER et al. 1986).

It is always the maximum extent of the side-effects during or after radiotherapy which is judged (SEEGENSCHMIEDT and SAUER 1993). If differing clinical parameters exist for judging an organ system, the worst form of the side-effects must be considered in each case (SEEGENSCHMIEDT and SAUER 1993). If side-effects occur within the first 90 days of starting radiotherapy, they are considered acute; thereafter they are regarded as chronic (Radiation Therapy Oncology Group 1984).

With grade 1 toxicity, negligible symptoms/deviations from laboratory parameters occur; they do not require therapy and spontaneously return to normal. With acute radiation morbidity grade 1, it is not necessary to interrupt the irradiation or to reduce the dose (SEEGENSCHMIEDT and SAUER 1993). Between grades 2 and 4, the severity of the symptoms/deviations from laboratory parameters increases and requires a more comprehensive therapy. If necessary, the irradiation must be interrupted and modified and, at grade 4, discontinued (SEEGENSCHMIEDT and SAUER 1993). Grade 5 toxicity causes the death of the patient (Radiation Therapy Oncology Group 1984).

Table 15.1. Acute radiation morbidity scoring schema.[a] (Modified from Radiation Therapy Oncology Group 1984)

Organ/tissue	Grade 1	Grade 2	Grade 3	Grade 4
Skin	Follicular, faint or dull erythema; epilation; dry desquamation; decreased sweating	Tender or bright erythema, patchy moist desquamation; moderate edema	Confluent, moist desquamation other than skin folds, pitting edema	Ulceration, hemorrhage, necrosis
Mucous membrane	Erythema; may experience mild pain not requiring analgesic	Patchy mucositis which may produce an inflammatory serosanguinous discharge; may experience moderate pain requiring analgesic	Confluent fibrinous mucositis; may include severe pain requiring narcotic	Ulceration, hemorrhage, necrosis
Upper gastrointestinal (GI)	Anorexia with ≤5% weight loss from pretreatment baseline; nausea not requiring antiemetics; abdominal discomfort not requiring parasympatholytic drugs or analgesics	Anorexia with ≤15% weight loss from pretreatment baseline; nausea and/or vomiting requiring antiemetics; abdominal pain requiring analgesics	Anorexia with >15% weight loss from pretreatment baseline or requiring nasogastric tube or parenteral support. Nausea and/or vomiting requiring nasogastric tube or parenteral support; abdominal pain severe despite medication; hematemesis or melena; abdominal distention (flat plate radiograph demonstrates distended bowel loops)	Ileus, subacute or acute obstruction, perforation, GI bleeding requiring transfusion; abdominal pain requiring tube decompression or bowel diversion

Table 15.1 *(continued)*

Organ/tissue	Grade 1	Grade 2	Grade 3	Grade 4
Lower GI, incluidng pelvis	Increased frequency or change in quality of bowel habits not requiring medication; rectal discomfort not requiring analgesics	Diarrhea requiring parasympatholytic drugs (e.g., Lomotil); mucous discharge not necessitating sanitary pads; rectal or abdominal pain requiring analgesics	Diarrhea requiring parenteral support; severe mucous or bloody discharge necessitating sanitary pads; abdominal distention (flat plate radiograph demonstrates distended bowel loops)	Acute or subacute obstruction, fistula or perforation, GI bleeding requiring transfusion, abdominal pain or tenesmus requiring tube decompression or bowel diversion
Genitourinary	Frequency of urination or nocturia twice pretreatment habit; dysuria, urgency not requiring medication	Frequency of urination or nocturia which is less frequent than every hour. Dysuria, urgency, bladder spasm requiring local anesthetic (e.g., Pyridium)	Frequency with urgency and nocturia hourly or more frequently; dysuria, pelvis pain, or bladder spasm requiring regular, frequent narcotic; gross hematuria with or without clot passage	Hematuria requiring transfusion; acute bladder obstruction not secondary to clot passage; ulceration or necrosis
CNS	Fully functional status (i.e. able to work) with minor neurological findings no medication needed	Neurological findings sufficient to require home care; nursing assistance may be required; medication including steroids; antiseizure agents may be required	Neurological findings requiring hospitalization for initial management	Serious neurological impairment which includes paralysis, coma, or seizures >3 per week despite medication; hospitalization required
Hemoglobin (g%)	11–9.5	<9.5–7.5	<7.5–5.0	–
Hematocrit (%)	28–<32	28	Packed cell transfusion required	–
WBC (×1000)	3.0–<4.0	2.0–<3.0	1.0–<2.0	<1.0
Neutrophils (×1000)	1.5–<1.9	1.0–<1.5	0.5–<1.0	<0.5 or sepsis
Platelets (×1000)	75–<100	50–<75	25–<50	<25 or spontaneous bleeding

Guidelines:
The acute morbidity criteria are used to score/grade toxicity from radiation therapy. The criteria are relevant from day 1 (the commencement of therapy) through day 90. Thereafter, the EORTC/RTOG criteria for late effects are to be utilized.
The evaluator must attempt to discriminate between disease and treatment-related signs and symptoms.
An accurate baseline evaluation prior to commencement of therapy is necessary.
[a] Any toxicity which causes death is graded 5.

15.3 Modification of Radiation Tolerance

The tolerance doses for serious side-effects (approximately grade 3 or 4 in the RTOG/EORTC radiation scoring system for late effects) which occur with a conventional fractionation schedule of 5 times 180–200 cGy per week, were assembled by Emami et al. and have been modified for the abdominal irradiation indicated in Table 15.3 (Emami et al. 1991). TD 5/5 and TD 50/5 signify the likelihood of 5% and 50% complications within 5 years of the treatment. In order to address volume dependency, the most clinical (i.e., severe) endpoint was chosen (Emami et al. 1991).

It is known that a number of factors can increase or decrease the tolerance of tumor-free tissue with respect to irradiation. With a reduction in tolerance, the risk of a radioreaction increases. By the use of "radioprotectors," on the other hand, the side-effects of the radiotherapy should be reduced.

Table 15.2. RTOG/EORTC late radiation morbidity scoring schema.[a] (Modified from Radiation Therapy Oncology Group 1984)

Organ/tissue	Grade 1	Grade 2	Grade 3	Grade 4
Skin	Slight atrophy Pigmentation change Some hair loss	Patchy atrophy Moderate telangiectasia Total hair loss	Marked atrophy Gross telangiectasia	Ulceration
Subcutaneous tissue	Slight induration (fibrosis) and loss of subcutaneous fat	Moderate fibrosis but asymptomatic; slight field contracture; <10% linear reduction	Severe induration and loss of subcutaneous tissue field contracture >10% linear measurement	Necrosis
Mucous membrane	Slight atrophy and dryness	Moderate atrophy and telangiectasia; little mucus	Marked atrophy with complete dryness; severe telangiectasia	Ulceration
Spinal cord	Mild Lhermitte's syndrome	Severe Lhermitte's syndrome	Objective neurological findings at or below cord level treated	Mono-, para-, or quadriplegia
Small/large intestine	Mild diarrhea; mild cramping; bowel movement 5 times daily; slight rectal discharge or bleeding	Moderate diarrhea and colic; bowel movement >5 times daily; excessive rectal mucus or intermittent bleeding	Obstruction or bleeding requiring surgery	Necrosis; perforation; fistula
Liver	Mild lassitude; nausea; dyspepsia; slightly abnormal liver function	Moderate symptoms; some abnormal liver function tests; serum albumin normal	Disabling hepatitic insufficiency; liver function tests grossly abnormal; low albumin; edema or ascites	Necrosis; hepatic coma or encephalopathy
Kidney	Transient albuminuria; no hypertension; mild impairment of renal function; urea 25–35 mg%, creatinine 1.5–2.0 mg%, creatinine clearance >75%	Persistent moderate albuminuria (2#); mild hypertension; no related anemia; moderate impairment of renal function; urea >35–60 mg%, creatinine >2.0–4.0 mg%, creatinine clearance 50%–74%	Severe albuminuria; severe hypertension; persistent anemia (<10 g%)/severe renal failure; urea >60 mg%, creatinine >4.0 mg%, creatinine clearance <50%	Malignant hypertension; uremic coma; urea >100%
Bladder	Slight epithelial atrophy; minor telangiectasia (microscopic hematuria)	Moderate frequency; generalized telangiectasia; intermittent macroscopic hematuria	Severe frequency and dysuria; severe generalized telangiectasia (often with petechiae); frequent hematuria; reduction in bladder capacity (<150 cc)	Necrosis; contracted bladder (capacity <100 cc); severe hemorrhagic cystitis
Bone	Asymptomatic; no growth retardation; reduced bone density	Moderate pain or tenderness; growth retardation irregular bone sclerosis	Severe pain or tenderness complete arrest bone growth Dense bone sclerosis	Necrosis; spontaneous fracture

[a] Any toxicity which causes death is graded 5.

15.3.1 Reduction of Radiation Tolerance

Age, diet, and performance status, a number of accompanying illnesses, hemoglobin, and protein content of the blood apparently all have an influence on the effectiveness of radiotherapy (Grant et al. 1989; Hübener et al. 1993; Teshima et al. 1987).

Thin and elderly patients have an increased amount of small intestine in the pelvis. Accordingly, these people have a higher risk of sustaining damage to the small intestine when exposed to pelvic radiotherapy (Galland and Spencer 1987; Green 1983; Potish et al. 1979). Schray et al. (1989) reported that all patients who were treated with irradiation of the whole abdomen who had their therapy stopped

Table 15.3. Normal adult tissue tolerance to irradiation. (EMAMI et al. 1991; SEEGENSCHMIEDT and SAUER 1993): tolerance doses (cGy) are shown for a conventional fractionation schedule of 5 × 180–200 cGy per week)

Partial organ volume:	TD 5/5[a]			TD 50/5[b]			Selected endpoint
	1/3	2/3	3/3	1/3	2/3	3/3	
Kidney	5000	3000[c]	2300[c]	–	4000[c]	2800[c]	Clinical nephritis
Bladder	–	8000	6500	–	8500	8000	Symptomatic bladder contracture and volume loss
Femoral head	–	–	5200	–	–	6500	Necrosis
Marrow pancytopenia	3000	–	250	4000	–	450	Aplasia
Skin	–	–	100 cm: 5000	–	–	100 cm: 6500	Telangiectasia
	10 cm: 7000	30 cm: 6000	1000 cm: 5500	–	–	100 cm: 7000	Necrosis, ulceration
Spinal cord	5 cm: 5000	10 cm: 5000	20 cm: 4700	5 cm: 7000	10 cm: 7000	–	Myelitis, necrosis
Cauda equina	No volume effect		6000	No volume effect		7500	Clinically apparent nerve damage
Stomach perforation	6000	5500	5000	7000	6700	6500	Ulceration
Small intestine	5000	–	4000[c]	6000	–	5000	Obstruction, perforation/fistula
Colon perforation/ ulceration	5500	–	4500	6500	–	5500	Obstruction, fistula
Rectum	Volume 100 cm^3 no volume effect		6000	Volume 100 cm^3 no volume effect		8000	Severe proctitis/ necrosis/fistula, stenosis
Liver	5000	3500	3000	5500	4500	4000	Liver failure

[a] TD 5/5, likelihood of 5% complications within 5 years of treatment.
[b] TD 50/5, likelihood of 50% complications within 5 years of treatment.
[c] <50% of volume does not induce a significant change.

on account of acute gastrointestinal complaints were older than 60 years. However, HUGUENIN et al. (1992) found only minimal acute toxicity in patients aged 75 years or more, and GREVEN et al. (1991) even found a reduced incidence of complications with increasing age.

Operations before irradiation increase the danger of a radiation-specific side-effect (DALY et al. 1989; GREEN 1983; JEREMIC et al. 1991; LOJUDICE et al. 1977; O'BRIEN et al. 1987; PERSSON et al. 1992; SCHELLHAMMER et al. 1986; STOCKBINE et al. 1970). After lymphadenectomy before the irradiation of cervical and endometrial carcinomas, there is a drastic increase in the incidence and seriousness of complications (BARTER et al. 1989; GREVEN et al. 1991; LEWANDOWSKI et al. 1990; STOCKBINE et al. 1970; WITHERSPOON et al. 1979). With complete abdominal irradiation of ovarian carcinomas, second-look laparotomy before the radiotherapy is associated with an increased risk of serious intestinal complications (WHELAN et al. 1992). The lack of movement of the intestine and the urinary system during the irradiation caused by operation-specific scars or inflammation of the pelvis (GRAHAM and ABAD 1967; GREEN 1983; PERSSON et al. 1992; STOCKBINE et al. 1970) can be considered as the main cause of this increase in risk.

A significant link apparently exists between hypertension, diabetes, and cardiovascular disease at the time of radiotherapy and subsequent development of radiation enteritis (DE COSSE et al. 1969; POTISH et al. 1979). Smoking also clearly increases the radiation toxicity (HÜBENER et al. 1993; RUGG et al. 1990). In particular, the healing of radiation-specific mucositis with continuous smoking takes 8–11 weeks longer than in nonsmokers (RUGG et al. 1990).

The incidence and severity of complications increases with the extent of the disease because of the high dose of radiation that is then required (STOCKBINE et al. 1970).

Some medicines increase the radiation sensitivity of the tissue; this is particularly true of cytostatic drugs (TESHIMA et al. 1985). With methotrexate, the tissue tolerance is considerably reduced (KIM et al. 1977; KRAMER 1975; SHEHATA and MEYER 1980). During cytostasis with cyclophosphamide and ifosfamide, active alkylating metabolites and acrolein are renally excreted, which are toxic to the urothelium (BISSETT et al. 1993). With irradiation of the pelvis, hemorrhaging from the bladder is a dreaded complication (BISSETT et al. 1993; JAYALAKSHMAMMA and PINKEL 1976; PRICE and KELDAHL 1990). The use of mesna, which renders the metabolic derivatives harmless to the urothelium by SH binding (BROCK and POHL 1983), is, therefore, definitely recommended for therapy which includes cyclophosphamide and ifosfamide (BISSETT et al. 1993).

15.3.2 Radioprotection

Several approaches have been adopted in an attempt to improve the therapeutic ratio by using substances which selectively protect the normal tissue (HOPEWELL et al. 1993). In both in vitro and in vivo studies, WR-2721, a sulfhydryl compound, has shown selective protection of normal tissues against the toxicity of radiation (COLEMAN et al. 1988; SCHUCHTER et al. 1992). In a random study of 100 rectal carcinoma patients, those who were treated with 340 mg of WR-2721/m^2 15 min before radiotherapy had statistically significantly fewer moderate or serious side-effects. The tumor response was equivalent in both groups. Hypotension and allergic reactions each affected three patients; 82% experienced a mostly mild or moderate vomiting (LIU et al. 1992).

Sucralfate has a beneficial influence on diarrhea, nausea, vomiting, and loss of appetite during irradiation. The incidence of intestinal reactions is reduced. These effects are explained by the protection of the mucosa denuded by the irradiation, the cytoprotective properties, and the binding of the gallbladder acids (HENRIKSSON et al. 1992a, 1990). Cimetidine also reduces the acute and subacute gastrointestinal side-effects of radiotherapy at doses of between 400 and 800 mg per day (TESHIMA et al. 1990).

BROHULT et al. (1979) found that the use of alkoxyglycerol during the treatment of cervical carcinomas reduced the radiation damage considerably. Rectovaginal and vesicovaginal fistulae were reduced by 47% and complex injuries with a high mortality were reduced by one-third when alkoxyglycerol was given prophylactically, in comparison with patients who received radiotherapy alone (BROHULT et al. 1979).

The use of orgotein is judged varyingly. Whereas a number of authors, both in animal experiments (CIVIDALLI et al. 1985) and in the field of clinical examinations (EDSMYR and MENANDER-HUBER 1981; GRIO et al. 1989), have observed a radioprotective effect, this could not be proved in a double-blind study (NIELSEN et al. 1987).

15.4 Prevention of Radiation Morbidity

For the prevention of radiation damage, both the planning and the performance of the irradiation must be given careful attention. The isodoses must be carefully adjusted to the tumor and tissue to be treated, assisted by sophisticated tumor localization systems and by computer-assisted dosimetry planning (COX et al. 1986; LAUGIER et al. 1968; REMY et al. 1986; STOCKBINE et al. 1970; VAHRSON and RÖMER 1988).

The use of a multidirectional, sharply collimated, high-energy photon and electron beam, strategically positioned bladder and rectum shields, and progressive "shrinking" of the radiation fields during the treatment (COX et al. 1986; GUNDERSON et al. 1985) allows concentration of the radiation dose in tumor-containing areas, thus avoiding normal structures (LAUGIER et al. 1968).

Due to the special radiation sensitivity of the small intestine, special procedures have been developed for use when treating the pelvis with radiation. This involves the shielding or displacing of the small intestine from the volume of treatment by positioning the patient during irradiation or by distension of the bladder (CASPERS and HOP 1983; GRANICK et al. 1993; KINSELLA and BLOOMER 1980), peritoneal insufflation (HINDLEY and COLE 1993), use of a tissue expander (HERBERT et al. 1993), or use of sling procedures (KAVANAH et al. 1985; TRIMBOS et al. 1991).

Measurement of the dose in the critical organs such as the bladder and rectum is necessary when combining percutaneous irradiation with brachytherapy in the pelvis (COX et al. 1986).

Critical analysis of extensive clinical experience has determined the optimal physical characteristics of implant systems and how best to integrate them with external irradiation to yield maximum tumor control with acceptable morbidity (Cox et al. 1986; Stockbine et al. 1970).

15.5 Radiation Morbidity at Diverse Locations

The acute side-effects of radiotherapy can completely return to normal. Ordinary medicinal therapy should alleviate the symptoms and accelerate the healing process. By definition, grade 1 side-effects require no treatment. By contrast, the later side-effects caused by damage to the vessels show a tendency to progression. Therapy is often only capable of alleviating the symptoms, and a return to normal is medicinally difficult to achieve.

With serious side-effects (grades 3 and 4), major surgery is sometimes necessary with its associated higher morbidity and mortality rates. Unavoidable operations must be individually planned and performed, and must take into consideration possible subsequent progression. If possible, the sutures should lie outside the irradiated areas. In particular, transplants for the repair of defects require a sufficient blood supply to the tissue.

Hyperbaric oxygen appears to be the only form of treatment that reverses the basic vascular pathophysiology induced by radiation (Kindwall 1993). In this way, neovascularization and growth of granulation tissue are encouraged (Williams et al. 1992). Protocols for hyperbaric oxygen treatment are at present mostly empirical. Much additional research is needed to better define the therapeutic indications.

15.5.1 Skin

In order to prevent acute radiation damage to the skin, it is necessary to treat the skin carefully during the irradiation. The application of powder several times a day to the irradiated areas gives a pleasant cooling feeling which is brought about by an increase in surface area. With very dry skin, on the other hand, care is based on the use of oils (Maiche et al. 1991). Warm and moist secretions should not be impaired by the dressing. With moist reactions greater than grade 2, powder and oil treatments should be stopped and the radiotherapy temporarily halted. Intertriginous folds can be protected from microbial infections by lightly tanning with an aqueous disinfectant. Physical irritations (pressure, rubbing of clothing, rubbing dry after washing, etc., chemical irritants (e.g., sprays, soaps), overheating, and also long cold periods should be avoided.

In the skin, the sebaceous glands are perhaps most affected (Fajardo 1989). For this reason, due to the radiation-specific dryness of the skin after radiotherapy, lengthy oil-based skin care is recommended.

Dermatophytic infections sometimes develop within the radiation field, worsening an acute radiation effect. Topical antimicrobial agents are then recommended. Depending on the seriousness, in certain circumstances analgesics and antiphlogistics must also be administered.

With wounds resulting from radiation, as with burns, the danger of bacterial contamination should be considered. The local application of antibiotics can lead to resistance, allergies, and the promotion of fungal infections. Analogous to the treatment of burns, such methods can be recommended as do not disturb wound healing, e.g., light tanning, application of colors, as are commonly used in dermatology, or the use of povidone-iodine (Steen 1993; Viljanto 1980). Pape et al. (1990) report the healing of radiation-induced epitheliolysis through the use of bandages consisting of hydrocolloids and polymers.

Cosmetically disturbing telangiectasia can be treated by laser therapy (dye or argon laser) (Polla et al. 1987; Landthaler et al. 1984). An alternative sclerosing treatment is use of a well-diluted sodium tetradecyl sulfate solution and benzyl alcohol (Gordon et al. 1987).

An additional possible cause of later skin reactions independent of obliterative endarteritis is possibly the significantly longer mean generation time of skin fibroblasts in radiation wounds (Rudolph et al. 1988). As the later damage in skin areas also has a tendency to progress, conservative measures are frequently without therapeutic effect, and with ulcerations, surgical grafting is necessary. The method as well as the degree of surgery in the treatment of skin lesions induced by radiation must be individually planned with consideration being given to the site and severity of the lesions (Salfeld and Huchzermeyer 1985). Wound debridement and simultaneous coverage using well-vascularized flaps with an independent source of circulation distant from the site of radiation damage is a useful and reliable method of repairing radiation necrosis and achieving good healing (Mathes and Hurwitz 1986; Galli et al. 1987; Salfeld and Huchzermeyer 1985).

15.5.2 Gastrointestinal Tract

Serious treatment complications primarily involve the bowel and bladder (Rubin et al. 1985). The small intestine is among the most radiation-sensitive organs of the body due to the high cell turnover of the mucosa. Tables 15.4 and 15.5 give an overview of the intestinal complications observed after the irradiation of cervical and endometrial carcinomas. A comparison of the results is made difficult by the sometimes differing assessment criteria.

After radiation treatment of cervical carcinomas, 4.3%–53.9% have been reported to show intestinal reactions, irrespective of their seriousness (Table 15.4). The incidence of rectal fistulae – grade 4 in the RTOG/EORTC system – lies between 0.2% and 6.3%. Most authors observe fewer serious complications after high-dose-rate (HDR) brachytherapy than after low-dose-rate (LDR) irradiation. After radiotherapy of endometrial carcinomas, rectal fistulae are observed in 0%–5.4% of cases (Table 15.5).

An important parameter for the development of complications in the small and large intestine is the strength of the external radiation dose, and in the case of the rectum, also the dose reaching point A (Montana et al. 1985). For the rectum, unlike the bladder, the correlation between the radiation dose and subsequent complications can be proved (Montana et al. 1985; Stryker et al. 1988; Teshima et al. 1985). Montana et al. (1985) found a mean dose of 6907 cGy in cases with the appearance of proctitis. The mean dose in cases without the development of proctitis, on the other hand, was 6381 cGy.

Symptomatology and classification of the radiation effects on the intestine are presented in Tables 15.1 and 15.2. Clinical symptoms of acute radiation enteritis include cramping diarrhea, mucous discharges, tenesmus, vomiting, and anorexia. Sometimes hemorrhage or bacterial infection results. Death may even occur due to loss of fluid and electrolytes (Behr et al. 1990; Kinsella and Bloomer 1980; Weijers et al. 1990). The severity of symptoms correlates with the volume of intestine which is irradiated (Piver and Barlow 1977). With the irradiation of the complete abdomen, 61%–79% of patients suffer from nausea and vomiting (Fyles et al. 1992; Schray et al. 1989; Whelan et al. 1992). Due to acute gastrointestinal complaints (mainly nausea and vomiting), 9% of patients must have their therapy interrupted.

It is often difficult to differentiate between cancer and chronic radiation damage (Deitel and To 1987). Radiologically, no individual feature is specific to radiation damage, neoplasia, inflammatory bowel disease, or infection. Weijers et al. (1990) found no radiation-induced changes in the jejunum, except for bowel dilatation signifying a distal obstruction, while in the ileum there was evidence of submucosal thickening.

Whilst the intrinsically inferior contrast resolution of CT compared with MRI reduces its ability to discriminate between tumor and radiation damage, there is some evidence that MRI can be used to dis-

Table 15.4. Complications of radiotherapy in cases of carcinoma of the cervix

Author	Ext. rad.	Int. rad.	No. of patients	Rect. fist.	Int. sten.	Int. react.	Ves. fist.	Uret. sten.	Blad. react.	Total react.
Kutzner et al. (1986)	Co	LDR	770	1.3%	4%	27%	0.8%	2.7%	18%	45%
Cikaric (1988)	Acc	HDR	140	2.9%		7.2%	0.7%		5%	12.1%
Cikaric (1988)	Acc	LDR	187	6.4%		16.6%	2.7%		9.6%	26.2%
Glaser (1988)		HDR	623	0.2%	0.4%	4.3%	0.1%	0.2%	3%	7.3%
Glaser (1988)		LDR	1131	6.3%	4.7%	53.9%	4.3%	3.8%	29.5%	83.4%
Kuipers (1988)		HDR	142	5.6%			3.5%			
Kuipers (1988)		LDR	152	4.6%			2.6%			
Vahrson and Römer (1988)	Co	HDR	147	3%			3%			
Vahrson and Römer (1988)	Co	LDR	835	2%			2%			
Stryker et al. (1988)	Acc		132			19%			8%	17%
Montana et al. (1985)			572			12.4%			8.1%	20.5%
Sinistrero et al. (1993)	Co/Acc		215			14%			7%	33%
Stockbine et al. (1970)	Acc	LDR	831	3.9%		17.3%	0%		0.7%	18%
Orton et al. (1991)		HDR	10887							9.05%
Orton et al. (1991)		LDR	4709							20.66%

Ext. rad, external irradiation; Co, cobalt –60; Acc, accelerator; Int. rad., intracavitary irradiation; HDR, high dose rate; LDR, low dose rate; Rect. fist., rectovaginal fistula; Int. sten., intestinal stenosis; Int. react., intestinal reaction; Ves. fist., vesicovaginal fistula; Uret. sten., ureter stenosis; Blad. react., bladder reaction; Total react., all reactions.

Table 15.5. Complications of radiotherapy in cases of endometrial carcinoma

Author	Ext. rad.	Int. rad.	No. of patients	Rect. fist.	Int. sten.	Int. react.	Ves. fist.	Uret. sten.	Blad. react.	Total react.
Bekerus et al. (1988)	Co/Acc	HDR	65	1.5%			0%			43.1%
Bekerus et al. (1988)	Co/Acc	LDR	74	5.4%			0%			51.4%
Rauthe et al. (1988)	Co/Acc	HDR	191	2%			1%			
Rauthe et al. (1988)	Co/Acc	LDR	577	1%			0.2%			
Rotte (1988)		HDR	227	0%		5.2%	0%		1.7%	6.9%
Rotte (1988)		LDR	106	0%		5.6%	0%		1.8%	7.4%

Ext. rad, External irradiation; Co, cobalt –60; Acc, accelerator; Int. rad., intracavitary irradiation; HDR, high dose rate; LDR, low dose rate; Rect. fist., rectovaginal fistula; Int. sten., intestinal stenosis; Int. react., intestinal reaction; Ves. fist., vesicovaginal fistula; Uret. sten., ureter stenosis; Blad. react., bladder reaction; Total react., all reactions.

tinguish between the two by measuring T1 and T2 relaxation times, analyzing the signal intensity appearing on T1- and T2-weighted images, and using gadolinium-DTPA (Johnson and Carrington 1992).

Endoscopically, the mucosa is seen to be inflamed, edematous, and friable following a radiation reaction. Later, the injury can vary from hyperemia and telangiectasia to ulceration, necrosis, and fibrous stenosis as the result of obliterating endarteritis of the small vessels in the intestinal wall (Kinsella and Bloomer 1980; Polson and Misiewicz 1992; Wellwood and Jackson 1973).

Histological abnormalities correlate poorly with symptoms and functional changes (Trier and Browning 1966). In some cases of radiation-induced colitis, aneuploid DNA profiles may be relevant to the increased risk of malignancy in the irradiated tissues (Pearson et al. 1992).

Grade 2 or 3 complaints are treated with antispasmodic, parasympatholytic, or anticholinergic drugs and codeine or lopiramide (Deitel and To 1987; Kinsella and Bloomer 1980; Yeoh and Horowitz 1987; Yeoh et al. 1993; Zentler-Munro and Bessell 1987). Opioids deliver pain relief as well as having the desirable side-effect of reducing intestine mobility (Kinsella and Bloomer 1980).

Bile acid malabsorption in the terminal ileum is probably the main cause of more chronic enteritis (Danielsson et al. 1991; Stryker et al. 1977; Zentler-Munro and Bessell 1987). However, other factors, such as bacteria which cause gallbladder acid deconjugation (Danielsson et al. 1991; Yeoh et al. 1984; Zentler-Munro and Bessell 1987) and lactose intolerance caused by mucosal damage (Yeoh et al. 1993; Zentler-Munro and Bessell 1987), also play a role. For this reason, in cases of diarrhea it has been recommended that cholestyramine (Arlow et al. 1987; Zentler-Munro and Bessell 1987) or lopiramide (Yeoh et al. 1993) be used, if necessary in combination with antibiotics and a reduced fat diet (Danielsson et al. 1991; Zentler-Munro and Bessell 1987) or even a lactose-free diet (Zentler-Munro and Bessell 1987). The nutrition should contain fat-soluble vitamins and vitamin B_{12} in order to prevent hypovitaminosis.

As a consequence of fibrosis and thickening, segments of the intestine become rigid and motionless, resulting in functional obstruction (Wittich et al. 1984). Cases of partial obstruction of the small intestine frequently respond to conservative therapy (Smith and De Cosse 1986). Helmkamp and Kimmel (1985) reported a 45% success rate in the resolution of small intestine obstructions by means of long tube decompression.

For the prevention of therapy-specific weight loss in serious cases, dietetic measures are also required. A nondistending, easily absorbable, calorie-rich diet is advisable. A semihydrolyzed, elemental, or similar diet (Bounous et al. 1975; Yeoh and Horowitz 1987) is recommended. In serious cases, even partial or total parenteral nutrition is necessary (Deitel and To 1987; Radiation Therapy Oncology Group 1984; Seegenschmiedt and Sauer 1993; Silvain et al. 1992).

One of the most common and most distressing side-effects of radiation is emesis. Emesis during and after radiotherapy depends on the site, field size, dose per fraction, age, and anxiety of the patient (Danjoux et al. 1979; Roberts and Priestman 1993). It causes some patients to refuse treatment, delay appointments, or discontinue therapy entirely, leads to anorexia, and seriously influences the quality of life (Fitch 1992). The pathophysiology of radiation-induced emesis remains incompletely understood (Roberts and Priestman 1993; Scarantino et al. 1992). It is probable that both peripheral and central effects are important in its etiology (STEWART 1990). A peripheral effect may be mediated by small intestine damage (STEWART 1990; YOUNG 1986), eliciting the release of serotonin from enterochromaffin cells (ANDREWS and BHANDARI 1993; HENRIKSSON et al. 1992b). 5-HT_3 binding sites are present in both the peripheral and the central nervous system (ANDREWS and BHANDARI 1993).

Combination antiemetic therapy appears to be superior to single-agent therapy. Combinations that contain metoclopramide plus a corticosteroid with or without benzodiazepine or diphenhydramine appear to be particularly effective (SAGAR 1991; STEWART 1990). Diarrhea is an inconvenient side-effect which can be caused by using metoclopramide during irradiation.

The 5-hydroxytryptamine-receptor antagonists are effective for the treatment of radiation-induced vomiting (ANDREWS and BHANDARI 1993). Ondansetron has proved to be very effective, with a good side-effect profile (ROBERTS 1992; ROBERTS and PRIESTMAN 1993; SAGAR 1991). With radiotherapy of the upper abdomen, emesis can be completely controlled in 79% of patients using 8 mg ondansetron t.i.d. Diarrhea does not occur. A third of the patients report mild constipation (HENRIKSSON et al. 1992b). The antiemetic effect of ondansetron can be increased further through the use of dexamethasone (SMITH et al. 1991). The effect of tropisetron during irradiation of ovarian carcinoma patients is just as promising. SORBE et al. (1992) found that vomiting occurred in less than 10% of patients who were treated with tropisetron. The overall ratings for quality of life were excellent or good in 75%–85% of cases. The drug was very well tolerated and no serious adverse effects were recorded despite long-term treatment.

Side-effects of radiation in the rectum and sigmoid colon can be managed by local therapy (POLSON and MISIEWICZ 1992). In a prospective randomized double-blind controlled study, radiation-induced proctosigmoiditis could be significantly improved with sucralfate enemas twice daily, as compared with a placebo group (KOCHHAR et al. 1991). The use of rectal steroid enemas, each with 20 mg prednisolone in combination with oral sulfasalazine medication, also yielded an improvement, but here the systemic side-effects must be considered (KOCHAR et al. 1991).

Patients with less serious complaints may find enemas containing cod liver oil to be very beneficial. The parallel infusion of protein-free hemolysate from calf's blood appears to support the effects.

In a group of 13 patients, only 9% failed to show an improvement of chronic radiation-induced proctitis when sodium pentosanpolysulfate was used (GRIGSBY et al. 1990).

Bleeding in radiation proctosigmoiditis occurs from the telangiectases and other mucosal abnormalities (HABOUBI et al. 1988). With light bleeding, the infusions described for the treatment of proctitis can be applied. If hemostasis is necessary, in addition to diathermy, laser treatment is seen as a safe method (ALEXANDER and DWYER 1988; BUCHI and DIXON 1987; VIGGIANO et al. 1993). Argon laser has a superficial penetration and is selectively absorbed by hemoglobin, effectively coagulating the mucosal vascular lesions without damaging the underlying submucosa or intestine wall (BUCHI and DIXON 1987). Nd:YAG laser penetrates deeper, as a consequence of which complications such as ileus and pain can arise sooner (ALEXANDER and DWYER 1988). VIGGIANO et al. (1993) reported a complication rate of 6% using Nd:YAG therapy for bleeding due to radiation proctopathy.

With deep-seated bleeding lesions, a tamponade such as a balloon catheter can achieve quick results (KATZEN et al. 1976). Especially serious bleeding can be rendered low risk through percutaneous arterial catheter embolization (BANASCHAK et al. 1985; CROWE and STELLATO 1985; SCHNUR and BOUMEA 1983). Otherwise, nonstaunchable life-threatening bleeding and other serious radiation damage of the intestine, such as ileus, perforations, and fistulae which cannot be rectified conventionally, necessitate surgery (ANSELINE et al. 1981; COVENS et al. 1991; MÄKELÄ et al. 1987; MOESCHL and MIHOLIC 1989; MORGENSTERN et al. 1977; ZOETMULDER et al. 1988). However, due to the higher operation-specific morbidity and mortality, all methods of conventional therapy should be exhausted before such operations are carried out (FENNER et al. 1989; MÄKELÄ et al. 1987; MORGENSTERN et al. 1977; YEOH and HOROWITZ 1987). The morbidity and mortality rates are reported to be 45%–47% and 14%–16% respectively (FENNER et al. 1989; MÄKELÄ et al. 1987). Major postoperative complications are intestinal, intra-abdominal, pelvic, and retroperitoneal perforations, enterocutaneous fistulae, anastomotic dehiscences, and serious wound infections (MORGENSTERN et al. 1977). Hypoalbuminemia, more than one laparotomy before the irradiation, and a short interval (less than 12 months) between the irradiation and surgical intervention increase the risk of complications (VAN HALTEREN et al. 1993). Mortality is especially high in patients who have more than just one site of localized radiation damage, such as coexistent injuries in the urinary tract (JAYALAKSHMAMMA and PINKEL 1976). The more aggressive the operation, the more likely are subsequent complications (JAO et al. 1986). The results can be improved by careful preoperative diagnosis and planning (MIHOLIC et al. 1987).

The controversy over resection of radiation-damaged bowel versus bypass is unresolved (COVENS et al. 1991; FENNER et al. 1989; MÄKELÄ et al. 1987; MOESCHL and MIHOLIC 1989; MIHOLIC et al. 1987). Both procedures have their own fields of indication (FENNER et al. 1989; GALLAND and SPENCER 1987; MÄKELÄ et al. 1987; VAN HALTEREN et al. 1993). In each case, where possible, the anastomosis should be outside the irradiated area (BRICKER et al. 1981; CROSS and FRAZEE 1992; DEITEL and TO 1987; GALLAND and SPENCER 1987; O'BRIEN et al. 1987; ZOETMULDER et al. 1988) in order to prevent postoperative healing difficulties. The disease may progress and relapses may appear years later in areas previously thought to be normal (LOCALIO et al. 1969).

In some cases, a proximal diversion is unavoidable (CRAM et al. 1977; CROSS and FRAZEE 1992; MOESCHL and MIHOLIC 1989; MIHOLIC et al. 1988; ZOETMULDER et al. 1988), especially in patients where the cure is unproven or where tumors persist.

After major or repeated surgery, a short gut syndrome can result. Parenteral nutrition may be necessary to improve this (MORGENSTERN et al. 1977).

Fistula closures should be restricted to carefully selected cases, as the long-term results are poor due to the progression of change (AARTSEN and SINDRAM 1988). Maintenance of normal vaginal function after local fistula repair is the exception (AARTSEN and SINDRAM 1988).

The low rate of side-effects and the healing achieved with hyperbaric oxygen in cases of fistulae and therapy-resistant bleeding are interesting (CHARNEAU et al. 1991; WILLIAMS et al. 1992).

15.5.3 Bladder and Ureter

The urinary bladder is also very vulnerable to radiation damage. Tables 15.4 and 15.5 contain details concerning the frequency of bladder complications after irradiation of cervical and endometrial carcinomas. Bladder reactions occur in 0.7%–29.5% of patients with cervical carcinomas following radiotherapy (Table 15.4). The incidence of vesicovaginal fistulae lies between 0% and 4.3%, which is lower than the incidence of rectovaginal fistulae. After the radiation treatment of endometrial carcinomas, the incidence of vesicovaginal fistulae may amount to 1% (Table 15.5).

As with the complications in the area of the rectum, those in the bladder correlate with the applied dose. MONTANA and FOWLER (1989) reported that the mean bladder dose in patients with cystitis was higher (6661 cGy) than that in patients without cystitis (6390 cGy), though it should be noted that determination of the exact bladder dose creates difficulties (STRYKER et al. 1988).

With the bladder, irradiation leads to early hyperemia, and later to sclerosing endarteritis, fibrosis, and tissue atrophy (Lancet Editorial 1987). Symptomatology and classifications of the radiation effects on the bladder are presented in Tables 15.1 and 15.2. Increased frequency of urination, urgency, nocturia, dysuria, and bladder spasms occur with early and late radiation damage of the bladder and greatly inconvenience patients. The diagnosis can be easily accomplished cystoscopically.

Acute radiation reactions are characterized by marked mucosal edema and diffuse erythema with prominent submucosal vascularity. In the more chronic stages, there are areas of extreme pallor separating areas of intense erythema with petechiae. Occasionally, ulceration is present (SCHELLHAMMER et al. 1986). Radiation ulcers typically lie in the region of the greatest radiation exposure. Biopsies should be avoided in order not to provoke fistulae through additional trauma. Fistulae present initially as radiation ulcers, punched out with a raised margin (SCHELLHAMMER et al. 1986).

The irradiated bladder is susceptible to infection and ulceration. Healing is slow (JOHNSON and CARRINGTON 1992; Lancet Editorial, 1987). The symptoms of bladder reaction and infection are similar, and can be moderated with local anesthetics, spasmolytics, anticholinergics, normal saline solution containing 100 mg hydrocortisone per liter, and α-adrenergic agents. The instillation of 50 ml of a 10% solution of DMSO yields an improvement in some patients (SCHELLHAMMER et al. 1986). Infections frequently occur simultaneously with the radiation reaction, and must be treated using specific therapy, whereby sufficient fluid intake is important.

The fibrotic tissue reaction after irradiation leads to a lower filling volume, increased bladder pressure, and a stronger urge to urinate. Together with lack of urethral function, this results in a clear increase in incontinence which is sometimes also induced by stress. Urge and urge incontinence, especially with cervical carcinomas, is considered to be among the most serious problems encountered after radiotherapy (Behr et al. 1990; Parkin et al. 1987, 1988; Zoubek et al. 1989).

The aforementioned symptoms can be alleviated through the introduction of bladder training (Behr et al. 1990). Depending on the severity of the incontinence, however, operative measures such as augmentative cystoplasty may also be necessary (Zoubek et al. 1989).

With acute reactions greater than grade 2 and late reactions greater than grade 1, macrohematuria frequently appears and, with grade 4, forces transfusions. Coagula which hinder the emptying of the bladder must be removed cystoscopically or by rinsing through a large-diameter catheter system (Livne et al. 1987).

As estrogen receptors are located in the bladder, systemic and local hormone therapy appears worthwhile, at least as an additional supporting measure. According to Liu et al. (1990), improvement in hematuria could be achieved by the twice daily intravenous administration of 1 mg conjugated estrogen per kg body weight followed by 5 mg daily. After the therapy, the bladder wall cystoscopically showed a stronger mechanical resistance capacity. Significant improvement in hematuria and dysuria has also been reported following bladder instillations of placental extract (Micic and Genbacev 1988), which fully corresponds with the effects of intravesical estrogen applications (Kurz et al. 1993). The timely infusion of a protein-free emulsion from calf's blood appears to support the effects.

A beneficial effect of orally administered sodium pentosanpolysulfate was described by Parsons (1986) in five patients.

Cystoscopic hemostasis is only possible at localized sources of bleeding with diathermy, laser, or the injection of sclerosing substances (Maier and Hofbauer 1986; Lancet Editorial 1987). Local submucosal bladder injection of orgotein has shown favorable results in the treatment of serious bladder symptoms such as macrohematuria, bladder tenesmus, and frequency (Maier and Hofbauer 1986; Maier and Zechner 1988; Mayer et al. 1984), but anaphylactic reactions are described as serious side-effects (Maier and Hofbauer 1986; Maier and Zechner 1988).

Diffuse bladder hemorrhage requires other procedures. Attempts at hydrostatic bladder distention are dangerous due to the possibility of perforation, interstitial and submucosal hemorrhage, and bladder contraction, these risks being especially pronounced after radiotherapy (Anderson et al. 1976). The instillation of 10% formalin into the bladder for hemostasis is very effective but, of course, must be carried out under narcosis and carries some risks (Donahue and Frank 1989; Schoenrock and Cianci 1986). Of lower risk is continuous intravesicular lavage with 1% aluminum potassium sulfate solution in sterile distilled water via a two-way catheter (Arrizabalaga et al. 1987). Using this technique to treat radiation-induced bladder hemorrhage, these authors reported complete success in 66% of the treated patients, and partial success in 15%. In most cases, suprapubic pain, vesical tenesmus, and spasms can be controlled using antispasmodics without narcosis. A low-risk, low-exposure therapy for immitigable hemorrhaging from the urogenital region is arterial embolization, as is palliatively used for hemorrhaging from tumors (Banaschak et al. 1985; Schellhammer et al. 1986; Schnur and Boumea 1983). The side-effects such as pain, temperature increase, and reflex-specific ileus symptoms are transitory. Complications ranging from circulatory disturbances to necrosis outside the area of embolization, as often occurs with operative ligation for hemostasis, are seldom (Andriole and Sugarbaker 1985; Banaschak et al. 1985; Berthrong 1986).

Urinary diversion and/or cystectomy only seldom needs to be undertaken due to hemorrhaging (Lapides 1970; Power et al. 1983).

Ulcerations and necrosis have a poor tendency to heal due to the frequently progressive vascular changes of the tissue. Radiation-induced fistulae also display no tendency to heal spontaneously. However, they affect the quality of life so severely that therapy almost always appears necessary.

Direct closure is not advisable due to a poor tendency to heal (Maier and Hofbauer 1986). For this reason, plastic surgical methods are recommended using nonirradiated tissue with intact blood supplies. Kiricuta achieved a 90% successful closure rate for radiation-induced vesicovaginal fistulae through the use of omentum. The peritonitis-specific mortality amounted to 10% (Kiricuta 1988).

Various operative techniques are suitable to the urinary system, in which bowel sections are generally inserted (Hendry et al. 1991; Maier and Hofbauer 1986; Morgan et al. 1993); even continence may be achieved by this means (Mundy 1988).

The application of hyperbaric oxygen is reported to yield good results, with low side-effects (Kindwall 1993, 1992; Rijkmans et al. 1989; Schoenrock and Cianci 1986; Weiss et al. 1985).

After only a few sessions for bladder hemorrhaging, there is a decrease in the transfusion frequency because of a reduction in the hemorrhaging sites and telangiectasia (RIJKMANS et al. 1989). Even the closure of a large radiation-induced vesicocutaneous fistula was reported by SCHOENROCK and CIANCI (1986). Protocols for the use of hyperbaric oxygen should be produced if other conservative therapies have failed.

Ureteral strictures are seldom caused purely by irradiation (SCHELLHAMMER et al. 1986); thus, the possibility of a tumor should always be excluded. In their group of 1749 cervical carcinomas treated with radiation therapy, SLATER and FLETCHER (1971) found only five unilateral ureteral strictures, which were attributable to postirradiation fibrosis. PARLIAMENT et al. (1989) reported that fibrosis-specific obstructive ureteropathy occurs in more than 3% of patients receiving radiation therapy for carcinoma of the cervix. The ureter in the pelvis is usually affected, especially the parametrial triangle (PARLIAMENT et al. 1989). Ureteral dilatation and hydronephrosis occur above the stenosis (JOHNSON and CARRINGTON 1992). Only 50% of patients show notable symptoms. Nonspecific symptoms such as pain in the lower pelvis, malaise, and tiredness are sometimes present. This insidious nature of ureteral strictures means that there is a real risk of failure to detect renal impairment (JOHNSON and CARRINGTON 1992).

Ureteral fistulae are extremely rare and difficult to diagnose. The best method for this purpose may be transvaginal visualization (RAUTHE et al. 1992).

Therapy for stenosis and fistulae is usually operative and must maintain the renal function (JOHNSON and CARRINGTON 1992; MICIC and GENBACEV 1988).

15.5.4 Vagina and Vulva

Particularly with brachytherapy of the genital region, the vagina is often exposed to extremely high radiation doses, as a consequence of which radiation-induced damage to the vagina is very frequent. Bacterial flora of the vagina, which is not stable throughout the course of therapy (GORDON et al. 1989), may play a role in the development of acute radiation reactions of the vagina. A radiation-induced lesion of the vaginal epithelium is made considerably worse through infection by bacteria or fungi.

In the early phase of radiation reaction, there is hyperemia of the vagina, frequently accompanied by symptoms of colpitis with fluorine and considerable discomfort.

As in other organs, in the vagina and vulva late radiation ulcerations are caused by vessel obliterations. Shrinking and shortening of the organs occur due to fibrosis. The epithelium becomes blanched and thin, and is easily damaged by telangiectases which bleed lightly. Excisions should only be undertaken very cautiously in order not to encourage the formation of fistulae.

Fistulae, as the greatest manifestation of vaginal radiation reactions after radiotherapy of cervical and endometrial carcinomas, occur in the rectum more frequently than in the bladder because the dorsal wall and the caudal part of the vagina have a lower tolerance to radiation than the rest of the organ (HINTZ et al. 1980; HIMMELMANN et al. 1985). The frequency of fistula lies between 0% and 10.6% (Tables 15.4, 15,5). The leakage of feces, urine, or both from the vagina quickly has pronounced adverse physical, psychological, and social effects on the patient.

Local antimicrobial treatment with douching, creams, or vaginal suppositories, which can also be used prophylactically, frequently achieves quick alleviation of acute radiation reactions. As the proliferation of the vaginal epithelium is estrogen dependent, local treatment has a clear use in the healing of the reactions. However, with serious disorders such as ulcerations, parenteral estrogen intake should also be considered.

After careful diagnosis (RAUTHE et al. 1992), fistulae must be rectified either by closure or by proximal diversion of feces or urine. Necrotic tissue is carefully removed (RHOMBERG and EITER 1988) or locally broken down with enzymes. In particular, deep-seated necrosis in the distal vaginal and vulvar region requires surgical treatment (ROBERTS et al. 1991). Perineal, vulval, or vaginoperineal reconstruction is successful using flaps with a good blood supply (GRANICK et al. 1993; MATHES and HURWITZ 1986; SKENE et al. 1990). Maintenance of normal vaginal function after fistula repair is the exception (AARTSEN and SINDRAM 1988).

Light bleeding of the vagina can be stopped through coagulation or hemostyptics. Serious bleeding requires a tamponade. Topical acetone, or the placing of an acetone-soaked pack, may be helpful if embolism techniques (BANASCHAK et al. 1985; CROWE and STELLATO 1985; SCHNUR and BOUMEA 1983) are not immediately available (PATSNER 1993).

Late irradiation-induced anatomical and functional changes, such as damaging light bleeding of the epithelium and a dry, stiff, shrivelled, and constricted vagina embedded in a fibrosed region, complicate the reestablishment of sexual intercourse. Between 66% and 78% of patients have considerable sexual dysfunction after irradiation of cervical carcinomas (ABITBOL and DAVENPORT 1974; BERTELSEN 1983; LOTZE 1990), which can only be treated with difficulty (ABITBOL and DAVENPORT 1974). Starting intercourse early, however, appears to be important in avoiding shrivelling. With dryness of the epithelium, water or oil-based lubricants can, with the addition of local anesthetics, bring relief in certain circumstances. Local estrogen applications have a positive influence on the resistibility of the epithelium.

In general, changes in the vulvar region caused by irradiation lead to more severe complaints than in the vaginal region, due to the good supply of sensory nerves. For this reason, pain relievers must be frequently administered. Local therapy of radiation damage in the vulva region is very similar to that carried out for the external skin and the vagina. Of course, powder treatment is not used in this damp region. Rather, disinfecting and/or light tanning hip baths and local or systemic antiphlogistics in the case of reactions greater than grade 1 alleviate the complaints. Severe inflammatory changes cause urination to be very painful, and temporary suprapubic bladder catheterization is then helpful.

Androgens promote the proliferation of the vulvar epithelium more strongly than estrogen and therefore may be employed locally when atrophic changes are present. Although with sparing application, symptoms of androgenization are not expected, this potential side-effect should be mentioned.

15.5.5 Ovaries

Radiation damage to the ovaries is only relevant to premenopausal women. The response of the ovaries to irradiation varies with age as well as dose and there is also a considerable variation in response between individuals (ASH 1980; GRADISHAR and SCHILSKY 1989). With additional cytostasis, the effect of irradiation on the female gonads is increased (HAIE-MEDER et al. 1993). There is no convincing evidence that concurrent administration of LHRH analogues or oral contraceptives during infradiaphragmatic irradiation can protect the gonads (KREUSER et al. 1993).

The dose required to destroy all oocytes in women over 40 years old and to induce the menopause lies between 400 and 600 cGy (DOLL and SMITH 1968; LUSHBAUGH and CASARETT 1976). With younger women who have a large number of oocytes, higher doses are necessary (ASH 1980; RAY et al. 1970). Sterility is inevitable at an ovarian dose greater than 800 cGy (BAKER 1971; GRADISHAR and SCHILSKY 1989).

The luteal function appears to be less susceptible to irradiation (JANSON et al. 1981). A radiation dose of about 1000–1500 cGy, however, is reported to disturb ovarian function in about 90% of patients (JOSLIN 1971).

While with the irradiation of nongynecological malignancies the gonads can be completely luxated from the radiation path through ovarian transpositions so that fertility remains intact (HAIE-MEDER et al. 1993; THOMAS et al. 1976), with radiotherapy of genital tumors the generative and hormonal function of the ovaries cannot generally be maintained. Even after only brachytherapy of cervical carcinomas in young women, hormone production in the ovaries is interrupted (JANSON et al. 1981).

With individually adapted, well-balanced, hormonal substitution, the castration complaints can be brought under control almost without exception. Estrogen substitution is not only important for the relief of physical and vegetative symptoms: with long-term follicular hormone treatment, morbidity and mortality through osteoporosis and heart/circulatory illnesses can be decidedly reduced (GRADY et al. 1992; WHITCROFT and STEVENSON 1992).

15.5.6 Bones

Insufficiency fractures occur when the elastic resistance of bone is inadequate to withstand the stress of normal activity (COOPER et al. 1985). With mature bones, irradiation leads to damage of the osteoblasts, which eventually causes osteoporosis (COX et al. 1986). Preexisting osteoporosis is a usual causative factor. The affected patients are, therefore, usually postmenopausal (ABE et al. 1992; COOPER et al. 1985).

In the patient group of ABE et al. (1992), 85% had more than one fracture; 62% were located close to the sacroiliac joint, 28% in the upper sacrum, 4% in the lower sacrum, 4% in the os pubis, and 3% in the os ischii. Eighty-four percent of the patients indicated that pain was a symptom (ABE et al. 1992).

If fractures are not accurately diagnosed, further irradiation to the pelvis might erroneously be instigated (RAFII et al. 1988). Diagnosis on plain films may be difficult in complex anatomical areas like the sacrum. Insufficiency fractures are especially likely to go undetected on x-ray films.

Radionuclide bone scan is invariably positive but nonspecific (Abe et al. 1992; Cooper et al. 1985). Increased bilateral activity in the upper sacrum is typical (Ries 1983).

Fractures can be accurately identified by CT (Cooper et al. 1985; Rafii et al. 1988). The soft tissue mass that might be expected in metastatic disease is missing (Cooper et al. 1985); biopsies are therefore unnecessary (Cooper et al. 1985).

Radiation-induced fractures are a repairable complication even though the healing process in irradiated bone is slow (Bragg et al. 1970; Rafii et al. 1988).

Osteoradionecrosis is an end-stage of tissue damage induced by irradiation. Vascular damage due to the highly radiosensitive endothelial cells results in hypoxic, hypovascular, and hypocellular tissue (Westermark et al. 1990). Necrosis of the head of the hip bone and fractures of the femoral neck have become less frequent due to current practices, including the use of megavoltage accelerators and hip-preserving irradiation methods (Parker and Berry 1976; Vahrson and Römer 1988). The frequency of femoral neck fractures is lower than 1:1000 (Parker and Berry 1976); with this complication, operations are generally performed.

Radiation necrosis may be difficult to differentiate from sarcoma arising in irradiated bone. A soft tissue mass favors the diagnosis of neoplasia, while its absence suggests radiation necrosis. Lack of pain favors necrosis. Calcification may occur in radiation necrosis and does not indicate neoplasia. A lack of progression shown on serial x-ray films favors necrosis (Dalinka and Mazzeo 1985).

15.5.7 Vessels

While late radiation damage of all organs and areas is mainly caused by changes to the small vessels, larger vessels are also affected. Side-effects of irradiation in the arteries appear in patients who also have radiation reactions in other organs (Pettersson and Swedenborg 1990). There are two main types of side-effect in the arteries: disruption and stenosis or occlusion (Himmel and Hassett 1986; McCready et al. 1983).

Radiotherapy acts synergistically with other atherogenic factors (Nylander et al. 1978; Pettersson and Swedenborg 1990). Smoking seems to increase the risk (Himmel and Hassett 1986; Nylander et al. 1978; Pettersson and Swedenborg 1990), and diabetes and high blood pressure are apparently further risk factors (Himmel and Hassett 1986).

Radiation-induced chronic arterial injuries can occur at any time between a few months and more than 20 years after irradiation (Himmel and Hassett 1986; Lawson 1985); a third of such injuries occur within the first 5 years. The incidence after the treatment of cervical and ovarian carcinomas has been reported to be 1:300 surviving patients (Pettersson and Swedenborg 1990), whereby the number of patients with arterial injuries but without symptoms is perhaps much greater (Himmel and Hassett 1986). Subclinical vascular damage, which could be induced by low radiotherapy doses, has been found to affect 5% of seminoma patients (Goodman et al. 1993). The changes in the arteries resemble those of arterial sclerosis. Characteristic of the radiation-specific genesis is limitation of the damage to the field of irradiation exposure (Himmel and Hassett 1986; Pettersson and Swedenborg 1990; von Paes et al. 1991).

The principal symptoms of arterial injury in the pelvic region are claudication or circulatory disturbances when resting (Himmel and Hassett 1986; Pettersson and Swedenborg 1990).

Treatment of the arterial changes is by arterial bypass, whereby the anastomosis should lie outside the irradiation field whenever possible (Lawson 1985).

15.5.8 Hematopoietic System

The bone marrow is the organ most sensitive to irradiation. However, irradiation of the bone marrow often cannot be avoided and the doses are often higher than its tolerance. After radiotherapy with 30 Gy or more, a lack of hematopoiesis results, independent of the patient's age and of the interval after radiotherapy (Kauczor et al. 1992). The irradiated bone marrow exhibits a homogeneous hyperintense pattern on T1-weighted MR images. This allows clear recognition of the former target volumes.

Interruption of large-volume abdominal irradiation is usually the consequence of myelosuppression (Fyles et al. 1992; Whelan et al. 1992); Schray et al. (1989) reported such interruption to be necessary in 27% of patients. The toxicity rises with an increasing irradiation volume and also commences earlier (Abrams et al. 1985). The myelotoxic effects of irradiation are increased by cytostatic drugs, as shown by the higher frequency of thrombocyte transfusions and the lower number of circulating granulocyte-monocyte precursor colony-forming units when using both methods (ABRAMS et al. 1985).

Granulocyte colony-stimulating factor (G-CSF), successfully introduced for cytostatic-induced leukocytopenia, is just as effective in combatting the effects of radiotherapy (MACMANUS et al. 1993; SAKATA et al. 1993; SCHMIDBERGER et al. 1993; KNOX et al. 1994). Different dosing methods have been described. When using extended field radiotherapy, MACMANUS et al. (1993) intermittently administered G-CSF subcutaneously for leukocyte values of ≤1500/µl in daily doses similar to those recommended for patients receiving chemotherapy. In this way, a rapid normalization of neutrophil granulocytes was achieved in all cases without toxicity. KNOX et al. (1994), on the other hand, adapted the daily G-CSF dose to the current leukocyte values. During subdiaphragmatic irradiation, patients received 3 µg G-CSF/kg daily. The dose was decreased to 2 µg/kg daily for ≥10000 neutrophil granulocytes/µl and 1 µg/kg daily for ≥15000 granulocytes/µl. It was discontinued for values of neutrophil granulocytes ≥20000. The optimal dose appeared to be 1 µg G-CSF/kg daily, if no other cytotoxic therapy was administered. With neither treatment method does the radiotherapy need to be interrupted.

Within the framework of a radiochemotherapy, just as successfully, a 2 µg/kg body weight dose of G-CSF was administered with no side-effects if the leukocyte value fell below 3000 per mm^3. With a 3- to 5-day treatment duration, a delay in the radiochemotherapy could be avoided using this method (SAKATA et al. 1993). The daily administration of 5 µg G-CSF/kg prophylactically, on the other hand, led to very high leukocyte values (SCHMIDBERGER et al. 1993).

The side-effects of G-CSF treatment are restricted to an increase in the alkaline phosphate level and temporary mild aching of the bones.

15.5.9 Nervous System

Radiation-induced lesions of the lumbosacral plexus are infrequent. Their frequency after the irradiation of cervical and endometrial carcinomas is cited as between 0.09% and 0.17% (GEORGIOU et al. 1993; ABE et al. 1992; KIMOSE et al. 1989). Observations from BLOSS et al. (1991) and COHEN et al. (1983) seem to suggest that concomitant chemotherapy could reduce the tolerance of the nerves to radiotherapy. This should be noted for multimodal therapy comprising the use of cytostatics and irradiation for gynecological malignancies.

Chronic progressive radiation myelopathy of the spinal cord leads to severe physical disability and eventually death due to secondary infections. There is no effective treatment (GRAU 1993).

15.5.10 Psyche

The relatively good prognosis of gynecological malignancies contrasts greatly with the psychological distress that women experience before, during, and after irradiation (ANDERSEN and ANDERSON 1986). For women, a malignant growth of the genitals represents an especially severe threat, including at a psychological level (HARRIS et al. 1982): the woman is affected at the center of her sexuality (FERVERS-SCHORRE 1987). Many patients are prepared neither for the treatment nor for the subsequent side-effects (LANCASTER 1993). Women whose sexual organs are attacked by cancer frequently develop a strong sense of guilt, which in many cases leads to self-incriminations or accusations levelled at their partners (FERVERS-SCHORRE 1987). In addition, fantasies and anxieties develop about the consequences of intercourse for the formation of gynecological tumors and relapses, and also about the consequences of the treatment for the patient and her partner (CAPONE et al. 1980; HARRIS et al. 1982). For this reason, some subjects choose to avoid sexual contact altogether (LANCASTER 1993; LASNIK and TATRA 1986), and Lasnik and Tatra found that only one-third of women receiving radiation treatment for cervical cancer had had their first intercourse by 3 months after the irradiation.

By contrast, the desire for bodily contact increases in cancer patients (HARRIS et al. 1982). Intimacy can be encouraged through nongenital contact during any stage of the woman's illness (HARRIS et al. 1982): It is a very narrow stereotype of sexuality and sexual activity that consists only of penis-vagina intercourse. Equating an erect penis or intact genitalia with the ability to experience sexual pleasure is unfortunate (BULLARD et al. 1980).

The least disturbance to intimate relationships has been found in women who had a harmonious family life and who were suitably well informed (LASNIK and TATRA 1986; LOTZE 1990). A decisive influence of counselling on the sexual rehabilitation of gynecological cancer patients could be shown by CAPONE et al. (1980). Of noncounselled women in the survey, more than three-quarters reported that intercourse had ceased or decreased at 3 and 6 months after their primary medical treatment, with over half still reporting absence of or less frequent intercourse 1 year after treatment. Reduction or cessation of intercourse among the counselled women, on the other hand, was reported by less than half the group at 3 months, one-third at 6 months, and one-fifth at 12 months after treatment (CAPONE et al. 1980).

It is important to assess the frequency of oral, anogenital, and masturbatory sexual activities and patients' attitudes in regard to these activities. If traditional sexual activities become difficult or impossible, these coital substitutes after gynecological treatment may be helpful (ANDERSEN 1987; CAPONE et al. 1980).

References

Aartsen EJ, Sindram IS (1988) Repair of the radiation induced rectovaginal fistulas without or with interposition of the bulbocavernosus muscle (Martius procedure). Eur J Surg Oncol 14:171–177

Abe H, Nakamura M, Takahashi S, Maruoka S, Ogawa Y, Sakamoto K (1992) Radiation-induced insufficiency fractures of the pelvis: evaluation with ^{99m}Tc-methylene diphosphonate scintigraphy. Am J Roentgenol 158:599–602

Abitbol MM, Davenport JH (1974) Sexual dysfunction after therapy of cervical carcinoma. Am J Obstet Gynecol 119:181–189

Abrams RA, Lichter AS, Bromer RH, Minna JD, Cohen MH, Deisseroth AB (1985) The hematopoietic toxicity of regional radiation therapy. Correlations for combined modality therapy with systemic chemotherapy. Cancer 55:1429–1435

Alexander TJ, Dwyer RM (1988) Endoscopic Nd:YAG laser treatment of severe radiation injury of the lower gastrointestinal tract: long-term follow-up. Gastrointest Endosc 34:407–411

Andersen BL (1987) Sexual functioning complications in women with gynecologic cancer. Outcomes and directions for prevention. Cancer 60:2123–2128

Andersen BL, Anderson B (1986) Psychosomatic aspects of gynecologic oncology: present status and future directions. J Psychosom Obstet Gynaecol 5:233–244

Anderson JD, England HR, Molland EA, Blandy JP (1976) The effects of overstretching on the structure and function of the bladder in relation to Helmstein's distension therapy. Br J Urol 47:835–840

Andrews PLR, Bhandari P (1993) The 5-hydroxytryptamine receptor antagonists as antiemetics: preclinical evaluation and mechanism of action. Eur J Cancer 29A(Suppl 1):11–16

Andriole GL, Sugarbaker PH (1985) Perineal and bladder necrosis following bilateral internal iliac artery ligation. Dis Colon Rectum 28:183–184

Anseline PF, Lavery IC, Fazio VW, Jagelman DG, Weakley FL (1981) Radiation injury of the rectum. Ann Surg 194:716–724

Arlow FL, Dekovich AA, Priest RJ, Beher WT (1987) Bile acids in radiation-induced diarrhea. South Med J 80:1259–1261

Arrizabalaga M, Extramiana J, Parra JL, Ramos C, Diaz-Gonzales R, Seiva O (1987) Treatment of massive haematuria with aluminous salts. Br J Urol 60:223–226

Ash P (1980) The influence of radiation on fertility in man. Br J Radiol 53:271–278

Baker TG (1971) Radiosensitivity of mammalian oocytes with particular reference to the human female. Am J Obstet Gynecol 110:746–761

Banaschak A, Stößlein F, Kielbach O, Bilek K, Elling D (1985) Transcatheter arterial embolisation in cases of life-threatening pelvic haemorrhage. Zentralbl Gynäkol 107:1050–1056

Barter JF, Soong SJ, Shingleton HM, Hatch KD, Orr JW (1989) Complications of combined radical hysterectomy-postoperative radiation therapy in women with early stage cervical cancer. Gynecol Oncol 32:292–296

Behr J, Winkler M, Willgeroth F (1990) Functional changes in the lower urinary tract following to irradiation of the cervix carcinoma. Strahlenther Onkol 166:135–139

Bekerus M, Durbaba M, Frim O, Vujnic V (1988) Comparison of HDR and LDR results in endometrium cancer. Sonderbd Strahlenther Onkol 82:222–227

Bertelsen K (1983) Sexual dysfunction after treatment of cervical cancer. Dan Med Bull 30(Suppl 2):31–34

Berthrong M (1986) Radiation-induced pathologic changes. World J Surg 10:155–170

Bissett D, Khan A, McLaughlin I, Davis JA, Symonds RP (1993) Haemorrhagic cystitis requiring cystectomy after cyclophosphamide and radiotherapy. Eur J Cancer 29A:1222–1223

Bloomer WD, Hellman S (1975) Normal tissue responses to radiation therapy. N Engl J Med 293:80

Bloss JD, DiSaia PJ, Mannel RS, Hyden EC, Manetta A, Walker JL, Berman ML (1991) Radiation myelitis: a complication of concurrent cisplatin and 5-fluorouracil chemotherapy with extended field radiotherapy for carcinoma of the uterine cervix. Gynecol Oncol 43:305–308

Bounous G, Le Bel E, Shuster J, Gold P, Tahan WT, Bastin E (1975) Dietary protection during radiation therapy. Strahlentherapie 149:476–483

Bragg DG, Shidnia H, Chu FCH, Higinbotham NL (1970) The clinical and radiographic aspects of radiation ostitis. Radiology 97:103–111

Bricker EM, Johnston WD, Patwardhan RV (1981) Repair of postirradiation damage to colorectum. A progress report. Ann Surg 193:555–564

Brock M, Pohl J (1983) The development of mesna for regional detoxification. Cancer Treat Rev (Suppl A) 10:33–44

Brohult A, Brohult J, Brohult S, Joelsson I (1979) Effect of alkoxyglycerols on the frequency of fistulas following radiation therapy for carcinoma of the uterine cervix. Acta Obstet Gynecol Scand 58:203–207

Buchi KN, Dixon JA (1987) Argon laser treatment of hemorrhagic radiation proctitis. Gastrointest Endosc 33:27–30

Bullard DG, Causey GG, Newman AB, Orloff R, Schanche K, Wallace DH (1980) Sexual health care and cancer: a needs assessment. Front Radiat Ther Oncol 14:55–58

Capone MA, Westie KS, Good RS (1980) Sexual rehabilitation of the gynecologic cancer patient: an effective counseling model. Front Radiat Ther Oncol 14:123–129

Caspers RJL, Hop WCJ (1983) Irradiation of true pelvis for bladder and prostatic carcinoma in supine, prone or Trendelenburg position. Int J Radiat Oncol Biol Phys 9:589–593

Charneau J, Bouachour G, Person B, Burtin P, Ronceray J, Boyer J (1991) Severe hemorrhagic radiation proctitis advancing to gradual cessation with hyperbaric oxygen. Dig Dis Sci 36:373–375

Cikaric S (1988) Radiation therapy of cervical carcinoma using either HDR or LDR afterloading: comparison of 5-year results and complications. Sonderbd Strahlenther Onkol 82:119–122

Cividalli A, Adami M, De Tomasi F, Palmisano L, Pardini MC, Spano M, Mauro F (1985) Orgotein as a radioprotector in normal tissues. Acta Radiol Oncol 24:273–277

Cohen ME, Duffner PK, Terplan KL (1983) Myelopathy with severe structural derangement associated with combined modality therapy. Cancer 52:1590–1596

Coleman CN, Bump EA, Kramer RA (1988) Chemical modifiers of cancer treatment. J Clin Oncol 6:709–733

Cooper KL, Beabout JW, Swee RG (1985) Insufficient fractures of the sacrum. Radiology 156:15–20

Covens A, Thomas G, DePetrillo A, Jamieson C, Myhr T (1991) The prognostic importance of site and type of radiation-induced bowel injury in patients requiring surgical management. Gynecol Oncol 43:270–274

Cox JD, Byhardt RW, Wilson JF, Haas JS, Komaki R, Olson LE (1986) Complications of radiation therapy and factors in their prevention. World J Surg 10:171–188

Cram AE, Pearlman NW, Jochimsen PR (1977) Surgical management of complications of radiation-injured gut. Am J Surg 133:551–553

Cross MJ, Frazee RC (1992) Surgical treatment of radiation enteritis. Am Surg 58:132–135

Crowe J, Stellato TA (1985) Radiation-induced solitary rectal ulcer. Dis Colon Rectum 28:610–612

Dalinka MK, Mazzeo VP (1985) Complications of radiation therapy. Crit Rev Diagn Imaging 23:235–267

Daly NJ, Izar F, Bachaud JM, Delannes M (1989) The incidence of severe chronic ileitis after abdominal and/or pelvic external irradiation with high energy photon beams. Radiother Oncol 14:287–295

Danielsson A, Nyhlin H, Persson H, Stendahl U, Stenling R, Suhr O (1991) Chronic diarrhoea after radiotherapy for gynecological cancer: occurrence and aetiology. Gut 32:1180–1187

Danjoux CE, Rider WD, Fitzpatrick PJ (1979) The acute radiation syndrome. Clin Radiol 30:581–584

De Cosse JJ, Rhodes RS, Wentz WB, Reagan JW, Dworken HJ, Holden WD (1969) The natural history and management of radiation induced injury of the gastrointestinal tract. Ann Surg 170:369–384

Deitel M, To TB (1987) Major intestinal complications of radiotherapy. Management and nutrition. Arch Surg 122:1421–1424

Doll R, Smith PG (1968) The long-term effects of x-irradiation in patients treated for metropathia haemorrhagica. Br J Radiol 41:362–368

Donahue LA, Frank IN (1989) Intravesical formalin for hemorrhagic cystitis: analysis of therapy. J Urol 141:809

Edsmyr F, Menander-Huber KB (1981) Orgotein efficacy in ameliorating side effects due to radiation therapy. Eur J Rheumatol Inflamm 4:228–236

Emami B, Lyman J, Brown A, et al. (1991) Tolerance of normal tissue to therapeutic irradiation. Int J Radiat Oncol Biol Phys 21:109–122

Fajardo LF (1989) Morphologic patterns of radiation injury. Front Radiat Ther Oncol 23:75–84

Fenner MN, Sheehan P, Nanavati PJ, Ross DS (1989) Chronic radiation enteritis: a community hospital experience. J Surg Oncol 41:246–249

Fervers-Schorre B (1987) Psychic problems in women with uterus carcinoma. In: Schulz KD, King RJB, Pollow K, Taylor RW (eds) Endometrial cancer. Zuckschwerdt, München, pp 136–139

Fitch MI (1992) Managing treatment-induced emesis: a nursing perspective. Oncology 49:312–316

Fletcher GH (1979) Parameters involved in radiotherapy complications. In: Libshitz HI (ed) Diagnostic roentgenology of radiotherapy change. Williams and Wilkins, Baltimore, pp 85–100, pp 123–135

Fyles AW, Dembo AJ, Bush RS, et al. (1992) Analysis of complications in patients treated with abdomino-pelvic radiation therapy for ovarian carcinoma. Int J Radiat Oncol Biol Phys 22:847–851

Galland RB, Spencer J (1987) Natural history and surgical management of radiation enteritis. Br J Surg 74:742–747

Galli A, Berrino P, Rainero ML, Santi P (1987) Present day role of plastic surgery in management of chronic radiation wounds: our experience. Eur J Surg Oncol 13:239–246

Georgiou A, Grigsby PW, Perez CA (1993) Radiation induced lumbosacral plexopathy in gynecologic tumors: clinical findings and dosimetric analysis. Int J Radiat Oncol Biol Phys 26:479–482

Glaser FH (1988) Comparison of HDR afterloading with ^{192}Ir versus conventional radium therapy in cervix cancer: 5-year results and complications. Sonderbd Strahlenther Onkol 82:106–113

Goodman MJ, Lalka SG, Reddy S (1993) Static and dynamic vascular impact of large artery irradiation. Int J Radiat Oncol Biol Phys 26:305–310

Gordon AB, Harmer CL, O'Sullivan M (1987) Treatment of post-radiotherapy telangiectasia by injection sclerotherapy. Clin Radiol 38:25–26

Gordon AN, Martens M, LaPread Y, Faro S (1989) Response of lower genital tract flora to external pelvic irradiation. Gynecol Oncol 35:233–235

Gradishar WJ, Schilsky RL (1989) Ovarian function following radiation and chemotherapy for cancer. Semin Oncol 16:425–436

Grady D, Rubin SM, Petitti DB, et al. (1992) Hormone therapy to prevent disease and prolong life in postmenopausal women. Ann Intern Med 117:1016–1037

Graham JB, Abad RS (1967) Ureteral obstruction due to radiation. Am J Obstet Gynecol 99:409–415

Granick MS, Solomon MP, Larson DL (1993) Management of radiation-associated pelvic wounds. Clin Plast Surg 20:581–587

Grant PT, Jeffrey JF, Fraser RC, Tompkins MG, Filbee JF, Wong OS (1989) Pelvic radiation therapy for gynecologic malignancy in geriatric patients. Gynecol Oncol 33:185–188

Grau C (1993) Damage to the spinal medulla caused by radiation. Ugeskr Laeger 155:208–211

Green M (1983) The avoidance of small intestine injury in gynecologic cancer. Int J Radiat Oncol Biol Phys 9:1385–1390

Greven KM, Lanciano RM, Herbert SH, Hogan PE (1991) Analysis of complications in patients with endometrial

carcinoma receiving adjuvant irradiation. Int J Radiat Oncol Biol Phys 21:919–923
Grigsby PW, Pilepich MV, Parsons CL (1990) Preliminary results of a phase I/II study of sodium pentosanpolysulfate in the treatment of chronic radiation-induced proctitis. Am J Clin Oncol 13:28–31
Grio R, Tamburrano F, Tetti M, et al. (1989) Use of orgotein in the treatment of reactive damage to the use of high-energy radiation. Minerva Ginecol 41:413–415
Gunderson LL, Russell AH, Llewellyn HJ, Doppke KP, Tepper JE (1985) Treatment planning for colorectal cancer: radiation and surgical techniques and value of small-bowel films. Int J Radiat Oncol Biol Phys 11:1379–1393
Haboubi NY, Schofield PF, Rowland PL (1988) The light and electron microscopic features of early and late phase radiation-induced proctitis. Am J Gastroenterol 83:1140–1144
Haie-Meder C, Mlika-Cabanne N, Michel G, et al. (1993) Radiotherapy after ovarian transposition: ovarian function and fertility preservation. Int J Radiat Oncol Biol Phys 25:419–424
Harris R, Good RS, Pollack L (1982) Sexual behavior of gynecologic cancer patients. Arch Sex Behav 11:503–510
Hasleton PS, Carr ND, Schofield PF (1985) Vascular changes in radiation bowel disease. Histopathology 9:517–534
Helmkamp BF, Kimmel J (1985) Conservative management of small bowel obstruction. Am J Obstet Gynecol 152:677–679
Hendry WF, Christmas TJ, Shepherd JH (1991) Anterior pelvic reconstruction with ileum after cancer treatment. J R Soc Med 84:709–713
Henriksson R, Arevärn M, Franzen L, Persson H, Stendahl U (1990) Beneficial effects of sucralfate in radiation induced diarrhea. Eur J Gynaecol Oncol 11:299–302
Henriksson R, Franzen L, Littbrand B (1992a) Effects of sucralfate on acute and late bowel discomfort following radiotherapy of pelvic cancer. J Clin Oncol 10:969–975
Henriksson R, Lomberg H, Israelsson G, Zackrisson B, Franzen L (1992b) The effect of ondansetron on radiation-induced emesis and diarrhoea. Acta Oncol 31:767–769
Herbert SH, Solin LJ, Hoffman JP, et al. (1993) Volumetric analysis of small bowel displacement from radiation portals with the use of a pelvic tissue expander. Int J Radiat Oncol Biol Phys 25:885–893
Himmel PD, Hassett JM (1986) Radiation-induced chronic arterial injury. Semin Surg Oncol 2:225–247
Himmelmann A, Notter G, Turesson I (1985) Normal tissue reactions to high dose-rate intracavitary irradiation of the vagina with different fractionation schedules and dose levels. Strahlentherapie 161:163–167
Hindley A, Cole H (1993) Use of peritoneal insufflation to displace the small bowel during pelvic and abdominal radiotherapy in carcinoma of the cervix. Br J Radiol 66:67–73
Hintz BL, Kagan AR, Chan P, Gilbert HA, Nussbaum H, Rao AR, Wollin M (1980) Radiation tolerance of the vaginal mucosa. Int J Radiat Oncol Biol Phys 6:711–716
Holthusen H (1921) Beiträge zur Biologie der Strahlenwirkung. Untersuchungen an Askarideneiern. Pflügers Arch 187:1
Hopewell JW, Robbins MEC, van den Aardweg GJMJ, et al. (1993) The modulation of radiation-induced damage to pig skin by essential fatty acids. Br J Cancer 68:1–7
Hübener KH, Baumann M, Krull A, Schwarz R (1993) Clinically important factors modifying the response of tumors and normal tissue to radiation therapy. Recent Results Cancer Res 130:41–47
Huguenin PU, Glanzmann C, Hammer F, Lütolf UM (1992) Endometrial carcinoma in patients aged 75 years or older: outcome and complications after postoperative radiotherapy or radiotherapy alone. Strahlenther Onkol 168:567–572
Janson PO, Jansson I, Skryten A, Damber JE, Lindstedt G (1981) Ovarian endocrine function in young women undergoing radiotherapy for carcinoma of the cervix. Gynecol Oncol 11:218–233
Jao SW, Beart RW Jr, Gunderson LL (1986) Surgical treatment of radiation injuries of the colon and rectum. Am J Surg 151:272–277
Jayalakshmamma BJ, Pinkel D (1976) Urinary bladder toxicity following pelvic irradiation and simultaneous cyclophosphamide therapy. Cancer 38:701–707
Jeremic B, Djuric LJ, Mijatovic LJ (1991) Severe late intestinal complications after abdominal and/or pelvic external irradiation with high energy photon beams. Clin Oncol R Coll Radiol 3:100–104
Johnson RJ, Carrington BM (1992) Pelvic radiation disease. Clin Radiol 45:4–12
Joslin CA (1971) The biological effects of radiation therapy in gynecological malignancy. In: MacDonald RR (ed) Scientific basis of obstetrics and gynaecology. Churchill, London, p 455
Katzen BT, Rossi P, Passariello R, Simonetti G (1976) Transcatheter therapeutic arterial embolization. Radiology 220:523–531
Kauczor HU, Dietl B, Kreitner KF, Brix G (1992) Bone marrow changes after radiotherapy. Assessment by MRI. Radiologe 32:516–522
Kavanah MT, Feldman MI, Devereux DF, Kondi ES (1985) New surgical approach to minimize radiation-associated small bowel injury in patients with pelvic malignancies requiring surgery and high-dose irradiation. Cancer 56:1300–1304
Kim YH, Aye MS, Fayos JV (1977) Radiation necrosis of the scalp: a complication of cranial irradiation and methotrexate. Radiology 124:813–814
Kimose HH, Fischer L, Spjeldnaes N, Wara P (1989) Late radiation injury of the colon and rectum. Surgical management and outcome. Dis Colon Rectum 32:684–689
Kindwall EP (1992) Uses of hyperbaric oxygen therapy in the 1990s. Cleve Clin J Med 59:517–528
Kindwall EP (1993) Hyperbaric oxygen treatment of radiation cystitis. Clin Plast Surg 20:589–592
Kinsella TJ, Bloomer WD (1980) Tolerance of the intestine to radiation. Surg Gynecol Obstet 151:273–284
Kiricuta I (1988) Treatment by omentoplasty of vesicorectovaginal and rectovaginal fistulae. J Urol (Paris) 94:289–293
Knox SJ, Fowler S, Marquez C, Hoppe RT (1994) Effect of Filgrastim (G-CSF) on Hodgkin's disease patients treated with radiation therapy. Int J Radiat Oncol Biol Phys 28:445–450
Kochhar R, Patel F, Dhar A, et al. (1991) Radiation-induced proctosigmoiditis. Prospective, randomized, double-blind controlled trial of oral sulfasalazine plus rectal steroids versus rectal sucralfate. Dig Dis Sci 36:103–107
Kramer S (1975) Methotrexate and radiation therapy in the treatment of advanced squamous cell carcinoma of the oral cavity, oropharynx, supraglottic larynx and hypopharynx. Can J Otolarnygol 4:213–218
Kreuser ED, Klingmüller D, Thiel E (1993) The role of LHRH-analogues in protecting gonadal functions during chemotherapy and irradiation. Eur Urol 23:157–164
Kuipers T (1988) Dosimetry and complication rate in the treatment of cervix carcinoma with external irradiation

and brachytherapy. Sonderbd Strahlenther Onkol 82:127–131

Kurz C, Nagele F, Sevelda P, Enzelsberger H (1993) Intravesical application of oestriol as therapy of sensory urge-incontinence – a prospective study. Geburtshilfe Frauenheilkd 53:535–538

Kutzner J, Knappstein T, Hager S, Koch H (1986) Radiotherapy results in cervix carcinoma with regard to side effects. Strahlenther Onkol 162:549–554

Lancaster J (1993) Women's experiences of gynaecological cancer treated with radiation. Curationis 16:37–42

Lancet, editorial (1987) Haemorrhagic cystitis after radiotherapy. Lancet 1(8528):304–306

Landthaler M, Haina D, Waidelich W, Braun-Falco O (1984) Laser therapy of venous lakes (Bean-Walsh) and telangiectasias. Plast Reconstr Surg 73:78–83

Lapides J (1970) Treatment of delayed intractable hemorrhagic cystitis following radiation or chemotherapy. J Urol 104:707–708

Lasnik E, Tatra G (1986) Sexual behavior following primary radiotherapy of cervix cancer. Geburtshilfe Frauenheilkd 46:813–816

Laugier A, Schlienger M, Le Fur R, Eschwege F (1968) La prévention des radiolésions digestive. Semin Hop Paris 44:449

Lawson JA (1985) Surgical treatment of radiation induced atherosclerotic disease of the iliac and femoral arteries. J Cardiovasc Surg 26:151–156

Lewandowski G, Torrisi J, Potkul RK, Holloway RW, Popescu G, Whitfield S, Delgado G (1990) Hysterectomy with extended surgical staging and radiotherapy versus hysterectomy alone and radiotherapy in stage I endometrial cancer: a comparison of complication rates. Gynecol Oncol 36:401–404

Liu T, Liu Y, He S, Zhang Z, Kligerman MM (1992) Use of radiation with or without WR-2721 in advanced rectal cancer. Cancer 69:2820–2825

Liu YK, Harty JI, Steinbock GS, Holt HA Jr, Goldstein DH, Amin M (1990) Treatment of radiation or cyclophosphamide induced hemorrhagic cystitis using conjugated estrogen. J Urol 144:41–43

Livne PM, Huben RP, Wolf RM, Pontes JE, Piver SM (1987) Simple method for the management of hematuria caused by radiation or cytoxan. Eur Urol 13:180–181

Localio SA, Stone A, Friedman M (1969) Surgical aspects of radiation enteritis. Surg Gynecol Obstet 129:1163–1172

LoJudice T, Baxter D, Balint J (1977) Effects of abdominal surgery on the development of radiation enteropathy. Gastroenterology 73:1093–1097

Lotze W (1990) Sexual rehabilitation in patients with carcinoma of the cervix. Geburtshilfe Frauenheilkd 50:781–784

Lushbaugh CC, Casarett GW (1976) The effects of gonadal irradiation in clinical radiation therapy: a review. Cancer 37:1111–1120

MacManus MP, Clarke J, McCormick D, Abram WP (1993) Use of recombinant granulocyte-colony stimulating factor to treat neutropenia occuring during craniospinal irradiation. Int J Radiat Oncol Biol Phys 26:845–850

Maiche AG, Gröhn P, Mäki-Hokkonen H (1991) Effect of chamomile cream and almond ointment on acute radiation skin reaction. Acta Oncol 30:395–396

Maier U, Hofbauer J (1986) Urological complications after curative irradiation of gynecologic carcinomas. Urologe [A] 25:33–37

Maier U, Zechner O (1988) Therapy of radiation injuries of the bladder with orgotein (Peroxinorm). Z Urol Nephrol 81:305–308

Mäkelä J, Nevasaari K, Kairaluoma MI (1987) Surgical treatment of intestinal radiation injury. J Surg Oncol 36:93–97

Mathes SJ, Hurwitz DJ (1986) Repair of chronic radiation wounds of the pelvis. World J Surg 10:269–280

Mayer P, Marx FJ, Schilling A (1984) Therapy of acute radiation cystitis. Urologe [A] 23:65–67

McCready RA, Hyde GL, Rivins BA, Mattingly SS, Griffin WO (1983) Radiation-induced arterial injuries. Surgery 93:306–312

Micic S, Genbacev O (1988) Post-irradiation cystitis improved by instillation of early placental extract in saline. Eur Urol 14:291–293

Miholic J, Schlappack O, Klepetko W, Kölbl H, Szepesi T, Moeschl P (1987) Surgical therapy of radiation-induced small-bowel lesions. Arch Surg 122:923–926

Miholic J, Schwarz C, Moeschl P (1988) Surgical therapy of radiation-induced lesions of the colon and rectum. Am J Surg 155:761–763

Moeschl P, Miholic J (1989) Ileus following radiotherapy: importance and therapeutic aspects of surgery for radiation-induced bowel injuries. Wien Klin Wochenschr 101:84–87

Montana GS, Fowler WC (1989) Carcinoma of the cervix: analysis of bladder and rectal radiation dose and complications. Int J Radiat Oncol Biol Phys 16:95–100

Montana GS, Fowler WC, Varia MA, Walton LA, Mack Y (1985) Analysis of results of radiation therapy for stage II carcinoma of the cervix. Cancer 55:956–962

Morgan PR, Murdoch JB, Lopes A, Piura B, Monaghan JM (1993) The Wallace technique of ureteroileal anastomosis and its use in gynecologic oncology: a study of 81 cases. Obstet Gynecol 82:594–597

Morgenstern L, Thompson R, Friedman NB (1977) The modern enigma of radiation enteropathy: sequelae and solutions. Am J Surg 134:166–169

Mundy AR (1988) A technique for total substitution of the lower urinary tract without the use of a prothesis. Br J Urol 62:334–338

Nielsen OS, Overgaard J, Overgaard M, Steenholdt S, Jakobsen A, Sell A (1987) Orgotein in radiation treatment of bladder cancer. Acta Oncologica 26:101–104

Nylander G, Pettersson F, Swedenborg J (1978) Localized arterial occlusions in patients treated with pelvic field radiation for cancer. Cancer 41:2158–2161

O'Brien PH, Jenrette III JM, Garvin JA (1987) Radiation enteritis. Am Surg 53:501–504

Orton CG, Seyedsadr M, Somnay A (1991) Comparison of high and low dose rate remote afterloading for cervix cancer and the importance of fractionation. Int J Radiat Oncol Biol Phys 21:1425–1434

Pape H, Schnabel T, Kölzer K, Schmitt G, Jung U (1990) Therapy of radiation induced epitheliolysis with a bandage consisting of hydrocolloids and polymeres (Biofilm^{R}). A report of clinical experiences. Strahlenther Onkol 166:714–717

Parker RG, Berry H (1976) Late effects of therapeutic irradiation on the skeleton and bone marrow. Cancer 37:1162

Parkin DE, Davis JA, Symonds RP (1987) Long-term bladder symptomatology following radiotherapy for cervical carcinoma. Radiother Oncol 9:195–199

Parkin DE, Davis JA, Symonds RP (1988) Urodynamic findings following radiotherapy for cervical carcinoma. Br J Urol 61:213–217

Parliament M, Genest P, Girard A, Gerig L, Prefontaine M (1989) Obstructive ureteropathy following radiation therapy for carcinoma of the cervix. Gynecol Oncol 33:237–240

Parsons CL (1986) Successful management of radiation cystitis with sodium pentosanpolysulfate. J Urol 136:813–814

Patsner B (1993) Topical acetone for control of life-threatening vaginal hemorrhage from recurrent gynecologic cancer. Eur J Gynaecol Oncol 14:33–35

Pearson JM, Kumar S, Butterworth DM, Schofield PF, Haboubi NY (1992) Flow cytometric DNA characteristics of radiation colitis – a preliminary study. Anticancer Res 12:1647–1650

Persson H, Hedberg B, Angquist KA (1992) Surgical management of intestinal complications of radiotherapy for gynecological malignancies. Eur J Gynaecol Oncol 13:419–422

Pettersson F, Swedenborg J (1990) Atherosclerotic occlusive disease after radiation for pelvic malignancies. Acta Chir Scand 156:367–371

Pilepich MV, Pajak T, George FW, et al. (1983) Preliminary report on phase III RTOG studies of extended-field irradiation in carcinoma of the prostate. Am J Clin Oncol 6:485

Piver MS, Barlow JT (1977) High dose irradiation to biopsy confirmed aortic node metastases from carcinoma of the uterine cervix. Cancer 39:1243–1246

Polla LL, Tan OT, Garden JM, Parrish JA (1987) Tunable pulsed dye laser for the treatment of benign cutaneous vascular ectasia. Dermatologica 174:11–17

Polson RJ, Misiewicz JJ (1992) Medical management of severe inflammatory disease of the rectum and distal colon: non-nutritional aspects. Baillieres Clin Gastroenterol 6:1–26

Potish RA, Jones TK, Levitt SH (1979) Factors predisposing to radiation-related small bowel damage. Radiology 132:479

Power S, Karcher G, Simon W (1983) Cutaneous ureterostomy as last resort treatment of intractable haemorrhagic cystitis following radiation. Br J Urol 55:392

Price WE, Keldahl LR (1990) Fatal hemorrhagic cystitis induced by pelvic irradiation and cyclophosphamide therapy. Case report and review. Minn Med 73:39–41

Radiation Therapy Oncology Group (1984) Acute and late radiation morbidity scoring.

Rafii M, Firooznia H, Golimbu C, Horner N (1988) Radiation induced fractures of sacrum: CT diagnosis. J Comput Assist Tomogr 12:231–235

Rauthe G, Vahrson H, Giers G (1988) Five-year results and complications in endometrium cancer: HDR afterloading vs. conventional radium therapy. Sonderb Strahlenther Onkol 82:240–245

Rauthe G, Bryxi V, Vahrson H (1992) Transvaginal fistula visualization. J Cancer Res Clin Oncol 118 (Suppl):R108

Ray GH, Trueblood HW, Enright LP, Kaplan HS, Nelson TS (1970) Oophoropexy: a means of preserving ovarian function following pelvic megavoltage radiotherapy for Hodgkin's disease. Radiology 96:175–180

Remy JC, Fruchter RG, Choi K, Rotman M, Boyce JG (1986) Complications of combined radical hysterectomy and pelvic radiation. Gynecol Oncol 24:317–326

Rhomberg W, Eiter H (1988) Radiogenic vaginal necroses. Strahlenther Onkol 164:527–530

Ries T (1983) Detection of osteoporotic sacral fractures with radionuclides. Radiology 146:783–785

Rijkmans BG, Bakker DJ, Dabhoiwala NF, Kurth KH (1989) Successful treatment of radiation cystitis with hyperbaric oxygen. Eur Urol 16:354–356

Roberts JT (1992) Ondansetron in the control of refractory emesis following radiotherapy. Clin Oncol 4:67–68

Roberts JT, Priestman TJ (1993) A review of ondansetron in the management of radiotherapy-induced emesis. Oncology 50:173–179

Roberts WS, Hoffman MS, La Polla JP, Ruas E, Fiorica JV, Cavenagh D (1991) Management of radionecrosis of the vulva and distal vagina. Am J Obstet Gynecol 164:1235–1238

Rotte K (1988) Long-time results of HDR afterloading in comparison with radium therapy in endometrium cancer in Würzburg. Sonderb Strahlenther Onkol 82:218–221

Rubin SC, Young J, Mikuta JJ (1985) Squamous carcinoma of the vagina: treatment, complications, and long-term follow-up. Gynecol Oncol 20:346–353

Rudolph R, Vande Berg J, Schneider JA, Fisher JC, Poolman WL (1988) Slowed growth of cultured fibroblasts from human radiation wounds. Plast Reconstr Surg 82:669–675

Rugg T, Saunders M, Dische S (1990) Smoking and mucosal reactions to radiotherapy. Br J Radiol 63:554–556

Russel JC, Welch JP (1979) Operative management of radiation injuries of the intestinal tract. Am J Surg 137:166–172

Sagar SM (1991) The current role of anti-emetic drugs in oncology: a recent revolution in patient symptom control. Cancer Treat Rev 18:95–135

Sakata K, Aoki Y, Muta N, et al. (1993) Effect of human granulocyte colony-stimulating factor on neutropenia induced by radiotherapy and chemotherapy. Oncology 50:238–240

Salfeld K, Huchzermeyer S (1985) Surgical treatment of skin damages induced by x-rays. Z Hautkr 60:438–452

Scarantino CW, Ornitz RD, Hoffman LG, Anderson RF (1992) Radiation-induced emesis: effects of ondansetron. Semin Oncol 19 (Suppl 15):38–43

Schellhammer PF, Jordan GH, El-Mahdi AM (1986) Pelvic complications after interstitial and external beam irradiation of urologic and gynecologic malignancy. World J Surg 10:259–268

Schmidberger H, Hess CF, Hoffmann W, Reuss-Borst MA, Bamberg M (1993) Granulocyte clony-stimulating factor treatment of leucopenia during fractionated radiotherapy. Eur J Cancer 29A:1927–1931

Schnur KH, Boumea J (1983) Palliative embolization in gynaecological patients. Eur J Radiol 3:9–11

Schoenrock GJ, Cianci P (1986) Treatment of radiation cystitis with hyperbaric oxygen. Urology 27:271–272

Schray MF, Martinez A, Howes AE (1989) Toxicity of open-field whole abdominal irradiation as primary postoperative treatment in gynecologic malignancy. Int J Radiat Oncol Biol Phys 16:397–403

Schuchter LM, Luginbuhl WE, Meropol NJ (1992) The current status of toxicity protectants in cancer therapy. Semin Oncol 19:742–751

Seegenschmiedt MH, Sauer R (1993) The systematics of acute and chronic radiation sequelae. Strahlenther Onkol 169:83–95

Shehata WM, Meyer RL (1980) The enhancement effect of irradiation by methotrexate. Cancer 46:1349–1352

Silvain C, Besson I, Ingrand P, et al. (1992) Long-term outcome of severe radiation enteritis treated by total parenteral nutrition. Dig Dis Sci 37:1065–1071

Sinistrero G, Sismondi P, Rumore A, Zola P (1993) Analysis of complications of cervix carcinoma treated by radiotherapy using the Franco-Italian glossary. Radiother Oncol 26:203–211

Skene AI, Gault DT, Woodhouse CRJ, Breach NM, Thomas JM (1990) Perineal, vulval and vaginoperineal reconstruction using the rectus abdominis myocutaneous flap. Br J Surg 77:635–637

Slater JM, Fletcher GH (1971) Ureteral strictures after radiotherapy for carcinoma of the uterine cervix. AJR 111:269

Smith DB, Newlands ES, Rustin GJS, Begent RHJ, Howells N, McQuade B, Bagshawe KD (1991) Comparison of ondansetron and ondansetron plus dexametasone as antiemectic prophylaxis during cisplatin-containing chemotherapy. Lancet 338:487–490

Smith DH, De Cosse JJ (1986) Radiation damage to the small intestine. World J Surg 10:189–194

Sorbe B, Berglind AM, de Bruijn K (1992) Tropisetron, a new 5-HT_3 receptor antagonist, in the prevention of radiation-induced emesis. Radiother Oncol 23:131–132

Steen M (1993) Review of the use of povidone-iodine (PVP-I) in the treatment of burns. Postgrad Med J 69 (Suppl 3):S84–S92

Stewart DJ (1990) Cancer therapy, vomiting, and antiemetics. Can J Physiol Pharmacol 68:304–313

Stockbine MF, Hancock JE, Fletcher GH (1970) Complications in 831 patients with squamous cell carcinoma of the intact uterine cervix treated with 3000 rads or more whole pelvis irradiation. AJR 108:293–304

Stryker JA, Hepner GW, Mortel R (1977) The effect of pelvic irradiation on ileal function. Radiology 124:213–216

Stryker JA, Bartholomew M, Velkley DE, Cunningham DE, Mortel R, Craycraft G, Shafer J (1988) Bladder and rectal complications following radiotherapy for cervix cancer. Gynecol Oncol 29:1–11

Teshima T, Chatani M, Hata K, Inoue T, Suzuki T (1985) Rectal complication after remote afterloading intracavitary therapy for carcinoma of the uterine cervix. Strahlentherapie 161:343–347

Teshima T, Chatani M, Hata K, Inoue T (1987) High-dose rate intracavitary therapy for carcinoma of the uterine cervix. I. General figures of survival and complication. Int J Radiat Oncol Biol Phys 13:1035–1041

Teshima T, Inoue T, Chatani M, et al. (1990) Radiation therapy of the para-aortic lymph nodes in carcinoma of the uterine cervix: the concurrent use of cimetidine to reduce acute and subacute side effects from radiation. Clin Ther 12:71–77

Thomas PRM, Winstanly D, Peckham MJ, Austin CDE, Murrary MAF, Jacobs HS (1976) Reproductive and endocrine function in patients with Hodgkin's disease: effects of oophoropexy and irradiation. Br J Cancer 33:226–231

Trier JS, Browning TH (1966) Morphologic response of the mucosa of the human small intestine to x-ray exposure. J Clin Invest 45:194–204

Trimbos JB, Snijders-Keilholz T, Peters AAW (1991) Feasibility of the application of a resorbable polyglycolic-acid mesh (dexon mesh) to prevent complications of radiotherapy following gynaecological surgery. Eur J Surg 157:281–284

Vahrson H, Römer G (1988) 5-year results with HDR afterloading in cervix cancer: dependence on fractionation and dose. Sonderbd Strahlenther Onkol 82:139–146

van Halteren HK, Gortzak E, Taal BG, Helmerhorst TJ, Aleman BM, Hart AA, Zoetmulder FA (1993) Surgical intervention for complications caused by late radiation damage of the small bowel: a retrospective analysis. Eur J Surg Oncol 19:336–341

Viggiano TR, Zighelboim J, Ahlquist DA, Gostout CJ, Wang KK, Larson MV (1993) Endoscopic Nd: Yag laser coagulation of bleeding from radiation proctopathy. Gastrointest Endosc 39:513–517

Viljanto J (1980) Disinfection of surgical wounds without inhibition of normal wound healing. Arch Surg 115:253–256

von Paes E, Treitschke F, Suhr P, Friedrich JM, Mickley V, Vollmar JF (1991) Arterial vascular damage after radiotherapy. Fortschr Röntgenstr 154:39–43

Weijers RE, van der Jagt EJ, Jansen W (1990) Radiation enteritis: an overview. Fortsch Röntgenstr 152:453–459

Weiss JP, Boland FP, Mori H, Gallagher M, Brereton H, Preate DL, Neville EC (1985) Treatment of radiation-induced cystitis with hyperbaric oxygen. J Urol 134:352–354

Wellwood JM, Jackson BT (1973) The intestinal complications of radiotherapy. Br J Surg 60:814–818

Westermark A, Sindet-Pedersen S, Jensen J (1990) Osteoradionecrosis, pathogenesis, treatment and prevention. Tandlaegebladet 94:669–673

Whelan TJ, Dembo AJ, Bush RS, et al. (1992) Complications of whole abdominal and pelvic radiotherapy following chemotherapy for advanced ovarian cancer. Int J Radiat Oncol Biol Phys 22:853–858

Whitcroft SI, Stevenson JC (1992) Hormone replacement therapy: risks and benefits. Clin Endocrinol (Oxf) 36:15–20

Williams JA, Clarke D, Dennis WA, Dennis EJ, Smith ST (1992) The treatment of pelvic soft tissue radiation necrosis with hyperbaric oxygen. Am J Obstet Gynecol 167:412–416

Witherspoon BJ, Marks RD, Moore TN, Underwood PB, Wilson W (1979) The role of radiation therapy in the management of the patient with IB carcinoma of the cervix. Int J Radiat Oncol Biol Phys 5:1757–1760

Wittich G, Salomonowitz E, Szepesi T, Czembirek H, Fruehwald F (1984) Small bowel double-contrast enema in stage III ovarian cancer. Am J Roentgenol 142:299–304

Yeoh EK, Horowitz M (1987) Radiation enteritis. Surg Gynecol Obstet 165:373–379

Yoeh EK, Lui D, Lee NY (1984) The mechanism of diarrhoea resulting from pelvic and abdominal radiotherapy; a prospective study using selenium-75 labeled conjugated bile acid and cobalt-58 labelled cyanocobalamin. Br J Radiol 57:1131–1136

Yeoh EK, Horowitz M, Russo A, Muecke T, Robb T, Chatterton BE (1993) Gastrointestinal function in chronic radiation enteritis – effects of loperamide-*N*-oxide. Gut 34:467–482

Young RW (1986) Mechanisms and treatment of radiation-induced nausea and vomiting. In: Davis CJ, Lake-Bakaar GV, Grahame-Smith DG (eds) Nausea and vomiting: mechanisms and treatment. Springer, Berlin Heidelberg New York, pp 94–109

Zentler-Munro PL, Bessell EM (1987) Medical management of radiation enteritis – an algorithmic guide. Clin Radiol 38:291–294

Zoetmulder FAN, Gortzak E, den Hartog-Jager FCA, Taal BG, Aartsen EJ, Heintz APM, van Bunningen BNFM (1988) Surgical repair of radiation damage of the rectum: a systematic approach to a difficult problem. Eur J Surg Oncol 14:179–186

Zoubek J, McGuire EJ, Noll F, DeLancey JOL (1989) The late occurrence of urinary tract damage in patients successfully treated by radiotherapy for cervical carcinoma. J Urol 141:1347–1349

16 Palliative Radiation Therapy in Female Genital Cancers

D. CARSTENS

CONTENTS

16.1 Distant Metastases

Compared with other solid neoplasms, distant metastases from gynecological neoplasms are relatively rare, and well-founded statistical material is scarce. A synopsis of the most frequent sites of distant metastases and their relative frequency in autoptic cases is given by NOLTENIUS (1987) (Table 16.1); data on distant metastases from malignancies of the vagina, vulva, and fallopian tube are not included since such metastases are of no clinical significance.

16.1.1 Brain Metastases

The absolute rate of brain metastases from gynecological neoplasms is about 1.5% (WRIGHT and DELANEY 1989). Rates of 3%–15% in autopsy studies and less than 1% in clinical studies have been reported (HENRIKSEN 1949; BADIB et al. 1968; PEEPLES et al. 1976; CARLSON et al. 1967; KISHI et al. 1982; VIETH and ODOM 1965; KOTTKE-MARCHANT et al. 1991). Similar results have been seen with carcinoma of the corpus uteri and ovarian carcinoma (BERGE and LUNDBERG 1977; GRAF et al. 1988).

The interval between treatment of the primary tumor and the diagnosis of brain metastases varies between 1 and 105 months. In general, brain metastases are a sign of disseminated disease.

The main clinical symptoms are headache (sometimes unilateral), weakness, cognitive or affective disorders, and seizures. Computed tomography (CT) or, better still, magnetic resonance imaging (MRI) is diagnostic, demonstrating the number and localization of the lesions as well as the perifocal edema. Multiple supratentorial lesions are more frequent than solitary metastases.

The treatment goal is to restore neurological function or to minimize progressive neurological dysfunction. The principal treatment regimens are: (a) surgery, (b) radiotherapy, (c) radiotherapy combined with chemotherapy, and (d) a combination of all these treatment modalities.

In the case of a solitary lesion, the possibility of neurosurgical treatment should be checked, especially when the performance status is good. A previously completed staging has to exclude distant metastases in other organs, which would imply a poor prognosis.

There are case reports of long-term survivors after resection of brain metastases followed by postoperative radiotherapy. SAWADA et al. (1990) reported on a 43-year-old woman who developed a solitary brain metastasis 7 years after primary treatment of an endometrial carcinoma. She was free of disease 82 months after resection of the lesion followed by postoperative radiotherapy. KUMAR et al. (1992) treated a patient with a solitary brain metastasis from a carcinoma of the uterine cervix with resection and postoperative radiotherapy, and found her to be free of disease 7 months after treatment. However, these reports concern only isolated cases; usually there are multiple lesions, and surgery will not be useful. In such circumstances palliative radiotherapy of the whole brain, perhaps in combination with chemotherapy, will be indicated.

D. CARSTENS, MD, Hermann-Holthusen-Institut für Strahlentherapie, Allgemeines Krankenhaus St. Georg, Lohmühlenstraße 5, D-20099 Hamburg, Germany

Table 16.1. Relative frequency of distant metastases from gynecological neoplasms. (Modified from NOLTENIVS 1987)

	Bones	Liver	Brain	Lung	Pleura	Omentum
Cervix uteri	22.1%	29.9%	6.5%	32.5%	20.8%	3.9%
Corpus uteri	5.4%	13.5%	2.7%	18.9%	16.2%	8.1%
Ovary	6.2%	30.9%	–	12.3%	17.3%	14.8%

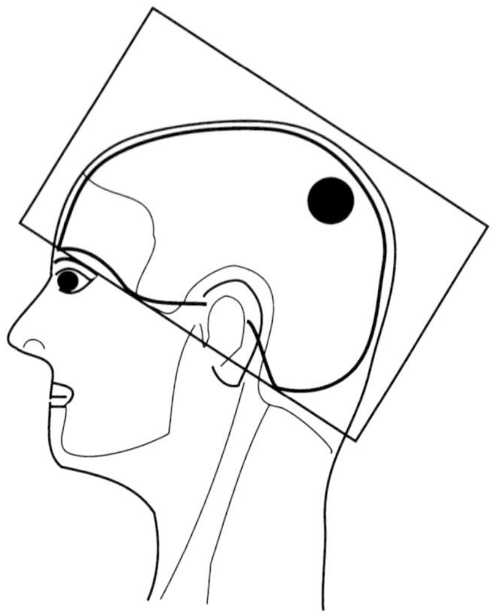

Fig. 16.1. Whole brain irradiation

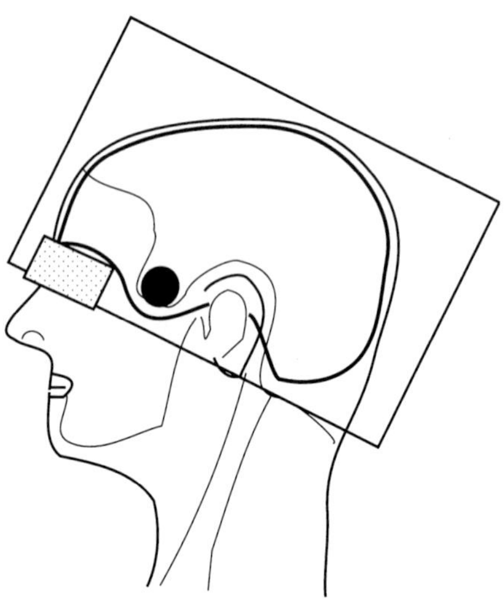

Fig. 16.2. Whole brain irradiation with orbital block

Glucocorticoids fight the effects of vasogenic edema secondary to brain metastases; alternatively, osmotherapy can be used for this purpose.

Irradiation of the whole brain with parallel opposing fields is a simple technique without any serious side-effects. The target volume comprises the whole skull with an inferior border from the supraorbital ridge to the tip of the mastoid (Fig. 16.1). If there are lesions at the base of the frontal or temporal lobe, the portal should include the infraorbital ridge and the external auditory meatus. In these cases an orbital block is necessary (Fig. 16.2). Because of the poor prognosis in most of these cases, the overall treatment time should be as short as possible. Different fractionation schedules are recommended: (a) 30 Gy in 2 weeks, (b) 30 Gy in 3 weeks, (c) 40 Gy in 3 weeks, or (d) 40 Gy in 4 weeks. None of these fractionation schedules seems to be superior to the others, as no substantial differences in duration of improvement of neurological function, time to progression, or survival were found in an RTOG study (BORGELT et al. 1980).

Bibliographic data show the median survival of patients with brain metastases to be 5–10 months, though it is perhaps possible to achieve prolonged survival when irradiation is combined with chemotherapy. SCHLECHTINGEN and LANGE (1985) treated 84 patients with brain metastases from different primary neoplasms with a combination of BCNU, ifosfamide, and irradiation of the whole brain. After a median follow-up of 16.5 months, 50% of the patients were still alive.

Radiotherapy alone usually results in a satisfactory palliation of brain metastases with significant relief of symptoms such as headache due to increased intracranial pressure, motor loss, or impaired mentation. According to bibliographic data, such palliation can be achieved in 60%–90% of cases.

16.1.2 Pulmonary Metastases

Pulmonary metastases from gynecological neoplasms are quite uncommon, but statistical data do exist for pulmonary metastases from carcinomas of the uterine cervix. The incidence is related to the stage of the primary tumor: more advanced primary lesions have a higher probability of metastasizing to the lungs.

IMACHI et al. (1989) found lung metastases in 50 of 817 (6.1%) patients with cancer of the uterine cervix; the incidence was 3.2% in stage FIGO I, 5% in stage FIGO II, 9.4% in stage FIGO III, and 20.9% in stage FIGO IV. TAKEMURA et al. (1990) reported lung metastases in 3.1% in a retrospective analysis of 1121 patients, with the incidence depending on the stage of the primary tumor, as mentioned above.

The chance of an early diagnosis is small because most of the lesions are located in the periphery of the lung and there are no early symptoms. Most of the metastases are found on routine follow-up x-rays of the chest.

The median interval between treatment of the primary tumor and diagnosis of metastases to the lung is 17 months, but cases with an extremely long interval of up to 105 months were reported by ZINK et al. (1990). Usually, the diagnosis of metastases is made within 2 years after detection of the primary tumor. Isolated lung metastases are a rare event, with synchronous metastases in other organs or local recurrences being much more typical.

Once pulmonary metastases have been found, the median survival is 4 months only according to our own results. There is no significant difference in respect of survival between pulmonary metastases from primary carcinomas of the cervix and endometrial carcinomas (Fig. 16.3).

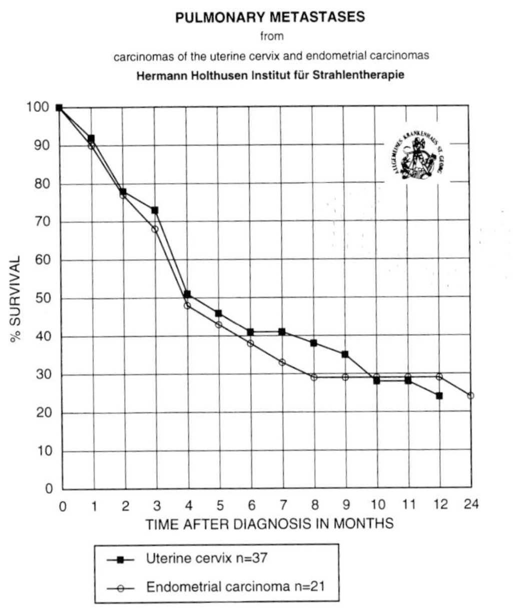

Fig. 16.3. Survival after diagnosis of pulmonary metastases

Rarely there are solitary pulmonary lesions, but lung metastases are more often multiple. In cases of solitary metastases surgical resection may be indicated. MORROW et al. (1980) and MOUNTAIN et al. (1982) reported on 22 and 31 patients, respectively, whose lung metastases were resected. The 5-year-survival rates were 6% and 19%, respectively. MATSUKUMA et al. (1989) reported seven patients who survived more than 2 years, including one who survived more than 4 years and another who survived more than 8 years.

ZINK et al. (1990) treated 61 patients with lung metastases from uterine cancer between 1976 and 1987. In the presence of a solitary lesion a resection was performed and no further adjuvant therapy was applied. When multiple lesions were found, chemotherapy and/or hormonal therapy was added. The 5-year survival was 57% for patients with solitary metastases and 27% for those with multiple lesions.

Chemotherapy can be considered, but treatment results are quite disappointing. The remission rates, especially in squamous cell carcinomas, are 20%–30%, and long-term results are poor (PARK and THIGPEN 1993).

Radiotherapy is only a second-line treatment in lung metastases from female genital cancers. It can be feasible in exceptional cases, when pain appears due to infiltration of pleura or chest wall.

16.1.3 Liver Metastases

Liver metastases from female genital cancer are a sign of advanced systemic dissemination and augur a very poor prognosis. Untreated liver metastases from solid tumors are lethal within a very short time. JAFFE et al. (1968) reported a median survival of 75 days and a 1-year survival of 6.6%.

The main symptoms of liver metastases are persistent nausea and vomiting and, in cases of a severely enlarged liver, there may be considerable pain caused by penetration or distension of Glisson's capsule.

The efficacy of liver irradiation is limited because of the relatively small threshold dose for whole liver radiation-induced hepatitis. A maximum of 25–30 Gy in 2.5–4 weeks (INGOLD et al. 1965; KAPLAN and BAGSHAW 1968) can be applied. Nevertheless, there are some reports of satisfying results in the palliative irradiation of liver metastases, mostly from gastrointestinal primaries (PHILLIPS et al. 1954; PRASAD et al. 1977; SHERMAN et al. 1978; TUREK-MAISCHEIDER and KASEM 1975).

A prospective, uncontrolled, nonrandomized RTOG study (BORGELT et al. 1981) was designed to gain information regarding the feasibility of hepatic irradiation for symptomatic liver metastases, most of them from carcinomas of the gastrointestinal tract and the lung. No significant differences were found for different fractionation schedules. The acute side-effects were relatively moderate. Only in 3% of cases was premature termination of treatment mandatory. Symptoms, especially nausea and pain, were relieved in about 50% of patients, the relief lasting for the remaining lifetime in 60%–80% of these. A total dose of 21 Gy in seven fractions is feasible in the treatment of liver metastases.

A recent study (RUSSELL et al. 1993) investigated the feasibility of hyperfractionated accelerated hepatic irradiation of liver metastases in patients with primary cancers of the gastrointestinal tract. Twice daily hepatic irradiation was employed in single fractions of 1.5 Gy separated by 4 h or longer. The total doses were 27 Gy, 30 Gy, and 33 Gy. There was no prolongation of survival, but more frequent side-effects were observed, which were mild to moderate in most cases. Superiority of this extended and burdensome treatment regimen compared with the common palliative treatment comprising 21 Gy in seven fractions could not be demonstrated.

In conclusion, palliative irradiation of the whole liver with 21 Gy in seven fractions is feasible in patients with advanced symptomatic liver metastases from female genital cancer.

16.1.4 Bone Metastases

Bone metastases from female genital cancer are quite uncommon. The incidence of bone metastases caused by cancer of the uterine cervix is 2%–8% in clinical studies (RATANATHARATHORN et al. 1994), while in autoptic studies it is about 20%. In endometrial cancer the rate of bone metastases is of a quite similar order of magnitude, while it is only 4% in ovarian cancer. Bone metastases from cancer of the vulva, the vagina, and the fallopian tube are extremely rare (ABDUL-KARIM et al. 1990).

The most common site of metastases is the vertebral column, especially the lumbar spine, followed by the pelvic bones. In principle all parts of the skeleton can be involved.

Most of the bone metastases arise hematogenously, since normal bone does not contain any lymphatic channels. BATSON (1940) described a complex network of vertebral, perivertebral, and epidural veins, which partially explains the frequency and distribution of metastases in the vertebral column, the shoulder girdle, and the pelvic bones.

Most of the metastases develop within 2.5 years after treatment of the primary tumor. The median survival after diagnosis of bone metastases is about 4–9 months, according to our own results (Fig. 16.4).

The hallmark of bone metastases is localized pain. Usually there are multiple lesions; therefore bone scintigraphy should be performed as a staging procedure. Plain radiographs of the suspicious regions should then be obtained, and if no definite sites of destruction can be demonstrated, CT or MRI can be added.

Bone metastases of gynecological malignancies are nearly always osteolytic; few metastases of cervical carcinomas are osteoblastic.

Frequently distant metastases in other organs are found when a complete staging is carried out.

Since life expectancy is limited, therapy should aim for the maximum benefit to the patient, especially in terms of relief of pain and the restoration of stability with minimum associated morbidity

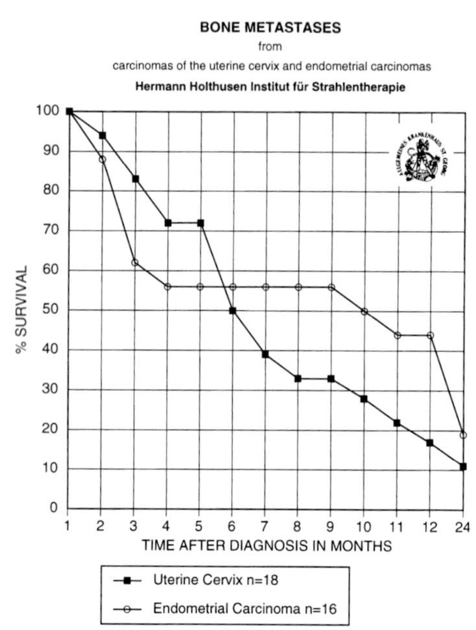

Fig. 16.4. Survival after diagnosis of bone metastases

and minimum disruption of the patient's remaining life.

16.1.4.1 Pain Reduction

Radiotherapy is a reliable method to reduce pain caused by bone metastases. Localized pain should correlate with a positive imaging study. If there is a solitary lesion after a disease-free interval of more than 2 years, percutaneous needle biopsy is recommended (MINK 1986). When a pathological fracture has already occurred, surgical fixation is required prior to radiotherapy, because otherwise bone healing cannot be expected. CT or MRI is recommended for lesions in the vertebral column to ensure that there is no compression of the spinal cord, which could necessitate a neurosurgical intervention.

The extent of the destruction must be clarified. The portals must encompass the whole area of destruction. If soft tissue tumor masses surround the destroyed bone, they should be included in the treatment portals. Treatment information should be complete as overlapping fields from prior treatment must be avoided in order not to seriously injure normal tissue structures.

There are many different fractionation schedules. An RTOG study (TONG et al. 1982) could not point out any significant differences among various schedules. For solitary lesions, 40.5 Gy in 3 weeks and 20 Gy in 1 week were analysed, as were 30 Gy in 2 weeks, 15 Gy in 1 week, 20 Gy in 1 week and 25 Gy in 1 week for multiple metastases. In a reanalysis of this study, BLITZER (1985) concluded that protracted dose-fractionation schedules are more effective than short-course schedules.

We prefer 40 Gy in 16 fractions, although smaller fractions are sometimes required, especially when larger parts of the small bowel or parts of the liver and the kidneys have to be included in the treatment volume. Since late reactions are dependent on the fraction size, this is of major importance in patients with solitary lesions, who have a longer life expectancy and can experience such complications. In cases of short-term survival, e.g., in disseminated disease, or when no risk organs are included in the treatment volume, a shorter overall treatment time is preferable, which means larger dose fractions.

Satisfying results are obtained in about 80%–90% of the treated patients, with complete pain relief being achieved in 50%. Usually pain will increase after 2 weeks of treatment, and it may take about 1–2 months before pain decreases. In most cases there will be no relapse of pain in the treated region because of the short life expectancy (TONG et al. 1982). At least 55%–65% of patients will have persistent pain relief in the first year after irradiation (GILBERT and KAGAN 1977).

Recalcification of the treated bones will not occur earlier than 2 months after termination of the treatment. Therefore radiographic examinations are not useful before this time.

16.1.4.2 Stabilizing Therapy

In some situations, radiotherapy is not recommended as first-line treatment. If there are lytic lesions of more than 2.5 cm in diameter in weight-bearing bones, e.g., midfemoral diaphysis, midhumeral metaphysis, or the subtrochanteric region of the hip, or cortical destruction of more than 50%, radiotherapy alone is unable to diminish the risk of pathological fractures (FIDLER 1981; SIM et al. 1992). Such lesions should be treated surgically.

The common surgical treatment methods for stabilization of metastatic bones are (FRIEDL 1990; HARDMAN et al. 1992):

1. Complete resection of the metastases with tumor-free margins followed by intramedullary rod fixation, or reconstruction with bone plates and screws.
2. Resection of joints, especially the hip joint, and reconstruction with an endoprosthesis.

Prior to surgery the extent of the destruction must be clearly defined in order not to omit other lesions in neighboring regions, which would need simultaneous fixation.

Indications for surgical treatment of spine lesions are progressive neurological symptoms, intractable pain, and progressive deformity. Radiotherapy alone might be too slowly effective to recover neurological deficiencies (LAPRESLE et al. 1991). With a laminectomy followed by plate fixation or transpedicular screw fixation, decompression and stabilization are achieved, and in many cases neurological function can be restored or at least progression avoided. A supporting corset allows early mobilization of the patient.

Postoperative radiotherapy is useful to destroy residual tumor and to diminish the possibility of local failure (FINDLAY 1984).

16.2 Combined Obstructive Edema of the Lower Limb

In about 10% of patients with advanced or recurrent gynecological neoplasms, edema of the lower limb will develop (Lotze and Richter 1989), owing to diminished lymphatic or venous return, or a combination of both factors. Vahrson (1976, 1985) reported the main cause to be a highly iliac or para-aortic lymphatic spread of disease. As a result a complete block of pelvic veins and a complete or incomplete block of lymphatic vessels occur, as verified by pertrochanteric intraosseous venography.

Edema following surgery alone is quite uncommon and is seen only after ultraradical resection of lymphatic tissues with complete removal of lymphatic collaterals or when larger lymphoceles develop. In general the lymphatic system has a great capability to develop superficial and deep lymphatic collaterals or lymphovenous anastomoses, maintaining a sufficient transport capacity. However, after lymphadenectomy and postoperative radiotherapy this transport capacity is reduced by additional cicatrization in the treated region, so that edema develops more frequently (Lotze and Richter 1989).

Sohn et al. (1993) reported alterations in the pelvic and leg venous system following intracavitary irradiation. Ultrasonographic examinations showed the veins to be much less clearly outlined, with thickening of the venous walls. Light reflection rheographic and occlusion plethysmographic measurements showed a deterioration in the venous function.

Kataoka et al. (1991) employed quantitative lymphoscintigraphy and observed a reduction in technetium-99m clearance following radiation, with a close correlation to the dose. Other methods of clarifying the etiology of edema are CT (Vaughan 1990), Doppler ultrasonography, plethysmography (Podhaisky et al. 1990), and MRI (Fujii et al. 1990).

There are different treatment modalities. If iliac and/or para-aortic lymph node metastases are detected and if a venous block exists, palliative irradiation of the metastases combined with diuretics and anticoagulative medication is recommended. With these treatments, Vahrson (1976) achieved significant relief of symptoms, with shrinkage of the swollen leg, pain reduction, and restitution of mobility. If tumor progression is not responsible for edema, surgical treatment may be possible. Baumeister and Siuda (1990) reported a microsurgical treatment method, i.e., bridging the defect with autologous lymphatic grafts. The transport index, measured by volume measurements and lymph scintiscans, showed an improvement of 30% with reduction of edema by up to 80% in the follow-up period of 3 years. Alternatively, complex physiotherapeutic treatment methods can be employed, such as manual lymphatic drainage according to Földi (1982, 1987), combined with elevation of the limbs and intermittent compression by different specially designed bandages and cryotherapy.

16.3 Recurrent Peritoneal and Pleural Effusions

Malignant ascites is a sign of advanced disease. With respect to gynecological neoplasms, it most often occurs in cases of ovarian carcinoma, in which it may be the first symptom.

The etiology of malignant ascites is multifactorial. Often there is delayed resorption of peritoneal fluid, caused by tumor-induced obstruction of infradiaphragmatic lymphatic vessels. In addition there can be excessive fluid production.

The principal symptoms are increase in weight with increasing abdominal girth, dyspnea due to diaphragmatic elevation, and deterioration of performance status. The diagnosis is easily made by clinical examination. Ultrasonography and/or CT may provide confirmation. Malignancy is proven by abdominal paracentesis and cytological examination.

The main goal of therapy must be a rapid improvement of quality of life, with minimal treatment-induced morbidity, since the average length of survival is only 2 months and the 1-year survival rate is merely 5%–10%. Diuretics have little impact on malignant ascites, although Greenway et al. (1982) reported success in 13 of 15 patients treated with large doses of spironolactone. Peritoneovenous shunting, primarily developed for the treatment of cirrhotic ascites, has also been used (Baker 1989). There is no prolongation of survival, but significant relief of symptoms is achieved. Shunt-induced tumor dissemination is a likely complication (Lacy et al. 1984; Souter et al. 1985), but the clinical course is rarely affected, as reported by Tarin et al. (1984a,b).

Repeated paracentesis is not a useful treatment of malignant ascites. In a catabolic state metabolism this would lead to further protein depletion and electrolyte disturbances, and infections of the peritoneal fluid might result.

There are several reports on the intracavitary application of chemotherapeutic agents (PREISS 1987). Prior to the application, complete removal of ascites is mandatory, otherwise drugs may develop an uncontrollable protein binding, e.g., cis-DDP and doxorubicin. In addition, the free distribution of the drugs in the peritoneal cavity must be proved by nuclear medical methods or CT. Bleomycin (OSTROWSKI and HALSTALL 1982; PALADINE et al. 1976), doxorubicin (MARKMAN et al. 1984), cis-DDP (LOPEZ et al. 1985; MARKMAN et al. 1984), and mitoxantrone have been investigated. There were partial or complete responses in about 60%, with a mean duration of 2–3 months; only rarely were remissions longlasting.

Some more recent reports have investigated the use of beta-interferon and TNF (CHERCHI et al. 1990; CAPPELLI and GOTTI 1992; GEBBIA et al. 1991). The remission rates were 35%–75%, remission lasting for 1–6 months. In some patients long-term remissions were observed, but the patient numbers were small.

The incidence of pleural effusions is particularly high (17%) in ovarian cancers (SEITZER 1990). Dyspnea, cough, and chest pain are the main symptoms. Dyspnea depends on the volume of effusion and resulting pulmonary compression. Cough is usually unproductive and is due to compression of the bronchial wall by fluid. Pain is caused by inflammatory irritation of the pleura or by tumor invasion of the pleural membranes.

Pleural effusions are a sign of advanced disease and curative treatment is impossible. Life expectancy is limited. The treatment goal is the most rapid possible relief of symptoms and avoidance of long-term hospitalization.

Chest radiographs show the extent of effusion. A lateral decubitus film determines whether or not effusions are free-flowing and whether or not loculations are present. Ultrasonography is useful in determining the most appropriate site for thoracentesis. Following thoracentesis, careful cytological and serological examination is mandatory. Tumor cells are usually found, the rate being 67% in the case of primary ovarian neoplasms (JÄRVI et al. 1972). Once the diagnosis has been established, the pleural effusion is drained with a chest tube inserted under local anesthesia. The evacuation may be spontaneous or be achieved by suction drainage. Only in a small proportion of cases does complete drainage of the pleural fluid and the resulting approximation of the visceral and parietal pleura lead to a pleurodesis.

In most cases, however, additional sclerotherapy is necessary to prevent reaccumulation of pleural fluid. If too much fluid remains in the pleural space, the efficiency of sclerotherapy might be reduced due to dilution of the sclerosing substances. Many different potential sclerosing substances have been tested, e.g., antibiotics, especially tetracyclines, quinicrine, talc, and antineoplastic agents. Radioactive isotopes like gold-198, yttrium-90, and phosphorus-32 have been applied in the interpleural space, too, but they are now only rarely used in view of the special precautions required for radiation protection and the high costs. Talc is effective in 90%–100% of cases, but it must be applied under general anesthesia and has a significant mortality of 5%–11% (SORENSEN et al. 1984; SHEDBALKAR et al. 1971).

Tetracyclines are widely used as a sclerosing substance. Pathophysiologically they induce an inflammatory reaction of the pleura with increasing permeability of pleural capillaries, which allows the accumulation of clotting factors, and especially fibrinogen, in the interpleural space. Reaction with thrombin leads to the formation of fibrin, resulting in fibrosis and sclerosis and finally an obliteration of the pleural space. The effectiveness is about 75%; the side-effects are only moderate and the treatment costs are low. After complete removal of the pleural fluid, tetracyclines in a dose of 1–3 g in 100 ml of normal saline solution are instilled via the chest tube, which is afterwards clamped. The patient is instructed to change positions in order to equally distribute the sclerosing agent throughout the pleural cavity. After 4 h, the fluid is drained and suction reestablished for about 24 h. When the daily amount of effluent is <100 ml, and the lungs remain expanded, the drainage can be removed. In recurrent effusions, patients can be retreated in the same manner. The main side-effects are localized pain and sometimes fever, which can be easily controlled by adequate medication.

Among the antineoplastic agents, mitoxantrone has relatively modest tissue toxicity and is under investigation for the treatment of malignant pleural effusions. Due to its high polarity and protein binding, it will be absorbed very slowly from the interpleural space. The achievable concentrations here are 100- to 200-fold higher compared with intravenous injection, and the systemic side-effects are negligible. TORSTEN et al. (1992) reported on the treatment of malignant pleural effusions caused by breast and ovarian cancer. After removal of pleural fluid, 30 mg mitoxantrone was instilled for 24 h. In 11 of 12 cases a complete remission was obtained, lasting for a mean of 3 months. Side-effects were localized pain and leukopenia (WHO grade II leukopenia was seen in 25% of cases). SEITZER et al. (1990) instilled mitoxantrone for 48h. In 23 of 28 patients with breast cancer and six of seven patients with ovarian neoplasms a complete remission was achieved. The side-effects were comparable to those reported by TORSTEN et al. (1992).

Recently, interferons have been under investigation for the treatment of malignant pleural effusions (GALOTTI et al. 1992; DAVIS et al. 1992; BHATIA et al. 1994). The reported rates of partial and complete remission are not, however, superior to those obtained with other methods; therefore routine clinical use of interferons cannot be recommended, especially in view of the high costs.

16.4 Care of Incurable Patients

In far advanced stages of disease, without any chance of cure, no aggressive treatment modalities are indicated. The response of endometrial carcinomas to chemotherapy is quite disappointing, even when aggressive combination chemotherapy has been applied: although reported response rates are as high as 46%, most responses have been only partial (CAMPORA et al. 1990; SUTTON et al. 1992; MUSS et al. 1991). Combination chemotherapy of cervical carcinomas shows similarly unsatisfying results (TAY et al. 1992; JUNOR et al. 1991; PARK and THIGPEN 1993). There may be various reasons for the poor efficiency of chemotherapy. First, most patients have previously undergone surgical and/or radiotherapeutic treatment, and the blood supply thus may be altered. Second, radiotherapy can induce decreased bone marrow reserves, and there is therefore less tolerance to dose-intensive chemotherapy. Third, advanced or recurrent female genital cancer is often associated with decreased renal function following ureteral obstruction. In conclusion, chemotherapy should be employed in clinical trials only.

One of the most important duties in the palliative treatment of terminally ill patients with gynecological neoplasms is achievement of sufficient analgesia. Pain may occur through (a) a local recurrence with invasion of adjacent structures, especially the lumbosacral nerval plexus, causing severe radicular pain, (b) metastases to bones, or (c) diffuse peritoneal involvement. As in other tumor entities, treatment of pain should be systematic, e.g., in accordance with the WHO (1986) three-step approach to analgesic drug therapy (Fig. 16.5).

The choice of drugs should be specific to the different types of pain. In cases of persistent pain, drugs must be administered on a regular basis, the time

Table 16.2. Dosages of nonsteroidal anti-inflammatory drugs

Drug	Single dose	Interval
Acetylsalicylic acid	500–1000 mg	4–6 h
Diclofenac	50–100 mg	6–8 h
Ibuprofen	400–600 mg	6–8 h
Acetaminophen	500–1000 mg	4–6 h
Metamizol	500–1000 mg	4–6 h

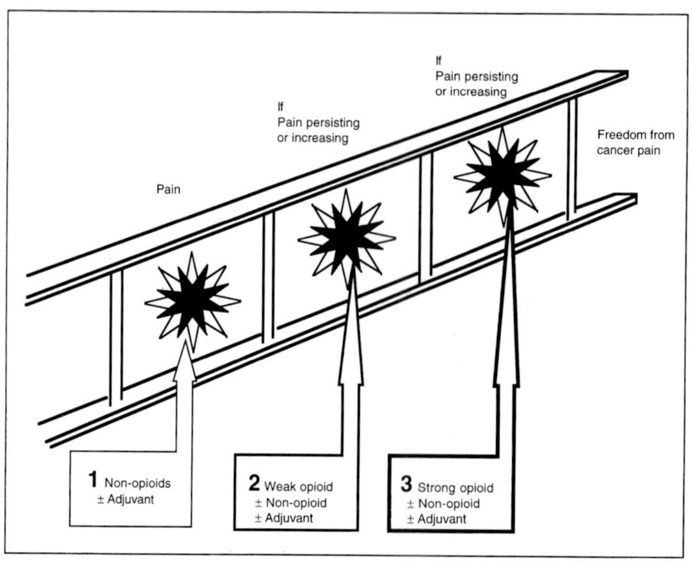

Fig. 16.5. The WHO three-step ladder approach to analgesic drug therapy

Table 16.3. Dosages of weak opioids

Drug	Single dose	Interval
Codeine	30–150 mg	4–6 h
Dextropropoxyphene	150 mg	6–8 h
Tramadol	50–100 mg	4–6 h
Tilidine naloxone	50–100 mg	4–6 h

Table 16.4. Dosages of strong opioids

Drug	Single dose	Interval
Morphine	5–500 mg	4 h
Morphine sulfate	10–500 mg	8–12 h
Buprenorphine	0.2–1.2 mg	6–8 h

Table 16.5. Adjuvants used in the management of cancer pain

Class	Drug	Indications	Dosage
Antidepressants	Amitriptyline Imipramine	Depression, neuropathic pain	3 × 10–50 mg 3 × 25–75 mg
Anticonvulsants	Phenytoin Carbamazepine	Neuropathic pain	1–3 × 100 mg 3–4 × 200 mg
Neuroleptics	Levomepromazine Haloperidol	Agitation, vomiting	3 × 5–30 mg 3 × 1–10 mg
Hypnotics	Bromazepam Flunitrazepam	Somnipathy	6 mg 2–4 mg
Steroids	Prednisone Dexamethasone	Somatic and deafferentation pain, lumbar plexopathy, cerebral edema	5–15 mg 2–8 mg

interval being determined in accordance with the pharmacokinetics of the applied drugs (Tables 16.2–16.4). Such regular administration is necessary to achieve a constant plasma level, and should be adhered to even when patients have to be awakened from their sleep. The oral route should be preferred, but if immediate pain relief is required, parenteral administration is the method of choice. Different additional drugs can be administered adjuvantly (Table 16.5).

When pain is increasing, or side-effects are severe, opioids ± local anesthetics can be administered via an epidural catheter with intermittent or continuous infusion (Shaves et al. 1991; Hassenbusch et al. 1990; Stamer and Maier 1992). There are few side-effects with this treatment, though in some cases catheter replacement is necessary due to occlusion. Infections are rare. Most patients can be discharged from hospital after a regimen for optimal pain relief has been found.

References

Abdul-Karim FW, Masatoshi K, Budd Wentz W, et al. (1990) Bone metastases from gynecological carcinomas: a clinicopathologic study. Gynecol Oncol 39:108–114

Badib AO, Kurohara SS, Webster JH, Pickren JW (1968) Metastasis to organs in carcinoma of the uterine cervix: influence of treatment on incidence and distribution. Cancer 21:434–439

Baker AR (1989) Treatment of malignant ascites. In: De Vita VT, Hellman S, Rosenberg SA (eds) Principles and Practice of oncology, 3rd edn. Lippincott, Philadelphia, p 2328

Batson OV (1940) The function of the vertebral veins and their role in the spread of metastases. Ann Surg 112:138–149

Baumeister RG, Siuda S (1990) Treatment of lymphedemas by microsurgical lymphatic grafting: what is proved? Plast Reconstr Surg 85:64–74

Berge T, Lundberg S (1977) Cancer in Malmö – an autopsy study. Acta Scand Pathol Microbiol Sect A Suppl 260

Bhatia A, Rice TW, McLain D, et al. (1994) A phase I trial of intrapleural recombinant human interferon alpha (rHuIFN alpha 2b) in patients with malignant pleural effusions. J Cancer Res Clin Oncol 120:169–172

Blitzer PH (1985) Reanalysis of the RTOG study of the palliation of symptomatic osseous metastasis. Cancer 55:1468–1472

Borgelt BB, Gelber R, Kramer S (1980) The palliation of brain metastases: final results of the first two studies by the Radiation Therapy Oncology Group. Int J Radiat Oncol Biol Phys 6:1–9

Borgelt BB, Gelber R, Brady LW, Griffin T, Hendrickson FR (1981) The palliation of hepatic metastases: results of the Radiation Therapy Oncology Group pilot study. Int J Radiat Oncol Biol Phys 7:587–591

Campora E, Vidali A, Mammoliti S, Ragni N, Conte PF (1990) Treatment of advanced or recurrent adenocarcinoma of the endometrium with doxorubucin and cyclophosphamide. Eur J Gynaecol Oncol 11:181–183

Cappelli R, Gotti G (1992) Trattamento locoregionale dell'ascite neoplastica con interferone beta. Recenti Prog Med 83:82–84

Carlson V, Delclos L, Fletcher GH (1967) Distant metastasis in squamous cell carcinoma of the uterine cervix. Radiology 88:961–966

Cherchi PL, Campiglio A, Rubattu A, Desole A, Andria G, Ambrosini A (1990) Endocavitary beta interferon in neoplastic effusions. Eur J Gynaecol Oncol 11:477–479

Davis M, Williford S, Muss HB, White DR, Cooper MR, Jackson DV, Barrett R (1992) A phase II study of recombinant intrapleural alpha interferon in malignant pleural effusions. Am J Clin Oncol 15:328–330

Fidler M (1981) Incidence of fracture through metastasis in long bones. Acta Orthop Scand 52:623–627

Findlay GFG (1984) Adverse effects of the management of spinal cord compression. J Neurol Neurosurg Psychiatry 47:761–768

Földi M (1982) Das chronische Lymphödem. Fortschr Med 100:877–880

Földi M (1987) Postoperatives und postaktinisches lymphödem gynäkologischer malignome. Speculum 4:18–23

Friedl W (1990) Indication, management and results of surgical therapy for pathological fractures in patients with bone metastases. Eur J Surg Oncol 16:380–396

Fujii K, Ishida O, Mabuchi N, et al. (1990) MRI of lymphedema using short TI-IR (STIR). Rinsho Hoshasen 35:77–82

Gallotti P, Natale G, Olgiati A, Bottaro G, Chiesa E, Zocco S (1992) Intracavitary alpha-2b interferon as palliative treatment in pleural malignant effusions (meeting abstract). Ann Oncol 3:182

Gebbia V, Russo A, Gebbia N, Valenza R, Testa A, Palmeri S, Rausa L (1991) Intracavitary beta-interferon for the management of pleural and/or abdominal effusions in patients with advanced cancer refractory to chemotherapy. In Vivo 5:579–581

Gilbert HA, Kagan HR (1977) Evaluation of radiation therapy for bone metastases: pain relief and quality of life. AJR 129:1095

Graf AH, Buchberger W, Langmayr H, Schmidt KW (1988) Site preference of metastatic tumours of the brain. Virchows Arch [A] 412:493–498

Gralow I, von Hornstein W, Behling H (1991) Schmerztherapie bei Patientinnen mit gynäkologischen Tumorerkrankungen. Zentralbl Gynäkol 113:1288–1297

Greenway B, Johnson PJ, Williams R (1982) Control of malignant ascites with spironolactone. Br J Surg 69:441–442

Hardman PD, Robb JE, Kerr GR, Rodger A, MacFarlane A (1992) The value of fixation and radiotherapy in the management of upper and lower limb bone metastases. Clin Oncol 4:244–248

Hassenbusch SJ, Pillay PK, Magdinec M, Currie K, Bay JW, Covington EC, Tomaszewski MZ (1990) Constant infusion of morphine for intractable cancer pain using an implanted pump. J Neurosurg 73:405–409

Henriksen E (1949) The lymphatic spread of carcinoma of the cervix and the body the uterus: a study of 420 necropsies. Am J Obstet Gynecol 58:924–940

Imachi M, Tsukamoto N, Matsuyama T, Nakano H (1989) Pulmonary metastasis from carcinoma of the uterine cervix. Gynecol Oncol 33:189–192

Ingold JA, Reed GB, Kaplan HS, Bagshaw MA (1965) Radiation hepatitis. Am J Roentgenol 93:200–208

Jaffe BM, Donegan WL, Watson F, Spratt JS Jr (1968) Factors influencing survival in patients with untreated hepatic metastases. Surg Gynecol Obstet 127:1–11

Järvi OH, Kunnas RJ, Laitio MT, Tyrköö JES (1972) The accuracy and significance of cytologic cancer diagnosis of pleural effusions. Acta Cytol 16:152–158

Junor E, Davies J, Habeshaw T, et al. (1991) Carboplatin based chemotherapy for advanced carcinoma of the cervix. Cancer Chemother Pharmacol 27:484–486

Kaplan HS, Bagshaw MA (1968) Radiation hepatitis: possible prevention by combined isotopic and external radiation therapy. Radiology 91:1214–1220

Kataoka M, Kawamura M, Hamada K, Itoh H, Nishiyama Y, Hamamoto K (1991) Quantitative lymphoscintigraphy using $^{99}Tc^{m}$ human serum albumin in patients with previously treated uterine cancer. Br J Radiol 64:1191–1121

Kishi K, Nomura K, Miki Y, Shibui S, Takakura K (1982) Metastatic brain tumour: a clinical and pathologic analysis of 101 cases with biopsy. Arch Pathol Lab Med 106:133–135

Kottke-Marchant K, Estes ML, Nunez C (1991) Early brain metastases in endometrial carcinoma. Gynecol Oncol 40:107–111

Kumar L, Tanwar RK, Singh SP (1992) Intracranial metastases from carcinoma cervix and review of literature. Gynecol Oncol 46:391–392

Lacy JH, Wieman TJ, Shively EH (1984) Management of malignant ascites. Surg Gynecol Obstet 159:397–412

Lapresle P, Roy-Camille R, Lazennec JY, Mariambourg G (1991) Traitement chirurgical des metastases vertebrales. Chirurgie 117:49–58

Lopez JA, Krikorian JG, Reich SD (1985) Clinical pharmacology of intraperitoneal cisplatin. Gynecol Oncol 20:1–9

Lotze W, Richter P (1989) Sekundäre Lymphödeme bei gynäkologischen Malignomen. Zentralbl Gynäkol 111:92–98

Markman M, Howell SB, Lucas WE, Pfeifle CE, Green MR (1984) Combined intraperitoneal chemotherapy with cisplatin, cytarabine and doxorubicin for refractory ovarian carcinoma and other malignancies principally confined to the peritoneal cavity. J Clin Oncol 2:1321–1326

Matsukuma K, Miyake M, Iino H, et al. (1989) Surgical management of pulmonary metastasis from carcinoma of the uterine cervix. Nippon Sanka Fujinka Gakkai Zasshi 41:1911–1915

Matthiesen H von (1991) Pain treatment in gynaecological cancer. Postgrad Med J 67:26–30

Mink J (1986) Percutaneous bone biopsy in the patient with known or suspected osseous metastases. Radiology 161:191–194

Morrow CE, Vassilopoulos P, Grage TB (1980) Surgical resection for metastatic neoplasms of the lung. Cancer 45:2981–2985

Mountain CF, Khalil KG, Hermes KE (1982) The contributions of surgery to the management of carcinomatous pulmonary metastases. Cancer 50:1057–1060

Muss HB, Bundy BN, Adcock L (1991) Teniposide (VM-26) in patients with advanced endometrial carcinoma. A phase II trial of the Gynecologic Oncology Group. Am J Clin Oncol 14:36–37

Noltenius H (1987) Tumorhandbuch, Pathologie und Klinik der menschlichen Tumoren, vol 3, 4th edn. Urban & Schwarzenberg, München

Ostrowski MJ, Halstall GM (1982) Intracavitary bleomycin in the management of malignant effusions: a multicenter study. Cancer Treat Rep 66:1903–1907

Paladine W, Cunningham PJ, Sponzo R, Donavan M, Olson K, Horton J (1976) Intracavitary bleomycin in the management of malignant effusions. Cancer 38:1903–1908

Park RC, Thigpen JT (1993) Chemotherapy in advanced and recurrent cervical cancer. Cancer 71:1446–1450

Peeples WJ, Inalsingh H, Hazra TA, Graft D (1976) The occurrence of metastasis outside the abdomen and retroperitoneal space in invasive carcinoma of the cervix. Gynecol Oncol 4:307–310

Phillips R, Karnofsky DA, Hamilton LD, Nickson JJ (1954) Roentgen therapy of hepatic metastases, Am J Roentgenol 71:826–834

Podhaisky H, Hansgen K, Lampe D, Methfessel G, Methfessel HD (1990) Angiologische Funktionsdiagnostik beim einseitigen Beinödem nach kombinierter Therapie des Zervixkarzinoms. Z Gesamte Inn Med 45:55–58

Prasad B, Lee MS, Hendrickson FR (1977) Irradiation of hepatic metastases. Int J Radiat Oncol Biol Phys 2:129–132

Preiss J (1987) Intraperitoneale Therapie. In: Schmoll HJ, Peters HD, Peters HD, Fink U (eds) Kompendium Internistische Onkologie. Springer, Berlin Heidelberg New York, p 1044

Ratanatharathorn V, Powers WE, Steverson N, Han I, Ahmad K, Grimm J (1994) Bone metastases from cervical cancer. Cancer 73:2372–2379

Russell AH, Clyde C, Wasserman TH, Turner SS, Rotman M (1993) Accelerated hyperfractionated hepatic irradiation in the management of patients with liver metastases: results of the RTOG dose escalating protocol. Int J Radiat Oncol Biol Phys 27:117–123

Sawada M, Inagaki M, Ozaki M, et al. (1990) Long-term survival after brain metastasis from endometrial cancer. Jpn J Clin Oncol 20:312–315

Schlechtingen J, Lange O (1985) Erste Ergebnisse bei der Behandlung von Hirnmetastasen maligner solider Tumoren durch kombinierten Einsatz von Strahlen- und zytostatischer Chemotherapie. In: Heilmann HP (ed) Palliative Therapie, Indikation, Probleme, Ergebnisse. Zuckschwerdt, München, pp 129–138

Seitzer D, Musch E, Kuhn W (1990) Die lokale Behandlung maligner Pleuraergüsse bei gynäkologischen Tumoren. Zentra bl Gynäkol 112:757–765

Shaves M, Barnhill D, Bosscher J, Remmenga S, Hahn M, Park R (1991) Indwelling epidural catheters for pain control in gynecologic cancer patients. Obstet Gynecol 77:642–644

Shedbalkar AR, Head JM, Head LR (1971) Evaluation of talc pleural symphysis in management of malignant pleural effusions. J Thorac Cardiovasc Surg 61:492

Sherman DM, Weichselbaum R, Eilber FR, Morton DL (1978) Palliation of hepatic metastases. Cancer 41:2013–2017

Sim FH, Frassica FJ, Frassica DA (1992) Metastatic bone disease: current concepts of clinicopathophysiology and modern surgical treatment. Ann Acad Med Singapore 21:274–279

Sohn C, Meyberg G, von Fournier D, Bastert G (1993) Einfluss der intrakavitären Bestrahlung auf das Becken-Beinvenensystem. Zentralbl Gynäkol 115:220–224

Sorensen PG, Svendsen TL, Enk B (1984) Treatment of malignant pleural effusions with drainage, with and without instillation of talc. Eur J Respir Dis 65:131

Sorge J, Lehmkuhl C, Lohse K, Herrmann H, Pichlmayr I (1990) Langzeittherapie von Tumorschmerzen mit Morphin-retard-Tabletten. Med Klin 85:523–528

Souter RG, Weels C, Tarin D (1985) Surgical and pathological complications associated with peritoneovenous shunts in the management of malignant ascites. Cancer 55:1973–1978

Stamer U, Maier C (1992) Ambulante Epiduralanalgesie bei Tumorpatienten. Ein überholtes Verfahren? Anaesthesist 41:288–296

Sutton GP, Blessing JA, Manetta A, Homesley H, McGuire W (1992) Gynecologic Oncology Group studies with ifosfamide. Semin Oncol 19:31–34

Takemura M, Yamasaki M, Shimizu H, et al. (1990) A clinicopathological study of pulmonary metastases in carcinoma of the uterine cervix. Nippon Gan Chiryo Gakkai Shi 25:776–780

Tarin D, Price JE, Kettlewell MGW (1984a) Mechanisms of human tumor metastasis studied in patients with peritoneovenous shunts. Cancer Res 44:3584–3592

Tarin D, Vass ACR, Kettlewell MGW (1984b) Absence of metastatic sequelae during long term treatment of malignant ascites by peritoneo-venous shunting. Invasion Metastasis 4:1–12

Tay SK, Lai FM, Soh LT, Ho TH, Ang PT, Au E (1992) Combined chemotherapy using cisplatin, ifosfamide and bleomycin (PIB) in the treatment of advanced and recurrent cervical carcinoma. Aust N Z J Obstet Gynaecol 32:263–266

Tong D, Gillick L, Hendrickson FR (1982) The palliation of symptomatic osseous metastases. Final results of the study by the Radiation Therapy Oncology Group. Cancer 50:893–899

Torsten U, Opri F, Weitzel H (1992) Local therapy of malignant pleural effusion with mitoxantrone. Anti-Cancer Drugs 3:17–18

Turek-Maischeider M, Kasem I (1975) Palliative irradiation for liver metastases. JAMA 232:625–628

Vahrson H (1976) Der Wert der Ossovenographie beim fortgeschrittenen Genitalkarzinom der Frau. Ein Beitrag zur diagnose des kombinierten Stauungsödems. Röntgenblätter 29:341–349

Vahrson H (1985) Probleme der Palliativtherapie bei der Behandlung weiblicher Genitalkarzinome. In: Heilmann HP (ed) Palliative Therapie, Indikation, Probleme, Ergebnisse. Zuckschwerdt, München, pp 35–51

Vaughan BF (1990) CT of swollen legs. Clin Radiol 41:24–30

Vieth RG, Odom GL (1965) Intracranial metastases and their neurosurgical treatment. J Neurosurg 23:375–383

Weiss GR, Cortez MC, Kuhn JG, Shaffer D (1991) Phase I trial of combined intraperitoneal (IP) cisplatin and mitoxantrone for peritoneal cancer (meeting abstract). Proc Annu Meet Am Soc Clin Oncol 10:A327

World Health Organization (1986) Cancer pain relief. Office of Publications, WHO, Geneva

Wright DC, Delaney TF (1989) Treatment of metastatic cancer to the brain. In: De Vita VT, Hellman S, Rosenberg SA (eds) Principles and practice of oncology, 3rd edn. Lippincott, Philadelphia, p 2245

Zink M, Greschuchna D, Niederle N, Stamatis G (1990) Interdisziplinäre Behandlungsmaßnahmen bei pulmonal metastasierendem Uteruskarzinom: Erste Ergebnisse bei 61 Patientinnen. Pneumologie 44 (Suppl 1):271–272

17 Radiation Treatment of Benign Gynecologic Diseases

R. Pfab

CONTENTS

17.1 Introduction

A correct indication is a prerequisite for successful radiotherapy. Often radiotherapy is not employed in cases where it is of proven efficacy while on the other hand many patients undergo radiotherapy although their radiation therapist knows well enough that radiotherapy is not indicated. The application of radiotherapy in patients with benign diseases has to be limited to those diseases which can be exposed to isolated irradiation and which have a higher radiosensitivity than the unaffected adjoining parts of the body. Furthermore, it is particularly important to completely exclude somatic damage and also genetic damage with maximum certainty according to state-of-the-art knowledge. Especially the skin should not be exposed to irradiation of more than 30 Gy per field in the course of life during radiation treatment of benign diseases (Hess 1987).

While antiphlogistic irradiation particularly aims at nonspecific stimulation, radiation treatment of benign hypertrophic processes emphasizes the cytocidal effect of irradiation. Efficacious radiation treatment of benign hypertrophic diseases necessitates radiation doses which are close to the tolerance limit of the skin and the connective tissue. Therefore, special care has to be taken that the unaffected adjoining tissue is protected from irradiation as well as possible. This can only be achieved to a limited degree in the case of internal diseases. Furthermore, before deciding on radiotherapy, it has to be taken into account that high radiation doses may cause late changes such as atrophy, pigmentation shifts, or telangiectases. The risk of such changes must always be in reasonable proportion to the functional and cosmetic significance of the benign disease. According to all we know today about the mutative effects of radiation, we have to reckon with the possibility that these effects are an important factor in carcino- and sarcomagenesis. Therefore, due to the risk of radiation-induced tumors, radiation treatment of benign diseases is only indicated in special cases.

The essential factor in stimulation irradiation is not the destruction of certain parts of the body, but the stimulating effect that the decomposition products caused by radiotherapy have on different organs (Glauner 1951). Clinical experience has shown that antiphlogistic irradiation may shorten the healing of acute, subacute, and chronic inflammation (Trott 1994). In the case of acute processes, pain and inflammatory tissue tension subside within a few hours, resulting either in immediate complete remission or, in advanced processes, in accelerated softening. Due to this development, it is soon possible to remove the pus by means of a stab incision, which causes an acceleration of the healing process. Radiation treatment of patients with chronic inflammations results in a more or less pronounced increase in inflammation with subsequent reduction of the symptoms. Even today, in spite of the success of medication therapy, antiphlogistic irradiation can be of value, especially in cases of local inflammation. The technical realization of antiphlogistic irradiation is simple because in most cases one irradiation field is sufficient. The required low doses do not cause any cutaneous lesion; the radiation dose is suited to the stage and the intensity of the inflammation. The

R. Pfab, MD, Professor, Komm. Leiter der Abteilung für Strahlentherapie, Klinikum der Philipps-Universität Marburg, Baldingerstraße, D-35043 Marburg, Germany fresher and the more violent the inflammation, the lower the dose must be. In general, a single dose of 0.5–1 Gy is applied to the surface of acute inflammations; for subacute inflammations, the surface dose is increased to a maximum of 2 Gy. Patients with chronic inflammations are administered the same dose; a surface dose of >2.5 Gy is not necessary (Scherer 1958, 1965). Fractionation of irradiation can be adjusted to the radiation effect. If necessary, this dose can be administered daily; in the case of chronic inflammations, irradiation-free intervals of several days are possible.

Radiation treatment of patients with acute inflammations must be started as soon as possible. The irradiation field always has to be larger than the focus of inflammation. In order to sufficiently reach the tissue around the focus of inflammation even deep in the body, the irradiation must not be too soft. Surface irradiation is only sufficient for very superficial inflammation; in all other cases, intermediate or deep radiotherapy is indicated.

17.2 Furunculosis Vulvae

Furunculosis vulvae is a purulent inflammation of hair follicles occurring only in the hair region. This disease should be irradiated 3–4 times with a single daily dose of 0.2–0.8 Gy. The doses depend on the stage of the disease. Daily doses of 0.2 Gy are indicated for fresh exudative processes where inflammatory softening has not yet started and complete remission of the infiltrates is still possible. Patients suffering from softening inflammation should be treated with daily doses of 0.5 Gy at intervals of 2–3 days. Radiation should be intermediate with a tissue half-value layer of 7.0–13.0 mm (half-value layer: 0.4–0.88 mm of aluminum; focal-skin distance: 15–30 cm).

17.3 Mastitis Puerperalis

The changes in the female breast due to lactation, with neoformation of glands and connective tissue as well as vascular changes, is likely to result in higher radiosensitivity and, thus, in an increased efficacy of radiotherapy (Kruchen 1973). Mastitis occurring at other times does not show such a prompt response to radiation treatment. At the initial stage of the disease, this is the fastest way to achieve healing without having to resort to incision: healing without incision was achieved in 96% of patients after radiation treatment within 24 h (Gászágo 1938), and in 88% after radiation treatment within 48 h (Rech 1943). Doses of 0.25–0.75 Gy used to be given at an early stage. The integral dose did not exceed 1.5 Gy (Böttger and Rumphorst 1956; Hess 1980). Before the antibiotic era, acute inflammation in the lactating breast was one of the most rewarding fields of application of radiotherapy; due to the fact that irradiated patients have been found to run a fourfold higher risk of subsequent breast cancer than a nonirradiated control group, radiotherapy can no longer be recommended (Hess 1980; Mettler 1969; Rausch 1982; Shore 1977; Trott 1994).

17.4 Pruritus Vulvae et Ani Sine Materia (True Pruritus Senilis)

Radiation treatment of pruritus, which can be persistent and therapy resistant, often has a surprisingly good though not always lasting effect (Braun-Falco and Lucacs 1973). Repeated irradiation is successful from time to time, though its effect decreases. Due to the risk of radiation-induced side-effects, radiation treatment is only indicated in patients who are not of a reproductive age. Doses of 0.5–1.5 Gy are recommended, with soft x-rays (20–30 kV); in the event of persistent affections, the dose may be increased to 2.0–4.0 Gy and irradiation may be repeated once. The irradiation field should cover the complete perineovulvar region.

17.5 Kraurosis Vulvae

Kraurosis vulvae, which is characterized by atrophy of the skin of all parts of the vulva due to a recession of adipose tissue and elastic fibers, is considered to be a facultative precancerosis. It is not advisable to treat kraurosis vulvae by means of irradiation.

17.6 Keloids

Keloids develop due to an individual proneness to skin injury with pathologically increased growth of connective tissue (Baensch 1937). The cause of a keloid is always a trauma (Allan and Keen 1954;

BAENSCH 1937; DALICHO 1949; SIMONS 1930). Even small, unnoticed traumas may result in a relatively large keloid. Keloids often occur after burns and acid erosion or – in susecptible patients – also in operation scars. The incidence of keloids is 3–4 times higher in female than in male individuals (RÖSLER et al. 1993). Only fresh keloids are radioresponsive. Irradiation treatment of keloids is not so much directed against mature tissue as against the regeneration layer from which keloids develop. Large, extensive keloids, particularly keloids caused by burns, narrow down the indication for radiation treatment as the integral dose and the strain on adjoining tissue become unjustifiably high. The size of the irradiation field corresponds to the area covered by the keloid. In the presence of irregular forms, the healthy adjoining tissue must be carefully covered with lead foil up to the keloid edge. The tissue half-value layer has to be adapted to the thickness of the keloid. If a single dose of 2.0 Gy is delivered at intervals of 2 days, an integral dose of 20 Gy is necessary (HESS 1987). Successful radiation treatment of keloids is possible if postoperative irradiation is started as early as possible after excision, with electrons of 5 MeV from a linear accelerator in a dose of 5 × 2 Gy per week up to a mean surface dose of 20 Gy (RÖSLER et al. 1993). Older keloids are irradiated in the same way as soon after excision as the condition of the wound permits and with the stitches still present. Instead of being excised, extensive keloids can also be ground down at high revolution or be levelled off with a snare loop before they are irradiated as described above (HESS 1987). There is general agreement that radiotherapy alone, a combination of surgery and radiotherapy, or intralesional treatment by injection of glucocorticoids with or without surgical measures can be employed in the treatment of keloids (BRAUN-FALCO and LUCACS 1973). Ablation alone is known to lead to more extensive recurrences. Interstitial radiotherapy (FRACOIS et al. 1993) and laser techniques (ABERGEL et al. 1984a,b; HENDERSON et al. 1984) are also increasingly employed in the treatment of keloids.

17.7 Radiotherapy to Arrest Uterine Bleeding Due to Benign Gynecologic Diseases

Radiation treatment of uterine bleeding is only indicated if the treatment is aimed at encouraging spontaneous arrest of bleeding. This is only possible in cases of (a) bleeding from small vessels and (b) so-called parenchymatous bleeding; by contrast, bleeding from medium or large vessels absolutely must be treated by mechanical surgery. Radiation treatment of bleeding in patients with benign gynecologic diseases is only employed today if other therapeutic measures cannot be employed instead. Inoperable uterine bleeding which cannot be arrested indicates the destruction of the uterine mucosa and possibly the suspension of ovarian function. For the destruction of the uterine mucosa, the administration of radioactive substances from the uterine cavity is most effective, leading to a fast arrest of bleeding.

Historically, radiotherapy of benign functional uterine bleedings was used for many years, but with decreasing frequency during the radium and x-ray era. Several different methods were employed according to age, constitution and operability of the patient, and amount and duration of blood loss (HOFMANN 1963):

1. Radium insertion with use of beta and gamma rays
2. Radium (cobalt-60, cesium-137) insertion with use of gamma rays
3. Percutaneous irradiation of the ovaries
4. Percutaneous irradiation of the spleen

Each of these methods is briefly discussed below:

1. Radium insertion with use of beta and gamma rays based on radium capsules filtered by 0.2-mm monel (a natural alloy containing nickel, copper, iron, and magnesium) and intrauterine plastic tubes (soft filter) allowed a high amount of beta rays to penetrate the tubes and destroy the endometrium while the amount of gamma rays reaching the ovaries was less, due to the short time of exposure, and did not stop their function. Three applicators with a 70-mg (30, 20, 20) radium element were typically inserted for 5 h into the uterine cavity (=350 mgeh), though 450 mgeh (SOOST 1958) seemed to give better results. This method produced prompt hemostasis and minor menopausal complaints. It was introduced by CZECH in 1951 and achieved a temporary menolysis for younger women, i.e., recurrence of bleeding was 40% in women aged 35–37 years and 3.5% in women aged 47–49 years.
2. Radium insertion with the usual use of gamma rays based on platinum or steel capsules and brass tubes as filters (hard filter) destroyed the endometrium and stopped the function of the ovaries. One insertion with a single tube of minimum 2000 mgeh (23.6 Gy to point A by a 3 × 3

tube with 90 mgeh) was effective in stopping the bleeding and achieving radiocastration, as the ovaries received a dose of more than 3 Gy (HOFMANN 1963). The postmenopausal complaints were less intensive than with castration by x-rays.
3. Percutaneous irradiation by x-rays used a castration dose of 3.6 Gy in the ovaries but this was reduced to 2.9 Gy in climacteric or 3.2 Gy in younger women; the treatment was applied by opposing pelvic fields in one or two sessions (HOFMANN 1963).
4. For the irradiation of the spleen by x-rays, a spleen dose of 0.6 Gy (from an 8 × 10 cm field with 180–200 kV and a 0.5-mm copper filter) was thought to be sufficient to influence uterine bleeding (KEPP 1949; KEPP et al. 1954). The mechanism of the hemostatic effect was unknown, and the method is now obsolete.

On account of the advances in the field of hormonal and hemostatic therapy, the aforementioned methods are only taken into consideration in exceptional cases. Intracavitary irradiation is performed with applicators in which the radioactive sources are embedded in a certain order. Such applicators are left in the cavity for a certain period until the desired dose is achieved. In intracavitary contact radiation treatment of the uterine corpus, threefold fractionation is recommended in all cases where an optimum dose distribution was not possible at the first insertion. In radium treatment of the uterine corpus, the clinical rule is that an upper dose limit of 90 Gy at the surface of the uterine serosa should not be exceeded (BUSCH 1987). The isodose course should ensure that a single dose of 7 Gy or an integral dose of 60 Gy is not exceeded either at the rectum or at the bladder mucosa. Each intrauterine radiation treatment with radioactive substances must be preceded by fractionated dilatation and curettage as well as by a histologic examination of the obtained tissue in order to rule out a malignant process, but also to reduce the distance from the radioactive source due to the ablation of the hyperplastic mucosa.

If fever of more than 38.5°C occurs during radiotherapy, the applicator has to be removed and antibiotic treatment started.

17.8 Menolysis (Radiocastration)

One further field of application of radiotherapy is the arrest of premenopausal benign gynecologic bleeding by stopping the normal hormonal ovarian function. This method is employed very rarely today because on the one hand, hormone therapy as conservative treatment is quite sufficient, and on the other hand, the women suddenly have to suffer from very severe menopausal complaints after radiotherapy. However, if in younger women an endocrine ablative therapy by castration is preferred and for some reason surgery is not possible, the small pelvis is irradiated with 9–12 Gy for 3–4 days from one large ventral field and one large dorsal field in the direction of the ovaries (SACK and THESEN 1987).

17.9 Conclusion

Radiotherapy no longer plays an important part in the treatment of the benign gynecologic diseases dealt with in this chapter. However, there are still special cases where this well-tried therapeutic measure can be employed with success.

References

Abergel RP, Dwyker RM, Meeker CA, Lask G, Kelly AP, Uitto I (1984a) Laser treatment of keloids: a clinical trial and in vitro study with Nd:YAG laser. Lasers Surg Med 4:91–95

Abergel RP, Meeker CA, Lam TS, Dwyer RM, Lesavoy MA, Uitto I (1984b) Control of connective tissue metabolism by lasers: recent developments and future prospects. J Am Acad Dermatol 11:1142–1150

Allan JG, Keen P (1954) The management of keloid in the South African Bantu. South Afr Med J 28:1034–1037

Baensch W (1937) Über die Strahlenbehandlung der Keloide. Strahlentherapie 60:204–209

Böttger H, Rumphorst K (1956) Die Röntgenentzündungsbestrahlung der Mastitis puerperalis. Dtsch Med Wochenschr 81:1124–1129

Braun-Falco O, Lucacs S (1973) Dermatologische Röntgentherapie. Springer, Berlin Heidelberg New York

Busch M (1987) Klinische applikationsverfahren mit umschlossenen nukliden. In: Scherer E (ed) Strahlentherapie – Radiologische Onkologie, 3rd edn. Springer, Berlin Heidelberg New York, pp 135–172

Czech A (1951) Über die Behandlung der klimakterischen Blutungen mit den Betastrahlen des Radiums. Geburtshilfe Frauenheilkd 11:867–877

Dalicho W (1949) Zur Therapie der Keloide mit besonderer Berücksichtigung der Radiumbehandlung. Strahlentherapie 78:87–92

Fracois H, Gosserez O, Michel M, et al. (1993) The treatment of 783 keloid scars by iridium 192 interstitial irradiation after surgical excision. Int J Radiat Oncol Biol Phys 26:245–251

Gaszago E (1938) Die Bedeutung der Röntgenschwachbestrahlung in der Gynäkologie. Strahlentherapie 62:167

Glauner R (1951) Die Entzündungsbestrahlung. Thieme, Stuttgart

Henderson DL, Cromwell TA, Mes LG (1984) Argon and carbon dioxide laser treatment of hypertrophic and keloid scars. Laser Surg Med 3:271–277

Heß F (1980) Die Strahlentherapie gutartiger Erkrankungen. Akute Entzündung in der laktierenden Mamma. In: Scherer E (ed) Strahlentherapie – Radiologische Onkologie, 2nd edn. Springer, Berlin Heidelberg New York, pp 353–368

Heß F (1987) Die Strahlentherapie gutartiger Erkrankungen. In: Scherer E (ed) Strahlentherapie – Radiologische Onkologie, 3rd edn. Springer, Berlin Heidelberg New York, pp 354–368

Hofmann D (1963) Die Strahlenbehandlung gutartiger gynäkologischer Erkrankungen. In: Klinik der gynäkologischen Strahlentherapie. Urban and Schwarzenberg, München

Kepp RK (1949) Die Milzbestrahlung. Geburtshilfe Frauenheilkd 9:24–30

Kepp RK, Oehlert G, Fuchs G (1954) Weitere Erfahrungen in der Behandlung präklimakterischer Blutungsstörungen mit schwach gefiltertem Radium. Geburtshilfe Frauenheilkd 14:310–317

Kruchen C (1973) Röntgenbestrahlung der puerperalen Mastitis. Strahlentherapie 73:464

Mettler FA (1969) Breast neoplasms in women treated with x-rays for acute postpartum mastitis. A pilot study. J Natl Cancer Inst 43:803

Rausch L (1982) Mensch und Strahlenwirkung. Piper, München

Rech U (1943) Unsere Erfahrungen mit der Röntgenbestrahlung der puerperalen Mastitis. Strahlentherapie 74:5

Rösler HP, Zapf S, Kuffner HD, Wissen-Siegert I, Kutzner J (1993) Strahlentherapie beim Narbenkeloid. Fortschr Med 111:46–49

Sack H, Thesen N (1987) Weibliche und männliche Mamma. In: Scherer E (ed) Strahlentherapie – Radiologische Onkologie, 3rd edn. Springer, Berlin Heidelberg New York, pp 863–891

Scherer E (1958) Die Röntgenreizbestrahlung als Mittel zur unspezifischen Anregung von Abwehrmaßnahmen des Körpers. In: Lehrbuch der Strahlenheilkunde v. R. du Mesnil de Rochemont. Ferdinand Enke, Stuttgart, pp 342–413

Scherer E (1965) Die Bedeutung der Strahlentherapie mit kleinen Dosen. Röntgenblätter 18:400–406

Shore RE (1977) Breast neoplasms in women treated with x-rays for acute postpartum mastitis. J Natl Cancer Inst 59:813

Simons A (1930) Zur Therapie der Keloide und Narbenhypertrophien. Strahlentherapie 78:87–92

Soost HJ (1958) Ergebnisse der Behandlung klimerakterischer Blutungen mit Radium-Beta-Strahlen. Zentralbl Gynäkol 80:1257–1267

Trott UR (1994) Therapeutic effects of low radiation doses. Strahlenther Onkol 170:1–12

Subject Index*

It is assumed that the reader will be searching for particular information in respect of a problem or situation regarding a known tumor entity. Therefore the list of contents at the front of each chapter is very detailed, including all of the principal subsections. In the Subject Index, tumor entities covered in the "Special Report" (Chaps. 5–14) are each accorded a separate section (e.g. "Cancer of the Cervix," "Cancer of the Endometrium," "Genital Soft Tissue Sarcomas") within which all of the indexed subjects in respect of the entity in question are to be found. There are no potentially distracting cross-references between the tumor chapters. Within the aforementioned sections, the main entries are Brachytherapy, Chemotherapy, Complications of treatment, Results of treatment (5-year survival), Surgery, and Teletherapy or External beam therapy. Each of these main entries subsumes a number of subentries which will provide the reader with further specific information.

The historical and basic chapters (1–4) and chapters 15–17, wich address topics of common relevance to all the tumor entities, are indexed together with occasional cross-references to the tumor chapters.

Used in conjunction, the lists of contents and Subject Index should enable the reader to locate quickly any subject of interest.

* Figures are designeated by the letter "f" following the page number; Tables are found on page numbers followed by the letter "t".

Index of Tumor Entities

Cancer of the Cervix

Cancer of the Endometrium

Cancer of the Fallopian Tube

Cancer of the Female Urethra

Cancer of the Vagina

Special Malignancies of the Vulva

List of Contributors

IRENÄUS A. ADAMIETZ, MD
Leitender Oberarzt
Abteilung für Strahlentherapie und Onkologie
Klinik und Poliklinik
Johann Wolfgang Goethe-Universität
Theodor-Stern-Kai 7
60590 Frankfurt, Germany

J. BAHNSEN, MD, Professor
Abteilung für Gynäkologische Radiologie
Frauenklinik
Universitätskrankenhaus Eppendorf
Martinistraße 52
20251 Hamburg, Germany

M.W. BECKMANN, MD
Universitäts-Frauenklinik
Moorenstraße 5
40225 Düsseldorf, Germany

H.G. BENDER, MD, Professor
Direktor, Universitäts-Frauenklinik
Moorenstraße 5
40225 Düsseldorf, Germany

HEINZ D. BÖTTCHER, MD, Professor
Leiter der Abteilung für Strahlentherapie
und Onkologie, Klinik und Poliklinik
Johann Wolfgang Goethe-Universität
Theodor-Stern-Kai 7
60590 Frankfurt, Germany

LUTHER W. BRADY, MD, Professor
Department of Radiation Oncology
Allegheny University of the Health Sciences
Broad and Vine Streets, Mail Stop 200
Philadelphia, PA 19102-1192, USA

DETLEF CARSTENS, MD
Hermann-Holthusen-Institut für Strahlentherapie
Allgemeines Krankenhaus St. Georg
Lohmühlenstraße 5
20099 Hamburg, Germany

G. CROMBACH, MD
Oberarzt, Universitäts-Frauenklinik
Moorenstraße 5
40225 Düsseldorf, Germany

R.G. DALE, PhD, FInstP, FIPEM
Department of Radiation Physics
and Radiobiology, Charing Cross Hospital
Fulham Palace Road
London W6 8RF, UK

MICHAEL F. DZEDA, MD
Department of Radiation Oncology
Allegheny University Hahnemann
Broad and Vine, Mail Stop 200
Philadelphia, PA 19102-1192, USA

GÜNTER EMONS, MD, Professor
Abteilung für Gynäkologie und Geburtshilfe
Klinikum der Philipps Universität Marburg
Pilgrimstraße 3
35037 Marburg, Germany

H.J. FRISCHBIER, MD, PhD, Professor
Klövensteenweg 64
22559 Hamburg-Rissen, Germany

A. GERBAULET, MD
Head of Brachytherapy Department
Institut Gustave-Roussy
39, rue Camillo Desmoulins
94805 Villejuif, France

C. HAIE-MEDER, MD
Brachytherapy Department
Institut Gustave-Roussy
39, rue Camillo Desmoulins
94805 Villejuif, France

M. Herbolsheimer, MD
Akademischer Oberrat
Institut für Radiologie
Klinikum Fulda
Pacelliallee 4
36043 Fulda, Germany

R.D. Hunter, MD
Christie Hospital
Holt-Radium Insitute
Wilmslow Road
Withington, Manchester M20 48X, UK

H. Jacobs, MD, Chefarzt
Klinik für Strahlentherapie und Radioonkologie
Saarbrücker Winterberg-Kliniken
Theodor-Heuss-Straße
66119 Saarbrücken, Germany

H. Junkermann, MD
Abteilung für Gynäkologische Radiologie
Radiologische Universitätsklinik
Bereich Frauenklinik
Voßstraße 9
69115 Heidelberg, Germany

Ulrich Karck, MD
Universitäts-Frauenklinik
Hugstetter Straße 55
79106 Freiburg, Germany

D. Kieback, MD, Professor
Department of Obstetrics and Gynecology
Baylor College of Medicine
6550 Fannin
Houston, TX 77030, USA

P.G. Knapstein, MD, Professor
Direktor, Frauenklinik
Universität Mainz
Langenbeckstraße 1
55101 Mainz, Germany

R. Kreienberg, MD, Professor
Ärztlicher Direktor
Universitäts-Frauenklinik und Poliklinik
Prittwitzstraße 43
89075 Ulm, Germany

H. Kucera, MD
I. Universitäts-Frauenklinik
Allgemeines Krankenhaus der Stadt Wien
Spitalgasse 23
1090 Wien, Austria

H.-A. Ladner, MD, Professor
Im Großacker 3
79249 Merzhausen, Germany

Stefan Ladner, MD
Zentrales Röntgeninstitut
Städtisches Klinikum Karlsruhe
Moltkestraße 14
76133 Karlsruhe, Germany

E. Lartigau, MD
Brachytherapy Department
Insitut Gustave-Roussy
39, rue Camillo Demoulins
94805 Villejuif, France

Wallace A. Longton, MD
Department of Radiation Oncology
Allegheny University Hospitals
Center City
Philadelphia, PA 19102-1192, USA

M. Maher, MD
Brachytherapy Department
Insitut Gustave-Roussy
39, rue Camillo Demoulins
94805 Villejuif, France

H. Marsiglia, MD
Brachytherapy Department
Insitut Gustave-Roussy
39, rue Camillo Demoulins
94805 Villejuif, France

Bizhan Micaily, MD
Department of Radiation Oncology
Allegheny University Hahnemann
Broad and Vine, Mail Stop 200
Philadelphia, PA 19102-1192, USA

Kozo Morita, MD
Director, Aichi Cancer Center Hospital
1-1 Kanokoden, Chikusa-ku
464 Nagoya, Japan

Richard F. Mould, MSc, PhD
CPhys, FinstP, FIPSM, FIMA, FIS
Scientific Consultant
41 Ewhurst Avenue
Sanderstead, South Croydon
Surrey CR2 0DH, UK

D. Niederacher, MD
Molekulargenetisches Labor
Universitäts-Frauenklinik
Gebäude 23.12.04
Moorenstraße 5
40225 Düsseldorf, Germany

U. Nitz, MD, PD
Oberärztin, Universitäts-Frauenklinik
Moorenstraße 5
40225 Düsseldorf, Germany

Diana M. Ostapovicz, MD
Department of Radiation Oncology
Altoona Hospital
620 Howard Avenue
Altoona, PA 16602, USA

Carlos A. Perez, MD
Director, Radiation Oncology Center
Mallinckrodt Institute of Radiology
Washington University Medical Center
4511 Forest Park, Suite 200
Saint Louis, MO 63108, USA

R. Pfab, MD, Professor
Komm. Leiter der Abteilung für Strahlentherapie
Klinikum der Philipps-Universität Marburg
Baldingerstraße
35043 Marburg, Germany

Albrecht Pfleiderer, MD, Professor(em.)
Universitäts-Frauenklinik
Hugstetter Straße 55
79106 Freiburg, Germany

G. Rauthe, MD, PD
Chefarzt, Schloßbergklinik
87534 Oberstaufen, Germany

Karsten Rotte, MD, Professor
Ziegelhütte 2-Oberdürrbach
97080 Würzburg

Bernhard Schopohl, MD
Oberarzt, Abteilung für Strahlentherapie
und Onkologie, Klinik und Poliklinik
Johann Wolfgang Goethe-Universität
Theodor-Stern-Kai 7
60590 Frankfurt, Germany

Ingrid Schreer, MD, PD
Machabäerstraße 19-27
50668 Köln, Germany

Klaus-Dieter Schulz, MD, Professor
Leiter, Abteilung für Gynäkologie
und Geburtshilfe
Klinikum der Philipps-Universität Marburg
Pilgrimstraße 3
35037 Marburg, Germany

V. Stelte, MD
Abteilung für Gynäkologische Radiologie
Frauenklinik
Universitätskrankenhaus Eppendorf
Martinistraße 52
20251 Hamburg, Germany

Dirk Timmerman, MD
Gynecologic Oncology
Department of Obstetrics and Gynecology
University Hospital of Leuven
Herestraat 49, Gasthuisberg
3000 Leuven, Belgium

Helmut W. Vahrson, MD, Professor
Leiter, Abteilung für Gynäkologische Onkologie
und Strahlentherapie, Frauenklinik
Klinikum der Justus-Liebig-Universität
Klinikstraße 32
35385 Gießen, Germany

Ignace B. Vergote, MD, PhD, Professor
Gynecologic Oncology
Department of Obstetrics and Gynecology
University Hospital of Leuven
Herestraat 49, Gasthuisberg
3000 Leuven, Belgium

Dietrich von Fournier, MD, Professor
Leiter, Abteilung für Gynäkologische Radiologie
Radiologische Universitätsklinik
Bereich Frauenklinik
Voßstraße 9
69115 Heidelberg, Germany

W. Weikel, MD
Universität Mainz
Langenbeckstraße 1
55101 Mainz, Germany

Medical Radiology
Diagnostic Imaging and Radiation Oncology

Titles in the series already published

Diagnostic Imaging

Innovations in Diagnostic Imaging
Edited by J.H. Anderson

Radiology of the Upper Urinary Tract
Edited by E.K. Lang

The Thymus - Diagnostic Imaging, Functions, and Pathologic Anatomy
Edited by E. Walter, E. Willich, and W.R. Webb

Interventional Neuroradiology
Edited by A. Valavanis

Radiology of the Pancreas
Edited by A.L. Baert, co-edited by G. Delorme

Radiology of the Lower Urinary Tract
Edited by E.K. Lang

Magnetic Resonance Angiography
Edited by I.P. Arlart, G.M. Bongartz, and G. Marchal

Contrast-Enhanced MRI of the Breast
S. Heywang-Köbrunner and R. Beck

Spiral CT of the Chest
Edited by M. Rémy-Jardin and J. Rémy

Radiological Diagnosis of Breast Diseases
Edited by M. Friedrich and E.A. Sickles

Radiology of the Trauma
Edited by M. Heller and A. Fink

Biliary Tract Radiology
Edited by P. Rossi

Radiation Oncology

Lung Cancer
Edited by C.W. Scarantino

Innovations in Radiation Oncology
Edited by H.R. Withers and L.J. Peters

Radiation Therapy of Head and Neck Cancer
Edited by G.E. Laramore

Gastrointestinal Cancer - Radiation Therapy
Edited by R.R. Dobelbower, Jr.

Radiation Exposure and Occupational Risks
Edited by E. Scherer, C. Streffer, and K.-R. Trott

Radiation Therapy of Benign Diseases - A Clinical Guide
S.E. Order and S.S. Donaldson

Interventional Radiation Therapy Techniques - Brachytherapy
Edited by R. Sauer

Radiopathology of Organs and Tissues
Edited by E. Scherer, C. Streffer, and K.-R. Trott

Medical Radiology
Diagnostic Imaging and Radiation Oncology

Titles in the series already published

Radiation Oncology

Concomitant Continuous Infusion Chemotherapy and Radiation
Edited by M. Rotman and C.J. Rosenthal

Intraoperative Radiotherapy – Clinical Experiences and Results
Edited by F.A. Calvo, M. Santos, and L.W. Brady

Radiotherapy of Intraocular and Orbital Tumors
Edited by W.E. Alberti and R.H. Sagerman

Interstitial and Intracavitary Thermoradiotherapy
Edited by M.H. Seegenschmiedt and R. Sauer

Non-Disseminated Breast Cancer
Controversial Issues in Management
Edited by G.H. Fletcher and S.H. Levitt

Current Topics in Clinical Radiobiology of Tumors
Edited by H.-P. Beck-Bornholdt

Practical Approaches to Cancer Invasion and Metastases
A Compendium of Radiation Oncologists' Responses to 40 Histories
Edited by A.R. Kagan with the Assistance of R.J. Steckel

Radiation Therapy in Pediatric Oncology
Edited by J.R. Cassady

Radiation Therapy Physics
Edited by A.R. Smith

Late Sequelae in Oncology
Edited by J. Dunst and R. Sauer

Mediastinal Tumors. Update 1995
Edited by D.E. Wood and C.R. Thomas, Jr.

Thermoradiotherapy and Thermochemotherapy
Volume 1: Biology, Physiology, and Physics
Volume 2: Clinical Applications
Edited by M.H. Seegenschmiedt, P. Fessenden, and C.C. Vernon

Carcinoma of the Prostate
Innovations in Management
Edited by Z. Petrovich, L. Baert, and L.W. Brady

Carcinoma of the Bladder
Innovations in Management
Edited by Z. Petrovich, L. Baert, and L.W. Brady

Radiation Oncology of Gynecological Cancers
Edited by H.W. Vahrson